PCF4

PALLIATIVE CARE FORMULARY

Published by palliativedrugs.com Ltd.

Palliativedrugs.com Ltd
Hayward House Study Centre
Nottingham University Hospitals NHS Trust, City Campus
Nottingham NG5 1PB
United Kingdom

www.palliativedrugs.com

PCF4 2011, reprinted 2012 (twice)
PCF3 2007, reprinted 2008, 2009
PCF2 2002, reprinted 2003
PCF1 1998

British Library Cataloguing in Publication Data

A catalogue record for this book is available from the British Library.

ISBN 978-0-9552547-5-8

Typeset by OKS Prepress Services Private Ltd, Chennai, India
Printed by Halstan Printing Group, Amersham, UK

DISCLAIMER

Every effort has been made to ensure the accuracy of this text, and that the best information available has been used. However, palliativedrugs.com Ltd neither represents nor guarantees that the practices described herein will, if followed, ensure safe and effective patient care. The recommendations contained in this book reflect the editors' judgement regarding the state of general knowledge and practice in the field as of the date of publication. Information in a book of this type can never be all-inclusive, and therefore will not cover every eventuality.

Thus, those who use this book must make their own determinations regarding specific safe and appropriate patient-care practices, taking into account the personnel, equipment, and practices available at the hospital or other facility at which they are located. Neither palliativedrugs.com Ltd nor the editors can be held responsible for any liability incurred as a consequence of the use or application of any of the contents of this book. Mention of specific product brands does not imply endorsement.

Particularly when prescribing a drug for the first time, a doctor (or other independent prescriber) should study the contents of the manufacturer's Summary of Product Characteristics (SPC), paying particular attention to indications, contra-indications, cautions, drug interactions, and undesirable effects.

EDITORIAL STAFF

Brian Creedon MB BCh BAO, MRCPI, MMedSci
Consultant in Palliative Medicine, Waterford Regional Hospital, Waterford, Ireland

Vincent Crosby FRCP
Consultant in Palliative Medicine, Hayward House Specialist Palliative Care Unit, Nottingham University Hospitals NHS Trust, Nottingham, UK

Andrew Davies MSc, MD, FRCP
Consultant in Palliative Medicine, St. Luke's Cancer Centre, Royal Surrey County Hospital, Guildford, UK

Mervyn Dean MB ChB, CCFP
Palliative Care Physician (rtd), Corner Brook, NL, Canada

Rebecca Dunn MB BS
Registrar in Dermatology, Oxford Radcliffe Hospitals NHS Trust, Oxford, UK Churchill Hospital, Oxford, UK

Ruth England MRCP
Registrar in Palliative Medicine, East Midlands Healthcare Workforce Deanery (North), UK

Marie Fallon MD, FRCP
St Columbas Hospice Chair of Palliative Medicine, University of Edinburgh and Edinburgh Cancer Centre, UK

Jeff Fry BSc, PhD
Associate Professor and Reader in Molecular Toxicology, School of Biomedical Sciences, University of Nottingham Medical School, Nottingham, UK

Vanessa Halliday PhD, RD
Lecturer in Clinical Nutrition and Dietetics, Division of Nutritional Sciences, University of Nottingham, UK

Janet Hardy BSc, MD, FRACP
Director, Department of Palliative and Supportive Care, Mater Health Services, Brisbane; Professor of Palliative Medicine, University of Queensland, Australia

Miriam Johnson MB ChB, MD, FRCP, MRCGP
Senior Lecturer in Palliative Medicine, Hull York Medical School, University of Hull, Hull, UK

Paul Keeley MB ChB, FRCP
Consultant in Palliative Medicine, Glasgow Royal Infirmary, Glasgow, Scotland, UK

Vaughan Keeley PhD, FRCP
Consultant in Palliative Medicine, Derby Hospitals NHS Trust, Derby, UK

Bruce Kennedy BSc(Pharm), MBA
Clinical Pharmacy Specialist Palliative Care, Palliative Care Program, Fraser Health, Surrey, BC, Canada

Samuel King BM, MRCP
Registrar in Palliative Medicine, Southmead Hospital, Bristol, UK

Susie Lapwood MA, BM BCh, MRCGP, DFSRH, DipPallMed
Lead Doctor, Helen and Douglas House Hospices for Children & Young Adults, Oxford UK

Mark Lee MD, MRCP
Consultant in Palliative Medicine, NHS South of Tyne and Wear Community Health Services and St Benedict's Hospice, Sunderland, UK

CONTENTS

PREFACE

Welcome to the fourth edition of the *Palliative Care Formulary* (*PCF*), written primarily for the UK. Regional adaptations include *Hospice and Palliative Care Formulary* (USA), *Canadian PCF*, and German and Polish editions. For details, see www.palliativedrugs.com.

The target audience comprises doctors, nurses and pharmacists involved in the care of patients receiving palliative/hospice care. *PCF* is a core textbook for medical registrars in Palliative Medicine in the UK. It is used in some areas to fulfil the NHS National Cancer Standards requirement for specialist palliative care services within a Cancer Centre and Network to have a core palliative care drug formulary. *PCF* also complements *Changing Gear: Guidelines for managing the last days of life in adults*, re-issued by the UK National Council for Palliative Care in 2006, and is referred to in many official healthcare documents.

Although written primarily with cancer patients in mind, *PCF* contains specific material relating to a number of other life-limiting diseases, e.g. COPD, congestive heart failure, renal failure, and Parkinson's disease. *PCF* also includes a number of *Quick Practice Guides*. To enhance user-friendliness, each *QPG* is limited to no more than two pages, and references are not included. We welcome feedback on these. We also encourage the donation of clinical guidance from other sources for posting on our website (e-mail copies to hq@palliativedrugs.com).

Information in a book of this type can never be all-inclusive, and therefore will not cover every eventuality. Thus, readers should satisfy themselves as to the appropriateness of the information before applying it in practice. Particularly when prescribing a drug for the first time, a doctor (or other independent prescriber) should study the contents of the manufacturer's Summary of Product Characteristics (SPC), paying particular attention to indications, contra-indications, cautions, drug interactions, and undesirable effects. *PCF* often refers to the use of drugs beyond the scope of their marketing authorization (product licence).The use of drugs in this way clearly has implications for the prescriber (see p.xiii).

As always, a cautious approach is necessary when prescribing for the frail, the elderly, and patients with hepatic impairment, renal impairment or respiratory insufficiency (see p.605). Further, if caring for a woman who is pregnant or breast-feeding, or for someone with porphyria, it is crucial to double-check a drug's suitability in both the *BNF* and SPC.

The production of a book of this nature depends partly on the help and advice of numerous colleagues, both past and present. We acknowledge with gratitude the support of clinical colleagues, and members of the palliativedrugs.com community who have provided feedback, particularly via surveys or by contributing to the Syringe Driver Survey Database.

We acknowledge with thanks the advice provided by numerous correspondents, including: Claudia Bausewein, James Beattie, June Frame, Ian Hogg, Sue Hollingsworth, Stephen Kirkham, Mary Mihalyo, Eric Prommer, Constanze Remi, John Shuster, Brian Stickle, and various Medical Information Departments in the pharmaceutical industry.

We are grateful to Karen Isaac for secretarial assistance.

Editors-in-chief
June 2011

ABOUT www.palliativedrugs.com

Readers of *PCF* are encouraged to register with the website, and to participate fully in this on-line community of some 20,000 members from >100 countries. The website provides a range of on-line information:

- ***Bulletin Board*** enables members to seek help and offer advice
- ***Latest additions*** informs members about the latest changes to the Formulary and website
- ***News*** informs members about drug-related news including changes in drug availability and/or formulation
- ***Document library*** acts as a repository for guidelines, policies and other documents donated by members
- ***Syringe Driver Survey Database*** has >1,000 observational compatibility reports of drug combinations given by continuous subcutaneous infusion (CSCI)
- ***Online bookshop*** enables members to purchase copies of *PCF* online.

On-line surveys

Surveys on aspects of palliative care and drug use are conducted through the website. Relevant information from these sources is included in *PCF*. We also encourage registrants to participate in occasional website satisfaction surveys.

Feedback

We are constantly striving to improve the site and its resources, and welcome feedback via hq@palliativedrugs.com.

HOW PCF IS CONSTRUCTED

The *Palliative Care Formulary (PCF)* is a unique independent professional publication which provides essential information for prescribers involved in palliative and hospice care. *PCF* brings together authoritative independent guidance on best practice with clinically validated drug information, and thus helps to ensure that drugs are used appropriately, safely, and optimally. Many changes are made for each edition, and a list of major new additions and deletions is included.

Drugs are included under their recommended International Non-proprietary Name (rINN) or, for several combination products, their British Approved Name (BAN). The order of the drug monographs broadly follows the same sequence as in the *British National Formulary (BNF).*

Editorial team

The *PCF* editorial team comprises doctors and pharmacists with an extensive understanding of how drugs are used in palliative care, co-ordinated by two medically qualified Editors-in-chief. For each edition, every section of *PCF* is reviewed and updated with the help of an Editorial Board. Suggestions for new monographs are discussed by the *PCF* editorial team, and experts identified to assist in the preparation of new documents in dialogue with the editorial team.

The Editorial Board

The Editorial Board is a group of mainly palliative care physicians appointed for each edition on the basis of their clinical knowledge and expertise. Editorial Board members have committed to reviewing one or more drug monographs or chapters, and work in liaison with the editorial team. Responsibilities include scrutinizing literature databases such as PubMed, and accessing and studying relevant new publications.

Correspondents

Correspondents are drawn from a range of medical specialties. They include doctors, pharmacists, nurses, and others who provide advice on the text by:

- checking amendments for scientific accuracy, and to enhance clarity
- providing additional expert opinion in areas of controversy or when reliable evidence is lacking
- advising on areas when the *PCF* diverges from a manufacturer's Summary of Product Characteristics (SPC)
- providing additional validation and clinical evidence about off-label use.

Sources of *PCF* information

PCF uses various sources for its information, including:

Summary of product characteristics (SPC)

PCF accesses the SPCs of all new products as well as revised SPCs for existing products. The SPCs are the principal source of product information and are carefully reviewed to ensure that *PCF* monographs are fully up-to-date in this respect.

Literature

Research papers and reviews relating to the drugs featured in *PCF* are carefully processed. When a difference between the advice in the *PCF* and a paper is noted, the new information is evaluated for reliability and relevance to UK clinical practice. If necessary, new text is drafted and thoroughly reviewed by the editorial team with support, as needed, from the Editorial Board and/or Correspondents.

PCF has access to many on-line information resources, including *Martindale, the complete drug reference, Stockley's Drug Interactions, BNF* and *British Pharmacopoeia*. Editors keep other team members informed of significant developments and shifts in the trends of drug usage.

Systematic reviews

PCF monitors various databases of systematic reviews, including the *Cochrane Library* and several other web-based resources. Reviews published in *Clinical Evidence* are used to validate *PCF* advice.

Consensus guidelines

The advice in *PCF* is checked against consensus guidelines produced by expert bodies including the National Institute for Health and Clinical Excellence (NICE), the Scottish Medicines Consortium (SMC), and the Scottish Intercollegiate Guidelines Network (SIGN).

PCF also takes note of other expert bodies which produce clinical guidelines relevant to palliative care, e.g. Association for Palliative Medicine, British Lymphology Society.

Statutory information

PCF routinely processes relevant information from various Government bodies, including Statutory Instruments and regulations affecting the Prescription only Medicines Order, Controlled Drugs and from the Medicines and Healthcare products Regulatory Agency (MHRA). Safety warnings issued by the Commission on Human Medicines (CHM) and guidelines on drug use issued by the UK health departments are routinely processed.

Relevant professional statements issued by the Royal Pharmaceutical Society, Nursing and Midwifery Council (NMC) and General Medical Council (GMC) are included in *PCF* as are guidelines from the medical Royal Colleges.

Pricing information

PCF provides information on prices of medicinal products and appliances from the *BNF*. *PCF* checks prices direct with suppliers for products not included in the *BNF*.

Comments from readers

Readers of *PCF*, and visitors to www.palliativedrugs.com, are invited to send in comments (see p.xii). Such feedback helps to ensure that *PCF* provides accurate and clinically relevant information.

Comments from industry

Manufacturers are contacted directly if there are queries about the content of an SPC.

Surveys

Relevant information from surveys conducted at regular intervals through www.palliativedrugs.com is included in *PCF*.

SUMMARY OF MAIN CHANGES IN PCF4

Since the publication of *PCF3* in 2007, every drug monograph has been extensively reviewed and updated. Several items have been withdrawn (e.g. mexiletine, epoetin, quinine, pharmacokinetic appendix) and new ones added, notably:

- Chapters:
  - ▷ 14, Guidance about prescribing in palliative care, now includes a section on prescribing for children and an expanded section on drugs and hepatic impairment
  - ▷ 16, Drug treatment in the imminently dying
  - ▷ 17, Pre-emptive prescribing in the community
- Monographs:
  - ▷ Anti-epileptic pre-synaptic calcium channel blockers
  - ▷ Anti-epileptic sodium channel blockers (membrane stabilizers)
  - ▷ Cannabis sativa extract
  - ▷ Carbamazepine
  - ▷ Celecoxib
  - ▷ Levetiracetam
  - ▷ Melatonin
  - ▷ Modafinil
  - ▷ Oxcarbazepine
  - ▷ Nortriptyline
  - ▷ Prochlorperazine
  - ▷ Quetiapine
  - ▷ SSRIs
  - ▷ Transmucosal fentanyl
  - ▷ Valproate
  - ▷ Zinc
- Drug inserts ('mini-monographs'):
  - ▷ Lidocaine patches
  - ▷ Methylnaltrexone
  - ▷ Oxycodone combined with naloxone (Targinact®)
  - ▷ Phenytoin
  - ▷ Tapentadol
  - ▷ Vasopressin receptor antagonists (VRAs, vaptans)
- Quick practice guides (formerly Guidelines):
  - ▷ Setting up a McKinley T34 syringe pump
  - ▷ Setting up a Graseby MS16A or MS26 syringe driver
  - ▷ Administration of drugs by enteral feeding tube.

MONOGRAPHS NOT IN PCF4 BUT AVAILABLE ELSEWHERE

The content of *PCF4* is mostly restricted to drugs currently available and used in palliative care in the UK. The following monographs are contained in *Hospice and Palliative Care Formulary* 2nd edition (*HPCFusa*):

- Pharmaco-economics in the USA
- Chapter 3 Respiratory system
  - ▹ N-acetylcysteine
- Chapter 4 CNS
  - ▹ Chloral hydrate
  - ▹ Desipramine
  - ▹ Dronabinol
- Chapter 5 Analgesics
  - ▹ Choline magnesium salicylate
  - ▹ Hydrocodone
  - ▹ Nalbuphine
- Appendix: Medicare/Medicaid conditions of hospice participation.

GETTING THE MOST OUT OF PCF

The literature on the pharmacology of pain and symptom management in end-stage disease is growing continually, and it is impossible for anyone to be familiar with all of it. This is where a book like *PCF* comes into its own as a major accessible resource for prescribing clinicians involved in palliative care.

PCF is not an easy read, indeed it was never intended that it would be read from cover to cover. It is essentially a reference book — to study the monograph of an individual drug, or class of drugs, with fairly specific questions in mind.

In Part 1, the sections generally follow the systematic order of the *British National Formulary* (*BNF*). Drugs marked with an asterisk (*) should generally be used only by, or after consultation with, a specialist palliative care service.

Part 2 and the appendices deal with themes that transcend the drug monographs, e.g. pre-emptive prescribing in the community, continuous SC infusions, administering drugs via enteral tubes, the use of nebulized drugs.

Information in a book of this type can never be all-inclusive, and therefore will not cover every eventuality. Particularly when prescribing a drug for the first time, a doctor (or other independent prescriber) should study the corresponding entry in the *BNF* and the contents of the manufacturer's Summary of Product Characteristics (SPC), paying particular attention to indications, contra-indications, cautions, drug interactions, and undesirable effects (see p.xx).

PCF often refers to the use of drugs beyond the scope of their marketing authorization (product licence).The use of drugs in this way clearly has implications for the prescriber (see p.xxiii). As always, readers should satisfy themselves as to the appropriateness of the information before applying it in practice.

Symptom Management in Advanced Cancer 4th edition (Twycross, Wilcock and Toller 2009, palliativedrugs.com Ltd, Nottingham) is the specific companion book to *PCF4*. Readers should also be aware of *Opioids in Cancer Pain 2nd edition* (Davis et al. 2009, OUP). This provides a wealth of additional data, and will be particularly useful for clinical teachers.

Reliable knowledge and levels of evidence

Research is the pursuit of reliable knowledge. The gold standard for drug treatment is the randomized controlled trial (RCT) or, better, a systematic review of homogeneous RCTs.

Over the last 20–30 years, numerous systems have been published for categorizing levels of evidence and the strength of the derived recommendations. Box A reproduces the system used by the British Medical Journal. This checklist is based on material published by three main sources, namely the US Agency for Health Care Policy and Research, the NHS Management Executive, and the North of England Guidelines Group.[1–3]

However, it is important to recognize that the RCT is *not* the only source of reliable knowledge. Broadly speaking, sources of knowledge can be conveniently grouped under three headings:

- *instrumental*, includes RCT data and data from other high-quality studies
- *interactive*, refers to anecdotal data (shared clinical experience), including retrospective and prospective surveys
- *critical*, data unique to the individual in question (e.g. personal choice) and societal/cultural factors (e.g. financial and logistic considerations).[5]

Relying on one type of knowledge alone is not good practice. All three sources must be exploited in the process of therapeutic decision-making.

Box A A scheme for categorizing evidence and grading recommendations[4]

Category	*Level of evidence*	*Grade*	*Strength of recommendations*
Ia	Evidence obtained from a meta-analysis of RCTs	A	Directly based on Category I evidence without extrapolation
Ib	Evidence from at least one RCT		
IIa	Evidence obtained from at least one well-designed controlled study without randomization	B	Directly based on Category II evidence or by extrapolation from Category I evidence
IIb	Evidence obtained from at least one other well-designed quasi-experimental study		
III	Evidence obtained from well-designed non-experimental descriptive studies, such as comparative studies, correlation studies and case studies	C	Directly based on Category III evidence or by extrapolation from Category I or II evidence
IV	Evidence obtained from expert committee reports or opinions and/or clinical experiences of respected authorities	D	Directly based on category IV evidence or by extrapolation from Category I, II, or III evidence. This grading indicates that directly applicable clinical studies of good quality are absent or not readily available

Pharmaceutical company information

Although the manufacturer's SPC is an important source of information about a drug, it is important to remember that many published studies are sponsored by the drug company in question. This can lead to a conflict of interest between the desire for objective data and the need to make one's own drug as attractive as possible.[6] It is thus best to treat information from company representatives as inevitably biased. The information provided by *PCF* is commercially independent, and should serve as a counterbalance to manufacturer bias.

Remember: it is often safer to stick with an 'old favourite', and not seek to be among the first to prescribe a newly released product — which may simply be a 'me-too' drug rather than true innovation.[6]

Generic drugs

PCF encourages generic prescribing.[7] Apart from occasional exceptions, e.g. m/r formulations of diltiazem, nifedipine and theophylline, there is little reliable evidence that different preparations of the same drug are significantly different in terms of bio-availability and efficacy.[8] However, particularly for oral morphine preparations, the Department of Health (London) recommends including the brand name of opioid analgesics on the prescription and dispensing label, to avoid unwittingly switching brands and confusing the patient.[9]

Contra-indications and cautions

Contra-indications and cautions listed in Summaries of Product Characteristics (SPCs) sometimes vary between different manufacturers of the same drug. Thus, a contra-indication in one SPC may be styled a caution in another, and *vice versa*.

In *PCF*, we do not include universal contra-indications (e.g. history of hypersensitivity to the drug), and have generally *not* included a contra-indication from the SPC if the use of the drug in the stated circumstance is accepted prescribing practice in palliative care.

Further, it is assumed that clinicians are aware of the risk of commonsense pharmacodynamic interactions, e.g. that the concurrent prescription of two or more drugs with sedative properties is likely to result in more sedation than when prescribed alone. However, pharmacokinetic interactions (leading to either increased or reduced effect) are generally covered in individual drug monographs and in the chapter on cytochrome P450 (see p.735).

As always, a cautious approach is necessary when prescribing for the frail, the elderly, and patients with hepatic impairment, renal impairment or respiratory insufficiency (see p.605). If caring for a woman who is pregnant or breast-feeding, or for someone with porphyria, it is crucial to check a drug's suitability in both the *BNF* and *SPC*.

Pharmacokinetics

Generally, pharmacokinetic data are taken from *Martindale: the complete drug reference*[10] or from a manufacturer's SPC. Other sources are referenced in the text.

Undesirable effects of drugs

In *PCF*, the term 'undesirable effect' is used rather than 'side effect' or 'adverse drug reaction', as recommended by the European Commission. Wherever possible, undesirable effects are categorized as:

- very common (>10%)
- common (<10%, >1%)
- uncommon (<1%, >0.1%)
- rare (<0.1%, >0.01%)
- very rare (≤0.01%).

PCF generally includes information on the very common and common undesirable effects. Selected other undesirable effects are also included, e.g. uncommon or rare ones which may have serious consequences. The manufacturer's SPC should be consulted for a full list of undesirable effects.

Drugs costs

Drug prices are net prices based on those in the *BNF* No. 60 (September 2010). Variation will occur, dependent upon local retail market conditions. Further, drugs bought on contract are generally much cheaper.

Costs under £5 have been rounded up to the next 50p; prices over £5 are rounded up to the next full pound. Further, because prices change over time, those given in *PCF* should be regarded only as a rough guide.

Literature references

In choosing references, articles in hospice and palliative care journals have frequently been selected preferentially. Such journals are likely to be more readily available to our readers, and often contain detailed discussion.

It is not feasible to reference every statement in *PCF*. However, readers are invited to enter into constructive dialogue with the Editors via the Bulletin Board on *www.palliativedrugs.com*. This is currently accessed by >18,000 health professionals worldwide.

Electronic sources of information

Several of the sources cited in *PCF* can be accessed free online by UK users. To facilitate access to the relevant documents, website details are given below:

- *Bandolier* (evidence-based articles for health professionals): available from www.medicine.ox.ac.uk/bandolier/
- *British National Formulary*: two editions/year, March and September, available from www.bnf.org.uk/bnf/ (free registration required in the UK, Channel Islands, Isle of Man and some developing countries; subscription required in other countries).
- *The Cochrane Library* (collection of evidence-based systematic reviews): available from www.thecochranelibrary.com/view/0/index.html (subscription required in some countries).
- *Current Problems in Pharmacovigilance* (now superseded by *Drug Safety Update, see below*): archive available via MHRA website at www.mhra.gov.uk/home/idcplg?IdcService=SS_GET_PAGE&nodeId=368
- Department of Health resources (various UK government health publications and medical advice for travellers): available from http://www.dh.gov.uk/en/Healthcare/index.htm

- *Drug Safety Update*: available via MHRA website at www.mhra.gov.uk/Safetyinformation/DrugSafetyUpdate/DrugSafetyUpdatePDFarchive/index.htm
- *MeReC Bulletin*: available via National Prescribing Centre website at www.npc.nhs.uk/merec/
- National Institute for Health and Clinical Excellence (NICE) guidelines: available from www.nice.org.uk/
- Scottish Intercollegiate Guidelines Network (SIGN) guidelines: available from www.sign.ac.uk/index.html
- UK manufacturers' SPCs: available from www.medicines.org.uk

Various other sources (e.g. *Clinical Knowledge Summaries*) and full-text core journals are available free to UK NHS staff with an Athens password through the NHS Evidence Health Information Resources website (formerly the National Library for Health; NLH) at www.library.nhs.uk/Default.aspx

Certain BMJ group publications (e.g. the *British Medical Journal, BMJ Supportive & Palliative Care*) are available free to UK NHS staff with an Athens password through the BMJ website at www.bmj.com

The Pharmaceutical Journal (the official weekly journal of the Royal Pharmaceutical Society) is available without extra cost to UK pharmacists who have subscribed to annual membership of this professional body: available from www.pjonline.com. Site also gives access to *Clinical Pharmacist online*.

1 Eccles M *et al.* (1996) North of England evidence based guidelines development project: methods of guideline development. *British Medical Journal*. **312**: 760–762.
2 DoH (1996) *Clinical Guidelines: Using Clinical Guidelines to Improve Patient Care Within the NHS. Department of Health: NHS* Executive, Leeds.
3 Agency for Health Care Policy and Research (1992) Acute pain management, operative or medical procedures and trauma 92-0032. In: *Clinical Practice Guideline Quick Ref Guide for Clinicians*. AHCPR Publications, Rockville, Maryland, USA, pp. 1–22.
4 BMJ Publishing Group (2009) Resources for authors. Checklists and forms: clinical management guidelines. Available from: http://resources.bmj.com/bmj/authors/checklists-forms/clinical-management-guidelines
5 Aoun SM and Kristjanson LJ (2005) Challenging the framework for evidence in palliative care research. *Palliative Medicine*. **19**: 461–465.
6 Angell M (2004) *The Truth About the Drug Companies: how they deceive us and what to do about it*. Random House, New York.
7 National Prescribing Centre (2011) Generic prescribing in primary care. *MeReC Bulletin*. **21 (February)**: 1–6.
8 National Prescribing Centre (2000) Modified-release preparations. *MeReC Bulletin*. **11**: 13–16.
9 Smith J (2004) Building a Safer NHS for Patients — Improving Medication Safety. pp.105–111. Department of Health, London. Available from: www.dh.gov.uk/assetRoot/04/08/49/61/04084961.pdf
10 Sweetman S (2011) Martindale: the Complete Drug Reference (online edition). Available from: www.medicinescomplete.com/mc/martindale/current/

THE USE OF DRUGS BEYOND (OFF-LABEL) AND WITHOUT (UNLICENSED) MARKETING AUTHORIZATION

The use of drugs for off-label purposes is widespread. Surveys suggest that up to 1/4 of all prescriptions in palliative care come into this category.[1,2] In *PCF*, the symbol † is used to indicate such use. However, it is impractical to highlight all cases of off-label use, particularly when it is simply a matter of the route or dose being different from those in the manufacturer's Summary of Product Characteristics (SPC).

It is important for prescribers to understand that *marketing authorization* for drugs regulates the *marketing activities* of pharmaceutical companies, and not the prescriber's clinical practice. Even so, off-label use does have implications for prescribers, and these are discussed in this section.

The situation has become more complicated now that mixing two or more *licensed* drugs in a syringe for administration by continuous infusion is officially considered to produce an *unlicensed* preparation. However, such use in palliative care is often appropriate and will generally represent standard practice.

Definitions

Marketing authorization

Marketing authorization (MA) means that a drug has been approved by a regulatory body for use in humans and licensed for specific indications, and can be marketed by the relevant pharmaceutical company.

Off-label use

Off-label describes the use of a drug beyond the specifications of its MA, e.g. for an unlicensed indication, or in doses, preparations, patient population or route not covered by the MA.

Unlicensed drug

There is no simple definition of an unlicensed drug. Essentially it is a drug which does not have MA for medicinal use in humans. Unlicensed drugs include:

- a mixture of two or more drugs in a syringe for administration by continuous infusion (see p.665)
- 'specials' obtained from a commercial company with a 'specials' manufacturing licence, e.g. alfentanil solution for nasal/buccal administration (see p.769)
- preparations made in a local pharmacy at the request of a prescriber for an individual named patient
- drugs from a licensed manufacturer in the UK without MA in the UK, e.g. new drugs awaiting MA, or drugs for which MA has been abandoned, suspended or revoked, e.g. cisapride, oxetacaine, thioridazine
- drugs with MA in another country but not the UK and are imported
- new drugs undergoing clinical trials.

The authorization (licensing) process

Before a drug can be marketed in the UK, it requires MA (previously product licence). There are four application procedures in the European Union:

- *centralized*, application evaluated by the European Medicines Agency (EMEA); the European Commission grants a single MA valid for the whole European Union

- *decentralized*, simultaneous application made by several member states, with one taking the lead; if successful, national MA then being granted in each state
- *mutual recognition*, application for authorization in a member state when MA exists in another member state; the new member state relies on the original member state's evaluation as a basis for its decision
- *national*, application for MA in only one member state; in the UK the application is evaluated by the Medicines and Healthcare products Regulatory Agency (MHRA) on behalf of the Licensing Authority, a body consisting of UK health ministers.[3]

Certain drugs, e.g. for HIV/AIDS, cancer, neurodegenerative diseases, must be licensed through the centralized procedure. The UK Parallel Import Licensing Scheme also allows a drug authorized in other European Union states to be imported and marketed in the UK, if it has labels and a Patient Information Leaflet (PIL) in English.

In the UK, the MHRA evaluation comprises an evaluation of the efficacy, safety and quality of the drug from a medical, pharmaceutical and scientific viewpoint to ensure that it satisfies predefined criteria. Advice is sought from the Commission on Human Medicines (CHM), an independent advisory body, which in turn is assisted by specialist expert advisory groups.

At a European level, the Committee for Medicinal Products for Human Use (CHMP) fulfils a similar role to the CHM. New drugs will have relatively limited safety information and the pharmaceutical company is generally required to outline a risk management plan.

Restrictions are imposed if evidence of safety and efficacy is unavailable in particular patient groups, e.g. children. MA is granted for up to 5 years and then renewed following re-evaluation of the risks and benefits.[3]

Thus, the process ensures that in relation to the drug's authorized uses, there has been due consideration of its efficacy, safety and quality, that the benefits outweigh the potential risks, and that there is appropriate accompanying product information and labelling.[4] The MA defines the conditions and patient groups for which a pharmaceutical company can market and supply the drug, with more information about the drug's authorized uses provided by the manufacturer in the Summary of Product Characteristics (SPC).

However, the MA does not limit what the drug could be used for (i.e. off-label use), and clinical experience may reveal other indications. For these to receive a MA, additional evidence would need to be gathered and submitted. The considerable expense of this, perhaps coupled with a small market for a new indication, often means that a revised application is not made.

Prescribing for off-label indications or unlicensed drugs

In the UK, the following may legally prescribe licensed drugs for off-label indications and unlicensed drugs:[5–7]

- doctors, specifically safeguarded in the UK Medicines Act 1968
- nurses, pharmacists, podiatrists, physiotherapists and radiographers who are registered as *supplementary prescribers*, provided it is done in the framework of an agreed Clinical Management Plan for a specific patient in partnership with a doctor or dentist
- nurses or pharmacists who are registered as *independent prescribers* if this is accepted clinical practice.

These prescriptions can be dispensed by pharmacists[8] and administered by nurses or midwives.[9]

In addition to clinical trials, such prescriptions may be justified:

- when prescribing generic formulations for which indications are not described
- with established drugs for proven but unlicensed indications
- with drugs for conditions for which there are no other treatments (even in the absence of strong evidence)
- when using drugs in individuals not covered by the MA, e.g. children
- when mixing drugs before administration, e.g. two or more drugs in a syringe for administration by continuous infusion.[10,11]

Any *independent prescriber*, including non-medical prescribers, can mix drugs and direct others to mix, as can *supplementary prescribers* when the preparation is part of the Clinical Management Plan for an individual patient. Legislation on mixing now extends to controlled drugs. Existing good practice recommendations should be followed in relation to mixing all drugs.[10] Preparations resulting from mixing drugs, other than when one product is a vehicle for the administration of the other, cannot be supplied or administered under Patient Group Direction arrangements.

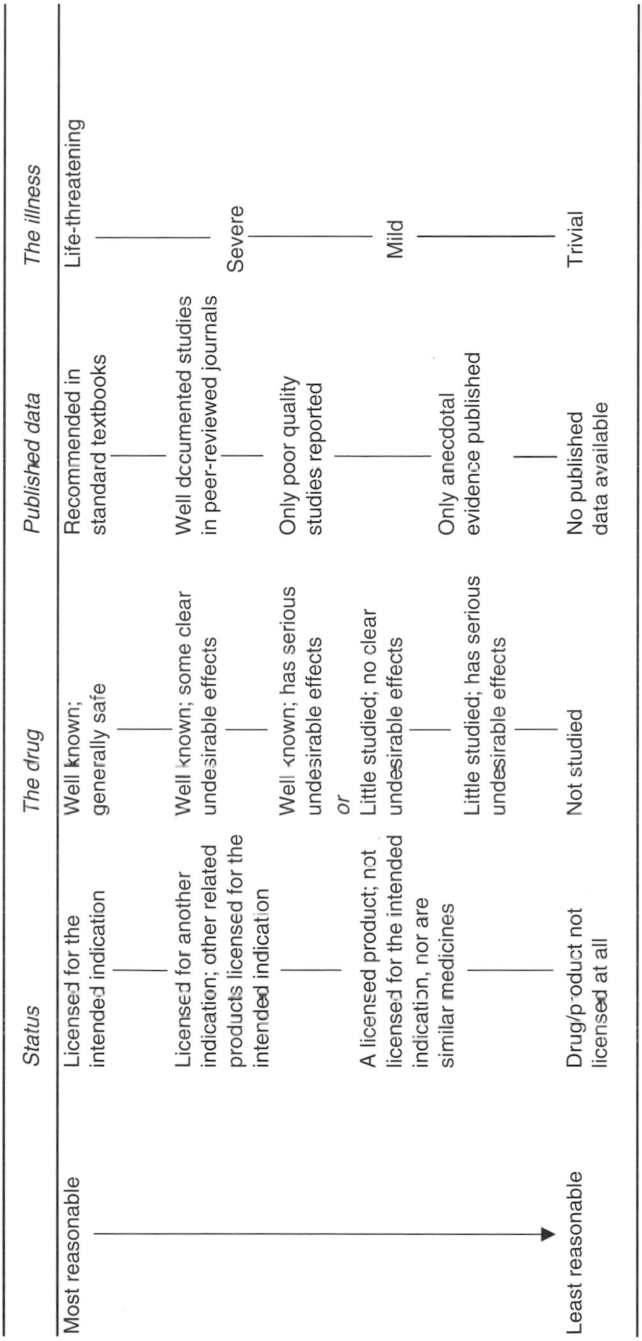

	Status	The drug	Published data	The illness
Most reasonable	Licensed for the intended indication	Well known; generally safe	Recommended in standard textbooks	Life-threatening
↓	Licensed for another indication; other related products licensed for the intended indication	Well known; some clear undesirable effects	Well documented studies in peer-reviewed journals	Severe
		Well known; has serious undesirable effects *or*	Only poor quality studies reported	
	A licensed product; not licensed for the intended indication, nor are similar medicines	Little studied; no clear undesirable effects		Mild
		Little studied; has serious undesirable effects	Only anecdotal evidence published	
Least reasonable	Drug/product not licensed at all	Not studied	No published data available	Trivial

Figure 1 Factors influencing the reasonableness of prescribing decisions.

The responsibility for the consequences of prescribing a drug under such circumstances lies with the prescriber, who must be competent, operate within the professional codes and ethics of their statutory bodies and the prescribing practices of their employers.[4-6] The prescriber must be fully informed about the actions and uses of the drug, be assured of the quality of the particular product, and in the light of published evidence, balance both the potential good and the potential harm which might ensue.

It is possible to draw a hierarchy of degrees of reasonableness relating to off-label and unlicensed drug use (Figure 1). The more dangerous the medicine and the more flimsy the evidence the more difficult it is to justify its prescription.

The PIL will not contain information about unlicensed indications. Thus, it is important that prescribers (or those authorizing treatment on their behalf) provide sufficient information to patients about the drug's expected benefits and potential risks (undesirable effects, drug interactions, etc.) to enable them to make an informed decision (Box B). The GMC also recommends that when prescribing a drug off-label, doctors should:

- be satisfied that such use would better serve the patient's needs than an authorized alternative (if one exists)
- be satisfied that there is sufficient evidence/experience of using the drug to show its safety and efficacy, seeking the necessary information from appropriate sources
- record in the patient's clinical notes the drug prescribed and, when not following common practice, the reasons for the choice
- take responsibility for prescribing the drug and for overseeing the patient's care, including monitoring the effects of the drug.

For off-label prescribing, monitoring can be delegated to another doctor, but not if the drug is completely unlicensed.[12]

Non-medical prescribers should ensure that they are familiar with their own profession's prescribing standards, e.g. NMC. Although the advice is broadly similar to that of the GMC, there are some differences.[13,14]

Box B Providing information for patients about the use of drugs beyond and without marketing authorization[12]

Some drugs are routinely used beyond their licence, e.g. when treating children. When current practice supports the use of a drug in this way, it may not be necessary to draw attention to the licence when recommending it.

However, it is good practice to give as much information as patients or those authorizing treatment on their behalf, require or which they may see as significant.

When patients, or their carers express concern, you should also explain in broad terms the reasons why the drug is not licensed for its proposed use. Such explanations may be supported by written information.

However, you must explain the reasons for prescribing a drug that is unlicensed or being used off-label when there is little research or other evidence of current practice to support its use, or when the use of the drug is innovative.

In palliative care, off-label drug use is so widespread that concerns have been expressed that a detailed explanation on every occasion is impractical, would be burdensome for the patient and increase anxiety, and could result in the refusal of beneficial treatment.[15] A recent UK survey of over 220 palliative medicine doctors showed that, when using a drug for a routine off-label indication, only 5% *always* mention this to their patients, and 31% *never* do. However, in situations where there is little evidence and limited clinical experience to support a drug's off-label use, these figures change to 57% and 7% respectively.[16]

This is a grey area and each clinician must decide how explicit to be; an appropriate level of counselling and a sensitive approach is essential. Some NHS Trusts and other institutions have policies in place and have produced information cards or leaflets for patients and caregivers (Box C). A position statement has also been produced by the Association for Palliative Medicine and the Pain Society (Box D).[17]

Box C Example of a patient information leaflet about the off-label use of a drug

Use of medicines beyond their licence (off-label)

This leaflet contains important information about your medicines, so please read it carefully.

Generally, medicines prescribed by your doctor or bought over-the-counter from a pharmacist are licensed for use by the Medicines and Healthcare products Regulatory Agency (MHRA).

The licence (or marketing authorization) specifies the conditions and patient groups for which the medicine should be used, and how it should be given.

Patient Information Leaflets (PILs) supplied with medicines reflect the licensed uses. When a medicine is used beyond its licence, the information in the PIL may not be relevant to your circumstances.

In palliative care, medicines are commonly used for conditions or in ways that are not specified on the licence.

Your doctor will use medicines beyond the licence only when there is research and experience to back up such use.

Medicines used very successfully beyond the licence include some antidepressants and anti-epileptics (anti-seizure drugs) when given to relieve some types of pain.

Also, instead of injecting into a vein or muscle, medicines are often given subcutaneously (under the skin) because this is more comfortable and convenient.

If you would like more information, please ask your doctor or pharmacist.

Alternatively, contact:

Dr/Nurse ....

Hospital ....

....

....

Tel ....

1 Atkinson C and Kirkham S (1999) Unlicensed uses for medication in a palliative care unit. *Palliative Medicine*. **13**: 145–152.
2 Todd J and Davies A (1999) Use of unlicensed medication in palliative medicine. *Palliative Medicine*. **13**: 466.
3 Anonymous (2009) The licensing of medicines in the UK. *Drug and Therapeutics Bulletin*. **47**: 45–48.
4 Anonymous (2009) Off-label or unlicensed medicines: prescribers' responsibilities. *MHRA Drug Safety Update*. **2 (9)**: 6–7.
5 Department of Health (2005) Supplementary prescribing by nurses, pharmacists, chiropodists/podiatrists, physiotherapists and radiographers within the NHS in England: a guide for implementation. HMSO, London. Available from: www.dh.gov.uk/en/Publicationsandstatistics/Publications/PublicationsPolicyAndGuidance/DH_4110032
6 Department of Health (2006) Improving patients' access to medicines: a guide to implementing nurse and pharmacist independent prescribing within the NHS in England. HMSO, London. Available from: www.dh.gov.uk/assetRoot/04/13/37/47/04133747.pdf
7 Department of Health (2010) Changes to medicines legislation to enable Mixing of Medicines prior to administration in clinical practice. Available from: www.dh.gov.uk/en/Healthcare/Medicinespharmacyandindustry/Prescriptions/TheNon-Medical-PrescribingProgramme/DH_110765
8 Royal Pharmaceutical Society of Great Britain (2007) Fitness to practise and legal affairs directorate fact sheet: five. The use of unlicensed medicines in pharmacy. Royal Pharmaceutical Society of Great Britain. Available from: www.rspgb.org/pdfs/factsheet5.pdf
9 Anonymous (1992) Prescribing unlicensed drugs or using drugs for unlicensed indications. *Drug and Therapeutics Bulletin*. **30**: 97–99.
10 Department of Health (2009) Mixing of medicines prior to administration in clinical practice: medical and non-medical prescribing. HMSO, London. Available from: www.dh.gov.uk/prod_consum_dh/groups/dh_digitalassets/@dh/@en/@ps/documents/digitalasset/dh_116360.pdf
11 National Prescribing Centre (2010) Mixing of medicines prior to administration in clinical practice — responding to legislative changes. Liverpool. Available from: www.npc.nhs.uk/improving_safety/mixing_meds/resources/mixing_of_medicines.pdf

Box D Recommendations of the Association for Palliative Medicine of Great Britain and Ireland and the British Pain Society[17]

Use of medicines beyond (off-label) and without (unlicensed) Marketing Authorization (MA) in palliative care and pain medicine

1 This statement should be seen as reflecting the views of a responsible body of opinion within the clinical specialties of palliative medicine and pain medicine

2 The use of medicines beyond and without a MA in palliative care and pain medicine practice is both necessary and common and should be seen as a legitimate aspect of clinical practice.

3 Organizations providing palliative care and pain medicine services should support therapeutic practices that are underpinned by evidence and advocated by a responsible body of professional opinion.

4 Health professionals involved in prescribing medicines beyond or without MA should select those medicines that offer the best balance of benefit against harm for any given patient.

5 Choice of treatment requires partnership between patients and health professionals, and informed consent should be obtained, whenever possible, before prescribing any medicine.

6 Patients should be offered accurate, clear and specific information that meets their needs about the use of medicines beyond or without a MA in accordance with professional regulatory body guidance. The information needs of carers and other health professionals involved in the care of the patient should also be considered and met as appropriate. The use of information cards or leaflets may help with this. It is often unnecessary to take additional steps when recommending medicines beyond or without MA.

7 Health professionals should inform, change and monitor their practice with regard to medicines beyond or without MA in the light of evidence from audit and published research.

8 The Department of Health should work with health professionals and the pharmaceutical industry to enable and encourage the extension of product licences where there is evidence of benefit in circumstances of defined clinical need.

12 General Medical Council (2008) Good practice in prescribing medicines. Available from: www.gmc-uk.org/guidance/ethical_guidance/prescriptions_faqs.asp

13 Nursing and Midwifery Council (2007) Standards for medicines managment. Available from: www.nmc-uk.org/Documents/Standards/nmcStandardsForMedicinesManagementBooklet.pdf

14 Royal Pharmaceutical Society of Great Britain (2010) Professional Standards and Guidance for Pharmacist Prescribers. Available from: www.rpharms.com/archived-documents/archived-documents.asp#law

15 Pavis H and Wilcock A (2001) Prescribing of drugs for use outside their licence in palliative care: survey of specialists in the United Kingdom. *British Medical Journal*. **323**: 484–485.

16 Wilcock A (2011) *Personal communication.*

17 British Pain Society (2011) Use of medicines beyond and without Marketing Authorization in palliative care and pain medicine. In press.

DRUG NAMES

All drugs marketed in Europe are now known by their recommended International Non-proprietary (generic) Name (rINN). In the past, most publications in the UK used the now outdated British Approved Name (BAN). To aid understanding of the older literature, significant differences between BANs and rINNs are listed in Table 1. However, when the difference is simply, e.g. 'f' instead of 'ph', 'e' instead of 'oe', or 't' instead of 'th', these generally have *not* been included.

In the USA, United States Adopted Names (USANs) take precedence over rINNs. USANs are also included in the Table where these differ significantly from rINNs.

With combination products such as codeine and paracetamol or diphenoxylate and atropine, the UK conventional names are shown in Table 2.

Table 1 Drug names relevant to palliative care for which the rINN, BAN and/or USAN differ

rINN	*BAN*	*USAN*
Alimemazine	Trimeprazine	Trimeprazine
Amobarbital	Amylobarbitone	
Bendroflumethiazide	Bendrofluazide	Bendroflumethiazide
Benzylpenicillin		Penicillin G
Calcitonin (salmon)	Salcatonin	Calcitonin
Carmellose		Carboxymethylcellulose
Chlorphenamine	Chlorpheniramine	Chlorpheniramine
Clomethiazole	Chlormethiazole	
Dexamfetamine	Dexamphetamine	Dextroamphetamine
Dextropropoxyphene		Propoxyphene
Dicycloverine	Dicyclomine	Dicyclomine
Diethylstilbestrol	Stilboestrol	Diethylstilbestrol
Dosulepin	Dothiepin	Dothiepin
Epinephrine	Adrenaline	Epinephrine
Glibenclamide		Glyburide
Glycerol	Glycerine	Glycerin
Glyceryl trinitrate		Nitroglycerin
Hyoscine		Scopolamine
Isoprenaline		Isoproterenol
	Ispaghula	Psyllium
Levomepromazine	Methotrimeprazine	
Levothyroxine	Thyroxine	
Liquid paraffin		Mineral oil
Methenamine hippurate	Hexamine hippurate	
Paracetamol		Acetaminophen
Pethidine		Meperidine
Phenobarbital	Phenobarbitone	
Phenoxymethylpenicillin		Penicillin V
Phytomenadione		Phytonadione
Retinol	Vitamin A	Vitamin A
Rifampicin		Rifampin
Salbutamol		Albuterol
Simeticone[a]	Simethicone	Simethicone
Sodium cromoglicate	Sodium cromoglycate	Cromolyn sodium
Tetracaine	Amethocaine	
Trihexyphenidyl	Benzhexol	Trihexyphenidyl

a. silica-activated dimeticone; known in some countries as activated dimethylpolysiloxane.

Table 2 Names of combination preparations

Contents	*UK name*
Amoxicillin-clavulanate	Co-amoxiclav
Diphenoxylate-atropine	Co-phenotrope
Magnesium hydroxide-aluminium hydroxide[a]	Co-magaldrox
Paracetamol-codeine phosphate	Co-codamol
Paracetamol-dextropropoxyphene[a]	Co-proxamol
Paracetamol-dihydrocodeine	Co-dydramol
Sulfamethoxazole-trimethoprim	Co-trimoxazole

a. no longer marketed in the UK.

ABBREVIATIONS

Drug administration
In 2005, the Joint Commission on Accreditation of Healthcare Organizations (JCAHO) in the USA published National Patient Safety Goals. These include a series of recommendations about ways in which confusion (and thus errors) can be reduced by avoiding the use of certain abbreviations on prescriptions. The full set of recommendations is available at www.jointcommission.org/PatientSafety/DoNotUseList.

Although some traditional abbreviations remain acceptable (e.g. Table 3), other commonly used ones are not. Thus, it is now recommended that the following are written in full:

- at bedtime
- once daily
- each morning
- every other day.

These four recommendations have also been adopted in *PCF*.

Although the following conventions have *not* been adopted in PCF, readers should be aware of the following recommendations for handwritten and printed prescriptions, and other printed medical matter, e.g. packaging, patient records:

- include a space between the drug dose and the unit of measure, e.g. 25 mg, not 25mg
- write 'per' instead of an oblique (mistaken for a figure 1), e.g. 200 mg per day, not 200mg/day
- use 'subcut' or 'subcutaneous' instead of SC (mistaken for SL)
- write 'less than' or 'greater than' instead of < and > (mistaken for a letter L or figure 7; or written the wrong way round and thus signifying the opposite of the intended meaning).

Further, although it has been recommended in the UK that 'PR' (prolonged-release) should become the generic term for 'slow-release', 'extended-release' etc., PR is a time-honoured abbreviation for 'per rectum'. It is in this latter sense that PR will be used in *PCF4*. As in earlier editions, 'm/r' (modified-release) will be used.

Table 3 Abbreviations used in *PCF* for the times of drug administration

Times	*UK*	*Latin*
Twice per day	b.d.	*bis die*
Three times per day	t.d.s.	*ter die sumendus*
Four times per day	q.d.s.	*quarta die sumendus*
Every 4 hours etc.	q4h	*quaque quarta hora*
Rescue medication(as needed/required)	p.r.n.	*pro re nata*
Give immediately	stat	

a.c. — ante cibum (before food)
amp — ampoule containing a single dose (cf. vial)
CD — preparation subject to prescription requirements under the Misuse of Drugs Act (UK); for regulations see BNF
CIVI — continuous intravenous infusion
CSCI — continuous subcutaneous infusion
e/c — enteric-coated (gastroresistant)

ED	epidural
IM	intramuscular
IT	intrathecal
IV	intravenous
IVI	intravenous infusion
m/r	modified-release; alternatives, controlled-release, extended-release, prolonged-release, slow-release, sustained-release
~~NHS~~	not prescribable on NHS prescriptions
OTC	over the counter (i.e. can be obtained without a prescription)
p.c.	post cibum (after food)
PO	per os, by mouth
POM	prescription-only medicine
PR	per rectum
PV	per vaginum
SC	subcutaneous
SL	sublingual
TD	transdermal
TM	transmucosal
vial	sterile container with a rubber bung containing either a single or multiple doses (cf. amp)
WFI	water for injections

General

*	specialist use only
†	unlicensed use
AHFS	American Hospital Formulary Service
BNF	British National Formulary
BP	British Pharmacopoeia
CHM	Commission on Human Medicines
CSM	Committee on Safety of Medicines (now part of CHM)
EMEA	European Medicines Agency
EORTC	European Organisation for Research and Treatment of Cancer
FDA	Food and Drug Administration (USA)
IASP	International Association for the Study of Pain
IDIS	International Drug Information Service
MCA	Medicines Control Agency (now MHRA)
MHRA	Medicines and Healthcare products Regulatory Agency (formerly MCA)
NICE	National Institute for Health and Clinical Excellence
NPF	Nurse Prescribers' Formulary
NYHA	New York Heart Association
PCS/PCU	palliative care service/unit
PEG	percutaneous endoscopic gastrostomy
PIL	Patient Information Leaflet
rINN	recommended International Non-proprietary Name
SPC	Summary of Product Characteristics
UK	United Kingdom
USA	United States of America
USP	United States Pharmacopoeia
VAS	visual analogue scale, 0–100mm
WHO	World Health Organization

Medical

ACE	angiotensin-converting enzyme
ADH	antidiuretic hormone (vasopressin)
ATP	adenosine triphosphate
AUC	area under the plasma concentration–time curve
β_2	beta 2 adrenergic (receptor)
CHF	congestive heart failure

C_{max}	maximum plasma drug concentration
CNS	central nervous system
COX	cyclo-oxygenase; alternative, prostaglandin synthase
COPD	chronic obstructive pulmonary disease
CKD	chronic kidney disease
CRP	C-reactive protein
CSF	cerebrospinal fluid
CT	computed tomography
δ	delta-opioid (receptor)
D_2	dopamine type 2 (receptor)
DIC	disseminated intravascular coagulation
DVT	deep vein thrombosis
ECG (EKG)	electrocardiogram
EFT	enteral feeding tube
FBC	full blood count
FEV_1	forced expiratory volume in 1 second
FRC	functional residual capacity
FSH	follicle-stimulating hormone
FVC	forced vital capacity of lungs
GABA	gamma-aminobutyric acid
GI	gastro-intestinal
Hb	haemoglobin
HIV	human immunodeficiency virus
H_1, H_2	histamine type 1, type 2 (receptor)
Ig	immunoglobulin
INR	international normalized ratio
κ	kappa-opioid (receptor)
LABA	long-acting β_2-adrenergic receptor agonist
LFTs	liver function tests
LH	luteinizing hormone
LMWH	low molecular weight heparin
MAOI	mono-amine oxidase inhibitor
MARI	mono-amine re-uptake inhibitor
MRI	magnetic resonance imaging
MSU	mid-stream specimen of urine
μ	mu-opioid (receptor)
NaSSA	noradrenergic and specific serotoninergic antidepressant
NDRI	noradrenaline (norepinephrine) and dopamine re-uptake inhibitor
NG	nasogastric
NJ	nasojejunal
NMDA	N-methyl D-aspartate
NNH	number needed to harm, i.e. the number of patients needed to be treated in order to harm one patient sufficiently to cause withdrawal from a drug trial
NNT	number needed to treat, i.e. the number of patients needed to be treated in order to achieve 50% improvement in one patient compared with placebo
NO	nitric oxide
NRI	noradrenaline (norepinephrine) re-uptake inhibitor
NSAID	non-steroidal anti-inflammatory drug
$PaCO_2$	arterial partial pressure of carbon dioxide
PaO_2	arterial partial pressure of oxygen
PCA	patient-controlled analgesia
PE	pulmonary embolus/embolism
PEF	peak expiratory flow
PG	prostaglandin
PPI	proton pump inhibitor
RCT	randomized controlled trial
RIMA	reversible inhibitor of mono-amine oxidase type A
RTI	respiratory tract infection
SaO_2	oxygen saturation

SNRI	serotonin and noradrenaline (norepinephrine) re-uptake inhibitor
SSRI	selective serotonin re-uptake inhibitor
TCA	tricyclic antidepressant
TIBC	total iron-binding capacity; alternative, plasma transferrin concentration
Tl_{CO}	transfer factor of the lung for carbon monoxide
T_{max}	time to reach C_{max}
UTI	urinary tract infection
VEGF	vascular endothelial growth factor
VIP	vaso-active intestinal polypeptide
WBC	white blood cell
w/v	weight of solute (g) per 100mL

Units

cm	centimetre(s)
cps	cycles per sec
dL	decilitre(s)
g	gram(s)
Gy	Gray(s), a measure of radiation
h	hour(s)
Hg	mercury
kcal	kilocalories
kg	kilogram(s)
L	litre(s)
mg	milligram(s)
microL	microlitre(s)
micromol	micromole(s)
mL	millilitre(s)
mm	millimetre(s)
mmol	millimole(s)
min	minute(s)
mosmol	milli-osmole(s)
msec	millisecond
nm	nanometre(s)
nmol	nanomole(s); alternative, nM
sec	second(s)

1: GASTRO-INTESTINAL SYSTEM

ANTACIDS — BNF 1.1.1

Antacids taken by mouth to neutralize gastric acid include:

- magnesium salts
- aluminium hydroxide
- hydrotalcite (aluminium magnesium carbonate hydroxide hydrate)
- calcium carbonate
- sodium bicarbonate.

***Magnesium salts** are laxative and can cause diarrhoea; **aluminium salts** constipate.* Most proprietary antacids contain a mixture of **magnesium salts** and **aluminium salts** so as to have a neutral impact on intestinal transit. With doses of 100–200mL/24h or more, the effect of **magnesium salts** tends to override the constipating effect of **aluminium**.[1]

The sodium content of some antacids may be detrimental in patients on salt-restricted diets, e.g. those with hypertension or heart failure; Gaviscon® Liquid, Acidex® liquid, Peptac® oral suspension (available OTC) and **magnesium trisilicate mixture BP** contain 6mmol/10mL. Gaviscon® Advance liquid contains 4.6mmol in 10 mL. This compares with 0.1 nmol/10mL in **co-magaldrox**.

Regular use of **sodium bicarbonate** may cause sodium loading and metabolic alkalosis. **Calcium carbonate** may cause rebound acid secretion about 2h after each dose, and regular use may cause hypercalcaemia, particularly if taken with **sodium bicarbonate**.

Aluminium hydroxide binds dietary phosphate. It is of benefit in patients with hyperphosphataemia in renal failure. Long-term complications of phosphate depletion and osteomalacia are not an issue in advanced cancer. **Hydrotalcite** binds bile salts and is of specific benefit in patients with bile salt reflux, e.g. after certain forms of gastroduodenal surgery.

In post-radiation oesophagitis and candidosis which is causing painful swallowing, an **aluminium hydroxide-magnesium hydroxide** suspension containing **oxetacaine**, a local anaesthetic, can be helpful; this is unlicensed in the UK. Give 5–10mL (without fluid) 15min a.c. & at bedtime., and p.r.n. before drinks. This should be regarded as short-term symptomatic treatment while time and specific treatment of the underlying condition permits healing of the damaged mucosa. Alternatively, plain **benzocaine** suspension can be used (locally prepared).

The following should be borne in mind:

- the administration of antacids should be separated from the administration of e/c tablets; direct contact between e/c tablets and antacids may result in damage to the enteric coating with consequential exposure of the drug to gastric acid, and of the stomach mucosa to the drug
- apart from **sodium bicarbonate**, antacids delay gastric emptying and may thereby modify drug absorption
- some proprietary products contain peppermint oil which masks the chalky taste of the antacid and helps belching by decreasing the tone of the lower oesophageal sphincter
- some proprietary products are fruit-flavoured, e.g. Tums® (chewable tablet)
- most antacid tablets feel gritty when sucked; some patients dislike this
- the cheapest single-ingredient products are **magnesium trisilicate mixture BP** and **aluminium hydroxide** capsules; if a combination is required, the cheapest liquid product is Mucogel®
- magnesium-containing antacids should be used with caution in patients with renal impairment (see p.49); **calcium carbonate** is preferable
- some antacids contain additional substances for specific situations, e.g. **alginates** (see p.3), **simeticone** (silica-activated **dimeticone**) (see p.3).

Nowadays, antacids are generally only used p.r.n. for occasional dyspepsia; H_2-receptor antagonists (see p.22) and PPIs (see p.27) are used when continuous gastric acid reduction is indicated.[2]

Supply

Also see **Simeticone**, p.3.

Aluminium hydroxide
Alucap® (Meda)
Capsules 475mg, 28 days @ 1 t.d.s. & at bedtime. = £3.50.

Magnesium trisilicate mixture BP (generic)
Oral suspension 28 days @ 10mL t.d.s. & at bedtime. = £5; *peppermint flavour.*

Co-magaldrox
Maalox® (Sanofi-Aventis)
Oral suspension (sugar-free) **co-magaldrox** 195/220 (**magnesium hydroxide** 195mg, **aluminium hydroxide** 220mg/5mL), 28 days @ 10mL t.d.s. & at bedtime. = £6; *low* Na^+.

Mucogel® (Forest)
Oral suspension (sugar-free) **co-magaldrox** 195/220 (**magnesium hydroxide** 195mg, **aluminium hydroxide** 220mg/5mL), 28 days @ 10mL t.d.s. & at bedtime. = £4; *low* Na^+.

Hydrotalcite (generic)
Oral suspension 500mg/5mL, 28 days @ 10mL t.d.s. & at bedtime. = £6; *low* Na^+.

With **oxetacaine**
Oral suspension **oxetacaine** 10mg, **aluminium hydroxide** 200mg, **magnesium hydroxide** 100mg/5mL, 28 days @ 10mL t.d.s. a.c. & at bedtime. = £147. (Unlicensed, available as a special order from Rosemont; see Obtaining unlicensed products, p.769). *Available as Mucaine® suspension (Wyeth) in some countries.*

1 Morrissey J and Barreras R (1974) Antacid therapy. *New England Journal of Medicine*. **290**: 550–554.
2 NICE (2004) Dyspepsia. Management of dyspepsia in adults in primary care. In: *Clinical Guideline 17*. National Institute for Clinical Excellence. Available from: www.nice.org.uk/page.aspx?o = CG017

COMPOUND ALGINATE PRODUCTS — BNF 1.1.2

Included for general information. Alginate products are generally *not recommended* as antacids for palliative care patients.

Class: Alginate.

Indications: Acid reflux ('heartburn').

Pharmacology

Antacid products containing alginic acid or sodium alginate prevent oesophageal reflux pain by forming an inert low-density raft on the top of the acidic stomach contents. Both acid and air bubbles are necessary to produce the raft. Compound alginate products may thus be less effective if used with drugs which reduce acid (e.g. an H_2-receptor antagonist or a PPI) or products which reduce air bubbles (i.e. an antifoaming agent/antiflatulent).

Gaviscon® products, Peptac® and Acidex® oral suspensions are sodium alginate products and weak antacids; most of the antacid content adheres to the alginate raft. This neutralizes acid which seeps into the oesophagus around the raft but does nothing to correct the underlying causes, e.g. lax lower oesophageal sphincter, hyperacidity, delayed gastric emptying, obesity. Indeed, alginate-containing products are no better than **simeticone**-containing antacids in the treatment of acid reflux.[1] Compound alginate products have been largely superseded by acid suppression with PPIs and H_2-receptor antagonists.
Onset of action <5min.
Duration of action 1–2h.

Cautions

Gaviscon® Liquid, Peptac® and Acidex® oral suspensions contain approximately Na^+ 6mmol/10mL. Gaviscon® Advance oral suspension and tablets contain Na^+4.6mmol/10mL and 2.3mmol/tablet, respectively. They should not be used in patients on a salt-restricted diet, e.g. those with fluid retention, heart failure or renal impairment.

Dose and use

Several products are available but none is recommended.

Supply

See BNF for products prescribable on the NHS. Gaviscon® products, Peptac® and Acidex® oral suspensions are available OTC.

1 Pokorny C *et al.* (1985) Comparison of an antacid/dimethicone mixture and an alginate/antacid mixture in the treatment of oesophagitis. *Gut.* **26**: A574.

SIMETICONE — BNF 1.1.1

Class: Antifoaming agent (antiflatulent).

Indications: Acid dyspepsia (including acid reflux), gassy dyspepsia, †hiccup (if associated with gastric distension).

Pharmacology

Simeticone (silica-activated dimeticone or dimethylpolysiloxane) is a mixture of liquid dimeticones with silicon dioxide. It is an antifoaming agent present in several proprietary combination antacids, e.g. Asilone®, Maalox Plus®. By facilitating belching, simeticone eases flatulence, distension and postprandial gastric discomfort. Simeticone-containing antacids are as effective as alginate-containing products in the treatment of acid reflux.[1] Asilone® or Maalox Plus® should be used in

preference to Gaviscon® Liquid, Gaviscon® Advance oral suspension or Peptac® oral suspension because they contain much less sodium and are cheaper.
Onset of action <5min.
Duration of action 1–2h.

Cautions

Although Asilone® and Maalox Plus® contain both **aluminium** and **magnesium**, at higher doses (e.g. >100–200mL/day) the laxative effect of **magnesium** tends to override the constipating effect of **aluminium**.[2]

Dose and use

- start with Asilone® or Maalox Plus® suspension 5mL p.r.n., or 5mL q.d.s. & p.r.n.
- if necessary, double dose to 10mL.

Supply

Asilone® (Thornton & Ross)
Oral suspension (sugar-free) simeticone 135mg, dried **aluminium hydroxide** 420mg, light **magnesium oxide** 70mg/5mL, 28 days @ 5mL q.d.s. = £2; *low* Na^+.

Maalox Plus® (Sanofi Aventis)
Oral suspension (sugar-free) simeticone 25mg, dried **aluminium hydroxide** 220mg, **magnesium hydroxide** 195mg/5mL, 28days @ 5mL q.d.s = .£3; *low* Na^+

1 Pokorny C *et al.* (1985) Comparison of an antacid/dimethicone mixture and an alginate/antacid mixture in the treatment of oesophagitis. *Gut.* **26**: A574.
2 Morrissey J and Barreras R (1974) Antacid therapy. *New England Journal of Medicine.* **290**: 550–554.

ANTIMUSCARINICS BNF 1.2, 4.6 & 15.1.3

Indications: Smooth muscle spasm (e.g. bladder, intestine), motion sickness (**hyoscine *hydrobromide*** TD), drying secretions (including surgical premedication, †sialorrhoea, †drooling, †death rattle/noisy respiratory secretions, †inoperable intestinal obstruction), †paraneoplastic pyrexia and sweating.

Contra-indications: See individual monographs.

Pharmacology

Antimuscarinics are classified chemically as tertiary amines or quaternary ammonium compounds. The naturally-occurring belladonna alkaloids, **atropine** and **hyoscine *hydrobromide***, are tertiary amines, whereas the numerous semisynthetic and synthetic derivatives fall into both categories. Thus, **dicycloverine**, **oxybutynin** and **tolterodine** are tertiary amines, and **glycopyrronium**, **propantheline** and **hyoscine *butylbromide*** are quaternary ammonium compounds.

Except for **hyoscine *hydrobromide***, which causes CNS depression at therapeutic doses, the tertiary amines stimulate the brain stem and higher centres, producing mild central vagal excitation and respiratory stimulation. At toxic doses, all the tertiary amines, including **hyoscine *hydrobromide*** cause CNS stimulation resulting in agitation and delirium. Synthetic tertiary amines generally cause less central stimulation than the naturally-occurring alkaloids. Quaternary ammonium compounds do not cross the blood-brain barrier in any significant amount, and accordingly do not have any central effects.[1] They are also less well absorbed from the GI tract.

Peripheral antimuscarinic effects are a class characteristic (Box 1.A), and have been summarized as:

'Dry as a bone, blind as a bat, red as a beet, hot as a hare, mad as a hatter.'

However, at least five different types of muscarinic receptors have been identified,[2] and newer drugs tend to be more selective in their actions. Thus, **oxybutynin** and **tolterodine** are relatively selective for muscarinic receptors in the urinary tract (see p.527).

Except when a reduction of oropharyngeal secretions is intended, dry mouth is an almost universal *undesirable* effect with this class of drugs. The secretion of saliva is mainly under the control of the autonomic nervous system. Food in the mouth causes reflex secretion of saliva, and so does stimulation by acid of afferent vagal fibres in the lower oesophagus. Stimulation of the parasympathetic nerves causes profuse secretion of watery saliva, whereas stimulation of the sympathetic nerve supply causes the secretion from only the submaxillary glands of small quantities of saliva rich in organic constituents.[3] If the parasympathetic supply is interrupted, the salivary glands atrophy, whereas interruption of the sympathetic supply has no such effect.

Box 1.A Peripheral antimuscarinic effects

Visual
Mydriasis
Loss of accommodation } blurred vision (and thus may impair driving ability)

Cardiovascular
Tachycardia, palpitations
Extrasystoles
Arrhythmias } also related to noradrenaline (norepinephrine) potentiation and a quinidine-like action

Gastro-intestinal
Dry mouth
Heartburn (relaxation of lower oesophageal sphincter)
Constipation

Urinary tract
Hesitancy of micturition
Retention of urine

Skin
Reduced sweating
Flushing

The muscarinic receptors in salivary glands are very responsive to antimuscarinics and inhibition of salivation occurs at lower doses than required for other antimuscarinic effects.[4] This reduces the likelihood of undesirable effects when antimuscarinics are given to reduce salivation. In some patients, a reduction in excess saliva results in improved speech.[5]

Antimuscarinics are widely used to prevent death rattle (noisy respiratory secretions) in those close to death (see Quick Practice Guide, p.8). Although debatable,[6] the general consensus is that their use is often beneficial.[7–9] The belladonna alkaloids are equally effective,[7] but **glycopyrronium** may sometimes be effective when the belladonna alkaloids have not been.[10] Death rattle is reduced in 1/2–2/3 of patients.[10,11] Although one study reported that **hyoscine *hydrobromide*** acts faster than **glycopyrronium**, there is no detectable difference between the two drugs 1 h after administration.[12]

To reduce the risk of undesirable effects, e.g. the development of an agitated delirium (central antimuscarinic syndrome), the concurrent use of two antimuscarinic drugs should generally be avoided (Box 1.B). Likewise, the concurrent use of an antimuscarinic and an opioid should be avoided as far as possible. Both cause constipation (by different mechanisms) and, if used together, will result in an increased need for laxatives, and may even result in a paralytic ileus. On the other hand, **morphine** and **hyoscine *butylbromide*** or **glycopyrronium** are sometimes purposely combined in terminally ill patients with inoperable intestinal obstruction in order to prevent colic and to reduce vomiting.[13]

Box 1.B Drugs with antimuscarinic effects used in palliative care

Analgesics pethidine (*not* recommended) nefopam (mostly postoperative) Antidepressants TCAs, e.g. amitriptyline, imipramine paroxetine (SSRI) Antihistamines, e.g. chlorphenamine cyclizine dimenhydrinate (not UK) promethazine Antiparkinsonians, e.g. orphenadrine procyclidine Antipsychotics (atypical) clozapine olanzapine	Antipsychotics (typical) phenothiazines, e.g. chlorpromazine levomepromazine prochlorperazine Antisecretory drugs belladonna alkaloids atropine hyoscine hyoscyamine (l-atropine, not UK)[a] glycopyrronium Antispasmodics, e.g. dicycloverine mebeverine oxybutynin propantheline tolterodine

a. because the d-isomer is virtually inactive, hyoscyamine is twice as potent as racemic atropine.

Antimuscarinics used as antispasmodics and/or antisecretory drugs differ in their pharmacokinetic characteristics (Table 1.1). Availability and fashion are probably the main influences in choice of drug.

Table 1.1 Pharmacokinetic details of antimuscarinic drugs used for death rattle (noisy respiratory secretions)

	Bio-availability	*Plasma halflife*	*Duration of action (antisecretory)*
Atropine	'readily absorbed' PO,SL	4h	no data
Glycopyrronium	<5% PO	1.7h	7h
Hyoscine *butylbromide*	8–10% PO	5–6h	<2h[a]
Hyoscine *hydrobromide*	60–80% SL	5–6h	1–9h

a. in volunteers; possibly longer in moribund patients.

Cautions

Use with caution in myasthenia gravis, conditions predisposing to tachycardia (e.g. thyrotoxicosis, heart failure, β agonists), and bladder outflow obstruction (prostatism). Use in hot weather or pyrexia may lead to heatstroke. Likely to exacerbate acid reflux. Narrow-angle glaucoma may be precipitated in those at risk, particularly the elderly.

Concurrent treatment with two antimuscarinic drugs will increase the likelihood of undesirable effects, and of central toxicity, i.e. restlessness, agitation, delirium. Children, the elderly, and patients with renal or hepatic impairment are more susceptible to the central effects of antimuscarinics.

Various drugs not generally considered antimuscarinic have been shown to have detectable antimuscarinic activity by means of a radioreceptor assay, including **codeine**, **digoxin**, **dipyridamole**, **isosorbide**, **nifedipine**, **prednisolone**, **ranitidine**, **theophylline**, **warfarin**.[14] Theoretically, these drugs could exacerbate toxicity, particularly in debilitated elderly patients.

The increased GI transit time produced by antimuscarinics may allow increased drug absorption from some formulations, e.g. **digoxin** and **nitrofurantoin** from tablets and **potassium** from m/r tablets, but reduced absorption from others, e.g. **paracetamol** tablets. Dissolution and absorption of SL tablets (e.g. **glyceryl trinitrate**) may be reduced because of decreased saliva production.

Drug interactions

Because antimuscarinics competitively block the final common (cholinergic) pathway through which prokinetics act,[15] concurrent prescription with **metoclopramide** and **domperidone** should be avoided if possible.

Dose and use

Antispasmodic

Antimuscarinics are used to relieve smooth muscle spasm in the bladder (see **oxybutynin**, p.527) and rectum.

Antispasmodic and antisecretory

Antimuscarinics are used to reduce intestinal colic and intestinal secretions, particularly gastric, associated with inoperable organic intestinal obstruction in terminally ill patients (Table 1.2).

Table 1.2 Antisecretory and antispasmodic drugs: typical SC doses

Drug	*Stat and p.r.n. doses*	*CSCI dose/24h*
Atropine	400microgram	1,200–2,000microgram
Glycopyrronium	200microgram	600–1,200microgram
Hyoscine *butylbromide*	20mg	20–300mg[a]
Hyoscine *hydrobromide*	400microgram	1,200–2,000microgram

a. death rattle 20–60mg, some centres use up to 120mg; intestinal obstruction 60–300mg.

Antisecretory

Drooling (and sialorrhoea)

Seen particularly in patients with ALS/MND, advanced Parkinson's disease or with various disorders of the head and neck. Several regimens have been recommended, including:

- **atropine** 1% ophthalmic solution, 4 drops SL q4h p.r.n. (Note: drop size varies with applicator and technique, dose per drop may vary from 200–500microgram, i.e. 800microgram–2mg/dose)
- **glycopyrronium** PO (see p.11)
- **hyoscine *hydrobromide*** 1mg/3 days TD.[16]

A regimen of **atropine** 1% 500microgram (1 drop) b.d. has been reported[17] but a controlled trial found 500microgram (2 drops) q.d.s. no better than placebo.[18]

When antimuscarinics are contra-indicated, not tolerated or ineffective, **botulinum toxin** injections (with ultrasound guidance) into the parotid and submandibular glands offer an alternative approach. Generally effective in ≤1–2 weeks, with benefit lasting 3–4 months.[19–23]

Death rattle (noisy respiratory secretions)

In the UK, antimuscarinic drugs for death rattle are generally given SC.[24] See Table 1.2 and Quick Practice Guide, p.8. In some countries the SL route is preferred, particularly in home care because it circumvents the need for injections. Treatment regimens, all unlicensed, are based mainly on local clinical experience, e.g.:

- **atropine** 1% ophthalmic solution, 4 drops SL q4h p.r.n. (Note: drop size varies with applicator and technique, dose per drop may vary from 200–500microgram, i.e. 800microgram–2mg/dose)
- **glycopyrronium** 100microgram SL q6h p.r.n. (see p.11).

Paraneoplastic pyrexia and sweating

Antimuscarinic drugs are used in the treatment of paraneoplastic pyrexia (Box 1.C).

Quick Practice Guide: Management of death rattle (noisy respiratory secretions)

Death rattle is a term used to describe noisy rattling breathing which occurs in about 50% of patients near the end of life. It is caused by fluid pooling in the hypopharynx which arises from one or more sources:

- saliva (most common)
- respiratory tract infection
- pulmonary oedema
- gastric reflux.

Rattling breathing can also occur in patients with a tracheostomy and infection. Because the patient is generally semiconscious or unconscious, drug treatment for death rattle is mainly for the benefit of relatives, other patients and staff.

Non-drug treatment

- ease the family's distress by explaining that the semiconscious/unconscious patient is not distressed by the rattle
- position the patient semiprone to encourage postural drainage; but upright or semirecumbent if the cause is pulmonary oedema or gastric reflux
- oropharyngeal suction but, because it is distressing to many moribund patients, generally reserve for unconscious patients.

Drug treatment

Saliva

Because they do not affect existing secretions, an antisecretory drug should be given SC (see Table) or SL (see Box) as soon as the onset of the rattle begins. SL use is unlicensed and less well supported by the literature.

Antimuscarinic antisecretory drugs for death rattle: typical SC doses

Drug	*Stat and p.r.n. SC dose*	*CSCI dose/24h*
Atropine	400microgram	1,200–2,000microgram
Glycopyrronium	200microgram	600–1,200microgram
Hyoscine *butylbromide*	20mg	20–120mg
Hyoscine *hydrobromide*	400microgram	1,200–2,000microgram
Hyoscyamine (l-atropine; not UK)	200microgram	600–1,000microgram

Antimuscarinic antisecretory drugs for death rattle: typical SL doses

Atropine 1% ophthalmic solution, 4 drops SL q4h p.r.n. (Note: drop size varies with applicator and technique, dose per drop may vary from 200–500microgram, i.e. 800microgram–2mg/dose).

Glycopyrronium 0.01% oral solution, 1mL (100microgram) SL q6h p.r.n.; can be prepared locally from glycopyrronium powder.

Hyoscyamine drops 125microgram/mL, 2mL (250microgram) SL q4h p.r.n. (not UK).

Note:

- by injection, the efficacy of the different drugs is broadly similar, and the rattle is reduced in 1/2–2/3 of patients
- hyoscine *hydrobromide* crosses the blood-brain barrier and possesses anti-emetic and sedative properties, but there is also a risk of developing or exacerbating delirium
- atropine and hyoscyamine also cross the blood-brain barrier but tend to stimulate rather than sedate; concurrent use with midazolam or haloperidol is more likely to be necessary.

Respiratory tract infection

Occasionally it is appropriate to prescribe an antibiotic in an imminently dying patient if death rattle is caused by profuse purulent sputum associated with an underlying chest infection:

- e.g. ceftriaxone, mix 1g ampoule with 2.1mL lidocaine 1% (total volume 2.6–2.8mL), and give 250–1000mg SC/IM once daily.
- some centres use larger volumes of lidocaine 1% (up to 4mL) and administer a divided dose at separate SC/IM sites once daily, or give b.d.

Pulmonary oedema

Consider furosemide 20–40mg SC/IM/IV q2h p.r.n.
Note: beware precipitating urinary retention.

Gastric reflux

Consider metoclopramide 20mg SC/IV q3h p.r.n., but do not use concurrently with an antimuscarinic because the latter blocks the prokinetic effect of the former.

Rattling breathing causing distress to a patient
In a semiconscious patient, if rattling breathing is associated with breathlessness, supplement the above with an opioid (e.g. morphine) ± an anxiolytic sedative (e.g. midazolam).

Box 1.C Symptomatic drug treatment of paraneoplastic pyrexia and sweating

Prescribe an antipyretic:

- paracetamol 500–1,000mg q.d.s. or p.r.n. (generally less toxic than an NSAID)
- NSAID, e.g. ibuprofen 200–400mg t.d.s. or p.r.n. (or the locally preferred alternative).

If the sweating does not respond to an NSAID, prescribe an antimuscarinic drug:

- amitriptyline 25–50mg at bedtime. (may cause sedation, dry mouth, and other antimuscarinic effects)
- hyoscine *hydrobromide* 1mg/3 days TD[25]
- glycopyrronium up to 2mg PO t.d.s.[26]

If an antimuscarinic fails, other options include:

- propranolol 10–20mg b.d.–t.d.s.
- cimetidine 400–800mg b.d.[27]
- olanzapine 5mg b.d.[28]
- thalidomide 100mg at bedtime.[29,30]

Thalidomide is generally seen as the last resort even though the response rate appears to be high.[29] This is because it can cause an irreversible painful peripheral neuropathy, and may also cause drowsiness (see p.519).

Overdose

In the past, **physostigmine**, a cholinesterase inhibitor, was sometimes administered to correct antimuscarinic toxicity/poisoning. This is no longer recommended because **physostigmine** itself can cause serious toxic effects, including cardiac arrhythmias and seizures.[31–33] A benzodiazepine can be given to control marked agitation and seizures. Phenothiazines should not be given because they will exacerbate the antimuscarinic effects, and could precipitate an acute dystonia (see Drug-induced movement disorders, p.745). Anti-arrhythmics are not advisable if arrhythmias develop; but hypoxia and acidosis should be corrected.

Supply

See individual monographs: **hyoscine *butylbromide*** (p.14), **hyoscine *hydrobromide*** (p.16), **glycopyrronium** (p.11), **propantheline** (p.18), **oxybutynin** (p.527).

Atropine sulphate (generic)
Ophthalmic solution 1%, 10mL bottle = £1.

Minims® atropine sulphate (Bausch & Lomb)
Ophthalmic solution (single-dose units) 1%, 0.5mL single-dose unit = £0.50.

1 Sweetman SC (ed) (2005) *Martindale: The Complete Drug Reference* (34e). Pharmaceutical Press, London, p. 475.
2 Caulfield M and Birdsall N (1998) International Union of Pharmacology. XVII. Classification of muscarinic acetylcholine receptors. *Pharmacological Review.* **50**: 279–290.
3 Ganong WF (1979) *Review of Medical Physiology* (9e). Lange Medical Publications, pp. 177–181.
4 Ali-Melkkila T *et al.* (1993) Pharmacokinetics and related pharmacodynamics of anticholinergic drugs. *Acta Anaesthesiologica Scandinavica.* **37**: 633–642.
5 Rashid H *et al.* (1997) Management of secretions in esophageal cancer patients with glycopyrrolate. *Annals of Oncology.* **8**: 198–199.
6 Wee B and Hillier R (2008) Interventions for noisy breathing in patients near to death. *Cochrane Database of Systematic Reviews.* **1**: CD005177.
7 Wildiers H *et al.* (2009) Atropine, hyoscine butylbromide, or scopolamine are equally effective for the treatment of death rattle in terminal care. *Journal of Pain and Symptom Management.* **38**: 124–133.
8 Likar R *et al.* (2008) Efficacy of glycopyrronium bromide and scopolamine hydrobromide in patients with death rattle: a randomized controlled study. *Wiener Klinische Wochenschrift.* **120**: 679–683.
9 Hugel H *et al.* (2006) Respiratory tract secretions in the dying patient: a comparison between glycopyrronium and hyoscine hydrobromide. *Journal of Palliative Medicine.* **9**: 279–284.
10 Mirakhur R and Dundee J (1980) A comparison of the effects of atropine and glycopyrollate on various end organs. *Journal of the Royal Society of Medicine.* **73**: 727–730.
11 Hughes A *et al.* (2000) Audit of three antimuscarinic drugs for managing retained secretions. *Palliative Medicine.* **14**: 221–222.
12 Back I *et al.* (2001) A study comparing hyoscine hydrobromide and glycopyrrolate in the treatment of death rattle. *Palliative Medicine.* **15**: 329–336.
13 Twycross RG and Wilcock A (2001) *Symptom Management in Advanced Cancer* (3e). Radcliffe Medical Press, Oxford, pp. 113–114.
14 Tune I *et al.* (1992) Anticholinergic effects of drugs commonly prescribed for the elderly; potential means of assessing risk of delirium. *American Journal of Psychiatry.* **149**: 1393–1394.
15 Schuurkes JAJ *et al.* (1986) Stimulation of gastroduodenal motor activity: dopaminergic and cholinergic modulation. *Drug Development Research.* **8**: 233–241.
16 Talmi YP *et al.* (1990) Reduction of salivary flow with transdermal scopolamine: a four-year experience. *Otolaryngology Head and Neck Surgery.* **103**: 615–618.
17 Hyson HC *et al.* (2002) Sublingual atropine for sialorrhea secondary to parkinsonism: a pilot study. *Movement Disorders.* **17**: 1318–1320.
18 De Simone GG *et al.* (2006) Atropine drops for drooling: a randomized controlled trial. *Palliative Medicine.* **20**: 665–671.
19 Lipp A *et al.* (2003) A randomized trial of botulinum toxin A for treatment of drooling. *Neurology.* **61**: 1279–1281.
20 Mancini F *et al.* (2003) Double-blind, placebo-controlled study to evaluate the efficacy and safety of botulinum toxin type A in the treatment of drooling in parkinsonism. *Movement Disorders.* **18**: 685–688.
21 Ellies M *et al.* (2004) Reduction of salivary flow with botulinum toxin: extended report on 33 patients with drooling, salivary fistulas, and sialadenitis. *Laryngoscope.* **114**: 1856–1860.
22 Jongerius P *et al.* (2004) Effect of botulinum toxin in the treatment of drooling: a controlled clinical trial. *Pediatrics.* **114**: 620–627.
23 Ondo WG *et al.* (2004) A double-blind placebo-controlled trial of botulinum toxin B for sialorrhea in Parkinson's disease. *Neurology.* **62**: 37–40.
24 Bennett M *et al.* (2002) Using anti-muscarinic drugs in the management of death rattle: evidence based guidelines for palliative care. *Palliative Medicine.* **16**: 369–374.
25 Mercadante S (1998) Hyoscine in opioid-induced sweating. *Journal of Pain and Symptom Management.* **15**: 214–215.
26 Klaber M and Catterall M (2000) Treating hyperhidrosis. Anticholinergic drugs were not mentioned. *British Medical Journal.* **321**: 703.
27 Pittelkow M and Loprinzi C (2003) Pruritus and sweating in palliative medicine. In: D Doyle *et al.* (eds) *Oxford Textbook of Palliative Medicine* (3e). Oxford University Press, Oxford, pp. 573–587.
28 Zylicz Z and Krajnik M (2003) Flushing and sweating in an advanced breast cancer patient relieved by olanzapine. *Journal of Pain and Symptom Management.* **25**: 494–495.
29 Deaner P (2000) The use of thalidomide in the management of severe sweating in patients with advanced malignancy: trial report. *Palliative Medicine.* **14**: 429–431.
30 Calder K and Bruera E (2000) Thalidomide for night sweats in patients with advanced cancer. *Palliative Medicine.* **14**: 77–78.
31 Aquilonius SM and Hedstrand U (1978) The use of physostigmine as an antidote in tricyclic anti-depressant intoxication. *Acta Anaesthesiologica Scandinavica.* **22**: 40–45.
32 Caine ED (1979) Anticholinergic toxicity. *New England Journal of Medicine.* **300**: 1278.
33 Newton RW (1975) Physostigmine salicylate in the treatment of tricyclic antidepressant overdosage. *Journal of the American Medical Association.* **231**: 941–943.

GLYCOPYRRONIUM BNF 15.1.3

Class: Antimuscarinic (anticholinergic).

Indications: Drying secretions (including surgical premedication, control of upper airway secretions, †sialorrhoea, †drooling, †death rattle (noisy respiratory secretions), †smooth muscle spasm (e.g. intestine, bladder), †inoperable intestinal obstruction), †paraneoplastic pyrexia and sweating, †hyperhidrosis.

Pharmacology

Glycopyrronium is a synthetic ionized quaternary ammonium antimuscarinic that penetrates biological membranes slowly and erratically.[1] In consequence it rarely causes sedation or delirium.[2,3] Absorption PO is poor and the IV to PO potency ratio is about 35:1.[4] Even so, glycopyrronium 200–400microgram PO t.d.s. produces plasma concentrations associated with an antisialogogic effect lasting up to 8h.[5–7] By injection, glycopyrronium is 2–5 times more potent than **hyoscine *hydrobromide*** as an antisecretory drug,[4] and may be effective in some patients who fail to respond to **hyoscine**. However, the efficacy of **hyoscine *hydrobromide***, **hyoscine *butylbromide*** and glycopyrronium as antisialogogues is generally similar, with death rattle reduced in 1/2–2/3 of patients.[8] The optimal parenteral single dose is 200microgram.[9,10] It has fewer cardiac effects because of a reduced affinity for muscarinic-type 2 receptors.[11–13] Although at standard doses glycopyrronium does not change ocular pressures or pupil size, it can precipitate narrow-angle glaucoma. It is excreted by the kidneys and lower doses are effective in patients with renal impairment.[1,14]

Glycopyrronium has also been used to reduce drooling in MND/ALS,[15] for paraneoplastic pyrexia and sweating, for localized hyperhidrosis[16,17] and as a bronchodilator (inhaled or nebulized).[18]

Bio-availability $<$5% PO.
Onset of action 1min IV; 30–40min SC, PO.
Time to peak plasma concentration immediate IV; no data SC, PO.
Plasma halflife 1.7h.
Duration of action 7h.

Cautions

Competitively blocks the prokinetic effect of **metoclopramide** and **domperidone**.[19] Increases the peripheral antimuscarinic toxicity of antihistamines, phenothiazines and TCAs (see Antimuscarinics, p.4). Use with caution in conditions predisposing to tachycardia (e.g. thyrotoxicosis, heart failure, concurrent β_2 agonists), and bladder outflow obstruction (prostatism). Likely to exacerbate acid reflux. Narrow-angle glaucoma may be precipitated in those at risk, particularly the elderly. Use in hot weather or pyrexia may lead to heatstroke.

Undesirable effects

Peripheral antimuscarinic effects (see Box 1.A, p.5). The US Product Information lists the following effects, which are not included in the UK SPC:
Very common (>10%): inflammation at the injection site.
Common (<10%, >1%): dysphagia, photosensitivity.

Dose and use

Glycopyrronium is an alternative to **hyoscine *hydrobromide***, **hyoscine *butylbromide*** and **atropine**.[20–22] For CSCI, dilute with WFI, 0.9% saline or 5% glucose.

CSCI compatibility with other drugs: There are 2-drug compatibility data for glycopyrronium in WFI with **alfentanil**, **clonazepam**, **diamorphine**, **levomepromazine**, **metoclopramide**, **midazolam**, **morphine sulphate** and **oxycodone**.

Glycopyrronium is *incompatible* with **dexamethasone** and **phenobarbital**. For more details and 3-drug compatibility data, see Appendix 3 (p.773).

Compatibility charts for mixing drugs in 0.9% saline can be found on *www.palliativedrugs.com* Syringe Driver Survey Database.

Drooling

Administer as a locally prepared solution PO:

- start with 200microgram PO stat and q8h
- if necessary, increase dose progressively every 2–3 days to 1mg q8h[23]
- occasionally doses of up to 2mg q8h are needed.

A subsequent reduction in dose may be possible, particularly when initial dose escalation has been rapid. Can be given by gastrostomy tube.[7]

Several formulas for locally prepared oral solutions are shown in Box 1.D.[24,25] It is much cheaper to use the powder than the injection; 10mg of glycopyrronium costs £15 using 50mL of injection from 3mL ampoules, but only £0.50 using powder.

Box 1.D Examples of locally prepared oral solutions of glycopyrronium

From glycopyrronium powder

Glycopyrronium concentrated solution 1mg/mL (0.1%)
Dissolve 100mg of glycopyrronium powder (obtainable from Anpharm) in 100mL of sterile or distilled water.

This concentrate is stable for approximately 28 days if stored in a refrigerator.

Dilute the required volume of the concentrate 1 part with 9 parts sterile or distilled water (i.e. for every 1mL of concentrate, add 9mL of water) (0.01%).

To avoid microbial contamination, store in a refrigerator and discard any unused diluted solution after 1 week.

Glycopyrronium 500microgram/mL (1mg/2mL)[24]
Add 5mL of glycerol to 50mg of glycopyrronium powder and mix to form a smooth paste. Add 50mL of Ora-Plus® in portions and mix well. Add sufficient Ora-Sweet® or Ora-Sweet SF® to make a total volume of 100mL.

This solution is stable for 90 days at room temperature or in a refrigerator.

From glycopyrronium injection

Glycopyrronium 100microgram/mL (1mg/10mL)[25]
Combine 25mL of Ora-Plus® and 25mL of Ora-Sweet®; add to 50mL of preservative-free glycopyrronium injection 200microgram/mL to make up to 100mL, and mix well.

Stable for 35 days at room temperature or in a refrigerator (refrigeration minimizes risk of microbial contamination).

In a taste test, this formulation masked the bitter taste of glycopyrronium better than water or syrup-based vehicles, and was preferred by 4/5 patients.

Death rattle (noisy respiratory secretions)

- 200microgram SC stat and p.r.n.[26] *or*
- 100microgram SL q6h p.r.n.
- ±600–1,200microgram/24h CSCI.

Antispasmodic and inoperable intestinal obstruction

- 200microgram SC stat and p.r.n. *or*
- ±600–1,200microgram/24h CSCI.

Paraneoplastic pyrexia and sweating

- for long-term use and higher doses, use a locally prepared aqueous solution (Box 1.D)
- start with 200microgram PO t.d.s.
- if necessary, increase progressively to 2mg PO t.d.s.

Localized hyperhidrosis

- apply topically as a 0.5–4% cream (Box 1.E) or aqueous solution once daily–b.d. avoiding the nose, mouth and particularly the eyes; do not wash treated skin for 3–4h[17,27]
- if severe, or if alternative treatments fail, 1–2mg PO b.d.–t.d.s., titrated to response.[16]

Box 1.E Locally prepared glycopyrronium cream 10mg/mL (1%)[28]

Mix 1g of glycopyrronium powder with propylene glycol to make a paste. Incorporate into a water-washable cream base until smooth, making a total of 100g. Refrigerate after preparation. Stable for 60 days.

Supply

Glycopyrronium bromide (generic)
Injection 200microgram/mL, 1mL amp = £0.50, 3mL amp = £1.

Robinul® (Anpharm)
Glycopyrronium bromide
Powder for local preparation of oral solutions and topical formulations (see Box 1.D and Box 1.E), 3g = £110.

1 Mirakhur R and Dundee J (1983) Glycopyrrolate pharmacology and clinical use. *Anaesthesia*. **38**: 1195–1204.
2 Gram D *et al.* (1991) Central anticholinergic syndrome following glycopyrrolate. *Anesthesiology*. **74**: 191–193.
3 Wigard D (1991) Glycopyrrolate and the central anticholinergic syndrome (letter). *Anesthesiology*. **75**: 1125.
4 Mirakhur R and Dundee J (1980) A comparison of the effects of atropine and glycopyrollate on various end organs. *Journal of the Royal Society of Medicine*. **73**: 727–730.
5 Ali-Melkkila T *et al.* (1989) Glycopyrrolate; pharmacokinetics and some pharmacodynamics findings. *Acta Anaesthesiologica Scandinavica*. **33**: 513–517.
6 Blasco P (1996) Glycopyrrolate treatment of chronic drooling. *Archives of Paediatric and Adolescent Medicine*. **150**: 932–935.
7 Olsen A and Sjogren P (1999) Oral glycopyrrolate alleviates drooling in a patient with tongue cancer. *Journal of Pain and Symptom Management*. **18**: 300–302.
8 Hughes A *et al.* (2000) Audit of three antimuscarinic drugs for managing retained secretions. *Palliative Medicine*. **14**: 221–222.
9 Mirakhur R *et al.* (1978) Evaluation of the anticholinergic actions of glycopyrronium bromide. *British Journal of Clinical Pharmacology*. **5**: 77–84.
10 Back I *et al.* (2001) A study comparing hyoscine hydrobromide and glycopyrrolate in the treatment of death rattle. *Palliative Medicine*. **15**: 329–336.
11 Scheinin H *et al.* (1999) Spectral analysis of heart rate variability as a quantitative measure of parasympatholytic effect-integrated pharmacokinetics and pharmacodynamics of three anticholinergic drugs. *Therapeutic Drug Monitoring*. **21**: 141–151.
12 Warren J *et al.* (1997) Effect of autonomic blockade on power spectrum of heart rate variability during exercise. *American Journal of Physiology*. **273**: 495–502.
13 Mirakhur R *et al.* (1978) Atropine and glycopyrronium premedication. A comparison of the effects on cardiac rate and rhythm during induction of anaesthesia. *Anaesthesia*. **33**: 906–912.
14 Ali-Melkkila T *et al.* (1993) Pharmacokinetics and related pharmacodynamics of anticholinergic drugs. *Acta Anaesthesiologica Scandinavica*. **37**: 633–642.
15 Strutt R *et al.* (2002) Nebulized glycopyrrolate for drooling in a motor neuron patient. *Journal of Pain and Symptom Management*. **23**: 2–3.
16 Solish N *et al.* (2007) A comprehensive approach to the recognition, diagnosis, and severity-based treatment of focal hyperhidrosis: recommendations of the Canadian Hyperhidrosis Advisory Committee. *Dermatologic Surgery*. **33**: 908–923.
17 Kim WO *et al.* (2008) Topical glycopyrrolate for patients with facial hyperhidrosis. *British Journal of Dermatology*. **158**: 1094–1097.
18 Hansel TT *et al.* (2005) Glycopyrrolate causes prolonged bronchoprotection and bronchodilatation in patients with asthma. *Chest*. **128**: 1974–1979.
19 Schuurkes JAJ *et al.* (1986) Stimulation of gastroduodenal motor activity: dopaminergic and cholinergic modulation. *Drug Development Research*. **8**: 233–241.
20 Rashid H *et al.* (1997) Management of secretions in esophageal cancer patients with glycopyrrolate. *Annals of Oncology*. **8**: 198–199.
21 Lucas V and Amass C (1998) Use of enteral glycopyrrolate in the management of drooling. *Palliative Medicine*. **12**: 207.
22 Davis M and Furste A (1999) Glycopyrrolate: a useful drug in the palliation of mechanical bowel obstruction. *Journal of Pain and Symptom Management*. **18**: 153–154.
23 Arbouw ME *et al.* (2010) Glycopyrrolate for sialorrhea in Parkinson disease: a randomized, double-blind, crossover trial. *Neurology*. **74**: 1203–1207.
24 Anonymous (2004) Glycopyrrolate 0.5mg/mL oral liquid. *International Journal of Pharmaceutical Compounding*. **8**: 218.
25 Landry C *et al.* (2005) Stability and subjective taste acceptability of four glycopyrrolate solutions for oral administration. *International Journal of Pharmaceutical Compounding*. **9**: 396–398.
26 Bennett M *et al.* (2002) Using anti-muscarinic drugs in the management of death rattle: evidence based guidelines for palliative care. *Palliative Medicine*. **16**: 369–374.
27 Kavanagh GM *et al.* (2006) Topical glycopyrrolate should not be overlooked in treatment of focal hyperhidrosis. *British Journal of Dermatology*. **155**: 477–500.
28 Glasnapp A and BJ S (2001) Topical therapy for localized hyperhidrosis. *International Journal of Pharmaceutical Compounding*. **5**: 28–29.

HYOSCINE BUTYLBROMIDE BNF 1.2

Class: Antimuscarinic.

Indications: Smooth muscle spasm (e.g. bladder, GI tract), †drying secretions (including †sialorrhoea, †drooling, †death rattle (noisy respiratory secretions) and †inoperable bowel obstruction), †paraneoplastic pyrexia and sweating.

Contra-indications: Narrow-angle glaucoma (unless moribund), myasthenia gravis (unless moribund).

Pharmacology

Hyoscine *butylbromide* is an antimuscarinic (see p.14) and has both smooth muscle relaxant (antispasmodic) and antisecretory properties. It is a quaternary compound and, unlike **hyoscine *hydrobromide***, it does not cross the blood-brain barrier. Consequently, it does not have a central anti-emetic effect or cause drowsiness.

Oral bio-availability, based on urinary excretion, is <1%.[1] Thus, any antispasmodic effect reported after PO administration probably relates to a local contact effect on the GI mucosa.[2] In an RCT, hyoscine *butylbromide* 10mg t.d.s. PO and **paracetamol** 500mg t.d.s. both significantly reduced the severity of intestinal colic by >50%.[3] However, the difference between the benefit from these two drugs (both given in suboptimal doses) and placebo was only 0.5 cm on a 10 cm scale of pain intensity. This is of dubious clinical importance.[4] Thus the therapeutic value of PO hyoscine *butylbromide* for intestinal colic remains debatable.[5]

The main uses for hyoscine *butylbromide* in palliative care are as an antispasmodic and antisecretory drug in inoperable GI obstruction, and as an antisecretory drug for death rattle (noisy respiratory secretions). In an open non-randomized trial of hyoscine *butylbromide* 60mg/24h CSCI vs. **octreotide** 300microgram/24h CSCI, **octreotide** resulted in a more rapid reduction in the volume of gastric aspirate (by 75% vs. 50%) and improvement in nausea, although it was possible to remove nasogastric tubes in both groups after about 5 days.[6,7] However, higher doses of hyoscine *butylbromide*, e.g. 120–200mg/24h, have not been compared with **octreotide**.

In healthy volunteers, a bolus injection of 20mg has a maximum antisecretory duration of action of 2h.[8] However, the same dose by CSCI is often effective for 1 day in death rattle. Hyoscine *butylbromide* and **hyoscine *hydrobromide*** act faster than **glycopyrronium** for this indication,[9,10] but the overall efficacy is generally the same[11] with death rattle reduced in 1/2–2/3 of patients.

Bio-availability <1% PO.[1]
Onset of action <10min SC/IM/IV; 1–2h PO.[12]
Time to peak plasma concentration 15min–2h PO.[1]
Plasma halflife 1–5h.[1]
Duration of action <2h in volunteers; probably longer in moribund patients.[8]

Cautions

Competitively blocks the prokinetic effect of **metoclopramide** and **domperidone**.[1,13] Increases the peripheral antimuscarinic effects of antihistamines, phenothiazines and TCAs (see Antimuscarinics, p.4).

Use with caution in conditions predisposing to tachycardia (e.g. thyrotoxicosis, heart failure, β agonists), and bladder outflow obstruction (prostatism). Likely to exacerbate acid reflux. Narrow-angle glaucoma may be precipitated in those at risk, particularly the elderly. Use in hot weather or pyrexia may lead to heatstroke.

Undesirable effects

Peripheral antimuscarinic effects (see p. 5).

Dose and use

For CSCI dilute with WFI, 0.9% saline or 5% glucose.

CSCI compatibility with other drugs: There are 2-drug compatibility data for hyoscine butylbromide in WFI with **alfentanil**, **clonazepam**, **dexamethasone**, **diamorphine**, **haloperidol**, **levomepromazine**, **midazolam**, **morphine sulphate**, **octreotide** and **oxycodone**.

Incompatibility may occur with **cyclizine**. For more details and 3-drug compatibility data, see Appendix 3 (p.773).

Compatibility charts for mixing drugs in 0.9% saline can be found on *www.palliativedrugs.com* Syringe Driver Survey Database.

Inoperable intestinal obstruction with colic[14,15]

- start with 20mg SC stat and 60mg/24h CSCI
- if necessary, increase to 120mg/24h
- maximum reported dose 300mg/24h.

Note: the maximum benefit from hyoscine *butylbromide* may be seen only after some 3 days.[6] Some centres add **octreotide** 300–500microgram/24h if hyoscine *butylbromide* 120mg/24h fails to relieve symptoms adequately.[16,17]

For patients with obstructive symptoms without colic, **metoclopramide** (see p.227) should be tried before an antimuscarinic drug because the obstruction is often more functional than organic.

Death rattle (noisy respiratory secretions)

- start with 20mg SC stat, 20–60mg/24h CSCI, and/or 20mg SC q1h p.r.n.
- some centres use higher doses, namely 60–120mg/24h CSCI[10]

For use of alternative antimuscarinics, see Quick Practice Guide, p.8.

Supply

Buscopan® (Boehringer Ingelheim)

Tablets 10mg, 28 days @ 20mg q.d.s. – £9. *Also available OTC as Buscopan®* IBS Relief.

Injection 20mg/mL, 1mL amp = £0.50.

1 Boehringer Ingelheim GmbH *Data on file*.

2 Tytgat GN (2007) Hyoscine butylbromide: a review of its use in the treatment of abdominal cramping and pain. *Drugs*. **67**: 1343–1357.

3 Mueller-Lissner S *et al.* (2006) Placebo- and paracetamol-controlled study on the efficacy and tolerability of hyoscine butylbromide in the treatment of patients with recurrent crampy abdominal pain. *Alimentary Pharmacology & Therapeutics*. **23**: 1741–1748.

4 Farrar JT *et al.* (2000) Defining the clinically important difference in pain outcome measures. *Pain*. **88**: 287–294.

5 Thompson DG and Wingate DL (1981) Oral hyoscine butylbromide does not alter the pattern of small intestinal motor activity. *British Journal of Pharmacology*. **72**: 685–687.

6 Mercadante S *et al.* (2000) Comparison of octreotide and hyoscine butylbromide in controlling gastrointestinal symptoms due to malignant inoperable bowel obstruction. *Supportive Care in Cancer*. **8**: 188–191.

7 Ripamonti C *et al.* (2000) Role of octreotide, scopolamine butylbromide, and hydration in symptom control of patients with inoperable bowel obstruction and nasogastric tubes: a prospective randomized trial. *Journal of Pain and Symptom Management*. **19**: 23–34.

8 Herxheimer A and Haefeli L (1966) Human pharmacology of hyoscine butylbromide. *Lancet*. **ii**: 418–421.

9 Back I *et al.* (2001) A study comparing hyoscine hydrobromide and glycopyrrolate in the treatment of death rattle. *Palliative Medicine*. **15**: 329–336.

10 Bennett M *et al.* (2002) Using anti-muscarinic drugs in the management of death rattle: evidence based guidelines for palliative care. *Palliative Medicine*. **16**: 369–374.

11 Hughes A *et al.* (2000) Audit of three antimuscarinic drugs for managing retained secretions. *Palliative Medicine*. **14**: 221–222.

12 Sanches Martinez J *et al.* (1988) Clinical assessment of the tolerability and the effect of IK-19 in tablet form on pain of spastic origin. *Investigacion Medica International*. **15**: 63–65.

13 Schuurkes JAJ *et al.* (1986) Stimulation of gastroduodenal motor activity: dopaminergic and cholinergic modulation. *Drug Development Research*. **8**: 233–241.

14 De-Conno F *et al.* (1991) Continuous subcutaneous infusion of hyoscine butylbromide reduces secretions in patients with gastrointestinal obstruction. *Journal of Pain and Symptom Management*. **6**: 484–486.

15 Ripamonti C *et al.* (2001) Clinical-practice recommendations for the management of bowel obstruction in patients with end-stage cancer. *Supportive Care in Cancer*. **9**: 223–233.

16 Ripamonti C and Mercadante S (2004) How to use octreotide for malignant bowel obstruction. *Journal of Supportive Oncology*. **2**: 357–364.

17 Ripamonti CI *et al.* (2008) Management of malignant bowel obstruction. *European Journal of Cancer*. **44**: 1105–1115.

HYOSCINE HYDROBROMIDE BNF 4.6 & 15.1.3

Class: Antimuscarinic.

Indications: Prevention of motion sickness (TD route), drying secretions (including surgical premedication, †sialorrhoea, †drooling, †death rattle (noisy respiratory secretions) and †inoperable intestinal obstruction), †paraneoplastic pyrexia and sweating, †smooth muscle spasm (e.g. intestine, bladder).

Contra-indications: Narrow-angle glaucoma, prostatic hyperplasia, pyloric obstruction, paralytic ileus.

Pharmacology

Hyoscine *hydrobromide* is a naturally occurring belladonna alkaloid with smooth muscle relaxant (antispasmodic) and antisecretory properties. In many countries it is available as both the *hydrobromide* and *butylbromide* salts. **Hyoscine *butylbromide*** is a quaternary compound which does not cross the blood-brain barrier and, unlike hyoscine *hydrobromide*, the *butylbromide* does not cause drowsiness and does not have a central anti-emetic action (see p.14). In contrast, repeated administration of hyoscine *hydrobromide* SC q4h may result in accumulation leading to sedation and delirium. However, a small number of patients are stimulated rather than sedated.

Despite hyoscine *hydrobromide* having a plasma halflife of several hours, the duration of the antisecretory effect in volunteers after a single dose is only about 2h.[1] However, particularly after repeated injections in moribund patients, a duration of effect of up to 9h has been observed.[2] Hyoscine *hydrobromide* relieves death rattle in 50–60% of patients.[3] However, provided that time is taken to explain the cause of the rattle to the relatives and there is ongoing support, relatives' distress is relieved in $>90\%$ of cases.[2] Hyoscine *hydrobromide* can also be used in other situations where an antimuscarinic effect is needed.

A TD patch is available as prophylactic treatment for motion sickness.[4] It has also been used to control opioid-induced nausea.[5,6] Other off-label uses include the management of sialorrhoea and drooling in patients with disorders of the head and neck.[7,8] Features of the patch include:

- an immediate-release priming dose of 140microgram
- a drug reservoir containing 1.5mg
- a rate-controlling membrane allowing the release of 5microgram/h (120microgram/24h)
- steady-state is reached after about 24h, and maintained for 72h[8]
- absorption is best when the patch is applied on hairless skin behind the ear.[4]

Bio-availability 60–80% SL.
Onset of action 3–5min IM, 10–15min SL.
Time to peak effect 20–60min SL/SC; 24h TD.
Plasma halflife 5–6h.
Duration of action IM 15min (spasmolytic), 1–9h (antisecretory).

Cautions

Interacts competitively to block prokinetic effect of **metoclopramide** and **domperidone**.[9] Increases the antimuscarinic toxicity of antihistamines, phenothiazines and TCAs (see p.6). Likely to exacerbate acid reflux. Use in hot weather or pyrexia may lead to heatstroke. Use with caution in myasthenia gravis, bladder outflow obstruction, and in conditions predisposing to tachycardia (e.g. thyrotoxicosis, heart failure and concurrent use with β agonists).

Undesirable effects

Antimuscarinic effects (see p.5), including central antimuscarinic syndrome, i.e. agitated delirium, drowsiness, ataxia.

TD patch: despite the relatively small dose, delirium has been reported;[10] local irritation ± rash occasionally occurs.

Dose and use

TD patches contain metal in the backing, and must be removed before MRI to avoid burns.[11,12] Wash hands after handling the TD patch (and the application site after removing it) to avoid transferring hyoscine *hydrobromide* into the eyes (may cause mydriasis and exacerbate narrow-angle glaucoma).

Drooling (and sialorrhoea)

- hyoscine *hydrobromide* 1mg/3 days TD; if necessary, use 2 patches concurrently.

Note: an alternative drug PO with antimuscarinic effects may be preferable in some patients because of convenience or concurrent symptom management, e.g. **amitriptyline** (see p.189).

Death rattle (noisy respiratory secretions)

With death rattle caused by excess secretions pooling in the pharynx, an antisecretory drug is best administered as soon as the rattle becomes evident because the drug cannot dry up the existing secretions:

- 400microgram SC stat
- continue with 1,200microgram/24h CSCI
- if necessary, increase to 2,000microgram/24h CSCI
- repeat 400microgram p.r.n.

For CSCI dilute with WFI, 0.9% saline or 5% glucose.

CSCI compatibility with other drugs: There are 2-drug compatibility data for hyoscine hydrobromide in WFI with **clonazepam**, **cyclizine**, **dexamethasone**, **diamorphine**, **haloperidol**, **levomepromazine**, **midazolam**, **morphine sulphate** and **oxycodone**.

For more details and 3-drug compatibility data, see Appendix 3 (p.773).

Compatibility charts for mixing drugs in 0.9% saline can be found on *www.palliativedrugs.com* Syringe Driver Survey Database.

Some centres use **hyoscine *butylbromide*** instead (see p.14).[13] Other options include **glycopyrronium** (see p.11) and **atropine** (see p.7).

Supply

Kwells® Bayer Consumer Care
Tablets chewable 150microgram, 300microgram available OTC.

Scopoderm TTS® (Novartis Consumer Health)
TD (post-auricular) patch 1mg/72h, 1 patch = £2. Also available OTC as Scopoderm®

Hyoscine *hydrobromide* (generic)
Injection 400microgram/mL, 1mL amp = £3; 600microgram/mL, 1mL amp = £3.

1 Herxheimer A and Haefeli L (1966) Human pharmacology of hyoscine butylbromide. *Lancet*. **ii**: 418–421.
2 Hughes A *et al.* (1997) Management of 'death rattle'. *Palliative Medicine*. **11**: 80–81.
3 Hughes A *et al.* (2000) Audit of three antimuscarinic drugs for managing retained secretions. *Palliative Medicine*. **14**: 221–222.
4 Clissold S and Heel R (1985) Transdermal hyoscine (scopolamine). A preliminary review of its pharmacodynamic properties and therapeutic efficacy. *Drugs*. **29**: 189–207.
5 Ferris FD *et al.* (1991) Transdermal scopolamine use in the control of narcotic-induced nausea. *Journal of Pain and Symptom Management*. **6**: 289–393.
6 Harris SN *et al.* (1991) Nausea prophylaxis using transdermal scopolamine in the setting of patient-controlled analgesia. *Obstetrics and Gynecology*. **78**: 673–677.
7 Gordon C *et al.* (1985) Effect of transdermal scopolamine on salivation. *Journal of Clinical Pharmacology*. **25**: 407–412.
8 Talmi YP *et al.* (1990) Reduction of salivary flow with transdermal scopolamine: a four-year experience. *Otolaryngology Head and Neck Surgery*. **103**: 615–618.
9 Schuurkes JAJ *et al.* (1986) Stimulation of gastroduodenal motor activity: dopaminergic and cholinergic modulation. *Drug Development Research*. **8**: 233–241.
10 Wilkinson J (1987) Side-effects of transdermal scopolamine. *Journal of Emergency Medicine*. **5**: 389–392.
11 Institute for Safe Medication Practices (2004) Medication Safety Alert. Burns in MRI patients wearing transdermal patches. Available from: www.ismp.org/Newsletters/acutecare/articles/20040408.asp?ptr = y
12 Health Canada (2005) Notice to hospitals. Health Canada endorsed important safety information on magnetic resonance imaging systems. Available from: www.hc-sc.gc.ca/dhp-mps/alt_formats/hpfb-dgpsa/pdf/medeff/mri-irm_patch-timbre_nth-ah_e.pdf
13 Bennett M *et al.* (2002) Using anti-muscarinic drugs in the management of death rattle: evidence based guidelines for palliative care. *Palliative Medicine*. **16**: 369–374.

PROPANTHELINE BNF 1.2 & 7.4.2

Class: Antimuscarinic.

Indications: Smooth muscle spasm (e.g. bladder, intestine), urinary frequency and incontinence, hyperhidrosis, †gustatory sweating in diabetic neuropathy, †paraneoplastic sweating.

Contra-indications: Narrow-angle glaucoma (unless moribund), myasthenia gravis (unless moribund), paralytic ileus.

Pharmacology

Propantheline is a quaternary antimuscarinic (see p.4); it does not cross the blood-brain barrier and thus does *not* cause central effects. It doubles gastric emptying half-time[1] and slows GI transit generally. It has variable effects on drug absorption (see Cautions). Propantheline is extensively metabolized in the small intestine before absorption. *If taken with food, the effect of propantheline by mouth is almost abolished.*[2]
Bio-availability <50% PO (much reduced if taken after food).
Onset of action 30–60min.
Time to peak plasma concentration 2h.
Plasma halflife 2–3h.
Duration of action 4–6h.

Cautions

Competitively blocks the prokinetic effect of **metoclopramide** and **domperidone**.[3] May reduce the rate, but not the extent, of absorption of **paracetamol**, thereby delaying the onset of analgesia. May increase the absorption of some formulations of **digoxin** and **nitrofurantoin**.[4]

Increases the peripheral antimuscarinic toxicity of antihistamines, phenothiazines and TCAs (see Antimuscarinics, p.4). Use with caution in conditions predisposing to tachycardia (e.g. thyrotoxicosis, heart failure, β agonists), and bladder outflow obstruction (prostatism). Likely to exacerbate acid reflux. Narrow-angle glaucoma may be precipitated in those at risk, particularly the elderly. Use in hot weather or pyrexia may lead to heatstroke.

Undesirable effects

Peripheral antimuscarinic effects (see p.5).

Dose and use

Intestinal colic

- start with 15mg t.d.s. 1h a.c. & 30mg at bedtime
- maximum dose 30mg q.d.s.

Urinary frequency

- same as for colic, but largely replaced by **oxybutynin** (see p.527), **amitriptyline** (see p.189) or **imipramine**.

Sweating

Used as one of several alternatives to reduce paraneoplastic sweating (for other options, see Box 1.C, p.9):

- 15–30mg b.d.–t.d.s.

Supply

Pro-Banthine® (Archimedes)
Tablets 15mg, 28 days @ 15mg t.d.s. & 30mg at bedtime = £18.

1 Hurwitz A *et al.* (1977) Prolongation of gastric emptying by oral propantheline. *Clinical Pharmacology and Therapeutics*. **22**: 206–210.
2 Ekenved G *et al.* (1977) Influence of food on the effect of propantheline and L-hyoscyamine on salivation. *Scandinavian Journal of Gastroenterology*. **12**: 963–966.
3 Schuurkes JAJ *et al.* (1986) Stimulation of gastroduodenal motor activity: dopaminergic and cholinergic modulation. *Drug Development Research*. **8**: 233–241.
4 Baxter K (ed) (2010) Stockley's Drug Interactions (online edition). The Pharmaceutical Press, London. Available from: www.medicinescomplete.com

PROKINETICS — BNF 1.2

Pharmacology

Prokinetics accelerate GI transit and include:

- D_2 antagonists, e.g. **domperidone, metoclopramide**
- $5HT_4$ agonists, acting predominantly on the:
  - upper GI tract, e.g. **metoclopramide**
  - lower GI tract, e.g. **prucalopride**
- motilin agonists, e.g. **erythromycin**.

The reason for the differing sites of action of $5HT_4$ agonists is unclear. Cholecystokinin-1 antagonists are also undergoing clinical trials.[1]

Drugs which enhance intestinal transit indirectly are not considered prokinetics (e.g. bulk-forming agents and other laxatives, drugs which cause diarrhoea by increasing GI secretions, e.g. **misoprostol**). Some drugs increase contractile motor activity but not in a co-ordinated fashion, and so do not reduce transit time, e.g. **bethanechol**. Such drugs are promotility but not prokinetic.[2]

D_2 antagonists and $5HT_4$ agonists act by triggering a cholinergic system in the wall of the GI tract (Table 1.3, Figure 1.1).[3] This action is impeded by opioids. Further, antimuscarinic drugs competitively block cholinergic receptors on the intestinal muscle fibres (and elsewhere).[4] Thus, all drugs with antimuscarinic properties reduce the impact of prokinetic drugs. The extent of this depends on several factors, including the respective doses of the interacting drugs and times of administration. Thus, generally, the concurrent administration of prokinetics and antimuscarinic drugs is best avoided. On the other hand, even if the peripheral prokinetic effect is completely blocked, **domperidone** and **metoclopramide** will still exert an anti-emetic effect at the dopamine receptors in the area postrema (see p.219).

Table 1.3 Comparison of gastric prokinetic drugs[5]

Drug	*Erythromycin*	*Domperidone*	*Metoclopramide*
Mechanism of action			
Motilin agonist	+	–	–
D_2 antagonist	–	+	+
$5HT_4$ agonist	–	–	+
Response to treatment[a]			
Gastric emptying (mean % acceleration)	45	30	20
Symptom relief (mean % improvement)	50	50	40

a. all percentages rounded to nearest 5%.

Erythromycin is reported to improve symptoms in about half of patients. A review suggested that, overall, its prokinetic effect was greater than that of **metoclopramide** (Table 1.3). However, studies (mainly in diabetic gastroparesis) were small and open to bias.[6] Further, it can cause intestinal colic and diarrhoea. There is concern about the possibility of bacterial resistance developing, and tolerance to its prokinetic effects may develop over time.[7] Thus, erythromycin is generally used second-line when **metoclopramide** and **domperidone** have been ineffective. Some patients have taken **erythromycin** 250mg b.d. for more than a year without apparent loss of its prokinetic effect.[8] Non-antibacterial motilin agonists are undergoing trials.

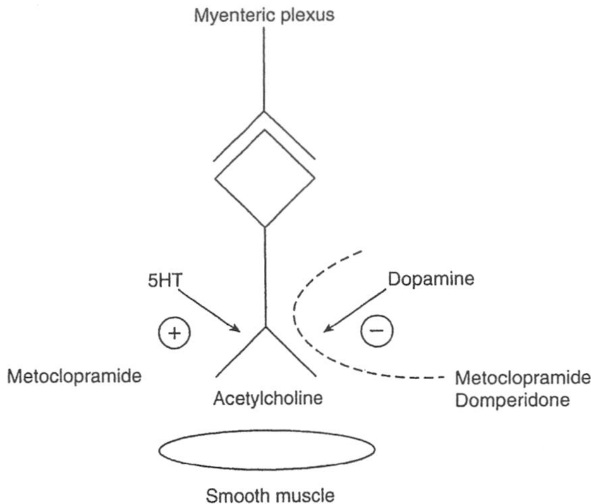

Figure 1.1 Schematic representation of drug effects on antroduodenal co-ordination via a postganglionic effect on the cholinergic nerves from the myenteric plexus.

⊕ stimulatory effect of 5HT triggered by metoclopramide; ⊖ inhibitory effect of dopamine;
- - - blockade of dopamine inhibition by metoclopramide and domperidone.

Use of prokinetics in palliative care

Prokinetics are used in various situations in palliative care (Box 1.F). D_2 antagonists block the dopaminergic 'brake' on gastric emptying induced by stress, anxiety, and nausea from any cause. In contrast, $5HT_4$ agonists have a direct excitatory effect which in theory gives them an advantage over the D_2 antagonists particularly for patients with gastric stasis or functional intestinal obstruction. However, when used for dysmotility dyspepsia, **metoclopramide** is no more potent than **domperidone** in standard doses.[9,10]

Box 1.F Indications for prokinetics in palliative care

Gastro-oesophageal reflux
Hiccup
Delayed gastric emptying
Gastroparesis
   dysmotility dyspepsia
   paraneoplastic autonomic neuropathy
   spinal cord compression
   diabetic autonomic neuropathy
Functional GI obstruction
   drug-induced, e.g. opioids
   cancer of head of pancreas
   linitis plastica (locally diffuse mural infiltration by cancer)

For patients with refractory symptoms, consider **clonidine** (see p.67) or specialist referral. Some patients benefit from intrapyloric **botulinum toxin** or gastric electrical pacing.[11]

Doses are given in individual monographs for **metoclopramide** (p.227) and **domperidone** (p.229). For **erythromycin**:

- start with 50–100mg q.d.s PO (use suspension)
- if necessary, increase every few days by 25–50mg to a maximum dose of 250mg q.d.s.[3]

Metoclopramide is also used to relieve hiccup associated with delayed gastric emptying and/or oesophageal reflux (Table 1.4).[12]

Table 1.4 Drug treatment of hiccup

Class of drug	*Drug*	*Acute relief*	*Maintenance regimen*
Reduce gastric distension ± gastro-oesophageal reflux			
Antiflatulent (carminative)	Peppermint water[a,b]	10mL	10–20mL b.d.
Antiflatulent (defoaming agent)	Simeticone, e.g. in Asilone®	10mL	10mL q.d.s.
Prokinetic	Metoclopramide[b,c]	10mg	10mg t.d.s.–q.d.s.
PPI	Lansoprazole	30mg	30mg each morning
Muscle relaxant (all of these also have central suppressant effects)			
GABA agonist	Baclofen	5mg PO	5–20mg t.d.s., occasionally more[13,14]
Calcium-channel blocker	Nifedipine	10mg PO/SL	10–20mg t.d.s., occasionally more[15,16]
Benzodiazepine	Midazolam	2mg IV, followed by 1–2mg increments every 3–5min	10–60mg/24h by CSCI if patient in last days of life[17]
Central suppression of the hiccup reflex			
Dopamine antagonist	Metoclopramide	As above	As above
	Haloperidol	5–10mg PO or IV if no response	1.5–3mg at bedtime[18,19]
	Chlorpromazine	10–25mg PO or IV if no response	25–50mg t.d.s.
	Methylphenidate	5mg PO	5–10mg b.d.[20]
GABA agonist	Baclofen	As above	As above
Anti-epileptic	Sodium valproate	200–500mg PO	15mg/kg/24h in divided doses[21]
	Gabapentin	'Burst gabapentin', i.e. 400mg t.d.s. for 3 days, then 400mg once daily for 3 days, then stop; repeat if necessary[d22]	400mg t.d.s.[d23,24]

a. facilitates belching by relaxing the lower oesophageal sphincter; an old-fashioned remedy, but can cause gastro-oesophageal reflux
b. peppermint water and metoclopramide should not be used concurrently because of their opposing actions on the gastro-oesophageal sphincter
c. tightens the lower oesophageal sphincter and hastens gastric emptying
d. a smaller dose advisable in elderly frail patients and those with renal impairment, e.g. start with 100mg t.d.s.

1 Di Nardo G *et al.* (2008) Review article: molecular, pathological and therapeutic features of human enteric neuropathies. *Alimentary Pharmacology and Therapeutics.* **28**: 25–42.
2 Rayner CK and Horowitz M (2005) New management approaches for gastroparesis. *Nature Clinical Practice Gastroenterology and Hepatology.* **2**: 454–462; quiz 493.
3 Patrick A and Epstein O (2008) Review article: gastroparesis. *Alimentary Pharmacology and Therapeutics.* **27**: 724–740.
4 Schuurkes JAJ *et al.* (1986) Stimulation of gastroduodenal motor activity: dopaminergic and cholinergic modulation. *Drug Development Research.* **8**: 233–241.
5 Sturm A *et al.* (1999) Prokinetics in patients with gastroparesis: a systematic analysis. *Digestion.* **60**: 422–427.
6 Maganti K *et al.* (2003) Oral erythromycin and symptomatic relief of gastroparesis: a systematic review. *American Journal of Gastroenterology.* **98**: 259–263.
7 Dhir R and Richter JE (2004) Erythromycin in the short- and long-term control of dyspepsia symptoms in patients with gastroparesis. *Journal of Clinical Gastroenterology.* **38**: 237–242.
8 Hunter A *et al.* (2005) The use of long-term, low-dose erythromycin in treating persistent gastric stasis. *Journal of Pain and Symptom Management.* **29**: 430–433.
9 Loose FD (1979) Domperidone in chronic dyspepsia: a pilot open study and a multicentre general practice crossover comparison with metoclopramide and placebo. *Pharmatheripeutica.* **2**: 140–146.
10 Moriga M (1981) A multicentre double blind study of domperidone and metoclopramide in the symptomatic control of dyspepsia. In: G Towse (ed) *International congress and symposium series: Progress with Domperidone, a gastrokinetic and anti-emetic agent* (No. 36). Royal Society of Medicine, London, pp. 77–79.
11 Haans JJ and Masclee AA (2007) Review article: The diagnosis and management of gastroparesis. *Alimentary Pharmacology and Therapeutics.* **26 (suppl 2)**: 37–46.
12 Twycross R *et al.* (2009) *Symptom Management in Advanced Cancer* (4e). palliativedrugs.com, Nottingham, pp. 174–177.
13 Ramirez FC and Graham DY (1992) Treatment of intractable hiccup with baclofen: results of a double-blind randomized, controlled, crossover study. *American Journal of Gastroenterology.* **87**: 1789–1791.
14 Guelaud C *et al.* (1995) Baclofen therapy for chronic hiccup. *European Respiratory Journal.* **8**: 235–237.
15 Lipps DC *et al.* (1990) Nifedipine for intractable hiccups. *Neurology.* **40**: 531–532.
16 Brigham B and Bolin T (1992) High dose nifedipine and fludrocortisone for intractable hiccups. *Medical Journal of Australia.* **157**: 70.
17 Wilcock A and Twycross R (1996) Case report: midazolam for intractable hiccup. *Journal of Pain and Symptom Management.* **12**: 59–61.
18 Scarnati RA (1979) Intractable hiccup (singultus): report of case. *Journal of the American Osteopathic Association.* **79**: 127–129.
19 Ives TJ *et al.* (1985) Treatment of intractable hiccups with intramuscular haloperidol. *American Journal of Psychiatry.* **142**: 1368–1369.
20 Marechal R *et al.* (2003) Successful treatment of intractable hiccup with methylphenidate in a lung cancer patient. *Support Care Cancer.* **11**: 126–128.
21 Jacobson P *et al.* (1981) Treatment of intractable hiccups with valproic acid. *Neurology.* **31**: 1458–1460.
22 Moretti R *et al.* (2004) Gabapentin as a drug therapy of intractable hiccup because of vascular lesion: a three-year follow up. *Neurologist.* **10**: 102–106.
23 Schuchmann JA and Browne BA (2007) Persistent hiccups during rehabilitation hospitalization: three case reports and review of the literature. *American Journal of Physical Medicine and Rehabilitation.* **86**: 1013–1018.
24 Tegeler ML and Baumrucker SJ (2008) Gabapentin for intractable hiccups in palliative care. *American Journal of Hospice and Palliative Care.* **25**: 52–54.

H_2-RECEPTOR ANTAGONISTS — BNF 1.3.1

Class: Gastroprotective drugs.

Indications: Chronic episodic dyspepsia, acid reflux, prevention and treatment of peptic ulceration (including NSAID-related ulceration), reduction of malabsorption and fluid loss in short bowel syndrome (**cimetidine**), prevention of degradation of pancreatin supplements (**cimetidine**).

Pharmacology

H_2-receptor antagonists (H_2 antagonists) reduce both gastric acid output and the volume of gastric secretions.[1] **Ranitidine** is a good choice in terms of convenience and safety. **Cimetidine**, alone among H_2 antagonists, can cause serious cytochrome P450-related drug interactions (see Cautions below, Table 1.5 and Cytochrome P450, p.735). None of the H_2 antagonists, including **cimetidine**, alters the metabolism of **morphine**.[2]

Prophylactic treatment with a standard dose of an H_2 antagonist reduces the incidence of NSAID-related *duodenal* ulcers.[3] Prevention of *gastric* erosions and ulcers is seen only with a double dose.[4,5] In patients taking NSAIDs, **ranitidine** (compared with **omeprazole**) is less effective and slower in *healing* gastroduodenal ulcers (63% vs. 80% at 8 weeks) and in *preventing* relapse (59% vs. 72% over 6 months).[3,6]

Bio-availability **ranitidine** 50% PO.

Onset of action < 1h.

Time to peak plasma concentration, **ranitidine** 2–3h PO, 15min IM.
Plasma halflife **ranitidine** 2–3h.
Duration of action **ranitidine** 8–12h.

Cautions

Serious drug interactions: the increase in gastric pH caused by all H_2 antagonists decreases the absorption of **itraconazole**, **ketoconazole** and **posaconazole**; an increased dose may be needed to avoid antifungal treatment failure.[7] There are inconsistent reports of **cimetidine** and **ranitidine** increasing the plasma concentration of **midazolam**.[7]

Hepatic impairment, renal impairment. The most relevant drug interactions with **cimetidine** are given in Table 1.5.

Table 1.5 Cimetidine Interactions[7,8]

Drug class	*Drug plasma levels increased*
Anti-epileptics	Carbamazepine (transient), phenytoin
Benzodiazepines	Alprazolam, diazepam, chlordiazepoxide, flurazepam, nitrazepam, triazolam (midazolam reports inconsistent)
Calcium antagonists	Potentially all, including diltiazem and nifedipine
Coumarin anticoagulants	e.g. warfarin
Local anaesthetics	Lidocaine (IV), procainamide
Opioids	Alfentanil, fentanyl, methadone
SSRIs	All
TCAs	Potentially all
Xanthines	Aminophylline, theophylline
Miscellaneous	Fluorouracil, mefloquine, mirtazapine, moclobemide, quinidine, tacrine, zolmitriptan

Undesirable effects

Cimetidine occasionally causes gynaecomastia.

Dose and use

Cochrane reviews: PPIs, H_2 antagonists and prokinetics are effective at *relieving symptoms* of non-ulcer dyspepsia and acid reflux, with PPIs having the greatest efficacy.[9,10] PPIs, **misoprostol** and double-dose H_2 antagonists are effective at *preventing* chronic NSAID-related endoscopic peptic ulcers.

Standard doses of H_2 antagonists reduce the risk of duodenal ulcers but not gastric ulcers. **Misoprostol** 400microgram/24h is less effective at preventing gastric ulcers than 800microgram/24h and is still associated with diarrhoea. Of all these treatments, only **misoprostol** 800microgram/24h has been definitely shown to reduce the overall incidence of ulcer *complications* (perforation, haemorrhage or gastric outlet obstruction).[4] PPIs significantly reduce rebleeding, need for surgery, and rate of ulcer recurrence. In high risk patients PPIs reduce mortality.[11] Additional bedtime dose of an H_2 antagonist to high dose PPI may improve night-time acid reflux but evidence is lacking.[12]

NICE guidance: PPIs are preferable to H_2 antagonists for the treatment of dyspepsia, gastro-oesophageal reflux disease and peptic ulcers, including NSAID-related peptic ulcers. Although PPIs are more effective in relieving uninvestigated dyspeptic symptoms, offer a trial of H_2 antagonists or a prokinetic if there has been an inadequate response to a PPI.

For patients taking an NSAID and at high risk of peptic ulcer disease, double-dose H_2 antagonists or PPIs significantly reduce endoscopically detected lesions. **Misoprostol** at low dose is less effective and has undesirable effects. When an NSAID-related ulcer is diagnosed, stop the NSAID if possible, treat *H pylori* infection if present (see p.464) and give double-dose H_2 antagonist or PPI. PPIs heal the majority of ulcers.[13]

If it is necessary to continue with the NSAID, treatments may be less effective. The rate of healing is higher and the risk of recurrence lower with PPIs and **misoprostol** compared with H_2 antagonists.[14]

H_2 antagonists are second-line treatment for gastro-oesophageal reflux disease, non-ulcer dyspepsia and uninvestigated dyspepsia, and are available as an OTC measure for mild dyspepsia.

Given that **cimetidine** is now more expensive than **ranitidine**, there is no justification for using the intrinsically more dangerous **cimetidine**. Accordingly, dose recommendations have been limited to **ranitidine**.

The dose and duration of treatment is least with duodenal ulceration and most with reflux oesophagitis and prophylaxis for NSAID-related peptic ulcer, although the dose for ulcer healing can be doubled if the initial response is poor (Table 1.6). **Ranitidine** is more effective if taken at bedtime rather than with the evening meal.[15]

Table 1.6 Treatment regimens for ranitidine

Indication	*Ranitidine*
Duodenal ulcer[a,b]	150mg b.d. or 300mg at bedtime for 4–8 weeks
Gastric ulcer[a,b]	150mg b.d. or 300mg at bedtime for 4–8 weeks
Prophylaxis for NSAID-associated peptic ulcer	150mg–†300mg b.d. indefinitely
Reflux oesophagitis	150mg b.d. or 300mg at bedtime for 8–12 weeks
Short bowel syndrome	†300mg at bedtime
To reduce degradation of pancreatin supplements	†150mg 1h a.c.

a. 8 weeks for NSAID-related ulcer
b. dose can be doubled if initial response is poor.

Parenteral formulations are available for IM and IV use if treatment is considered necessary in a patient with severe nausea and vomiting (see BNF section 1.3.1). Some centres use 50mg SC b.d.–q.d.s. (unlicensed route) without evidence of local inflammation.

In severe renal impairment (creatinine clearance $<$50mL/min), the dose of **ranitidine** should be reduced to 150mg at bedtime but increased to 150mg b.d. if an ulcer fails to respond at the lower dose.

Supply

Ranitidine (generic)

Tablets 150mg, 300mg, 28 days @ 150mg b.d. or 300mg at bedtime = £2.

Tablets effervescent 150mg, 300mg, 28 days @ 150mg b.d. = £18 or 300mg at bedtime = £17 (*Tablets may contain* Na^+).

Oral solution 75mg/5mL, 28 days @ 150mg b.d. = £38; *may contain alcohol.*

Injection 25mg/mL, 2mL amp = £0.50.

Zantac® (GSK)
Tablets 75mg, 150mg, 300mg, 28 days @ 150mg b.d. or 300mg at bedtime = £1.
Tablets effervescent 150mg, 300mg, 28 days @ 150mg b.d. or 300mg at bedtime = £23; 150mg tablets contain 14.3mmol Na^+/tablet, 300mg tablets contain 20.8mmol Na^+/tablet.
Oral solution (sugar-free) 75mg/5mL, 28 days @ 150mg b.d. = £39; contains 8% alcohol, mint flavour.
Injection 25mg/mL, 2mL amp = £0.50.

1 Williams JG and Strunin L (1985) Pre-operative intramuscular ranitidine and cimetidine. Double blind comparative trial, effect on gastric pH and volume. *Anaesthesia*. **40**: 242–245.
2 Mojaverian P *et al.* (1982) Cimetidine does not alter morphine disposition in man. *British Journal of Clinical Pharmacology*. **14**: 809–813.
3 Hollander D (1994) Gastrointestinal complications of nonsteroidal anti-inflammatory drugs: prophylactic and therapeutic strategies. *American Journal of Medicine*. **96**: 274–281.
4 Rostom A *et al.* (2002) Prevention of NSAID-induced gastroduodenal ulcers. *Cochrane Database of Systematic Reviews*. **4**: CD002296.
5 Leontiadis GI *et al.* (2007) Systematic reviews of the clinical effectiveness and cost-effectiveness of proton pump inhibitors in acute upper gastrointestinal bleeding. *Health Technology Assessment*. **11**: iii–iv, 1–164.
6 Yeomans N *et al.* (1998) A comparison of omeprazole with ranitidine for ulcers associated with nonsteroidal anti-inflammatory drugs. Acid suppression trial. *New England Journal of Medicine*. **338**: 719–726.
7 Baxter K (ed) (2010) Stockley's Drug Interactions (online edition). The Pharmaceutical Press, London. Available from: www.medicinescomplete.com
8 Sorkin E and Ogawa C (1983) Cimetidine potentiation of narcotic action. *Drug Intelligence and Clinical Pharmacy*. **17**: 60–61.
9 Moayyedi P (2006) Pharmacological interventions for non-ulcer dyspepsia. *Cochrane Database of Systematic Reviews*. **4**: CD001960.
10 van Pinxteren B *et al.* (2006) Short term treatment with proton pump inhibitors, H2-receptor antagonists and prokinetics for gastro-oesophageal reflux disease-like symptoms and endoscopy negative reflux disease. *Cochrane Database of Systematic Reviews*. **3**: CD002095.
11 Leontiadis G *et al.* (2010) Proton pump inhibitor treatment for acute peptic ulcer bleeding. *Cochrane Database of Systematic Reviews*. **5**: CD002094.
12 Wang Y *et al.* (2009) Additional bedtime H2 receptor antagonist for control of nocturnal gastirc acid breakthrough. *Cochrane Database of Systematic Reviews*. **4**: CD004275.
13 NICE (2004) Dyspepsia. Management of dyspepsia in adults in primary care. In: *Clinical Guideline 17*. National Institute for Clinical Excellence. Available from: www.nice.org.uk/page.aspx?o = CG017
14 Frech EJ and Go MF (2009) Treatment and chemoprevention of NSAID-associated gastrointestinal complications. *Therapeutics and Clinical Risk Management*. **5**: 65–73.
15 Johnston DA and Wormsley KG (1988) The effect of food on ranitidine-induced inhibition of nocturnal gastric secretion. *Alimentary Pharmacology and Therapeutics*. **2**: 507–511.

MISOPROSTOL — BNF 1.3.4

Class: Prostaglandin (PG) analogue, gastroprotective drug.

Indications: Healing of gastric and duodenal ulcers, prevention and healing of NSAID-related ulcers.

Contra-indications: Women of childbearing potential should not be started on misoprostol until pregnancy is excluded (misoprostol increases uterine tone).

Pharmacology

Misoprostol is a synthetic PG analogue with gastric antisecretory and protective properties. The protective effects occur at doses lower than those required to inhibit acid secretion.[1] After oral administration, misoprostol is rapidly converted to an active free acid.

Misoprostol helps to both prevent and heal NSAID-related gastroduodenal erosions and ulcers.[2–5] For NSAID-related ulcers, the rate of healing is higher and the risk of recurrence lower with PPIs and misoprostol compared with H_2 antagonists.[6]

PPIs are more effective than misoprostol at healing and preventing the recurrence of duodenal ulcers.[6–8] Misoprostol is as effective as PPIs in preventing relapse of gastric ulcers and, in one RCT when compared with **lansoprazole**, ulcer-free intervals were longer.[9] Overall, the risk of serious GI complications are significantly reduced by misoprostol.[4,5] However, its use is limited by its tendency to cause diarrhoea and intestinal colic.

Bio-availability 90% PO.
Onset of action <30min.
Time to peak plasma concentration 30min.
Plasma halflife 1–2h for free acid.
Duration of action 2–4h.

Cautions

Women of childbearing age should use effective contraception.
Conditions where hypotension might precipitate severe complications, e.g. cerebrovascular disease, cardiovascular disease.

Undesirable effects

Diarrhoea (may necessitate stopping treatment), colic, dyspepsia, flatulence, nausea and vomiting, abnormal vaginal bleeding (intermenstrual, menorrhagia, postmenopausal), rashes, dizziness.

Dose and use

Cochrane reviews: PPIs, H_2 antagonists and prokinetics are effective at *relieving symptoms* of non-ulcer dyspepsia and acid reflux, with PPIs having the greatest efficacy.[10,11] PPIs, misoprostol and double-dose H_2 antagonists are effective at *preventing* chronic NSAID-related endoscopic peptic ulcers.

Standard doses of H_2 antagonists reduce the risk of duodenal ulcers but not gastric ulcers. Misoprostol 400microgram/24h is less effective at preventing gastric ulcers than 800microgram/24h, and is still associated with diarrhoea. Of all these treatments, only misoprostol 800microgram/24h has been definitely shown to reduce the overall incidence of ulcer *complications* (perforation, haemorrhage or gastric outlet obstruction).[5] PPIs significantly reduce rebleeding, need for surgery, and rate of ulcer recurrence. In high risk patients PPIs reduce mortality.[12]

NICE guidance: PPIs are preferable to H_2 antagonists for the treatment of dyspepsia, gastro-oesophageal reflux disease and peptic ulcers, including NSAID-related peptic ulcers. Although PPIs are more effective in relieving uninvestigated dyspeptic symptoms, offer a trial of H_2 antagonists or prokinetic if there has been an inadequate response to a PPI.

For patients taking an NSAID and at high risk of peptic ulcer disease, double-dose H_2 antagonists or PPIs significantly reduce endoscopically detected lesions. Misoprostol at low dose is less effective and has undesirable effects. When an NSAID-related ulcer is diagnosed, stop the NSAID if possible, treat *H pylori* infection if present (see p.464) and give double-dose H_2 antagonist or a PPI. PPIs heal the majority of ulcers.[13]

If it is necessary to continue with the NSAID, treatments may be less effective. The rate of healing is higher and the risk of recurrence lower with PPIs and misoprostol compared with H_2 antagonists.[6] Misoprostol 800microgram/24h is as effective as PPIs for preventing symptomatic and complicated gastric ulcers, but less effective in preventing duodenal ulcers.[7]

Prophylaxis against NSAID-related ulcers

200microgram b.d.–q.d.s. taken with the NSAID.

NSAID-related ulceration

- 200microgram t.d.s. with meals & at bedtime *or*
- 400microgram b.d. (breakfast and bedtime) for 4–8 weeks.[3]

If it causes diarrhoea, give 200microgram t.d.s. with meals & at bedtime and avoid **magnesium salts**.

Supply

Cytotec® (Pharmacia)
Tablets 200microgram, 28 days @ 200microgram b.d. = £9.

1 Monk JP and Clissold SP (1987) Misoprostol. A preliminary review of its pharmacodynamic and pharmacokinetic properties, and therapeutic efficacy in the treatment of peptic ulcer disease. *Drugs*. **33**: 1–30.
2 Silverstein FE *et al.* (1995) Misoprostol reduces serious gastrointestinal complications in patients with rheumatoid arthritis receiving nonsteroidal anti-inflammatory drugs. *Annals of internal medicine*. **123**: 241–249.
3 Bardhan KD *et al.* (1993) The prevention and healing of acute NSAID-associated gastroduodenal mucosal damage by misoprostol. *British Journal of Rheumatology*. **32**: 990–995.
4 Hooper L *et al.* (2004) The effectiveness of five strategies for the prevention of gastrointestinal toxicity induced by non steroidal anti-inflammatory drugs: systematic review. *British Medical Journal*. **329**: 948.
5 Rostom A *et al.* (2002) Prevention of NSAID-induced gastroduodenal ulcers. *Cochrane Database of Systematic Reviews*. **4**: CD002296.
6 Frech EJ and Go MF (2009) Treatment and chemoprevention of NSAID-associated gastrointestinal complications. *Therapeutics and Clinical Risk Management*. **5**: 65–73.
7 Leontiadis GI *et al.* (2007) Systematic reviews of the clinical effectiveness and cost-effectiveness of proton pump inhibitors in acute upper gastrointestinal bleeding. *Health Technology Assessment*. **11**: iii–iv, 1–164.
8 Hawkey C *et al.* (1998) Omeprazole compared with misoprostol for ulcers associated with nonsteroidal anti-inflammatory drugs. *New England Journal of Medicine*. **338**: 727–734.
9 Graham DY *et al.* (2002) Ulcer prevention in long-term users of nonsteroidal anti-inflammatory drugs: results of a double-blind, randomized, multicenter, active- and placebo-controlled study of misoprostol vs lansoprazole. *Archives of Internal Medicine*. **162**: 169–175.
10 Moayyedi P (2006) Pharmacological interventions for non-ulcer dyspepsia. *Cochrane Database of Systematic Reviews*. **4**: CD001960.
11 van Pinxteren B *et al.* (2006) Short term treatment with proton pump inhibitors, H2-receptor antagonists and prokinetics for gastro-oesophageal reflux disease-like symptoms and endoscopy negative reflux disease. *Cochrane Database of Systematic Reviews*. **3**: CD002095.
12 Leontiadis G *et al.* (2010) Proton pump inhibitor treatment for acute peptic ulcer bleeding. *Cochrane Database of Systematic Reviews*. **5**: CD002094.
13 NICE (2004) Dyspepsia. Management of dyspepsia in adults in primary care. In: *Clinical Guideline 17*. National Institute for Clinical Excellence. Available from: www.nice.org.uk/page.aspx?o = CG017

PROTON PUMP INHIBITORS — BNF 1.3.5

Class: Gastroprotective drugs

Indications: Licensed indications vary between products; consult the manufacturers' SPCs for details; they include acid dyspepsia, acid reflux, peptic ulceration, prevention and treatment of NSAID-related ulceration and eradication of *Helicobacter pylori* (with antibacterials).

Pharmacology

Proton pump inhibitors (PPIs) reduce gastric acid output but, unlike H_2 antagonists, they do *not* reduce the volume of gastric secretions. Because they are all rapidly degraded by acid, they are formulated as e/c granules or tablets. These dissolve in the duodenum where the drug is rapidly absorbed to be selectively taken up by gastric parietal cells and converted into active metabolites. These irreversibly inhibit the proton pump (H^+/K^+-ATPase) and thereby block gastric acid secretion. Elimination is predominantly by metabolism in the liver to inactive derivatives excreted mainly in the urine. The plasma halflives of PPIs are mostly <2h but, because they irreversibly inhibit the proton pump, the antisecretory activity continues for several days until new proton pumps are synthesized.

PPIs are effective in treating acid-related disorders. They provide symptomatic relief, help prevent and heal peptic ulcers (including those associated NSAIDs), and reduce the risk of recurrent ulceration and rebleeding.[1–3]

When treating peptic ulceration **lansoprazole** 30mg daily is as effective as **omeprazole** 40mg daily, and **pantoprazole** 40mg daily is as effective as **omeprazole** 20mg daily.[4] However, **omeprazole** shows a dose-response curve above the standard dose of 20mg daily, whereas no further benefit is seen by increasing the dose of **lansoprazole** and **pantoprazole** above 30mg and 40mg daily respectively.[5,6] Thus, **omeprazole** 40mg daily is superior to **lansoprazole** 60mg daily and **pantoprazole** 80mg daily in the management of severe gastro-oesophageal reflux disease (oesophagitis and stricture).[7]

Comparative studies with newer PPIs show **esomeprazole** (the S-enantiomer of **omeprazole**) 40 mg once daily and **rabeprazole** 20mg once daily cause rapid relief of reflux symptoms and suppress acid for longer periods. However, the endoscopic healing rate of ulcers and reflex oesophagitis is similar to other PPIs.[8–10] **Esomeprazole** and **rabeprazole** may be more effective in patients who have not responded to other PPIs. Whereas **omeprazole**, **lansoprazole** and **pantoprazole** are metabolized mainly via CYP2C19, this is not so with **esomeprazole** and **rabeprazole**. Thus, in CYP2C19 extensive metabolizers, the plasma concentrations of the former three PPIs are reduced, but not **esomeprazole** and **rabeprazole**.[9]

The bio-availability of **lansoprazole** is reduced by food and the manufacturer recommends that it should be given each morning 1h before breakfast. However, the reduced bio-availability appears not to reduce efficacy.[11–13] In one study comparing **lansoprazole** given either before or after food, acid suppression was comparable with both regimens after 1 week (although on day 1 it was significantly less when taken after food).[14] Pharmacokinetic data are shown in Table 1.7.
Onset of action $<$2h.
Duration of action $>$24h.

Table 1.7 Pharmacokinetic details of PPIs given PO

	Bio-availability (%)	*Time to peak plasma concentration (h)*	*Plasma halflife (h)*
Esomeprazole	68 (20mg dose) 89 (40mg dose)	1–2	1.3
Lansoprazole	80–90	1.5–2	1–2
Omeprazole	60	3–6	0.5–3
Pantoprazole	77	2–2.5	1[a]
Rabeprazole	52	1.6–5	1[b]

a. increases to 3–6h in cirrhosis
b. increases to 2–3h in hepatic impairment.

Cautions

Serious undesirable drug reactions: ocular damage,[15] impaired hearing, angina, hypertension. Most cases of ocular damage have been reported with IV **omeprazole**.[16] PPIs possibly cause vasoconstriction by blocking H^+/K^+-ATPase. Because the retinal artery is an end-artery, anterior ischaemic optic neuropathy may result. If the PPI is stopped, visual acuity may improve. Some patients have become permanently blind, in some instances after 3 days. Impaired hearing and deafness have also been reported, again mostly with IV **omeprazole**. A similar mechanism may be responsible for the angina and hypertension included in the US manufacturer's list of undesirable effects for **omeprazole**.

The dose should be reduced in severe hepatic impairment (see Dose and use). Concern about serious cardiac events (infarction, death) with **omeprazole** and **esomeprazole** is now considered to be groundless.[17]

PPIs are an independent risk factor for *Clostridium difficile* infection; and the association is stronger than for other acid-reducing agents. Patients are at risk of recurrent *Clostridium difficile* colitis, up to nearly 5 times more likely.[18–23] Although the spores of *Clostridium difficile* are resistant to gastric acid, reduced acidity allows bacteria to survive. Counts of *Clostridium difficile* organisms, which cannot survive at normal stomach pH, increase when the pH is $>$5, and go on to infect the bowel. Further, the cells can live up to 6h on moist surfaces, long enough to allow transmission between patients.[24]

All PPIs increase gastric pH, and this can affect the absorption of other drugs. Because of reduced trough plasma concentrations and AUC, it is recommended that PPIs should not be used concurrently with **atazanavir** and **indinavir**.[25,26] **Omeprazole** and **rabeprazole** decrease the absorption of **ketoconazole**; and **esomeprazole** decreases the absorption of **posaconazole**.[26] **Omeprazole** also reduces the absorption of **itraconazole** from capsules but not oral solution. Increased azole doses may be necessary to avoid treatment failure. Alternatively, giving the azole with an acidic drink, e.g. cola, minimizes the interaction.[26]

Increased gastric pH with **omeprazole** increases the bio-availability of **digoxin** by 10%.[26]

PPIs are metabolized by the cytochrome P450 family of liver enzymes (see Cytochrome P450, p.735). However, clinically important interactions are rare with PPIs.[27,28] Sedation and gait disturbances have been reported when **omeprazole** was given with **diazepam**, **flurazepam** or **lorazepam**. **Omeprazole** levels are increased by some macrolides (**clarithromycin**, **erythromycin**) and azole antifungals (**fluconazole**, **ketoconazole**, **voriconazole**).[26] No other significant CYP450 drug-drug interactions have been identified with **pantoprazole** or **rabeprazole**.[26,29]

A minor pharmacokinetic interaction between **omeprazole** and **warfarin**, resulting in a less than 15% rise in **R-warfarin** levels (the less active enantiomer) is of limited clinical relevance. However, isolated cases of raised INRs have been reported with all PPIs.[26] It is recommended that, in patients taking **warfarin**, the INR is monitored if **omeprazole** or **esomeprazole** is started or stopped.[30]

The antithrombotic effect of **clopidogrel** (a pro-drug activated by CYP2C19) can be reduced by the concurrent administration of **omeprazole**, **esomeprazole** and **rabeprazole**.[31–33] Although the evidence for the other PPIs is inconsistent,[31,32,34] it would seem wise to avoid concurrent prescription with any PPI, and use an H_2 antagonist (e.g. **ranitidine**) instead.

Undesirable effects

Common (<10%, >1%): headache, abdominal pain, nausea, vomiting, diarrhoea or constipation, flatulence.

Dose and use

Cochrane reviews: PPIs, H_2 antagonists and prokinetics are effective at *relieving symptoms* of non-ulcer dyspepsia and acid reflux, with PPIs having the greatest efficacy.[35,36] PPIs, **misoprostol** and double-dose H_2 antagonists are effective at *preventing* chronic NSAID-related endoscopic peptic ulcers.

Standard doses of H_2 antagonists reduce the risk of duodenal ulcers but not gastric ulcers. **Misoprostol** 400microgram/24h is less effective at preventing gastric ulcers than 800microgram/24h and is still associated with diarrhoea. Of all these treatments, only **misoprostol** 800microgram/24h has been definitely shown to reduce the overall incidence of ulcer *complications* (perforation, haemorrhage or gastric outlet obstruction)[37] PPIs significantly reduce rebleeding, need for surgery and rate of ulcer recurrence. In high risk patients PPIs reduce mortality.[38] Additional bedtime dose of an H_2 antagonist to high dose PPI may improve night-time acid reflux but evidence is lacking.[39]

NICE guidance: PPIs are preferable to H_2 antagonists for the treatment of dyspepsia, gastro-oesophageal reflux disease and peptic ulcers, including NSAID-related peptic ulcers. Although PPIs are more effective in relieving uninvestigated dyspeptic symptoms, offer a trial of an H_2 antagonists or a prokinetic if there has been an inadequate response to a PPI.

For patients taking an NSAID and at high risk of peptic ulcer disease, double-dose H_2 antagonists or PPIs significantly reduce endoscopically detected lesions. **Misoprostol** at low dose is less effective and has undesirable effects. When an NSAID-related ulcer is diagnosed, stop the NSAID if possible, treat *H pylori* infection if present (see p.464) and give double-dose H_2 antagonist or PPI. PPIs heal the majority of ulcers.[40,41]

PPIs are used together with antibacterials for the eradication of *Helicobacter pylori* (see p.464).

Lansoprazole

The SPC for **lansoprazole** states that administration should be 1h before breakfast each morning in order to achieve 'optimal acid inhibition'. However, this precaution is unnecessary.[11,14]

- 30mg each morning for 4–8 weeks for treatment of ulcers and reflux oesophagitis
- 15mg each morning for prophylaxis of ulcers and reflux oesophagitis, increase to 30mg daily if necessary
- 30mg b.d. when used with antibacterials to eradicate *Helicobacter pylori* (see p.464).

Omeprazole

- 20mg each morning for both treatment and prevention of ulcer recurrence
- 40mg each morning in reflux oesophagitis if poor response to standard dose
- 20mg b.d. or 40mg each morning when used with antibacterials to eradicate *Helicobacter pylori* (see p.464).

In severe hepatic impairment, the dose should be limited to **lansoprazole** 30mg/day and **omeprazole** 20mg/day.

For patients who cannot safely swallow tablets, **lansoprazole** and **omeprazole** can be given as orodispersible or dispersible tablets (Zoton Fastabs® and Losec MUPS® respectively), or the capsules can be opened and the e/c granules swallowed with water or fruit juice, or mixed with apple sauce or yoghurt. Specific procedures are available from the manufacturers for administration by enteral feeding tubes (see p.693). For patients with obstructive dysphagia and acid dyspepsia or with severe gastritis and vomiting, the rectal route has also been used.

Omeprazole has been used in the management of acute bleeding from an endoscopically proven peptic ulcer, either PO or IV.[3] **Omeprazole** and **esomeprazole** have been used parenterally in palliative care to treat painful reflux oesophagitis in patients too ill or unable to take PO medication.[41,42] Although not licensed for SC administration, it has been used successfully by this route for ≤4 days. After reconstitution, PPI injections/infusions are alkaline (pH 9–10.5) and should not be mixed with other drugs.

Supply

Esomeprazole
Nexium® (Astra Zeneca)
Tablets 20mg, 40mg, 28 days @ 20mg each morning = £18.
Granules e/c 10mg per sachet, 28 days at 20mg each morning = £50.
Injection (powder for reconstitution in 5mL 0.9% saline for bolus injection over 5min, or further dilute to 100mL for infusion over 10–30min), 40mg vial = £3.

Lansoprazole (generic)
Capsules enclosing e/c granules 15mg, 30mg, 28 days @ 30mg each morning = £3.

Zoton® (Wyeth)
Tablets orodispersible (FasTab®) 15mg, 30mg, 28 days @ 30mg each morning = £5.

Omeprazole (generic)
Capsules enclosing e/c granules 10mg, 20mg, 40mg, 28 days @ 20mg each morning = £2.
Tablets e/c 10mg, 20mg, 40mg, 28 days @ 20mg each morning = £8.
Infusion (powder for reconstitution in 5mL of infusion fluid (0.9% saline or 5% glucose). Further dilute to 100mL and give as an IV infusion over 20–30min or continuous) 40mg vial = £5.

Losec® (AstraZeneca)
Capsules enclosing e/c granules 10mg, 20mg, 40mg, 28 days @ 20mg each morning = £12.
Tablets dispersible (multiple-unit pellet system, MUPS®) ***enclosing e/c pellets*** 10mg, 20mg, 40mg, 28 days @ 20mg each morning = £12.
Injection (powder for reconstitution in 10mL of diluent provided. Give as a slow IV injection over 5min) 40mg vial with diluent = £5.
Infusion (powder for reconstitution in 5mL of infusion fluid (0.9% saline or 5% glucose). Further dilute to 100mL and give as an IV infusion over 20–30min or continuous) 40mg vial = £5.

Pantoprazole (generic)
Tablets e/c 20mg, 40mg, 28 days @ 40mg each morning = £4.

Protium® (Nycomed)
Injection (powder for reconstitution with 0.9% saline and use as an IV injection/infusion) 40mg vial = £5.

Rabeprazole
Pariet® (Janssen-Cilag, Eisai)
Tablets e/c 10mg, 20mg, 28 days at 20mg each morning = £20.

1 Frech EJ and Go MF (2009) Treatment and chemoprevention of NSAID-associated gastrointestinal complications. *Therapeutics and Clinical Risk Management.* **5**: 65–73.
2 Leontiadis GI *et al.* (2007) Systematic reviews of the clinical effectiveness and cost-effectiveness of proton pump inhibitors in acute upper gastrointestinal bleeding. *Health Technology Assessment.* **11**: iii–iv, 1–164.
3 Leontiadis GI *et al.* (2005) Systematic review and meta-analysis of proton pump inhibitor therapy in peptic ulcer bleeding. *British Medical Journal.* **330**: 568.
4 DTB (1997) Pantoprazole — a third proton pump inhibitor. *Drug and Therapeutics Bulletin.* **35**: 93–94.
5 Dammann H *et al.* (1993) The effects of lansoprazole, 30 or 60mg daily, on intragastric pH and on endocrine function in healthy volunteers. *Alimentary Pharmacology and Therapeutics.* **7**: 191–196.
6 Koop H *et al.* (1996) Intragastric pH and serum gastrin during administration of different doses of pantoprazole in healthy subjects. *European Journal of Gastroenterology and Hepatology.* **8**: 915–918.
7 Jaspersen D *et al.* (1998) A comparison of omeprazole, lansoprazole and pantoprazole in the maintenance treatment of severe reflux oesophagitis. *Alimentary Pharmacology and Therapeutics.* **12**: 49–52.
8 Zheng N (2009) Comparative study of omeprazole, lansoprazole, pantoprazole and esomeprazole for the system relief in patients with reflux oesophagitis. *World Journal of Gastroenterology.* **28**: 900–995.
9 Shi S and Klotz U (2008) Proton pump inhibitors: an update of their clinical use and pharmacokinetics. *European Journal of Clinical Pharmacology.* **64**: 935–951.
10 Pace F *et al.* (2007) A review of rabeprazole in the treatment of acid-related diseases. *Therapeutics and Clinical Risk Management.* **3**: 363–379.
11 Moules I *et al.* (1993) Gastric acid inhibition by the proton pump inhibitor lansoprazole is unaffected by food. *British Journal of Clinical Research.* **4**: 153–161.
12 Delhotal-Landes B *et al.* (1991) The effect of food and antacids on lansoprazole absorption and disposition. *European Journal of Drug Metabolism and Pharmacokinetics.* **3**: 315–320.
13 Andersson T (1990) Bioavailability of omeprazole as enteric coated (EC) granules in conjunction with food on the first and seventh days of treatment. *Drug Investigations.* **2**: 184–188.
14 Brummer RJM and Geerling BJ (1995) Acute and chronic effect of lansoprazole and omeprazole in relation to food intake. *Gut.* **37**: 127
15 Schonhofer P *et al.* (1997) Ocular damage associated with proton pump inhibitors. *British Medical Journal.* **314**: 1805.
16 Schonhofer P (1994) Intravenous omeprazole and blindness. *Lancet.* **343**: 665.
17 Health Canada (2008). Available from: www.hc-sc.gc.ca/ahc-asc/media/advisories-avis/_2008/2008_34-eng.php
18 Garey KW *et al.* (2008) Meta-analysis to assess risk factors for recurrent Clostridium difficile infection. *Journal of Hospital Infection.* **70**: 298–304.
19 Cadle RM *et al.* (2007) Association of proton-pump inhibitors with outcomes in Clostridium difficile colitis. *American Journal of Health System Pharmacy.* **64**: 2359–2363.
20 Dial S *et al.* (2005) Use of gastric acid suppressive agents and the risk of community acquired Clostridium difficile-associated diarrhoea. *Journal of the American Medical Association.* **294**: 2984–2995.
21 Yearsley KA *et al.* (2006) Proton pump inhibitor therapy is a risk factor for Clostridium difficile-associated diarrhoea. *Alimentary Pharmacology and Therapeutics.* **24**: 613–619.
22 Cunningham R and Dial S (2008) Is over-use of proton pump inhibitors fuelling the current epidemic of Clostridium difficile-associated diarrhoea? *Journal of Hospital Infection.* **70**: 1–6.
23 Kim JW *et al.* (2010) Proton pump inhibitors as a risk factor for recurrence of Clostridium-difficile-associated diarrhea. *World Journal of Gastroenterology.* **16**: 3573–3577.
24 Jump RL *et al.* (2007) Vegetative Clostridium difficile survives in room air on moist surfaces and in gastric contents with reduced acidity: a potential mechanism to explain the association between proton pump inhibitors and C. difficile-associated diarrhea? *Antimicrobial Agents and Chemotherapy.* **51**: 2883–2887.
25 European Agency for the Evaluation of Medicinal Products (2004) Important new pharmacokinetic data demostrating that REYATAZ (atazanavir sulphate) combined with NORVIR (ritonavir) and omeprazole should not be co-administered.. In: *EMEA public statement.* Available from: www.emea.europa.eu/pdfs/human/press/pus/20264904en.pdf
26 Baxter K (ed) (2010) Stockley's Drug Interactions (online edition). The Pharmaceutical Press, London. Available from: www.medicinescomplete.com
27 Andersson T (1996) Pharmacokinetics, metabolism and interactions of acid pump inhibitors. Focus on omeprazole, lansoprazole and pantoprazole. *Clinical Pharmacokinetics.* **31**: 9–28.
28 Tucker G (1994) The interaction of proton pump inhibitors with cytochrome P450. *Alimentary Pharmacology and Therapeutics.* **8**: 33–38.
29 Steinijans W (1996) Lack of pantoprazole drug interactions in man: an updated review. *International Journal of Clinical Pharmacology and Therapeutics.* **34**: S31–S50.
30 MHRA (2009) Public assessment report. Warfarin: changes to product safety information December 2009. Available from: www.mhra.gov.uk/home/groups/pl-p/documents/websiteresources/con065506.pdf
31 Juurlink DN *et al.* (2009) A population-based study of the drug interaction between proton pump inhibitors and clopidogrel. *Canadian Medical Association Journal.* **180**: 713–718.
32 Ho M *et al.* (2009) Risk of adverse outcomes associated with concomitant use of clopidogrel and proton pump inhibitors following acute coronary syndrome. *Journal of the American Medical Association.* **301**: 937–944.
33 Society for Cardiovascular Angiography and Interventions (2009) A national study of the effect of individual proton pump inhibitors on cardiovascular outcomes in patients treated with clopidogrel following coronary stenting: The Clopidrogrel Medco Outcomes Study. Available from: www.scai.org/drlt1.aspx?PAGE_ID = 5870
34 MHRA (2010) Clopidogrel and proton pump inhibitors: interaction — updated advice. Drug Safety Update 3 (Sept) 4. Available from: www.mhra.gov.uk/home/idcplg?IdcService = GET_FILE&dDocName = CON084657&RevisionSelectionMethod = LatestReleased
35 Moayyedi P (2006) Pharmacological interventions for non-ulcer dyspepsia. *Cochrane Database of Systematic Reviews.* **4**: CD001960.
36 van Pinxteren B *et al.* (2006) Short term treatment with proton pump inhibitors, H2- receptor antagonists and prokinetics for gastro-oesophageal reflux disease-like symptoms and endoscopy negative reflux disease. *Cochrane Database of Systematic Reviews.* **3**: CD002095.
37 Rostom A *et al.* (2002) Prevention of NSAID-induced gastroduodenal ulcers. *Cochrane Database of Systematic Reviews.* **4**: CD002296.

38 Leontiadis GI *et al.* (2010) Proton pump inhibitor treatment for acute peptic ulcer bleeding. *Cochrane Database of Systematic Reviews.* **5**: CD002094.
39 Wang Y *et al.* (2009) Additional bedtime H2 receptor antagonist for control of nocturnal gastirc acid breakthrough. *Cochrane Database of Systematic Reviews.* **4**: CD004275.
40 NICE (2004) Dyspepsia. Management of dyspepsia in adults in primary care. In: *Clinical Guideline 17*. National Institute for Clinical Excellence. Available from: www.nice.org.uk/page.aspx?o = CG017
41 Desmidts T and Constans T (2009) Subcutaneous infusion of esomeprazole in elderly patients in palliative care: A report of two cases. *Journal of the American Geriatrics Society.* **57**: 1724–1725.
42 Agar M *et al.* (2004) The use of subcutaneous omeprazole in the treatment of dyspepsia in palliative care patients. *Journal of Pain and Symptom Management.* **28**: 529–531.

LOPERAMIDE BNF 1.4.2

Class: Antimotility drug.

Indications: Acute and chronic diarrhoea, †ileostomy (to improve faecal consistency).

Contra-indications: Colitis (ulcerative, infective, or antibiotic-associated).

Pharmacology

Loperamide is a potent μ-opioid receptor agonist (μ agonist).[1] Although well absorbed from the GI tract, loperamide is almost completely extracted and metabolized by cytochrome P450 in the liver (particularly CYP3A4) where it is conjugated, and the conjugates excreted in the bile. Because of this, little loperamide reaches the systemic circulation.

The antidiarrhoeal action of loperamide results from direct absorption into the gut wall. Like **morphine** and other μ agonists, loperamide increases intestinal transit time by decreasing propulsive activity and increasing non-propulsive activity via its effect on the myenteric plexus in the longitudinal muscle layer.[2,3] Loperamide also increases anal sphincter tone and improves night-time continence in patients with ileo-anal pouches.[4]

Loperamide also modifies the intestinal transport of water and electrolytes by stimulating absorption,[5] and by an anti-secretory action mediated by calmodulin antagonism, a property not shared by other opioids.[6–8]

Paradoxically, loperamide reduces the sodium-dependent uptake of glucose and other nutrients from the small bowel.[9] The development of tolerance to the GI effects of loperamide has been demonstrated in animal studies.[10] However, loperamide has been successfully used in patients with chronic diarrhoea for several years without evidence of tolerance.[11]

Loperamide is a substrate for P-glycoprotein, the efflux membrane transporter in the blood-brain barrier, and, although highly lipophilic,[3] loperamide is actively excluded from the CNS.[12,13] Consequently, unlike **morphine** which has both central and peripheral constipating effects, loperamide generally acts only peripherally[1] (but see Drug interactions and Undesirable effects).

Loperamide has an effect on peripheral μ-opioid receptors activated by inflammation, and has been investigated as a possible *topical analgesic* for painful ulcers of the skin or mouth.[14,15] There are preliminary reports of the successful use of orodispersible tablets (e.g. Imodium Instants) 2mg q2–3h p.r.n. as an adjuvant analgesic for oral pain from mucositis or cancer.[16] (Note: Imodium® *oral solution* contains alcohol and should *not* be used). However, these formulations are only available OTC and are relatively expensive (see Supply). Thus, oral **morphine** solution (without alcohol) may be a better option, particularly long-term.

Unlike other drugs used for diarrhoea, e.g. **diphenoxylate** (in **co-phenotrope**) and **codeine**, loperamide has no analgesic effect in therapeutic and supratherapeutic doses. The lack of CNS effects is one reason why loperamide is a popular first-line choice for the control of diarrhoea, including when secondary to surgery, radiotherapy or chemotherapy.[17,18]

However, **octreotide** (see p.507) is recommended first-line for chemotherapy or radiotherapy-induced diarrhoea when severe (i.e. an increase of ⩾7 stools/24h over baseline, hospital admission and IV fluids required for >24h), and second-line for less severe diarrhoea which does not respond to loperamide 16–24mg/24h.[17–19]

As an antidiarrhoeal, loperamide is about 3 times more potent mg for mg than **diphenoxylate** and 50 times more potent than **codeine**.[20] It is longer acting and, if used regularly, generally needs to be given only b.d. However, its maximum therapeutic impact may not manifest for 16–24h; this has implications for initial dosing.[13] The following regimens are approximately equivalent:

- loperamide 2mg b.d.
- **diphenoxylate** 2.5mg q.d.s. (in **co-phenotrope**)
- **codeine phosphate** 60mg q.d.s.

Loperamide is available in a range of formulations. Orodispersible tablets, which melt on the tongue, are bio-equivalent to the capsules and are preferred by some patients. A combination product with **simeticone** provides more rapid relief of diarrhoea and abdominal discomfort from bloating in acute non-specific diarrhoea than either loperamide or **simeticone** alone.[21,22] One suggested explanation is that the surfactant effect of **simeticone** enhances the contact of loperamide with the gut mucosa. However, both these formulations are only available OTC and are relatively expensive (see Supply).

Bio-availability $<2\%$.
Onset of action about 1h; maximum effect 16–24h.[23]
Time to peak plasma concentration 2.5h (oral solution); 5h (capsules).[24]
Plasma halflife 11h.[24]
Duration of action up to 3 days.[11]

Cautions

Severe hepatic impairment could increase plasma concentrations of loperamide and the risk of undesirable effects.[25]

Drug interactions

CYP3A4 inhibitors (e.g. **erythromycin**, **fluconazole**, **ketoconazole**, **quinidine**, **ritonavir**) can increase plasma concentrations of loperamide.[25]

Inhibitors of P-glycoprotein (e.g. **ciclosporin**, **clarithromycin**, **erythromycin**, **intraconazole**, **ketoconazole**, **quinidine**, **ritonavir**, **verapamil**) could potentially allow more loperamide to cross the blood-brain barrier and cause central opioid effects. Although one study in healthy volunteers of **quinidine** with loperamide found a blunted respiratory response to CO_2 (indicating respiratory depression),[13] others have failed to demonstrate significant CNS effects.[26]

However, with typical doses of loperamide, it is unlikely that these interactions are clinically relevant.[26]

Undesirable effects

Ileus, faecal impaction, urinary retention. CNS effects can occur in children <2 years who receive excessive doses,[27,28] or in children after unintentional overdose (e.g. drowsiness).[29] If necessary, use **naloxone** to reverse these effects (see **naloxone**, p.435).

A patient on **clozapine** (an atypical antipsychotic) died of toxic megacolon after taking loperamide during an episode of food poisoning. Additive inhibition of intestinal motility was considered the precipitating cause.[30]

Dose and use

Ensure that the diarrhoea is not secondary to faecal impaction.

Acute diarrhoea

- start with 4mg PO stat
- continue with 2mg after each loose bowel action for up to 5 days
- maximum recommended dose 16mg/24h.

Chemotherapy- or radiotherapy-induced diarrhoea

- if mild–moderate, give 4mg stat and 2mg after each loose bowel action
- if not responding to doses of 24mg/24h, switch to **octreotide** (see p.507)
- if severe, use **octreotide** first-line (see p.507).

Chronic diarrhoea

If symptomatic treatment is appropriate, the same initial approach is used for 2–3 days, after which a prophylactic b.d. regimen is instituted based on the needs of the patient during the previous 24h, plus 2mg after each loose bowel action. The effective dose varies widely. In palliative care, it is occasionally necessary to increase the dose to as much as 32mg/24h; *this is twice the recommended maximum daily dose.*

Supply

Loperamide (generic)
Capsules 2mg, 28 days @ 2mg q.d.s. = £4.50.
Tablets 2mg, 28 days @2mg q.d.s. = £8.

Imodium® (Janssen-Cilag)
Capsules 2mg, 28 days @ 2mg q.d.s. = £4.
Oral solution (sugar-free) 1mg/5mL, 28 days @ 2mg q.d.s. = £11; *contains alcohol.*

Imodium® Instants (McNeil)
Orodispersible tablet 2mg, 6 tablets = £4.50 OTC.

Imodium® Instant Melts (McNeil)
Orodispersible tablet 2mg, 12 tablets = £7 OTC.

With **simeticone**
Imodium® Plus (McNeil)
Caplets (capsule shaped tablets) containing loperamide 2mg, **simeticone** 125mg, 28 days @ 1 q.d.s. = £33.

1 Shannon H and Lutz E (2002) Comparison of the peripheral and central effects of the opioid agonists loperamide and morphine in the formalin test in rats. *Neuropharmacology.* **42**: 253–261.
2 Van Nueten JM *et al.* (1979) Distribution of loperamide in the intestinal wall. *Biochemical Pharmacology.* **28**: 1433–1434.
3 Ooms L *et al.* (1984) Mechanisms of action of loperamide. *Scandinavian Journal of Gastroenterology.* **19 (suppl 96)**: 145–155.
4 Hallgren T *et al.* (1994) Loperamide improves anal sphincter function and continence after restorative proctocolectomy. *Digestive Diseases and Sciences.* **39**: 2612–2618.
5 Dashwood MR *et al.* (1990) Autoradiographic demonstration of [3H] loperamide binding to opioid receptors in rat and human small intestine. *Progress in Clinical and Biological Research.* **328**: 165–169.
6 Merritt J *et al.* (1982) Loperamide and calmodulin. *Lancet.* **1**: 283.
7 Zavecz J *et al.* (1982) Relationship between anti-diarrheal activity and binding to calmodulin. *European Journal of Pharmacology.* **78**: 375–377.
8 Daly J and Harper J (2000) Loperamide: novel effects on capacitative calcium influx. *Celluar and Molecular Life Sciences.* **57**: 149–157.
9 Klaren P *et al.* (2000) Effect of loperamide on Na+/D-glucose cotransporter activity in mouse small intestine. *Journal of Pharmacy and Pharmacology.* **52**: 679–686.
10 Tan-No K *et al.* (2003) Development of tolerance to the inhibitory effect of loperamide on gastrointestinal transit in mice. *European Journal of Pharmaceutical Sciences.* **20**: 357–363.
11 Heel R *et al.* (1978) Loperamide: A review of its pharmacological properties and therapeutic efficacy in diarrhoea. *Drugs.* **15**: 33–52.
12 Heykants J *et al.* (1974) Loperamide (R 18553), a novel type of antidiarrheal agent. Part 5: The pharmacokinetics of loperamide in rats and man. *Arzneimittel-Forschung.* **24**: 1649–1653.
13 Sadeque A *et al.* (2000) Increased drug delivery to the brain by P-glycoprotein inhibition. *Clinical Pharmacology and Therapeutics.* **68**: 231–237.
14 Nozaki-Taguchi N *et al.* (2008) Potential utility of peripherally applied loperamide in oral chronic graft-versus-host disease related pain. *Japan Journal of Clinical Oncology.* **38**: 857–860.
15 Nozaki-Taguchi N and Yaksh TL (1999) Characterization of the antihyperalgesic action of a novel peripheral mu-opioid receptor agonist—loperamide. *Anesthesiology.* **90**: 225–234.
16 Regnard C (2011) *Personal communication. St Oswald's Hospice, Newcastle.*
17 Benson AB *et al.* (2004) Recommended Guidelines for the Treatment of Cancer Treatment-Induced Diarrhea. *Journal of Clinical Oncology.* **22**: 2918–2926.
18 Maroun JA *et al.* (2007) Prevention and management of chemotherapy-induced diarrhea in patients with colorectal cancer: a consensus statement by the Canadian Working Group on Chemotherapy-Induced Diarrhea. *Current Oncology.* **14**: 13–20.
19 Bhattacharya S (2009) Octreotide in chemotherapy induced diarrhoea in colorectal cancer: a review article. *Acta Gastroenterologica Belgica.* **72**: 289–295.
20 Schuermans V *et al.* (1974) Loperamide (R18553), a novel type of antidiarrhoeal agent. Part 6: clinical pharmacology. Placebo-controlled comparison of the constipating activity and safety of loperamide, diphenoxylate and codeine in normal volunteers. *Arzneimittel-Forschung Drug Research.* **24**: 1653–1657.
21 Kaplan MA *et al.* (1999) Loperamide-simethicone vs loperamide alone, simethicone alone, and placebo in the treatment of acute diarrhea with gas-related abdominal discomfort. A randomized controlled trial. *Archives of Family Medicine.* **8**: 243–248.

22 Hanauer SB *et al.* (2007) Randomized, double-blind, placebo-controlled clinical trial of loperamide plus simethicone versus loperamide alone and simethicone alone in the treatment of acute diarrhea with gas-related abdominal discomfort. *Current Medical Research Opinion*. **23**: 1033–1043.
23 Dreverman JWM and van der Poel AJ (1995) Loperamide oxide in acute diarrhoea: a double-blind placebo-controlled trial. *Alimentary Pharmacology and Therapeutics*. **9**: 441–446.
24 Killinger J *et al.* (1979) Human pharmacokinetics and comparative bioavailability of loperamide hydrochloride. *Journal of Clinical Pharmacology*. **19**: 211–218.
25 Baker DE (2007) Loperamide: a pharmacological review. *Reviews in Gastroenterological Disorders*. **7 (suppl 3)**: S11–18.
26 Vandenbossche J *et al.* (2010) Loperamide and P-glycoprotein inhibition: assessment of the clinical relevance. *Journal of Pharmacy and Pharmacology*. **62**: 401–412.
27 Friedli G and Haenggeli CA (1980) Loperamide overdose managed by naloxone. *Lancet*. **ii**: 1413.
28 Minton N and Smith P (1987) Loperamide toxicity in a child after a single dose. *British Medical Journal*. **294**: 1383.
29 Litovitz T *et al.* (1997) Surveillance of loperamide ingestions: an analysis of 216 poison center reports. *Journal of Toxicology and Clinical Toxicology*. **35**: 11–19.
30 Eronen M *et al.* (2003) Lethal gastroenteritis associated with clozapine and loperamide. *American Journal of Psychiatry*. **160**: 2242–2243.

LAXATIVES — BNF 1.6

The prescription of laxatives is influenced by fashion, availability and cost, and there is wide variation in their use between clinicians and countries.[1,2] However, it is important that clinicians develop a simple and logical approach based on an appreciation of how different laxatives work and of the underlying pathophysiology of constipation, particularly opioid-induced.[3,4] This would include ensuring that the dose of a stimulant laxative is always optimized and that the concurrent prescription of multiple different types of laxatives is avoided as far as possible.

Constipation is common in advanced cancer.[5,6] The key feature is reduced water in the faeces which results in the passage of hard faeces infrequently and with difficulty. Faecal dehydration occurs because of prolonged bowel transit time (allowing more absorption of water by the GI tract), or a reduced ability of the stool to retain water (because of reduced fibre intake). Constipation is more common in immobile patients with small appetites and those receiving constipating drugs, particularly opioids.[7,8]

The management of constipation aims to restore the amount of water in the faeces by:

- reducing bowel transit time (stimulant laxatives, exercise)
- increasing faecal water (hyperosmolar laxatives)
- increasing the ability of the faeces to retain water (fibre, **docusate**, iso-osmolar laxatives).

In palliative care, exercise and increased dietary fibre are rarely feasible options.[9] Although some strong opioids are less constipating than **morphine** (e.g. **buprenorphine**, **fentanyl**, **methadone**), most patients receiving any opioid regularly will need a laxative concurrently.[6,10] Thus, as a general rule, all patients prescribed **morphine** (or other opioid) should also be prescribed a laxative (see p.38).

About one third of patients also need rectal measures[11,12] either because of failed oral treatment or electively, e.g. in bedbound frail elderly patients, or patients with paralysis (see p.40).

Laxatives can be classified according to their primary action (Box 1.G).[13,14] However, many laxatives also have a secondary action. For example **lactulose** is a hyperosmolar osmotic laxative, but is converted by colonic fermentation to organic acids which act as contact stimulants in the large bowel.[15] At doses commonly used, **docusate sodium** acts mainly by lowering surface tension (enabling water and fats to penetrate into the substance of the faeces) but at higher doses it also acts as a stimulant laxative (see p.45).

Opioids are a major contributory factor for constipation in palliative care patients, reducing quality of life, and sometimes resulting in opioid discontinuation.[16–18] Opioids cause constipation by increasing ring contractions, decreasing propulsive intestinal activity, and by enhancing the resorption of fluid and electrolytes;[7,19] tolerance does not develop to these effects.[20] Stimulant

Box 1.G Classification of commonly used laxatives

Bulk-forming agents (fibre)
Ispaghula (psyllium) husk (e.g. Fybogel®, Regulan®)
Methylcellulose (e.g. Celevac®)
Sterculia (e.g. Normacol®)

Faecal softeners
Surface-wetting agents
Docusate sodium
Poloxamer 188 (in co-danthramer)

Lubricants
Liquid paraffin
Arachis oil

Osmotic laxatives
Iso-osmolar (when mixed with recommended quantity of water)
Macrogols (e.g. Movicol®)

Hyperosmolar
Lactulose syrup
Liquid paraffin and magnesium hydroxide oral emulsion BP
Magnesium hydroxide suspension (Milk of Magnesia®)
Magnesium sulphate (Epsom Salts)

Stimulant laxatives
Acting on small and large bowel
Bisacodyl
Dantron (in co-danthramer and co-danthrusate)

Acting on large bowel
Senna
Sodium picosulfate

laxatives reduce intestinal ring contractions and thus facilitate propulsive activity. Consequently, they provide a logical approach to the correction of opioid-induced constipation. Indeed, both **senna** and **sodium picosulfate** given alone are sufficient to treat opioid-induced constipation.[21,22] However, in practice, a combination of a stimulant laxative and a faecal softener is often prescribed (see p.38).[4,6,23,24]

Several RCTs of laxatives have been completed in palliative care patients:
- **senna** vs. **lactulose**[25]
- **senna** vs. **misrakasneham** (an Ayurvedic herbal remedy)[26]
- **senna** and **lactulose** vs. **co-danthramer** (dantron and poloxamer)[27]
- **senna** and **lactulose** vs. **magnesium hydroxide** and **liquid paraffin**.[28]

A significant difference between treatments was seen only in the third RCT.[27] The combination of **senna** and **lactulose** was significantly better at relieving constipation than **co-danthramer**. However, *PCF* generally discourages the use of **lactulose** because of its relative expense and its propensity for causing GI discomfort (see p.46). *PCF* also discourages the use of **macrogols** as first-line treatment of constipation in palliative care (see p.47).

Methylnaltrexone, a peripherally-acting opioid antagonist, represents an alternative (and potentially more specific) approach to the management of opioid-induced constipation (see p.38 and p.433). A recent Cochrane review concluded that there is some evidence that, compared with placebo, **methylnaltrexone** is effective in patients taking opioids who have not had a good response to conventional laxatives.[29]

1 Laugsand EA *et al.* (2009) Intensity and treatment of symptoms in 3,030 palliative care patients: a cross-sectional survey of the EAPC Research Network. *Journal of Opioid Management.* **5**: 11–21.
2 Borgsteede SD *et al.* (2009) Prescribing of pain medication in palliative care. A survey in general practice. *Pharmacoepidemiol Drug Safety.* **18**: 16–23.

3 Clemens KE and Klaschik E (2008) Management of constipation in palliative care patients. *Current Opinion in Supportive and Palliative Care*. **2**: 22–27.
4 Larkin PJ *et al.* (2008) The management of constipation in palliative care: clinical practice recommendations. *Palliative Medicine*. **22**: 796–807.
5 Droney J *et al.* (2008) Constipation in cancer patients on morphine. *Supportive Care in Cancer*. **16**: 453–459.
6 Miles CL *et al.* (2006) Laxatives for the management of constipation in palliative care patients. *Cochrane Database of Systematic Reviews*. CD003448.
7 Kurz A and Sessler DI (2003) Opioid-induced bowel dysfunction: pathophysiology and potential new therapies. *Drugs*. **63**: 649–671.
8 Pappagallo M (2001) Incidence, prevalence, and management of opioid bowel dysfunction. *American Journal of Surgery*. **182 (suppl 5A)**: 11s–18s.
9 Mancini IL *et al.* (2000) Opioid type and other clinical predictors of laxative dose in advanced cancer patients: a retrospective study. *Journal of Palliative Medicine*. **3**: 49–56.
10 Radbruch L *et al.* (2000) Constipation and the use of laxatives: a comparison between transdermal fentanyl and oral morphine. *Palliative Medicine*. **14**: 111–119.
11 Twycross RG and Lack SA (1986) *Control of Alimentary Symptoms in Far Advanced Cancer*. Churchill Livingstone, Edinburgh, pp. 173–174.
12 Twycross RG and Harcourt JMV (1991) The use of laxatives at a palliative care centre. *Palliative Medicine*. **5**: 27–33.
13 Tramonte S *et al.* (1997) The treatment of chronic constipation in adults. A systematic review. *Journal of General Internal Medicine*. **12**: 15–24.
14 Kamm MA (2003) Constipation and its management. *British Medical Journal*. **327**: 459–460.
15 Jouet P *et al.* (2008) Effects of therapeutic doses of lactulose vs. polyethylene glycol on isotopic colonic transit. *Alimentary Pharmacology and Therapeutics*. **27**: 988–993.
16 Sykes N (1998) The relationship between opioid use and laxative use in terminally ill cancer patients. *Palliative Medicine*. **12**: 375–382.
17 Bell T *et al.* (2009) Opioid-induced constipation negatively impacts pain management, productivity, and health-related quality of life: findings from the National Health and Wellness Survey. *Journal of Opioid Management*. **5**: 137–144.
18 Candrilli SD *et al.* (2009) Impact of constipation on opioid use patterns, health care resource utilization, and costs in cancer patients on opioid therapy. *Journal of Pain and Palliative Care Pharmacotherapy*. **23**: 231–241.
19 Beubler E (1983) Opiates and intestinal transport: in vivo studies. In: LA Turnberg (ed) *Intestinal secretion*. Smith Kline and French, Hertfordshire, pp. 53–55.
20 Ross GR *et al.* (2008) Morphine tolerance in the mouse ileum and colon. *Journal of Pharmacology and Experimental Therapeutics*. **327**: 561–572.
21 Hawley PH and Byeon JJ (2008) A comparison of sennosides-based bowel protocols with and without docusate in hospitalized patients with cancer. *Journal of Palliative Medicine*. **11**: 575–581.
22 Twycross RG *et al.* (2006) Sodium picosulfate in opioid-induced constipation: results of an open-label, prospective, dose-ranging study. *Palliative Medicine*. **20**: 419–423.
23 McMillan SC (2004) Assessing and managing opiate-induced constipation in adults with cancer. *Cancer Control*. **11**: 3–9.
24 Avila JG (2004) Pharmacologic treatment of constipation in cancer patients. *Cancer Control*. **11**: 10–18.
25 Agra Y *et al.* (1998) Efficacy of senna versus lactulose in terminal cancer patients treatment with opioids. *Journal of Pain and Symptom Management*. **15**: 1–7.
26 Ramesh P *et al.* (1998) Managing morphine-induced constipation: a controlled comparison of an Ayurvedic formulation and senna. *Journal of Pain and Symptom Management*. **16**: 240–244.
27 Sykes N (1991) A clinical comparison of laxatives in a hospice. *Palliative Medicine*. **5**: 307–314.
28 Sykes N (1991) A clinical comparison of lactulose and senna with magnesium hydroxide and liquid paraffin emulsion in a palliative care population. [cited in Miles CL *et al.* (2006) Laxatives for the management of constipation in palliative care patients. *The Cochrane Database of Systematic Reviews*. CD003448]
29 Candy B *et al.* (2011) Laxatives or methylnaltrexone for the management of constipation in palliative care patients. *Cochrane Database of Systematic Reviews*. **19**: CD003448.

Quick Practice Guide: Opioid-induced constipation

Generally, all patients prescribed an opioid should also be prescribed a stimulant laxative, with the aim of achieving a regular bowel movement, without straining, every 1–3 days. A standardized protocol aids management. However, occasionally, rather than automatically changing to senna or dantron, it may be more appropriate to optimize a patient's existing regimen.

These guidelines also provide a suitable approach to managing constipation in patients who are not on opioids. However, in these circumstances, smaller doses of laxatives may well suffice.

1. Ask about the patient's past and present bowel habit and use of laxatives; record the date of last bowel action.
2. Palpate for faecal masses in the line of the colon; examine the rectum digitally if the bowels have not been open for ⩾3 days or if the patient reports rectal discomfort or has diarrhoea suggestive of faecal impaction with overflow.
3. For inpatients, keep a daily record of bowel actions.
4. Encourage fluids generally, and fruit juice and fruit specifically.
5. When an opioid is prescribed, prescribe senna (see below) or dantron-containing stimulant laxative (see overleaf), and titrate the dose according to response.
6. During dose titration and subsequently, if ⩾3 days since last bowel action, give suppositories, e.g. bisacodyl 10mg and glycerol 4g, or a micro-enema. If these are ineffective, administer a phosphate enema and possibly repeat the next day.
7. If the maximum dose of the stimulant laxative is ineffective, halve the dose and add an osmotic laxative, then titrate as necessary, e.g.
   - macrogols (e.g. Movicol®) 1 sachet each morning *or*
   - lactulose 15mL once daily–b.d.
8. Alternatively, prescribe SC methylnaltrexone (see overleaf).
9. If the stimulant laxative causes intestinal colic, divide the total daily dose into smaller more frequent doses. Alternatively, change to an osmotic laxative (see above), then titrate as necessary.
10. An osmotic laxative may be preferable in patients with a history of colic with stimulant laxatives, e.g. bisacodyl, dantron, senna.

Dose schedule for senna

- if *not* constipated:
  - ▹ generally start with 15mg at bedtime
  - ▹ if no response after 24–48h, increase to 15mg at bedtime and each morning
- if already constipated
  - ▹ generally start with 15mg at bedtime and each morning
  - ▹ if no response after 24–48h, increase to 22.5mg at bedtime and each morning
- if no response after a further 24–48h, consider adding a third daytime dose
- if necessary, consider increasing to a maximum of 30mg t.d.s.

continued

Dose schedule for dantron-containing laxatives[a,b]

	Co-danthramer strong capsules	*Co-danthramer strong suspension*	*Co-danthrusate capsules*	*Co-danthrusate suspension*
Dantron content	37.5mg/capsule	75mg/5mL	50mg/capsule	50mg/5mL
Start with:				
• prophylactic	1 at bedtime	2.5mL at bedtime	1 at bedtime	5mL at bedtime
• if constipated	2 at bedtime	5mL at bedtime	2 at bedtime	10mL at bedtime
If necessary, adjust every 2–3 days up to:				
	3 t.d.s.	10mL b.d. *or* 20mL at bedtime	3 b.d.	15mL b.d.
Total daily dose	337.5mg	300mg	300mg	300mg

a. because dantron has been linked with liver and bowel tumours in rodents, dantron-containing laxatives are licensed for use only in the 'terminally ill'

b. in patients with urinary or faecal incontinence, dantron-containing laxatives are best avoided because of the risk of a contact skin burn in the perineum and surrounding areas.

Methylnaltrexone

Methylnaltrexone is relatively expensive (£21 per 12mg vial) and should be considered only when the optimum use of laxatives is ineffective. Because constipation in advanced disease is generally multifactorial in origin, methylnaltrexone is likely to augment rather than replace laxatives.

- marketed as a SC injection for use in patients with 'advanced illness' and opioid-induced constipation despite treatment with laxatives
- about 1/3–1/2 of patients given methylnaltrexone have a bowel movement within 4h, without loss of analgesia or the development of opioid withdrawal symptoms
- dose recommendations:
  - ▷ for patients weighing 38–61kg, start with 8mg on alternate days
  - ▷ for patients weighing 62–114kg, start with 12mg on alternate days
  - ▷ outside this range, give 150microgram/kg on alternate days
  - ▷ the interval between administrations can be varied, either extended or reduced, but not more than once daily
- in severe renal impairment (creatinine clearance <30mL/min) reduce the dose:
  - ▷ for patients weighing 62–114kg, reduce to 8mg
  - ▷ outside this range, reduce to *75microgram/kg*, rounding up the dose volume to the nearest 0.1mL
- methylnaltrexone is contra-indicated in cases of known or suspected bowel obstruction. It should be used with caution in patients with conditions which may predispose to perforation. Common undesirable effects include abdominal pain/colic, diarrhoea, flatulence, and nausea; these generally resolve after a bowel movement; postural hypotension can also occur.

Quick Practice Guide: Bowel management in paraplegia and tetraplegia

Theoretically, management is determined by the level of the spinal cord lesion:

- above T12–L1 = cauda equina intact → spastic GI tract with preserved sacral reflex; generally responds to digital stimulation of the rectum; the presence of an anal reflex suggests an intact sacral reflex
- below T12–L1 = cauda equina involved → flaccid GI tract; generally requires digital evacuation of the rectum
- a lesion at the level of the conus medullaris (the cone shaped distal end of the spinal cord, surrounded by the sacral nerves) may manifest a mixture of clinical features.

However, in practice, management tends to follow a common pathway.

Aims

1 Primary: to achieve the controlled regular evacuation of normal formed faeces:
  - every day in long-term paraplegia/tetraplegia, e.g. post-traumatic
  - every 1–3 days in advanced cancer.

2 Secondary: to prevent both incontinence (faeces too soft, over-treatment with laxatives) and an anal fissure (faeces too hard, under-treatment with laxatives).

Oral measures

3 In debilitated patients with a poor appetite, a bulking agent is unlikely to be helpful, and may result in a soft impaction.

4 Particularly if taking morphine or another constipating drug, an oral stimulant laxative should be prescribed, e.g. senna 15mg b.d., bisacodyl tablets 5–10mg b.d. The dose should be carefully titrated to a level which results in normal faeces *in the rectum* but without causing an uncontrolled evacuation.

5 In relatively well patients with a good appetite (probably the minority):
  - maintain a high fluid intake
  - encourage a high roughage diet, e.g. wholegrain cereals, wholemeal foods, greens, bran or a bulk-forming laxative, e.g. ispaghula.

6 Beware:
  - the prescription of docusate sodium, a faecal softener, may result in a soft faecal impaction of the rectum, and faecal leakage through a patulous anus
  - oral bisacodyl in someone not on opioids may cause multiple uncontrolled evacuations, at the wrong time and in the wrong place.

Rectal measures

7 Initially, if impacted with faeces, empty the rectum digitally. Then, develop a daily routine:
  - as soon as convenient after waking up in the morning, insert 2 glycerol suppositories, or 1–2 bisacodyl suppositories (10–20mg), or an osmotic micro-enema deep into the rectum, and wait for 1.5–2 hours
  - because the bisacodyl acts only after absorption and biotransformation, bisacodyl suppositories must be placed against the rectal wall, and not into faeces
  - the patient should be encouraged to have a hot drink after about 1h in the hope that it will stimulate a gastro-colonic reflex
  - if there is a strong sacral reflex, some faeces will be expelled as a result of the above two measures
  - to ensure complete evacuation of the rectum and sigmoid colon, digitally stimulate the rectum:
  - insert gloved and lubricated finger (either soap or gel)
    - ▹ rotate finger 3–4 times
    - ▹ withdraw and wait 5min

  - ▹ if necessary, repeat 3–4 times
  - ▹ check digitally that rectum is fully empty.

8 Patients who are unable to transfer to the toilet or a commode will need nursing assistance. Sometimes it is easiest for a patient to defaecate onto a pad while in bed in a lateral position.

9 If the above measures do not achieve complete evacuation of the rectum and sigmoid colon, proceed to digital evacuation (more likely with a flaccid bowel). A pattern will emerge for each patient, allowing the rectal measures to be adjusted to the individual patient's needs and response.

ISPAGHULA (PSYLLIUM) HUSK — BNF 1.6.1

Ispaghula husk is *not recommended* for patients taking constipating drugs, and in those with decreasing dietary intake and activity. However, it can be helpful in regulating the consistency of faeces (making them more formed) in a patient with a colostomy/distal ileostomy.

Class: Bulk-forming laxative.

Indications: Colostomy/ileostomy regulation, anal fissure, haemorrhoids, diverticular disease, irritable bowel syndrome, ulcerative colitis.

Contra-indications: Dysphagia, bowel obstruction, colonic atony, faecal impaction.

Pharmacology

Ispaghula (psyllium) is derived from the husks of an Asian plant, *Plantago ovata*. It has very high water-binding capacity, is partly fermented in the colon, and increases bacterial cell mass, thereby further increasing faecal bulk. Like other bulk-forming laxatives, ispaghula stimulates peristalsis by increasing faecal mass. Its water-binding capacity also helps to make loose faeces more formed in some patients with a colostomy/distal ileostomy.

Onset of action full effect obtained only after several days.

Duration of action best taken regularly to obtain a consistent ongoing effect; may continue to act for 2–3 days after the last dose.

Cautions

Adequate fluid intake should be maintained to avoid bowel obstruction.

Undesirable effects

Flatulence, abdominal distension, faecal impaction, bowel obstruction.

Dose and use

Ispaghula swells in contact with fluid and needs to be drunk quickly before it absorbs water. Stir the granules or powder briskly in 150mL of water and swallow immediately; carbonated water can be used if preferred. Alternatively, the granules can be swallowed dry, or mixed with a vehicle such as jam, but must be followed by 100–200mL of water. Give 1 sachet each morning–t.d.s., preferably after meals; not immediately before going to bed.

Supply

Fybogel® (Reckitt Benckiser)

Oral powder 3.5g/sachet, 28 days @ 1 sachet b.d. = £3.50; *low Na^+; sugar- and gluten-free; plain, lemon or orange flavour.*

Regulan® (Procter & Gamble)

Oral powder 3.4g/sachet, 28 days @ 1 sachet b.d. = £4.50; *sugar- and gluten-free; orange or lemon-lime flavour.*

This is not a complete list; see BNF for more information.

STIMULANT LAXATIVES BNF 1.6.2

Indications: Prevention and treatment of constipation.

Contra-indications: Large bowel obstruction.

Pharmacology

The laxative effect is through direct contact with the submucosal (Meissner's) plexus and the deeper myenteric (Auerbach's) plexus, resulting in both a secretory and a motor effect in the large intestine. The motor effect precedes the secretory effect, and is the more important laxative action. There is a decrease in segmenting muscular activity and an increase in propulsive waves.

Senna (sennosides) is a naturally-occurring plant-derived anthranoid. It is an inactive glycoside which passes unabsorbed and unchanged through the small intestine and is hydrolyzed by *bacterial glycosidases* in the large intestine to yield active compounds.[1] Thus, **senna** has no effect on the small intestine but becomes active in the large intestine. Differences in bacterial flora may be partly responsible for differences in individual responses.

Dantron, a synthetic anthranoid, is not a glycoside and has a direct action on the small intestine as well as the large intestine.[2] Whereas systemic absorption of **senna** or its metabolites is small, **dantron** is absorbed to some extent from the small intestine with subsequent significant urinary excretion.

Phenolics such as **bisacodyl** and **sodium picosulfate** are also pro-drugs. They are hydrolyzed to the same active metabolite but the mode of hydrolysis differs.[1] **Bisacodyl** is hydrolyzed by *intestinal enzymes* and thus acts on both the small and large intestines. When applied directly to the intestinal mucosa in normal subjects, **bisacodyl** induces powerful propulsive motor activity within minutes.[3] **Bisacodyl** is often given by suppository. The laxative effect is the result of local direct contact with the rectal mucosa after dissolution of the suppository, and after activation by hydrolysis. Thus the minimum time for response is generally $>$20min.[4] In contrast, **sodium picosulfate** is hydrolyzed by *colonic bacteria* and its action is thus confined to the large intestine. Its activity is potentially more uncertain because it depends on bacterial flora.

Phenolphthalein is another stimulant laxative, and is present in some proprietary laxatives. **Phenolphthalein** exists in two forms: white and yellow. The yellow form contains several impurities produced during manufacture. These impurities enhance the laxative effect of **phenolphthalein** so that the comparable dose of the yellow form is only two thirds that of the pure white form. The active constituent of **phenolphthalein** is released in two stages: by metabolism in the liver and subsequently in the colon, and it probably undergoes enterohepatic circulation.[5] Some people respond to small doses. However, it can cause a drug rash (see Undesirable effects) and is generally not considered a first-line laxative.

Several RCTs of stimulant laxatives have been completed in palliative care patients:[6]

- **senna** vs. **lactulose**[7]
- **senna** vs. **misrakasneham** (an Ayurvedic herbal remedy)[8]
- **senna** and **lactulose** vs. **co-danthramer** (**dantron** and **poloxamer**)[9]
- **senna** and **lactulose** vs. **magnesium hydroxide** and **liquid paraffin**.[10]

A significant difference between treatments was seen only in the third RCT.[9] The combination of **senna** and **lactulose** was significantly better at relieving constipation than **co-danthramer**.

Two non-blinded dose-ranging studies are also of interest. In cancer patients on an oncology unit mostly receiving opioids, a bowel protocol based on **senna** alone was as effective as one based on **senna** and **docusate** (and more so in patients admitted for palliative care).[11] For opioid-induced constipation in palliative care patients, **sodium picosulfate** alone yielded a satisfactory result in 15/20 patients (normal stool consistency, no need for enemas, suppositories or manual evacuation, and no significant undesirable effects).[12] Thus, for opioid-induced constipation in palliative care, a reasonable approach would be to optimize the dose of a stimulant laxative before adding a surface wetting agent or osmotic laxative.

Onset of action

Bisacodyl tablets 6–12h; suppositories 20min–3h (mean 1h).[4]
Dantron 6–12h.
Senna 6–12h.
Sodium picosulfate 6–24h (median 12h).[12]

Cautions

Because very high doses in rodents revealed a carcinogenic risk,[13–15] UK licences for laxatives containing **dantron** are limited to constipation in terminally ill patients.

Undesirable effects

Intestinal colic, diarrhoea. **Bisacodyl** suppositories may cause local rectal inflammation. **Dantron** discolours urine, typically red but sometimes green or bluish. Prolonged contact with skin (e.g. in urinary or faecally incontinent patients) may cause a **dantron** burn (a red erythematous rash with a definite edge); if ignored, this may cause painful excoriation. **Phenolphthalein** occasionally causes a drug rash or photosensitivity. Rarely, it causes encephalitis which can be fatal.

Dose and use

The doses recommended here for opioid-induced constipation are often higher than those featured in the BNF and SPCs. For frail patients not receiving opioids or other constipating drugs, the PO starting doses of a stimulant laxative will generally be lower.

Because round-the-clock opioids constipate, b.d. or t.d.s. laxatives may well be necessary, rather than the traditional once daily dose (at bedtime or each morning). Requirements do not correlate closely with the opioid dose; individual titration is necessary.

All palliative care services should have a protocol for the management of opioid-induced constipation (see Quick Practice Guide, p.38).[16–19] Likewise, there is need for a protocol for patients with paraplegia and tetraplegia (see Quick Practice Guide, p.40).

Bisacodyl

- start with 10–20mg PO at bedtime
- if necessary, increase by stages to 20mg PO t.d.s.
- by suppository: 10–20mg PR once daily.

Dantron

Variable, according to preparation, individual need and patient acceptance (see Quick Practice Guide p.38).

Senna

- start with 15mg at bedtime or, if taking opioids, 15mg b.d.
- if necessary, increase progressively to 15mg→22.5mg→30mg t.d.s.

Sodium picosulfate

- start with 5–10mg at bedtime; 10mg if taking regular opioids
- if necessary, increase daily by 5mg until a satisfactory result is achieved
- median satisfactory dose = 15mg at bedtime
- typical maximum dose = 30mg.[12]

Supply

Bisacodyl (generic)
Tablets e/c 5mg, 28 days @ 10mg at bedtime = £2.
Suppositories 10mg, 28 days @ 10mg once daily = £3.

Dantron
Co-danthramer (**dantron** and **poloxamer 188**) (generic)

Co-danthramer suspension 5mL = 1 **co-danthramer** capsule.
Co-danthramer suspension 15mL = 5mL *strong* **co-danthramer** suspension.
Strong **co-danthramer** suspension 5mL = 2 *strong* **co-danthramer** capsules.

Capsules **co-danthramer** 25/200 (**dantron** 25mg, **poloxamer 188** 200mg), 28 days @ 2 at bedtime = £12.

Strong capsules **co-danthramer** 37.5/500 (**dantron** 37.5mg, **poloxamer 188** 500mg), 28 days @ 2 at bedtime = £15.
Oral suspension **co-danthramer** 25/200 in 5mL (**dantron** 25mg, **poloxamer 188** 200mg/5mL), 28 days @ 10mL at bedtime = £11.
Strong oral suspension **co-danthramer** 75/1000 in 5mL (**dantron** 75mg, **poloxamer 188** 1g/5mL), 28 days @ 5mL at bedtime = £14.

Co-danthrusate (**dantron** and **docusate sodium**) (generic)
Capsules **co-danthrusate** 50/60 (**dantron** 50mg, **docusate sodium** 60mg), 28 days @ 2 at bedtime = £13.
Oral suspension **co-danthrusate** 50/60 in 5mL (**dantron** 50mg, **docusate sodium** 60mg/5mL), 28 days @ 10mL at bedtime = £12.

Senna (generic)
Tablets total sennosides/tablet 7.5mg, 28 days @ 15mg at bedtime = £2.

Senokot® (Reckitt Benckiser)
Tablets total **sennosides**/tablet 7.5mg (~~NHS~~).
Oral solution (sugar-free) total **sennosides** 7.5mg/5mL, 28 days @ 10mL at bedtime = £1.50.

Senokot Max Strength® (Reckitt Benckiser)
Tablets total sennosides/tablet 15mg (~~NHS~~).

Sodium picosulfate (generic)
Oral syrup 5mg/5mL, 28 days @ 10mL at bedtime = £5.

Sodium picosulfate oral syrup 5mg/5mL was previously available as Laxoberal® liquid but was rebranded in 2008 as Dulcolax® Pico liquid. The proprietary name Dulcolax® (~~NHS~~) is also used for **bisacodyl** tablets and suppositories.

1 Jauch R *et al.* (1975) Bis-(p-hydroxyphenyl)-pyridyl-2-methane: the common laxative principle of bisacodyl and sodium picosulfate. *Arzneimittel-Forschung Drug Research.* **25**: 1796–1800.
2 Lennard-Jones J (1994) Clinical aspects of laxatives, enemas and suppositories. In: M Kamm and J Lennard-Jones (eds) *Constipation.* Wrightson Biomedical Publishing, Petersfield, pp. 327–341.
3 De Schryver AM *et al.* (2003) Effects of a meal and bisacodyl on colonic motility in healthy volunteers and patients with slow-transit constipation. *Digestive Diseases Sciences.* **48**: 1206–1212.
4 Flig E *et al.* (2000) Is bisacodyl absorbed at all from suppositories in man? *International Journal of Pharmaceutics.* **196**: 11–20.
5 Godding EW (1975) Constipation and allied disorders: 3. Therapeutic agents-chemical laxatives (section 2). *Pharmaceutical Journal.* **215**: 60–62.
6 Miles CL *et al.* (2006) Laxatives for the management of constipation in palliative care patients. *Cochrane Database of Systematic Reviews.* CD003448.
7 Agra Y *et al.* (1998) Efficacy of senna versus lactulose in terminal cancer patients treatment with opioids. *Journal of Pain and Symptom Management.* **15**: 1–7.
8 Ramesh P *et al.* (1998) Managing morphine-induced constipation: a controlled comparison of an Ayurvedic formulation and senna. *Journal of Pain and Symptom Management.* **16**: 240–244.
9 Sykes N (1991) A clinical comparison of laxatives in a hospice. *Palliative Medicine.* **5**: 307–314.
10 Sykes N (1991) A clinical comparison of lactulose and senna with magnesium hydroxide and liquid paraffin emulsion in a palliative care population. [cited in Miles CL *et al.* (2006) Laxatives for the management of constipation in palliative care patients. *The Cochrane Database of Systematic Reviews.* CD003448]
11 Hawley PH and Byeon JJ (2008) A comparison of sennosides-based bowel protocols with and without docusate in hospitalized patients with cancer. *Journal of Palliative Medicine.* **11**: 575–581.
12 Twycross RG *et al.* (2006) Sodium picosulfate in opioid-induced constipation: results of an open-label, prospective, dose-ranging study. *Palliative Medicine.* **20**: 419–423.
13 Mori H *et al.* (1985) Induction of intestinal tumours in rats by chrysazin. *British Journal of Cancer.* **52**: 781–783.
14 Mori H *et al.* (1986) Carcinogenicity of chrysazin in large intestine and liver of mice. *Japanese Journal of Cancer Research (Gann).* **77**: 871–876.
15 CSM (Committee on Safety of Medicines and Medicines Control Agency) (2000) Danthron restricted to constipation in the terminally ill. *Current Problems in Pharmacovigilance.* **26 (May)**: 4.
16 Levy MH (1996) Pharmacologic treatment of cancer pain. *New England Journal of Medicine.* **335**: 1124–1132.
17 Pappagallo M (2001) Incidence, prevalence, and management of opioid bowel dysfunction. *American Journal of Surgery.* **182 (suppl 5A)**: 11s–18s.
18 Bouvy ML *et al.* (2002) Laxative prescribing in relation to opioid use and the influence of pharmacy-based intervention. *Journal of Clinical Pharmacy and Therapeutics.* **27**: 107–110.
19 Herndon CM *et al.* (2002) Management of opioid-induced gastrointestinal effects in patients receiving palliative care. *Pharmacotherapy.* **22**: 240–250.

DOCUSATE SODIUM — BNF 1.6.2

Class: Surface-wetting agent (faecal softener).

Indications: Constipation, haemorrhoids, anal fissure, bowel preparation before abdominal radiography, †partial bowel obstruction.

Pharmacology

Although sometimes classified as a stimulant laxative, docusate sodium is principally an emulsifying and wetting agent and has a relatively weak effect on GI transit. Other wetting agents include **poloxamer 188** (in **co-danthramer**). Docusate lowers surface tension, thereby allowing water and fats to penetrate hard, dry faeces. It also stimulates fluid secretion by the small and large intestines.[1,2] Docusate does not interfere with protein or fat absorption.[3] Docusate has been evaluated in several groups of elderly patients; frequency of defaecation increased and the need for enemas decreased almost to zero.[4–6] Given these clinical results, it is surprising that, in a study in normal subjects, docusate did not increase faecal weight.[7]

In palliative care, docusate is generally not recommended as the sole laxative except in patients with partial bowel obstruction.[8] The routine combination of docusate (or alternative surface-wetting agent) and a stimulant laxative has been criticized because of a lack of published data supporting such a regimen.[9] A non-blinded dose-ranging study in cancer patients failed to show any benefit when docusate was added to **senna**.[10]

Onset of action 12–72h.

Cautions

Docusate enhances the absorption of **liquid paraffin**;[11] combined preparations of these substances are prohibited in some countries.

Undesirable effects

Diarrhoea, nausea, abdominal cramp, rashes. Docusate solution may cause a bitter aftertaste or burning sensation, minimized by drinking plenty of water after taking the solution.

Dose and use

At many centres, docusate is used in combination with a stimulant laxative, e.g. **senna**, **bisacodyl** or **dantron** (in **co-danthrusate**) (see Quick Practice Guide, p.38). Docusate is often used alone for patients with persistent partial bowel obstruction. Dose varies according to individual need:

- generally start with 100mg b.d.
- if necessary, increase to 200mg b.d.–t.d.s.; *the latter is higher than the BNF maximum dose of 500mg/day.*

Docusate can also be used as an enema (see Rectal products, p.50).

Supply

Dioctyl® UCB Pharma

Capsules 100mg, 28 days @ 100mg b.d. = £3.50.

Docusol® (Typharm)

Oral solution 1% (sugar-free) 50mg/5mL, 28 days @ 10mL b.d. = £10.

1 Donowitz M and Binder H (1975) Effect of dioctyl sodium sulfosuccinate on colonic fluid and electrolyte movement. *Gastroenterology*. **69**: 941–950.

2 Moriarty K *et al.* (1985) Studies on the mechanism of action of dioctyl sodium sulphosuccinate in the human jejunum. *Gut*. **26**: 1008–1013.

3 Wilson J and Dickinson D (1955) Use of dioctyl sodium sulfosuccinate (aerosol O.T.) for severe constipation. *Journal of the American Medical Association*. **158**: 261–263.

4 Cass L and Frederik W (1956) Doxinate in the treatment of constipation. *American Journal of Gastroenterology*. **26**: 691–698.

5 Harris R (1957) Constipation in geriatrics. *American Journal of Digestive Diseases*. **2**: 487–492.

6 Hyland C and Foran J (1968) Dicotyl sodium sulphosuccinate as a laxative in the elderly. *Practitioner*. **200**: 698–699.

7 Chapman R *et al.* (1985) Effect of oral dioctyl sodium sulfosuccinate on intake-output studies of human small and large intestine. *Gastroenterology*. **89**: 489–493.

8 Twycross R *et al.* (2009) *Symptom Management in Advanced Cancer* (4e). palliativedrugs.com, Nottingham.
9 Hurdon V *et al.* (2000) How useful is docusate in patients at risk for constipation? A systematic review of the evidence in the chronically ill. *Journal of Pain and Symptom Management.* **19**: 130–136.
10 Hawley PH and Byeon JJ (2008) A comparison of sennosides-based bowel protocols with and without docusate in hospitalized patients with cancer. *Journal of Palliative Medicine.* **11**: 575–581.
11 Godfrey H (1971) Dangers of dioctyl sodium sulfosuccinate in mixtures. *Journal of the American Medical Association.* **215**: 643.

LACTULOSE — BNF 1.6.4

Class: Osmotic laxative.

Indications: Constipation, hepatic encephalopathy.

Contra-indications: Intestinal obstruction, galactosaemia.

Pharmacology

Lactulose is a synthetic disaccharide, a combination of galactose and fructose, which is not absorbed by the small intestine.[1] It is a 'small bowel flusher', i.e. through an osmotic effect, lactulose deposits a large volume of fluid into the large intestine. Lactulose is fermented in the large intestine to acetic, formic and lactic acids, hydrogen and carbon dioxide, with an increase in faecal acidity, which also stimulates peristalsis.

The low pH discourages the proliferation of ammonia-producing organisms and thus reduces the absorption of ammonium ions and other nitrogenous compounds; hence its use in hepatic encephalopathy.[2]

Lactulose has been shown to be more effective than increasing dietary fibre.[3] It also increases colonic bacterial flora, i.e. is prebiotic (whereas **macrogols** are not).[4] Lactulose does not affect the management of diabetes mellitus; 15mL of Duphalac® contains 14 calories. However, because bio-availability is negligible, the number of calories absorbed is negligible. (Note: other generic products may differ.)

Several RCTs of lactulose have been completed in palliative care patients:

- lactulose vs. **senna**[5]
- lactulose and **senna** vs. **co-danthramer** (**dantron** and **poloxamer**)[6]
- lactulose and **senna** vs. **magnesium hydroxide** and **liquid paraffin**.[7]
- lactulose vs. **macrogols** (specifically in opioid-induced constipation).[8]

A significant difference between treatments was seen only in the second RCT; lactulose plus **senna** was significantly better at relieving constipation than **co-danthramer**.[6]

A Cochrane review of lactulose and **macrogols** for chronic constipation concluded that **macrogols** are better than lactulose in terms of bowel movements per week, faecal consistency, relief of abdominal pain, and the need for additional products.[9] An earlier systematic review also favoured **macrogols**.[10] However, the volume per dose of **macrogols** is 5–10 times greater than lactulose (see p.47), and will be unacceptable to many seriously ill patients. Lactulose is also cheaper.

Bio-availability negligible.

Onset of action up to 48h.

Cautions

Lactose intolerance.

Undesirable effects

Abdominal bloating, flatulence, nausea, intestinal colic.

Dose and use

Lactulose can be used in patients who experience intestinal colic with stimulant laxatives, or who fail to respond to stimulant laxatives alone:

- start with 15mL b.d. and adjust according to need
- in hepatic encephalopathy, start with 30–50mL t.d.s. and adjust the dose to produce 2–3 soft evacuations per day.

Supply

Lactulose (generic)

Oral solution 10g/15mL, 28 days @ 15mL b.d. = £5.

1 Schumann C (2002) Medical, nutritional and technological properties of lactulose. An update. *European Journal of Nutrition*. **41 (suppl 1)**: 117–25.
2 Zeng Z *et al.* (2006) Influence of lactulose on the cognitive level and quality of life in patients with minimal hepatic encephalopathy. *Chinese Journal of Clinical Rehabilitation*. **10**: 165–167.
3 Quah HM *et al.* (2006) Prospective randomized crossover trial comparing fibre with lactulose in the treatment of idiopathic chronic constipation. *Techniques in Coloproctology*. **10**: 111–114.
4 Bouhnik Y *et al.* (2004) Prospective, randomized, parallel-group trial to evaluate the effects of lactulose and polyethylene glycoly-4000 on colonic flora in chronic idiopathic constipation. *Alimentary Pharmacology and Therapeutics*. **19**: 889–899.
5 Agra Y *et al.* (1998) Efficacy of senna versus lactulose in terminal cancer patients treatment with opioids. *Journal of Pain and Symptom Management*. **15**: 1–7.
6 Sykes N (1991) A clinical comparison of laxatives in a hospice. *Palliative Medicine*. **5**: 307–314.
7 Sykes N (1991) A clinical comparison of lactulose and senna with magnesium hydroxide and liquid paraffin emulsion in a palliative care population. [cited in Miles CL *et al.* (2006) Laxatives for the management of constipation in palliative care patients. *The Cochrane Database of Systematic Reviews*. CD003448]
8 Freedman MD *et al.* (1997) Tolerance and efficacy of polyethylene glycol 3350/electrolyte solution versus lactulose in relieving opiate induced constipation: a double-blinded placebo-controlled trial. *Journal of Clinical Pharmacology*. **37**: 904–907.
9 Lee-Robichaud H *et al.* (2010) Lactulose versus polyethylene glycol for chronic constipation. *Cochrane Database of Systematic Reviews*. **7**: CD007570.
10 Ramkumar D and Rao SS (2005) Efficacy and safety of traditional medical therapies for chronic constipation: systematic review. *American Journal of Gastroenterology*. **100**: 936–971.

MACROGOLS (POLYETHYLENE GLYCOLS) BNF 1.6.4

Class: Osmotic laxative.

Indications: Constipation, faecal impaction.

Contra-indications: Severe inflammatory bowel conditions, bowel obstruction.

Pharmacology

Macrogol 3350 and 4000 are available in the UK (the numbers refer to their respective molecular weights). They act by virtue of an osmotic action in the intestines, thereby producing an increase in faecal volume which induces a laxative effect. Macrogols are unchanged in the GI tract, virtually unabsorbed and have no known pharmacological activity. Any absorbed macrogols are excreted via the urine; no reduction is required in renal impairment. Macrogols reduce colonic bacterial flora, whereas the use of **lactulose** causes an increase.[1]

Most studies have used isotonic solutions. Adding more water to make a hypotonic (dilute) solution of macrogols is as effective as an isotonic solution in treating constipation but causes hyponatraemia.[2] There are no data on the effect on appetite of the volume of fluid needed with macrogols.

There are no studies in chronic constipation comparing macrogols with stimulant laxatives. However, when clearing the colon before colonoscopy, macrogols are inferior to stimulant laxatives.[3,4]

In an RCT in opioid-induced constipation, macrogols were found to be no better than **lactulose**.[5] On the other hand, a Cochrane review of macrogols and **lactulose** for chronic constipation in adults and in children concluded that macrogols are better than **lactulose** in terms of bowel movements per week, faecal consistency, relief of abdominal pain (children only), and the need for additional products.[6] An earlier systematic review also favoured macrogols.[7] However, the volume per dose of macrogols is 5–10 times greater than **lactulose** (see p.46); this will be unacceptable to many seriously ill patients.

In a second systematic review limited to chronic constipation in children, macrogols were found to be little better than other treatments.[8] Further, in childhood faecal impaction, they are

no better than enemas, and cause more faecal incontinence.[9] Children also find macrogols less palatable than **lactulose**.[10] Macrogols are also more expensive.
Onset of action 1–2 days for constipation; 1–3 days for faecal impaction.

Undesirable effects

Uncommon (<1%, >0.1%): abdominal bloating, discomfort, borborygmi, hyponatraemia (when used as a hypotonic solution), nausea.
Very rare (<0.01%): severe electrolyte shift (oedema, shortness of breath, dehydration and heart failure).

Dose and use

Macrogols are supplied as powder in sachets. Each sachet is dissolved in water:
- macrogol 3350 (with electrolytes), dissolve in half a glass of water (about 125mL)
- macrogol 4000 (without electrolytes), dissolve in a glass of water (about 250mL).

A half-strength macrogol 3350 product (with electrolytes) is available for fine-tuning the dose.

Constipation

The solution is used immediately after reconstitution:
- start with 1 sachet daily
- if necessary, increase to:
  - 1 sachet b.d.–t.d.s. (macrogol 3350)
  - 2 sachets each morning. or 1 sachet b.d. (macrogol 4000).

Faecal impaction

Macrogol 3350:
- start with 8 sachets on day 1, each dissolved in 125mL of water, and taken in <6h (total 1L)
- *patients with cardiovascular impairment should restrict intake to 2 sachets/h, i.e. 250mL/h*
- if necessary, repeat on days 2 and 3; most patients do not need the full dose on the second day.

For convenience, all 8 sachets can be made up together in 1L of water and kept in a refrigerator for a maximum of 6h, after which any remaining solution should be discarded.

Supply

Macrogol 3350
Movicol® (Norgine)
Oral powder macrogol 3350 13.125g, sodium bicarbonate 178.5mg, sodium chloride 350.7mg, potassium chloride 46.6mg/sachet, 28 days @ 1sachet once daily = £6; *lime-lemon flavour.*

Movicol-Half® (Norgine)
Oral powder macrogol 3350 6.563g, sodium bicarbonate 89.3mg, sodium chloride 175.4mg, potassium chloride 23.3mg/sachet, 28 days @ 1sachet once daily = £4; *lime-lemon flavour.*

Laxido® (Galen)
Oral powder macrogol 3350 13.125g, sodium bicarbonate 178.5mg, sodium chloride 350.7mg, potassium chloride 46.6mg/sachet, 28 days @ 1sachet once daily = £6; *orange flavour.*

Macrogol 4000
Dulcobalance® (Boehringer Ingelheim)
Oral powder macrogol 4000 10g/sachet, 28 days @ 1 sachet once daily = £13; *orange-grapefruit flavour. Available OTC.*

1 Bouhnik Y *et al.* (2004) Prospective, randomized, parallel-group trial to evaluate the effects of lactulose and polyethylene glycol-4000 on colonic flora in chronic idiopathic constipation. *Alimentary Pharmacology and Therapeutics.* **19**: 889–899.
2 Seinela L *et al.* (2009) Comparison of polyethylene glycol with and without electrolytes in the treatment of constipation in elderly institutionalized patients: a randomized, double-blind, parallel-group study. *Drugs and Aging.* **26**: 703–713.
3 Radaelli F *et al.* (2005) High-dose senna compared with conventional PEG-ES lavage as bowel preparation for elective colonoscopy: a prospective, randomized, investigator-blinded trial. *American Journal of Gastroenterology.* **100**: 2674–2680.
4 Valverde A *et al.* (1999) Senna vs polyethylene glycol for mechanical preparation the evening before elective colonic or rectal resection: a multicenter controlled trial. French Association for Surgical Research. *Archives of Surgery.* **134**: 514–519.
5 Freedman MD *et al.* (1997) Tolerance and efficacy of polyethylene glycol 3350/electrolyte solution versus lactulose in relieving opiate induced constipation: a double-blinded placebo-controlled trial. *Journal of Clinical Pharmacology.* **37**: 904–907.

6 Lee-Robichaud H *et al.* (2010) Lactulose versus polyethylene glycol for chronic constipation. *Cochrane Database of Systematic Reviews.* **7**: CD007570.
7 Ramkumar D and Rao SS (2005) Efficacy and safety of traditional medical therapies for chronic constipation: systematic review. *American Journal of Gastroenterology.* **100**: 936–971.
8 Pijpers MA *et al.* (2009) Currently recommended treatments of childhood constipation are not evidence based: a systematic literature review on the effect of laxative treatment and dietary measures. *Archives of Disease in Childhood.* **94**: 117–131.
9 Bekkali NL *et al.* (2009) Rectal fecal impaction treatment in childhood constipation: enemas versus high doses oral PEG. *Pediatrics.* **124**: e1108–1115.
10 Voskuijl W *et al.* (2004) PEG 3350 (Transipeg) versus lactulose in the treatment of childhood functional constipation: a double blind, randomised, controlled, multicentre trial. *Gut.* **53**: 1590–1594.

MAGNESIUM SALTS — BNF 1.6.4

Class: Osmotic laxative.

Indications: Constipation, particularly in patients who experience intestinal colic with stimulant laxatives, or who fail to respond to the latter.

Pharmacology

Magnesium ions are poorly absorbed from the gut. Their action is mainly osmotic but other factors may be important, e.g. the release of cholecystokinin.[1,2] Magnesium ions also decrease absorption or increase secretion in the small bowel. Total faecal PGE_2 increases progressively as the dose of magnesium hydroxide is raised from 1.2 to 3.2g/24h.[3] Also see Magnesium, p.545.
Magnesium hydroxide mixture BP contains about 8% of hydrated magnesium oxide. Magnesium sulphate is more potent and tends to produce a large volume of liquid faeces. In patients with idiopathic constipation, magnesium salts often lead to a sense of distension and the sudden passage of offensive liquid faeces which is socially inconvenient; it is difficult to adjust the dose to produce a normal soft result. However, when used as an osmotic laxative in conjunction with a stimulant laxative in opioid-induced constipation, this is not generally a problem.

An RCT of magnesium hydroxide and **liquid paraffin** vs. **senna** and **lactulose** failed to differentiate between the two combination treatments.[4]

Cautions

Risk of hypermagnesaemia in patients with renal impairment.

Dose and use

Magnesium hydroxide mixture BP

For opioid-induced constipation (see Quick Practice Guide p.38), as an alternative to **lactulose** when an osmotic laxative is indicated:

- if the maximum dose of a stimulant laxative (e.g. **dantron**, **senna**) is ineffective, halve the dose and add magnesium hydroxide 15–30mL b.d., and titrate as necessary
- alternatively, switch completely to magnesium hydroxide 15–60mL b.d.

Magnesium hydroxide (or **lactulose**) may be preferable in patients with a history of colic with stimulant laxatives (see p.42).

Magnesium sulphate

A typical dose is 5–10g of crystals once daily *before breakfast*; dissolve in warm water and take with extra fluid.

Supply

All the preparations below are available OTC.

Magnesium Hydroxide Mixture BP

Oral suspension contains about 8% hydrated magnesium oxide 415mg (7.1mmol elemental magnesium)/5mL, available OTC as Milk of Magnesia®; *do not store in a cold place.*

Magnesium sulphate
Oral powder (Epsom Salts), also Andrew's Liver Salts® (magnesium sulphate, citric acid, sodium bicarbonate).
Oral solution magnesium sulphate (Epsom Salts) 5g/10mL, locally prepared.

1 Donowitz M (1991) Magnesium-induced diarrhea and new insights into the pathobiology of diarrhea. *New England Journal of Medicine*. **324**: 1059–1060.
2 Harvey R and Read A (1975) Mode of action of the saline purgatives. *American Heart Journal*. **89**: 810–813.
3 Donowitz M and Rood R (1992) Magnesium hydroxide: new insights into the mechanism of its laxative effect and the potential involvement of prostaglandin E2. *Journal of Clinical Gastroenterology*. **14**: 20–26.
4 Sykes N (1991) A clinical comparison of lactulose and senna with magnesium hydroxide and liquid paraffin emulsion in a palliative care population. [cited in Miles CL *et al.* (2006) Laxatives for the management of constipation in palliative care patients. *The Cochrane Database of Systematic Reviews*. CD003448]

RECTAL PRODUCTS BNF 1.6.2, 1.6.3 & 1.6.4

Indications: Constipation and faecal impaction if oral laxatives are ineffective or not feasible.

Pharmacology

The evidence base for laxative suppositories and enemas in palliative care is generally limited to clinical experience and retrospective studies. Survey data indicate that about one third of palliative care patients receiving opioids require rectal measures (laxative suppositories, enemas and/or digital evacuation) either regularly and electively, or intermittently and p.r.n., generally in addition to laxatives PO (Box 1.H).[1] However, the need for enemas and digital evacuation has decreased since the introduction of **macrogols** (see p.47).[2,3]

There is evidence supporting the use of **bisacodyl** suppositories in postoperative ileus,[5] and in pre-colonoscopy preparations[6] and of **docusate sodium** enemas in spinal injury patients.[7]

In the UK, most patients needing laxative suppositories receive both **glycerol** and **bisacodyl**. The laxative effect of **bisacodyl** is the result of local direct contact with the rectal mucosa after dissolution of the suppository and after activation by enteric enzymes (see p.42). The minimum time for response is thus generally >20min, and may be up to 3h.[8] Defaecation a few minutes after the insertion of a **bisacodyl** suppository is the result of ano-rectal stimulation. **Bisacodyl** suppositories occasionally cause faecal leakage, even after a successful evacuation.

Osmotic *micro-enemas* contain mainly **sodium citrate** and **sodium lauryl sulphoacetate** with several excipients, including **glycerol** and **sorbitol**. **Sodium lauryl sulphoacetate** is a faecal softener (surface-wetting agent) similar to **docusate sodium** (see p.45), whereas **sodium citrate** draws fluid into the intestine by osmosis, an action enhanced by **sorbitol**. Osmotic *standard enemas* contain phosphates.

Box 1.H Rectal measures for the relief of constipation or faecal impaction

A PR examination is required to ensure the most appropriate intervention is used. Warm enemas to room temperature before use.

Suppositories (place in contact with rectal mucosa)
Glycerol 4g, has a hygroscopic and lubricant action; also said to be a rectal stimulant but this is unsubstantiated.

Bisacodyl 10mg, stimulates propulsive activity after hydrolysis by enteric enzymes.[4]

Micro-enemas
Osmotic 5mL, contains sodium citrate, sodium lauryl sulphoacetate, glycerol and sorbitol.

Faecal softener (surface-wetting agent), 10g contains docusate sodium 120mg.

Standard enemas
Osmotic 118–128mL, contain phosphates.

When treating a hard faecal impaction, a **docusate sodium** micro-enema will help to soften the faecal mass. This should be instilled into the rectum and retained overnight before giving a stimulant suppository (**bisacodyl**) or an osmotic enema (either micro or **phosphate**).

Other rectal products include:

- Carbalax®, a mixture of anhydrous **sodium acid phosphate** and **sodium bicarbonate** which reacts in the rectum, releasing 200mL of carbon dioxide and stimulating evacuation by rectal distension. Potentially useful in some patients with paraplegia/tetraplegia
- **arachis (peanut) oil** retention enema, sometimes used in patients with a hard faecal impaction; instil and leave overnight before giving a stimulant laxative suppository or an osmotic enema. *Do not use in patients with peanut allergy.*

Digital evacuation is the ultimate approach to faecal impaction but is a distressing procedure which may need sedation. Distress can be reduced by explaining the procedure, using plenty of lubrication, and encouraging the patient to respond to any urge to defaecate.

Supply

Suppositories
Glycerol BP 700mg, gelatin 140mg/1g, adult suppositories 4g, 28 days @ 4g once daily = £3.50.

Bisacodyl (generic) 10mg, 28 days @ 10mg once daily. = £3.
Dulcolax® (Boehringer Ingelheim) 10mg, 28 days @ 10mg once daily = £4.50 (~~NHS~~).

Sodium acid phosphate
Carbalax® (Forest) **sodium acid phosphate** (anhydrous) 1.3g, **sodium bicarbonate** 1.08g, 28 days @ 1 once daily = £4.50.

Micro-enemas
Osmotic, **sodium citrate**, **sodium lauryl sulphoacetate**, **glycerol** and **sorbitol**, supplied in 5mL single-dose disposable packs with nozzle:
Micolette® (Pinewood), Micralax® (UCB Pharma), Relaxit® (Crawford), 5mL = £0.50.

Faecal softener, Norgalax® (Norgine), **docusate sodium** 120mg in 10g single-use disposable pack, 1 enema = £0.50.

Standard enemas
Phosphate enema BP Formula B (generic), **sodium acid phosphate** 12.8g, **sodium phosphate** 10.24g in 128mL, 1 enema with standard tube = £3, 1 enema with long rectal tube = £4.
Fleet® Ready-to-use enema (De Witt), **sodium acid phosphate** 21.4g, **sodium phosphate** 9.4g in 118mL, 1 enema with standard tube = £0.50.

Arachis Oil retention enema (generic), **arachis (peanut) oil** in 130mL single-dose disposable pack, 130mL = £8; *do not use in patients with peanut allergy.*

---

1 Twycross RG and Harcourt JMV (1991) The use of laxatives at a palliative care centre. *Palliative Medicine*. **5**: 27–33.
2 Goldman M (1993) Hazards of phosphate enemas. *Gastroenterology Today*. **3**: 16–17.
3 Culbert P *et al.* (1998) Highly effective oral therapy (polyethylene glycol/electrolyte solution) for faecal impaction and severe constipation. *Clinical Drug Investigation*. **16**: 355–360.
4 von Roth W and von Beschke K (1988) Pharmakokinetik und laxierende wirkung von bisacodyl nach gabe verschiedener zubereitungsformen. *Arzneimittel Forschung Drug Research*. **38**: 570–574.
5 Wiriyakosol S *et al.* (2007) Randomized controlled trial of bisacodyl suppository versus placebo for postoperative ileus after elective colectomy for colon cancer. *Asian Journal of Surgery*. **30**: 167–172.
6 Rapier R and Houston C (2006) A prospective study to assess the efficacy and patient tolerance of three bowel preparations for colonoscopy. *Gastroenterology Nursing*. **29**: 305–308.
7 Amir I *et al.* (1998) Bowel care for individuals with spinal cord injury: comparison of four approaches. *Journal of Spinal Cord Medicine*. **21**: 21–24.
8 Flig E *et al.* (2000) Is bisacodyl absorbed at all from suppositories in man? *International Journal of Pharmaceutics*. **196**: 11–20.

PRODUCTS FOR HAEMORRHOIDS BNF 1.7 & 15.2

Because haemorrhoids can be more troublesome if associated with the evacuation of hard faeces, constipation must be corrected (see Laxatives, p.35).

Peri-anal pruritus, soreness and excoriation are generally best treated by the application of a bland ointment or cream. Suppositories are often not effective because they are inserted into the rectum, bypassing the anal canal where the medication is needed.

For haemorrhoids, products containing mild astringents (e.g. **bismuth subgallate**, **zinc oxide**, **hamamelis** (**witch hazel**) often provide symptomatic relief. Some products, not featured here, also contain vasoconstrictors and/or antiseptics.

Lidocaine ointment is used mainly to relieve pain associated with an anal fissure, but will also relieve pruritus ani. Alternative local anaesthetics include **pramocaine** (**pramoxine**) and **cinchocaine** (**dibucaine**). Painful spasm of the internal anal sphincter is often eased by topical **glyceryl trinitrate** ointment (see p.70).

Local anaesthetic ointments are absorbed through the anal mucosa but, given the amount of ointment likely to be used, there is no realistic risk of systemic toxicity.[1] However, local anaesthetic ointments should be used for only a few days because all 'caines' can cause contact dermatitis.

Corticosteroids may be helpful if local inflammation is exacerbating discomfort. Infection (e.g. *Herpes simplex*) must first be excluded, and treatment limited to 7–10 days.

Dose and use

Topical products should be applied:

- t.d.s.–q.d.s. for the first 24h
- then b.d. and after defaecation for 5–7 days, or longer if necessary
- then daily for 3–5 days after symptoms have cleared.

Products containing a local anaesthetic (to ease painful defaecation) are best applied 15–20min before defaecation, and p.r.n.

Supply

The following list is highly selective. Other OTC products are also available.

Astringent
Anusol® (McNeil)
Ointment **zinc oxide, bismuth subgallate, Peru balsam, bismuth oxide** 25g. (Available OTC).

Local anaesthetic
Lidocaine (generic)
Ointment 5%, 15g = £1.

Corticosteroid plus astringent
Anusol HC® (McNeil)
Ointment **hydrocortisone acetate** 0.25%, **zinc oxide**, **benzyl benzoate**, **bismuth oxide**, **bismuth subgallate**, **Peru balsam** 30g = £3.50. (Available OTC).

Corticosteroid plus local anaesthetic
Scheriproct® (Valeant)
Ointment **cinchocaine** 0.5%, **prednisolone hexanoate** 0.19%, 30g = £3.

Corticosteroid plus local anaesthetic and astringent
Xyloproct® (Astra Zeneca)
Ointment (water miscible) **aluminium acetate**, **hydrocortisone acetate** 0.275%, **lidocaine** 5%, **zinc oxide**, 20g (with applicator) = £2.50.

1 Brosh-Nissimov T *et al.* (2004) Central nervous system toxicity following topical skin application of lidocaine. *European Journal of Clinical Pharmacology.* **60**: 683–684.

PANCREATIN BNF 1.9.4

Class: Enzyme supplement.

Indications: †Symptomatic steatorrhoea caused by biliary and/or pancreatic obstruction, e.g. cancer of the pancreas.

Pharmacology

Steatorrhoea (the presence of undigested faecal fat) typically results in pale, bulky, offensive, frothy and greasy faeces which flush away only with difficulty; associated with abdominal distension, increased flatus, loss of weight, and mineral and vitamin deficiency (A, D, E and K).

Pancreatin is a standardized preparation of porcine lipase, protease and amylase. Pancreatin hydrolyzes fats to glycerol and fatty acids, degrades protein into amino acids, and converts starch into dextrin and sugars. Because it is inactivated by gastric acid, pancreatin is best taken with food (or immediately before or after food).

Gastric acid may be reduced by prescribing a PPI concurrently; this leads to improved pancreatin efficacy.[1] With gastro-resistant (e/c) granules, acid reduction is generally unnecessary provided the granules are swallowed whole without chewing.[2] However, in patients who are not adequately controlled on high-dose gastro-resistant pancreatin (e.g. ⩾120,000 units of lipase/24h), concurrent prescription of a PPI generally leads to improvement.[3,4]

Cautions

Fibrotic strictures of the colon have developed in children with cystic fibrosis who have used certain high-strength pancreatin products. This has not been reported in adults or in patients without cystic fibrosis; Creon® has not been implicated.

Undesirable effects

Very common (>10%): abdominal pain.
Common (<10%, >1%): nausea and vomiting, constipation or diarrhoea, allergic skin reactions.

Dose and use

There are several different pancreatin products, of which Creon® is a good choice. Capsule strength denotes lipase unit content, e.g. Creon® 10,000 contains 10,000 units. The dose is adjusted upwards according to faecal size, consistency, and frequency:

- generally start with Creon® 10,000 1–2 capsules with each meal
- if a smaller dose is required, use Creon® Micro; this contains 5,000 units of lipase in 100mg of granules
- if necessary, change to a higher strength capsule.

Extra capsules may be needed if snacks are taken between meals. If the pancreatin continues to be ineffective, prescribe a PPI or H_2-receptor antagonist concurrently, and review.

The granules in the capsules are gastro-resistant (e/c) and, if preferred, may be added to fluid or soft food and *swallowed without chewing*. If mixing with food or drinks:

- avoid very hot food or drinks because heat inactivates pancreatin
- do not mix the capsule contents with alkaline foods or drinks, e.g. dairy products, because this degrades the gastro-resistant coating
- take immediately after mixing because the gastro-resistant coating dissolves if left to stand.

Supply

Creon® (Solvay)

A standardized preparation obtained from pigs; *there is no non-porcine alternative.*

Capsules enclosing gastro-resistant granules Creon® 10,000, lipase 10,000 units, amylase 8,000 units, protease 600 units, 28 days @ 2 t.d.s. = £22.

Creon® 25,000, lipase 25,000 units, amylase 18,000 units, protease 1,000 units, 28 days @ 2 t.d.s. = £47.

Creon® 40,000, lipase 40,000 units, amylase 25,000 units, protease 1,600 units, 28 days @ 2 t.d.s. = £101.

If smaller doses are required:
Gastro-resistant granules Creon® Micro, lipase 5,000 units, amylase 3,600 units, protease 200 units in 100mg, (measuring scoop provided). 28 days @ 200mg t.d.s. = £26.

1 Vecht J *et al.* (2006) Efficacy of lower than standard doses of pancreatic enzyme supplementation therapy during acid inhibition in patients with pancreatic exocrine insufficiency. *Journal of Clinical Gastroenterology.* **40**: 721–725.
2 Stead RJ *et al.* (1988) Treatment of steatorrhoea in cystic fibrosis: a comparison of enteric-coated microspheres of pancreatin versus non-enteric-coated pancreatin and adjuvant cimetidine. *Alimentary Pharmacology and Therapeutics.* **2**: 471–482.
3 Proesmans M and De Boeck K (2003) Omeprazole, a proton pump inhibitor, improves residual steatorrhoea in cystic fibrosis patients treated with high dose pancreatic enzymes. *European Journal of Pediatrics.* **162**: 760–763.
4 Dominguez-Munoz JE *et al.* (2006) Optimising the therapy of exocrine pancreatic insufficiency by the association of a proton pump inhibitor to enteric coated pancreatic extracts. *Gut.* **55**: 1056–1057.

2: CARDIOVASCULAR SYSTEM

This chapter features cardiovascular drugs used in palliative *cancer* care. It does *not* include guidance about the drug treatment of end-stage congestive heart failure (CHF). *For guidance about simplifying medication in patients with end-stage CHF who appear to be imminently dying,* *see p.642.*

More detailed guidance about caring for patients with end-stage CHF is available from NICE[1] and various other authorities.[2–4] Additional resources include:

- *Supportive Care in Heart Failure*[5]
- *Heart Failure and Palliative Care: a team approach*[6]
- *Heart Improvement Programme (website).*[7]

Unlike cancer, where disease-specific treatment tends to become increasingly burdensome and futile (and possibly counterproductive), the continued disease-specific treatment of CHF continues to be essential for symptom management even when end-stage.

Note: CHF can be a concurrent cause of breathlessness in some cancer patients, which needs to be recognized and treated appropriately.

1 NICE (2010) Clinical Guideline 108. Chronic heart failure: management of chronic heart failure in adults in primary and secondary care. Available from: www.nice.org.uk

2 Arnold JM *et al.* (2006) Canadian Cardiovascular Society consensus conference recommendations on heart failure 2006: diagnosis and management.[erratum appears in Canadian Journal of Cardiology. 2006 Mar 1;22(3):271]. *Canadian Journal of Cardiology.* **22**: 23–45.

3 Swedberg K *et al.* (2005) Guidelines for the diagnosis and treatment of chronic heart failure: full text (update 2005). European Heart Journal. Available from: 10.1093/eurheartj/ehi205

4 Hunt SA *et al.* (2005) Guideline Update for the Diagnosis and Management of Chronic Heart Failure in the Adult. ACC/AHA. Available from: http://circ.ahajournals.org/cgi/content/full/112/12/e154

5 Beattie J and Goodlin S (eds) (2008) *Supportive Care in Heart Failure.* Oxford University Press, Oxford.

6 Johnson MJ and Lehman R (eds) (2006) *Heart Failure and Palliative Care: a team approach.* Radcliffe Publishing Ltd., Oxford.

7 NHS (2007) Supportive and Palliative Care in Heart Failure. In: *Heart Improvement Programme.* Available from: http://www.heart.nhs.uk/endoflifecare/hip.htm

FUROSEMIDE — BNF 2.2.2

Class: Loop diuretic.

Indications: Oedema, †malignant ascites associated with portal hypertension and hyper-aldosteronism (with **spironolactone**), †bronchorrhoea.

Contra-indications: Hepatic encephalopathy, anuric renal failure.

Pharmacology

Furosemide inhibits Na^+ (and hence water) resorption from the ascending limb of the loop of Henlé in the renal tubule. It also increases urinary excretion of K^+, H^+, Cl^- and Mg^{2+}. Diuretics such as furosemide are the standard first-line therapy for the treatment of fluid overload in CHF and improve both symptoms and survival.[1–3]

In ascites caused by a *transudate* associated with cirrhosis, extensive liver metastases and portal hypertension, furosemide alone has little effect, even when used in total daily doses of 100–200mg PO.[4,5] Thus the use of furosemide in ascites is best limited to concurrent use with **spironolactone**, when the latter alone is insufficient (see p.59).

A diuretic-induced reduction in plasma volume can activate several neurohumoral systems, e.g. renin-aldosterone-angiotensin, resulting in impaired renal perfusion and increased Na^+ and water resorption. These changes reduce the effect of the diuretic and contribute to renal impairment. **Octreotide** 300microgram SC b.d. (see p.507) can suppress this diuretic-induced activation of the renin-aldosterone-angiotensin system and its addition has improved renal function and Na^+ and water excretion in patients with cirrhosis and ascites receiving furosemide and **spironolactone**.[6,7]

There is current interest in the use of *nebulized* furosemide for the treatment of breathlessness (Box 2.A). However, a review of 42 trials concluded that there was insufficient evidence to currently support its routine use.[8] Further, in one study,[9] 5/7 patients reported a deterioration in their breathing after furosemide. It is thus recommended that the use of nebulized furosemide is restricted to closely controlled circumstances. Anecdotally, nebulized furosemide is of benefit in bronchorrhoea.[10]

Box 2.A Nebulized furosemide for breathlessness

Nebulized furosemide 20–40mg attenuates experimentally-induced cough and breathlessness,[11,12] and also allergen-induced asthma,[13] possibly via an effect on vagal sensory nerve endings. The reduction in breathlessness may result from increasing sensory traffic to the brain stem from sensitized slowly adapting pulmonary stretch receptors. However, the effect:

- has not been demonstrated consistently
- shows wide interindividual variability
- is of short duration (generally <2h)
- systemic absorption can be sufficient to induce a diuresis.[8,14,15]

In moderate–severe COPD, compared with placebo, nebulized furosemide has reduced breathlessness ± increased exercise time during endurance testing,[16,17] but *not* incremental exercise testing.[16] The mechanism underlying the benefit is unclear, but improvements are seen in airway function (e.g. slow vital capacity at rest) and dynamic ventilatory mechanics (e.g. inspiratory capacity and breathing pattern).[17] Although small but significant bronchodilation was seen in one study,[16] this is unlikely to be a direct effect of nebulized furosemide.

Nebulized furosemide has been used to relieve severe breathlessness in patients with cancer.[18,19] However, RCTs have failed to show benefit.[9,20]

In heart failure, compared with bolus IV doses, furosemide by CIVI appears to provide a greater diuresis and a better safety profile.[21] Furosemide is effective when given by SC injection. Diuresis persists for about 4h, reaching a maximum at 2–3h, and urine output is significantly increased.[22,23] Furosemide has been successfully given by CSCI as a means of avoiding hospital admission or of continuing its use after oral medication becomes problematic in the last days of life. In a report of 47 episodes of the use of furosemide CSCI in 37 patients, the majority benefited (>80%), with mild or severe site reactions seen in one quarter and one episode respectively.[24]

Furosemide may also be given SL. The bio-availability of Lasix® (Sanofi-Aventis) 20mg tablet by this route is at least as good as PO, if not better.[25] However, this may be formulation-dependent.

Some centres use **bumetanide** as their preferred loop diuretic. It is chemically distinct but pharmacologically very similar to furosemide; 1mg is equivalent to 40mg of furosemide.[26] It has better bio-availability (80–95%), and may thus be preferable in end-stage CHF.

Bio-availability 60–70% PO, but may be reduced by GI oedema in CHF.
Onset of action 30–60min PO; 2–5min IV; 30min SC.[22]
Time to peak plasma concentration 1.5h PO/SL.[25]

Plasma halflife 30–120min in healthy subjects, 50min–6h in heart failure, 10h in end-stage renal disease.
Duration of action 4–6h PO; 2h IV; 4h SC.[22]

Cautions

Serious drug interaction: Sudden deaths, probably from cardiac arrhythmias secondary to QT prolongation, have occurred in patients taking high doses (40mg t.d.s.) of **ketanserin** (not UK) with potassium-depleting diuretics, including furosemide. Lower **ketanserin** doses (20mg b.d.) have less effect on the QT interval and may be used cautiously with furosemide, provided that adequate plasma K^+ concentrations are maintained.[27]

Increased risk of hypokalaemia with corticosteroids, β_2 agonists, **theophylline**, **amphotericin** and **carbenoxolone**; increased risk of hyponatraemia with **carbamazepine**; increased risk of hypotension with ACE inhibitors and TCAs; increased risk of nephrotoxicity with NSAIDs, **cefaloridine** and **cefalotin** (not UK); increased risk of **lithium** toxicity. Furosemide-induced hypokalaemia increases the risk of **digoxin** toxicity and may also increase the toxicity of other drugs which prolong the QT interval; maintain adequate plasma K^+ concentrations during concurrent use.[27]

Reduced diuretic effect of furosemide with **phenytoin** (up to 50% reduction), **indometacin** and possibly other NSAIDs; may need to increase the furosemide dose. **Colestyramine** and **colestipol** decrease absorption of furosemide; give furosemide 2–3h before the resin.[27]
Withdrawal: Some patients receive long-term diuretic therapy for hypertension, or non-heart failure ankle oedema. This often becomes inappropriate as physical deterioration progresses, and may lead to postural hypotension and prerenal failure. In such circumstances the dose of furosemide should be reduced and possibly discontinued altogether. However, the withdrawal of diuretics requires careful monitoring to prevent the subsequent insidious onset of CHF.[28]

Undesirable effects

Transient pain at the site of SC injection.[22]
Frequency not stated: dyspepsia, thirst, dizziness, dehydration, drowsiness, weakness, muscle cramps.
Rare: tinnitus and deafness (generally after rapid injection; may be permanent).
Biochemical disturbances: hyperglycaemia, hyperuricaemia, hypocalcaemia, hypokalaemia, hypomagnesaemia, hyponatraemia, metabolic alkalosis.

Dose and use

CHF

PO
- start with 40mg PO each morning
- if necessary, increase the dose progressively in 40mg increments
- usual maximum dose 160mg, generally given as 80mg each morning and noon
- usual maintenance dose 40–80mg each morning.

CSCI

Incompatibility: Furosemide injection is alkaline. It should not be mixed or diluted with glucose solutions or other acidic fluids. When given by CSCI, furosemide injection should be diluted with 0.9% saline. It should not be mixed in the same syringe with any other drugs.[29,30]

Some palliative care services use CSCI furosemide as a means of managing decompensated CHF in the community:[24]
- start with the same dose CSCI as the PO dose
- weigh the patient daily
- after 48h, if the daily weight loss is not ≥1kg/day, consider obtaining cardiologist/heart failure nurse specialist advice; options include:
  - ▹ increasing the furosemide dose by 50%

  - ▷ adding a thiazide diuretic, e.g. **metolazone**
  - ▷ adding or increasing the dose of an aldosterone antagonist, e.g. **spironolactone**
- because furosemide injection is 10mg/mL, a practical dose limit for a syringe driver is about 150mg/24h; higher doses can be delivered if syringe changes every 12h are possible
- if the maximum dose possible via a syringe driver fails to provide the necessary weight loss, admission to hospital/hospice for IV furosemide may be unavoidable.

Ascites

Use only as a supplement to **spironolactone** (see p.59):
- start with 40mg PO each morning
- usual maintenance dose 20–40mg each morning
- usual maximum dose 160mg each morning.

Supply

Furosemide (generic)
Tablets 20mg, 40mg, 500mg, 28 days @ 20mg, 40mg each morning = £1.
Oral solution (sugar-free) 20mg/5mL, 40mg/5mL, 50mg/5mL, 28 days @ 40mg each morning = £17.
Injection 10mg/mL, 2mL amp = £0.50, 5mL amp = £0.50, 25mL amp = £2.50

Lasix® (Sanofi-Aventis)
Injection 10mg/mL, 2mL amp = £1.

1 NICE (2010) Chronic heart failure: management of chronic heart failure in adults in primary and secondary care. Clinical Guideline 108. Available from: www.guidance.nice.org.uk'CG108
2 Faris R *et al.* (2006) Diuretics for heart failure. *Cochrane Database of Systematic Reviews.* CD003838.
3 McMurray JJ and Pfeffer MA (2005) Heart failure. *Lancet.* **365**: 1877–1889.
4 Fogel M *et al.* (1981) Diuresis in the ascitic patient: a randomized controlled trial of three regimens. *Journal of Clinical Gastroenterology.* **3**: 73–80.
5 Amiel S *et al.* (1984) Intravenous infusion of frusemide as treatment for ascites in malignant disease. *British Medical Journal.* **288**: 1041.
6 Kalambokis G *et al.* (2005) Renal effects of treatment with diuretics, octreotide or both, in non-azotemic cirrhotic patients with ascites. *Nephrology, Dialysis, Transplantation.* **20**: 1623–1629.
7 Kalambokis G *et al.* (2006) The effects of treatment with octreotide, diuretics, or both on portal hemodynamics in nonazotemic cirrhotic patients with ascites. *Journal of Clinical Gastroenterology.* **40**: 342–346.
8 Newton PJ *et al.* (2008) Nebulized furosemide for the management of dyspnea: does the evidence support its use? *Journal of Pain and Symptom Management.* **36**: 424–441.
9 Stone P *et al.* (2002) Re: nebulized furosemide for dyspnea in terminal cancer patients. *Journal of Pain and Symptom Management.* **24**: 274–275; author reply 275–276.
10 Twycross R *et al.* (2009) *Symptom Management in Advanced Cancer* (4e). palliativedrugs.com, Nottingham, pp. 160–166.
11 Ventresca P *et al.* (1990) Inhaled furosemide inhibits cough induced by low-chloride solutions but not by capsaicin. *American Review of Respiratory Disease.* **142**: 143–146.
12 Bianco S *et al.* (1989) Protective effect of inhaled furosemide on allergen-induced early and late asthmatic reactions. *New England Journal of Medicine.* **321**: 1069–1073.
13 Nishino T *et al.* (2000) Inhaled furosemide greatly alleviates the sensation of experimentally induced dyspnea. *American Journal of Respiratory and Critical Care Medicine.* **161**: 1963–1967.
14 Laveneziana P *et al.* (2008) Inhaled furosemide does not alleviate respiratory effort during flow-limited exercise in healthy subjects. *Pulmonary Pharmacology and Therapeutics.* **21**: 196–200.
15 Moosavi SH *et al.* (2006) Effect of inhaled furosemide on air hunger induced in healthy humans. *Respiritory Physiology and Neurobiology.* **156**: 1–8.
16 Ong KC *et al.* (2004) Effects of inhaled furosemide on exertional dyspnea in chronic obstructive pulmonary disease. *American Journal of Respiratory and Critical Care Medicine.* **169**: 1028–1033.
17 Jensen D *et al.* (2008) Mechanisms of dyspnoea relief and improved exercise endurance after furosemide inhalation in COPD. *Thorax.* **63**: 606–613.
18 Shimoyama N and Shimoyama M (2002) Nebulized furosemide as a novel treatment for dyspnea in terminal cancer patients. *Journal of Pain and Symptom Management.* **23**: 73–76.
19 Kohara H *et al.* (2003) Effect of nebulized furosemide in terminally ill cancer patients with dyspnea. *Journal of Pain and Symptom Management.* **26**: 962–967.
20 Wilcock A *et al.* (2008) Randomised, placebo-controlled trial of nebulised furosemide for breathlessness in patients with cancer. *Thorax.* **63**: 872–875.
21 Salvador DR *et al.* (2005) Continuous infusion versus bolus injection of loop diuretics in congestive heart failure. *Cochrane Database of Systematic Reviews.* CD003178.
22 Verma AK *et al.* (2004) Diuretic effects of subcutaneous furosemide in human volunteers: a randomized pilot study. *Annals of Pharmacotherapy.* **38**: 544–549.
23 Goenaga MA *et al.* (2004) Subcutaneous furosemide. *Annals of Pharmacotherpy.* **38**: 1751.
24 Zacharias H *et al.* (2011) Is there a role for subcutaneous furosemide in the community and hospice management of end-stage heart failure? *Palliative Medicine.* Epub ahead of print.

25 Haegeli L *et al.* (2007) Sublingual administration of furosemide: new application of an old drug. *British Journal of Clinical Pharmacology*. **64**: 804–809.
26 Ward A and Heel RC (1984) Bumetanide. A review of its pharmacodynamic and pharmacokinetic properties and therapeutic use. *Drugs*. **28**: 426–464.
27 Baxter K (2011) Stockley's Drug Interactions (online edition). Pharmaceutical Press, London. Available from: www.medicinescomplete.com
28 Walma E *et al.* (1997) Withdrawal of long term diuretic medication in elderly patients: a double blind randomised trial. *British Medical Journal*. **315**: 464–468.
29 Chiu MF and Schwartz ML (1997) Visual compatibility of injectable drugs used in the intensive care unit. *American Journal of Health System Pharmacy*. **54**: 64–65.
30 Trissel LA *et al.* (1997) Compatibility of parenteral nutrient solutions with selected drugs during simulated Y-site administration. *American Journal of Health System Pharmacy*. **54**: 1295–1300.

SPIRONOLACTONE BNF 2.2.3 & 2.5.5

Class: Potassium-sparing diuretic; aldosterone antagonist.

Indications: Ascites and peripheral oedema associated with portal hypertension and hyperaldosteronism (i.e. cirrhosis, hepatocellular cancer, massive hepatic metastases), CHF, nephrotic syndrome, primary hyperaldosteronism.

Contra-indications: Hyperkalaemia, Addison's disease, anuria, severe renal impairment.

Pharmacology

Spironolactone and two metabolites (7α-thiomethyl-spironolactone and canrenone) bind to cytoplasmic mineralocorticoid receptors and function as aldosterone antagonists. In the distal tubules of the kidney, this results in a potassium-sparing diuretic effect. Hyperaldosteronism is a concomitant of ascites associated with portal hypertension (a *transudate* with a relatively low albumin concentration, best indicated by a serum-ascites albumin difference or gradient of ≥11g/L), i.e. cirrhosis, hepatocellular cancer, massive hepatic metastases.[1,2] Most evidence comes from cirrhosis, but spironolactone in a median daily dose of 200–300mg is successful in the majority of patients with these conditions (90% in cirrhosis).[1–6] Spironolactone alone is the initial drug of choice, it is as safe and effective as spironolactone + **furosemide**, and requires less frequent dose adjustments.[4,5] In contrast, treatment with even large PO doses of a loop diuretic alone, e.g. **furosemide** 200mg, generally fails to reduce ascites.[7] Even if paracentesis becomes necessary, diuretics should be continued as they reduce the rate of recurrence.[4] Note: paracentesis is generally preferable for patients with predominantly peritoneal (an *exudate* with relatively high albumin concentration, best indicated by a serum–ascites albumin gradient of ≤11g/L) or chylous ascites as these are unlikely to respond to diuretics,[3,6] and also for patients with a tense distended abdomen in need of rapid relief, and those unable to tolerate spironolactone.

A diuretic-induced reduction in plasma volume can increase the activity of various closely related neurohumoral systems, e.g. the renin-aldosterone-angiotensin system, sympathetic nervous system, ADH secretion, which results in impaired renal perfusion and increased Na^+ and water resorption. These changes reduce the effect of the diuretic and contribute to renal impairment. In patients with cirrhosis receiving spironolactone ± **furosemide**, improved renal function and diuresis is seen with co-administration of **octreotide** 300microgram SC b.d. (see p.507) or **clonidine** 75microgram PO b.d. (see p.67) due to inhibition of the renin-aldosterone-angiotensin (**octreotide** and **clonidine**) and sympathetic nervous (**clonidine**) systems.[8–10] Patients in the **clonidine** study were considered to have an overactive sympathetic nervous system based on a higher than normal serum noradrenaline (norepinephrine) level.[10]

Spironolactone is also added in low dose (12.5–50mg daily) to standard treatment for patients with severe symptomatic CHF.[11–13] Its aldosterone antagonist action helps reduce vascular and myocardial fibrosis, sympathetic nervous system activation, baroreceptor dysfunction and K^+ and Mg^{2+} depletion.[14]

The non-specific binding of spironolactone to various steroid receptors can result in undesirable effects such as menstrual disorders and, in men, gynaecomastia, breast pain or impotence. **Eplerenone**, an aldosterone antagonist with greater selectively for the mineralocorticoid receptor, has been used as an alternative in these circumstances.[15]

Spironolactone (but not its metabolites) has several other actions independent of the mineralocorticoid receptor, including an anti-inflammatory effect. This involves the inhibition of the nuclear factor-κB pathway involved in the production of pro-inflammatory cytokines.[16] Longer-acting analogues of spironolactone may thus be developed as anti-inflammatory drugs.
Bio-availability about 90%.
Onset of action 2–4h; maximum effect 7h (single dose), 2–3 days (multiple doses).
Time to peak plasma concentration 2–3h; active metabolites 3–4.5h PO.
Plasma halflife 1–1.5h; active metabolites 14–16.5h (multiple doses).
Duration of action >24h (single dose), 2–3 days (multiple doses).

Cautions

Serious drug interactions: risk of hyperkalaemia with potassium supplements (avoid concurrent use), table salt substitutes (contain both potassium and sodium chlorides), potassium-sparing diuretics, ACE inhibitors and angiotensin II receptor antagonists, particularly if other risk factors also present, e.g. elderly, renal impairment, diabetes.[17]

Elderly; hepatic impairment, renal impairment. Initial drowsiness and dizziness (may impair driving). May induce hyponatraemia, particularly if used with other diuretics. May induce reversible hyperchloraemic metabolic acidosis in patients with decompensated hepatic cirrhosis. Natriuretic effect reduced by **aspirin**, **indometacin** and possibly other NSAIDs. Spironolactone increases the plasma concentration of **digoxin** by up to 25% and can interfere with **digoxin** plasma concentration assays; measure free **digoxin** levels using a chemiluminescent assay.[17]

Undesirable effects

Very common (>10%): CNS disturbances (drowsiness, lethargy, confusion, headache, fever, ataxia, fatigue), GI disturbances (anorexia, dyspepsia, nausea, vomiting, peptic ulceration, colic).
Common (<10%, >1%): gastritis, hyperkalaemia, gynaecomastia, breast pain.[18]

Dose and use

Cirrhotic or malignant ascites

Elimination of ascites may take 10–28 days:

- monitor body weight and renal function
- start with 100–200mg each morning with food; give in divided doses if it causes nausea and vomiting
- if necessary, increase by 100mg every 3–7 days to achieve a weight loss of 0.5–1kg/24h (<0.5kg/24h when peripheral oedema absent)
- a typical maintenance dose is 200–300mg/24h; maximum dose 400–600mg/24h[1,2,5,7]
- if not achieving the desired weight loss with spironolactone 300–400mg/24h, consider adding **furosemide** 40–80mg each morning
- in cirrhosis, **furosemide** is generally increased in 40mg steps every 3 days to a maximum of 160mg/24h[4,5,19,20]
- if Na^+ falls to <120mmol/L, temporarily stop diuretics
- if K^+ falls to <3.5mmol/L, temporarily stop or decrease the dose of **furosemide**; if it rises to >5.5mmol/L, halve the dose of spironolactone; if >6mmol/L, temporarily stop spironolactone
- if creatinine rises to >150micromol/L, temporarily stop diuretics.[4]

Severe CHF (NYHA class III or IV disease)

The following is based on several sets of published guidelines:

- do *not* prescribe spironolactone unless serum K^+ <5mmol/L and creatinine <200micromol/L
- start with 12.5–25mg once daily; check serum K^+ and creatinine after 4–7 days
- if necessary, *after 1 month*, increase to 50mg once daily; check serum K^+ and creatinine after 1 week
- if K^+ rises to >5mmol/L, halve the dose; if >5.5mmol/L, stop spironolactone completely
- it is particularly important to monitor potassium levels when spironolactone and an ACE inhibitor are prescribed concurrently.[13,14,21]

Supply

Spironolactone (generic)

Tablets 25mg, 50mg, 100mg, 28 days @ 200mg each morning = £6.

Oral suspension (sugar-free) 5mg/5mL, 10mg/5mL, 25mg/5mL, 50mg/5mL, 100mg/5mL; 28 days @ 200mg each morning = £270. (Unlicensed, available as a special order from Rosemont; see Obtaining unlicensed products, p.769.)

Aldactone® (Pharmacia)

Tablets 25mg, 50mg, 100mg, 28 days @ 200mg each morning = £20.

Spironolactone suspension can also be prepared locally for individual patients.[22]

1 Greenway B *et al.* (1982) Control of malignant ascites with spironolactone. *British Journal of Surgery.* **69**: 441–442.

2 Fernandez-Esparrach G *et al.* (1997) Diuretic requirements after therapeutic paracentesis in non-azotemic patients with cirrhosis. A randomized double-blind trial of spironolactone versus placebo. *Journal of Hepatology.* **26**: 614–620; erratum 1430.

3 Pockros P *et al.* (1992) Mobilization of malignant ascites with diuretics is dependent on ascitic fluid characteristics. *Gastroenterology.* **103**: 1302–1306.

4 Moore KP *et al.* (2003) The management of ascites in cirrhosis: report on the consensus conference of the International Ascites Club. *Hepatology.* **38**: 258–266.

5 Santos J *et al.* (2003) Spironolactone alone or in combination with furosemide in the treatment of moderate ascites in nonazotemic cirrhosis. A randomized comparative study of efficacy and safety. *Journal of Hepatology.* **39**: 187–192.

6 Becker G *et al.* (2006) Malignant ascites: systematic review and guideline for treatment. *European Journal of Cancer.* **42**: 589–597.

7 Fogel M *et al.* (1981) Diuresis in the ascitic patient: a randomized controlled trial of three regimens. *Journal of Clinical Gastroenterology.* **3**: 73–80.

8 Kalambokis G *et al.* (2005) Renal effects of treatment with diuretics, octreotide or both, in non-azotemic cirrhotic patients with ascites. *Nephrology, Dialysis, Transplantation.* **20**: 1623–1629.

9 Kalambokis G *et al.* (2006) The effects of treatment with octreotide, diuretics, or both on portal hemodynamics in nonazotemic cirrhotic patients with ascites. *Journal of Clinical Gastroenterology.* **40**: 342–346.

10 Lenaerts A *et al.* (2006) Effects of clonidine on diuretic response in ascitic patients with cirrhosis and activation of sympathetic nervous system. *Hepatology.* **44**: 844–849.

11 Veterans Health Administration (2003) The Pharmacologic Management of Chronic Heart Failure. Department of Veterans Affairs, Washington DC. Available from: www.guideline.gov/summary/summary.aspx?doc_id = 5184

12 McMurray JJ and Pfeffer MA (2005) Heart failure. *Lancet.* **365**: 1877–1889.

13 NICE (2010) Chronic heart failure: management of chronic heart failure in adults in primary and secondary care. Clinical Guideline 108. Available from: www.guidance.nice.org.uk/CG108

14 Swedberg K *et al.* (2005) Guidelines for the diagnosis and treatment of chronic heart failure: full text (update 2005). European Heart Journal. Available from: 10.1093/eurheartj/ehi205

15 Barnes BJ and Howard PA (2005) Eplerenone: a selective aldosterone receptor antagonist for patients with heart failure. *Annals of Pharmacotherapy.* **39**: 68–76.

16 Sonder SU *et al.* (2006) Effects of spironolactone on human blood mononuclear cells: mineralocorticoid receptor independent effects on gene expression and late apoptosis induction. *British Journal of Pharmacology.* **148**: 46–53.

17 Baxter K (2011) Stockley's Drug Interactions (online edition). Pharmaceutical Press, London. Available from: www.medicinescomplete.com

18 Williams EM *et al.* (2006) Use and side-effect profile of spironolactone in a private cardiologist's practice. *Clinical Cardiology.* **29**: 149–153.

19 Gines P *et al.* (1987) Comparison of paracentesis and diuretics in the treatment of cirrhotics with tense ascites. *Gastroenterology.* **93**: 234–241.

20 Sharma S and Walsh D (1995) Management of symptomatic malignant ascites with diuretics: two case reports and a review of the literature. *Journal of Pain and Symptom Management.* **10**: 237–242.

21 Arnold JM *et al.* (2006) Canadian Cardiovascular Society consensus conference recommendations on heart failure 2006: diagnosis and management.[erratum appears in Canadian Journal of Cardiology. 2006 Mar 1;22(3):271]. *Canadian Journal of Cardiology.* **22**: 23–45.

22 Allen LV Jr and Erickson MA 3rd (1996) Stability of ketoconazole, metolazone, metronidazole, procainamide hydrochloride, and spironolactone in extemporaneously compounded oral liquids. *American Journal of Health System Pharmacy.* **53**: 2073–2078.

SYSTEMIC LOCAL ANAESTHETICS BNF 2.3.2 & 4.7.3

Local anaesthetics and their orally administered congeners are sometimes useful as third- or fourth-line drugs in the treatment of neuropathic pain. An analgesic effect has been reported when such drugs have been administered systemically:[1]

- **lidocaine** TD, CSCI, IVI[2,3]
- **flecainide** PO (see p.65)
- **mexiletine** PO (not UK; may be imported as a special order/ named patient supply through IDIS)
- **tocainide** PO (not UK).

The mechanism by which they provide relief is not fully understood, but probably includes blockade of sodium channels. This stabilizes the nerve membrane and thus suppresses injury-induced hyperexcitability in the peripheral and central nervous systems. Antidepressants and anti-epileptics which benefit neuropathic pain also have membrane stabilizing properties, e.g. **carbamazepine**, **amitriptyline**.[4]

A systematic review of 32 RCTs, mostly of IV **lidocaine** and PO **mexiletine**, for neuropathic pain of various causes concluded that systemic local anaesthetics are better than placebo and as effective as **amantadine**, **carbamazepine**, **gabapentin**, **morphine** (Box 2.B).[1] Even so, despite the occasional impressive anecdotal account, RCT evidence of benefit is not overwhelming. Thus, the overall degree of improvement is small, and some studies suggest that not all components of neuropathic pain are relieved, e.g. constant pain and allodynia to touch improve but cold-induced allodynia does not.[5,6] Benefit is inconsistent in some types of pain, e.g. diabetic neuropathy, and absent in others, e.g. cancer-related neuropathic pain.[1,7,8] Further, in a study of elderly patients (mean age 77 years), **lidocaine** 5mg/kg IVI over 2h provides no greater analgesic benefit than 1mg/kg, despite producing higher serum levels which were potentially toxic in some patients.[9]

Box 2.B Systemic local anaesthetics and neuropathic pain[1]

Of overall benefit in:
- trigeminal neuralgia
- post-herpetic neuralgia
- diabetic neuropathy
- lumbosacral radiculopathy
- post-stroke pain
- chronic post-surgery pain
- chronic post-trauma pain
- spinal cord injury pain
- complex regional pain syndrome.

Not of benefit in:
- cancer-related neuropathy (but see main text)
- HIV-related neuropathy.

Lidocaine dose used ranged from 1mg/kg IV over 2–3min to 1–5mg/kg IVI over 30min–2h.

Mexiletine median dose 600mg/24h (range 300–1200mg/24h).

Improvement equivalent to a reduction of 10mm on a 100mm VAS, but about 50% of patients achieve an improvement of ⩾30%.

Although improvement lasting 8–20 weeks following a single dose of IV **lidocaine** has been reported in patients with central pain syndrome, generally benefit is limited to a few hours.[10,11] Thus, the need for ongoing relief will necessitate CIVI or CSCI **lidocaine** or the use of an oral analogue, e.g. **mexiletine** (not UK). However, the response to IV **lidocaine** does not reliably predict subsequent benefit from **mexiletine** and undesirable effects can limit its chronic use.[5,12] For example, in a cohort of patients with non-cancer neuropathic pain treated with **mexiletine**, the median time to discontinuation (for any reason) was 6 weeks with only 20% persisting with its use > 1 year.[13]

There are case reports of patients with cancer-related neuropathic pain benefiting from **lidocaine**:
- IV, e.g. 1–2mg/kg over 15–20min[14]
- CIVI, e.g. 0.5–1mg/kg/h[14,15]
- CSCI, e.g. 4 or 10% **lidocaine** hydrochloride solution, generally 10–80mg/h; 100–160mg/h reported in younger patients (age ~ 60 years).[15,16]

Continuous infusions have been given for up to 6 months.[16] As a minimum, some suggest monitoring serum levels 1–3 days after commencement or dose escalation and when toxicity is suspected.[15]

Analgesia is generally seen with serum levels of 1.5–5microgram/mL and severe neurotoxicity with levels ⩾10microgram/mL.[3,17] However, there is large interindividual variation and the beneficial/toxic effect relates more to the amount of free local anaesthetic (unbound to protein), rather than the total serum level (bound plus unbound).[18]

With a continuous infusion, accumulation of **lidocaine** and its active metabolites, e.g. monoethylglycinexylidide and glycinexylidide, can occur and lead to toxicity. Particular caution is required in the elderly in whom clearance is already reduced.[18–20] For example, two elderly patients (≥70 years) despite normal renal/liver function and receiving a relatively small dose of **lidocaine** (200–300mg/day), developed severe drowsiness after 10 days.[21]

Generally, developing toxicity should be clinically obvious because as serum levels rise, there is a progressive worsening of neurotoxicity:

- lightheadedness, dizziness
- circumoral numbness
- tinnitus
- visual changes
- dysarthria
- muscle spasm
- seizures
- coma
- respiratory arrest.

However, the monitoring of serum levels is the most effective way of maintaining a consistent and safe **lidocaine** dose.[3,19,21]

Prolonged toxicity has also been reported when 10mL of 2% viscous **lidocaine** (not UK) was used hourly for a painful mouth ulcer (twice the recommended daily dose), and was probably partly caused by accumulation of metabolites.[20]

Lidocaine medicated plasters, licensed for post-herpetic neuralgia, are available (Box 2.C). Sufficient high-quality data are lacking to recommend them for first-line use for post-herpetic neuralgia.[22] NICE guidance regards them as third-line treatment, to be tried as a temporary measure in patients with localized neuropathic pain who are unable to take oral medication pending referral to a specialist pain service.[23]

Thus, in cancer-related neuropathic pains, systemic local anaesthetics should generally be considered only when the combination of a strong opioid + NSAID + TCA + anti-epileptic is ineffective or poorly tolerated. Even so, **ketamine** (see p.593) may be preferable because:

- the serum level does not need to be monitored
- it can be given PO
- it is more effective than **lidocaine** in spinal cord injury pain.[34]

Box 2.C Lidocaine 5% medicated plaster

Lidocaine 5% medicated plaster (Lidoderm®) containing 700mg lidocaine is approved for post-herpetic neuralgia.

A recommended maximum of three plasters are applied to the painful area on a 12h on–12h off basis. The plasters can be cut if required but must not be applied close to the eyes or mouth, or on inflamed/broken skin or wounds.

Similar considerations apply as for other medical transdermal products, e.g. skin hair should be clipped rather than shaved, fold plasters in half and dispose of safely (≥665mg remains in the plasters).

Only about 5% of the plaster dose is absorbed. Steady-state is achieved after three days. Maximum concentrations (0.07–0.19microgram/mL) are well below systemic analgesic (1.5–5microgram/mL) and serious toxic levels (≥10microgram/mL). The analgesic effect is thus considered a local one.

The 12h off periods are to help reduce the risk of skin reactions, but these still occur in about 15% of patients. The skin can be rested for longer when necessary, but up to 5% of patients have to discontinue. Anaphylaxis is a very rare complication (≤1:10,000).

Generally, high quality data are lacking. A recent study of post-herpetic neuralgia suggests that overall <50% of patients will obtain sufficient benefit to warrant continuing with the plasters.[24] For those who respond, sustained benefit (≥1 year) has been reported.[25] The magnitude of the benefit appears similar to that obtained with pregabalin but the plasters are better tolerated.[26]

continued

Box 2.C Continued

Use of the plasters in other settings include:

- diabetic polyneuropathy[26]
- post-surgical scar pain[2,27,28]
- osteoarthritis[29]
- carpal tunnel syndrome[30]
- erythromelalgia[31]
- cancer-related.[32]

These have mostly been low-quality open studies, case series or reports, with mixed results. A survey of palliative care practitioners revealed the main use of the plasters to be neuropathic pain resulting from invasion of the chest wall by mesothelioma, breast or lung cancer. They were considered acceptable, well tolerated and beneficial to most patients. On the other hand, there were concerns about an unpredictable or variable response and high cost.[33]

1 Challapalli V *et al.* (2005) Systemic administration of local anesthetic agents to relieve neuropathic pain. *Cochrane Database of Systematic Reviews.* CD003345.

2 Meier T *et al.* (2003) Efficacy of lidocaine patch 5% in the treatment of focal peripheral neuropathic pain syndromes: a randomized, double-blind, placebo-controlled study. *Pain.* **106**: 151–158.

3 Devulder J *et al.* (1993) Neuropathic pain in a cancer patient responding to subcutaneously administered lignocaine. *The Clinical Journal of Pain.* **9**: 220–223.

4 Devor M (2006) Sodium channels and mechanisms of neuropathic pain. *Journal of Pain.* **7**: S3–S12.

5 Attal N *et al.* (2000) Intravenous lidocaine in central pain: a double-blind, placebo-controlled, psychophysical study. *Neurology.* **54**: 564–574.

6 Attal N *et al.* (2004) Systemic lidocaine in pain due to peripheral nerve injury and predictors of response. *Neurology.* **62**: 218–225.

7 Ellemann K *et al.* (1989) Trial of intravenous lidocaine on painful neuropathy in cancer patients. *Clinical Journal of Pain.* **5**: 291–294.

8 Bruera E *et al.* (1992) A randomized double-blind crossover trial of intravenous lidocaine in the treatment of neuropathic cancer pain. *Journal of Pain and Symptom Management.* **7**: 138–140.

9 Baranowski AP *et al.* (1999) A trial of intravenous lidocaine on the pain and allodynia of postherpetic neuralgia. *Journal of Pain and Symptom Management.* **17**: 429–433.

10 Backonja M and Gombar KA (1992) Response of central pain syndromes to intravenous lidocaine. *Journal of Pain and Symptom Management.* **7**: 172–178.

11 Tremont-Lukats IW *et al.* (2006) A randomized, double-masked, placebo-controlled pilot trial of extended IV lidocaine infusion for relief of ongoing neuropathic pain. *Clinical Journal of Pain.* **22**: 266–271.

12 Chong S *et al.* (1997) Pilot study evaluating local anesthetics administered systemically for treatment of pain in patients with advanced cancer. *Journal of Pain and Symptom Management.* **13**: 112–117.

13 Carroll IR *et al.* (2008) Mexiletine therapy for chronic pain: survival analysis identifies factors predicting clinical success. *Journal of Pain and Symptom Management.* **35**: 321–326.

14 Thomas J *et al.* (2004) Intravenous lidocaine relieves severe pain: results of an inpatient hospice chart review. *Journal of Palliative Medicine.* **7**: 660–667.

15 Ferrini R (2000) Parenteral lidocaine for severe intractable pain in six hospice patients continued at home. *Journal of Palliative Medicine.* **3**: 193–200.

16 Massey GV *et al.* (2002) Continuous lidocaine infusion for the relief of refractory malignant pain in a terminally ill pediatric cancer patient. *Journal of Pediatric Hematology/Oncology.* **24**: 566–568.

17 Ferrante FM *et al.* (1996) The analgesic response to intravenous lidocaine in the treatment of neuropathic pain. *Anesthesia and Analgesia.* **82**: 91–97.

18 Rosenberg PH *et al.* (2004) Maximum recommended doses of local anesthetics: a multifactorial concept. *Regional Anesthesia and Pain Medicine.* **29**: 564–575; discussion 524.

19 Brose W and Cousins M (1991) Subcutaneous lidocaine for treatment of neuropathic pain. *Pain.* **45**: 145–148.

20 Yamashita S *et al.* (2002) Lidocaine toxicity during frequent viscous lidocaine use for painful tongue ulcer. *Journal of Pain and Symptom Management.* **24**: 543–545.

21 Tei Y *et al.* (2005) Lidocaine intoxication at very small doses in terminally ill cancer patients. *Journal of Pain and Symptom Management.* **30**: 6–7.

22 Khaliq W *et al.* (2007) Topical lidocaine for the treatment of postherpetic neuralgia. *Cochrane Database of Systematic Reviews.* CD004846.

23 NICE (2010) Clinical Guideline 96. Neuropathic pain: the pharmacological management of neuropathic pain in adults in non-specialist settings.

24 Binder A *et al.* (2009) Topical 5% lidocaine (lignocaine) medicated plaster treatment for post-herpetic neuralgia: results of a double-blind, placebo-controlled, multinational efficacy and safety trial. *Clinical Drug Investigation.* **29**: 393–408.

25 Hans G *et al.* (2009) Efficacy and tolerability of a 5% lidocaine medicated plaster for the topical treatment of post-herpetic neuralgia: results of a long-term study. *Current Medical Research Opinion.* **25**: 1295–1305.

26 Baron R *et al.* (2009) 5% lidocaine medicated plaster versus pregabalin in post-herpetic neuralgia and diabetic polyneuropathy: an open-label, non-inferiority two-stage RCT study. *Current Medical Research and Opinion.* **25**: 1663–1676.
27 Nayak S and Cunliffe M (2008) Lidocaine 5% patch for localized chronic neuropathic pain in adolescents: report of five cases. *Paediatric Anaesthesia.* **18**: 554–558.
28 Cheville AL *et al.* (2009) Use of a lidocaine patch in the management of postsurgical neuropathic pain in patients with cancer: a phase III double-blind crossover study (N01CB). *Supportive Care in Cancer.* **17**: 451–460.
29 Burch F *et al.* (2004) Lidocaine patch 5% improves pain, stiffness, and physical function in osteoarthritis pain patients. A prospective, multicenter, open-label effectiveness trial. *Osteoarthritis and Cartilage.* **12**: 253–255.
30 Nalamachu S *et al.* (2006) A comparison of the lidocaine patch 5% vs naproxen 500 mg twice daily for the relief of pain associated with carpal tunnel syndrome: a 6-week, randomized, parallel-group study. *Medscape General Medicine.* **8**: 33.
31 Davis MD and Sandroni P (2005) Lidocaine patch for pain of erythromelalgia: follow-up of 34 patients. *Archives of Dermatology.* **141**: 1320–1321.
32 Fleming JA and O'Connor BD (2009) Use of lidocaine patches for neuropathic pain in a comprehensive cancer centre. *Pain Research and Management.* **14**: 381–388.
33 Palliativedrugs com (2009) Survey. Lidocaine 5% medicated plasters—What is your experience? Available from: www.palliativedrugs.com/download/090731_lidocaine_survey_sc.pdf
34 Kvarnstrom A *et al.* (2004) The analgesic effect of intravenous ketamine and lidocaine on pain after spinal cord injury. *Acta Anaesthesiologica Scandinavica.* **48**: 498–506.

*FLECAINIDE — BNF 2.3.2

Class: 1C anti-arrhythmic.

Indications: Cardiac arrhythmias, †neuropathic pain.

Contra-indications: Include history of myocardial infarction, heart failure, cardiac conduction defects (*see manufacturer's SPC for details*). Do not use concurrently with **ritonavir**, **lopinavir**, **indinavir**, **fosamprenavir**, **artemether**, **lumefantrine** or **mizolastine**.

Pharmacology

Flecainide is a chemical congener of **lidocaine**. It is a membrane stabilizer, i.e. it inhibits sodium ion channels in nerve membranes, thereby suppressing injury-induced hyperexcitability in the peripheral and central nervous systems.[1] Flecainide is licensed for use primarily in the prevention and treatment of ventricular and supraventricular arrhythmias but, like **mexiletine** (not UK; may be imported as a special order/ named patient supply through IDIS), it is sometimes used to treat nerve injury pain, generally after treatment failure with a combination of strong opioid + NSAID + TCA + anti-epileptic (see Systemic local anaesthetics, p.61). Response rate in non-controlled studies in cancer and AIDS patients varies between 30–60%.[2–5] Flecainide has a narrow therapeutic index, and some patients experience psychoneurological and cardiac toxicity within the recommended therapeutic range (see p.63).[6,7]

When used as prophylaxis against arrhythmias after myocardial infarction (<2 years), flecainide was associated with an increased incidence of sudden death.[8] Thus, when used as an anti-arrhythmic, the manufacturer recommends that treatment is started in hospital. However, at some centres, flecainide for neuropathic pain is started on an outpatient basis without an ECG provided the patient is in normal rhythm, is not in heart failure and has no history of myocardial infarction. Alternative treatments include **ketamine** (see p.593), **methadone** (see p.416) and spinal analgesia (see p.681).
Bio-availability 90–95% PO.
Onset of action 0.5–2h as an anti-arrhythmic.
Time to peak plasma concentration 1.5–6h PO.
Plasma halflife 12–27h.
Duration of action 15–23h as an anti-arrhythmic.

Cautions

Correct electrolyte disturbances, e.g. of K^+, Ca^{2+}, Mg^{2+}, before starting treatment. Hepatic and renal impairment. Risk of myocardial depression increased by β antagonists (β-blockers), calcium-channel blockers and hypokalaemia; risk of arrhythmia if used with a pro-arrhythmic drug, e.g. TCAs, **saquinavir**.[9]

Flecainide is metabolized by, and inhibits, CYP2D6 (see Cytochrome P450, p.735). Plasma concentration increased by **amiodarone** (halve flecainide dose and monitor plasma concentrations), **cimetidine**, **propranolol** and **quinine** and decreased by smoking.[10] In contrast, flecainide elimination may be increased by about 30% by **phenytoin**, **phenobarbital** and **carbamazepine** but this is unlikely to require a dose change.

Undesirable effects

Very common (>10%): dizziness, dyspnoea.
Common (<10%, >1%): headache, fatigue, malaise, drowsiness or insomnia, vertigo, anxiety, depression, fever, hypaesthesia, ataxia, tremor, weakness, paraesthesia, double/blurred vision, tinnitus, palpitations, tachycardia, sinus node dysfunction, chest pain, nausea, vomiting, anorexia, abdominal pain, constipation or diarrhoea, rash, abnormal LFTs.

Dose and use

Flecainide is not a first-line adjuvant analgesic (see Systemic local anaesthetics, p.61). *Generally, antidepressants should be stopped at least 48h before starting flecainide.* Initial doses are comparable to those used in cardiology:

- start with 50mg b.d.
- usual dose 100mg b.d.
- maximum dose 200mg b.d.

The use of a test dose of **lidocaine** 2–5mg/kg IVI has been suggested as a means of predicting whether flecainide or **mexiletine** (not UK) will be of benefit.[11] However, this is not a reliable guide.[12] Further, in cancer patients, **lidocaine** 5mg/kg IV over 30min is no more effective than placebo.[13–15]

Overdose

A single dose of 800mg, i.e. twice the maximum recommended daily dose, is potentially life-threatening.[6] Symptoms of overdose include sedation, delirium, coma, seizures, respiratory arrest, hypotension, sinus arrest, AV block, and asystole. Treatment is supportive and may necessitate the use of anti-epileptic and anti-arrhythmic drugs. **Sodium bicarbonate** may reverse QRS prolongation, bradycardia and hypotension. Haemodialysis is not of benefit.

Supply

Flecainide (generic)
Tablets 50mg, 100mg, 28 days @ 100mg b.d. = £10.

Tambocor® (Meda)
Tablets 50mg, 100mg, 28 days @ 100mg b.d. = £15.

1 Devor M (2006) Sodium channels and mechanisms of neuropathic pain. *Journal of Pain*. **7**: S3–S12.
2 Dunlop R *et al.* (1988) Analgesic effects of oral flecainide. *Lancet*. **1**: 420–421.
3 Sinnott C *et al.* (1991) Flecainide in cancer nerve pain. *Lancet*. **337**: 1347.
4 Chong S *et al.* (1997) Pilot study evaluating local anesthetics administered systemically for treatment of pain in patients with advanced cancer. *Journal of Pain and Symptom Management*. **13**: 112–117.
5 von Gunten CF *et al.* (2007) Flecainide for the treatment of chronic neuropathic pain: a Phase II trial. *Palliative Medicine*. **21**: 667–672.
6 Nestico PF *et al.* (1988) New antiarrhythmic drugs. *Drugs*. **35**: 286–319.
7 Bennett M (1997) Paranoid psychosis due to flecainide toxicity in malignant neuropathic pain. *Pain*. **70**: 93–94.
8 Cardiac arrhythmia suppression trial (CAST) (1989) Investigators' preliminary report: effect of encainide and flecainide on mortality in a randomized trial of arrhythmia suppression after myocardial infarction. *New England Journal of Medicine*. **321**: 406–412.
9 MHRA (2010) Saquinavir: effects on QT and PR interval prolongation. Article A1.Drug safety update.4(1, August): 2–3. Available from: www.mhra.gov.uk?publications/Safetyguidance/index.htm
10 Baxter K (ed) (2006) *Stockley's Drug Interactions* (7e). Pharmaceutical Press, London.
11 Galer B *et al.* (1996) Response to intravenous lidocaine infusion predicts subsequent response to oral mexiletine: a prospective study. *Journal of Pain and Symptom Management*. **12**: 161–167.
12 Jarvis B and Coukell AJ (1998) Mexiletine. A review of its therapeutic use in painful diabetic neuropathy. *Drugs*. **56**: 691–707.
13 Ellemann K *et al.* (1989) Trial of intravenous lidocaine on painful neuropathy in cancer patients. *Clinical Journal of Pain*. **5**: 291–294.
14 Challapalli V *et al.* (2005) Systemic administration of local anesthetic agents to relieve neuropathic pain. *Cochrane Database of Systematic Reviews*. CD003345.
15 Bruera E *et al.* (1992) A randomized double-blind crossover trial of intravenous lidocaine in the treatment of neuropathic cancer pain. *Journal of Pain and Symptom Management*. **7**: 138–140.

*CLONIDINE BNF 2.5.2

Class: α-adrenergic receptor agonist (α agonist).

Indications: Hypertension, migraine prophylaxis, menopausal flushing, †pain poorly responsive to epidural or intrathecal **diamorphine/morphine** and **bupivacaine**, †spasticity, †diarrhoea or †gastroparesis related to autonomic dysfunction in diabetes mellitus, †sweating.

Contra-indications: Cardiac conduction defects.

Pharmacology

Clonidine is a mixed α_1 and α_2 agonist (mainly α_2). It reduces the responsiveness of peripheral blood vessels to vasoconstrictor and vasodilator substances, and to sympathetic nerve stimulation.[1] Clonidine can cause a reduction in venous return and mild bradycardia, resulting in a reduced cardiac output.

Clonidine attenuates the opioid withdrawal syndrome, indicating an interaction with the opioid system. It appears to have synergistic analgesic effects with opioids.[2,3] In surgical patients, clonidine also enhances the analgesic effect and duration of block produced by local anaesthetics administered IT or peripherally (single nerve or plexus blocks).[4–6] Clonidine also reduces post-operative nausea and vomiting; in patients undergoing laparoscopic surgery, the incidence of vomiting was approximately halved with PO clonidine compared to placebo.[7]

Clonidine provides reproducible pain relief in some patients with neuropathic pain, particularly when given via the ED or IT routes.[8–12] ED clonidine is effective in cancer-related neuropathic pain, generally as an 'add-on' drug (see Spinal analgesia, p.681). It is particularly useful for patients who do not respond to high-dose systemic opioids or who tolerate them poorly, and for those who fail to respond to spinal **morphine** plus **bupivacaine**.[13,14] Although a typical dose is 150–300microgram/24h ED, benefit has been reported in some patients with IT doses of ≤1mg/day.[12] Further, solo treatment with high-dose ED clonidine, i.e. a bolus of 10microgram/kg followed by an infusion of 6microgram/kg/h, provides effective postoperative analgesia.[15] Benefit has also been reported in patients receiving clonidine by CSCI, with increasing benefit in a few patients with doses of up to 1.5mg/24h.[16]

ED clonidine is absorbed into the systemic circulation producing significant plasma concentrations (reflected clinically by drowsiness and cardiovascular effects), reaching a peak after 20min. IT clonidine produces similar effects; sedation occurs within 15–30min and lasts 1–2h.[12,17,18] The analgesic effect of clonidine can be reversed by α antagonists but not by **naloxone**.[11] Clonidine can thus be used in the management of unexpected acute pain in addicts receiving **naltrexone** (see p.438). It is probable that clonidine analgesia is mediated by an effect at α_2-receptors or imidazoline receptors resulting in:

- peripheral and/or central suppression of sympathetic transmitter release[11,19]
- presynaptic inhibition of nociceptive afferents[20]
- post-synaptic inhibition of spinal cord neurones[21,22]
- facilitation of brain stem pain modulating systems.[23]

In patients with spinal cord injury, the addition of clonidine reduces muscle spasticity which has failed to respond to maximal doses of **baclofen**.[24,25] In healthy volunteers, clonidine induces muscular relaxation and reduces pain caused by distension in the stomach, colon and rectum.[26,27] In patients with diabetic-related intestinal autonomic neuropathy, clonidine improves symptoms of gastroparesis and chronic diarrhoea.[28–30] The improvement in diarrhoea is due partly to the stimulation of α_2-adrenergic receptors on enterocytes, which promotes intestinal fluid and electrolyte absorption, inhibits anion secretion and may also modify intestinal motility.[29,30]

There is RCT evidence that clonidine relieves sweating in menopausal women (with or without hot flushes), and sweating in both men and women resulting from hormonal manipulation by drugs (e.g. **tamoxifen**) or surgery (e.g. castration).[31,32] However, some trials have found no difference from placebo.[33,34] More recent trials in patients with breast cancer and hot flushes have found **venlafaxine** (p.195) to be as effective or more so than clonidine.[35,36] However, clonidine appears better tolerated than **venlafaxine**, with undesirable effects leading to discontinuation in 9% vs. 24% of patients respectively.[35]

In patients with cirrhosis receiving **spironolactone** ± **furosemide**, improved renal function and diuresis is seen with co-administration of clonidine 75microgram PO b.d. (see p.59) due to inhibition of the renin-aldosterone-angiotensin and sympathetic nervous systems.[37,38] Patients were considered to have an overactive sympathetic nervous system based on a higher than normal serum noradrenaline (norepinephrine) level.[38]

About half of a dose of clonidine is excreted unchanged by the kidneys, and most of the remainder is metabolized by the liver to inactive metabolites. Accumulation occurs in renal impairment, extending its halflife up to 40h.

Bio-availability 75–100% PO; 60% TD.[39]

Onset of action 30–60min IV, PO; 2–3 days TD.

Time to peak plasma concentration 1.5–5h PO; 20min ED; 2 days TD.

Plasma halflife 12–16h.

Duration of action 8–24h PO; 24h TD.

Cautions

Severe coronary insufficiency, recent myocardial infarction, stroke, peripheral vascular disease. May precipitate depression in susceptible patients. Occasionally precipitates delirium in susceptible patients.[40] Abrupt curtailment of long-term treatment likely to cause agitation, sympathetic overactivity, rebound hypertension; therefore withdraw treatment progressively over 2–4 days (ED) or 1 week (PO).

Effects reduced or abolished by drugs with α antagonist activity, e.g. **mirtazapine**, TCAs (e.g. **amitriptyline**, **clomipramine**, **desipramine** (not UK), **imipramine**), and antipsychotic drugs, although the hypotensive effects of the phenothiazines can be additive.[41]

TD patches (not UK) contain metal in the backing and must be removed before MRI to avoid burns.[42]

Undesirable effects

Very common (>10%): sedation and dry mouth (initially), dizziness, orthostatic hypotension, transient pruritus and erythema (TD route).

Common (<10%, >1%): headache, fatigue, depression (long-term use), disturbed sleep, nausea, vomiting, constipation, erectile dysfunction, salivary gland pain, local reactions with TD route (e.g. rash, hyperpigmentation, excoriation).

Dose and use

Clonidine can be given as a TD patch (not UK, but see Supply),[10,43] PO, by CSCI, and spinally. TD is generally better tolerated than PO, but the relationship between effective doses of PO and TD clonidine is not predictable. Start with a patch delivering 100microgram/24h applied once every 7 days and review.

Spinal analgesia

ED clonidine is generally given with **diamorphine/morphine** and **bupivacaine** (see Spinal analgesia, p.681). A typical ED regimen would be:

- a test bolus dose of 50–150microgram in 5mL saline injection over 5min
- if relief obtained, 150–300microgram/24h by infusion.

Clonidine is also used IT. A typical IT regimen would be:

- a test bolus dose of 50microgram in 5mL saline injection over 5min
- if relief obtained, 50–150microgram/24h by infusion.

Spasticity

Generally used as an adjunct to maximum dose of **baclofen**:

- start with 50microgram PO b.d.
- if necessary, increase by 50microgram every 3–7 days
- usual maximum dose 200microgram b.d.

Gastroparesis or diarrhoea related to autonomic dysfunction in diabetes mellitus

- start with 50microgram PO b.d.
- if necessary, increase by 50microgram every 24h
- usual maintenance dose 150microgram b.d.

- usual maximum dose for diabetic gastroparesis 300microgram b.d.
- usual maximum dose for diabetic diarrhoea 600microgram b.d.

Hormonal/menopausal sweating

- start with 50microgram PO b.d.
- after 2 weeks, if necessary, increase to 75microgram b.d.
- for some patients, the optimum dose is 100microgram b.d.

Supply

Dixarit® (Boehringer Ingelheim)
Tablets 25microgram, 28 days @ 50microgram b.d. = £7.

Catapres® (Boehringer Ingelheim)
Tablets 100microgram, 28 days @ 100microgram b.d. = £3.
Injection 150microgram/mL, 1mL amp = £0.50.

Catapres® TTS
Transdermal patch 2.5mg (100microgram/24h), 5mg (200microgram/24h) 7.5mg (300microgram/24hr) 1 patch (7 days treatment) = £8, £63, £200 respectively. (Unlicensed, available as a named patient supply from IDIS, but cost can be prohibitive; see Obtaining unlicensed products, p.769).

1 Hieble JP and Ruffolo RR (1991) Therapeutic applications of agents interacting with alpha-adrenoceptors. In: RR Ruffolo (ed) *Alpha-adrenoceptors: molecular biology, biochemistry and pharmacology* Vol 8. Karger, Basel, pp. 180–220.
2 Siddall PJ *et al.* (2000) The efficacy of intrathecal morphine and clonidine in the treatment of pain after spinal cord injury. *Anesthesia and Analgesia.* **91**: 1493–1498.
3 Nader ND *et al.* (2009) Adjuvant therapy with intrathecal clonidine improves postoperative pain in patients undergoing coronary artery bypass graft. *Clinical Journal of Pain.* **25**: 101–106.
4 Elia N *et al.* (2008) Clonidine as an adjuvant to intrathecal local anesthetics for surgery: systematic review of randomized trials. *Regional Anesthesia and Pain Medicine.* **33**: 159–167.
5 Popping DM *et al.* (2009) Clonidine as an adjuvant to local anesthetics for peripheral nerve and plexus blocks: a meta-analysis of randomized trials. *Anesthesiology.* **111**: 406–415.
6 Ya Deau JT *et al.* (2008) Clonidine and analgesic duration after popliteal fossa nerve blockade: Randomized, double-blind, placebo-controlled study. *Anesthesia and Analgesia.* **106**: 1916–1920.
7 Javaherfroosh F *et al.* (2009) Clonidine reduces post operative nausea and vomiting in laparoscopic gynecological surgery. *Pakistan Journal of Medical Sciences.* **25**: 782–785.
8 Glynn C *et al.* (1988) A double-blind comparison between epidural morphine and epidural clonidine in patients with chronic noncancer pain. *Pain.* **34**: 123–128.
9 Max MB *et al.* (1988) Association of pain relief with drug side effects in postherpetic neuralgia: a single-dose study of clonidine, codeine, ibuprofen and placebo. *Clinical Pharmacology and Therapeutics.* **43**: 363–371.
10 Zeigler D *et al.* (1992) Transdermal clonidine versus placebo in painful diabetic neuropathy. *Pain.* **48**: 403–408.
11 Quan D *et al.* (1993) Clonidine in pain management. *Annals of Pharmacotherapy.* **27**: 313–315.
12 Ackerman LL *et al.* (2003) Long-term outcomes during treatment of chronic pain with intrathecal clonidine or clonidine/opioid combinations. *Journal of Pain and Symptom Management.* **26**: 668–677.
13 Eisenach JC *et al.* (1995) Epidural clonidine analgesia for intractable cancer pain. The Epidural Clonidine Study Group. *Pain.* **61**: 391–399.
14 Chen H *et al.* (2004) Contemporary management of neuropathic pain for the primary care physician. *Mayo Clinic Proceedings.* **79**: 1533–1545.
15 deKock M *et al.* (1999) Epidural clonidine or bupivacaine as the sole analgesic agent during and after abdominal surgery. [Erratum appears in *Anesthesiology* (1999) **91**:602.]. *Anesthesiology.* **90**: 1354–1362.
16 Glynn C (1997) Personal communication.
17 Wells J and Hardy P (1987) Epidural clonidine. *Lancet.* **1**: 108.
18 Malinovsky JM *et al.* (2003) Sedation caused by clonidine in patients with spinal cord injury. *British Journal of Anaesthesia.* **90**: 742–745.
19 Langer SZ *et al.* (1980) Recent developments in noradrenergic neurotransmission and its relevance to the mechanism of action of certain antihypertensive agents. *Hypertension.* **2**: 372–382.
20 Calvillo O and Ghignone M (1986) Presynaptic effect of clonidine on unmyelinated afferent fibers in the spinal cord of the cat. *Neuroscience Letters.* **64**: 335–339.
21 Yaksh T (1985) Pharmacology of spinal adrenergic systems which modulate spinal nociceptive processing. *Pharmacology, Biochemistry and Behaviour.* **22**: 845–858.
22 Michel MC and Insel PA (1989) Are there multiple imidazoline binding sites? *TIPS.* **10**: 342–344.
23 Sagen J and Proudfit H (1985) Evidence for pain modulation by pre- and postsynaptic noradrenergic receptors in the medulla oblongata. *Brain Research.* **331**: 285–293.
24 Weingarden S and Belen J (1992) Clonidine transdermal system for treatment of spasticity in spinal cord injury. *Archives of Physical Medicine and Rehabilitation.* **73**: 876–877.
25 Yablon S and Sipski M (1993) Effect of transdermal clonidine on spinal spasticity: a case series. *American Journal of Physical Medicine and Rehabilitation.* **72**: 154–156.
26 Thumshirn M *et al.* (1999) Modulation of gastric sensory and motor functions by nitrergic and alpha2-adrenergic agents in humans. *Gastroenterology.* **116**: 573–585.

27 Viramontes BE *et al.* (2001) Effects of an alpha(2)-adrenergic agonist on gastrointestinal transit, colonic motility, and sensation in humans. *American Journal of Physiology Gastrointestinal and Liver Physiology.* **281**: G1468–1476.
28 Rosa-Silva L *et al.* (1995) Treatment of diabetic gastroparesis with oral clonidine. *Alimentary Pharmacology and Therapeutics.* **9**: 179–183.
29 Fedorak R *et al.* (1985) Treatment of diabetic diarrhea with clonidine. *Annals of internal medicine.* **102**: 197–199.
30 Fedorak R and Field M (1987) Antidiarrheal therapy prospects for new agents. *Digestive Diseases and Science.* **32**: 195–205.
31 Goldberg R *et al.* (1994) Transdermal clonidine for ameliorating tamoxifen-induced hot flashes. *Journal of Clinical Oncology.* **12**: 155–158.
32 Pandya K *et al.* (2000) Oral clonidine in postmenopausal patients with breast cancer experiencing tamoxifen-induced hot flashes: a university of Rochester Cancer Centre community clinical oncology program study. *Annals of internal medicine.* **132**: 788–793.
33 Salmi T and Punnonen R (1979) Clonidine in the treatment of menopausal symptoms. *International Journal of Gynaecology and Obstetrics.* **16**: 422–461.
34 Loprinzi C *et al.* (1994) Transdermal clonidine for ameliorating post-orchidectomy hot flashes. *Journal of Urology.* **151**: 634–636.
35 Buijs C *et al.* (2009) Venlafaxine versus clonidine for the treatment of hot flashes in breast cancer patients: a double-blind, randomized cross-over study. *Breast Cancer Research and Treatment.* **115**: 573–580.
36 Loibl S *et al.* (2007) Venlafaxine is superior to clonidine as treatment of hot flashes in breast cancer patients—a double-blind, randomized study. *Annals of Oncology.* **18**: 689–693.
37 Kalambokis G *et al.* (2005) Renal effects of treatment with diuretics, octreotide or both, in non-azotemic cirrhotic patients with ascites. *Nephrology, Dialysis, Transplantation.* **20**: 1623–1629.
38 Lenaerts A *et al.* (2006) Effects of clonidine on diuretic response in ascitic patients with cirrhosis and activation of sympathetic nervous system. *Hepatology.* **44**: 844–849.
39 Toon S *et al.* (1989) Rate and extent of absorption of clonidine from a transdermal therapeutic system. *Journal of Pharmacy and Pharmacology.* **41**: 17–21.
40 Delaney J *et al.* (2006) Clonidine-induced delirium. *International Journal of Cardiology.* **113**: 276–278.
41 Baxter K (2011) Stockley's Drug Interactions (online edition). Pharmaceutical Press, London. Available from: www.medicinescomplete.com
42 Institute for Safe Medication Practices (2004) Medication Safety Alert. Burns in MRI patients wearing transdermal patches. Available from: www.ismp.org/Newsletters/acutecare/articles/20040408.asp?ptr = y
43 Davis K *et al.* (1991) Topical application of clonidine relieves hyperalgesia in patients with sympathetically maintained pain. *Pain.* **47**: 309–317.

GLYCERYL TRINITRATE — BNF 1.7.4 & 2.6.1

Class: Nitrate.

Indications: Angina, left ventricular failure, anal fissure, †smooth muscle spasm pain (particularly of the oesophagus, rectum and anus or cutaneous leiomyomas),[1] †biliary and †renal colic, †painful diabetic neuropathy,[2,3] †symptomatic relief of breathlessness in acute pulmonary oedema (in conjunction with opioids and diuretics)[4] or paroxysmal nocturnal dyspnoea.

Contra-indications: Severe hypotension (systolic <90mmHg), or severe aortic or mitral stenosis, cardiac tamponade, constrictive pericarditis, hypertrophic obstructive cardiomyopathy, marked anaemia, severe hypovolaemia, raised intracranial pressure, narrow-angle glaucoma. Concurrent use of **sildenafil**, **tadalafil** and **vardenafil** (may precipitate hypotension and myocardial infarction).[5]

Pharmacology

Glyceryl trinitrate relaxes smooth muscle in blood vessels and the GI tract, and may thus improve dysphagia and odynophagia associated with oesophagitis and oesophageal spasm.[6,7]

In patients with anal fissure, glyceryl trinitrate relieves pain, improves quality of life and aids healing. It is more effective than **botulinum toxin** but less effective than surgery.[8–12] In chronic anal fissure, glyceryl trinitrate ointment 0.2–0.4% applied b.d. to the anal canal is as effective as m/r **nifedipine** 20mg PO b.d. (see p.73).[13] It also relieves painful rectal spasm. However, most patients experience headache which, although this may be transient, is severe in ≤25%.[14] Thus, for topical symptomatic treatment of anal fissure, **diltiazem** cream is a better choice; it is as effective but causes less headache and less anal irritation.[15] Alternatively, use PO **nifedipine**, as described above.

Glyceryl trinitrate produces its smooth muscle relaxant effects via its metabolism to nitric oxide (NO), which stimulates guanylate cyclase. This results in an increase in cyclic guanosine monophosphate which reduces the amount of intracellular calcium available for muscle contraction.[16] NO appears to have an important role in the regulation of distal oesophageal peristalsis and relaxation of the lower oesophageal sphincter. A wider role of NO in pain is evident but is yet to be clarified. NO is produced when the NMDA-receptor is stimulated by excitatory amino acids (see **ketamine**, p.593) and may be important in the development of opioid tolerance as NO synthase inhibitors attenuate the development of analgesic tolerance.[17]

TD glyceryl trinitrate enhances pain relief in cancer patients and, as a topical gel, reduces local pain and inflammation.[18–23] In a placebo-controlled RCT in diabetic neuropathic pain affecting the feet, locally applied glyceryl trinitrate spray reduced mean pain scores significantly from 7.5 to 4.6 (NNT = 4).[2] In a second RCT, the concurrent use of PO **sodium valproate** provided no additional benefit.[3]

In patients with lung cancer, a TD patch for 5 days with each cycle of chemotherapy increases the frequency and duration of response. This may reflect improved perfusion of the tumour, thereby increasing drug delivery or decreasing hypoxia (a factor associated with drug resistance).[24]

Nitrates cause venous then arterial dilation in a dose-related manner. Nitrates such as glyceryl trinitrate and **isosorbide dinitrate** are thus used SL or IVI in acute pulmonary oedema to reduce pre- and after-load, which, in conjunction with opioids and diuretics, helps to relieve breathlessness. This is not suitable for patients with hypotension (systolic <90mmHg), severe obstructive valvular disease, or long-term use (nitrate tolerance generally develops after 24–48h).[4] Also because of tolerance, the chronic use of nitrates in cardiovascular disease is best reserved for specific circumstances, such as nocturnal angina or paroxysmal nocturnal dyspnoea. In this setting, p.r.n. glyceryl trinitrate spray SL may be helpful or, if a frequent occurrence, a regular bedtime dose of a longer-acting nitrate PO. In those unable to swallow tablets, a bedtime application of TD glyceryl trinitrate can be used. All these approaches permit a reasonable daily nitrate-free period.

Glyceryl trinitrate is rapidly absorbed through the buccal mucosa but orally it is inactivated by extensive first-pass metabolism in the GI mucosa and liver. Many patients on long-acting or TD nitrates develop tolerance, i.e. experience a reduced therapeutic effect. Tolerance is generally prevented if nitrate levels are allowed to fall for 4–8h in every 24h (a 'nitrate holiday'). This may not be possible for patients with persistent pain. If tolerance develops, it will be necessary to increase the dose to restore efficacy.

Bio-availability 40% SL.
Onset of action 1–3min SL; 30–60min ointment or TD patch.
Time to peak plasma concentration 3–6min SL; 2h TD.
Plasma halflife 1–3min SL; 2–4min TD.
Duration of action 30–60min SL; 8h ointment; 24h TD patch.

Cautions

Severe hepatic or renal impairment, hypothyroidism, malnutrition, hypovolaemia, hypoxaemia, hypothermia, recent myocardial infarction.

Exacerbates the hypotensive effect of other drugs. Drugs causing dry mouth may reduce the effect of sublingual nitrates. Topically applied glyceryl trinitrate can be absorbed in sufficient quantities to cause undesirable systemic effects.

TD patches which contain metal in the backing, e.g. Transiderm-Nitro® must be removed before MRI to avoid burns.[25]

Undesirable effects

Very common (>10%): headache.
Common (<10%, >1%): flushing, dizziness, postural hypotension, tachycardia (paradoxical bradycardia also reported), nausea, local stinging, itching or burning sensation after SL spray or rectal administration.
These effects generally settle with continued use.

Dose and use

Intermittent dysphagia and/or odynophagia

- start with 400–500microgram SL 5–15min a.c.
- if necessary, increase to a maximum single dose of 1mg

- instruct the patient to swallow or spit out tablet once pain relief is obtained
- repeat p.r.n.

Persistent spasm
Consider:
- glyceryl trinitrate TD patches *or*
- orally active nitrates, e.g. **isosorbide mononitrate**.

Anal fissure pain
- use 0.2–0.4% rectal ointment (see Supply)
- apply a pea-sized quantity or 2.5 cm length of ointment to the anal rim b.d. for 6–8 weeks.[8]

Painful diabetic neuropathy
- apply glyceryl trinitrate spray locally to the painful extremity: 1 puff/sole of foot/day.

Acute pulmonary oedema in conjunction with diuretics and opioids
Use under the guidance of a cardiologist. Give by SL tablet or spray, or in more severe cases by IVI, e.g.:
- 400microgram SL every 5–10min, *or*
- 10–20microgram/min IVI, titrate every 3–5min as needed in 5–10microgram/min increments, up to a maximum of 200microgram/min.

Supply

Because glyceryl trinitrate is an explosive substance, spray formulations contain additives (e.g. medium chain partial glycerides or alcohol) to stabilize the solution and minimize the potential for explosion (see below).

Glyceryl trinitrate (generic)
Tablets SL 300microgram, 500microgram, 600microgram, 100 = £2.50, £2.50 and £14 respectively; *store in the original glass container; because of degradation, unused tablets should be discarded after 8 weeks.*
Aerosol spray 400microgram/metered dose, 200-dose unit = £3, *contains alcohol.*

Coro-Nitro Pump Spray® (Ayrton Saunders)
Aerosol spray 400microgram/metered dose, 200-dose unit = £3, *contains alcohol and medium chain partial triglycerides.*

Glytrin Spray® (Sanofi-Aventis)
Aerosol spray 400microgram/metered dose, 200-dose unit = £3.50, *contains alcohol.*

Nitrolingual Pumpspray® (Merck Serono)
Aerosol spray 400microgram/metered dose, 200-dose unit = £3.50; *contains alcohol and medium chain partial glycerides.*

Nitromin® (Egis)
Aerosol spray 400microgram/metered dose, 200-dose unit = £2.50, *contains alcohol.*

TD products
Deponit® (UCB)
TD patch 5mg/24h, 10mg/24h, 28 days @ 1 patch daily = £13 and £14 respectively.

Minitran® (Meda)
TD patch 5mg/24h, 10mg/24h, 15mg/24h, 28 days @ 1 patch daily = £12, £13 and £14 respectively.

Nitro-Dur® (Schering-Plough)
TD patch 200microgram/h (approx 5mg/24h), 400microgram/h (approx 10mg/24h), 600microgram/h (approx 15mg/24h), 28 days @ 1 patch daily = £11, £12 and £13 respectively.

Transiderm-Nitro® (Novartis)
TD patch 5mg/24h, 10mg/24h, 28 days @ 1 patch daily = £17 and £19 respectively.

Rectal ointments
Rectogesic® (ProStrakan)
Rectal ointment 0.4%, 30g = £35.

Rectal ointment 0.2%, 20g = £33. (Unlicensed, available as a special order from Queens Medical Centre Pharmacy, Nottingham; see Obtaining unlicensed products, p.769). Can be locally prepared by diluting 2% glyceryl trinitrate ointment (Percutol®, Teva, 60g = £10) 1:10 with white soft paraffin.[26]

1 George S *et al.* (1997) Pain in multiple leiomyomas alleviated by nifedipine. *Pain.* **73**: 101–102.
2 Agrawal RP *et al.* (2007) Glyceryl trinitrate spray in the management of painful diabetic neuropathy: a randomized double blind placebo controlled cross-over study. *Diabetes Research and Clinical Practice.* **77**: 161–167.
3 Agrawal RP *et al.* (2009) Management of diabetic neuropathy by sodium valproate and glyceryl trinitrate spray: a prospective double-blind randomized placebo-controlled study. *Diabetes Research and Clinical Practice.* **83**: 371–378.
4 Dickstein K *et al.* (2008) ESC Guidelines for the diagnosis and treatment of acute and chronic heart failure 2008: the Task Force for the Diagnosis and Treatment of Acute and Chronic Heart Failure 2008 of the European Society of Cardiology. Developed in collaboration with the Heart Failure Association of the ESC (HFA) and endorsed by the European Society of Intensive Care Medicine (ESICM). *European Heart Journal.* **29**: 2388–2442.
5 Baxter K (ed) (2009) Stockley's Drug Interactions (online edition). Pharmaceutical Press, London. Available from: www.medicinescomplete.com/mc/stockley/current/ (subscription required)
6 McDonnell F and Walsh D (1999) Treatment of odynophagia and dysphagia in advanced cancer with sublingual glyceryl trinitrate. *Palliative Medicine.* **13**: 251–252.
7 Tutuian R and Castell DO (2006) Review article: oesophageal spasm — diagnosis and management. *Alimentary Pharmacology and Therapeutics.* **23**: 1393–1402.
8 Lund J and Scholefield J (1997) A randomised, prospective, double-blind, placebo-controlled trial of glyceryl trinitrate ointment in treatment of anal fissure. *Lancet.* **349**: 11–14.
9 Griffin N *et al.* (2004) Quality of life in patients with chronic anal fissure. *Colorectal Disease.* **6**: 39–44.
10 Solomon M and Smith S (2004) Review: medical therapies are less effective than surgery for anal fissure. Available from: http://ebm.bmjjournals.com/cgi/reprint/9/4/112
11 Thornton MJ *et al.* (2005) Manometric effect of topical glyceryl trinitrate and its impact on chronic anal fissure healing. *Diseases of the Colon and Rectum.* **48**: 1207–1212.
12 Fruehauf H *et al.* (2006) Efficacy and safety of botulinum toxin a injection compared with topical nitroglycerin ointment for the treatment of chronic anal fissure: a prospective randomized study. *American Journal of Gastroenterology.* **101**: 2107–2112.
13 Mustafa NA *et al.* (2006) Comparison of topical glyceryl trinitrate ointment and oral nifedipine in the treatment of chronic anal fissure. *Acta Chirurgica Belgica.* **106**: 55–58.
14 Fenton C *et al.* (2006) 0.4% nitroglycerin ointment: in the treatment of chronic anal fissure pain. *Drugs.* **66**: 343–349.
15 Sajid MS *et al.* (2008) The efficacy of diltiazem and glyceryltrinitrate for the medical management of chronic anal fissure: a meta-analysis. (Review). *International Journal of Colorectal Disease.* **23**: 1–6.
16 Hashimoto S and Kobayashi A (2003) Clinical pharmacokinetics and pharmacodynamics of glyceryl trinitrate and its metabolites. *Clinical Pharmacokinetics.* **42**: 205–221.
17 Elliott K *et al.* (1994) The NMDA receptor antagonists, LY274614 and MK-801, and the nitric oxide synthase inhibitor, NG-nitro-L-arginine, attenuate analgesic tolerance to the mu-opioid morphine but not to kappa opioids. *Pain.* **56**: 69–75.
18 Ferreira S *et al.* (1992) Blockade of hyperalgesia and neurogenic oedema by topical application of nitroglycerin. *European Journal of Pharmacology.* **217**: 207–209.
19 Berrazueta J *et al.* (1994) Local transdermal glyceryl trinitrate has an antiinflammatory action on thrombophlebitis induced by sclerosis of leg varicose veins. *Angiology.* **5**: 347–351.
20 Lauretti G *et al.* (1999) Oral ketamine and transdermal nitroglycerin as analgesic adjuvants to oral morphine therapy and amitriptyline for cancer pain management. *Anesthesiology.* **90**: 1528–1533.
21 Lauretti GR *et al.* (2002) Double blind evaluation of transdermal nitroglycerine as adjuvant to oral morphine for cancer pain management. *Journal of Clinical Anesthesia.* **14**: 83–86.
22 El-Sheikh SM and El-Kest E (2004) Transdermal nitroglycerine enhanced fentanyl patch analgesia in cancer pain management. *Egyptian Journal of Anaesthesia.* **20**: 291–294.
23 Paoloni JA *et al.* (2004) Topical glyceryl trinitrate treatment of chronic noninsertional achilles tendinopathy. A randomized, double blind, placebo-controlled trial. *Journal of Bone and Joint Surgery American Volume.* **86-A**: 916–922.
24 Yasuda H *et al.* (2006) Randomized phase II trial comparing nitroglycerin plus vinorelbine and cisplatin with vinorelbine and cisplatin alone in previously untreated stage IIIB/IV non small-cell lung cancer. *Journal of Clinical Oncology.* **24**: 688–694.
25 Institute for Safe Medication Practices (2004) Medication Safety Alert. Burns in MRI patients wearing transdermal patches. Available from: www.ismp.org/Newsletters/acutecare/articles/20040408.asp?ptr = y
26 DTB (1998) Glyceryl trinitrate for anal fissure? *Drug and Therapeutics Bulletin.* **36**: 55–56.

NIFEDIPINE — BNF 2.6.2

Class: Calcium-channel blocker.

Indications: Prophylaxis of stable angina, hypertension, Raynaud's phenomenon (normal-release only licensed formulation), †severe smooth muscle spasm pain (particularly of the oesophagus, rectum and anus, cutaneous leiomyomas),[1–5] †intractable hiccup.[6,7]

Contra-indications: Cardiogenic shock, severe aortic stenosis, acute or unstable angina (normal-release capsules PO or SL may cause hypotension and reflex tachycardia precipitating myocardial or cerebrovascular ischaemia). *Do not use within one month of myocardial infarction.*

Pharmacology

Calcium-channel blockers inhibit the influx of calcium into cells, thereby modifying cell function, e.g. smooth muscle contraction and neural transmission.[8] They have an antinociceptive effect and augment opioid analgesia. Nifedipine may help hiccup by relieving oesophageal spasm or by interference with neural pathways involved in hiccup.[6,7,9] In chronic anal fissure, m/r nifedipine 20mg PO b.d. is as effective as **glyceryl trinitrate** ointment 0.2–0.4% applied b.d. to the anal canal but causes much less headache (see p.70).[10]

Nifedipine exhibits most of its effects on blood vessels, less on the myocardium and has no anti-arrhythmic activity. It rarely precipitates heart failure because any negative inotropic effect is offset by a reduction in left ventricular work. Nifedipine undergoes extensive first-pass metabolism in the liver to inactive metabolites which are excreted in the urine. Higher plasma concentrations are seen in slow metabolizers, which are more prevalent in South American, South Asian and black African populations.[11,12] Hepatic impairment increases bio-availability and halflife.

Bio-availability 45–75% PO (normal-release capsules).
Onset of action 15min (normal-release capsules); 1.5h (m/r tablets, Adalat® Retard).
Time to peak plasma concentration 30min PO (normal-release capsules).
Plasma halflife about 2h (normal-release capsules); 2–2.5h (m/r tablets, Adalat® Retard).
Duration of action 8h (normal-release capsules); 12 or 24h (m/r tablets, depending on brand).

Cautions

Serious drug interactions: augments the hypotensive and negative inotropic effects of other drugs, e.g. α and β antagonists, **chlorpromazine**.[13]

May exacerbate angina; discontinue nifedipine if angina occurs 30–60min after the first dose. Rarely, it may precipitate or worsen heart failure; avoid in patients with significantly impaired cardiac function or heart failure. Hepatic impairment. May impair glucose tolerance and worsen diabetes mellitus.

Nifedipine is metabolized by and inhibits CYP3A4 and CYP2D6; it also inhibits CYP1A2 and CYP2C8/9. Plasma concentration increased by grapefruit juice, protease inhibitors**, cimetidine** (reduce nifedipine dose by 50%), **fluoxetine**, **fluconazole** and **itraconazole**; reduced by **carbamazepine**, **phenobarbital**, **phenytoin** and **rifampicin**. Nifedipine increases plasma concentrations of **sertindole**, **tacrolimus** and **theophylline**; may increase or reduce plasma concentrations of **quinidine** (see Cytochrome P450, p.735).[13]

Undesirable effects

Common (<10%, >1%): headache, dizziness, vasodilation, peripheral oedema, nausea.
Uncommon (<1%, >0.1%): asthenia, lethargy, malaise, agitation, nervousness, sleep disorder, tremor, vertigo, abnormal vision, chest pain, tachycardia, palpitations, postural hypotension, oedema, dyspnoea, dry mouth, dyspepsia, abdominal pain, diarrhoea or constipation, rash, pruritus, sweating.

Dose and use

Patients with angina should not bite into or use a normal-release capsule SL because of the risk of rapid-onset hypotension and reflex tachycardia, which could lead to myocardial or cerebrovascular ischaemia.

- start with 10mg PO/SL stat, and 10–20mg t.d.s. with food, or m/r 20mg b.d. or 30–60mg once daily.
- in achalasia, use 10–20mg SL 30min a.c.
- usual maximum dose 60–80mg/24h.

Up to 160mg/24h has been used for intractable hiccup with concurrent **fludrocortisone** 0.5–1mg to overcome associated orthostatic hypotension.[7]

Supply

Because of their different dosing regimens and concern over possible non-bio-equivalence, the National Prescribing Centre recommends that m/r formulations of nifedipine should be prescribed by brand name.[14]

Nifedipine (generic)
Capsules 5mg, 10mg, 28 days @ 10mg t.d.s. = £6.
Oral solution (drops) 20mg/mL, 30mL = £34. (Unlicensed, available as a special order from The Specials Lab; see Obtaining unlicensed products, p.769.)

Adalat® (Bayer)
Capsules 5mg, 10mg, 28 days @ 10mg t.d.s. = £7.

Modified-release
Adalat Retard (Bayer)
Tablets m/r 10mg, 20mg, 28 days @ 20mg b.d. = £9.

Adalat LA (Bayer)
Tablets m/r 20mg, 30mg, 60mg, 28 days @ 30mg once daily = £7.

Adipine® MR (Chiesi)
Tablets m/r 10mg, 20mg, 28 days @ 20mg b.d. = £5.

Adipine® XL (Chiesi)
Tablets m/r 30mg, 60mg, 28 days @ 30mg once daily = £5.

This is not a complete list; see BNF for more information.

1 Cargill G *et al.* (1982) Nifedipine for relief of esophageal chest pain. *New England Journal of Medicine.* **307**: 187–188.
2 Al-Waili N (1990) Nifedipine for intestinal colic. *Journal of the American Medical Association.* **263**: 3258.
3 Celik A *et al.* (1995) Hereditary proctalgia fugax and constipation: report of a second family. *Gut.* **36**: 581–584.
4 George S *et al.* (1997) Pain in multiple leiomyomas alleviated by nifedipine. *Pain.* **73**: 101–102.
5 McLoughlin R and McQuillan R (1997) Using nifedipine to treat tenesmus. *Palliative Medicine.* **11**: 419–420.
6 Lipps DC *et al.* (1990) Nifedipine for intractable hiccups. *Neurology.* **40**: 531–532.
7 Brigham B and Bolin T (1992) High dose nifedipine and fludrocortisone for intractable hiccups. *Medical Journal of Australia.* **157**: 70.
8 Castell DO (1985) Calcium-channel blocking agents for gastrointestinal disorders. *American Journal of Cardiology.* **55**: 210B–213B.
9 Williams M (2004) The management of hiccups in advanced cancer. *CME Cancer Medicine.* **2**: 68–70.
10 Mustafa NA *et al.* (2006) Comparison of topical glyceryl trinitrate ointment and oral nifedipine in the treatment of chronic anal fissure. *Acta Chirurgica Belgica.* **106**: 55–58.
11 Sowunmi A *et al.* (1995) Ethnic differences in nifedipine kinetics: comparisons between Nigerians, Caucasians and South Asians. *British Journal of Clinical Pharmacology.* **40**: 489–493.
12 Castaneda-Hernandez G *et al.* (1996) Interethnic variability in nifedipine disposition: reduced systemic plasma clearance in Mexican subjects. *British Journal of Clinical Pharmacology.* **41**: 433–434.
13 Baxter K (2011) Stockley's Drug Interactions (online edition). Pharmaceutical Press, London. Available from: www.medicinescomplete.com
14 National Prescribing Centre (2000) Modified-release preparations. *MeReC Bulletin.* **11**: 13–16.

LOW MOLECULAR WEIGHT HEPARIN (LMWH) BNF 2.8.1

Indications: Surgical thromboprophylaxis (**bemiparin, dalteparin, enoxaparin, tinzaparin**), medical thromboprophylaxis (**dalteparin, enoxaparin**), initial treatment of thrombo-embolism (**dalteparin, enoxaparin, tinzaparin**), treatment of cancer associated thrombosis (**dalteparin**), prevention of clotting in extracorporeal circuits during haemodialysis (**bemiparin, dalteparin, enoxaparin, tinzaparin**), unstable angina and non-Q wave myocardial infarction (**dalteparin, enoxaparin**), †thrombophlebitis migrans, †disseminated intravascular coagulation (DIC).

Contra-indications: Active major bleeding, suspected or confirmed immune-mediated heparin-induced thrombocytopenia (HIT) with a LMWH, known bleeding diathesis, severe uncontrolled hypertension, haemorrhagic stroke, diabetic or haemorrhagic retinopathy, bacterial

endocarditis, injury or surgery involving the brain, spinal cord, eyes or ears, spinal analgesia (if *treatment* dose of LMWH, increased risk of spinal haematoma), IM use (risk of haematoma at the injection site).
Note: variation exists in what manufacturers consider to be a contra-indication or a caution; see SPCs.

Pharmacology

Several varieties of low molecular weight heparin (LMWH) are now available, e.g. **bemiparin**, **certoparin** (not UK), **dalteparin**, **enoxaparin**, **nadroparin** (not UK), **parnaparin** (not UK), **reviparin** (not UK), and **tinzaparin**. All LMWH is derived from porcine heparin and some patients may need to avoid it because of hypersensitivity, or for religious or cultural reasons. The most appropriate non-porcine alternative is **fondaparinux**.[1–3]

LMWH acts by potentiating the inhibitory effect of antithrombin III on factor Xa and thrombin. It has a relatively higher ability to potentiate factor Xa inhibition than to prolong plasma clotting time (APTT), which cannot be used to guide dosing.[1] Anti-factor Xa activity levels can be measured if necessary, e.g. if a patient is at increased risk of bleeding, but routine monitoring is not generally required because the dose is determined by the patient's weight.

LMWH is as effective as unfractionated heparin for the treatment of DVT and pulmonary embolism (PE) and is now considered the initial treatment of choice.[1] Other advantages include a longer duration of action which allows administration once daily, and possibly a better safety profile, e.g. fewer major haemorrhages.[4,5]

Compared with non-cancer patients, those with cancer are about three times more likely to experience recurrent thrombo-embolism, *despite* optimal oral anticoagulant treatment (e.g. 21% vs. 7% of patients).[6] The increased risk results from the cancer-related pro-inflammatory state, activation of the coagulation cascade by procoagulant proteins expressed by the cancer, damage to blood vessel walls and venous stasis in addition to other general risk factors (Box 2.D). Major bleeding is also more likely in patients with cancer, irrespective of the INR.[7] In patients with cancer, LMWH is more effective than **warfarin**, with a similar (or reduced) risk of bleeding.[8–11] Thus, LMWH is considered superior to **warfarin** for the treatment of thrombo-embolism in patients with cancer (UK specialist guidelines)[12] and is recommended for at least the first 3–6 months of indefinite anticoagulation for thrombo-embolism in patients with cancer (USA specialist guidelines).[13] It has also been recommended as the treatment of choice in the management of thrombo-embolism in the advanced cancer setting.[14]

Box 2.D Main risk factors for thrombo-embolism in medical patients[2,15–22]

Age ⩾40 years, particularly >60 years
Immobility
Dehydration
Obesity
Cancer, particularly metastatic, especially of the pancreas, stomach, bladder, ovary, uterus, kidney or lung; also haematological
Chronic respiratory or cardiac disease
Other serious medical conditions, e.g. sepsis, lower limb weakness (including spinal cord compression), inflammatory bowel disease, collagen disorder
Varicose veins/chronic venous insufficiency
Previous thrombo-embolism
Cancer chemotherapy, e.g. platinum compounds, 5-FU, mitomycin-C, thalidomide
Growth factors, e.g. granulocyte colony stimulating factor, erythropoietin
Radiation therapy, e.g. to the pelvis
Hormone therapy, e.g. oral contraceptives, hormone replacement, tamoxifen, anastrozole, and possibly progestins
Thrombophilia

LMWH is the preferred choice for indefinite anticoagulation in patients for whom maintaining a stable INR is likely to be, or turns out to be, difficult (risking either therapeutic failure or haemorrhagic complications) or those who have recurrent thrombo-embolism despite a therapeutic INR.

LMWH is also the treatment of choice for *chronic* DIC; this commonly presents as recurrent thromboses in both superficial and deep veins which do not respond to **warfarin**. Antifibrinolytic drugs, e.g. **tranexamic acid** and **aminocaproic acid** (not UK), should not be used in DIC because they increase the risk of end-organ damage from microvascular thromboses. For recurrent thrombo-embolism despite LMWH, exclude HIT, check patient adherence and seek the advice of a haematologist.

LMWH interacts with growth factors, other blood components and vascular cells. An anticancer effect has been seen, possibly via inhibiting cancer-cell growth, angiogenesis and metastasis.[23–26] Survival is improved in cancer patients receiving LMWH compared with unfractionated heparin, or when LMWH is given in addition to chemotherapy compared with chemotherapy alone. This effect cannot be attributed to differences in thrombosis or complications of bleeding and the improvement was greatest in those whose life expectancy was >6 months at the outset of treatment. However, such use of LMWH is not currently recommended outside of a clinical trial.[1]

For pharmacokinetic details, see Table 2.1. It is possible that LMWH will be superseded by direct thrombin inhibitors, e.g. **dabigatran** or specific factor Xa inhibitors, e.g. **fondaparinux**.[1–3] Some of these need be administered only once weekly, e.g. **idraparinux** (not UK).[27]

Table 2.1 Selected pharmacokinetic details for dalteparin, enoxaparin and tinzaparin[28–31]

	Dalteparin	*Enoxaparin*	*Tinzaparin*
Bio-availability SC[a]	87%	100%	87%
Onset of action	3min IV 2–4h SC	5min IV 3h SC	5min IV 2–3h SC
Time to peak plasma activity[a]	4h SC	2–6h SC	4–5h SC
Plasma activity halflife[a]	2h IV 3–5h SC	2–4.5h IV 4.5–7h SC	1.5h IV 3–4h SC
Duration of action	10–24h SC	>24h SC	24h

a. based on anti-factor Xa activity.

Cautions

Note: variation exists in what manufacturers consider to be a contra-indication or a caution; see SPCs.

Serious drug interactions: enhanced anticoagulant effect with anticoagulant/antiplatelet drugs, e.g. NSAIDs (particularly **ketorolac**).

Increased risk of haemorrhage if underlying bleeding diathesis (e.g. thrombocytopenia), recent cerebral haemorrhage, recent neurological or ophthalmic surgery, uncontrolled hypertension, diabetic or hypertensive retinopathy, current or past peptic ulcer.

Risk of spinal (intrathecal or epidural) haematoma in patients undergoing spinal puncture or with an indwelling spinal catheter, particularly if concurrently receiving a drug which affects haemostasis. Spinal analgesia may be used in patients on *thromboprophylactic* doses of LMWH but monitor for neurological impairment.

Severe hepatic impairment: reduced synthesis of clotting factors increases the risk of bleeding. Caution (e.g. consider dose reduction) is recommended for **dalteparin**, **enoxaparin** (also possible risk of accumulation) and **tinzaparin**. Dose reduction is recommended for **tinzaparin** in patients with severe hepatic impairment who are also undergoing haemodialysis.

Severe renal impairment: dose reduction is recommended for **enoxaparin** and may be necessary for **dalteparin** and **tinzaparin** (see below).

Inhibition of aldosterone secretion by heparin/LMWH may cause hyperkalaemia. The risk increases with duration of therapy and is higher in patients with diabetes mellitus, chronic renal failure, acidosis and those taking potassium supplements or potassium-sparing drugs. The CSM recommends measuring plasma potassium in such patients before starting heparin and regularly thereafter, particularly if heparin is to be continued for > 1 week.

Undesirable effects

Common (<10%, >1%): headache, dizziness, pain at the injection site, minor bleeding (generally haematoma at the injection site), major bleeding in surgical patients receiving thromboprophylaxis and patients being treated for DVT or PE, tachycardia, chest pain, peripheral oedema, hypotension, hypertension, anaemia, nausea, constipation, reversible increases in liver transaminase enzymes, back pain, haematuria.
Uncommon (<1%, >0.1%): major bleeding in patients receiving thromboprophylaxis, thrombocytopenia (see below), abdominal pain, diarrhoea.

Heparin-induced thrombocytopenia

Both standard heparin and LMWH can cause thrombocytopenia (platelet count $< 100 \times 10^9$/L). An early (<4 days) mild fall in platelet count is often seen after starting heparin therapy, particularly after surgery. This corrects spontaneously despite the continued use of heparin and is asymptomatic.[32] However, in <1% of patients, immune HIT develops, associated with heparin-dependent IgG antibodies (Box 2.E).[32–34] The antibodies form a complex with platelet factor 4 and bind to the platelet surface, causing disruption of the platelets and a release of procoagulant material. HIT manifests as venous or arterial thrombo-embolism which may be fatal.

Box 2.E Diagnosis and management of heparin-induced thrombocytopenia (HIT)[33–35]

High clinical suspicion for HIT
- platelet count fall below the normal range or by >50%, generally after >4 days of heparin use, sometimes sooner and occasionally several days after heparin has been stopped
- new thrombotic or thrombo-embolic event (routine lower-limb ultrasonography is recommended, whether or not there is clinical evidence of DVT)
- necrosis or erythematous plaques at injection sites.

If any of the above occur, evaluate probability of HIT and obtain advice from a haematologist.

Diagnosis
Based on both the clinical probability (see Table 2.2) and laboratory tests, e.g.:
- platelet activation assay using washed platelets if available, *or*
- antigen-based high-sensitivity assay of platelet factor 4/heparin IgG antibodies.

Therapeutic approach
If high probability of HIT, while awaiting results of laboratory test:
- stop heparin or LMWH
- start treatment with a non-heparin anticoagulant, e.g. danaparoid, lepirudin, whether or not there is clinical evidence of a DVT.

Do not:
- use warfarin alone because this may increase the risk of venous limb gangrene
- prescribe warfarin until the platelet count has recovered, i.e. $\geq 150 \times 10^9$/L
- give prophylactic platelet transfusions.

The non-heparin anticoagulant should be continued until:
- the platelet count has stabilized
- the INR has reached a therapeutic level
- warfarin has been taken for ≥5 days (i.e. overlapping with the non-heparin anticoagulant).

Preventing recurrence
- record the diagnosis in the patient's notes as a serious allergy
- warn the patient to avoid the future use of heparin and LMWH
- issue an antibody card.

HIT is less common with prophylactic regimens (low doses) than with therapeutic ones (higher doses) and with LMWH rather than unfractionated heparin. Cross-reactivity between unfractionated heparin and LMWH is rare. HIT typically develops 5–10 days after starting heparin, but rarely >15 days. Routine monitoring of the platelet count is recommended (see p.80). *LMWH should be stopped immediately if there is a fall in the platelet count below the normal range or by >50% and the advice of a haematologist obtained.*

Because the procoagulant material released by the disintegrating platelets increases the risk of thrombosis, anticoagulation should be continued with a non-heparin anticoagulant, such as **danaparoid** (a heparinoid) or **lepirudin** (a hirudin derivative) even if there is no clinically evident thrombosis.[34,35]

The risk of HIT with **fondaparinux** (a synthetic factor Xa inhibitor) is also likely to be low.[34] If possible, surgery should be avoided in patients with HIT for at least 3 months, after which they generally become antibody negative. Even so, for patients with a history of HIT, if subsequent thromboprophylaxis or anticoagulation for a thrombo-embolism is required, a non-heparin anticoagulant should be used.[34] For patients requiring dialysis with HIT or a history of HIT, seek specialist advice.

Table 2.2 Estimating the pre-laboratory-test probability of HIT: the 'four Ts' (adapted from[36])

	Score		
	2	*1*	*0*
Feature present			
Thrombocytopenia	>50% fall or platelet nadir 20–100 × 10^9/L	30–50% fall or platelet nadir 10–19 × 10^9/L	<30% fall or platelet nadir <10 × 10^9/L
Timing of platelet count fall or other sequelae	Clear onset after 5–10 days; or <1 day if heparin exposure within past 100 days	Onset of thrombocytopenia after 10 days, or unclear due to missing counts	Platelet count fall too early (without recent heparin exposure)
Thrombosis or other sequelae	New thrombosis, skin necrosis or post-heparin bolus acute systemic reaction	Progressive or recurrent thrombosis, erythematous skin lesions or suspected thrombosis not yet proven	None
Other cause of thrombocytopenia present	None	Possible	Definite
Combine the scores for the four individual features to obtain a total score			
Probability of HIT	6–8 high	4–5 intermediate	0–3 low

Dose and use

There are no UK guidelines for the *treatment* of venous thrombo-embolism specific to patients with incurable cancer. More specific guidelines are available in the USA.[13] Anticoagulation should be considered for those who:

- develop a DVT (indefinite anticoagulation, using LMWH for at least 3–6 months)[13]
- sustain a PE (indefinite anticoagulation, using LMWH for at least 3–6 months)[13]
- are hospitalized and bedbound as a result of an acute medical illness for ⩾3 days (see Thromboprophylaxis below).[18,22]

Currently, only **dalteparin** is licensed for extended treatment of DVT, PE and prevention of recurrence. Generally, indefinite anticoagulation is discontinued only if contra-indications develop, or when the patient reaches the stage when symptom relief alone is appropriate, e.g. in the last few weeks of life.

If patients undergoing curative treatment for cancer experience thrombo-embolism and are deemed to have only a transient risk factor, duration of treatment is generally 3 months (DVT) or 6 months (PE). Long-term anticoagulation should be considered following a second episode of thrombo-embolism, or for those with a first episode considered to have a significant ongoing risk factor. Thrombo-embolism in a 'cured' cancer patient may be related to disease recurrence. If truly idiopathic, a minimum of 6–12 months of anticoagulation is recommended but long-term anticoagulation should be considered.

In patients at high risk of recurrent thrombo-embolism for whom anticoagulation is contra-indicated, an inferior vena caval filter may be an option, but requires careful patient selection.

SC injections

May cause transient stinging and local bruising.[37] Rotate injection sites daily, e.g. between left and right anterolateral and left and right posterolateral abdominal wall; introduce the total length of the needle vertically into the thickest part of a skin fold produced by squeezing the skin between the thumb and forefinger. Do not rub the injection site.

For the manufacturers' recommended sites for injection, see respective SPCs and **dalteparin** and **enoxaparin** monographs (p.84 and p.89). The long-term use of SC injections is not acceptable to some patients with cancer (about 15% in one survey).[38]

Severe renal impairment (creatinine clearance <30mL/min)

Clearance of **enoxaparin** is reduced by up to 65% and **tinzaparin** clearance is decreased by up to 25%. The manufacturers recommend dose reduction for **enoxaparin** (see p.89). The anti-factor Xa activity halflives of **dalteparin** and **tinzaparin** are prolonged, and specialist guidelines suggest monitoring anti-factor Xa activity to guide dosing in severe renal impairment.[1] For example, the dose of **tinzaparin** should be reduced if anti-factor Xa activity exceeds 1.5 units/mL (usual range 1–1.2 units/mL).[39]

During haemodialysis, the IV or extracorporeal circuit dose of **dalteparin** should be reduced in patients with acute renal failure, or with chronic renal failure and an increased risk of bleeding. The dose of **tinzaparin** should be reduced in patients with severe hepatic impairment who require haemodialysis (see respective SPCs).

Specialist guidelines suggest using unfractionated heparin IV instead of LMWH in severe renal impairment but the evidence is grade 2C; i.e. not based on RCT.[1,13,22]

Routine platelet count monitoring

All patients should have a baseline platelet count before starting LMWH. Those who have received unfractionated heparin in the last 3 months should have a repeat platelet count after 24h to exclude rapid-onset HIT due to pre-existing antibodies. Subsequently, and for all patients, a platelet count should be monitored every 2–4 days from days 4–14.[34]

Thromboprophylaxis

For **dalteparin** and **enoxaparin** monographs, see p.84 and p.89 respectively.

Patients with cancer undergoing surgery

Patients with cancer undergoing major surgery are at high risk of thrombo-embolism; they have twice the risk of developing a DVT and three times the risk of a fatal PE.[40] Abdominal and pelvic surgery is particularly high-risk.[41,42]

The dose of **tinzaparin** in high-risk surgical patients is:

- 50 units/kg 2h before surgery, then 50 units/kg every 24h for 7–10 days *or*
- 4,500 units 12h before surgery, then 4,500 units every 24h for 7–10 days.

However, 4 weeks of thromboprophylaxis is more effective than 1 week and thromboprophylaxis should be continued for 2–4 weeks after hospital discharge in patients with cancer (and in non-cancer patients >60 years old or with a history of thrombo-embolism).[18,43,44]

Patients with cancer with indwelling venous catheters

The presence of a central (subclavian) or peripheral indwelling venous catheter can lead to catheter-related thrombosis. It occurs in up to two thirds of patients and is symptomatic in 10–30%, although more recent figures suggest the incidence is falling (5–15%), possibly as a result of improved catheter materials and placement. Routine thromboprophylaxis with LMWH is not recommended because RCTs have shown no benefit from their use (e.g. **enoxaparin** 40mg daily), or from low-dose **warfarin** (1mg daily).[18,22,45–47]

Patients with cancer who are immobile or confined to bed because of a concurrent acute medical illness

Compared with surgical patients, thromboprophylaxis is underused in medical patients, even though mortality and morbidity from thrombo-embolism (major/fatal PE) and its treatment (major/fatal haemorrhage) are higher in medical patients.[48]

Hospitalized cancer patients will be at high risk of venous thrombo-embolism, and specialist guidelines recommend that thromboprophylaxis should be considered if an acute medical illness is likely to render them bedbound for ⩾3 days, particularly in the presence of one or more additional risk factors (Box 2.D).[1,22,41] Duration of treatment is generally ⩽2 weeks.[20]

If anticoagulation is contra-indicated, the use of graduated compression stockings or intermittent pneumatic compression is recommended.[18] However, the evidence base in medical patients is limited and in some populations there have been reports of harm.[49]

Thromboprophylaxis appears acceptable to palliative care inpatients,[50] and should be considered for patients meeting the above criteria. The decision to use thromboprophylaxis should take into account the views of patients, family/informal carers and the multiprofessional team, and be reviewed every few days. (Note: NICE guidance suggests reviewing daily, but this seems excessive and will often be impractical.[22])

However, thromboprophylaxis is less relevant for cancer patients with a poor performance status in their last few weeks–days of life, e.g. when admitted for terminal care or started on an end-of-life care pathway;[22] in other words, when symptom relief alone would be the most appropriate treatment for any new thrombo-embolic episode.

Patients with cancer undertaking long-distance air travel

The evidence for an association between prolonged travel and venous thrombo-embolism is controversial.[18] The risk appears greatest in journeys of >6h and in those travellers with one or more pre-existing risk factors (see Box 2.D). Although there is insufficient evidence to support routine thromboprophylaxis in any group, all travellers should follow some general recommendations (Box 2.F). The need for additional measures in those deemed to be at an increased risk (e.g. patients with cancer) should be made on an individual basis (Box 2.F).

Box 2.F Recommendations for preventing thrombo-embolism in long-distance travel (>6h)[18]

General recommendations for all travellers

Avoid constrictive clothing around the waist and lower limbs.

Avoid dehydration.

Frequently stretch the calf muscles by moving the feet up and down.

Additional recommendations for travellers with one or more risk factors for thrombo-embolism (see Box 2.D)

Properly fitted, below-knee graduated compression stockings, providing 15–30mmHg of pressure at the ankle *or*

A single prophylactic dose of LMWH (e.g. enoxaparin 40mg) 2–4h before departure.

Treatment

For **dalteparin** and **enoxaparin** monographs, see p.84 and p.89 respectively.

DVT and PE

Uncomplicated DVT or PE are increasingly treated on an outpatient basis.[51] Some centres use a fixed-dose regimen (see Box 2.G, p.87):[52]

- general guidance is to give **tinzaparin**, 175 units/kg SC once daily for at least 6 days, or until the INR has been in the therapeutic range for two successive days
- USA guidelines specific to patients with cancer advise giving LMWH, e.g. **tinzaparin** 175 units/kg SC once daily, for at least the first 3–6 months, followed by LMWH or warfarin indefinitely, or until the cancer is cured[13]

If **warfarin** is used, the LMWH should be continued until the INR is ≥2 on two consecutive days.

In palliative care, LMWH is preferable because haemorrhagic complications with **warfarin** occur in nearly 50% (possibly related to a poor performance status, drug interactions and hepatic impairment). Those patients agreeing to the indefinite use of LMWH have found it acceptable.[37,50,53,54] Compared with **warfarin**, treatment with LMWH is more straightforward (no blood tests or need for frequent dose adjustments).

Disseminated intravascular coagulation (DIC)

- confirm the diagnosis:
  - ▹ thrombocytopenia (platelet count $<150 \times 10^9$/L in 95% of cases)
  - ▹ decreased plasma fibrinogen concentration
  - ▹ elevated plasma D-dimer concentration, a fibrin degradation product (85% of cases)
  - ▹ prolonged prothrombin time and/or partial thromboplastin time.[55]

A normal plasma fibrinogen concentration (200–250mg/100mL) is also suspicious because fibrinogen levels are generally raised in cancer (e.g. 450–500mg/100mL) unless there is extensive liver disease. Infection and cancer both may be associated with an increased platelet count which likewise may mask an evolving thrombocytopenia.

- do not use **warfarin** because it is ineffective
- for chronic DIC presenting with recurrent thromboses, give LMWH as for treatment of DVT
- for chronic or acute DIC presenting with haemorrhagic manifestations (e.g. ecchymoses, haematomas), seek specialist advice.

Thrombophlebitis migrans

- do not use **warfarin** because it is ineffective
- generally responds rapidly to small doses of LMWH
- if necessary, titrate dose to maximum allowed according to weight
- continue treatment indefinitely.[56]

Overdose

In emergencies, **protamine sulphate** can be used to reverse the effects of **tinzaparin**:

- for each 100 units of **tinzaparin**, give 1mg of **protamine sulphate**
- give a maximum of 50mg by IV injection over 10min.

Note: the anti-factor Xa activity of **tinzaparin** cannot be completely neutralized even by high doses of **protamine sulphate** (maximum reversal ~60%).

In three patients who bled after surgery or an invasive procedure, a single dose of recombinant activated **factor VIIa** concentrate 20–30microgram/kg IV successfully reversed anticoagulation from LMWH. It did not precipitate thrombosis, despite all patients having risk factors for hypercoagulation, e.g. protein S deficiency, antiphospholipid antibody syndrome, cancer-related surgery.[57]

Supply

Dalteparin and **enoxaparin**: see respective monographs, p.84 and p.89.

Tinzaparin

Innohep® (Leo)

Injection 10,000 units/mL, 0.25mL (2,500 unit) syringe = £2, 0.35mL (3,500 unit) syringe = £3, 0.45mL (4,500 unit) syringe = £4, 2mL (20,000 unit) vial = £11.

Injection 20,000 units/mL, 0.5mL (10,000 unit) syringe = £8, 0.7mL (14,000 unit) syringe = £12, 0.9mL (18,000 unit) syringe = £15, 2mL (40,000 unit) vial = £34.

---

1 Baglin T *et al.* (2006) Guidelines on the use and monitoring of heparin. *British Journal of Haematology.* **133**: 19–34.

2 Blann AD and Lip GY (2006) Venous thromboembolism. *British Medical Journal.* **332**: 215–219.

3 Cohen AT *et al.* (2006) Efficacy and safety of fondaparinux for the prevention of venous thromboembolism in older acute medical patients: randomised placebo controlled trial. *British Medical Journal.* **332**: 325–329.

4 Van Dongen CJ *et al.* (2004) Fixed dose subcutaneous low molecular weight heparins versus adjusted dose unfractionated heparin for venous thromboembolism. *Cochrane Database of Systematic Reviews.* **4**: CD001100.

5 Quinlan D *et al.* (2004) Low-molecular weight heparin compared with intravenous unfractionated heparin for treatment of pulmonary embolism. *Annals of internal medicine.* **140**: 175–183.

6 Prandoni P *et al.* (2002) Recurrent venous thromboembolism and bleeding complications during anticoagulant treatment in patients with cancer and venous thrombosis. *Blood.* **100**: 3484–3488.

7 Streiff MB (2006) Long-term therapy of venous thromboembolism in cancer patients. *Journal of the National Comprehensive Cancer Network.* **4**: 903–910.

8 Meyer G *et al.* (2002) Comparison of low-molecular-weight heparin and warfarin for the secondary prevention of venous thromboembolism in patients with cancer: a randomized controlled study. *Archives of Internal Medicine.* **162**: 1729–1735.

9 Lee A *et al.* (2003) Low molecular weight heparin versus a coumarin for the prevention of recurrent venous thromboembolism in patients with cancer. *New England Journal of Medicine.* **349**: 146–153.

10 Iorio A *et al.* (2003) Low-molecular-weight heparin for the long-term treatment of symptomatic venous thromboembolism: meta-analysis of the randomized comparisons with oral anticoagulants. *Journal of Thrombosis and Haemostasis.* **1**: 1906–1913.

11 Hull RD *et al.* (2006) Long-term low-molecular-weight heparin versus usual care in proximal-vein thrombosis patients with cancer. *American Journal of Medicine.* **119**: 1062–1072.

12 Keeling D *et al.* (2011) Guidelines on oral anticoagulation with warfarin: fourth edition. *British Journal of Haematology.* Epub ahead of print. doi:10.1111/j.1365-2141.2011.08753.x

13 Kearon C *et al.* (2008) Antithrombotic therapy for venous thromboembolic disease: American College of Chest Physicians Evidence-Based Clinical Practice Guidelines (8th Edition). *Chest.* **133 (suppl 6)**: 454S–545S.

14 Noble SI *et al.* (2008) The management of venous thromboembolism in advanced cancer: a systematic review and meta-analysis by the thrombosis task group, on behalf of the Association for Palliative Medicine Science Committee. *Lancet Oncology.* **9**: 577–584.

15 Samama MM *et al.* (1999) A comparison of enoxaparin with placebo for the prevention of venous thromboembolism in acutely ill medical patients. Prophylaxis in Medical Patients with Enoxaparin Study Group. *New England Journal of Medicine.* **341**: 793–800.

16 De Cicco M (2004) The prothrombotic state in cancer: pathogenic mechanisms. *Critical Reviews in Oncology Hematology.* **50**: 187–196.

17 Deitcher SR and Gomes MP (2004) The risk of venous thromboembolic disease associated with adjuvant hormone therapy for breast carcinoma: a systematic review. *Cancer.* **101**: 439–449.

18 Geerts WH *et al.* (2008) Prevention of venous thromboembolism: American College of Chest Physicians Evidence-Based Clinical Practice Guidelines (8th Edition). *Chest.* **133 (suppl 6)**: 381S–453S.

19 Leizorovicz A *et al.* (2004) Randomized, placebo-controlled trial of dalteparin for the prevention of venous thromboembolism in acutely ill medical patients. *Circulation.* **110**: 874–879.

20 Leizorovicz A and Mismetti P (2004) Preventing venous thromboembolism in medical patients. *Circulation.* **110**: IV13–19.

21 Chew HK *et al.* (2006) Incidence of venous thromboembolism and its effect on survival among patients with common cancers. *Archives of Internal Medicine.* **166**: 458–464.

22 NICE (2010) Clinical Guideline 92: Reducing the risk of venous thromboembolism (deep vein thrombosis and pulmonary embolism) in patients admitted to hospital. London. Available from: www.nice.org.uk/guidance/CG92

23 Hettiarachchi RJ *et al.* (1999) Do heparins do more than just treat thrombosis? The influence of heparins on cancer spread. *Journal of Thrombosis and Haemostasis.* **82**: 947–952.

24 Khorana AA and Fine RL (2004) Pancreatic cancer and thromboembolic disease. *Lancet Oncology.* **5**: 655–663.

25 Klerk CP *et al.* (2005) The effect of low molecular weight heparin on survival in patients with advanced malignancy. *Journal of Clinical Oncology.* **23**: 2130–2135.

26 Cunningham RS (2006) The role of low-molecular-weight heparins as supportive care therapy in cancer-associated thrombosis. *Seminars in Oncology.* **33**: S17–25.

27 Prandoni P (2004) Toward the simplification of antithrombotic treatment of venous thromboembolism. *Annals of internal medicine.* **140**: 925–926.

28 Bara L and Samama M (1990) Pharmacokinetics of low molecular weight heparins. *Acta Chirurgica Scandinavica Supplementum.* **556 (suppl)**: 57–61.

29 Dawes J (1990) Comparison of the pharmacokinetics of enoxaparin (Clexane) and unfractionated heparin. *Acta Chirurgica Scandinavica Supplementum.* **556 (suppl)**: 68–74.

30 Fareed J *et al.* (1990) Pharmacologic profile of a low molecular weight heparin (enoxaparin): experimental and clinical validation of the prophylactic antithrombotic effects. *Acta Chirurgica Scandinavica Suppl.* **556 (suppl)**: 75–90.

31 Fossler MJ *et al.* (2001) Pharmacodynamics of intravenous and subcutaneous tinzaparin and heparin in healthy volunteers. *American Journal of Health System Pharmacy.* **58**: 1614–1621.

32 Warkentin T *et al.* (1995) Heparin-induced thrombocytopenia in patients treated with low molecular weight heparin or unfractionated heparin. *New England Journal of Medicine.* **332**: 1330–1335.

33 Hirsh J *et al.* (2001) Heparin and low-molecular-weight heparin: mechanisms of action, pharmacokinetics, dosing, monitoring, efficacy, and safety. *Chest.* **119 (suppl)**: 64S–94S.

34 Keeling D *et al.* (2006) The management of heparin-induced thrombocytopenia. *British Journal of Haematology.* **133**: 259–269.

35 Warkentin TE and Greinacher A (2008) Treatment and prevention of heparin-induced thrombocytopenia: American College of Chest Physicians Evidence-Based Clinical Practice Guidelines (8th Edition). *Chest.* **133 (suppl 6)**: 340S–380S.

36 Warkentin TE and Heddle NM (2003) Laboratory diagnosis of immune heparin-induced thrombocytopenia. *Current Hematology Reports.* **2**: 148–157.

37 Noble SI and Finlay IG (2005) Is long-term low-molecular-weight heparin acceptable to palliative care patients in the treatment of cancer related venous thromboembolism? A qualitative study. *Palliative Medicine.* **19**: 197–201.
38 Wittkowsky AK (2006) Barriers to the long-term use of low-molecular weight heparins for treatment of cancer-associated thrombosis. *Journal of Thrombosis and Haemostasis.* **4**: 2090–2091.
39 Leo Laboratories *Personal communication.*
40 Kakkar AK and Williamson RC (1999) Prevention of venous thromboembolism in cancer patients. *Seminars in Thrombosis and Hemostasis.* **25**: 239–243.
41 Cunningham MS *et al.* (2006) Prevention and management of venous thromboembolism in people with cancer: a review of the evidence. *Clinical Oncology (Royal College of Radiologists).* **18**: 145–151.
42 Negus JJ *et al.* (2006) Thromboprophylaxis in major abdominal surgery for cancer. *European Journal of Surgical Oncology.* **32**: 911–916.
43 Bergqvist D *et al.* (2002) Duration of prophylaxis against venous thromboembolism with enoxaparin after surgery for cancer. *New England Journal of Medicine.* **346**: 975–980.
44 Kher A and Samama MM (2005) Primary and secondary prophylaxis of venous thromboembolism with low-molecular-weight heparins: prolonged thromboprophylaxis, an alternative to vitamin K antagonists. *Journal of Thrombosis and Haemostasis.* **3**: 473–481.
45 Tesselaar ME *et al.* (2004) Risk factors for catheter-related thrombosis in cancer patients. *European Journal of Cancer.* **40**: 2253–2259.
46 Couban S *et al.* (2005) Randomized Placebo-Controlled Study of Low-Dose Warfarin for the Prevention of Central Venous Catheter-Associated Thrombosis in Patients With Cancer. *Journal of Clinical Oncology.* **23**: 4063–4069.
47 Verso M *et al.* (2005) Enoxaparin for the Prevention of Venous Thromboembolism Associated With Central Vein Catheter: A Double-Blind, Placebo-Controlled, Randomized Study in Cancer Patients. *Journal of Clinical Oncology.* **23**: 4057–4062.
48 Monreal M *et al.* (2004) The outcome after treatment of venous thromboembolism is different in surgical and acutely ill medical patients. Findings from the RIETE registry. *Journal of Thrombosis and Haemostasis.* **2**: 1892–1898.
49 Dennis M *et al.* (2009) Effectiveness of thigh-length graduated compression stockings to reduce the risk of deep vein thrombosis after stroke (CLOTS trial 1): a multicentre, randomised controlled trial. *Lancet.* **373**: 1958–1965.
50 Noble SI *et al.* (2006) Acceptability of low molecular weight heparin thromboprophylaxis for inpatients receiving palliative care: qualitative study. *British Medical Journal.* **332**: 577–580.
51 Wells PS *et al.* (2005) A randomized trial comparing 2 low-molecular-weight heparins for the outpatient treatment of deep vein thrombosis and pulmonary embolism. *Archives of Internal Medicine.* **165**: 733–738.
52 Monreal M *et al.* (2004) Fixed-dose low-molecular-weight heparin for secondary prevention of venous thromboembolism in patients with disseminated cancer: a prospective cohort study. *Journal of Thrombosis and Haemostasis.* **2**: 1311–1315.
53 Johnson M (1997) Problems of anticoagulation within a palliative care setting: an audit of hospice patients taking warfarin. *Palliative Medicine.* **11**: 306–312.
54 Johnson M and Sherry K (1997) How do palliative physicians manage venous thromboembolism? *Palliative Medicine.* **11**: 462–468.
55 Spero J *et al.* (1980) Disseminated intravascular coagulation: findings in 346 patients. *Journal of Thrombosis and Haemostasis.* **43**: 28–33.
56 Walsh-McMonagle D and Green D (1997) Low-molecular weight heparin in the management of Trousseau's syndrome. *Cancer.* **80**: 649–655.
57 Firozvi K *et al.* (2006) Reversal of low-molecular-weight heparin-induced bleeding in patients with pre-existing hypercoagulable states with human recombinant activated factor VII concentrate. *American Journal of Hematology.* **81**: 582–589.

DALTEPARIN BNF 2.8.1

Class: Low molecular weight heparin (LMWH).

Indications: Prevention of DVT and PE in surgical patients and bedbound medical patients (including cancer patients), initial treatment of DVT and PE, treatment of cancer associated thrombosis, prevention of clotting in extracorporeal circuits during haemodialysis or haemofiltration, unstable angina, non-Q wave myocardial infarction, †thrombophlebitis migrans, †disseminated intravascular coagulation (DIC).

Contra-indications: Active major bleeding, active peptic ulcer, cerebral haemorrhage, haemorrhagic pericardial or pleural effusion, known bleeding diathesis, confirmed or suspected immune-mediated heparin-induced thrombocytopenia (HIT), subacute bacterial endocarditis, injury or surgery to the CNS, eyes or ears, spinal analgesia (if on *treatment* dose of dalteparin, increased risk of spinal haematoma), IM use (risk of haematoma at the injection site).

Pharmacology

Dalteparin acts by potentiating the inhibitory effect of antithrombin III on factor Xa and thrombin. It has a relatively higher ability to potentiate factor Xa inhibition than to prolong plasma clotting time (APTT) which cannot be used to guide dosing. Anti-factor Xa levels can be measured if necessary, e.g. if a patient is at increased risk of bleeding, but routine monitoring is not generally required because the dose is determined by the patient's weight. LMWH is as effective as

unfractionated heparin for the treatment of DVT and PE and is now the initial treatment of choice.[1–3] Other advantages include a longer duration of action which allows administration once daily and possibly a better safety profile, e.g. fewer major haemorrhages.[2–6] LMWH is the treatment of choice for *chronic* DIC; this commonly presents as recurrent thromboses in both superficial and deep veins which do not respond to **warfarin**. Antifibrinolytic drugs, e.g. **tranexamic acid** and **aminocaproic acid** (not UK), should not be used in DIC because they increase the risk of end-organ damage from microvascular thromboses. All LMWH is derived from porcine heparin and some patients may need to avoid it because of hypersensitivity, or for religious or cultural reasons. The most appropriate non-porcine alternative is **fondaparinux**.[7,8]
Bio-availability 87% SC (based on plasma anti-factor Xa activity).
Onset of action 3min IV; 2–4h SC.
Time to peak plasma anti-factor Xa activity 4h SC.
Plasma anti-factor Xa activity halflife 2h IV; 6h IV in haemodialysis patients; 3–5h SC.
Duration of action 10–24h SC.

Cautions

Serious drug interactions: enhanced anticoagulant effect with anticoagulant/antiplatelet drugs, e.g. NSAIDs.

Risk of spinal (intrathecal or epidural) haematoma in patients undergoing spinal puncture or with an indwelling spinal catheter, particularly if concurrently receiving a drug which affects haemostasis; spinal analgesia may be used cautiously in patients on *thromboprophylactic* doses of dalteparin but monitor for neurological impairment.

Increased risk of haemorrhage if underlying bleeding diathesis (e.g. thrombocytopenia), recent cerebral haemorrhage, recent trauma, recent neurological or ophthalmic surgery, uncontrolled hypertension, diabetic or hypertensive retinopathy, previous peptic ulcer. Other risk factors for bleeding include serious concurrent illness, chronic heavy consumption of alcohol, use of platelet inhibiting drugs, renal failure, age, and possibly female gender. In severe liver disease, the manufacturer recommends dose reduction but gives no definite guidance. In severe renal impairment, the anti-factor Xa activity halflife of dalteparin is prolonged in patients requiring haemodialysis and the manufacturers recommend reduced IV doses in patients with acute renal failure or with chronic renal failure and an increased risk of bleeding who are undergoing haemodialysis. Specialist guidelines suggest using IV unfractionated heparin instead of LMWH in severe renal impairment but the evidence is not strong (grade 2C, i.e. not based on RCT).[9]

Inhibition of aldosterone secretion by heparin/LMWH may cause hyperkalaemia. The risk appears to increase with duration of treatment; patients with diabetes mellitus, chronic renal failure, acidosis and those taking potassium supplements or potassium-sparing drugs are more susceptible. The CSM recommends that plasma potassium should be measured in such patients before starting heparin and monitored regularly thereafter, particularly if heparin is to be continued for more than 1 week.

Undesirable effects

Common (<10%, >1%): haematoma at the injection site, mild thrombocytopenia which reverses with continued treatment.
Uncommon (<1%, >0.1%): major bleeding (e.g. GI, retroperitoneal, intracranial, surgical sites), thrombocytopenia during prophylaxis.

Both standard heparin and LMWH can cause thrombocytopenia (platelet count $< 100 \times 10^9$/L). An early (<4 days) mild fall in platelet count is often seen after starting heparin treatment, particularly after surgery. This corrects spontaneously despite the continued use of heparin and is asymptomatic.[10] However, occasionally, an immune heparin-induced thrombocytopenia (HIT) develops, associated with heparin-dependent IgG antibodies (see LMWH, p.78).[6,10] Dalteparin should be stopped immediately if there is a fall in the platelet count of >50% and the advice of a haematologist obtained. Anticoagulation should be continued with a either a hirudin derivative, e.g. **lepirudin**, or a heparinoid, e.g. **danaparoid**, even if there is no clinically evident thrombosis (see LMWH, p. 78).[11]

Dose and use

All patients should have a baseline platelet count before starting LMWH. Those who have received unfractionated heparin in the last 3 months should have a repeat platelet count after 24h to exclude rapid-onset HIT due to pre-existing antibodies. Subsequently, for all patients, the platelet count should be monitored every 2–4 days from days 4–14.[12]

May cause transient stinging and local bruising. Inject SC, rotate sites daily between the left and right anterolateral abdominal wall, posterolateral abdominal wall and lateral thigh; introduce the total length of the needle vertically into the thickest part of a skin fold produced by squeezing the skin between the thumb and forefinger. Do not rub the injection site.

The anti-factor Xa activity halflife of dalteparin is prolonged in patients with severe renal impairment requiring haemodialysis. The manufacturer recommends a reduced IV dose in patients with acute renal failure or with chronic renal failure and an increased risk of bleeding who are undergoing haemodialysis (see SPC for Fragmin®–haemodialysis/haemofiltration for details). No guidelines for reduced SC doses in other patients are given. Specialist guidelines suggest using IV unfractionated heparin instead of LMWH in severe renal impairment but the evidence is not strong (grade 2C, i.e. not based on RCT).[9,13]

Thromboprophylaxis

Patients with cancer undergoing surgery

- give 5,000 units SC once daily, starting the evening before surgery
- continue for 2–4 weeks;[14] 4 weeks is more effective than 1 week[15,16]
- consider additional mechanical measures such as graduated compression stockings or intermittent pneumatic compression.[14]

Patients with cancer who are immobile or confined to bed because of a concurrent acute medical illness

- give 5,000 units SC once daily (see LMWH, p.80)
- duration of therapy is generally ≤2 weeks[17,18]
- if anticoagulation is contra-indicated, the use of graduated compression stockings may be considered although the evidence base in medical patients is limited and in some populations has demonstrated increased episodes of harm.[19]

Thromboprophylaxis appears acceptable to palliative care inpatients,[20] and should be considered in patients meeting the recommended criteria (see p.80). The decision to use thromboprophylaxis should take into account the views of patients, family/informal carers and the multiprofessional team, and be reviewed every few days. (Note: NICE guidance suggests reviewing daily, but this seems excessive and will often be impractical.[13])

However, thromboprophylaxis is less relevant for cancer patients with a poor performance status in their last few weeks–days of life, e.g. when admitted for terminal care or started on an end-of-life care pathway;[13] in other words, when symptom relief alone would be the most appropriate treatment for any new thrombo-embolic episode.

Patients with cancer undertaking long-distance air travel

- if a LMWH is deemed necessary (see p.81), prescribe three injections (one each for the outward and return journeys, and one spare)
- provide training in the correct administration of the injection (see the information on self-administration included in the patient information leaflet)
- self-administer 5,000 units SC 2–4h before departure
- if there is a stop over, followed by another long flight, another injection is not necessary unless the second flight is more than 24h after the first.

Treatment

DVT and PE in patients with cancer: initial treatment

Confirm the diagnosis radiologically (ultrasound, venogram, V/Q scan, CT pulmonary angiography). General guidance is to treat for 3–6 months:

- 200 units/kg SC once daily for the first month
- then 150 units/kg SC once daily for 2–5 months
- followed by LMWH or **warfarin** indefinitely or until the cancer is cured (see below).

DVT and PE in patients with cancer: ongoing treatment

Indefinite anticoagulation should be considered for patients who have a DVT, a sudden severe PE, or a persistent major risk factor for thrombo-embolism such as cancer[9] (see Box 2.D, p.76). In patients with cancer, long-term LMWH appears more effective than **warfarin**, with a similar (or reduced) risk of bleeding.[21–23] **Warfarin** should be reserved for those patients whose cancer is relatively stable. When switching to **warfarin**, LMWH should be continued until a therapeutic INR has been achieved on two consecutive days. Patients undergoing anticancer treatments should receive LMWH.

In palliative care, because haemorrhagic complications with **warfarin** occur in nearly 50% (possibly related to drug interactions and hepatic impairment), LMWH (e.g. dalteparin 150 units/kg SC once daily) is preferable. It has been used indefinitely and is acceptable to patients.[24,25] Generally, indefinite anticoagulation is stopped only if contra-indications develop, or when the patient reaches the stage when symptom relief alone is appropriate, e.g. in the last weeks of life.

Some centres use a fixed low-dose regimen, independent of body weight (Box 2.G). With this regimen, 15% of patients did not complete the first week (6% experienced a major bleed, 5% required a smaller dose of dalteparin due to abnormal coagulation and 2% had massive recurrent PE). Subsequently, almost 80% of patients received chemotherapy, 27% experienced transient thrombocytopenia (generally related to chemotherapy) and 23% required surgery or an invasive procedure. Major bleeding occurred in 5% (fatal in 3%) and minor bleeding in 8%. Recurrent thrombo-embolism in 9%. Complications were no higher in patients with liver or brain metastases, thrombocytopenia, or undergoing surgical or invasive procedures.[25]

Box 2.G Modified dalteparin regimen in patients with metastatic cancer and venous thrombo-embolism[26]

First week
Give dalteparin in a dose according to body weight (see DVT and PE, p.86).

Subsequent weeks (continue indefinitely)
Dalteparin in a fixed dose of 10,000 units SC once daily

If DVT recurs
Increase the fixed-dose of dalteparin to 12,500 units SC once daily.

If PE occurs/recurs
Treat with an inferior vena caval filter.

Dose modifications
Thrombocytopenia
If the platelet count falls below 50×10^9/L reduce the dose of dalteparin to 5,000 units SC once daily.

If the platelet count falls below 10×10^9/L reduce the dose of dalteparin to 2,500 units SC once daily.

Surgical procedures
Give dalteparin 5,000 units SC once daily for the first 4 days postoperatively and then return to the patient's usual dose.

Other invasive procedures (e.g. biopsy)
Give dalteparin 5,000 units SC on the day of the procedure and then return to the patient's usual dose.

Disseminated intravascular coagulation (DIC)

- confirm the diagnosis (see p.82)
- *do not use **warfarin** because it is ineffective*
- *for chronic* DIC presenting with recurrent thromboses, give dalteparin as for treatment of DVT
- *for chronic or acute* DIC presenting with haemorrhagic manifestations (e.g. ecchymoses and haematomas), seek specialist advice.

Thrombophlebitis migrans

- *do not use **warfarin** because it is ineffective*
- generally responds rapidly to small doses, e.g. 2,500–5,000 units SC once daily
- continue treatment indefinitely[3,27]
- if necessary, titrate dose to maximum allowed according to weight, i.e. 200 units/kg.

Overdose

In emergencies, **protamine sulphate** can be used to reverse the effects of dalteparin:

- for each 100 units of dalteparin, give 1mg of **protamine sulphate**
- give a maximum of 50mg by IV injection over 10min.

Note: the anti-factor Xa activity of dalteparin is not completely neutralized by **protamine sulphate** (maximum reversal about 50%).

Supply

Fragmin® (Pharmacia)

Injection (prefilled single-dose graduated syringe for SC injection) 10,000 units/mL, 1mL (10,000 units) = £6.

Injection (prefilled single-dose syringe for SC injection) 12,500 units/mL, 0.2mL (2,500 units) = £2; 25,000 units/mL, 0.2mL (5,000 units) = £3, 0.3mL (7,500 units) = £4, 0.4mL (10,000 units) = £6, 0.5mL (12,500 units) = £7, 0.6mL (15,000 units) = £8, 0.72mL (18,000 units) = £10.

Injection (for SC or IV use) 2,500 units/mL, 4mL amp (10,000 units) = £5; 10,000 units/mL, 1mL amp (10,000 units) = £5.

Injection (multiple dose vial for SC injection) 25,000 units/mL, 4mL (100,000 units) = £49.

---

1 Baglin T *et al.* (2006) Guidelines on the use and monitoring of heparin. *British Journal of Haematology.* **133**: 19–34.
2 Quinlan D *et al.* (2004) Low-molecular weight heparin compared with intravenous unfractionated heparin for treatment of pulmonary embolism. *Annals of internal medicine.* **140**: 175–183.
3 Van Dongen CJ *et al.* (2004) Fixed dose subcutaneous low molecular weight heparins versus adjusted dose unfractionated heparin for venous thromboembolism. *Cochrane Database of Systematic Reviews.* **4**: CD001100.
4 Fareed J *et al.* (2003) Pharmacodynamic and pharmacokinetic properties of enoxaparin: implications for clinical practice. *Clinical Pharmacokinetics.* **42**: 1043–1057.
5 Prandoni P (2001) Heparins and venous thromboembolism: current practice and future directions. *Journal of Thrombosis and Haemostasis.* **86**: 488–498.
6 Hirsh J *et al.* (2001) Heparin and low-molecular-weight heparin: mechanisms of action, pharmacokinetics, dosing, monitoring, efficacy, and safety. *Chest.* **119 (suppl)**: 64s–94s.
7 Blann AD and Lip GY (2006) Venous thromboembolism. *British Medical Journal.* **332**: 215–219.
8 Cohen AT *et al.* (2006) Efficacy and safety of fondaparinux for the prevention of venous thromboembolism in older acute medical patients: randomised placebo controlled trial. *British Medical Journal.* **332**: 325–329.
9 Kearon C *et al.* (2008) Antithrombotic therapy for venous thromboembolic disease: American College of Chest Physicians Evidence-Based Clinical Practice Guidelines (8th Edition). *Chest.* **133 (suppl 6)**: 454S–545S.
10 Warkentin T *et al.* (1995) Heparin-induced thrombocytopenia in patients treated with low molecular weight heparin or unfractionated heparin. *New England Journal of Medicine.* **332**: 1330–1335.
11 Warkentin TE and Greinacher A (2004) Heparin-induced thrombocytopenia: recognition, treatment, and prevention: the seventh ACCP Conference on Antithrombotic and Thrombolytic Therapy. *Chest.* **126 (suppl)**: 311s–337s.
12 Keeling D *et al.* (2006) The management of heparin-induced thrombocytopenia. *British Journal of Haematology.* **133**: 259–269.
13 NICE (2010) Clinical Guideline 92: Reducing the risk of venous thromboembolism (deep vein thrombosis and pulmonary embolism) in patients admitted to hospital. London. Available from: www.nice.org.uk/guidance/CG92
14 Geerts WH *et al.* (2008) Prevention of venous thromboembolism: American College of Chest Physicians Evidence-Based Clinical Practice Guidelines (8th Edition). *Chest.* **133 (suppl 6)**: 381S–453S.
15 Kher A and Samama MM (2005) Primary and secondary prophylaxis of venous thromboembolism with low-molecular-weight heparins: prolonged thromboprophylaxis, an alternative to vitamin K antagonists. *Journal of Thrombosis and Haemostasis.* **3**: 473–481.
16 Bergqvist D *et al.* (2002) Duration of prophylaxis against venous thromboembolism with enoxaparin after surgery for cancer. *New England Journal of Medicine.* **346**: 975–980.
17 Leizorovicz A and Mismetti P (2004) Preventing venous thromboembolism in medical patients. *Circulation.* **110**: IV13–19.
18 Leizorovicz A *et al.* (2004) Randomized, placebo-controlled trial of dalteparin for the prevention of venous thromboembolism in acutely ill medical patients. *Circulation.* **110**: 874–879.
19 Dennis M *et al.* (2009) Effectiveness of thigh-length graduated compression stockings to reduce the risk of deep vein thrombosis after stroke (CLOTS trial 1): a multicentre, randomised controlled trial. *Lancet.* **373**: 1958–1965.
20 Noble SI *et al.* (2006) Acceptability of low molecular weight heparin thromboprophylaxis for inpatients receiving palliative care: qualitative study. *British Medical Journal.* **332**: 577–580.
21 Hull RD *et al.* (2006) Long-term low-molecular-weight heparin versus usual care in proximal-vein thrombosis patients with cancer. *American Journal of Medicine.* **119**: 1062–1072.
22 Lee A *et al.* (2003) Low molecular weight heparin versus a coumarin for the prevention of recurrent venous thromboembolism in patients with cancer. *New England Journal of Medicine.* **349**: 146–153.

23 Meyer G *et al.* (2002) Comparison of low-molecular-weight heparin and warfarin for the secondary prevention of venous thromboembolism in patients with cancer: a randomized controlled study. *Archives of Internal Medicine.* **162**: 1729–1735.
24 Noble SI *et al.* (2008) The management of venous thromboembolism in advanced cancer: a systematic review and meta-analysis by the thrombosis task group, on behalf of the Association for Palliative Medicine Science Committee. *Lancet Oncology.* **9**: 577–584.
25 Noble SI and Finlay IG (2005) Is long-term low-molecular-weight heparin acceptable to palliative care patients in the treatment of cancer related venous thromboembolism? A qualitative study. *Palliative Medicine.* **19**: 197–201.
26 Monreal M *et al.* (2004) Fixed-dose low-molecular-weight heparin for secondary prevention of venous thromboembolism in patients with disseminated cancer: a prospective cohort study. *Journal of Thrombosis and Haemostasis.* **2**: 1311–1315.
27 Walsh-McMonagle D and Green D (1997) Low-molecular weight heparin in the management of Trousseau's syndrome. *Cancer.* **80**: 649–655.

ENOXAPARIN — BNF 2.8.1

Class: Low molecular weight heparin (LMWH).

Indications: Prevention of DVT and PE in surgical patients and bedbound medical patients, initial treatment of DVT and PE, prevention of clotting in extracorporeal circuits during haemodialysis, unstable angina, non-Q wave myocardial infarction, †thrombophlebitis migrans, †disseminated intravascular coagulation (DIC).

Contra-indications: Active major bleeding, thrombocytopenia with positive aggregation test in the presence of enoxaparin, known bleeding diathesis, acute bacterial endocarditis, spinal analgesia if on *treatment* dose of enoxaparin (increased risk of spinal haematoma), IM use (risk of haematoma at the injection site).

Pharmacology

Enoxaparin acts by potentiating the inhibitory effect of antithrombin III on factor Xa and thrombin. It has a relatively higher ability to potentiate factor Xa inhibition than to prolong plasma clotting time (APTT) which cannot be used to guide dosing. Anti-factor Xa levels can be measured if necessary, e.g. if a patient is at increased risk of bleeding, but routine monitoring is not generally required because the dose is determined by the patient's weight. In renal impairment excretion of enoxaparin is reduced and increased bleeding can occur. LMWH is as effective as unfractionated heparin for the treatment of DVT and PE and is now the initial treatment of choice.[1–3] Other advantages include a longer duration of action which allows administration once daily and possibly a better safety profile, e.g. fewer major haemorrhages.[2–6] LMWH is the treatment of choice for *chronic* DIC; this commonly presents as recurrent thromboses in both superficial and deep veins which do not respond to **warfarin**. Antifibrinolytic drugs, e.g. **tranexamic acid** and **aminocaproic acid** (not UK), should not be used in DIC because they increase the risk of end-organ damage from microvascular thromboses. All LMWH is derived from porcine heparin and some patients may need to avoid it because of hypersensitivity, or for religious or cultural reasons. The most appropriate non-porcine alternative is **fondaparinux**.[7,8]
Bio-availability 100% SC (based on plasma anti-factor Xa activity).
Onset of action 5min IV; 3h SC.[9]
Time to peak plasma anti-factor Xa activity 2–6h SC.
Plasma anti-factor Xa activity halflife 2–4.5h IV;[10,11] 4.5–7h SC.
Duration of action >24h SC.[6]

Cautions

Serious drug interactions: enhanced anticoagulant effect with anticoagulant/antiplatelet drugs, e.g. NSAIDs.

Risk of spinal (intrathecal or epidural) haematoma in patients undergoing spinal puncture or with indwelling spinal catheter, particularly if concurrently receiving a drug which affects haemostasis; spinal analgesia may be used cautiously in patients on *thromboprophylactic* doses of enoxaparin but monitor for neurological impairment.

Increased risk of haemorrhage if underlying bleeding diathesis (e.g. thrombocytopenia), recent cerebral haemorrhage, recent neurological or ophthalmic surgery, uncontrolled hypertension, diabetic or hypertensive retinopathy, current or past peptic ulcer, severe liver disease. Severe renal impairment: the clearance of enoxaparin is decreased by 65% and dose reduction is required if creatinine clearance <30mL/min. Specialist guidelines suggest using IV unfractionated heparin instead of LMWH but the evidence is not strong (grade 2C, i.e. not based on RCT).[12]

Inhibition of aldosterone secretion by heparin/LMWH may cause hyperkalaemia. The risk appears to increase with duration of therapy; patients with diabetes mellitus, chronic renal failure, acidosis and those taking potassium supplements or potassium-sparing drugs are more susceptible. The CSM recommends that plasma potassium should be measured in such patients before starting heparin and monitored regularly thereafter, particularly if heparin is to be continued for more than 1 week.

Undesirable effects

Frequency not stated: mild, transient, asymptomatic thrombocytopenia; pain, haematoma and mild irritation at the injection site; transient, asymptomatic increases in LFTs.

Both standard heparin and LMWH can cause thrombocytopenia (platelet count $< 100 \times 10^9$/L). An early (<4 days) mild fall in platelet count is often seen after starting heparin therapy, particularly after surgery. This corrects spontaneously despite the continued use of heparin and is asymptomatic.[13] However, occasionally, an immune heparin-induced thrombocytopenia (HIT) develops associated with heparin-dependent IgG antibodies (see LMWH, p.78).[4,13] Enoxaparin should be stopped immediately if there is a fall in the platelet count >50% and the advice of a haematologist obtained. Anticoagulation should be continued with a hirudin derivative, e.g. **lepirudin**, or a heparinoid, e.g. **danaparoid**, even if there is no clinically evident thrombosis (see LMWH, p.78).[14]

Dose and use

All patients should have a baseline platelet count before starting LMWH. Those who have received unfractionated heparin in the last 3 months should have a repeat platelet count after 24h to exclude rapid-onset HIT due to pre-existing antibodies. Subsequently, for all patients, the platelet count should be monitored every 2–4 days from days 4–14.[15]

May cause transient stinging and local bruising. Inject SC; rotate injection sites between left and right anterolateral and left and right posterolateral abdominal wall; introduce the total length of the needle vertically into the thickest part of a skin fold produced by squeezing the skin between the thumb and forefinger. Do not rub the injection site.

In severe renal impairment (creatinine clearance <30mL/min), the dose of enoxaparin should be reduced to a maximum of 20mg SC once daily (thromboprophylaxis) or 1mg/kg SC once daily (treatment). Although the evidence is not strong (grade 2C, i.e. not based on RCT), specialist guidelines suggest using IV unfractionated heparin instead of LMWH in severe renal impairment.[12–16]

Thromboprophylaxis

Patients with cancer undergoing surgery

- give 40mg SC once daily, starting 12h before surgery
- continue for 2–4 weeks;[17] 4 weeks is more effective than 1 week[18,19]
- consider additional mechanical measures such as graduated compression stockings or intermittent pneumatic compression.[17]

Patients with cancer who are immobile or confined to bed because of a concurrent acute medical illness

- give 40mg SC once daily (see LMWH, p.81)
- duration of therapy is generally ≤2 weeks[20,21]
- if anticoagulation is contra-indicated, the use of graduated compression stockings may be considered although the evidence base in medical patients is limited and in some populations have demonstrated increased episodes of harm.[22]

Thromboprophylaxis appears acceptable to palliative care inpatients,[23] and should be considered in patients meeting the recommended criteria (see p.80). The decision to use thromboprophylaxis should take into account the views of patients, family/informal carers and the multiprofessional team, and be reviewed every few days. (Note: NICE guidance suggests reviewing daily, but this seems excessive and will often be impractical.[16])

However, thromboprophylaxis is less relevant for cancer patients with a poor performance status in their last few weeks–days of life, e.g. when admitted for terminal care or started on an end-of-life care pathway;[16] in other words, when symptom relief alone would be the most appropriate treatment for any new thrombo-embolic episode.

Patients with cancer undertaking long-distance air travel

- if a LMWH is deemed necessary (see p.81), prescribe three injections (one each for the outward and return journeys, and one spare)
- provide training in the correct administration of the injection (see the information on self-administration included in the patient information leaflet)
- self-administer 40mg SC 2–4h before departure
- if there is a stop over followed by another long flight, another injection is not necessary unless the second flight is more than 24h after the first.

Treatment

DVT and PE in patients with cancer: initial treatment

Confirm diagnosis radiologically (ultrasound, venogram, V/Q scan, CT pulmonary angiography). General guidance is to treat with 1.5mg/kg SC once daily for 3–6 months, followed by LMWH or **warfarin** indefinitely or until the cancer is cured (see below).

DVT and PE in patients with cancer: ongoing treatment

Indefinite anticoagulation should be considered for patients who have a DVT, a sudden severe PE, or a persistent major risk factor such as cancer[12] (see Box 2.D, p.76). In patients with cancer, long-term LMWH appears more effective than **warfarin**, with a similar (or reduced) risk of bleeding.[24–26] **Warfarin** should be reserved for those patients whose cancer is relatively stable. When switching to **warfarin**, LMWH should be continued until a therapeutic INR has been achieved on two consecutive days. Patients undergoing anticancer treatments should receive LMWH.

In palliative care, because haemorrhagic complications with **warfarin** occur in nearly 50% (possibly related to drug interactions and hepatic impairment), LMWH is preferable. It has been used indefinitely and is acceptable to patients.[27–29] Generally, indefinite anticoagulation is discontinued only if contra-indications develop, or when the patient reaches the stage when symptom relief alone is appropriate, e.g. in the last few weeks of life.

Some centres use a fixed low-dose regimen, independent of body weight (see Box 2.G, p.87).

Disseminated intravascular coagulation (DIC)

- confirm the diagnosis (see LMWH, p.82)
- *do not use **warfarin** because it is ineffective*
- *for chronic* DIC presenting with recurrent thromboses, give enoxaparin as for treatment of DVT
- *for chronic or acute* DIC presenting with haemorrhagic manifestations (e.g. ecchymoses and haematomas), seek specialist advice.

Thrombophlebitis migrans

- *do not use **warfarin** because it is ineffective*
- generally responds rapidly to small doses, e.g. ≤60mg/day
- continue treatment indefinitely[30]
- if necessary, titrate dose to maximum allowed according to weight, i.e. 1.5mg/kg SC once daily.

Overdose

In emergencies, **protamine sulphate** can be used to reverse the effects of enoxaparin:

- for each 1mg (100 units) of enoxaparin, give 1mg of **protamine sulphate**
- give a maximum of 50mg by slow IV injection over 10min.

Note: even with high doses of **protamine sulphate**, the anti-factor Xa activity of enoxaparin is not completely neutralized (maximum reversal ~60%).

Supply

Clexane® (Sanofi-Aventis)

Injection (single dose syringe for SC injection) 100mg/mL, 0.2mL (20mg, 2,000 units) = £3, 0.4mL (40mg, 4,000 units) = £4, 0.6mL (60mg, 6,000 units) = £5, 0.8mL (80mg, 8,000 units) = £6, 1mL (100mg, 10,000 units) = £8.

Clexane® Multidose (Sanofi-Aventis)
Injection (Multiple dose vial for SC or IV use) 100mg/mL, 3mL (300mg, 30,000 units) = £21.

Clexane® Forte (Sanofi-Aventis)
Injection (single dose syringe for SC injection) 150mg/mL, 0.8mL (120mg, 12,000 units) = £10, 1mL (150mg, 15,000 units) = £11.

---

1 Baglin T *et al.* (2006) Guidelines on the use and monitoring of heparin. *British Journal of Haematology.* **133**: 19–34.
2 Quinlan D *et al.* (2004) Low-molecular weight heparin compared with intravenous unfractionated heparin for treatment of pulmonary embolism. *Annals of internal medicine.* **140**: 175–183.
3 Van Dongen CJ *et al.* (2004) Fixed dose subcutaneous low molecular weight heparins versus adjusted dose unfractionated heparin for venous thromboembolism. *Cochrane Database of Systematic Reviews.* **4**: CD001100.
4 Hirsh J *et al.* (2001) Heparin and low-molecular-weight heparin: mechanisms of action, pharmacokinetics, dosing, monitoring, efficacy, and safety. *Chest.* **119 (suppl)**: 64s–94s.
5 Prandoni P (2001) Heparins and venous thromboembolism: current practice and future directions. *Journal of Thrombosis and Haemostasis.* **86**: 488–498.
6 Fareed J *et al.* (2003) Pharmacodynamic and pharmacokinetic properties of enoxaparin: implications for clinical practice. *Clinical Pharmacokinetics.* **42**: 1043–1057.
7 Blann AD and Lip GY (2006) Venous thromboembolism. *British Medical Journal.* **332**: 215–219.
8 Cohen AT *et al.* (2006) Efficacy and safety of fondaparinux for the prevention of venous thromboembolism in older acute medical patients: randomised placebo controlled trial. *British Medical Journal.* **332**: 325–329.
9 Fareed J *et al.* (1990) Pharmacologic profile of a low molecular weight heparin (enoxaparin): experimental and clinical validation of the prophylactic antithrombotic effects. *Acta Chirurgica Scandinavica Suppl.* **556 (suppl)**: 75–90.
10 Bara L and Samama M (1990) Pharmacokinetics of low molecular weight heparins. *Acta Chirurgica Scandinavica Supplementum.* **556 (suppl)**: 57–61.
11 Dawes J (1990) Comparison of the pharmacokinetics of enoxaparin (Clexane) and unfractionated heparin. *Acta Chirurgica Scandinavica Supplementum.* **556 (suppl)**: 68–74.
12 Kearon C *et al.* (2008) Antithrombotic therapy for venous thromboembolic disease: American College of Chest Physicians Evidence-Based Clinical Practice Guidelines (8th Edition). *Chest.* **133 (suppl 6)**: 454S–545S.
13 Warkentin T *et al.* (1995) Heparin-induced thrombocytopenia in patients treated with low molecular weight heparin or unfractionated heparin. *New England Journal of Medicine.* **332**: 1330–1335.
14 Warkentin TE and Greinacher A (2008) Treatment and prevention of heparin-induced thrombocytopenia: American College of Chest Physicians Evidence-Based Clinical Practice Guidelines (8th Edition). *Chest.* **133 (suppl 6)**: 340S–380S.
15 Keeling D *et al.* (2006) The management of heparin-induced thrombocytopenia. *British Journal of Haematology.* **133**: 259–269.
16 NICE (2010) Clinical Guideline 92: Reducing the risk of venous thromboembolism (deep vein thrombosis and pulmonary embolism) in patients admitted to hospital. London. Available from: www.nice.org.uk/guidance/CG92
17 Geerts WH *et al.* (2008) Prevention of venous thromboembolism: American College of Chest Physicians Evidence-Based Clinical Practice Guidelines (8th Edition). *Chest.* **133 (suppl 6)**: 381S–453S.
18 Kher A and Samama MM (2005) Primary and secondary prophylaxis of venous thromboembolism with low-molecular-weight heparins: prolonged thromboprophylaxis, an alternative to vitamin K antagonists. *Journal of Thrombosis and Haemostasis.* **3**: 473–481.
19 Bergqvist D *et al.* (2002) Duration of prophylaxis against venous thromboembolism with enoxaparin after surgery for cancer. *New England Journal of Medicine.* **346**: 975–980.
20 Leizorovicz A and Mismetti P (2004) Preventing venous thromboembolism in medical patients. *Circulation.* **110**: IV13–19.
21 Samama MM *et al.* (1999) A comparison of enoxaparin with placebo for the prevention of venous thromboembolism in acutely ill medical patients. Prophylaxis in Medical Patients with Enoxaparin Study Group. *New England Journal of Medicine.* **341**: 793–800.
22 Dennis M *et al.* (2009) Effectiveness of thigh-length graduated compression stockings to reduce the risk of deep vein thrombosis after stroke (CLOTS trial 1): a multicentre, randomised controlled trial. *Lancet.* **373**: 1958–1965.
23 Noble SI *et al.* (2006) Acceptability of low molecular weight heparin thromboprophylaxis for inpatients receiving palliative care: qualitative study. *British Medical Journal.* **332**: 577–580.
24 Meyer G *et al.* (2002) Comparison of low-molecular-weight heparin and warfarin for the secondary prevention of venous thromboembolism in patients with cancer: a randomized controlled study. *Archives of Internal Medicine.* **162**: 1729–1735.
25 Lee A *et al.* (2003) Low molecular weight heparin versus a coumarin for the prevention of recurrent venous thromboembolism in patients with cancer. *New England Journal of Medicine.* **349**: 146–153.
26 Hull RD *et al.* (2006) Long-term low-molecular-weight heparin versus usual care in proximal-vein thrombosis patients with cancer. *American Journal of Medicine.* **119**: 1062–1072.
27 Johnson M and Sherry K (1997) How do palliative physicians manage venous thromboembolism? *Palliative Medicine.* **11**: 462–468.
28 Noble SI and Finlay IG (2005) Is long-term low-molecular-weight heparin acceptable to palliative care patients in the treatment of cancer related venous thromboembolism? A qualitative study. *Palliative Medicine.* **19**: 197–201.
29 Noble SI *et al.* (2008) The management of venous thromboembolism in advanced cancer: a systematic review and meta-analysis by the thrombosis task group, on behalf of the Association for Palliative Medicine Science Committee. *Lancet Oncology.* **9**: 577–584.
30 Walsh-McMonagle D and Green D (1997) Low-molecular weight heparin in the management of Trousseau's syndrome. *Cancer.* **80**: 649–655.

ETAMSYLATE BNF 2.11

Class: Haemostatic agent.

Indications: Menorrhagia, †surface bleeding from ulcerating tumours, nasal cavity and other organs (bladder, uterus, rectum, stomach and lungs).

Contra-indication: Porphyria.

Pharmacology

Etamsylate acts by increasing capillary vascular wall resistance and platelet adhesiveness in the presence of a vascular lesion. This is achieved by inhibiting the biosynthesis and actions of those PGs which cause platelet disaggregation, vasodilation and increased capillary permeability, thereby promoting platelet activation and aggregation, and also by increasing communication between platelets, leucocytes and endothelial cells via the cell adhesion molecule P-selectin.[1] Etamsylate does not cause vasoconstriction, nor does it affect normal coagulation; it has no effect on prothrombin time, fibrinolysis, or platelet count.

Studies have mainly explored the use of etamsylate for menorrhagia or peri-ventricular haemorrhage in premature infants.[1] In palliative care, it is used for surface bleeding ± **tranexamic acid** (see p.93). Rarely, parenteral use may be necessary, e.g. in patients with bleeding and complete dysphagia due to oesophageal cancer. Etamsylate is excreted in the urine mainly unchanged.

Bio-availability completely absorbed PO.
Onset of action 30min IV.
Time to peak plasma concentration 4h PO; 1h IV.
Plasma halflife 5–17h PO; 1.7–2.5h IM; 1.8–2h IV.
Duration of action no data.

Undesirable effects

Fever, headache, nausea, vomiting, diarrhoea, rash.

Dose and use

Etamsylate is generally one part of a multimodal approach to the management of surface bleeding (see Box 2.H Management of surface bleeding, p.94):

- 500mg q.d.s. either indefinitely or until 1 week after cessation of bleeding
- if it causes nausea, vomiting or diarrhoea, take p.c.

Supply

Dicynene® (Sanofi-Aventis)
Tablets 500mg, 28 days @ 500mg q.d.s. = £9.
Injection 125mg/mL, 2mL amp = £1. (Unlicensed, available as a special order from IDIS; see Obtaining unlicensed products, p.769.)

1 Garay RP *et al.* (2006) Therapeutic efficacy and mechanism of action of ethamsylate, a long-standing hemostatic agent. *American Journal of Therapeutics.* **13**: 236–247.

ANTIFIBRINOLYTIC DRUGS BNF 2.11

Indications: Prevention of bleeding after dental extraction in haemophilia or postoperatively, haemorrhagic complications after thrombolytic treatment, menorrhagia, epistaxis, hereditary angioedema, †subarachnoid haemorrhage, †surface bleeding from ulcerating tumours on the skin, in the nose, mouth, pharynx and other hollow organs (lungs, stomach, rectum, bladder, uterus).

Contra-indications: Active thrombo-embolic disease, e.g. recent thrombo-embolism, DIC.

Pharmacology

Tranexamic acid and **aminocaproic acid** (not UK) are structurally related synthetic antifibrinolytic drugs which block the binding of plasminogen and plasmin to fibrin, thereby preventing dissolution of haemostatic plugs.[1] **Tranexamic acid** is also a weak direct inhibitor of plasmin. Both drugs have been used in various circumstances either PO, IV or topically; e.g. in coronary artery by-pass graft surgery, **aminocaproic acid** applied into the pericardial space reduces post-operative bleeding and transfusion requirements.[2] Both drugs are used in cancer patients to control surface bleeding. **Tranexamic acid** is preferable to **aminocaproic acid**; it is more potent and may be more effective. It has a longer duration of action, and is less likely to cause undesirable GI effects.[3] Both **tranexamic acid** and **aminocaproic acid** are excreted in the urine mainly unchanged. Because of accumulation, dose reduction is necessary in renal impairment. Although the SPC gives severe renal impairment as a contra-indication to **tranexamic acid**, there are reports of its use in reduced doses (Table 2.4).[4,5]

Antifibrinolytic drugs should *not* be used in DIC, even when haemorrhagic manifestations (ecchymoses, haematomas) are predominant, because clot formation is the trigger for further intravascular coagulation and platelet consumption, and there is an increased risk of end-organ damage from microvascular thromboses.

Pharmacokinetic details are listed in Table 2.3.

Table 2.3 Pharmacokinetics of antifibrinolytic drugs

	Tranexamic acid	*Aminocaproic acid*
Bio-availability PO	30–50%[a]	'complete'
Onset of action (route-dependent)	1–3h	1–3h
Time to peak plasma concentration	3h PO	2h
Plasma halflife	2h	2h
Duration of action	24h	12–18h

a. systemic bio-availability minimal with oral rinse.

Cautions

Serious drug interactions: increased risk of thrombosis with other thrombogenic drugs.

History of thrombo-embolism, renal impairment. In both microscopic and macroscopic haematuria there is a risk of clot formation causing ureteric obstruction or urinary retention.[6]

Undesirable effects

Nausea, vomiting, abdominal pain, diarrhoea (generally settle if the dose is reduced).
Tranexamic acid: disturbances in colour vision (discontinue drug).

Dose and use

Box 2.H summarizes the clinical management of surface bleeding.

Tranexamic acid

The following recommendations are taken mainly from anecdotal reports.

As an oral rinse for local bleeding
As a mouthwash, **tranexamic acid** can be used as a 4–5% aqueous solution, 10mL q.d.s.[14]

Surface bleeding from any site[12,15]
- 1.5g PO stat and 1g t.d.s.
- if bleeding not subsiding after 3 days, increase dose to 1.5–2g t.d.s.
- manufacturer's recommended maximum dose = 1.5g t.d.s.
- in practice, doses of ≤2g q.d.s. have been used
- discontinue 1 week after cessation of bleeding or reduce to 500mg t.d.s.
- restart if bleeding occurs, and possibly continue indefinitely.

Box 2.H Management of surface bleeding

Physical
Gauze applied with pressure for 10min soaked in:
- adrenaline (epinephrine) (1 in 1,000) 1mg in 1mL *or* } use standard ampoules.
- tranexamic acid 500mg in 5mL. }

Silver nitrate sticks applied to bleeding points in the nose and mouth, and on skin nodules and fungating tumours.

Haemostatic dressings, i.e. alginate (e.g. Kaltostat®, Sorbsan®).

Diathermy.

Specialist therapy:
- cryotherapy
- LASER
- embolization.[7,8]

Drugs
Review existing medication
Discontinue aspirin and/or other platelet-impairing NSAID.

Prescribe an NSAID which does not impair platelet function (see Table 5.5, p.297) or paracetamol.

Topical
Sucralfate paste 2g (two 1g tablets crushed in 5mL KY jelly).[9]

Sucralfate suspension 2g in 10mL b.d. for the mouth and rectum.[10]

Tranexamic acid 5g in 50mL warm water b.d. for rectal bleeding[11] (e.g. 10 ampoules of undiluted injection).

1% alum solution.

Systemic
Antifibrinolytic drug, e.g. tranexamic acid.[12] *Do not use if DIC suspected.*

Etamsylate (see p.93).

Desmopressin (augments platelet function; see p.496).[13]

Radiation therapy
Teletherapy and brachytherapy are both used to control haemorrhage from:
- skin
- lungs
- oesophagus
- rectum
- bladder
- uterus
- vagina

Parenteral use may occasionally be indicated, e.g. in patients with bleeding and complete dysphagia due to oesophageal cancer:
- 10mg/kg IV over 5–10min t.d.s.–q.d.s.

Note: in renal impairment the dose should be reduced (Table 2.4).

Table 2.4 Tranexamic acid doses in renal impairment[5]

Creatinine clearance (mL/min)	*PO dose*	*IV dose*
50–80	15mg/kg b.d.	10mg/kg b.d.
10–50	15mg/kg once daily	10mg/kg once daily
<10	15mg/kg every 2 days	5mg/kg once daily or 10mg/kg every 2 days

Topical solution for bleeding from fungating cancer in the skin[16]
- solution (10%): use injection, 500mg in 5mL, soak into gauze and apply with pressure for 10min, then leave *in situ* with a dressing *or*
- paste (3.3%): use tablets, 2g crushed in 60g base (e.g. *hydrophilic* soft paraffin) and apply b.d.; cover with a dressing.[17]

Topical solution for bleeding from cancer in rectum, bladder or pleura[11,18]
Generally used only if PO **tranexamic acid** has failed:
- 5g in 50mL of water, instilled at body temperature once daily–b.d. (e.g. 10 ampoules of undiluted injection).

Aminocaproic acid (not UK)
In oliguria or end-stage renal disease, give 15–25% of the normal dose.[5]

Acute bleeding syndromes due to elevated fibrinolytic activity
- stat dose of 5g PO (or 4–5g IVI in 250mL of diluent) during the first hour of treatment, then 1.25g/h PO (or 1g/h IVI in 50mL of diluent) for 8h or until bleeding stops; suitable diluents for IVI are 0.9% saline or 5% glucose
- manufacturer's maximum recommended dose = 30g/24h PO/IV.

Chronic bleeding tendency
- 5–30g daily in divided doses at 3–6h intervals, adjusted to the lowest dose that controls the bleeding.

Bleeding from oral cancers[19]
- 500mg PO q.d.s. until bleeding stops
- discontinue by tapering dose frequency every 2–3 days.

Supply
Tranexamic acid (generic)
Tablets 500mg, 28 days @ 500mg t.d.s. = £10.

Cyklokapron® (Meda)
Tablets 500mg, 28 days @ 500mg t.d.s. = £20.

Cyklokapron® (Pfizer)
Injection 100mg/mL, 5mL amp = £1.50.

1 Verstraete M (1985) Clinical application of inhibitors of fibrinolysis. *Drugs*. **29**: 236–261.
2 Breda JR *et al.* (2009) Topical use of antifibrinolytic agent to reduce postoperative bleeding after coronary artery bypass surgery. *Revista Brasileira de Cirurgia Cardiovascular*. **24**: 341–345.
3 Okamoto S *et al.* (1964) An active stereoisomer (trans form) of AMCHA and its antifibrinolytic (antiplasminic) action in vitro and in vivo. *Keio Journal of Medicine*. **13**: 177–185.
4 Andersson L *et al.* (1978) Special considerations with regard to the dosage of tranexamic acid in patients with chronic renal diseases. *Urological Research*. **6(2)**: 83–88.
5 Lacy C *et al.* (eds) (2003) *Lexi-Comp's Drug Information Handbook* (11e). Lexi-Comp and the American Pharmaceutical Association, Hudson, Ohio.
6 Schultz M and van der Lelie H (1995) Microscopic haematuria as a relative contraindication for tranexamic acid. *British Journal of Haematology*. **89**: 663–664.
7 Rankin E *et al.* (1988) Transcatheter embolisation to control severe bleeding in fungating breast cancer. *European Journal of Surgical Oncology*. **14**: 27–32.
8 Broadley K *et al.* (1995) The role of embolization in palliative care. *Palliative Medicine*. **9**: 331–335.
9 Regnard C and Makin W (1992) Management of bleeding in advanced cancer: a flow diagram. *Palliative Medicine*. **6**: 74–78.
10 Kochhar R *et al.* (1988) Rectal sucralfate in radiation proctitis. *Lancet*. **332**: 400.
11 McElligott E *et al.* (1991) Tranexamic acid and rectal bleeding. *Lancet*. **337**: 431.
12 Dean A and Tuffin P (1997) Fibrinolytic inhibitors for cancer-associated bleeding problems. *Journal of Pain and Symptom Management*. **13**: 20–24.
13 Hedges SJ *et al.* (2006) Evidence-based treatment recommendations for uremic bleeding. *Nature Clinical Practice Oncology*. **3**: 138–153.
14 Dunn CJ and Goa KL (1999) Tranexamic acid: a review of its use in surgery and other indications. *Drugs*. **57**: 1005–1032.
15 Seto AH and Dunlap DS (1996) Tranexamic acid in oncology. *Annals of Pharmacology*. **30**: 868–870.
16 Twycross R *et al.* (2009) *Symptom Management in Advanced Cancer* (4e). palliativedrugs.com, Nottingham, p. 236.
17 Kennedy B *Personal Communication*.
18 deBoer W *et al.* (1991) Tranexamic acid treatment of haemothorax in two patients with malignant mesothelioma. *Chest*. **100**: 847–848.
19 Setla J (2004) Duration of aminocaproic acid therapy in bleeding for malignant wounds. In: *Bulletin Board*. Palliativedrugs.com Ltd. Available from: www.palliativedrugs.com

3: RESPIRATORY SYSTEM

BRONCHODILATORS BNF 3.1

Palliative care clinicians caring for patients with end-stage COPD need to be aware of the latest management guidelines. Further, some patients with cancer also suffer from COPD or asthma, and occasionally both. Concurrent COPD can be a major cause of breathlessness, notably in lung cancer, but may be unrecognized, and so go untreated.

The guidelines provided here (Box 3.A–Box 3.C, Table 3.1) for the use of bronchodilators in patients with asthma and COPD are based on the recommendations of the British Thoracic Society/Scottish Intercollegiate Guidelines Network Guidelines on Asthma[1] and the National Institute for Health and Clinical Excellence COPD Guidelines.[2] These have much in common with international guidelines produced by the Global Initiative for Asthma (GINA) and the Global Initiative for Chronic Obstructive Lung Disease (GOLD), although there are some differences in emphasis.[3,4]

Generally, the guidelines should be followed. However, for patients in the last weeks or days of life, particularly those having difficulties with metered-dose inhalers (MDIs), the regular use of short-acting nebulized bronchodilators may be preferable. Further, if a patient is receiving long-term PO corticosteroids for another indication (see p.483), it is often possible to discontinue inhaled corticosteroids.

Inhalation delivers the drug directly to the bronchi and enables a smaller dose to work more quickly and with fewer undesirable systemic effects. β_2-Adrenergic receptor agonists (β_2 agonists), e.g. **salbutamol** (p.106) and **salmeterol** (p.108), act directly on bronchial smooth muscle to cause bronchodilation whereas antimuscarinics, e.g. **ipratropium** (p.103) and **tiotropium** (p.105), act by reducing the vagal tone to the airways. Both classes of drug improve breathlessness by airway bronchodilation and/or reducing air-trapping at rest (static hyperinflation) and on exertion (dynamic hyperinflation). A reduction in hyperinflation probably explains why clinical benefit may be seen in patients with COPD with little or no change in the FEV_1.

β_2 Agonists are used in both asthma and COPD; antimuscarinic drugs in COPD and *acute* asthma. Their use is often combined in *acute* asthma and COPD (Table 3.1, Box 3.B). In asthma and in severe COPD, bronchodilators are generally combined with inhaled corticosteroids (Box 3.A, Table 3.1; also see p.114).

In asthma and COPD, if the optimal use of inhaled therapy provides inadequate relief, a third class of bronchodilators, the methylxanthines, are sometimes used systemically, e.g. PO m/r **theophylline** (p.112). Because of a narrow therapeutic index, their use requires careful monitoring to avoid toxicity.

β-Adrenergic receptor blocking drugs (β-blockers), both cardioselective and non-selective, are contra-indicated in patients with asthma. They should also be avoided in patients with COPD, unless there are compelling reasons for their use, e.g. severe glaucoma. In such circumstances, a cardioselective β-blocker should be used with extreme caution under specialist guidance.

Table 3.1 Summary of the immediate management of acute exacerbations of asthma in adults[1, a]

	Severity of exacerbation		
	Moderate	*Severe*	*Life-threatening*[b]
Assessment			Any of the following:
PEF[c]	>50–75%	33–50%	<33%
SpO_2 (pulse oximeter)	No features of severe asthma	⩾92%	<92%; check blood gases
Speech		Unable to complete sentence in one breath	Silent chest, poor respiratory effort, cyanosis, PaO_2 <8kPa, normal or raised $PaCO_2$[d], arrhythmia, hypotension, exhaustion, altered consciousness
Respiration (breaths/min)		⩾25	
Heart rate (beats/min)		⩾110	
Chest radiograph	When pneumothorax, pneumomediastinum or consolidation suspected, life-threatening asthma, failure to respond to treatment or ventilation required		
Place of care	Hospital for life-threatening; severe or moderate when, e.g. failure to respond to treatment or psychosocial concerns. Intensive care for life-threatening or severe when failure to respond to treatment or ventilation required		
Treatment			
Oxygen	Not applicable	via face/venturi mask or nasal cannulae at flow rate which maintains SpO_2 94–98%	
Bronchodilators[e]	Salbutamol or terbutaline MDI 4 puffs via spacer (give one puff at a time), followed by 2 puffs every 2min, up to maximum of 10 *or* salbutamol 5mg or terbutaline 10mg via oxygen-driven nebulizer		β_2 agonist as for moderate–severe plus ipratropium 500microgram via oxygen-driven nebulizer; use spacer only if nebulizer unavailable
	If inadequate response after 15min, give nebulized β_2 agonist		Repeat above
	If inadequate response after 15min:	Use nebulized β_2 agonist + ipratropium (if not already given) or consider continuous nebulization of salbutamol 5–10mg/h (requires specific nebulizer)	
Corticosteroid[f]	Prednisolone 40–50mg PO stat & once daily for 5 days or until recovery		
Other treatments[g]		IV magnesium sulphate 1.2–2g over 20min IV aminophylline 5mg/kg over 20min, followed by 500–700microgram/kg/h[h]	

a. full guidance available on www.brit-thoracic.org.uk/guidelines/asthma-guidelines.aspx
b. obtain senior/intensive care unit help as soon as life-threatening asthma recognized
c. percentage of best peak expiratory flow (PEF) within last two years or, if unavailable, predicted PEF
d. termed near-fatal asthma when $PaCO_2$ is raised and/or mechanical ventilation is required with raised inflation pressures
e. IV β_2 agonists are reserved for patients in whom inhaled route unreliable (see full guidance)
f. the earlier corticosteroids are given, the better the outcome; where PO not possible, give hydrocortisone 100mg IV stat & q.d.s.
g. when poor response to standard bronchodilator therapies; requires guidance from senior/experienced staff (see full guidance)
h. monitor plasma levels daily (aim for 10–20mg/L or 55–110micromol/L); in patients already taking regular PO theophylline, omit loading dose and measure plasma level on admission.

Box 3.A Summary of the management of chronic asthma in adults[1]

Start at the step most appropriate to the initial severity of asthma. The aim is to achieve control as soon as possible, defined as:

- no daytime symptoms
- no night-time awakening due to asthma
- no exacerbations
- no limitation of physical activity
- normal lung function, i.e. $FEV_1 \pm$ PEF $>$80% predicted or best.

This aim is balanced against the potential undesirable effects or inconvenience of drug treatment. Before initiating a new drug, check adherence, inhaler technique and eliminate trigger factors.

Step 1: mild intermittent asthma
Inhaled short-acting β_2-adrenergic receptor agonist (β_2 agonist) p.r.n., e.g. salbutamol.

Move to Step 2 if:

- symptomatic/inhaler needed $\geqslant$3 times a week
- night-time symptoms $\geqslant$1 times a week
- exacerbation of asthma requiring PO corticosteroids in the last 2 years.

Step 2: regular preventer therapy
Regular inhaled corticosteroid[a,b]

+ inhaled short-acting β_2 agonist p.r.n.

Consider a move to Step 3 if asthma not controlled on beclometasone 400–800microgram/24h or equivalent. (Note: an absolute threshold does not exist and individual patient factors are also taken into account.)

Step 3: initial add-on therapy
Regular inhaled long-acting β_2 agonist (LABA), e.g. salmeterol 50microgram b.d. or formoterol 12microgram b.d.[c]

+ regular inhaled corticosteroid[a,b]

+ inhaled short-acting β_2 agonist p.r.n.

If there is:

- *insufficient response*, continue the LABA and increase the inhaled corticosteroid to beclometasone 800microgram/24h or equivalent; *if control remains poor go to Step 4*
- *no response*, discontinue the LABA and increase inhaled corticosteroid to beclometasone 800microgram/24h or equivalent; *if control remains poor consider therapeutic trials of:*
  - ▷ PO leukotriene receptor antagonist
  - ▷ PO m/r theophylline
  - ▷ PO m/r β_2 agonist.

If control remains poor go to Step 4.

Step 4: persistent poor control
Regular moderate-dose inhaled corticosteroid, i.e. beclometasone 800microgram/24h or equivalent

+ regular inhaled LABA (when of known benefit)[c]

+ inhaled short-acting β_2 agonist p.r.n.

If above inadequate, consider sequential therapeutic trials of the following:

- regular high-dose inhaled corticosteroid, i.e. beclometasone 2,000microgram/day or equivalent (via a spacer device with MDIs)
- PO leukotriene receptor antagonist
- PO m/r theophylline
- PO m/r β_2 agonist (use with caution if already on inhaled LABA).

If add-on drug ineffective, discontinue, except for the inhaled corticosteroid (reduce back to moderate dose).

continued

Box 3.A Continued

If asthma not controlled, consider referral to asthma clinic before proceeding to Step 5.

Step 5: continuous or frequent use of oral corticosteroids
Regular high-dose inhaled corticosteroid, i.e. beclometasone 2,000microgram/24h or equivalent

+ one or more long-acting bronchodilator (see Step 4)

+ regular PO prednisolone at lowest effective dose once daily (monitor blood/urine glucose, blood pressure, cholesterol and bone mineral density)

+ inhaled short-acting β_2 agonist p.r.n.

Refer to asthma clinic.

Moving up or stepping down
Review treatment regularly, moving up a step if control inadequate. Conversely, if control good, consider going down a step. The most appropriate drug to reduce first may be influenced by individual patient circumstances. Reduce dose of inhaled corticosteroid slowly, e.g. $\leqslant$50% every 3 months.

a. typical starting doses are beclometasone or budesonide 200microgram b.d. or fluticasone 100microgram b.d., but up to double these doses can be used according to the severity of the asthma; ultimately, the dose is titrated to the lowest which provides effective control, at which point giving the total daily dose once daily can be considered
b. less well-established inhaled corticosteroids include mometasone and ciclesonide (see full guidance)
c. inhaled LABAs should not be used without inhaled corticosteroids because of concern over an increase in severe asthma exacerbations and asthma-related deaths.

Box 3.B Summary of palliative drug therapy in COPD[2]

Smoking and β-blockers may cause bronchoconstriction and should be avoided.

The choice of drug(s) is informed by the degree of benefit obtained from a therapeutic trial, patient preference, undesirable effects, potential to reduce exacerbations and cost. Assess benefit in terms of improvement in symptoms, activities of daily living, exercise capacity, and rapidity of symptom relief; discontinue if ineffective.

Breathlessness and/or exercise limitation
Short-acting β_2 agonist, e.g. salbutamol, or short-acting antimuscarinic bronchodilator, e.g. ipratropium, p.r.n.

Exacerbations or persistent breathlessness
Short-acting β_2 agonist p.r.n. +

- *if* $FEV_1 \geqslant 50\%$, regular LABA *or* long-acting antimuscarinic bronchodilator, e.g. tiotropium
- *if* $FEV_1 < 50\%$, regular LABA + corticosteroid combination inhaler *or,* if corticosteroid declined or not tolerated, LABA + long-acting antimuscarinic bronchodilator, *or* long-acting antimuscarinic bronchodilator.

Persistent exacerbations or breathlessness (irrespective of FEV_1)
Short-acting β_2 agonist p.r.n. +

- if previously only on LABA, regular LABA + corticosteroid combination inhaler, *or,* if corticosteroid declined or not tolerated, LABA + long-acting antimuscarinic bronchodilator, *or ultimately*
- regular LABA + corticosteroid combination inhaler + long-acting antimuscarinic bronchodilator.

Patients with distressing or disabling breathlessness despite maximal use of inhalers (with spacer if appropriate) should be considered for nebulizer therapy.

continued

Box 3.B Continued

Other drugs
Reserved for patients with distressing symptoms despite maximal inhaled therapy:
- oral corticosteroids; when unavoidable in advanced COPD keep dose to a minimum and in patients >65 years provide routine osteoporosis prophylaxis; in those <65 years, monitor for osteoporosis and treat if required
- theophylline; requires caution, particularly in the elderly, monitoring of serum concentration and for risk of drug–drug interaction; can be used earlier in patients unable to use inhaled therapy
- mucolytics; can be considered in patients with chronic productive cough
- for the role of oxygen in COPD, see p.118
- for the role of opioids and benzodiazepines for breathlessness in advanced COPD and the last days of life, see p.368 and p.635.

Box 3.C Summary of the initial management of exacerbations of COPD[2]

Diagnosis
A sustained worsening of symptoms of acute onset, beyond the normal day-to-day variation experienced by the patient. Commonly reported symptoms are:
- worsening breathlessness, cough
- increased sputum volume
- change in sputum colour.

Management
Optimize bronchodilator use (see Box 3.B); for patients with distressing or disabling breathlessness despite maximal use of inhalers:
- consider use of a nebulizer
- oral corticosteroid, e.g. prednisolone 30mg once daily for 1–2 weeks
- antibacterials if purulent sputum.

Admission to hospital should be considered if:
- rapid onset of symptoms
- acute confusion or impaired consciousness
- severe breathlessness, cyanosis, SpO_2 <90%, PaO_2 <7kPa, arterial pH <7.35
- already receiving long-term oxygen
- increasing peripheral oedema
- living alone or unable to cope at home
- poor ± deteriorating general condition and level of activity
- significant co-morbidity (particularly cardiac disease, insulin-dependent diabetes mellitus)
- changes on chest radiograph.

For those requiring hospitalization, investigations will include:
- chest radiograph, ECG
- arterial blood gases
- serum theophylline concentration, if already taking theophylline
- if sputum purulent, sputum microscopy and culture
- if pyrexial, blood cultures.

For those requiring hospitalization, management will also include:
- oxygen to keep SaO_2 within an individualized target range, according to local protocols
- consideration of the need for:
  - IV aminophylline if poor response to other bronchodilators
  - non-invasive ventilation (NIV)
  - a respiratory stimulant, e.g. doxapram (if NIV unavailable)
  - intubation.

Diagnosing asthma and COPD

The diagnosis of asthma or COPD is based mainly on the history and examination, supported by objective tests and, ultimately, the response to treatment.

In asthma, objective tests are recommended to try to confirm the diagnosis before long-term therapy is started, i.e. the demonstration of variable airflow obstruction over short periods of time using spirometry preferably or peak expiratory flow rate. Patients with airflow obstruction and a high probability of asthma can be given a trial of treatment. Those with an intermediate probability can be offered either a trial of treatment or reversibility testing. In those with obstruction, asthma is strongly suggested by an improvement in symptoms and FEV_1 >400mL in response to either:[1]

- inhaled **salbutamol** 400microgram *or when there is incomplete response*
- corticosteroids, either inhaled, e.g. **beclometasone** 200microgram b.d. or equivalent for 6–8 weeks, or PO, e.g. **prednisolone** 30mg once daily for 2 weeks.

Further tests are recommended for patients without obstruction and an intermediate probability of asthma, and when there is only a low probability of asthma.[1]

In suspected COPD, post-bronchodilator spirometry is generally sufficient to indicate the presence of airflow obstruction ($FEV_1/FVC < 0.7$) and its severity. COPD is now classified as stage I (mild; $FEV_1 \geqslant 80\%$ of predicted), stage 2 (moderate; FEV_1 50–79%), stage 3 (severe; FEV_1 30–49%) and stage 4 (very severe; $FEV_1 < 30\%$).[2]

In palliative care, when airflow obstruction is suspected, evaluating the impact on symptoms of a 1–2 week trial of a bronchodilator is probably the most pragmatic and relevant approach.

Delivery devices

Pressurized metered-dose inhalers (MDIs) are the most commonly prescribed delivery device and the correct inhaler technique should be carefully explained to the patient and subsequently checked.[1] The patient should be instructed to inhale slowly and then, if possible, hold their breath for 10sec. With an MDI, even with a good technique, 80% of a dose is deposited in the mouth and oropharynx.

If inhaler technique does not improve with training or in patients with poor respiratory effort, consider using an MDI plus a large-volume (650–850mL) spacer device to deliver single-dose actuations. There should be minimal delay between actuation and inhalation, but normal (tidal) breathing is as effective as taking a single breath. Build up of static on plastic and polycarbonate spacers attracts drug particles and reduces drug delivery. To reduce static, spacers should be washed once a month with detergent, rinsed and left to dry without wiping.[1] Spacers should be replaced every 6–12 months.[5]

Dry powder inhalers, e.g. Turbohalers® and breath-actuated MDIs, are other options. Patients generally prefer Turbohalers® over an MDI ± a spacer, but they are not suited to patients with poor inspiratory effort. Breath-actuated MDIs are triggered at low inspiratory flow rates, are popular with patients and are the easiest to use correctly.[6]

Nebulizers are more expensive and less convenient than an MDI but may be preferable in patients with a poor inhaler technique, e.g. children, the frail, and patients with end-stage disease. Because of improved drug delivery, there may be better symptom relief.[7] However, the higher doses administered can increase the risk of undesirable effects and their use should be carefully monitored (also see Nebulized drugs, p.721).

There is no evidence to suggest that a nebulizer is superior to any inhaler device for the delivery of a β_2 agonist or corticosteroid for the treatment of stable asthma, or to an MDI + spacer in the initial treatment of acute asthma, unless there are life-threatening features.[1] In patients with COPD and a good inhaler technique, nebulized bronchodilator therapy is only indicated in severe acute exacerbations or when there is distressing or disabling breathlessness despite maximal therapy using inhalers.[2]

In patients with lung cancer, concurrent COPD can be a major cause of breathlessness but may be unrecognized and so go untreated.[8] Breathlessness can be improved in most patients with lung cancer and COPD by a combination of a β_2 agonist and an antimuscarinic bronchodilator; this is equally effective when given by an MDI + a spacer or by nebulizer (see Nebulized drugs, p.721).[8]

Propellants

In the UK, hydrofluoroalkane-134a (HFA) has now replaced chlorofluorocarbons (CFC) as the propellant in all MDIs containing bronchodilators. Compared with CFC, 'clogging' is more likely with HFA because of a reduced exit velocity, and weekly cleaning of the nozzle is recommended, particularly with drugs suspended rather than dissolved in the propellant, e.g. **salbutamol**.

Supply

Inhaler and spacer devices
Haleraid® (A&H) to aid operation of manually actuated pressurized MDIs by patients with impaired strength in hands, available for 120 and 200-dose inhalers = £1. NHS

AeroChamber Plus® (GSK) medium-volume spacer for use with all pressurized MDIs, standard adult device = £4.50, with mask = £8.

PARI Vortex Spacer® (Pari) medium-volume spacer for use with pressurized MDIs, spacer with mouthpiece = £6, with adult mask = £10. NHS

Optichamber® (Respironics) spacer for use with all pressurized MDIs, standard adult device = £4, with mask = £7.

Volumatic® (A&H) large-volume spacer for use with **salbutamol** (*Ventolin*®), **beclometasone** (*Clenil Modulite*®), **fluticasone** (*Flixotide*®) and **salmeterol** (*Seretide*®, *Serevent*®) pressurized MDIs = £3.

1 BTS/SIGN (2011) British Guideline on the Management of Asthma. A National Clinical Guideline. Revised edition May 2011. British Thoracic Society and Scottish Intercollegiate Guidelines Network. Available from: www.sign.ac.uk/pdf/sign101.pdf
2 NICE (2010) Chronic obstructive pulmonary disease: management of chronic obstructive pulmonary disease in adults in primary and secondary care. London: National Clinical Guideline Centre. Available from: http://guidance.nice.org.uk/CG101/Guidance
3 NHLBI/WHO (2009) Global Initiative for Chronic Obstructive Lung Disease. Global strategy for the diagnosis, management and prevention of chronic obstructive pulmonary disease. Available from: www.goldcopd.com
4 NHLBI/WHO (2009) Global Initiative for Asthma (GINA). Pocket guide for asthma management and prevention. Available from: www.ginasthma.com
5 DTB (2000) Inhaler devices for asthma. *Drug and Therapeutics Bulletin*. **38**: 9–14.
6 Lenney J *et al.* (2000) Inappropriate inhaler use: assessment of use and patient preference of seven inhalation devices. *Respiratory Medicine*. **94**. 496–500.
7 Tashkin DP *et al.* (2007) Comparing COPD treatment: nebulizer, metered dose inhaler, and concomitant therapy. *American Journal of Medicine*. **120**: 435–441.
8 Congleton J and Muers MF (1995) The incidence of airflow obstruction in 8bronchial carcinoma, its relation to breathlessness, and response to bronchodilator therapy. *Respiratory Medicine*. **89**: 291–296.

IPRATROPIUM BROMIDE — BNF 3.1.2

Class: Quaternary ammonium antimuscarinic bronchodilator.

Indications: Reversible airways obstruction, particularly in COPD.

Pharmacology

Ipratropium is a short-acting antimuscarinic. In patients with COPD, cholinergic vagal efferent nerves to the airways activate muscarinic receptors, resulting in increased resting bronchial tone and mucus secretion.[1] Antimuscarinics block these effects and cause bronchodilation. Short-acting antimuscarinics increase FEV_1 but have less consistent benefit on breathlessness, need for rescue medication, walking distance and quality of life.[2]

For patients with COPD-related breathlessness and exercise limitation, an inhaled short-acting antimuscarinic bronchodilator *or* a short-acting β_2 agonist are recommended as initial treatment on a p.r.n. basis. However, a short-acting β_2 agonist is generally preferred as it has a more rapid onset of action and, unlike a short-acting antimuscarinic bronchodilator, can also be prescribed concurrently with a long-acting antimuscarinic bronchodilator (**tiotropium**, p.105), which subsequently may be required (see Box 3.B, p.100). In acute exacerbations of COPD when there is insufficient relief with an inhaled short-acting β_2 agonist, a short-acting antimuscarinic bronchodilator is often added despite limited evidence to support this (also see Box 3.C, p.101).[3]

Antimuscarinic bronchodilators have no role in the management of chronic asthma, but nebulized ipratropium bromide is used in severe or life-threatening exacerbations (see Table 3.1, p.98).[4]

Bio-availability most of the 10–30% of the inhaled dose which reaches the lower airways is absorbed.
Onset of action 3–30min asthma; 15min COPD.
Peak response 1.5–3h asthma; 1–2h COPD.
Plasma halflife 2.3–3.8h.
Duration of action 4–8h.

Cautions

Nebulized solution reaching the eye may precipitate narrow-angle glaucoma in susceptible patients; bladder neck obstruction, prostatic hypertrophy.

Undesirable effects

Common (<10%, >1%): headache, dizziness, dry mouth, oropharyngeal irritation, cough, bronchoconstriction, vomiting, GI motility changes.
Uncommon (<1%, >0.1%): visual accommodation changes, tachycardia.
Rare (<0.1%, >0.01%): cardiac arrhythmia, e.g. atrial fibrillation, laryngospasm, nausea, urinary retention.

Nebulized drug droplets may reach the eye and there have been uncommon reports of precipitation of narrow-angle glaucoma and rare reports of eye pain, mydriasis and increased intra-ocular pressure.

Dose and use

In most patients, administration t.d.s. is sufficient.

Aerosol inhalation

- 20–40microgram (1–2 puffs) p.r.n. up to t.d.s.–q.d.s.
- 20–40microgram (1–2 puffs) before exercise in exercise-induced bronchoconstriction.

Nebulizer solution

- use with a mouthpiece to minimize any nebulized drug entering the eye
- 250–500microgram p.r.n. up to t.d.s.–q.d.s in COPD; generally given q.d.s. in an exacerbation of COPD
- 500microgram q6h–q4h in acute exacerbation of asthma (see Table 3.1, p.98).[4]

Supply

Ipratropium bromide (generic)
Nebulizer solution (single-dose units) 250microgram/mL, 20 × 1mL (250microgram) = £7, 20 × 2mL (500microgram) = £7; *may be diluted with sterile 0.9% saline.*

Atrovent® (Boehringer Ingelheim)
Aerosol inhalation (CFC-free) 20microgram/metered inhalation, 28 days @ 40microgram (2 puffs) t.d.s. = £4.
Nebulizer solution (single-dose units) 250microgram/mL, 20 × 1mL (250microgram) = £4, 20 × 2mL (500microgram) = £5; *may be diluted with sterile 0.9% saline.*

Ipratropium Steri-Neb® (IVAX)
Nebulizer solution (single-dose units) 250microgram/mL, 20 × 1mL (250microgram) = £9, 20 × 2mL (500microgram) = £10; *may be diluted with sterile 0.9% saline.*

Respontin® (A&H)
Nebulizer solution (single-dose units) 250microgram/mL, 20 × 1mL (250microgram) = £5, 20 × 2mL (500microgram) = £6; *may be diluted with sterile 0.9% saline.*

With **salbutamol** (generic)
Nebulizer solution (single-dose units for use with nebulizer) ipratropium bromide 500microgram, **salbutamol** 2.5mg /2.5mL, 60 × 2.5mL = £24.

Combivent® (Boehringer Ingelheim)
Nebulizer solution (single-dose units for use with nebulizer) ipratropium bromide 500microgram, **salbutamol** 2.5mg /2.5mL, 60 × 2.5mL = £24.

1 Gross NJ *et al.* (1989) Cholinergic bronchomotor tone in COPD. Estimates of its amount in comparison with that in normal subjects. *Chest.* **96**: 984–987.
2 NICE (2010) Chronic obstructive pulmonary disease: management of chronic obstructive pulmonary disease in adults in primary and secondary care. London: National Clinical Guideline Centre. Available from: http://guidance.nice.org.uk/CG101/Guidance
3 McCrory D and Brown CD (2008) Anticholinergic bronchodilators versus beta2-sympathomimetic agents for acute exacerbations of chronic obstructive pulmonary disease. *Cochrane Database of Systematic Reviews.* **4**: CD003900.
4 BTS/SIGN (2011) British Guideline on the Management of Asthma. A National Clinical Guideline. Revised edition May 2011. British Thoracic Society and Scottish Intercollegiate Guidelines Network. Available from: www.sign.ac.uk/pdf/sign101.pdf

TIOTROPIUM BNF 3.1.2

Class: Quaternary ammonium antimuscarinic bronchodilator.

Indications: Maintenance treatment of airways obstruction in COPD.

Contra-indications: Hypersensitivity to **atropine** or its derivatives, including **ipratropium**, lactose intolerance.

Pharmacology

Tiotropium bromide is structurally related to **ipratropium bromide** but is longer acting and thus has the convenience of once daily administration.[1–3] Its main effect is to inhibit muscarinic M_3-receptors in airway smooth muscle and mucous glands, and M_1-receptors in parasympathetic ganglia. Because it is a quaternary compound, relatively little tiotropium is absorbed into the systemic circulation. However, a small amount of tiotropium is excreted renally unchanged and, theoretically at least, accumulation could occur in patients with moderate–severe renal impairment.

In patients with COPD, tiotropium is more effective than **ipratropium** in improving lung function, relieving breathlessness, reducing exacerbations, exacerbation-related hospitalizations, and improving quality of life.[4] It improves lung function significantly more than **salmeterol**, but the difference is unlikely to be clinically important.[5] It is cost-effective, although not cost-saving.[4] Tiotropium can be introduced and used alone when symptoms are unrelieved by the use of p.r.n. short-acting bronchodilators, or as an add-on therapy when other regular long-acting bronchodilator approaches are insufficient (see Box 3.B, p.100).[6]

Tiotropium has a relatively slow onset of bronchodilation and it should not be used as rescue therapy for acute bronchospasm.[7] Patients receiving tiotropium should use a short-acting β_2 agonist, e.g. **salbutamol**, as a rescue bronchodilator; **ipratropium** should *not* be used as it has a slower onset of action and the muscarinic receptors will already be occupied by tiotropium.[8]
Bio-availability 20% dry powder inhalation, 33% solution for inhalation (soft mist inhaler).
Onset of action ≤30min.
Peak response 1–3h.
Plasma halflife 5–6 days.
Duration of action >24h.

Cautions

Powder accidentally sprayed into the eye may precipitate narrow-angle glaucoma in susceptible patients; cardiac arrhythmia, bladder neck obstruction, prostatic hypertrophy, moderate–severe renal impairment (creatinine clearance ≤50mL/min).

Undesirable effects

Common (<10%, >1%): dry mouth (generally mild and improves with continued use).
Uncommon (<1%, >0.1%): dizziness, headache, cardiac arrhythmia, e.g. atrial fibrillation, tachycardia, epistaxis, oropharyngeal candidosis, pharyngitis, cough, dysphagia, dysphonia, constipation, dysuria, urinary retention, pruritus, rash.
Rare (<0.1%, >0.01%): blurred vision, increased intra-ocular pressure, glaucoma, oropharyngeal irritation, bronchoconstriction, gastro-oesophageal reflux, dry skin.

Dose and use

Dry powder inhalation

- regular administration of 1 capsule once daily via the HandiHaler® inhalation device.

Solution for inhalation (soft mist inhaler)

- regular administration of 5microgram (2 puffs) once daily via the Respimat® inhalation device.

Supply

Spiriva® (Boehringer Ingelheim)

Dry powder inhalation capsules for use with the HandiHaler® device, 18microgram/capsule, 28 days @ 1 capsule once daily = £30; *contain lactose.*

Solution for inhalation (soft mist inhaler) cartridges for use with the Respimat® device, 2.5microgram/metered inhalation, 28 days @ 5microgram (2 puffs) once daily = £34.

1 Barnes PJ (2000) The pharmacological properties of tiotropium. *Chest.* **117 (suppl)**: 63s–66s.

2 Hvizdos KM and Goa KL (2002) Tiotropium bromide. *Drugs.* **62**: 1195–1203; discussion 1204–1195.

3 Gross NJ (2004) Tiotropium bromide. *Chest.* **126**: 1946–1953.

4 Barr RG *et al.* (2006) Tiotropium for stable chronic obstructive pulmonary disease: A meta-analysis. *Thorax.* **61**: 854–862.

5 Brusasco V *et al.* (2003) Health outcomes following treatment for six months with once daily tiotropium compared with twice daily salmeterol in patients with COPD. *Thorax.* **58**: 399–404.

6 NICE (2010) Chronic obstructive pulmonary disease: management of chronic obstructive pulmonary disease in adults in primary and secondary care. London: National Clinical Guideline Centre. Available from: http://guidance.nice.org.uk/CG101/Guidance

7 Calverley PMA (2000) The timing and dose pattern of bronchodilation with tiotropium in stable COPD [abstract P523]. *European Respiratory Journal.* **16 (suppl 31)**: 56s.

8 Sutherland ER and Cherniack RM (2004) Management of chronic obstructive pulmonary disease. *New England Journal of Medicine.* **350**: 2689–2697.

SALBUTAMOL BNF 3.1.1.1

Class: β_2-Adrenergic receptor agonist (β_2 agonist, sympathomimetic).

Indications: Asthma and other conditions associated with reversible airways obstruction.

Pharmacology

Short-acting β_2 agonists (salbutamol, **terbutaline**) have an important role in the management of chronic asthma and COPD and acute exacerbations of both (see Bronchodilators, p.97).[1,2] At low doses, they have predominantly a β_2 agonist bronchodilator effect and no major impact on the heart. However, with increasing dose, tachycardia can occur and rarely prolongation of the QT interval, which may predispose to *torsade de pointes*, a ventricular tachyarrhythmia (see Prolongation of the QT interval in palliative care, p.727).

In chronic asthma, short-acting β_2 agonists should be used only p.r.n.[1] They are not recommended for regular use because little benefit has been shown in RCTs. Further, regular use has also been associated with poorer asthma control.[3] Thus, p.r.n. use ⩾3 times a week is one indication for the need for prophylactic therapy with an inhaled corticosteroid (see Box 3.A, p.99).[1]

In chronic COPD, for breathlessness and exercise limitation, either a short-acting β_2 agonist or a short-acting antimuscarinic bronchodilator can be used p.r.n. If symptoms persist, a regular long-acting bronchodilator is recommended (see Box 3.B, p.100).[2] Thus, for p.r.n. symptom relief, a short-acting β_2 agonist is generally preferred; it has a more rapid onset of action and, unlike a short-acting antimuscarinic bronchodilator, can also be prescribed concurrently with a long-acting antimuscarinic bronchodilator (see **tiotropium**, p.105).

Plasma potassium concentration should be monitored in severe asthma because β_2 agonists, particularly in combination with **theophylline** and inhaled corticosteroids, can cause *hypokalaemia* which further increases the QT interval and risk of arrhythmia.

For details of the use of salbutamol in the treatment of *hyperkalaemia*, see **Potassium**, p.543.

Bio-availability 10–20% of the dose reaches the lower airways.

Onset of action 5min inhaled; 3–5min nebulized.

Peak response 0.5–2h inhaled; 1.2h nebulized.
Plasma halflife 4–6h inhaled and nebulized.
Duration of action 4–6h inhaled and nebulized.

Cautions

Serious drug interaction: increased risk of hypokalaemia with corticosteroids, diuretics, **theophylline**.[4]

Hyperthyroidism, myocardial insufficiency, hypertension, diabetes mellitus (risk of keto-acidosis if given by CIVI).

Undesirable effects

Common (<10%, >1%): tremor, headaches, tachycardia.
Uncommon (<1%, >0.1%): mouth and throat irritation from dry powder inhalation.

Dose and use

Asthma

In moderate–severe exacerbations of asthma, β_2 agonists can be given by MDI + spacer or nebulizer, and repeated until symptoms improve. In life-threatening asthma, they should be nebulized and combined with **ipratropium** (see Table 3.1, p.98).

Aerosol inhalation
Chronic asthma:
- 100–200microgram (1–2 puffs). p.r.n. up to q.d.s.
- 200microgram (2 puffs) before exercise in exercise-induced bronchoconstriction.

Acute asthma (see Table 3.1, p.98):
- 4 puffs via a spacer, given one at a time and inhaled separately, followed by 2 puffs every 2min, up to a maximum of 10 puffs.[1]

Nebulizer solution
Chronic asthma:
- 2.5–5mg p.r.n. up to q.d.s. in patients for whom inhalers are unsuitable.

Acute asthma (see Table 3.1, p.98):
- 5mg up to every 15–30min via an oxygen-driven nebulizer
- 5–10mg/h by continuous nebulization (requires specific nebulizer).[1]

COPD

In acute exacerbations of COPD, bronchodilator use should be optimized (see Box 3.B, p.100); both nebulizers and inhalers can be used to administer inhaled therapy during exacerbations (see Box 3.B, p.100 and Box 3.C, p.101).

In stable COPD, patients with distressing or disabling breathlessness despite maximal bronchodilator therapy using inhalers should be considered for nebulizer therapy (also see Delivery devices, p.102).[2]

Aerosol inhalation
- 100–200microgram (1–2 puffs) p.r.n. up to q.d.s.

Nebulizer solution
- 2.5–5mg p.r.n. up to q.d.s. via an oxygen-driven nebulizer, unless the patient is hypercapnic or acidotic, when compressed air should be used. If oxygen therapy is required by such patients, administer simultaneously by nasal cannulae.

Supply

Salbutamol (generic)
Aerosol inhalation (CFC-free) 100microgram/metered inhalation, 28 days @ 200microgram (2 puffs) p.r.n. up to q.d.s. = £3.50.

Dry powder inhalation 100microgram, 200microgram/metered inhalation; for both, 28 days @ 200microgram p.r.n. up to q.d.s. = £4.
Dry powder inhalation capsules for use in Cyclohaler® device, 200microgram, 400microgram, 28 days @ 200microgram p.r.n. up to q.d.s. = £8.
Nebulizer solution (single-dose units) 1mg/mL, 20 × 2.5mL (2.5mg) = £2; 2mg/mL, 20 × 2.5mL (5mg) = £4; *may be diluted with sterile 0.9% saline.*

Airomir® (IVAX)
Aerosol inhalation (CFC-free) 100microgram/metered inhalation, 28 days @ 200microgram (2 puffs) p.r.n. up to q.d.s. = £2.
Breath-actuated aerosol inhalation (CFC-free) Autohaler®, 100microgram/metered inhalation, 28 days @ 200microgram (2 puffs) p.r.n. up to q.d.s. = £7.

Salamol Easi-Breathe® (IVAX)
Breath-actuated aerosol inhalation (CFC-free) 100microgram/metered inhalation, 28 days @ 200microgram (2 puffs) p.r.n. up to q.d.s. = £7.

Salbulin Novolizer® (Meda)
Dry powder inhalation 100microgram/metered inhalation, 28 days @ 200microgram p.r.n. up to q.d.s. = £6 (using entire refillable units), £3 (using refill packs only).

Ventolin® (A&H)
Aerosol inhalation (CFC-free) Evohaler®, 100microgram/metered inhalation, 28 days @ 200microgram (2 puffs) p.r.n. up to q.d.s. = £1.50.
Dry powder inhalation blisters for use with Accuhaler® device, 200microgram/blister, 28 days @ 200microgram (1 blister) p.r.n. up to q.d.s = £9.
Nebulizer solution (multiple-dose bottle for use with a nebulizer or ventilator) 5mg/mL, 20mL = £2.50; *only available for use in hospitals, may be diluted with sterile 0.9% saline.*
Nebulizer solution (single-dose units for use with nebulizer) Nebules®, 1mg/mL, 20 × 2.5mL (2.5mg) = £2; 2mg/mL, 20 × 2.5mL (5mg) = £3; *may be diluted with sterile 0.9% saline if administration time > 10min is required.*

With **ipratropium bromide** (generic)
Nebulizer solution (single-dose units for use with nebulizer) salbutamol 2.5mg, **ipratropium bromide** 500microgram/2.5mL, 60 × 2.5mL = £24.

Combivent® (Boehringer Ingelheim)
Nebulizer solution (single-dose units for use with nebulizer) salbutamol 2.5mg, **ipratropium bromide** 500microgram/2.5mL, 60 × 2.5mL = £24.

---

1 BTS/SIGN (2011) British Guideline on the Management of Asthma. A National Clinical Guideline. Revised edition May 2011. British Thoracic Society and Scottish Intercollegiate Guidelines Network. Available from: www.sign.ac.uk/pdf/sign101.pdf
2 NICE (2010) Chronic obstructive pulmonary disease: management of chronic obstructive pulmonary disease in adults in primary and secondary care. London: National Clinical Guideline Centre. Available from: http://guidance.nice.org.uk/CG101/Guidance
3 Sears M (2000) Short-acting inhaled B-agonists: to be taken regularly or as needed? *Lancet.* **355**: 1658–1659.
4 Baxter K (2011) Stockley's Drug Interactions (online edition). Pharmaceutical Press, London. Available from: www.medicinescomplete.com

INHALED LONG-ACTING β_2 AGONISTS (LABAS) BNF 3.1.1.1

Class: β_2-Adrenergic receptor agonist (β_2 agonist, sympathomimetic).

Indications: Reversible airways obstruction in patients requiring long-term regular bronchodilator therapy. *In selected patients only* (see Pharmacology): relief of acute asthma symptoms (licensed for Oxis® and Symbicort®) or prevention of exercise-induced bronchospasm (licensed for Foradil®, Oxis® and Serevent®).

Contra-indications: Salmeterol should not be used for the relief of acute asthma because of its slow onset of action.

Pharmacology

The selective LABAs **salmeterol** and **formoterol** have a bronchodilating effect which lasts for 12h.[1] **Salmeterol** has a relatively slow onset of action; **formoterol** has an onset of action similar to **salbutamol** and can thus also be used as an alternative reliever inhaler in patients with asthma. However, because of safety concerns (see below), **formoterol** should be used as a reliever inhaler *only* in patients already on regular maintenance treatment with an inhaled corticosteroid and **formoterol**, given either via separate inhalers, or via the **formoterol + budesonide** combination inhaler, Symbicort®. The need for ≥1 dose for symptom relief on a daily basis should prompt a treatment review.[2] This approach has not been studied with the **formoterol + beclometasone** combination inhaler (Fostair®).

LABAs can also be used regularly to prevent exercise-induced bronchospasm in patients whose asthma is otherwise well controlled on an inhaled corticosteroid. They provide longer protection than short-acting β_2 agonists, although tolerance can occur, resulting in a reduced duration of action. For use immediately before exercise, a short-acting β_2 agonist is preferred.[2]

In patients with asthma, inhaled LABAs are added when symptoms are inadequately relieved by a regular standard-dose inhaled corticosteroid (see Box 3.A, p.99).[2] The addition of inhaled LABAs to inhaled corticosteroids improves lung function, symptoms, and decreases exacerbations more effectively than increasing the dose of inhaled steroids alone.[3,4] However, the findings of post-marketing studies generally have been less impressive and safety concerns have been identified when LABAs have been used *without* an inhaled corticosteroid, i.e. increased life-threatening and fatal exacerbations of asthma.[5,6] *Thus inhaled LABAs should not be used without inhaled corticosteroids* (see Cautions).[7,8]

Inhalers are available which combine a LABA and a corticosteroid. There is no difference in efficacy compared with the use of separate inhalers.[2] However, reducing the number of inhalations and inhalers required may aid patient adherence, and guarantees that inhaled LABAs are not used alone without corticosteroids.[1]

In patients with COPD, a LABA can be introduced and used alone when symptoms are unrelieved by the use of p.r.n. short-acting bronchodilators, or as an add-on therapy when other regular long-acting bronchodilator approaches are insufficient (see Box 3.B, p.100).[9] Unlike asthma, the combined use of LABAs with an inhaled corticosteroid is not essential in COPD, but is recommended for patients with a predicted FEV_1 <50%, or when other approaches are inadequate (see Box 3.B, p.100). Inhaled LABAs and long-acting antimuscarinic bronchodilators are equally effective in terms of improving lung function, relieving breathlessness, reducing exacerbations and hospitalizations, and improving quality of life.[9] For pharmacokinetic details see Table 3.2.

Table 3.2 Pharmacokinetics of inhaled LABAs

	Formoterol	*Salmeterol*
Bio-availability	30–50% of the delivered dose reaches the lungs (Turbohaler®)	Approximately 10% of the delivered dose reaches the lungs (aerosol)[10]
Onset of action	1–3min	10–20min
Peak response	5–10min	≤30min[10]
Plasma halflife	≤8h	≤8h (plasma concentration low or undetectable after therapeutic doses)[10]
Duration of action	About 12h	12–16h[10]

Cautions

In asthma, inhaled LABAs should *not* be used without inhaled corticosteroids because of concern over an increase in life-threatening and fatal exacerbations. To ensure safe use, the MHRA/CHM advise that in chronic asthma:[6]

- patients receiving **formoterol** or **salmeterol** should always be prescribed an inhaled corticosteroid
- adherence will be aided by the use of a combination LABA + corticosteroid inhaler.

Hyperthyroidism, cardiovascular disease, arrhythmias, susceptibility to QT prolongation or concurrent use of drugs which prolong the QT interval (see p.727), hypertension, paradoxical bronchoconstriction (discontinue and use alternative treatment), severe liver cirrhosis (**formoterol**), diabetes mellitus (may cause hyperglycaemia; monitor blood glucose).

Increased risk of hypokalaemia with systemic corticosteroids, diuretics, **theophylline**.

Undesirable effects

Common (<10%, >1%): headache, tremor, palpitations, muscle cramps.
Uncommon (<1%, >0.1%): tachycardia.
Rare (<0.1%) or very rare (<0.01%): arrhythmias, e.g. atrial fibrillation, supraventricular tachycardia, QT interval prolongation, paradoxical bronchoconstriction.

Dose and use

Asthma

An inhaled LABA should be added *only* if p.r.n. treatment with a short-acting β_2 agonist *and* regular prophylactic therapy with an inhaled corticosteroid is insufficient to control symptoms (see Box 3.A, Step 3, p.99). Use of a combination inhaler will help ensure the concurrent use of a LABA + a corticosteroid (see Supply).

COPD

An inhaled LABA is one option when exacerbations or persistent symptoms occur despite short-acting bronchodilators p.r.n. Combined use with an inhaled corticosteroid is recommended for patients with a predicted FEV_1 <50%, or when other approaches are inadequate (see Box 3.B, p.100).

Formoterol

The dose varies with formulation and indication (Table 3.3). In selected patients with asthma regularly using a **formoterol + budesonide** combination inhaler, extra doses may be used on a p.r.n. basis instead of a short-acting β_2 agonist. However, such use ≥1/day should prompt a treatment review.[2]

Table 3.3 Adult doses of formoterol (all in *microgram*)

Formulation	*Formoterol (dry powder)*	*Atimos Modulite® (aerosol)[a]*	*Foradil® (dry powder)*	*Oxis® (turbohaler)[b]*
Asthma				
Starting dose	12 b.d.	10.1 b.d.	12 b.d.	4.5–9 once daily–b.d.
Maximum dose	24 b.d.	20.2 b.d.	24 b.d.	Generally 18 b.d.; on exceptional occasions 27 b.d.
COPD				
Starting dose	12 b.d.	10.1 b.d.	12 b.d.	9 once daily–b.d.
Maximum dose	12 b.d.	20.2 b.d.[c]	12 b.d.	18 b.d.
Relief of bronchospasm or use before exercise				
	n/a		n/a	4.5–9 p.r.n. for relief of bronchospasm[d] 9 before exercise

a. each nominal 12microgram metered inhalation delivers 10.1microgram of formoterol fumarate
b. each nominal 6microgram or 12microgram metered inhalation delivers 4.5microgram or 9microgram of formoterol fumarate respectively
c. maximum total dose 40.4microgram daily, including regular treatment and any extra doses taken for additional symptom relief
d. maximum of 27microgram for any single dose; maximum total dose generally 36microgram daily, on exceptional occasions 54microgram daily.

Formoterol + budesonide combination inhaler

For all strengths in the maintenance of asthma (*without* extra doses for symptom relief):

- start with 1–2 puffs b.d.
- if necessary, increase to a maximum of 4 puffs b.d.
- gradually reduce to 1 puff once daily if control maintained.

Single maintenance and reliever therapy (SMART), using Symbicort® 100/6 or Symbicort® 200/6:

- for regular maintenance:
  - ▹ start with 1 puff b.d. or 2 puffs once daily
  - ▹ if necessary, increase to 2 puffs b.d.
- extra doses for relief of symptoms:
  - ▹ 1 puff p.r.n. up to a maximum of 6 puffs at a time
- maximum dose generally 8 puffs daily, but on exceptional occasions 12 puffs daily.

Salmeterol

Available in aerosol and dry powder formulations (see Supply):

- start with 50microgram b.d. (maximum dose in COPD)
- if necessary, in asthma, can increase to a maximum of 100microgram b.d.

Supply

Formoterol fumarate (generic)
Dry powder inhalation 12microgram/metered inhalation, 28 days @ 1 puff b.d. = £11.

Atimos Modulite® 12 (Chiesi)
Aerosol inhalation (CFC-free) each nominal 12microgram metered inhalation delivers 10.1microgram of formoterol fumarate, 28 days @ 1 puff b.d. = £17.

Foradil® (Novartis)
Dry powder inhalation capsules for use with the inhaler device supplied, 12microgram/capsule, 28 days @ 1 capsule b.d. = £22.

Oxis® (AstraZeneca)
Dry powder inhalation Oxis® 6 Turbohaler® each nominal 6microgram metered inhalation delivers 4.5microgram of formoterol fumarate, 28 days @ 2 puffs b.d. = £46; Oxis® 12 Turbohaler®, each nominal 12microgram metered inhalation delivers 9microgram of formoterol fumarate, 28 days @ 1 puff b.d. = £23.

With **beclometasone dipropionate**
Fostair 100/6® (Chiesi)
Solution for inhalation (CFC-free) formoterol fumarate 6microgram, **beclometasone dipropionate** 100microgram/metered dose, 28 days @ 2 puffs b.d. = £27.

With **budesonide**
Symbicort® (AstraZeneca)
Dry powder inhalation Symbicort® 100/6 Turbohaler®, formoterol fumarate 6microgram, **budesonide** 100microgram/metered inhalation, 28 days @ 2 puffs b.d. = £31; Symbicort® 200/6 Turbohaler®, formoterol fumarate 6microgram, **budesonide** 200microgram/metered inhalation, 28 days @ 2 puffs b.d. = £35; Symbicort® 400/12 Turbohaler®, formoterol fumarate 12microgram, **budesonide** 400microgram/metered inhalation, 28 days @ 1 puff b.d. = £35.

Salmeterol
Serevent® (A&H)
Aerosol inhalation (CFC-free) Evohaler®, salmeterol (as xinafoate) 25microgram/metered inhalation, 28 days @ 50microgram (2 puffs) b.d. = £27.
Dry powder inhalation blisters for use with Accuhaler® device, salmeterol (as xinafoate) 50microgram/blister, 28 days @ 50microgram (1 blister) b.d. = £27.
Dry powder inhalation disks of blisters for use with Diskhaler® device, salmeterol (as xinafoate) 50microgram/blister, 50microgram (1 blister) b.d. = £33.

With **fluticasone propionate**
Seretide® (A&H)
Aerosol inhalation (CFC-free) Seretide 50 Evohaler®, salmeterol (as xinafoate) 25microgram, **fluticasone propionate** 50microgram/metered inhalation, 28 days @ 2 puffs b.d. = £17;

Seretide 125 Evohaler®, salmeterol (as xinafoate) 25microgram, **fluticasone propionate** 125microgram/metered inhalation, 28 days @ 2 puffs b.d. = £33; Seretide 250 Evohaler®, salmeterol (as xinafoate) 25microgram, **fluticasone propionate** 250microgram/metered inhalation, 28 days @ 2 puffs b.d. = £56.
Dry powder inhalation blisters for use with Accuhaler® device, Seretide 100 Accuhaler®, salmeterol (as xinafoate) 50microgram, **fluticasone propionate** 100microgram/blister, 28 days @ 1 blister b.d. = £29; Seretide 250 Accuhaler®, salmeterol (as xinafoate) 50microgram, **fluticasone propionate** 250microgram/blister, 28 days @ 1 blister b.d. = £33; Seretide 500 Accuhaler®, salmeterol (as xinafoate) 50microgram, **fluticasone propionate** 500microgram/blister, 28 days @ 1 blister b.d. = £38.

1 Kips JC and Pauwels RA (2001) Long-acting inhaled beta(2)-agonist therapy in asthma. *American Journal of Respiratory and Critical Care Medicine*. **164**: 923–932.
2 BTS/SIGN (2011) British Guideline on the Management of Asthma. A National Clinical Guideline. Revised edition May 2011. British Thoracic Society and Scottish Intercollegiate Guidelines Network. Available from: www.sign.ac.uk/pdf/sign101.pdf
3 Pauwels RA *et al.* (1997) Effect of inhaled formoterol and budesonide on exacerbations of asthma. Formoterol and Corticosteroids Establishing Therapy (FACET) International Study Group. *New England Journal of Medicine*. **337**: 1405–1411.
4 Shrewsbury S *et al.* (2000) Meta-analysis of increased dose of inhaled steroid or addition of salmeterol in symptomatic asthma (MIASMA). *British Medical Journal*. **320**: 1368–1373.
5 Nelson HS *et al.* (2006) The Salmeterol Multicenter Asthma Research Trial: a comparison of usual pharmacotherapy for asthma or usual pharmacotherapy plus salmeterol. *Chest*. **129**: 15–26.
6 MHRA (2008) Long-acting B2-agonists for asthma: review. *Drug Safety Update*. **1 (January)**: 9.
7 National Prescribing Centre (2008) Current issues in the drug treatment of asthma. *MeReC Bulletin*. **19 (September)**: 3–4.
8 Cates CJ and Cates MJ (2010) Regular treatment with salmeterol for chronic asthma: serious adverse events. *Cochrane Database of Systematic Reviews*. **1**: CD006363.
9 NICE (2010) Chronic obstructive pulmonary disease: management of chronic obstructive pulmonary disease in adults in primary and secondary care. London: National Clinical Guideline Centre. Available from: http://guidance.nice.org.uk/CG101/Guidance
10 Cazzola M *et al.* (2002) Clinical pharmacokinetics of salmeterol. *Clinical Pharmacokinetics*. **41**: 19–30.

THEOPHYLLINE — BNF 3.1.3

Class: Methylxanthine.

Indications: Reversible airways obstruction; given by injection as **aminophylline** for severe or life-threatening exacerbations of asthma (see below).

Contra-indications: Uncontrolled arrhythmias, seizure disorders.

Pharmacology

In patients with asthma and COPD, because of its inferior safety and efficacy, theophylline should generally be considered only after the use of an inhaled corticosteroid and one or more inhaled long-acting bronchodilators (see Box 3.A, p.99 and Box 3.B, p.100).[1–3]

Theophylline is given by injection as **aminophylline**, a mixture of theophylline with ethylenediamine; it is 20 times more soluble than theophylline alone. **Aminophylline** must be given by slow IV injection over 20–30min; it is too irritant for IM use and is a potent gastric irritant PO. **Aminophylline** should be used only with guidance from senior/experienced staff. It has a limited role in patients with life-threatening or near fatal asthma or an exacerbation of COPD who are not responding to initial therapy (see Table 3.1, p.98 and Box 3.C, p.101).[1,2]

Theophylline shares the actions of the other xanthine alkaloids (e.g. caffeine) on the CNS, myocardium, kidney and smooth muscle. It has a relatively weak CNS effect but a more powerful relaxant effect on bronchial smooth muscle. It probably acts by inhibiting cyclic nucleotide phosphodiesterase. This leads to an accumulation of cyclic AMP which prevents the use of intracellular calcium for muscle contraction. In addition, an immunomodulator effect on cells important in airway inflammation has been shown at plasma concentrations as low as 5mg/L.[4,5] Other effects include an improvement in respiratory muscle strength, the release of catecholamines from the adrenal medulla, inhibition of catechol-O-methyl transferase and blockade of adenosine receptors, all of which may play a part in the beneficial effect of theophylline.

Theophylline is metabolized by the liver. Its therapeutic index is narrow and some patients experience toxic effects even in the therapeutic range. Plasma concentrations of theophylline are influenced by infection, hypoxia, smoking, various drugs, hepatic impairment, thyroid disorders, and heart failure; all these can make the use of theophylline difficult. Steady-state theophylline levels are attained within 3–4 days of adjusting the dose of a m/r preparation. Blood for theophylline levels should be taken 4–6h after the last dose.
Bio-availability ⩾90%; 80% m/r.
Onset of action 40–60min PO; immunomodulation ⩽3 weeks.
Plasma halflife 6–12h, but wide interindividual variation.
Duration of action 12h m/r theophylline PO; immunomodulation several days.

Cautions

Elderly, cardiac disease, hypertension, hyperthyroidism and hypothyroidism, peptic ulcer, hepatic impairment, pyrexia. May potentiate hypokalaemia associated with β_2 agonists, corticosteroids, diuretics and hypoxia.[6,7] High-dose **loperamide** (32mg/24h) reduces the absorption of PO theophylline.

Theophylline is metabolized mainly by CYP1A2, and to some extent by CYP3A4 and CYP2E1 and there are numerous interactions (Box 3.D; also see Cytochrome P450, p.735).

Box 3.D Interactions between theophylline and other drugs involving CYP450[7]

Plasma concentrations of theophylline

Increased by	**Decreased by**
Aciclovir	Smoking
Allopurinol	Heavy alcohol intake
β-blockers	Carbamazepine
Barbiturates	Isoprenaline
Cimetidine	Phenytoin
Clarithromycin	Rifampicin
Diltiazem	Ritonavir
Erythromycin	St John's wort
Fluconazole	Sulfinpyrazone
Fluvoxamine	
Leukotriene inhibitors/antagonists	
Mexiletine	
Oral contraceptives	
Quinolone antibacterials	
Troleandomycin (not UK)	
Verapamil	

Undesirable effects

Common (<10%, >1%): headache, dyspepsia, nausea, vomiting; risk of seizures and arrhythmias increases as plasma levels increase; hyperpnoea (fast breathing) when given IV.

Dose and use

Because it is not possible to ensure bio-equivalence between different m/r theophylline products, they should be prescribed by brand name and not interchanged.

An m/r formulation should be used,[1] but an unlicensed normal-release oral liquid can be imported for patients who require it, e.g. those being fed by enteral feeding tube (see p.693). For m/r products:
- starting dose varies between brands; see individual SPCs
- maintain on a single brand because absorption rates vary between products

- titrate dose according to response and plasma theophylline level
- in patients whose symptoms manifest diurnal fluctuation, a larger evening or morning dose is appropriate to ensure maximum therapeutic benefit when symptoms are most severe
- samples for drug plasma concentration monitoring should be taken 4–6h after a PO dose of theophylline m/r, and at least 5 days after the dose was started/adjusted
- the recommended therapeutic range is 10–20mg/L (55–110micromol/L).

However, some patients may experience unacceptable undesirable effects even within the recommended therapeutic range and for them a lower range may suffice, e.g. 5–15mg/L (28–83micromol/L). Ultimately, the clinical response, rather than the plasma level, will determine the need for dose adjustment.

Give IV **aminophylline** in acute severe asthma or exacerbation of COPD only with guidance from senior/experienced staff:[1,2]

- loading dose 250–500mg (maximum 5mg/kg) IV over 20min; omit if already on regular PO theophylline and check theophylline levels stat
- maintenance dose 500–700microgram/kg/h CIVI; check blood levels 4–6h after starting CIVI and then daily; adjust dose to achieve a level of 10–20mg/L (55–110micromol/L).

Supply

Modified-release

Uniphyllin Continus® (Napp)

Tablets m/r 200mg, 300mg, 400mg, 28 days @ 200mg, 300mg b.d. = £3 and £5 respectively.

Normal-release

Oral liquid (elixir) 80mg/15mL, 28 days @ 100mg t.d.s. = £77. (Unlicensed, available as a named patient supply from IDIS; see Obtaining unlicensed products, p.769).

Aminophylline (generic)

Injection 25mg/mL, 10mL amp = £1.

This is not a complete list; see BNF for full details.

1 BTS/SIGN (2011) British Guideline on the Management of Asthma. A National Clinical Guideline. Revised edition May 2011. British Thoracic Society and Scottish Intercollegiate Guidelines Network. Available from: www.sign.ac.uk/pdf/sign101.pdf

2 NICE (2010) Chronic obstructive pulmonary disease: management of chronic obstructive pulmonary disease in adults in primary and secondary care. London: National Clinical Guideline Centre. Available from: http://guidance.nice.org.uk/CG101/Guidance

3 Tee A *et al.* (2009) Long-acting beta2-agonists versus theophylline for maintenance treatment of asthma. *Cochrane Database of Systematic Reviews.* **3**: CD001281.

4 Sullivan P *et al.* (1994) Anti-inflammatory effects of low-dose oral theophylline in atopic asthma. *Lancet.* **343**: 1006–1008.

5 Kidney J *et al.* (1995) Immunomodulation by theophylline in asthma. Demonstration by withdrawal of therapy. *American Journal of Respiratory and Critical Care Medicine.* **151**: 1907–1914.

6 Sweetman S (2011) Martindale: the Complete Drug Reference (online edition). Available from: www.medicinescomplete.com/mc/martindale/current/

7 Baxter K (2011) Stockley's Drug Interactions (online edition). Pharmaceutical Press, London. Available from: www.medicinescomplete.com

INHALED CORTICOSTEROIDS — BNF 3.2

Indications: Reversible and irreversible airways obstruction, †stridor, †lymphangitis carcinomatosa, †radiation pneumonitis, †cough after insertion of a bronchial stent (see Nebulized drugs, p.721).

Pharmacology

Inhaled corticosteroids reduce airway inflammation. **Fluticasone** is given in a smaller dose because it is twice as potent as **beclometasone** and **budesonide**, which are considered approximately equivalent. However, variations with different formulations can occur. For example, one of the hydrofluoroalkane-134a (HFA) formulations of **beclometasone** (Qvar®) delivers a greater fraction of smaller particles to the lung, approximately doubling its potency compared with other formulations (see Dose and use, Table 3.5). This is also true for the combined **beclometasone + formoterol** inhaler, Fostair®.[1] **Ciclesonide** and **mometasone** are relatively new and less well-established inhaled corticosteroids.

Inhaled corticosteroids reach the systemic circulation via both the pulmonary circulation and the GI tract. Long-term high-dose inhaled corticosteroids have been associated with adrenal suppression, and deaths from Addisonian crisis (acute adrenal failure) have occurred rarely (see Cautions).[2] Daily doses of **budesonide** ≤1,500microgram or equivalent do not generally lead to adrenal suppression. However, there is significant variation amongst individuals, and formulation and duration of treatment are also important. Systemic corticosteroids (see p.483) should therefore be considered to cover stressful periods (e.g. infection, surgery) in patients receiving long-term high-dose inhaled corticosteroids, i.e. **budesonide** >800microgram/day or equivalent.[3]

Inhaled corticosteroids are the most effective preventer drug in asthma and there is a low threshold for their use (see Box 3.A, p.99).[4] Improvement in symptoms generally occurs within 3–7 days, but maximal improvement in airway inflammation may take weeks. If standard doses fail to improve symptoms, it is recommended that an inhaled long-acting β_2 agonist (LABA), e.g. **salmeterol** (p.108), is added before using higher doses of an inhaled corticosteroid (see Box 3.A, p.99).[4] If high-dose inhaled corticosteroids are subsequently used, they should be continued only if they have clear benefit over the lower dose. If there is insufficient response to higher-dose inhaled corticosteroids, alternatives include PO leukotriene-receptor antagonists (**montelukast**, **zafirlukast**), which complement the anti-inflammatory effect of inhaled corticosteroids (see Box 3.A, p.99).

In COPD, inhaled corticosteroids are recommended in conjunction with an inhaled LABA for patients with a predicted FEV_1 <50%, or when other approaches are inadequate (see Box 3.B, p.100).[5] It should be noted that studies in COPD have generally used high-dose inhaled corticosteroids, e.g. **fluticasone** 1,000microgram/day. Despite this, the overall clinical benefit of inhaled corticosteroids is relatively small.[6–8] For example, although the annual exacerbation rate is reduced by about 20% compared with placebo, in absolute terms this represents a reduction from 1.1 to 0.9 per patient, with NNTs of 4 and 32 to prevent one exacerbation and one exacerbation requiring hospitalization per year respectively.[6] This relatively small benefit must be balanced on an individual patient basis against the undesirable effects of using inhaled corticosteroids.

The only evidence to support the other indications for inhaled or nebulized corticosteroids listed above is clinical experience.

For pharmacokinetic details, see Table 3.4.

Table 3.4 Pharmacokinetics of inhaled corticosteroids in asthma

	Beclometasone dipropionate[9–11]	*Budesonide*[a,12]	*Fluticasone propionate*[a,12]
Bio-availability	62%[b] CFC-containing and CFC-free aerosol inhalers	39% Turbohaler® 6% Respules®	30% aerosol inhaler 14% powder inhaler
Onset of action	Days to weeks	Days to weeks	Days to weeks
Time to peak plasma concentration	30–60min[b] CFC-containing and CFC-free aerosol inhalers	5–10min Turbohaler® 10–30min Respules®	1–2h powder inhaler
Plasma halflife	3h[b] CFC-containing and CFC-free aerosol inhalers	2–3h	8h

a. data from Micromedex

b. values for beclometasone *17-monopropionate*, the form to which most of the dipropionate is converted before reaching the circulation.

Cautions

Active or quiescent tuberculosis, mycetoma, immunosuppression.

Because of the risk of adrenal suppression, patients receiving the following should be warned not to abruptly stop treatment, and should be given a steroid card (see Box 7.H, p.489):[13]

- long-term high-dose inhaled corticosteroids (e.g. doses higher than the licensed maximum, such as **beclometasone** >2,000microgram/24h)
- inhaled corticosteroids with drugs which may inhibit their metabolism by cytochrome P450 (e.g. protease inhibitors).

Despite concern about corticosteroid-induced osteoporosis, a recent study concluded that, even before starting **fluticasone** 1,000microgram/24h, osteoporosis is common in patients with COPD and, after 3 years, **fluticasone** had no greater effect on bone mineral density than placebo.[14]

Undesirable effects

Oropharyngeal candidosis, sore throat, hoarse voice, paradoxical bronchospasm, hypersensitivity reactions (e.g. rash).

Prolonged use of inhaled corticosteroids is associated with increased risk of glaucoma and cataract, particularly in those aged >40 years.[15–17] Increased risk of onset and worsening of diabetes, particularly in patients receiving the equivalent of **fluticasone** ≥1,000microgram/day.[18]

In COPD, inhaled corticosteroids are associated with a small increase in the frequency of non-fatal pneumonia;[19] patients should be informed of this if inhaled corticosteroids are considered.[5]

Dose and use

Aerosol inhalation

MDIs are most commonly prescribed, alternatives include breath-actuated and dry powder inhalers.

- check the patient's inhaler technique
- use a large-volume spacer device if patient on an MDI, particularly when they:
  - have a poor inhaler technique
  - are using a high dose (Table 3.5)
  - develop a hoarse voice, sore throat or oral candidosis
- instruct patient to rinse mouth after use to reduce systemic availability and oral candidosis
- in asthma, start with a dose appropriate to severity, e.g. **beclometasone** 100–400microgram b.d. or equivalent (Table 3.5), and titrate to the lowest dose effective against symptoms (see Box 3.A, p.99); b.d. dosing is generally preferred (except for **ciclesonide** which is always given once daily);[4] however, if subsequently the asthma is controlled on a low dose, e.g. 200–400microgram/day, once daily administration could be considered[4,20]
- in COPD, inhaled corticosteroids, e.g. **fluticasone** 1,000microgram/day, are recommended in conjunction with an inhaled LABA for patients with a predicted FEV_1 <50%, or when other approaches are inadequate (see Box 3.B, p.100).[5]

Nebulizer solution

- **budesonide** 1–2mg b.d.; occasionally more.

Table 3.5 Approximate equivalent doses for inhaled corticosteroids in adults with asthma[4]

Corticosteroid and examples of formulations	*Equivalent dose (microgram)*
Beclometasone	
Pulvinal®, Easyhaler®, Asmabec Clickhaler®, Becodisks®, Cyclohaler®, Clenil Modulite®	400
Qvar®[a]	200–300
Fostair®[a]	200
Budesonide	
Easyhaler®, Pulmicort Turbohaler®, Cyclohaler®, Budelin Novolizer®	400
Ciclesonide	200–300
Fluticasone	
Flixotide Evohaler®, Flixotide Accuhaler®	200
Mometasone	200

a. approximately twice as potent as other beclometasone inhalers.

Supply

Because of their differing potency and doses, CFC-free aerosol inhalers containing **beclometasone** should be prescribed by brand name and not interchanged.[1]

Beclometasone (generic)
Dry powder inhalation 100microgram, 200microgram, 400microgram/metered inhalation, 28 days @ 200microgram (1 puff) b.d. = £4.
Dry powder inhalation capsules for use in Cyclohaler® device, 100microgram, 200microgram, 400microgram, 28 days @ 200microgram (1 capsule) b.d. = £12.

Asmabec® (UCB)
Dry powder inhalation Clickhaler®, 50microgram, 100microgram, 250microgram/metered inhalation, 28 days @ 200microgram (2 puffs) b.d. = £5, 28 days @ 250microgram (1 puff) b.d. = £7.

Becodisks (A&H)
Dry powder inhalation blisters for use with Diskhaler® device, 100microgram, 200microgram, 400microgram/blister, 28 days @ 200microgram (1 blister) b.d. = £20.

Clenil Modulite® (Chiesi)
Aerosol inhalation (CFC-free) 50microgram, 100microgram, 200microgram, 250microgram/metered inhalation, 28 days @ 200microgram (1 puff) b.d. = £4.50.

Qvar® (Teva)
Aerosol inhalation (CFC-free) 50microgram, 100microgram/metered inhalation, 28 days @ 100microgram (1 puff) b.d. = £5.
Breath-actuated aerosol inhalation (CFC-free) Autohaler®, 50microgram, 100microgram/metered inhalation, 28 days @ 100microgram (1 puff) b.d. = £5.
Breath-actuated aerosol inhalation (CFC-free) Easi-Breathe®, 50microgram, 100microgram/metered inhalation, 28 days @ 100microgram (1 puff) b.d. = £5.
Qvar® is approximately twice as potent as Clenil Modulite®

Budesonide (generic)
Dry powder inhalation 100microgram, 200microgram, 400microgram/metered inhalation, 28 days @ 200microgram (1 puff) b.d. = £5.
Dry powder inhalation capsules for use in Cyclohaler® device, 200microgram, 400microgram, 28 days @ 200microgram (1 capsule) b.d. = £9.

Budelin® (Meda)
Dry powder inhalation cartridges for use in refillable Novolizer® device, 200microgram, 28 days @ 200microgram (1 puff) b.d. = £5.

Pulmicort® (AstraZeneca)
Dry powder inhalation Turbohaler®, 100microgram, 200microgram, 400microgram/metered inhalation, 28 days @ 200microgram (1 puff) b.d. = £7.
Nebulizer solution (single-dose units) Respules®, 250microgram/mL, 20 x 2mL (500microgram) = £20; 500microgram/mL, 20 x 2mL (1,000microgram) = £30.

Fluticasone
Flixotide® (A&H)
Aerosol inhalation (CFC-free) Evohaler®, 50microgram, 125microgram, 250microgram/metered inhalation, 28 days @ 100microgram (2 puffs) b.d. = £5.
Dry powder inhalation blisters for use with Accuhaler® device, 50microgram, 100microgram, 250microgram, 500microgram/blister, 28 days @ 100microgram (1 blister) b.d. = £8.

Ciclesonide
Alvesco® (Nycomed)
Aerosol inhalation (CFC-free) 80microgram, 160microgram/metered inhalation, 28 days @ 160microgram (1 puff) once daily = £9.

Mometasone
Asmanex® (Schering-Plough)
Dry powder inhalation Twisthaler®, 200microgram, 400microgram, 28 days @ 200microgram (1 puff) once daily = £11.

For combination products containing inhaled corticosteroids and LABAs, see Inhaled long-acting β_2 *agonists (LABAs), p.111.*

1 MHRA (2008) Inhaled products that contain corticosteroids. *Drug Safety Update.* **1 (July)**: 6.
2 Tattersfield AE *et al.* (2004) Safety of inhaled corticosteroids. *Proceedings of the American Thoracic Society.* **1**: 171–175.
3 DTB (2000) The use of inhaled corticosteroids in adults with asthma. *Drug and Therapeutics Bulletin.* **38**: 5–8.
4 BTS/SIGN (2011) British Guideline on the Management of Asthma. A National Clinical Guideline. Revised edition May 2011. British Thoracic Society and Scottish Intercollegiate Guidelines Network. Available from: www.sign.ac.uk/pdf/sign101.pdf
5 NICE (2010) Chronic obstructive pulmonary disease: management of chronic obstructive pulmonary disease in adults in primary and secondary care. London: National Clinical Guideline Centre. Available from: http://.guidance.nice.org.uk/CG101/Guidance
6 Calverley PM *et al.* (2007) Salmeterol and fluticasone propionate and survival in chronic obstructive pulmonary disease. *New England Journal of Medicine.* **356**: 775–789.
7 Kardos P *et al.* (2007) Impact of salmeterol/fluticasone propionate versus salmeterol on exacerbations in severe chronic obstructive pulmonary disease. *American Journal of Respiratory and Critical Care Medicine.* **175**: 144–149.
8 Niewoehner DE and Wilt TJ (2007) Inhaled corticosteroids for chronic obstructive pulmonary disease: a status report. *American Journal of Respiratory and Critical Care Medicine.* **175**: 103–104.
9 Daley-Yates PT *et al.* (2001) Beclomethasone dipropionate: absolute bioavailability, pharmacokinetics and metabolism following intravenous, oral, intranasal and inhaled administration in man. *British Journal of Clinical Pharmacology.* **51**: 400–409.
10 Harrison LI *et al.* (2002) Pharmacokinetics of beclomethasone 17-monopropionate from a beclomethasone dipropionate extrafine aerosol in adults with asthma. *European Journal of Clinical Pharmacology.* **58**: 197–201.
11 Woodcock A *et al.* (2002) Modulite technology: pharmacodynamic and pharmacokinetic implications. *Respiratory Medicine.* **96 (Suppl D)**: S9–15.
12 Harrison TW and Tattersfield AE (2003) Plasma concentrations of fluticasone propionate and budesonide following inhalation from dry powder inhalers by healthy and asthmatic subjects. *Thorax.* **58**: 258–260.
13 CHM (2006) High dose inhaled steroids: new advice on supply of steroid treatment cards. *Current Problems in Pharmacovigilance.* **31 (May)**: 5.
14 Ferguson GT *et al.* (2009) Prevalence and progression of osteoporosis in patients with COPD: results from the TOwards a Revolution in COPD Health study. *Chest.* **136**: 1456–1465.
15 Cumming R and Mitchell P (1999) Inhaled corticosteroids and cataract. Prevalence, prevention and management. *Drug Safety.* **20**: 77–84.
16 Carnahan M and Goldstein D (2000) Ocular complications of topical, peri-ocular, and systemic corticosteroids. *Current Opinion in Ophthalmology.* **11**: 478–483.
17 Jick S *et al.* (2001) The risk of cataract among users of inhaled steroids. *Epidemiology.* **12**: 229–234.
18 Suissa S *et al.* (2010) Inhaled corticosteroids and the risks of diabetes onset and progression. *American Journal of Medicine.* **123**: 1001–1006.
19 Crim C *et al.* (2009) Pneumonia risk in COPD patients receiving inhaled corticosteroids alone or in combination: TORCH study results. *European Respiratory Journal.* **34**: 641–647.
20 Chisholm S *et al.* (1998) Once-daily budesonide in mild asthma. *Respiratory Medicine.* **92**: 421–425.

OXYGEN

Oxygen should be prescribed only after careful consideration, particularly if for home use.[1,2] Used inappropriately, oxygen can have serious effects, or even be fatal (see Cautions and Box 3.E).[3]

Indications: Acute and chronic hypoxaemia; breathlessness unrelieved by other measures in, for example, severe COPD, pulmonary fibrosis, heart failure, or cancer.

Pharmacology

Oxygen is prescribed for hypoxaemic patients to increase alveolar oxygen tension and decrease the work of breathing necessary to maintain a given arterial oxygen tension. The appropriate concentration varies with the underlying condition. Examples of established short- and long-term uses include severe exacerbation of asthma and selected patients with COPD (see Prescribing oxygen below). On the other hand, despite the widespread use of oxygen to relieve breathlessness *per se*, most of the available evidence does not support this.[4–7] Breathlessness is a complex sensation which does not simply relate to oxygen tension. Thus, there is great variation in the response to oxygen which cannot be reliably predicted by the level of oxygen saturation at rest, the degree of desaturation on exercise or by the degree of improvement in oxygen saturation.[8–10]

One short-term study in cancer-related breathlessness suggests that oxygen is generally better than piped air in severe hypoxaemia (SpO_2 <90%).[11] However, short and long-term (7 days) studies in patients mainly with lesser degrees of hypoxaemia/normoxia have found no significant difference in the benefit achieved with oxygen or piped air delivered by nasal prongs.[6,8–10] This suggests that a sensation of airflow is an important determinant of benefit.[12–16] Thus, these patients should be encouraged to test the benefit of a cool draught (open window or fan) before being offered oxygen.

Ideally, patients should undergo a formal assessment, e.g. shuttle walk test, symptom scores/ diaries, to examine the benefit of oxygen, e.g. on breathlessness, exercise capacity and quality of life.[2] The assessment should be tailored to the circumstances of each patient. As a minimum, for those breathless at rest, a trial of oxygen therapy can be given for 10–15min and the degree of breathlessness assessed. Initial oxygen saturation is a poor predictor of who will benefit subjectively, and the degree of symptom relief should be used to help guide the dose of oxygen ultimately given. However, a pulse oximeter will help identify those patients who are severely hypoxaemic for whom it appears reasonable to give sufficient oxygen to achieve an $SpO_2 > 90\%$. If benefit is obtained, review again after a longer period of use, e.g. 3–4 days. If the patient has persisted in using the oxygen and has found it useful, it can be continued but, if the patient has any doubts about its benefit, it should be discontinued.[6]

Helium 79%-oxygen 21% mixture (Heliox®) is less dense and viscous than air.[17] Its use helps to reduce the respiratory work required to overcome upper airway obstruction.[18–20] It can be used as a temporary measure in patients breathless at rest while more definitive therapy is arranged. A high concentration non-rebreathing mask must be used for optimal benefit, and the patient's voice will be squeaky. Mixtures containing higher concentrations of oxygen are also available, e.g. **helium** 72%-oxygen 28%. This improves exercise capacity, oxygen saturation and breathlessness in patients with lung cancer.[21] However, this approach is expensive (each cylinder lasts only 2–3h) and limited by the practical difficulties of transporting a large cylinder. Nonetheless, there appears to be increasing interest in **helium**-oxygen mixtures, e.g. in acute exacerbations of asthma or COPD, or to improve exercise capacity in patients with COPD.[22,23]

Cautions

Patients with hypercapnic ventilatory failure who are dependent upon hypoxia for their respiratory drive. Patients should be advised of the fire risks of oxygen therapy:

- no smoking in the vicinity of the cylinder
- no open flames, including candles, matches and gas stoves
- keep away from sources of heat, e.g. radiators and direct sunlight.

Patients should notify the fire brigade and their home insurer that they have oxygen at home.

Undesirable effects (see Box 3.E)

Patients who benefit from oxygen under the care of a home palliative care service report that the advantages outweigh the disadvantages.[24]

Box 3.E Undesirable effects of oxygen therapy[2]

Psychological dependence:

- increased anxiety
- increased likelihood of excessive use
- excessive restriction of normal activities
- withdrawal difficult.

Apparatus restricts activities.

Oxygen mask may cause claustrophobia.

Nasal prongs may cause dryness and soreness of the nasal mucosa.

If necessary, humidification is noisy and not always effective.

Impaired communication.

Social stigmatization.

Cost.

Equipment

Masks are either constant or variable performance masks. Constant supply masks provide an almost constant supply of 28% oxygen over a wide range of oxygen supply (generally 4L/min) irrespective of the patient's breathing pattern. The flow rate should be adjusted for optimal patient comfort and symptom relief. *Constant supply masks should be used when an accurate delivery of oxygen is necessary, i.e. in patients at risk of hypercapnic respiratory failure.* With variable performance masks, the concentration of oxygen supplied to the patient varies with the rate of flow of the oxygen (2L/min is recommended and provides 24% oxygen) and with the patient's breathing pattern.

Nasal cannulae permit talking, eating and drinking and are thus better suited to chronic use. However, they are the least accurate, with the concentration of oxygen delivered dependent on factors other than flow rate. At 2L/min, oxygen concentrations can vary from 24–35%.[25]

Oxygen can be provided via a cylinder (large and small for home or ambulatory use respectively), oxygen concentrator, or liquid oxygen system. It is more economical to use an oxygen concentrator for long-term oxygen therapy, and other situations where use is likely to exceed 3 cylinders/month. Modern concentrators are compact, quiet and cheap to run (2p per hour; reimbursed to the patient). If necessary, two concentrators can be linked by tubing and a Y-connector to deliver higher flow rates (6–8L/min). A 'back up' oxygen cylinder is provided to all patients using a concentrator.

Liquid oxygen systems make use of the fact that 1L of liquid oxygen produces 860L of gaseous oxygen. Relatively compact base units can provide home oxygen, or be used to fill portable units to provide ambulatory oxygen; these are lighter and last longer than a portable cylinder, e.g. about 8h vs. 2h at 2L/min. Liquid oxygen systems are the most expensive, but are quiet, and require no electric power; the base unit is refilled as required.

Oxygen-conserving devices significantly increase the duration of use of an oxygen cylinder or liquid oxygen system. These permit gas flow during inspiration only, generally either as a fixed volume per breath (pulsed devices), or as a variable volume according to the length of inspiration (demand devices).

Prescribing oxygen

Oxygen is generally poorly prescribed. Ideally, there should be a specific oxygen prescription chart which includes details of:[26–28]

- target SpO_2 range
- name of delivery device
- flow rate/oxygen concentration
- duration of use
- method for monitoring the effect of oxygen treatment.

For domiciliary use, the home oxygen order form (HOOF) used in England and Wales requires the prescriber to specify:

- number of hours per day that oxygen will be used
- whether nasal cannulae or a mask
- flow rate
- oxygen concentration (if using a mask)
- need for humidification.

Completion of a home oxygen record form (HORF) is also recommended to document initial and ongoing assessments. Generally, these will be required unless home oxygen is provided on a palliative basis.

Short-term/intermittent

Emergency oxygen therapy

This is primarily used to treat hypoxaemia resulting from acute illness, e.g. pneumonia, pulmonary embolism and severe exacerbation of asthma. Specialty guidelines exist.[28] In brief, for patients not at risk of hypercapnic respiratory failure, initial oxygen therapy is via:

- preferably nasal cannulae at 2–6L/min *or*
- simple face mask at 5–10L/min *or*
- when $SpO_2 < 85\%$, a high concentration reservoir (non-rebreathe) mask at 10–15L/min.

Subsequently the delivery device and flow rate are adjusted to maintain the SpO_2 within a specified target range, typically 94–98%. Avoid flow rates <5L/min with a simple face mask because this may result in carbon dioxide rebreathing.

Greater caution is required in patients at risk of hypercapnic respiratory failure; oxygen treatment should commence using a 24% Venturi mask (2–4L/min) or 28% Venturi mask (4L/min) with a target SpO_2 of 88–92% pending urgent blood gas results:

- if $PaCO_2$ normal:
  - ▹ + no past history of hypercapnic respiratory failure requiring ventilation, adjust oxygen therapy to achieve SpO_2 target of 94–98%
  - ▹ + past history of hypercapnic respiratory failure requiring ventilation, maintain SpO_2 target of 88–92%
- if $PaCO_2$ raised, but pH ⩾7.35, maintain SpO_2 target of 88–92%
- for all of the above, recheck blood gases after 30–60min
- if at any time $PaCO_2$ raised and pH <7.35, consider non-invasive ventilation (seek experienced help urgently).

In the emergency setting, humidification is generally reserved for patients:

- with a tracheostomy or artificial airway
- with difficulty clearing viscous airway secretions (nebulized 0.9% saline is an alternative)
- needing high-flow oxygen >24h with upper airway discomfort because of dryness.

Humidification requires the use of an oxygen cylinder and cold nebulizer; *bubble bottles should not be used because they are ineffective and pose an infection risk.*

Short-burst oxygen therapy

This can be considered for episodic breathlessness not relieved by other treatments in patients with advanced cancer, COPD, interstitial lung disease and heart failure.[1,2] For exercise-induced breathlessness some patients use oxygen before the exercise and others afterwards to aid recovery. However, studies have shown inconsistent benefit from this strategy in patients with COPD.[29–33] Ideally, oxygen should be prescribed only after a formal evaluation has shown benefit in breathlessness and/or exercise tolerance (see Pharmacology).[1,2]

Ambulatory oxygen

This can be considered for patients who are not hypoxaemic at rest but desaturate on exertion to a level <90%, and whose walking distance and/or breathlessness improves when using oxygen to keep SpO_2 >90% in a formal evaluation, e.g. shuttle walk test.[1,2,34] It can also be prescribed in patients who fulfil the criteria for long term oxygen therapy who are mobile and wish to leave the home (see below).

Long-term/continuous

Long-term oxygen (⩾15h/day) can be considered for use in patients with severe disabling breathlessness because of cancer and other life-threatening diseases.[1] More specifically with:

- COPD or cystic fibrosis with PaO_2 <7.3kPa or ⩽8kPa with either secondary polycythaemia or nocturnal hypoxaemia (SaO_2 below 90% for at least 30% of the night) or peripheral oedema or evidence of pulmonary hypertension
- interstitial lung disease and PaO_2 ⩽8kPa
- pulmonary hypertension, without parenchymal lung involvement and PaO_2 ⩽8kPa
- obstructive sleep apnoea who remain hypoxic during sleep despite nasal continuous positive airway pressure (CPAP)
- heart failure and PaO_2 <7.3kPa or nocturnal hypoxaemia
- neuromuscular or skeletal disorders causing inspiratory muscle weakness, either alone or in combination with ventilatory support.

The oxygen is used overnight, and for several hours during the day. Evidence of benefit from such use relates mainly to patients with COPD, where correction of severe hypoxaemia improves survival (especially at 20h/day use), breathlessness and quality of life.[35] The precise mechanism for the improved survival is unknown, but possibilities include a reduction in pulmonary vascular resistance and the subsequent load on the right side of the heart.

Ideally, the assessment for long-term oxygen therapy should be undertaken by a respiratory specialist. For example, in patients with COPD, blood gas tensions should be measured before treatment when the patient's condition is stable (e.g. ⩾4 weeks after an exacerbation) on two occasions at least 3 weeks apart to ensure the criteria are met (see first bullet above). When treatment is commenced, ongoing evaluation is required to ensure the oxygen prescribed is achieving a PaO_2 of >8kPa without an unacceptable rise in $PaCO_2$. Generally, these should be detailed on the home oxygen record form (see Prescribing oxygen).

There is less need for as rigorous an evaluation when home oxygen is purely palliative.

Travel by aeroplane

Patients with lung conditions who wish to travel by air should be given specific advice (Box 3.F).

Box 3.F Air travel and oxygen[36]

Air travel exacerbates hypoxaemia in patients with lung disease and may cause compensatory hyperventilation and tachycardia.

Aeroplane cabins are pressurized, generally to reflect an altitude of about 8,000ft. This is equivalent to breathing a PO_2 of 15% instead of 21% at sea level. Even in the healthy, blood oxygen levels (PaO_2) will fall to about 7–8.5kPa (55–65mmHg).

Low risk

Patients who can walk 50m on the level at a steady pace without oxygen, breathlessness or needing to stop are unlikely to experience problems with reduced cabin pressure.

High risk

- severe COPD or asthma
- cystic fibrosis
- severe restrictive disease (including chest wall and respiratory muscle disease), particularly with blood gas abnormalities
- previous air travel intolerance with respiratory symptoms (breathlessness, chest pain, confusion or syncope)
- co-morbidity worsened by hypoxaemia (cerebrovascular disease, coronary artery disease, heart failure)
- <6 weeks since hospital discharge for acute respiratory illness.

Evaluation

If in doubt, or a hypoxic challenge required, refer to a respiratory specialist.

Generally, the following is recommended:

- clinical, history and examination (previous flying experience, breathlessness, cardio-respiratory disease)
- spirometry, FEV_1% predicted
- pulse oximetry (place the probe on a warm ear or finger long enough to obtain a stable reading)
- blood gases are preferable if hypercapnia is known or suspected:

SaO_2 when breathing air	Recommendation
>95%	Oxygen *not* required
92–95% with no risk factor[a]	Oxygen *not* required
92–95% with risk factor[a]	Hypoxic challenge test with arterial or capillary measurements[b]
<92%	In-flight oxygen required (2–4L/min)
On long-term oxygen therapy	Increase flow rate, e.g. by 2–4L/min

a. see list above; also if hypercapnia, FEV_1 <50% predicted, lung cancer, ventilator support, <6 weeks since hospital discharge for an exacerbation of chronic lung or cardiac disease

b. patient breathes 15% oxygen at sea level to mimic air cabin conditions; interpretation: PaO_2 >7.4kPa (>55mmHg), oxygen not required; PaO_2 <6.6kPa (<50mmHg), in-flight oxygen 2L/min required; PaO_2 6.6–7.4kPa (50–55mmHg) borderline result, consider a walk test.

In-flight oxygen provision

- generally airlines charge for providing in-flight oxygen (fees and services vary considerably)
- passengers may carry their own small, full oxygen cylinders with them as hand luggage for medical use, provided they have airline approval; a charge may be made for this service, in addition to a charge for in-flight oxygen
- the airline must be informed at the time of the booking, and at least one month before the flight
- the airline will issue a form to be completed by the patient and GP/hospital specialist; the airline's Medical Officer then evaluates the patient's needs
- in-flight oxygen is usually prescribed at a rate of 2–4L/min and given by nasal cannulae to be used when the plane is at cruising altitude; can be switched off at the start of descent.

For guidance on specific diseases, patients oxygen-dependent at sea level, and those requiring ventilation, see the full guidance.[36]

General advice

- *medical insurance*, travel with a European Health Insurance Card (if visiting a European Economic Area country) and ensure fully covered for medical costs that may arise related to the lung disease, including the cost of an air ambulance
- *documentation,* have a medical letter on their person detailing condition and medication
- *medication*, take a full supply of all medication as hand luggage, e.g. well-filled reliever and preventer inhalers
- *equipment,* e.g. portable battery-operated nebulizers may be used at the discretion of the cabin crew, but the airline must be notified in advance (an inhaler + spacer is an alternative)
- *ground transportation,* airports can usually provide transport assistance
- *DVT prophylaxis,* see Box 2.F, p.81.

Supply

England and Wales

Oxygen (and Heliox®) are ordered from regional suppliers using a home oxygen order form (HOOF). The doctor must also obtain the patient's consent to pass on their details to the supplier using the home oxygen consent form (HOCF).

The following types of oxygen treatment can be ordered:

- short-burst (intermittent) oxygen
- long-term oxygen
- ambulatory oxygen.

Standard delivery is generally within 3 days of receipt of order, during working hours. Other delivery services can also be specified:

- urgent response (4-hour delivery)
- next day (clinical assessment services and hospital discharges only).

HOOFs, HOCFs, home oxygen patient record forms and guidance on filling in the HOOF can be downloaded from the NHS Primary Care Commissioning website at: www.pcc.nhs.uk/217. Further information is available on the Home Oxygen Service website for health professionals at: www.homeoxygen.nhs.uk/15.php

The completed HOOF should be faxed to the appropriate regional supplier (Table 3.6). Copies should be sent to the Primary Care Trust Home Oxygen Service lead (England) or the Local Health Board (Wales), or to the patient's GP if appropriate, and placed in the patient's notes.

The supplier will ensure that the appropriate equipment is provided (cylinder or oxygen concentrator), contact the patient to arrange its delivery, installation and maintenance, and train the patient in its use. The supplier will continue the service until a revised order is received, or until notified that the patient no longer requires home oxygen.

Table 3.6 Regional suppliers of home oxygen in England and Wales

Supplier	*Region covered*	*Fax number for orders*	*Freephone number for enquiries*
Air Liquide South	South London, South Central, South East Coast	0800 781 4610	0500 823 773
Air Liquide	North East, South West	0191 497 4340	0808 202 2229
Air Products	North West, Yorkshire and Humberside, East Midlands, West Midlands, North London, Wales	0800 214 709	0800 373 580
BOC Healthcare	East of England	0800 169 9989	0800 136 603

Scotland

Oxygen *concentrators* are generally prescribable only by a respiratory or paediatric consultant. However, for palliative care patients, direct requests from palliative care consultants or other health professionals, e.g. GPs, are accepted. Concentrators, some types of cylinders, liquid oxygen systems and Heliox® are all ordered through Health Facilities Scotland, working in partnership with Dolby Medical. For enquiries contact:

Oxygen Therapy Service,
Health Facilities Scotland,
Gyle Square,
1 South Gyle Crescent,
Edinburgh
EH12 9EB.
Tel: 0131 275 6860
Fax: 0131 314 0724
e-mail: nss.oxycon@nhs.net

Certain ambulatory oxygen *cylinders* (2L/min and 4L/min) and accessories are prescribed by GPs using a standard prescription form (GP10), and are dispensed by pharmacists.

Northern Ireland

Oxygen concentrators and cylinders are prescribed by GPs on form HS21. The regional supplier of concentrators and back up cylinders is Air Liquide (customer services: 0500 526 007). Pharmacists dispense all other cylinders and accessories, including Heliox®. Liquid oxygen systems are not available in Northern Ireland.

For further assistance contact the Business Services Organisation (tel: 02890 535613).

Temporary supplies at other UK addresses

Patients travelling to other parts of the UK, e.g. for holidays, can obtain a temporary supply at the alternative address through reciprocal arrangements between the various UK authorities and oxygen suppliers. This is generally organized as a holiday order on a HOOF, even for Scottish or Northern Irish residents. (Arrangements can be made for Scottish patients who obtain oxygen cylinders on prescription to do so in Northern Ireland, and vice versa.) For patients from:

- England or Wales, a second HOOF needs to be filled in and sent to the usual home supplier
- Scotland, holiday supplies are arranged through the Oxygen Therapy Service (see contact details above)
- Northern Ireland, holiday supplies are arranged through the Business Services Organisation (tel: 02890 535613).

Ideally, at least 2 weeks notice should be given, but up to 4 weeks may be needed during peak holiday periods in popular tourist destinations or remote areas such as the Scottish Isles.

Patients travelling outside the UK (including the Isle of Man, the Channel Islands, and on cruises which start in the UK) need to arrange a private supply with their local oxygen supplier.

1 Royal College of Physicians of London (1999) *Domiciliary oxygen therapy services: clinical guidelines and advice for prescribers.* Royal College of Physicians, London.
2 Booth S *et al.* (2004) The use of oxygen in the palliation of breathlessness. A report of the expert working group of the scientific committee of the association of palliative medicine. *Respiratory Medicine.* **98**: 66–77.
3 Lamont T *et al.* (2010) Improving the safety of oxygen therapy in hospitals: summary of a safety report from the National Patient Safety Agency. *British Medical Journal.* **340**: C187.
4 Uronis HE *et al.* (2008) Oxygen for relief of dyspnoea in mildly- or non-hypoxaemic patients with cancer: a systematic review and meta-analysis. *British Journal of Cancer.* **98**: 294–299.
5 Cranston JM *et al.* (2008) Oxygen therapy for dyspnoea in adults. *Cochrane Database of Systematic Reviews.* **3**: CD004769.
6 Abernethy AP *et al.* (2010) Effect of palliative oxygen versus room air in relief of breathlessness in patients with refractory dyspnoea: a double-blind, randomised controlled trial. *Lancet.* **376**: 784–793.
7 Currow DC *et al.* (2009) Does palliative home oxygen improve dyspnoea? A consecutive cohort study. *Palliative Medicine.* **23**: 309–316.
8 Booth S *et al.* (1996) Does oxygen help dyspnea in patients with cancer? *American Journal of Respiratory and Critical Care Medicine.* **153**: 1515–1518.
9 Bruera E *et al.* (2003) A randomized controlled trial of supplemental oxygen versus air in cancer patients with dyspnea. *Palliative Medicine.* **17**: 659–663.
10 Philip J *et al.* (2006) A randomized, double-blind, crossover trial of the effect of oxygen on dyspnea in patients with advanced cancer. *Journal of Pain and Symptom Management.* **32**: 541–550.
11 Bruera E *et al.* (1993) Effects of oxygen on dyspnoea in hypoxaemic terminal cancer patients. *Lancet.* **342**: 13–14.
12 Schwartzstein R *et al.* (1987) Cold facial stimulation reduces breathlessness induced in normal subjects. *American Review of Respiratory Disease.* **136**: 58–61.
13 Burgess K and Whitelaw W (1988) Effects of nasal cold receptors on pattern of breathing. *Journal of Applied Physiology.* **64**: 371–376.
14 Freedman S (1988) Cold facial stimulation reduces breathlessness induced in normal subjects. *American Review of Respiratory Diseases.* **137**: 492–493.
15 Kerr D (1989) A bedside fan for terminal dyspnea. *American Journal of Hospice Care.* **89**: 22
16 Liss H and Grant B (1988) The effect of nasal flow on breathlessness in patients with chronic obstructive pulmonary disease. *American Review of Respiratory Disease.* **137**: 1285–1288.
17 Boorstein J *et al.* (1989) Using helium-oxygen mixtures in the emergency management of acute upper airway obstruction. *Annals of Emergency Medicine.* **18**: 688–690.
18 Lu T-S *et al.* (1976) Helium-oxygen in treatment of upper airway obstruction. *Anesthesiology.* **45**: 678–680.
19 Rudow M *et al.* (1986) Helium-oxygen mixtures in airway obstruction due to thyroid carcinoma. *Canadian Anaesthesiology Society Journal.* **33**: 498–501.
20 Khanlou H and Eiger G (2001) Safety and efficacy of heliox as a treatment for upper airway obstruction due to radiation-induced laryngeal dysfunction. *Heart and Lung.* **30**: 146–147.
21 Ahmedzai SH *et al.* (2004) A double-blind, randomised, controlled Phase II trial of Heliox28 gas mixture in lung cancer patients with dyspnoea on exertion. *British Journal of Cancer.* **90**: 366–371.
22 Laude EA and Ahmedzai SH (2007) Oxygen and helium gas mixtures for dyspnoea. *Current Opinion in Supportive and Palliative Care.* **1**: 91–95.
23 Chiappa GR *et al.* (2009) Heliox improves oxygen delivery and utilization during dynamic exercise in patients with chronic obstructive pulmonary disease. *American Journal of Respiratory and Critical Care Medicine.* **179**: 1004–1010.
24 Jaturapatporn D *et al.* (2010) Patients' experience of oxygen therapy and dyspnea: a qualitative study in home palliative care. *Supportive Care in Cancer.* **18**: 765–770.
25 Bazuaye E *et al.* (1992) Variability of inspired oxygen concentration with nasal cannulas. *Thorax.* **47**: 609–611.
26 Bateman NT and Leach RM (1998) ABC of oxygen. Acute oxygen therapy. *British Medical Journal.* **317**: 798–801.
27 Dodd ME *et al.* (2000) Audit of oxygen prescribing before and after the introduction of a prescription chart. *British Medical Journal.* **321**: 864–865.
28 O'Driscoll BR *et al.* (2008) BTS guideline for emergency oxygen use in adult patients. *Thorax.* **63 (Suppl 6)**: vi1–68.
29 McKeon JL *et al.* (1988) Effects of breathing supplemental oxygen before progressive exercise in patients with chronic obstructive lung disease. *Thorax.* **43**: 53–56.
30 Killen J and Corris P (2000) A pragmatic assessment of the placement of oxygen when given for exercise induced dyspnoea. *Thorax.* **55**: 544–546.
31 Nandi K *et al.* (2003) Oxygen supplementation before or after submaximal exercise in patients with chronic obstructive pulmonary disease. *Thorax.* **58**: 670–673.
32 Roberts CM (2004) Short burst oxygen therapy for relief of breathlessness in COPD. *Thorax.* **59**: 638–640.
33 Stevenson NJ and Calverley PM (2004) Effect of oxygen on recovery from maximal exercise in patients with chronic obstructive pulmonary disease. *Thorax.* **59**: 668–672.
34 Bradley J *et al.* (2005) Short-term ambulatory oxygen for chronic obstructive pulmonary disease. *Cochrane Database of Systematic Reviews.* **4**: CD004356.
35 NICE (2010) Chronic obstructive pulmonary disease: management of chronic obstructive pulmonary disease in adults in primary and secondary care. London: National Clinical Guideline Centre. Available from: http://guidance.nice.org.uk/CG101/Guidance
36 BTS Standards of Care Committee (2004) Managing passengers with respiratory disease planning air travel. British Thoracic Society. Available from: www.brit-thoracic.org.uk/Portals/0/Clinical%20Information/Air%20Travel/Guidelines/FlightRevision04.pdf

DRUGS FOR COUGH BNF 3.7–3.9

General strategy

Coughing helps clear the central airways of foreign matter, secretions or pus and should generally be encouraged.[1] It is pathological when:

- ineffective
- it adversely affects sleep, rest, eating, or social activities
- it causes other symptoms such as muscle strain, rib fracture, vomiting, syncope, headache, or urinary incontinence.

The primary aim is to identify and treat the cause of the distressing cough but, when this is not possible or is inappropriate, an antitussive is generally indicated (Figure 3.1). There is a wide range of available antitussives (Box 3.G) but few of these are in common use (for details of the latter, see p.128).

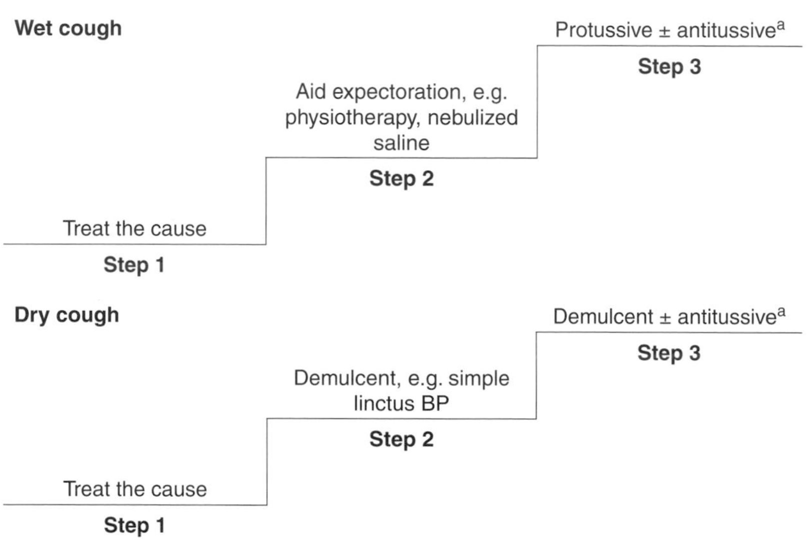

Figure 3.1 Treatment ladders for cough.

a. antitussives reduce the intensity and frequency of coughing; protussives make coughing more effective and less distressing.

Box 3.G Examples of drugs for cough (modified from[2])

Protussives (expectorants)

Topical mucolytics
Nebulized 0.9% saline
Chemical inhalations
  compound benzoin tincture (Friars' balsam)
  menthol and eucalyptus

Irritant mucolytics[a]
Ammonium chloride
Capsicum
Guaifenesin
Ipecacuanha
Potassium iodide

Antitussives

Peripheral
Simple linctus BP
Benzonatate (not UK)
Levocloperastine (not UK)
Levodropropizine (not UK)
Local anaesthetics (nebulized)
Mogusteine (not UK)
Sodium cromoglicate

Central
GABA agonists
  baclofen

continued

Box 3.G Continued

Chemical mucolytics	Opioids
Carbocisteine	codeine
Erdosteine	diamorphine
Mecysteine	dihydrocodeine
	hydrocodone (not UK)
	hydromorphone
	morphine
	methadone
	Opioid derivatives
	dextromethorphan
	pholcodine

a. generally found as constituents in OTC cough products.

Protussives (expectorants) make sputum less tenacious, and thus easier to expectorate. A wide range of protussives also exists (Box 3.G). Generally, nebulized 0.9% saline is the protussive of choice but sometimes an irritant mucolytic (e.g. **guaifenesin**) or a chemical mucolytic (e.g. **carbocisteine**, p.127) may be preferable. Generally, the evidence supporting the use of protussives or antitussives in acute or chronic cough is low-level.[3–5]

1 Twycross R *et al.* (2009) *Symptom Management in Advanced Cancer* (4e). palliativedrugs.com, Nottingham, pp. 160–166.
2 Homsi J *et al.* (2001) Important drugs for cough in advanced cancer. *Supportive Care in Cancer.* **9**: 565–574.
3 Smith SM *et al.* (2010) Over-the-counter (OTC) medications for acute cough in children and adults in ambulatory settings. *Cochrane Database of Systematic Reviews.* **9**: CD001831.
4 Molassiotis M *et al.* (2010) Interventions for cough in cancer. *Cochrane Database of Systematic Reviews.* **9**: CD007881.
5 Molassiotis A *et al.* (2010) Pharmacological and non-pharmacological interventions for cough in adults with respiratory and non-respiratory diseases: A systematic review of the literature. *Respiratory Medicine.* **104**: 934–944.

MUCOLYTICS — BNF 3.7

Class: Chemical mucolytic.

Indications: Reduction of sputum viscosity.

Contra-indications: Active peptic ulceration. **Erdosteine**: severe hepatic or renal impairment.

Pharmacology

The mucolytics **carbocisteine**, **erdosteine** and **mecysteine** reduce the viscosity of bronchial secretions and facilitate expectoration. They alter the physical and chemical characteristics of the mucin components of sputum to a more 'normal' pattern by reducing fructose and sulphate content and increasing the proportion of sialomucins. The role of mucolytics in patients with COPD is controversial; they reduce the frequency of exacerbations and days of illness, but have no effect on the need for hospitalization nor improve quality of life.[1,2] UK guidelines recommend that they should be considered for patients with a chronic productive cough, and continued only when there is symptomatic benefit.[1] Other guidelines acknowledge that a few patients with viscous sputum may benefit from mucolytics, but consider the overall benefit too small to recommend widespread use.[3]

Cautions

History of peptic ulcer disease (mucolytics can disrupt the gastric mucosal barrier). **Erdosteine**: limit dose to 300mg/24h in mild–moderate hepatic impairment.

Undesirable effects

Occasional dyspepsia, GI haemorrhage, rash.

Dose and use

Carbocisteine

- start with 750mg t.d.s.
- reduce to 750mg b.d. once satisfactory response obtained, i.e. reduction in cough and sputum production.

Erdosteine

- 300mg b.d. for up to 10 days.

Mecysteine

- start with 200mg q.d.s. for 2 days
- reduce to 200mg t.d.s. for 6 weeks
- reduce further to 200mg b.d.

Supply

Carbocisteine (Sanofi-Aventis)
Capsules 375mg, 28 days @ 750mg t.d.s. = £23.
Oral liquid 250mg/5mL, 28 days @ 750mg t.d.s. = £24; *cinnamon with rum flavour.*

Erdosteine
Erdotin® (Galen)
Capsules 300mg, 28 days @ 300mg b.d. = £16.

Mecysteine
Visclair® (Ranbaxy)
Tablets e/c 100mg, 28 days @ 200mg t.d.s. = £30.

1 NICE (2010) Chronic obstructive pulmonary disease: management of chronic obstructive pulmonary disease in adults in primary and secondary care. London: National Clinical Guideline Centre. Available from: http://guidance.nice.org.uk/CG101/Guidance
2 Poole P and Black P (2010) Mucolytic agents for chronic bronchitis or chronic obstructive pulmonary disease. *Cochrane Database of Systematic Reviews.* **2**: CD001287.
3 NHLBI/WHO (2009) Global Initiative for Chronic Obstructive Lung Disease. Global strategy for the diagnosis, management and prevention of chronic obstructive pulmonary disease. Available from: www.goldcopd.com

ANTITUSSIVES — BNF 3.9

Antitussives can be divided into peripherally-acting and centrally-acting agents. The former include local pharyngeal soothing agents (demulcents) and local anaesthetics and their derivatives.[1] The centrally-acting antitussives are almost exclusively opioids or opioid derivatives. Because in palliative care the opioid antitussives are generally used in preference to local anaesthetics and their derivatives, they are given precedence in this section. Generally, the evidence supporting the use of antitussives in acute or chronic cough is low-level.[2–4]

Demulcents

These contain soothing substances such as syrup or **glycerol**. The high sugar content stimulates the production of saliva and soothes the oropharynx. The associated swallowing may also interfere with the cough reflex. The sweet taste itself may be antitussive by stimulating the release of endogenous opioids in the brain stem, and this may contribute to the large placebo effect seen in controlled trials of demulcents.[5] However, the antitussive effect of demulcents is generally short-lived and there is no evidence that combination products are better than **simple linctus BP** (5mL t.d.s.–q.d.s.). Thus, if **simple linctus BP** is ineffective, there is little point in trying combination products.

Opioids

Opioids act primarily by suppressing the cough reflex centre in the brain stem. Opioids appear less effective for cough due to upper airway disorders, e.g. upper respiratory tract infection, possibly because laryngeal cough involves opioid-insensitive central mechanisms and/or reflects a different reflex (i.e. an expiration reflex).[6] **Codeine**, **pholcodine** and **dextromethorphan** are common ingredients in combination antitussive products but often in small and probably ineffective doses.[7] Thus, the benefit of combination products may reside mainly in the sugar content (see Demulcents above).[5] Nonetheless, the MHRA has recently advised against the use of OTC cough products containing **codeine** for under 18 year-olds.[8]

In palliative care, **codeine** is generally preferred to **pholcodine**, which has little analgesic effect (negligible amounts converted to **morphine**). If **codeine** or **hydrocodone** (not UK)[9] is ineffective, **morphine** should be prescribed.

For patients already receiving strong opioids, if a p.r.n. dose relieves the cough, continue to use it in this way or increase the regular dose of the opioid. However, if no benefit is obtained from a p.r.n. dose, there is little point in further regular dose increments. Some patients with cough but no pain benefit from a bedtime dose of **morphine** to prevent cough disturbing sleep. *If a patient is already receiving a strong opioid for pain relief it is a nonsense to prescribe* ***codeine*** *as well.*

Local anaesthetics

Nebulized local anaesthetics have been used as antitussives in patients with cough caused by cancer. They probably act locally by inhibiting the sensory nerves in the airways involved in the cough reflex but there could be a central effect as well. However, their use has not been formally evaluated; thus they should be considered only when other avenues have failed, including nebulized 0.9% saline.

Suggested doses are 5mL of either 2% **lidocaine** or 0.25% **bupivacaine** t.d.s.–q.d.s. Use is limited by:

- unpleasant taste
- oropharyngeal numbness → reduced gag/cough reflex; patients should be advised not to eat or drink for 1h after treatment
- risk of bronchoconstriction → pretreat asthmatic patients with **salbutamol**[10,11]
- a short duration of action (10–30min).[7]

Even so, there are anecdotal reports of patients with chronic lung disease, sarcoidosis or cancer, in whom a single treatment with nebulized **lidocaine** 400mg relieved cough for 1–8 weeks.[12–14] Also see Nebulized drugs, p.721.

Benzonatate

Benzonatate (not UK) is chemically related to the **procaine** class of local anaesthetics. It acts peripherally by inhibiting the stretch receptors in the lower respiratory tract, lungs and pleura. It acts in 15–20min, and the effect lasts 3–8h. It is used at some centres in the USA when opioids such as **hydrocodone** fail to relieve a dry irritating cough, or if opioid antitussives are poorly tolerated.[15]

Management strategy

Correct the correctable

If possible, the cause of the cough should be treated specifically, e.g. antibacterials for infection. However, when the cause of the cough is not amenable to specific treatment or is unknown, measures should be taken to suppress the cough (see Figure 3.1, p.126).

Drug treatment

If a locally soothing demulcent (e.g. **simple linctus BP** 5mL t.d.s.–q.d.s.) is inadequate, consider a centrally-acting opioid antitussive:

- **codeine** linctus 15–30mg (5–10mL) t.d.s.–q.d.s.
- if not effective, switch to **morphine**, starting with:
  - ▹ a *normal-release* formulation 5–10mg q.d.s.–q4h (but 2.5–5mg q.d.s.–q4h if not switching from **codeine**) *or*
  - ▹ a *modified-release* formulation 10–20mg b.d. (but 5–10mg b.d. if not switching from **codeine**)

- if necessary, increase the dose until the cough is relieved or until undesirable effects prevent further escalation (see p.362).

If a patient is already receiving a strong opioid for pain relief it is a nonsense to prescribe **codeine** or a second strong opioid for cough suppression.

If opioid antitussives are unsatisfactory, other possible treatments include:

- **sodium cromoglicate** 10mg inhaled q.d.s. improves cough in patients with lung cancer within 36–48h[16]
- **baclofen** 10mg PO t.d.s. or 20mg PO once daily has an antitussive effect in healthy volunteers and in patients with ACE inhibitor cough; maximum effect is seen after 2–4 weeks[1,17]
- **gabapentin** 100mg PO b.d. up to 800mg PO b.d. is reported to have an antitussive effect in idiopathic chronic cough[18]
- **levodropropizine** 75mg PO t.d.s. (not UK) is as effective as **dihydrocodeine** 10mg PO t.d.s. in patients with lung cancer and causes less drowsiness[19]
- **benzonatate** 100mg t.d.s. (not UK); if necessary, increase to 200mg t.d.s.

Supply

Simple linctus BP

Oral syrup 28 days @ 5mL q.d.s. = £1.50.

Codeine linctus BP

Oral solution 15mg/5mL, 28 days @ 15mg q.d.s. = £4.
Diabetic oral solution 15mg/5mL, 28 days @ 15mg q.d.s. = £2.
All of the above products are available OTC.

Morphine

Oramorph® (Boehringer Ingelheim)
Oral solution 10mg/5mL, 28 days @ 5mg q.d.s. = £4.
Also see **morphine**, p.369 for other products.

1 Dicpinigaitis PV (2006) Current and future peripherally-acting antitussives. *Respiratory Physiology and Neurobiology.* **152**: 356–362.
2 Molassiotis A *et al.* (2010) Pharmacological and non-pharmacological interventions for cough in adults with respiratory and non-respiratory diseases: A systematic review of the literature. *Respiratory Medicine.* **104**: 934–944.
3 Molassiotis M *et al.* (2010) Interventions for cough in cancer. *Cochrane Database of Systematic Reviews.* **9**: CD007881.
4 Smith SM *et al.* (2010) Over-the-counter (OTC) medications for acute cough in children and adults in ambulatory settings. *Cochrane Database of Systematic Reviews.* **9**: CD001831.
5 Eccles R (2006) Mechanisms of the placebo effect of sweet cough syrups. *Respiratory Physiology and Neurobiology.* **152**: 340–348.
6 Bolser DC (2006) Current and future centrally acting antitussives. *Respiratory Physiology and Neurobiology.* **152**: 349–355.
7 Fuller R and Jackson D (1990) Physiology and treatment of cough. *Thorax.* **45**: 425–430.
8 MHRA (2010) Codeine-containing liquid over-the-counter medicines: should not be used for cough under 18 years. *Drug Safety Update.* **4 (October)**: H3.
9 Homsi J *et al.* (2002) A phase II study of hydrocodone for cough in advanced cancer. *American Journal of Hospice and Palliative Care.* **19 (1)**: 49–56.
10 McAlpine L and Thomson N (1989) Lidocaine-induced bronchoconstriction in asthmatic patients. Relation to histamine airway responsiveness and effect of preservative. *Chest.* **96**: 1012–1015.
11 Groeben H *et al.* (2000) Combined lidocaine and salbutamol inhalation for airway anesthesia markedly protects against reflex bronchoconstriction. *Chest.* **118**: 509–515.
12 Howard P *et al.* (1977) Lignocaine aerosol and persistent cough. *British Journal of Diseases of the Chest.* **71**: 19–24.
13 Stewart C and Coady T (1977) Suppression of intractable cough. *British Medical Journal.* **1**: 1660–1661.
14 Sanders RV and Kirkpatrick MB (1984) Prolonged suppression of cough after inhalation of lidocaine in a patient with sarcoid. *Journal of the American Medical Association.* **252**: 2456–2457.
15 Doona M and Walsh D (1998) Benzonatate for opioid-resistant cough in advanced cancer. *Palliative Medicine.* **12**: 55–58.
16 Moroni M *et al.* (1996) Inhaled sodium cromoglycate to treat cough in advanced lung cancer patients. *British Journal of Cancer.* **74**: 309–311.
17 Dicpinigaitis P *et al.* (1998) Inhibition of capsaicin-induced cough by the gamma-aminobutyric acid agonist baclofen. *Journal of Clinical Pharmacology.* **38**: 364–367.
18 Mintz S and Lee JK (2006) Gabapentin in the treatment of intractable idiopathic chronic cough: case reports. *American Journal of Medicine.* **119**: e13–15.
19 Luporini G *et al.* (1998) Efficacy and safety of levodropropizine and dihydrocodeine on nonproductive cough in primary and metastatic lung cancer. *European Respiratory Journal.* **12**: 97–101.

4: CENTRAL NERVOUS SYSTEM

PSYCHOTROPICS — BNF 4

Psychotropic drugs are primarily used to alter a patient's psychological state. Generally, smaller doses should be used in debilitated patients than in those who are physically fit, particularly if they are already receiving a strong opioid or another psychotropic drug.[1] Close supervision is essential, particularly during the first few days. Either a reduction in dose because of drug accumulation or a further increase because of a lack of response may be needed.

A few patients respond paradoxically when prescribed psychotropic drugs, e.g. **diazepam** (become more distressed) or **amitriptyline** (become wakeful and restless at night). Other patients derive little benefit from a benzodiazepine, e.g. **diazepam**, but are helped by an antipsychotic, e.g. **haloperidol**. Tricyclic antidepressants (TCAs) are widely used to relieve neuropathic pain; dose escalation is often limited by undesirable effects.

Although prescribers will be influenced by local formularies and fashions, it is better to learn to use a small number of drugs well than to have limited experience with all possible alternatives (Box 4.A).

Box 4.A Psychotropic drugs: *PCF* preferred drugs[a]

Benzodiazepines
Diazepam (universally available but cannot be given SC, cheap)
Midazolam (used SC, mainly in imminently dying patients)
Clonazepam (anti-epileptic, adjuvant analgesic)
Lorazepam (status epilepticus, quick-acting SL)
Temazepam (night sedative)

Antipsychotics
Haloperidol
Prochlorperazine
Levomepromazine (if drowsiness desirable; also used for intractable vomiting)
Olanzapine (also used for intractable vomiting)
Quetiapine
Risperidone

Antidepressants
Methylphenidate (if prognosis <2–4 weeks)
Sertraline or citalopram
Mirtazapine
Amitriptyline or nortriptyline
Trazodone

a. for other classes of psychotropics, see respective generic monographs.

1 Wagner B and O'Hara D (1997) Pharmacokinetics and pharmacodynamics of sedatives and analgesics in the treatment of agitated critically ill patients. *Clinical Pharmacokinetics*. **33**: 426–453.

BENZODIAZEPINES BNF 4.1, 4.8, 10.2.2 & 15.1.4.1

Class: GABAmimetics, anxiolytic sedatives.

Indications: Licensed indications vary between products; consult the manufacturers' SPCs for details; they include insomnia, anxiety and panic disorder, status epilepticus, refractory epilepsy, myoclonus, skeletal muscle relaxant, alcohol withdrawal. Other indications include †acute psychotic agitation, †terminal agitation, †neuropathic pain, †nausea and vomiting, †intractable pruritus, †intractable hiccup.

Contra-indications: (unless in the imminently dying) Acute or severe pulmonary insufficiency, sleep apnoea syndrome, severe liver disease, myasthenia gravis. Also see individual monographs.

Pharmacology

GABA is the major inhibitory neurotransmitter of the nervous system. Several drug classes enhance its action (GABAmimetics):

- $GABA_A$ modulators: benzodiazepines, Z drugs (e.g. **zopiclone**), barbiturates (see p.270), some general anaesthetics (e.g. **propofol**, see p.600), alcohol
- $GABA_B$ agonists: **baclofen** (see p.563)
- inhibitors of GABA transaminase, e.g. **vigabatrin** or re-uptake, e.g. **tiagibine** (see p.237).

The $GABA_A$ receptor is a chloride channel formed by 5 subunits comprising varying subtypes (Figure 4.1). $GABA_A$ modulators bind to sites distinct from GABA itself (allosteric modulation), increasing the receptor's affinity for GABA (benzodiazepines) or prolonging channel opening (barbiturates).[1] The α subunit determines benzodiazepine affinity and function (Table 4.1). Thus, α-selective modulators are under investigation (e.g. $\alpha2/\alpha3$-selective non-sedating anxiolytics).[2]

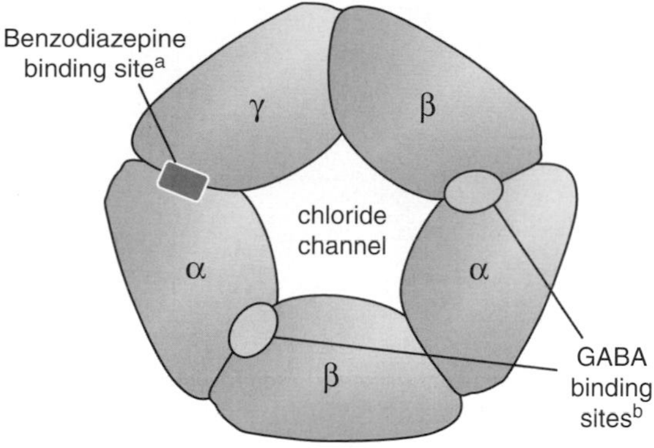

Figure 4.1 Structure of the $GABA_A$ receptor.

a. The binding sites for barbiturates, ethanol, neurosteroids and other allosteric modulators are less well characterized

b. The central chloride channel is opened by the concurrent binding of 2 GABA molecules.

Table 4.1 $GABA_A$ α-subunit function and selected binding affinities.[2–5]

Alpha subunit[a]	*1*	*2*	*3*	*4*[c]	*5*	*6*[c]
Function[b]	*Sleep*	*Anxiolysis*	*Anxiolysis*		*Amnesia*	
Clonazepam	+++	+++	+++	−		−
Diazepam	++	++	++	−	+++	−
Flunitrazepam	+++	+++	+++	−	+++	−
Midazolam	+++		+++	−	+++	−
Zolpidem	++	+	−	−	−	−
Zopiclone	+	+	−/+[d]	−	+	−
Pentobarbital[e]	++	+++	++	+++	+++	

Affinity: +++ high, ++ moderate, + low, − negligible or none; blank = no data.

a. affinities relate to α-subunit combinations with γ2-subunits

b. subunits influencing seizures and muscle tone are less well characterized

c. benzodiazepines do not bind to α4- and α6-subunits, or to receptors lacking α and γ subunits (benzodiazepine-insensitive $GABA_A$ receptors)

d. conflicting data

e. binding affinity extrapolated from a functional assay.

The use of non-selective GABA antagonists is precluded by their anxiogenic and pro-seizure properties. However, the memory-enhancing properties of α5-selective inverse agonists are being investigated. **Flumazenil** is a specific benzodiazepine antagonist, and can be used to reverse the sedative effects of benzodiazepines. Because of fatal iatrogenic overdoses of **midazolam**, the NPSA recommends that **flumazenil** is available for emergency use wherever **midazolam** is used clinically.[6] Endogenous ligands for the benzodiazepine binding site include peptide and neurosteroid molecules, but their physiological function is not yet understood.

Although the relationship is non-linear, the plasma halflife of a benzodiazepine and its pharmacologically active metabolites reflect duration of action (Figure 4.2); those with long halflives can be taken once daily, preferably at bedtime. Intermediate-acting agents (e.g. **oxazepam** and **temazepam**) are used mainly for night sedation; they are metabolized in one step to inactive compounds. Some long-acting agents (e.g. **diazepam** and **chlordiazepoxide**) are converted to a long-lasting active metabolite (nordiazepam). Differences in the pharmacological profile of different benzodiazepines are relatively minor (Table 4.1) but potency varies considerably (Table 4.2). Compared with its other properties, **clonazepam** has relatively more antiseizure activity.

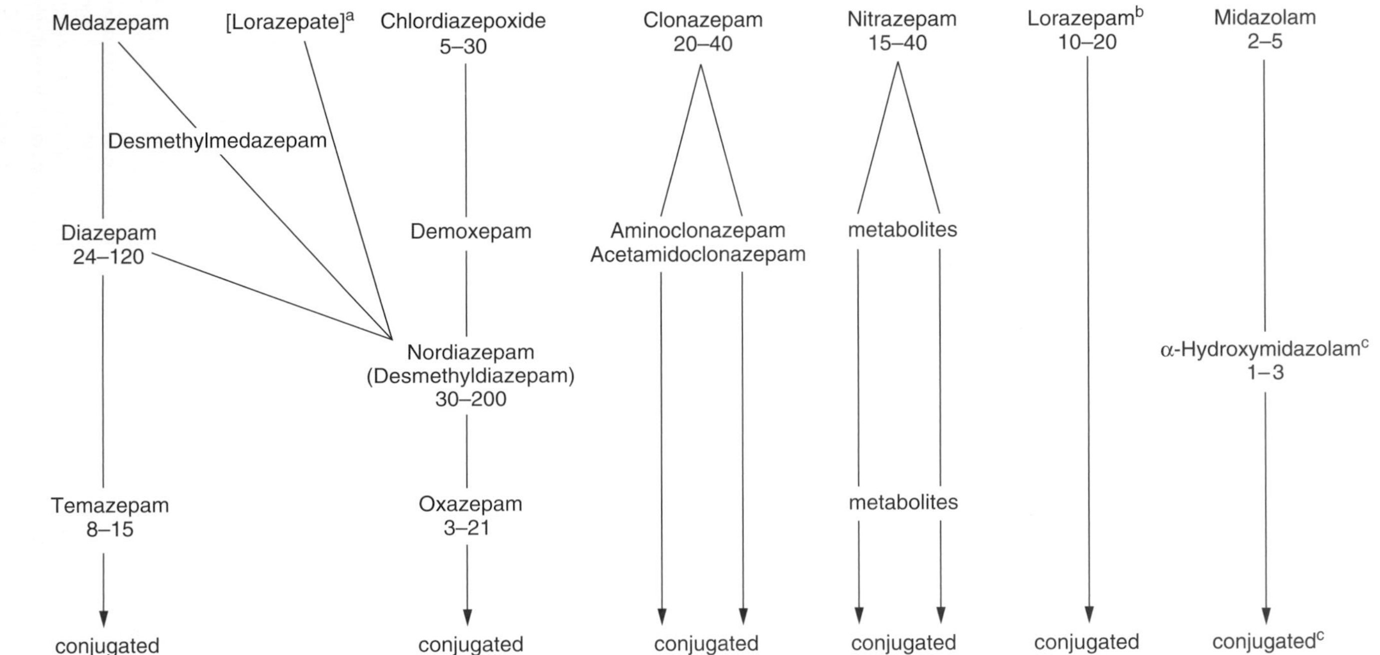

Figure 4.2 Metabolic pathways for selected benzodiazepines. Figures refer to plasma elimination halflives in hours of pharmacologically active substances.

a. lorazepate is a pro-drug
b. lorazepam does not use the P450 hepatic metabolic pathway and avoids interactions relating to competitive inhibition of metabolism
c. α-hydroxymidazolam glucuronide is an active substance, about 10 times less potent than both the unconjugated form and midazolam; accumulation in severe renal failure may lead to prolonged sedation.

Table 4.2 Approximate equivalent anxiolytic-sedative doses[7,8]

Drug	*Dose*
Clonazepam	250microgram
Lorazepam	500microgram
Midazolam	1.5–2mg
Diazepam	5mg
Nitrazepam	5mg
Temazepam	10mg
Chlordiazepoxide	15mg
Oxazepam	15mg

Cautions

Benzodiazepines with long halflives accumulate when given repeatedly and undesirable effects may manifest only after several days or weeks. Caution is required in mild–moderate hepatic impairment and renal impairment. Because their central depressant effect can depress respiration, caution is required in chronic respiratory disease. However, they are relatively safe in overdose.

Because benzodiazepines can cause physical and psychological dependence, patients with a history of substance abuse should be monitored closely. Further, if treatment is discontinued, taper gradually to avoid withdrawal symptoms, e.g. by one eighth of the daily dose every 2 weeks.

Undesirable effects

The main undesirable effects of benzodiazepines are dose-dependent drowsiness, impaired psychomotor skills (e.g. impaired driving ability), daytime fatigue, cognitive impairment and hypotonia (manifesting as unsteadiness/ataxia), with an increased (almost double) risk of femoral fracture in the elderly.[9]

Less commonly, complex actions while apparently asleep (e.g. driving, eating, cooking, conversations) occur both with benzodiazepines and Z drugs.[10]

Use of benzodiazepines in palliative care

Benzodiazepines are essential drugs in palliative care. Tolerance and dependence may occur with long-term use, e.g. ≥4 weeks. Further, palliative care patients may be particularly susceptible to their undesirable effects. Thus alternatives should be considered, particularly where long-term use is anticipated.

Choice of benzodiazepine will depend on several factors, including:

- indication for use
- availability, either of the drug itself or of a suitable formulation for the intended route of administration, e.g. SL, SC
- efficacy
- cost
- fashion (Box 4.B).

Box 4.B Benzodiazepines commonly used in palliative care

Diazepam (universally available but cannot be given SC, cheap)
Midazolam (used SC, mainly in imminently dying patients; buccally in seizures)
Clonazepam (anti-epileptic, adjuvant analgesic)
Lorazepam (status epilepticus, quick-acting SL)
Oxazepam or temazepam (night sedative)

Alprazolam is widely used in some countries for the short-term management of anxiety, particularly panic attacks.[11,12] Tolerance commonly occurs, necessitating dose escalation. Its relatively short duration of action means that tolerant patients may experience break-through (episodic) panic attacks during the night. These resolve if the patient is switched to a long-acting benzodiazepine such as **diazepam** or **clonazepam**, possibly combined with an SSRI such as **sertraline** (with a view to phasing out the benzodiazepine after 1–2 months). However, there are no hard data that **alprazolam** has a greater abuse liability than other benzodiazepines.[13] Despite claims of benefit in depression, **alprazolam** has no place as an antidepressant in palliative care.[14]

Insomnia

Initial treatment includes:

- correcting contributory factors if possible:
  - ▹ pain
  - ▹ delirium
  - ▹ depression
  - ▹ obstructive sleep apnoea
- non-drug measures.[15–19]

Where drug treatment is required, use a short-halflife benzodiazepine or a Z drug for <4 weeks; their efficacy is comparable. A tolerability advantage associated with the greater α-subunit selectivity of Z drugs (see above) is questionable because most undesirable effects are direct consequences of sedation. However, their halflives are shorter (except for **midazolam**). Indirect comparisons find fewer (mostly minor) undesirable effects.[20]

A meta-analysis confirmed that, in people >60 years of age, benzodiazepines and Z drugs had an NNT of 13 but an NNH of 6.[21] The undesirable effects were cognitive impairment, day-time drowsiness, ataxia and falls. Even low doses of short halflife benzodiazepines increase the risk of falls.[22] Alternatives include sedating antidepressants (e.g. TCAs, **trazodone**, **mirtazapine**, see p.182) and **melatonin** (see p.148).[23]

Short-acting drugs

- **midazolam** (halflife 2–5h)
- **zopiclone** (halflife 2–5h).

Intermediate-acting drug

- **temazepam** (halflife 8–15h) 10–30mg PO at bedtime.

Anxiety and panic disorder

The rapid onset of benzodiazepines makes them useful adjuncts for short-term relief (2–4 weeks) of *severe anxiety which is disabling to the individual*. However, for prolonged treatment, an SSRI is preferable (see p.182). The place of **gabapentin** and **pregabalin** in the management of anxiety is uncertain (see p.245).

Intermediate-acting drug

- **lorazepam** (halflife 10–20h) 1–2mg PO or SL b.d.–t.d.s.

SL **lorazepam** is used at some centres for episodes of acute severe distress, e.g. respiratory panic attacks. For regular use, give at bedtime or b.d. Specific SL tablets are not available in the UK. However, the generic tablets made by Genus dissolve easily enough in the mouth to be given SL. Alternatively, the injection can be used SL.

Long-acting drugs

- **diazepam** (halflife 24–120h) 2–20mg PO at bedtime
- **clonazepam** (halflife 20–40h) 500microgram–1mg at bedtime.

Although manufacturers often recommend administration in divided doses for **diazepam** and **clonazepam**, their long plasma halflives mean that administration once daily at bedtime will generally be equally effective, and easier for the patient.

Acute psychotic agitation

Surprisingly, **lorazepam** is as effective as **haloperidol** 5mg every 30min.[24]

- **lorazepam** 2mg PO/IM every 30min until the patient is settled.

Terminal agitation

- start with **midazolam** 2.5–10mg SC p.r.n. and 10mg/24h CSCI

- if necessary, increase both the as needed dose and CSCI until the patient is settled (commonly 10–60mg/24h CSCI, with ≤240mg/24h reported on occasion)
- however, if **midazolam** is poorly effective, or if >30mg/24h needed, consider adding an antipsychotic (e.g. **haloperidol** (p.159) or **levomepromazine** (p.164))
- if **midazolam** plus an antipsychotic are poorly effective despite titration, consider switching to **phenobarbital** (p.270) or **propofol** (p.600).

Skeletal muscle relaxant

- **diazepam** 2–10 mg PO at bedtime, occasionally more.

Baclofen (see p.563) is a useful non-benzodiazepine alternative, particularly if **diazepam** is too sedative and anxiety is not an associated problem, or if long-term use is anticipated.

Anti-epileptic

Benzodiazepines are first line treatments for acute seizures, including status epilepticus. However, their long-term use is hampered by the development of tolerance; thus they are used only for epilepsy refractory to other measures.

Acute treatment[25](see p.244)

- **lorazepam** 4mg IV over 2min *or*
- **clonazepam** 1mg IV/SC over 30sec *or*
- **diazepam** 10mg IV over 2–4min; can also be given rectally in status epilepticus (see p.140 and p.244) *or*
- **midazolam** 10mg IV over 2min or SC/buccal; the injection can be given buccally in status epilepticus.

If necessary, give two more doses at 10min intervals.[26]

Chronic treatment refractory to conventional anti-epileptic drugs

- start with **clonazepam** 500microgram–1mg PO at bedtime
- if necessary, increase by 500microgram every 3–5 days up to 2–4mg, occasionally more
- doses above 2mg can be divided, e.g. 2mg at bedtime and 1mg each morning.

End of life care; see Drug treatment in the imminently dying, p.633.

Myoclonus

If opioid-induced, consider dose reduction or switching to an alternative opioid. Otherwise, a benzodiazepine should be used, e.g.:

- **diazepam** 5mg PO at bedtime
- **midazolam** 5mg SC stat and 10mg/24h CSCI in moribund patients.

If necessary, give as needed doses and consider increasing the regular dose.

Neuropathic pain

Clonazepam is sometimes used as a second or third choice, or when a parenteral adjuvant is required (see p.144 and p.281).

Nausea and vomiting

Benzodiazepines are often of benefit in anticipatory nausea before chemotherapy, and in some cases of refractory nausea and vomiting, both after chemotherapy[27,28] and postoperatively.[29] Alternative approaches to anticipatory nausea include relaxation, hypnosis and other psychological approaches.[30,31]

- **lorazepam** 0.5mg SL p.r.n.
- **midazolam** 10–20mg/24h CSCI.

Alcohol withdrawal

The choice is as for seizures (see above) with dose and route dependent on severity of withdrawal syndrome.[32,33]

Intractable pruritus

The role of benzodiazepines in the management of intractable pruritus is debatable.[34] There are contradictory reports in relation to **diazepam**[35,36] and **nitrazepam**.[36,37] In one patient with cancer of the pancreas and cholestatic pruritus, a CSCI of **midazolam** was effective 'within a few hours' (2mg bolus followed by 1mg/h, increasing by 1mg/h every 15min 'as needed for itching'), whereas **lorazepam** 1mg q6h or 2mg at bedtime (and several other psychotropic drugs) was ineffective.[38] The affinity of **midazolam** for the GABA-receptor is 5–6 times greater than that of **lorazepam**,[39] and it is possible that this is the explanation for the difference in the response to the two benzodiazepines.[40] (For alternative approaches to the management of cholestatic pruritus, see Table 5.29, p.431 and Table 5.30, p.432).

Intractable hiccup

The use of **midazolam** (see p.141) is described for hiccup refractory to other measures (see Table 1.4, p.21).

---

1 Rudolph U and Mohler H (2006) GABA-based therapeutic approaches: GABAA receptor subtype functions. *Current Opinion in Pharmacology.* **6**: 18–23.

2 Mohler H (2011) The rise of a new GABA pharmacology. *Neuropharmacology.* **60**: 1042–1049.

3 Graham D *et al.* (1996) Pharmacological profile of benzodiazepine site ligands with recombinant GABAA receptor subtypes. *European Neuropsychopharmacology.* **6**: 119–125.

4 Pritchett DB *et al.* (1989) Type I and type II GABAA-benzodiazepine receptors produced in transfected cells. *Science.* **245**: 1389–1392.

5 Smith AJ *et al.* (2001) Effect of alpha subunit on allosteric modulation of ion channel function in stably expressed human recombinant gamma-aminobutyric acid(A) receptors determined using (36)Cl ion flux. *Molecular Pharmacology.* **59**: 1108–1118.

6 NPSA (National Patient Safety Agency) (2008) Reducing risk of overdose with midazolam injection in adults. Rapid response report 11. Available from: www.nrls.npsa.nhs.uk/resources/?entryid45 = 59896

7 BNF (2011) Section 4.1. Hypnotics and anxiolytics. In: *British National Formulary* (No. 61). British Medical Association and Royal Pharmaceutical Society of Great Britain, London. Current BNF available from: www.bnf.org.

8 AHFS (2009) Benzodiazepines general statement (pharmacokinetics). AHFS Drug Information 2009 (online edition). Available from: www.ahfsdruginformation.com/ (subscription required).

9 Grad R (1995) Benzodiazepines for insomnia in community-dwelling elderly: a review of benefit and risk. *Journal of Family Practice.* **41**: 473–481.

10 Dolder CR and Nelson MH (2008) Hypnosedative-induced complex behaviours: incidence, mechanisms and management. *CNS Drugs.* **22**: 1021–1036.

11 Pollack MH *et al.* (1993) Long-term outcome after acute treatment with alprazolam or clonazepam for panic disorder. *Journal of Clinical Psychopharmacology.* **13**: 257–263.

12 Woodman CL *et al.* (1994) Predictors of response to alprazolam and placebo in patients with panic disorder. *Journal of Affective Disorders.* **30**: 5–13.

13 Rush CR *et al.* (1993) Abuse liability of alprazolam relative to other commonly used benzodiazepines: a review. *Neuroscience and Biobehavioral Reviews.* **17**: 277–285.

14 Kravitz HM *et al.* (1993) Alprazolam and depression: a review of risks and benefits. *Journal of Clinical Psychiatry.* **54 Suppl**: 78–84; discussion 85.

15 Morin CM *et al.* (1994) Nonpharmacological interventions for insomnia: a meta-analysis of treatment efficacy. *American Journal of Psychiatry.* **151**: 1172–1180.

16 Murtagh DR and Greenwood KM (1995) Identifying effective psychological treatments for insomnia: a meta-analysis. *Journal of Consulting and Clinical Psychology.* **63**: 79–89.

17 Smith MT *et al.* (2002) Comparative meta-analysis of pharmacotherapy and behavior therapy for persistent insomnia. *American Journal of Psychiatry.* **159**: 5–11.

18 Hugel H *et al.* (2004) The prevalence, key causes and management of insomnia in palliative care patients. *Journal of Pain and Symptom Management.* **27**: 316–321.

19 Twycross R *et al.* (2009) *Symptom Management in Advanced Cancer* (4e). palliativedrugs.com, Nottingham, pp. 203–204.

20 Buscemi N *et al.* (2007) The efficacy and safety of drug treatments for chronic insomnia in adults: a meta-analysis of RCTs. *Journal of General Internal Medicine.* **22**: 1335–1350.

21 Glass J *et al.* (2005) Sedative hypnotics in older people with insomnia: meta-analysis of risks and benefits. *British Medical Journal.* **331**: 1169.

22 Wang PS *et al.* (2001) Hazardous benzodiazepine regimens in the elderly: effects of half-life, dosage, and duration on risk of hip fracture. *American Journal of Psychiatry.* **158**: 892–898.

23 Wilson SJ *et al.* (2010) British Association for Psychopharmacology consensus statement on evidence-based treatment of insomnia, parasomnias and circadian rhythm disorders. *Journal of Psychopharmacology.* **24**: 1577–1601.

24 Foster S *et al.* (1997) Efficacy of lorazepam and haloperidol for rapid tranquilization in the psychiatric emergency room setting. *International Clinical Psychopharmacology.* **12**: 175–179.

25 Rey E *et al.* (1999) Pharmacokinetic optimization of benzodiazepines therapy for acute seizures. Focus on delivery routes. *Clinical Pharmacokinetics.* **36**: 409–424.

26 BNF (2011) Section 4.8.2 Drugs used in status epilepticus. In: *British National Formulary* (No. 61). British Medical Association and Royal Pharmaceutical Society of Great Britain, London. Current BNF available from: www.bnf.org.

27 Maher J (1981) Intravenous lorazepam to prevent nausea and vomiting associated with cancer chemotherapy. *Lancet.* **1**: 91–92.

28 Bishop J *et al.* (1984) Lorazepam: a randomized, double-blind, crossover study of a new antiemetic in patients receiving cytotoxic chemotherapy and prochlorperazine. *Journal of Clinical Oncology.* **2**: 691–695.

29 Di Florio T and Goucke CR (1999) The effect of midazolam on persistent postoperative nausea and vomiting. *Anaesthesia and Intensive Care.* **27**: 38–40.

30 Mandala M *et al.* (2005) Midazolam for acute emesis refractory to dexamethasone and granisetron after highly emetogenic chemotherapy: a phase II study. *Supportive Care in Cancer.* **13**: 375–380.

31 Aapro MS *et al.* (2005) Anticipatory nausea and vomiting. *Supportive Care in Cancer.* **13**: 117–121.

32 Peppers M (1996) Benzodiazepines for alcohol withdrawal in the elderly and in patients with liver disease. *Pharmacotherapy.* **16**: 49–57.

33 Chick J (1998) Review: benzodiazepines are more effective than neuroleptics in reducing delirium and seizures in alcohol withdrawal. *Evidence-Based Medicine.* **3**: 11.

34 Twycross RG *et al.* (2003) Itch: scratching more than the surface. *Quarterly Journal of Medicine.* **96**: 7–26.

35 Hagermark O (1973) Influence of antihistamines, sedatives, and aspirin on experimental itch. *Acta Dermato-Venereologica.* **53**: 363–368.

36 Muston H *et al.* (1979) Differential effect of hypnotics and anxiolytics on itch and scratch. *Journal of Investigative Dermatology*. **72**: 283.
37 Ebata T *et al.* (1998) Effects of nitrazepam on nocturnal scratching in adults with atopic dermatitis: a double-blind placebo-controlled crossover study. *British Journal of Dermatology*. **138**: 631–634.
38 Prieto LN (2004) The use of midazolam to treat itching in a terminally ill patient with biliary obstruction. *Journal of Pain and Symptom Management*. **28**: 531–532.
39 Hanley DF and Kross JF (1998) Use of midazolam in the treatment of refractory status epilepticus. *Clinical Therapeutics*. **20**: 1093–1105.
40 Prommer E (2005) Re: Pruritus in patients with advanced cancer. *Journal of Pain and Symptom Management*. **30**: 201–202.

DIAZEPAM — BNF 4.1, 4.8, 10.2.2 & 15.1.4.1

Class: Benzodiazepine.

Indications: Insomnia, anxiety and †panic disorder, acute psychotic agitation, refractory epilepsy, status epilepticus, myoclonus, skeletal muscle relaxant, alcohol withdrawal.

Contra-indications: (unless in the imminently dying) Acute or severe pulmonary insufficiency, sleep apnoea syndrome, severe liver disease, myasthenia gravis. Do not use alone for depression, mixed anxiety-depression or psychosis.

Pharmacology

Diazepam is a typical benzodiazepine GABAmimetic (see p.132). In high doses, it induces hepatic metabolism. Standard parenteral products are oil-based or an oil-in-water emulsion, and absorption from muscle after IM injection is slower and more variable than after PO and PR administration. Diazepam has a long plasma halflife and several active metabolites, one of which has a plasma halflife of up to 120h in the elderly. Because of marked interindividual variation, the effects of a constant dose will vary greatly. Doses for individual patients are determined empirically.

Bio-availability almost 100% PO; 81% PR (rectal solution); 67–84% PR (suppository).[1]
Onset of action 15min PO; 1–5min IV (oil-based injection).[1]
Time to peak plasma concentration 30–90min PO; 10–30min PR (rectal solution); ≤15min IV (oil-based injection), ≥15min IV (Diazemuls®); 1–1.5h IM (oil based injection), 2h IM (Diazemuls®).
Plasma halflife 24–48h; active metabolite nordiazepam 48–120h.
Duration of action 3–30h, situation dependent; may be only 15min–1h after a single IV dose.[1]

Cautions

Old age, debilitation, chronic respiratory disease, mild–moderate hepatic impairment, renal impairment. If given IV can cause hypotension and transient apnoea. Accumulation of active metabolites may necessitate a dose reduction after several days. History of alcohol or drug abuse.

Drug Interactions

Diazepam is metabolized via the cytochrome P450 group of liver enzymes (see Cytochrome P450, p.735). Thus, **amiodarone**, **cimetidine**, **fluconazole**, **metronidazole**, **omeprazole**, **sodium valproate** all inhibit the clearance of diazepam, resulting in an enhanced and more prolonged effect.[2,3] Genetic polymorphism occurs and some people are slow metabolizers (whites 3–5%, Asians 20%); this also results in an enhanced and more prolonged effect (see Cytochrome P450, p.735).

Undesirable effects

Dose-dependent drowsiness, impaired psychomotor skills (e.g. impaired driving ability), daytime fatigue, cognitive impairment and hypotonia (manifesting as unsteadiness/ataxia), with an increased (almost double) risk of femoral fracture in the elderly. When given IV, the oil-based solution may cause painful thrombophlebitis.

Paradoxical reactions have been reported: insomnia, anxiety, excitement, rage, hallucinations, increased muscle spasticity.

Dose and use

Typical doses for diazepam are shown in Table 4.3. The initial dose will depend on the patient's age, general condition, previous use of diazepam and other benzodiazepines, the intensity of distress, and the urgency of relief. Generally, elderly and debilitated patients should be started on low doses.

Table 4.3 Dose recommendations for diazepam

Indication	*Stat & p.r.n. doses*	*Common range*
Anxiety[a]	2–10mg PO	2–20mg PO o.n.
Muscle spasm[b] Multifocal myoclonus	2–5mg PO	2–10mg PO o.n.
Anti-epileptic[c,d]	10mg PR/IV	10–30mg o.n.

a. given as an adjunct to non-drug approaches, e.g. relaxation therapy and massage
b. if localized, consider injection of a trigger point with local anaesthetic or acupuncture
c. acute use but in the moribund can be used as a convenient substitute for long-term oral anti-epileptic therapy (also see Midazolam p.141)
d. to reduce the risk of thrombophlebitis, inject IV diazepam slowly (rate not exceeding 5mg (1mL)/min) into a large vein, e.g. the antecubital vein.

Although the manufacturers of diazepam recommend giving it in divided doses, its long plasma halflife means that administration at bedtime will generally be equally effective, and easier for the patient. In an agitated moribund patient, b.d.–t.d.s. dosing is sometimes indicated so as to reduce the number of hours awake. Rectal diazepam is an alternative to buccal/SC midazolam in a crisis, or if the patient is moribund:

- rectal solution 5–10mg in 2.5mL
- suppositories 10mg
- if the above are unavailable, the parenteral formulation can be administered with a blunt (needle-free) cannula.

Patients occasionally react paradoxically, i.e. become more distressed; if this happens, **haloperidol** (see p.159) or **olanzapine** (see p.166) should be given instead.

Midazolam (see p.141), **clonazepam** (see p.144) or **lorazepam** (*not* CSCI; see p.146) are used if SC injections are necessary.

If using IM/IV diazepam, the emulsion formulation is preferable because it is less irritant.

Supply

Diazepam (generic)
Tablets 2mg, 5mg, 10mg, 28 days @ 5mg at bedtime = £1.
Oral solution 2mg/5mL, 28 days @ 5mg at bedtime = £21.
Strong oral solution 5mg/5mL, 28 days @ 5mg at bedtime = £9.
Injection (oil-based solution) 5mg/mL, 2mL amp = £0.50; *excipients include ethanol and propylene glycol.*
Injection (emulsion) 5mg/mL, 2mL amp = £1.
Rectal solution 2mg/mL, 1.25mL (2.5mg) tube = £1, 2.5mL (5mg) tube = £1.50; 4mg/mL, 2.5mL (10mg) tube = £2.
Suppositories 10mg, pack of 6 = £10.

1 AHFS (2009) Benzodiazepines general statement (pharmacokinetics). AHFS Drug Information 2009 (online edition). Available from: www.ahfsdruginformation.com/ (subscription required).
2 Klotz U and Reimann I (1980) Delayed clearance of diazepam due to cimetidine. *New England Journal of Medicine*. **302**: 1012–1014.
3 Wagner B and O'Hara D (1997) Pharmacokinetics and pharmacodynamics of sedatives and analgesics in the treatment of agitated critically ill patients. *Clinical Pharmacokinetics*. **33**: 426–453.

MIDAZOLAM   BNF 4.8.2 & 15.1.4.1

Class: Benzodiazepine.

Indications: Anaesthetic premedication/induction/maintenance agent, sedative for minor procedures, ICU sedation, †insomnia; †anxiety and panic disorder; †acute psychotic agitation; †terminal agitation;[1,2] †skeletal muscle relaxant; †status epilepticus; †refractory epilepsy; †myoclonus; †nausea and vomiting;[3,4] †alcohol withdrawal, †intractable pruritus, †intractable hiccup.[5]

Contra-indications: (unless in the imminently dying) Acute or severe pulmonary insufficiency, sleep apnoea syndrome, severe liver disease.

Pharmacology

Midazolam is a short-acting, water-soluble benzodiazepine GABAmimetic. In single doses for sedation, midazolam is 3 times more potent than **diazepam**; as an anti-epileptic, it is twice as potent. With multiple doses, **diazepam** will gain in potency because of its prolonged plasma halflife, i.e. 24–120h versus 2–5h for midazolam. In the elderly, the plasma halflife of midazolam is prolonged up to 3 times and in some intensive care patients having CIVI for sedation, the plasma halflife may be prolonged up to 6 times. It also may be prolonged in hepatic impairment and heart failure. An active metabolite, α-hydroxymidazolam glucuronide, has a receptor affinity about one tenth that of midazolam. In severe renal impairment (creatinine clearance <10mL/min) accumulation can result in prolonged sedation.[6] The main advantage of midazolam in palliative care is that it is water-soluble and is compatible with most of the drugs commonly given by CSCI. Intravenously, it does not cause thrombophlebitis, and can also be given by the buccal route as an alternative to SL **lorazepam**.[7]

When used in typical doses (see Table 4.5) in imminently dying patients, tolerance is not a practical problem. However, if much higher doses are used (e.g. >10–15mg/h CSCI), then a lack of response may be seen if the dose is further escalated. This relates in part to the fact that at these doses, maximum GABA-ergic inhibition has been reached.[8]

For severe terminal breathlessness, the combination of regular **morphine** and midazolam appears more effective than either drug alone (see p.368).[9]

In contrast to other benzodiazepines, midazolam may be of benefit in intractable (central) pruritus.[10,11] In one patient with cancer of the pancreas and cholestatic pruritus, a CSCI of midazolam was effective 'within a few hours' (2mg bolus followed by 1mg/h, increasing by 1mg/h every 15min 'as needed for itching'), whereas **lorazepam** 1mg q6h or 2mg at bedtime (and several other psychotropic drugs) was ineffective.[11] The affinity of midazolam for the GABA-receptor is 5–6 times greater than that of **lorazepam**,[12] and it is possible that this is the explanation for the difference in the response to the two benzodiazepines.[13] (For alternative approaches to the management of cholestatic pruritus, see Table 5.29, p.431 and Table 5.30, p.432).

Bio-availability >90% IM; 75% buccal; 35–44% PO.
Onset of action 5–10min SC; 2–3min IV; 15min buccal.
Time to peak plasma concentration 30min IM; 30min buccal; 60min PO.
Plasma halflife 2–5h; increased to about 10h by CSCI.
Duration of action 5mg <4h, interindividual variation.[14]

Cautions

Fatalities from oversedation or cardiorespiratory depression have occurred after *concurrent use with higher than approved doses of* ***olanzapine*** (see p.167).

Chronic respiratory disease, mild–moderate hepatic impairment, renal impairment, impaired cardiac function or low cardiac output, myasthenia gravis. If given IV can cause hypotension, reduced myocardial contractility and transient apnoea. History of alcohol or drug abuse.

Drug interactions

Midazolam is a substrate of CYP3A4 (see Cytochrome P450, p.735). Table 4.4 lists selected drugs which have clinically important drug interactions with midazolam.

Table 4.4 Clinically significant cytochrome P450 interactions with midazolam resulting in changed drug plasma concentrations[15]

Midazolam plasma concentration	
Increased by	*Decreased by*
Aprepitant (initially, e.g. 3–5 days after starting the usual 3-day aprepitant course)[a,b]	Aprepitant (transient induction of midazolam metabolism may occur 3–5 days after the end of the usual 3-day aprepitant course)
Clarithromycin[a,c]	Carbamazepine
Diltiazem[a,d]	Phenytoin
Erythromycin[a,c]	Rifampicin
Fluconazole[a,c]	
Grapefruit juice[a]	
Itraconazole[a,e]	
Ketoconazole[a,e]	
Nefazodone[b]	
Posaconazole[b]	
Propofol	
Protease inhibitors, e.g. lopinavir, saquinavir[a,f]	
Verapamil[a,d]	
Voriconazole[a,e]	

a. more pronounced with PO midazolam
b. monitor for excessive sedation and titrate midazolam dose accordingly (any route)
c. reduce PO midazolam dose by 50%; monitor patients on midazolam infusions for excessive sedation and titrate midazolam dose accordingly
d. reduce midazolam dose by 50% (any route)
e. reduce PO midazolam dose by 75%; monitor patients on midazolam infusions for excessive sedation and titrate midazolam dose accordingly
f. avoid concurrent use with PO midazolam; reduce dose of midazolam infusion by 50%.

Undesirable effects

Dose-dependent drowsiness, impaired psychomotor skills, daytime fatigue, cognitive impairment and hypotonia (manifesting as unsteadiness/ataxia), with an increased (almost double) risk of femoral fracture in the elderly. Paradoxical reactions have been reported: insomnia, anxiety, excitement, rage, hallucinations, increased muscle spasticity.

Dose and use

Typical doses for midazolam are shown in Table 4.5. In practice, midazolam is mostly used in the terminal phase. If given IV rather than SC, smaller stat doses are generally used. The minimal interval between p.r.n. doses is typically 1h if SC, and 10–15min if IV.

A liquid is available as a special order for *buccal administration* (see Supply). Alternatively, the contents of an ampoule for injection can be used.

Table 4.5 Dose recommendations for SC midazolam

Indication	*Stat & p.r.n. doses*	*Common range*
Muscle tension/spasm Multifocal myoclonus	5mg SC	10–30mg/24h CSCI
Terminal agitation Terminal breathlessness Intractable hiccup	2.5–10mg SC	10–60mg/24h CSCI[a]
Anti-epileptic	10mg SC/buccal[b]	30–60mg/24h CSCI
Nausea and vomiting	2.5–5mg SC	10–20mg/24h CSCI

a. reported upper dose range 120mg for hiccup; 240mg for agitation
b. repeated after 10min if needed.

Nausea and vomiting
Particularly used for anticipatory nausea or refractory post-chemotherapeutic and postoperative nausea and vomiting (see p.219).[3,4,16]

Status epilepticus
See Anti-epileptics, p.244.

Terminal agitation
If an agitated patient does not settle on 30mg/24h, an antipsychotic (e.g. **haloperidol**) is best introduced before further increasing the dose of midazolam.

Intractable hiccup
Generally limited to patients in whom persistent distressing hiccup is contributing to terminal restlessness at a time when sedation is acceptable to aid symptom relief.

Supply
All products are schedule 3 **CD**.
Midazolam (generic)
Injection 1mg/mL, 2mL amp, 5mL amp, 50mL vial = £0.50, £0.50 and £8 respectively; 2mg/mL, 5mL amp = £0.50; 5mg/mL, 2mL, 10mL amp = £0.50 and £2.50 respectively.

Epistatus® (Special Products)
Buccal liquid 10mg/mL, 5mL bottle + 4x1mL oral syringes = £56 (community pharmacies), £40 (hospital). Prices are exclusive of VAT but inclusive of postage and packing. (Unlicensed, available as a special order from Special Products Ltd; see Obtaining unlicensed products, p.769.)
Buccal liquid (prefilled oral syringe) 2.5mg/0.25mL; 5mg/0.5mL; 7.5mg/0.75mL; 10mg/1mL; 10mg/1mL syringe = £25 (community pharmacies), £23 (hospital). Prices are exclusive of VAT but inclusive of postage and packing. (Unlicensed, available as a special order from Special Products Ltd; see Obtaining unlicensed products, p.769.)

Hypnovel® (Roche)
Injection 2mg/mL, 5mL amp = £1; 5mg/mL, 2mL amp = £1.

1 Bottomley DM and Hanks GW (1990) Subcutaneous midazolam infusion in palliative care. *Journal of Pain and Symptom Management.* **5**: 259–261.
2 McNamara P *et al.* (1991) Use of midazolam in palliative care. *Palliative Medicine.* **5**: 244–249.
3 Mandala M *et al.* (2005) Midazolam for acute emesis refractory to dexamethasone and granisetron after highly emetogenic chemotherapy: a phase II study. *Supportive Care in Cancer.* **13**: 375–380.
4 Di Florio T and Goucke CR (1999) The effect of midazolam on persistent postoperative nausea and vomiting. *Anaesthesia and Intensive Care.* **27**: 38–40.
5 Wilcock A and Twycross R (1996) Case report: midazolam for intractable hiccup. *Journal of Pain and Symptom Management.* **12**: 59–61.
6 Bauer T *et al.* (1995) Prolonged sedation due to accumulation of conjugated metabolites of midazolam. *Lancet.* **346**: 145–147.
7 McIntyre J *et al.* (2005) Safety and efficacy of buccal midazolam versus rectal diazepam for emergency treatment of seizures in children: a randomised controlled trial. *Lancet.* **366**: 205–210.
8 Cheng C *et al.* (2002) When midazolam fails. *Journal of Pain and Symptom Management.* **23**: 256–265.
9 Navigante AH *et al.* (2006) Midazolam as adjunct therapy to morphine in the alleviation of severe dyspnea perception in patients with advanced cancer. *Journal of Pain and Symptom Management.* **31**: 38–47.

10 Thomsen JS *et al.* (2002) Suppression of spontaneous scratching in hairless rats by sedatives but not by antipruritics. *Skin Pharmacology and Applied Skin Physiology.* **15**: 218–224.
11 Prieto LN (2004) The use of midazolam to treat itching in a terminally ill patient with biliary obstruction. *Journal of Pain and Symptom Management.* **28**: 531–532.
12 Hanley DF and Kross JF (1998) Use of midazolam in the treatment of refractory status epilepticus. *Clinical Therapeutics.* **20**: 1093–1105.
13 Prommer E (2005) Re: Pruritus in patients with advanced cancer. *Journal of Pain and Symptom Management.* **30**: 201–202.
14 Schwagmeier R *et al.* (1998) Midazolam pharmacokinetics following intravenous and buccal administration. *British Journal of Clinical Pharmacology.* **46**: 203–206.
15 Baxter K (2011) Stockley's Drug Interactions (online edition). Pharmaceutical Press, London. Available from: www.medicinescomplete.com
16 Aapro MS *et al.* (2005) Anticipatory nausea and vomiting. *Supportive Care in Cancer.* **13**: 117–121.

CLONAZEPAM — BNF 4.8.1 & 4.8.2

Class: Benzodiazepine.

Indications: anxiety and panic disorder,[1,2] status epilepticus, refractory epilepsy, myoclonus, †neuropathic pain; †restless legs syndrome.[3,4]

Contra-indications: (unless in the imminently dying) Acute or severe pulmonary insufficiency, sleep apnoea syndrome, severe liver disease, myasthenia gravis.

Pharmacology

Clonazepam is a typical benzodiazepine GABAmimetic. Clonazepam is extensively metabolized to inactive metabolites, and the cytochrome CYP3A pathway may be important (see Cytochrome P450, p.735).
Bio-availability 90% PO.
Onset of action 20–60min PO; 5–10min SC.
Time to peak plasma concentration 1–4h.
Halflife 20–40h (mean 30h).
Duration of action 12h.

Cautions

Chronic respiratory disease, mild–moderate hepatic impairment, renal impairment, elderly or debilitated patients (may require dose reduction). Spinal or cerebellar ataxia. History of alcohol or drug abuse. Avoid abrupt withdrawal in epileptic patients (may precipitate status epilepticus). Anti-epileptic drugs are associated with suicidal thoughts or behaviour (see p.240).

Drug interactions

Clonazepam and **phenytoin** have unpredictable effects on each other's plasma concentrations, possibly because of changes in hepatic metabolism or in the volume of distribution. Clonazepam may increase, decrease, or leave **phenytoin** plasma concentrations unchanged, whereas **phenytoin** can decrease the plasma concentration of clonazepam. Monitor the **phenytoin** plasma concentration and adjust dose if necessary.[5]

Undesirable effects

Dose-dependent drowsiness, impaired psychomotor skills (e.g. impaired driving ability), daytime fatigue, cognitive impairment and hypotonia (manifesting as unsteadiness/ataxia), with an increased (almost double) risk of femoral fracture in the elderly. These effects can be minimized by starting with low doses at bedtime.

In children, clonazepam has been associated with salivary hypersecretion and drooling.

Dose and use

See Table 4.6. Because of the development of tolerance to its anti-epileptic effect, clonazepam is generally reserved for the treatment of refractory tonic-clonic or partial seizures.[1–3]

Clonazepam has also been used successfully in some patients with neuropathic pain, including phantom limb,[6–8] post-herpetic,[9] diabetic,[10] and cancer-related,[11] although there is no supporting RCT evidence.[6]

In countries where a parenteral formulation is available, clonazepam can be administered by CSCI as an alternative to **midazolam** (see p.141). However, if the infusion tubing is made of PVC, up to 50% of the infused clonazepam is adsorbed onto the tubing.[12] Thus, if clonazepam is given by CSCI, non-PVC tubing should be used (e.g. IVAC®). Alternatively, because it has a long halflife, clonazepam can be administered as a bolus injection once daily, preferably at bedtime.

Table 4.6 Dose recommendations for clonazepam

Indication	*Stat & p.r.n. doses*	*Common range*
Epilepsy	1mg PO/SC/IV[a,b,c]	1mg[b] at bedtime–8mg/24h in divided doses PO; 1–8mg/24h CSCI[d]
Panic disorder	250microgram PO	500microgram–4mg at bedtime PO
Restless legs	250microgram PO	500microgram–2mg at bedtime PO
Neuropathic pain	500microgram PO	500microgram at bedtime–8mg/24h in divided doses PO
Terminal sedation	500microgram SC[c]	2–8mg/24h CSCI[d]

a. for use in acute seizures, including status epilepticus, see p.137
b. because the elderly are more sensitive to central depressant effects, the manufacturer recommends a starting dose of 500microgram/24h for PO clonazepam in the elderly
c. for SC/IV bolus doses, dilute each 1mg/mL amp with 1mL WFI
d. see text above about adsorption onto PVC tubing

Supply

Rivotril® (Roche)

Tablets 500microgram, 2mg, 28 days @ 2mg once daily = £1.50.

Injection 1mg/mL, 1mL amp = £0.50; *dilute with 1mL WFI before SC/IV bolus injection.*

1 Davidson J and Moroz G (1998) Pivotal studies of clonazepam in panic disorder. *Psychopharmacology Bulletin.* **34**: 169–174.
2 Wulsin L *et al.* (1999) Clonazepam treatment of panic disorder in patients with recurrent chest pain and normal coronary arteries. *International Journal of Psychiatry and Medicine.* **29**: 97–105.
3 Joy M (1997) Clonazepam: benzodiazepine therapy for the restless legs syndrome. *ANNA Journal.* **24**: 686–689.
4 Vignatelli L *et al.* (2006) EFNS guidelines on management of restless legs syndrome and periodic limb movement disorder in sleep. *European Journal of Neurology.* **13**: 1049–1065.
5 Baxter K (2011) Stockley's Drug Interactions (online edition). Pharmaceutical Press, London. Available from: www.medicinescomplete.com
6 McQuay H *et al.* (1995) Anticonvulsant drugs for the management of pain: a systematic review. *British Medical Journal.* **311**: 1047–1052.
7 Reddy S and Patt R (1994) The benzodiazepines as adjuvant analgesics. *Journal of Pain and Symptom Management.* **9**: 510–514.
8 Bartusch S *et al.* (1996) Clonazepam for the treatment of lancinating phantom limb pain. *Clinical Journal of Pain.* **12**: 59–62.
9 Mamdani FS (1994) Pharmacologic management of herpes zoster and postherpetic neuralgia. *Canadian Family Physician.* **40**: 321–326, 329–332.
10 Young JP and Clarke BF (1985) Pain relief in diabetic neuropathy: the effectiveness of imipramine and related drugs. *Diabetic Medicine.* **2**: 363–366.
11 Hugel H *et al.* (2003) Clonazepam as an adjuvant analgesic in patients with cancer-related neuropathic pain. *Journal of Pain and Symptom Management.* **26**: 1073–1074.
12 Schneider JJ *et al.* (2006) Effect of tubing on loss of clonazepam administered by continuous subcutaneous infusion. *Journal of Pain and Symptom Management.* **31**: 563–567.

LORAZEPAM BNF 4.1.2, 4.8.2 & 15.1.4.1

Class: Benzodiazepine.

Indications: Insomnia; anxiety and panic disorder; †acute psychotic agitation; status epilepticus; refractory epilepsy; myoclonus; †nausea and vomiting; alcohol withdrawal.[1]

Contra-indications: (unless in the imminently dying) Acute or severe pulmonary insufficiency, sleep apnoea syndrome, severe liver disease, myasthenia gravis. Do not use alone for depression, anxiety-depression, psychosis, or delirium (unless alcohol withdrawal).[2]

Pharmacology

Lorazepam is a typical benzodiazepine GABAmimetic.[3] Like other benzodiazepines, lorazepam can cause amnesia. Lorazepam is rapidly absorbed PO. Although the tablets are marketed for PO use, lorazepam is sometimes given SL, generally when a rapid onset of effect is required and/or the patient cannot reliably swallow tablets. However, although one pharmacokinetic study suggested more rapid absorption SL than PO, others have found no difference.[4–7] Thus, it is likely that the amount of lorazepam absorbed SL is variable and formulation-dependent. Because of this, the patient will generally still need to be able to swallow and to have a patent upper GI tract. When the latter is not the case, parenteral administration should be considered.

Despite being 85% protein-bound, lorazepam quickly reaches the CNS.[8] It is glucuronidated in the liver to an inactive compound and is excreted by the kidneys and in the bile (cytochrome P450 is *not* involved). The conjugated metabolite undergoes enterohepatic circulation. Duration of action does not correlate with plasma concentrations, and can be up to 3 days.

Bio-availability 90% PO.
Onset of action 5min SL; 10–15min PO.
Time to peak plasma concentration 1h SL; 2h PO, IM.
Plasma halflife 10–20h.
Duration of action 6–72h.

Cautions

Fatalities from oversedation or cardiorespiratory depression have occurred after *concurrent use with higher than approved doses of* ***olanzapine*** (see p.167).

History of alcohol or drug abuse, renal impairment, mild–moderate hepatic impairment, chronic lung disease, e.g. COPD.

Elderly and debilitated patients are more susceptible to the central depressant effects of lorazepam, e.g. on respiration, and generally require lower doses than those recommended for adults in the SPC.

The metabolism of lorazepam is inhibited by **valproate**.[9] It has less interaction with **dextropropoxyphene** than other benzodiazepines.[10] **Carbamazepine** and **rifampicin** may decrease lorazepam levels.[11]

Although it has been used successfully as a sole agent in acute psychotic agitation (mania),[12,13] lorazepam should not be used alone in an agitated delirium because it is likely to exacerbate the condition.[2,14] May unmask or worsen pre-existing depression.

Undesirable effects

Drowsiness, fatigue, impaired co-ordination, blurred vision, lightheadedness, memory impairment, insomnia, dysarthria, anxiety, decreased libido, depression, headaches, tachycardia, chest pain, dry mouth, increased or decreased appetite, nausea, vomiting, constipation, diarrhoea, sweating, rash.

Dose and use

Lorazepam can be given SL, PO, PR, SC, IM, or IV. In some countries, specific SL tablets are available, *but not in the UK*. Thus, in the UK, proprietary tablets which dissolve more easily should be used SL, e.g. the generic tablets made by Genus, and the manufacturer's name should be stipulated on the prescription to ensure this.

Tablets will not dissolve SL in the absence of saliva. In patients with a dry mouth, the tablet should be dissolved in a few drops of warm water, drawn up in a 1mL oral syringe and put between the patient's cheek and gum (i.e. given buccally).[15]

Alternatively, the injection can be used SL; this is useful when a rapid onset of action is required but injection is impractical, e.g. in the crisis management of catastrophic haemorrhage (see Pre-emptive prescribing in the community, p.649).

If given by CSCI, there is a risk of precipitation.[16] Accidental intra-arterial administration or extravasation close to an artery has been associated with thrombosis and gangrene.

Status epilepticus

Lorazepam is widely regarded as the benzodiazepine of choice in the control of status epilepticus (see p.244).[17]

Insomnia

- 0.5–1mg PO at bedtime.

Anxiety and panic disorder

For short-term relief of severe anxiety (see p.136)
- 0.5–1mg SL/PO stat and b.d.
- if necessary, increase to 2–6mg/24h.[18]

Acute psychotic agitation

Use with **haloperidol** or **risperidone** to control psychotic agitation,[19] although some centres use lorazepam alone:[12,13]
- give 2mg PO every 30min until the patient is settled.[12]

Sedation in the imminently dying

Used at some centres instead of **midazolam**.[16,20] Generally use with an antipsychotic:
- 1–4mg IV stat
- 4–20mg/24h CIVI or 1–2mg SC q6–8h.

Supply

Lorazepam (generic)

Tablets 1mg, 2.5mg, 28 days @ 2mg b.d. = £22.

Injection 4mg/mL, 1mL amp = £0.50; *for IM injection, dilute with an equal volume of WFI or 0.9% saline and administer deep into muscle mass.*

1 Peppers M (1996) Benzodiazepines for alcohol withdrawal in the elderly and in patients with liver disease. *Pharmacotherapy.* **16**: 49 57.

2 Breitbart W *et al.* (1996) A double-blind trial of haloperidol, chlorpromazine, and lorazepam in the treatment of delirium in hospitalized AIDS patients. *American Journal of Psychiatry.* **153**: 231–237.

3 Ziemann U *et al.* (1996) The effect of lorazepam on the motor cortical excitability in man. *Experimental Brain Research.* **109**: 127–135.

4 Caille G *et al.* (1983) Pharmacokinetics of two lorazepam formulations, oral and sublingual, after multiple doses. *Biopharmaceutics and Drug Disposition.* **4**: 31–42.

5 Greenblatt DJ *et al.* (1982) Pharmacokinetic comparison of sublingual lorazepam with intravenous, intramuscular, and oral lorazepam. *Journal of Pharmaceutical Sciences.* **71**: 248–252.

6 Spenard J *et al.* (1988) Placebo-controlled comparative study of the anxiolytic activity and of the pharmacokinetics of oral and sublingual lorazepam in generalized anxiety. *Biopharmaceutics and Drug Disposition.* **9**: 457–464.

7 Gram-Hansen P and Schultz A (1988) Plasma concentrations following oral and sublingual administration of lorazepam. *International Journal of Clinical Pharmacology Therapy and Toxicology.* **26**: 323–324.

8 Wagner B and O'Hara D (1997) Pharmacokinetics and pharmacodynamics of sedatives and analgesics in the treatment of agitated critically ill patients. *Clinical Pharmacokinetics.* **33**: 426–453.

9 Samara E *et al.* (1997) Effect of valproate on the pharmacokinetics and pharmacodynamics of lorazepam. *Journal of Clinical Pharmacology.* **37**: 442–450.

10 Abernethy D *et al.* (1985) Interaction of propoxyphene with diazepam, alprazolam and lorazepam. *British Journal of Clinical Pharmacology.* **19**: 51 57.

11 Bachmann KA and Jauregui L (1993) Use of single sample clearance estimates of cytochrome P450 substrates to characterize human hepatic CYP status in vivo. *Xenobiotica.* **23**: 307–315.

12 Foster S *et al.* (1997) Efficacy of lorazepam and haloperidol for rapid tranquilization in the psychiatric emergency room setting. *International Clinical Psychopharmacology.* **12**: 175–179.

13 Lenox R *et al.* (1992) Adjunctive treatment of manic agitation with lorazepam versus haloperidol: a double-blind study. *Journal of Clinical Psychiatry.* **53**: 47–52.
14 Salzman C *et al.* (1991) Parenteral lorazepam versus parenteral haloperidol for the control of psychotic disruptive behavior. *Journal of Clinical Psychiatry.* **52**: 177–180.
15 Nicholson A (2007) Lorazepam. In: *Bulletin board.* Palliativedrugs.com Ltd. Available from: www.palliativedrugs.org/forum/read.php?f = 1&i = 11203&t = 11203
16 McCollam J *et al.* (1999) Continuous infusions of lorazepam, midazolam and propofol for sedation of the critically ill surgery trauma patient: a prospective, randomized comparison. *Critical Care Medicine.* **27**: 2454–2458.
17 Rey E *et al.* (1999) Pharmacokinetic optimization of benzodiazepines therapy for acute seizures. Focus on delivery routes. *Clinical Pharmacokinetics.* **36**: 409–424.
18 MacLaren R *et al.* (2000) A prospective evaluation of empiric versus protocol-based sedation and analgesia. *Pharmacotherapy.* **20**: 662–672.
19 Currier G and Simpson G (2001) Risperidone liquid concentrate and oral lorazepam versus intramuscular haloperidol and intramuscular lorazepam for treatment of psychotic agitation. *Journal of Clinical Psychiatry.* **62**: 153–157.
20 Fainsinger R *et al.* (2000) Sedation for delirium and other symptoms in terminally ill patients in Edmonton. *Journal of Palliative Care.* **16 (2)**: 5–10.

MELATONIN BNF 4.1.1

Class: Melatonin-receptor agonist.

Indications: Primary insomnia in adults >55yrs, †secondary insomnia, †sleep phase disorders.

Pharmacology

Melatonin is a pineal gland hormone which acts predominantly on the suprachiasmatic nucleus, the circadian pacemaker in the hypothalamus. The circadian sleep-wake cycle is modified by light and melatonin, released during darkness and acting through MT_2 receptors. During darkness, melatonin suppresses the wakefulness-promoting activity of the nucleus, through MT_1 receptors (Figure 4.3). Its other actions include immunomodulation[1] and a beneficial effect on cancer survival.[2,3] The function of MT_3, a **quinine** reductase, is uncertain.

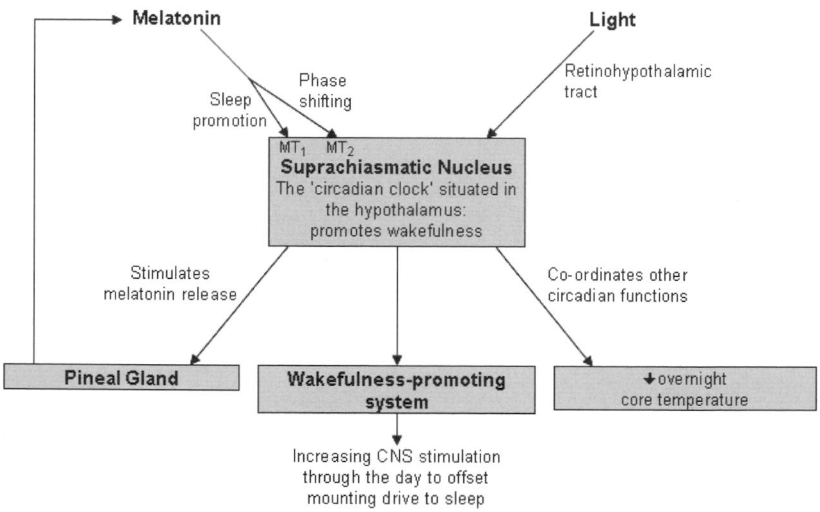

Figure 4.3 Action of melatonin.

Oral bio-availability is limited by extensive first pass hepatic metabolism. It is 60% protein bound and is metabolised by CYP1A1 and 1A2 to an inactive sulphatoxy metabolite, which is renally excreted.

Primary insomnia
Melatonin 2mg m/r (Circadin®) has been evaluated in adults aged >55 years using sleep diaries. The NNT for improvements of ≥1/10 in both quality of sleep and behaviour the following morning is 5 to 9 (and NNH for any adverse event ≥33).[4,5] The NNT for any subjective improvement in sleep quality in older adults with benzodiazepines and related hypnotics is 13 (and NNH for any adverse event 6).[6]

However, a meta-analysis of trials using objective measures of insomnia (polysomnography or actigraphy) found benefits of doubtful clinical significance (improved sleep latency, total sleep duration and sleep efficiency of 4min, 13min and 2.2% respectively).[7] Head-to-head comparisons found no clinically significant differences between doses[8] or formulations (normal-release vs. m/r).[9,10] Reduced melatonin production does not predict response.[11] Melatonin m/r is effective in patients using long-term benzodiazepine hypnotics.[12] Results of RCTs examining a possible role for melatonin in facilitating benzodiazepine discontinuation are conflicting.[13–15]

Insomnia in specific groups
Brain injury is associated with reduced evening melatonin production.[16] In individuals (mostly children) with various intellectual disabilities, a meta-analysis found melatonin improved sleep latency (35min), total sleep duration (50min) and sleep efficiency. The dose, timing and preparation of melatonin varied.[17]

Melatonin reduced sleep latency by 30min and improved sleep efficiency in haemodialysis patients with insomnia.[18] It is effective for jet lag,[19] shift work-related insomnia,[20] and delayed sleep phase syndrome.[21]

Sleep-wake cycle disturbance is common in dementia and delirium. Evening agitation and insomnia associated with dementia improved with melatonin in several case series and 2/4 RCTs.[22] Hyperactive delirium is associated with reduced, and hypoactive delirium with increased, urinary melatonin metabolites.[23] Disordered metabolism of tryptophan, the precursor of serotonin and melatonin, is hypothesised to underlie delirium.[24] Melatonin is reported to improve postoperative delirium refractory to **haloperidol** and **lorazepam**.[25]

Bio-availability 15% (because of first-pass hepatic metabolism).

Time to peak plasma concentration 3h (with food), 45min (empty stomach).

Plasma halflife 3.5–4h.

Cautions
Despite its focused mode of action, melatonin may enhance the sedative effect of sedative drugs.

Auto-immune disease; although there are no data in humans, melatonin causes deleterious immunostimulation in animals with auto-immunity.[2]

Drug interactions
Melatonin levels increased by inhibitors of CYP1A2 (e.g. **fluvoxamine**, quinolones; see p.735). Melatonin can increase or decrease INR (consider increased monitoring).

Undesirable effects
No undesirable effects occurred in >1% for melatonin m/r (Circadin®). In RCTs, adverse event rates were comparable to placebo.[4,5]

Uncommon (<1%, >0.1%): Restlessness, irritability, abnormal dreams, dizziness, somnolence, constipation, dry mouth, hyperbilirubinaemia.

Rare (<0.1%, >0.01%): Laboratory changes (leukopenia, thrombocytopenia, altered LFTs), rashes, mood alteration, vertigo, blurred vision, nausea and vomiting.

Dose and use
Sleep disturbance is common in palliative care. Treatment involves non-drug approaches (e.g. relaxation techniques), the correction of underlying causes (sleep-disturbing symptoms, fears, concurrent depression, delirium) and psychological therapies.

The efficacy of both conventional hypnotics and melatonin is modest. Further, it may not be possible to extrapolate the results of RCTs for primary insomnia to the palliative care setting because:

- of melatonin's propensity to alter cognition

- falls risk and fatigue have not been examined in a relevant patient group
- insomnia is more commonly secondary.

Thus, the place of melatonin for sleep problems in palliative care remains uncertain. It could be considered where other options have failed or lack of tolerability limits the use of conventional hypnotics:

- melatonin m/r 2mg 1–2h before bedtime for 3 weeks.

Supply

Circadin® (Lundbeck)

Tablets m/r 2mg, 21 days @ 2mg once daily (1–2h before bedtime) = £11.

1 Srinivasan V *et al.* (2005) Melatonin, immune function and aging. *Immunity and Ageing.* **2**: 17.
2 Carrillo-Vico A *et al.* (2005) A review of the multiple actions of melatonin on the immune system. *Endocrine.* **27**: 189–200.
3 Mills E *et al.* (2005) Melatonin in the treatment of cancer: a systematic review of randomized controlled trials and meta-analysis. *Journal of Pineal Research.* **39**: 360–366.
4 Lemoine P *et al.* (2007) Prolonged-release melatonin improves sleep quality and morning alertness in insomnia patients aged 55 years and older and has no withdrawal effects. *Journal of Sleep Research.* **16**: 372–380.
5 Wade AG *et al.* (2007) Efficacy of prolonged release melatonin in insomnia patients aged 55–80 years: quality of sleep and next-day alertness outcomes. *Current Medical Research Opinion.* **23**: 2597–2605.
6 Glass J *et al.* (2005) Sedative hypnotics in older people with insomnia: meta-analysis of risks and benefits. *British Medical Journal.* **331**: 1169.
7 Brzezinski A *et al.* (2005) Effects of exogenous melatonin on sleep: a meta-analysis. *Sleep Medicine Reviews.* **9**: 41–50.
8 Zhdanova IV *et al.* (2001) Melatonin treatment for age-related insomnia. *Journal of Clinical Endocrinology and Metabolism.* **86**: 4727–4730.
9 Haimov I *et al.* (1995) Melatonin replacement therapy of elderly insomniacs. *Sleep.* **18**: 598–603.
10 Hughes RJ *et al.* (1998) The role of melatonin and circadian phase in age-related sleep-maintenance insomnia: assessment in a clinical trial of melatonin replacement. *Sleep.* **21**: 52–68.
11 Wade AG *et al.* (2010) Nightly treatment of primary insomnia with prolonged release melatonin for 6 months: a randomized placebo controlled trial on age and endogenous melatonin as predictors of efficacy and safety. *BMC Medicine.* **8**: 51.
12 Garfinkel (1995) Improvement of sleep quality by controlled-release melatonin in benzodiazepine-treated elderly insomniacs. *Archives of Gerontology and Geriatrics.* **24**: 223–231.
13 Cardinali (2002) A double blind placebo controlled study of melatonin efficacy to reduce anxiolytic benzodiazepine use in the elderly. *Neuro Endocrinology Letters.* **23**: 55–60.
14 Vissers FH *et al.* (2007) Is melatonin helpful in stopping the long-term use of hypnotics? A discontinuation trial. *Pharmacy World and Science.* **29**: 641–646.
15 Garfinkel D *et al.* (1999) Facilitation of benzodiazepine discontinuation by melatonin: a new clinical approach. *Archives of Internal Medicine.* **159**: 2456–2460.
16 Shekleton JA *et al.* (2010) Sleep disturbance and melatonin levels following traumatic brain injury. *Neurology.* **74**: 1732–1738.
17 Braam W *et al.* (2009) Exogenous melatonin for sleep problems in individuals with intellectual disability: a meta-analysis. *Developmental Medicine and Child Neurology.* **51**: 340–349.
18 Koch BC *et al.* (2009) The effects of melatonin on sleep-wake rhythm of daytime haemodialysis patients: a randomized, placebo-controlled, cross-over study (EMSCAP study). *British Journal of Clinical Pharmacology.* **67**: 68–75.
19 Herxheimer A (2002) Melatonin for the prevention and treatment of jet lag. *Cochrane Database of Systematic Reviews.* **2**: CD001520.
20 Sadeghniiat-Haghighi (2008) Efficacy and hypnotic effects of melatonin in shift-work nurses. *Journal of Circadian Rhythms.* **6**: 6–10.
21 Kayumov L *et al.* (2001) A randomized, double-blind, placebo-controlled crossover study of the effect of exogenous melatonin on delayed sleep phase syndrome. *Psychosomatic Medicine.* **63**: 40–48.
22 de Jonghe A *et al.* (2010) Effectiveness of melatonin treatment on circadian rhythm disturbances in dementia. Are there implications for delirium? A systematic review. *International Journal of Geriatric Psychiatry.* **25**: 1201–1208.
23 Balan S *et al.* (2003) The relation between the clinical subtypes of delirium and the urinary level of 6-SMT. *Journal of Neuropsychiatry and Clinical Neurosciences.* **15**: 363–366.
24 Lewis MC and Barnett SR (2004) Postoperative delirium: the tryptophan dyregulation model. *Medical Hypotheses.* **63**: 402–406.
25 Hanania M and Kitain E (2002) Melatonin for treatment and prevention of postoperative delirium. *Anesthesia and Analgesia.* **94**: 338–339.

ANTIPSYCHOTICS — BNF 4.2.1

Indications: Acute psychotic symptoms, mania and bipolar disorders, schizophrenia, †agitation, †delirium, †nausea and vomiting, intractable hiccup, †treatment-resistant depression.

Neurophysiology of dopamine

Dopamine has a central role in arousal, motivation, attention, the extrapyramidal motor system and other pathways (Table 4.7). Although the exact mechanism is uncertain, dopamine dysregulation plays a role in several symptoms, e.g. nausea, hallucinations, low mood, and restlessness. Thus, the neurophysiology of dopamine underpins an understanding of the numerous therapeutic uses and undesirable effects of dopamine modulators, i.e. antipsychotics, psychostimulants (see p.205), and D_2 agonists.

Table 4.7 Dopaminergic pathways

Pathway	*Function*	*Symptoms of dysregulation*
Mesolimbic Midbrain reticular formation → limbic cortex	Pleasure, motivation and reward[a]	↑Dopamine: 'positive' symptoms of psychosis (delusions, hallucinations)
Mesocortical system Midbrain reticular formation → prefrontal cortex	Affect, executive function, concentration	↓Dopamine: depression; 'negative' symptoms of psychosis (apathy, anhedonia and cognitive blunting)
Nigrostriatal system Substantia nigra → corpus striatum	Extrapyramidal motor system	↓Dopamine: Parkinson's disease, drug-induced parkinsonism, akathisia, dystonia, restless legs ↑Dopamine: dyskinesia
Tubero-infundibular system	Dopaminergic inhibition of prolactin secretion	↓Dopamine: hyperprolactinaemia
Thalamic dopamine pathway[a] Multiple origins → thalamus	Sleep and arousal through sensory gating	
Area postrema	Emetogenesis	↑Dopamine: nausea and vomiting

a. Both the mesolimbic and thalamic dopamine pathways affect thalamic sensory gating. Mesolimbic dysregulation is best characterized in the formation of 'positive' psychotic symptoms (see text).

Psychotic symptoms arise from opposing dopamine imbalances:
- 'positive' symptoms (delusions and hallucinations) result from dopamine *excess* in the mesolimbic system
- 'negative' symptoms (apathy, anhedonia and cognitive blunting) result from dopamine *deficit* in the mesocortical system.

Arousal, motivation and attention are regulated by a 2-way loop between the prefrontal/limbic cortex and the thalamus. The prefrontal/limbic cortex identifies situations requiring attention and the thalamus is directed to allow relevant information to pass through to the cerebral cortex while filtering out the rest. This thalamic sensory filter is formed by GABAergic neurones which are switched off by dopamine to allow salient information through. In psychosis, dopamine overactivity leads to excessive information throughput, resulting in hallucinations and delusions (the 'salience hypothesis'). D_2 antagonist antipsychotics help to correct this overactivity, and improve these symptoms.[1–3]

Conversely, D_2 antagonists augment dopaminergic underactivity in the mesocortical system, which causes, or exacerbates, 'negative' symptoms.[1,3] D_2 antagonism can also disrupt other pathways unaffected by psychosis:
- nigrostriatal system, part of the extrapyramidal motor system:
  - ▷ D_2 antagonists initially cause underactivity, similar to Parkinson's disease → acute extrapyramidal symptoms
  - ▷ subsequent adaptation to D_2 antagonism leads to D_2 receptor upregulation → tardive dyskinesia
- tubero-infundibular system; D_2 antagonists cause hyperprolactinaemia → sexual dysfunction.

The newer 'atypical' antipsychotics have been developed in an attempt to overcome some of the above limitations of 'typical' D_2 antagonists.

Pharmacology

Conventionally, antipsychotics are divided into two classes:
- typical:
  - ▷ phenothiazines, e.g. **chlorpromazine**, **levomepromazine**, **prochlorperazine**

  - butyrophenones, e.g. **haloperidol**
- atypical, **aripipazole**, **clozapine**, **olanzapine**, **quetiapine**, **risperidone**.

However, there is much variation within, and overlap between, these classes. Although all antipsychotics are characterized by D_2 antagonism, differences in receptor profile result in clinical differences between them (Table 4.8).[4] Antipsychotics are variably associated with antagonistic effects at the following receptors:

- muscarinic, causing dry mouth, constipation, etc (see Box 1.A, p.5)
- adrenergic, causing postural hypotension
- histaminic, causing drowsiness
- serotoninergic (type 2), causing weight gain.

In contrast, the D_2-specific action of **haloperidol** avoids such problems, but increases the risk of extrapyramidal effects.

Table 4.8 Receptor affinities for selected antipsychotics[4–7]

	D_2	$5HT_{2A}$	$5HT_{2C}$	$5HT_3$	H_1	α_1	α_2	ACh_M
Aripiprazole	+++PA	+++	+++	–	+++	+++	++	–
Chlorpromazine	+++	+++	++	–	+++	+++	+	++
Clozapine	+	+++	++	+	+++	+	+	+++
Haloperidol	+++	+	–	–	–	++	–	–
Levomepromazine	++	+++			+++	+++	+	++
Perphenazine	+++	+++	+		+++	++	+	–
Prochlorperazine	+++	++	+	–	++	++	–	+
Olanzapine	++	+++	+	+	+	++	+	++
Quetiapine	+	+	+	–	++	+	++	–
Risperidone	+++	+++	++	–	++	+	+++	–

Affinity: +++ high, ++ moderate, + low, – negligible or none; blank = no data.
PA = partial agonist.

Atypical antipsychotics carry a lower risk of extrapyramidal effects and improved efficacy for negative symptoms. This relates to:[1,8,9]

- $5HT_2$ antagonism
- D_2 partial agonism
- lower affinity and shorter duration D_2 antagonism.

$5HT_2$ receptors inhibit dopaminergic neurones of the nigrostriatal and mesocortical systems. Thus, $5HT_2$ antagonist antipsychotics increase activity in these pathways, countering the extrapyramidal impact of D_2 antagonism and improving 'negative' symptoms.[10] 'Negative' symptoms overlap with depressive symptoms and can respond to antidepressants.[11] Conversely, some $5HT_2$ antagonist antipsychotics are beneficial in refractory depression (e.g. **olanzapine**).[12,13] It is noteworthy that increased prefrontal dopamine release through $5HT_2$ antagonism is also an important action of some antidepressants, e.g. **mirtazapine** (see p.200).

An antipsychotic which acts as a D_2 partial agonist will function as a D_2 antagonist in the presence of excessive dopamine (e.g. as in the mesolimbic system in psychosis), because partial activation of the D_2 receptor will reduce overall transmission. However, when there is dopamine depletion, the partial D_2 receptor activation is sufficient to increase overall transmission, and it functions as a D_2 agonist, e.g. in the nigrostriatal and mesocortical systems. In consequence, a D_2 partial agonist antipsychotic can potentially improve both 'positive' and 'negative' symptoms and limit undesirable extrapyramidal effects.

However, the extent to which atypical antipsychotics succeed *in practice* in reducing extrapyramidal effects and 'negative' symptoms is unclear. The relatively lower doses of atypicals used in RCTs with typicals may partly explain some of the observed differences. Further, the properties purported to account for such differences are also shared by some typical antipsychotics, e.g. $5HT_2$ antagonism. On the other hand, the higher incidence of other undesirable effects (particularly metabolic) with atypicals limits improvement in overall tolerability.

Direct comparisons suggest that acute extrapyramidal effects would be avoided in one patient for every 3–6 patients treated with an atypical rather than a typical antipsychotic.[14,15] However, the difference is greatest relative to **haloperidol**. Further, in an RCT, although extrapyramidal effects accounted for more discontinuations of **perphenazine** compared with several atypicals (8% vs. 2–4%), overall discontinuation rates for undesirable effects or lack of efficacy were comparable.[16] All treatment groups experienced some degree of involuntary movement (13–17%), akathisia (5–9%) or extrapyramidal signs (4–8%). Most studies are too short to evaluate the risk of tardive dyskinesia. Available data suggest a 5 times lower risk with atypicals compared with **haloperidol** in the first year of use, although **haloperidol** doses were relatively higher.[17] Among atypicals, **risperidone** carries the highest risk of extrapyramidal effects, and **clozapine** and **quetiapine** the lowest.[18]

Acquisition costs for atypicals are higher than for typicals. Suggested reductions in costs from the long-term use of atypicals may be less relevant in palliative care if drugs are used at lower doses and for shorter periods.[19]

Pharmacokinetic details of selected antipsychotics are summarized in Table 4.9.

Table 4.9 Pharmacokinetic details for selected antipsychotics.[20,21]

	Oral bio-availability (%)	*Time to peak plasma concentration*	*Halflife (h)*	*Metabolism (predominant P450 isoenzyme)*
Chlorpromazine	10–25	2–4h (PO)	30	CYP2D6
Clozapine	50–60	2h	12	CYP1A2, CYP3A4
Haloperidol	60–70	2–6h (PO) 10–20min (SC)	13–35	Multiple
Levomepromazine	40	1–3h (PO) 30–90min (SC)	15–30	Multiple[a]
Olanzapine	60	5–8h	34[b] (52[c])	CYP1A2, CYP2D6
Prochlorperazine	6 14 (buccal)	4h (PO) 4–8h (buccal); shorter with multiple doses	15–20	Multiple
Quetiapine	100	1.5h	7[d] (10–14[c]) (12[e])	CYP3A4
Risperidone	99	1–2h	24[f,g]	CYP2D6[h]

a. P450 iso-enzymes not fully characterized; some metabolites are active
b. unaffected by hepatic or renal impairment
c. in the elderly
d. clearance reduced by both renal and hepatic impairment
e. of active metabolite
f. for risperidone + active 9-hydroxy metabolite
g. clearance reduced by renal impairment
h. activity of 9-hydroxyrisperidone, the predominant CYP2D6 metabolite, is comparable to risperidone; thus overall clinical effect is not altered by CYP2D6 polymorphisms or inhibitors.

Cautions

Several pharmacodynamic interactions (additive sedation, hypotension and QT prolongation; reduced effect of antiparkinsonian drugs) can be predicted from the receptor profile of antipsychotics.

Stroke risk

Meta-analysis of RCTs in the elderly with dementia has shown that the risk of stroke with **olanzapine** and **risperidone** is 2–3 times higher compared with placebo,[22–25] with a doubling of all-cause mortality with **olanzapine**.[23] The mechanism of this association is not known, but it is regarded as a class effect. Subsequent findings indicate an increased risk in all elderly patients for both typicals and atypicals,[18,26–28] greatest in those with dementia,[29] within the first month of starting treatment, and with higher doses. The relative risk with individual drugs has not yet been determined.

Epilepsy

Similar to many other psychotropic medications, antipsychotics cause a dose-dependent reduction in seizure threshold. The risk for individual agents approximates to the degree of sedation: **chlorpromazine** and **clozapine** carry a higher risk and **haloperidol** a lower risk. To minimize the risk, use the lowest risk antipsychotic (e.g. **haloperidol**) at the lowest effective dose. In palliative care, depot formulations are best avoided because they cannot be withdrawn quickly if problems occur.

Parkinsonism and Parkinson's disease

All antipsychotics, through D_2 antagonism, can cause parkinsonism or worsen existing parkinsonism of any cause. The risk is lower with **clozapine** and **quetiapine**. In patients with parkinsonism, alternatives to antipsychotics should be used where possible, e.g. for agitation, consider **trazodone** (see p.202) or a benzodiazepine, for nausea and vomiting consider:

- **domperidone** (available as a suppository)
- **ondansetron**
- **hyoscine *hydrobromide***, but may cause delirium.

Nonetheless, at the end of life, despite being D_2 antagonists, it may be necessary to prescribe small doses of **levomepromazine**, **olanzapine** or **quetiapine** if all else fails.

Where delirium or psychotic symptoms occur in the context of Parkinson's disease or Lewy Body dementia:

- look for potentially reversible causes of delirium, e.g. sepsis
- consider a trial reduction of antiparkinsonian medication:
  - ▹ reduce D_2 agonists and antimuscarinic agents initially
  - ▹ dopamine precursors, e.g. **levodopa**, are less likely to cause psychosis.[30]

If the above measures are unhelpful, commence **quetiapine** 12.5–25mg/24h; if not tolerated, seek specialist advice. Options include switching to **clozapine**.[30]

Drug interactions

Potentially serious interactions may result from induction or inhibition of hepatic metabolism (see p.735). CYP3A4 inhibitors (e.g. **aprepitant**, **cimetidine**, macrolide antibiotics, **ketoconazole**) can significantly increase plasma levels of **aripiprazole**, **pimozide** and **quetiapine**. **Carbamazepine** and protease inhibitors exhibit varied interactions.

Antipsychotics are one of several classes of drugs which can prolong the QT interval, and at least theoretically increase the risk of cardiac tachyarrthymias, including potentially fatal *torsade de pointes*. Generally, concurrent prescribing of two drugs which can significantly prolong the QT interval should be avoided (see p.727 and www.azcert.org).

Undesirable effects

A summary is given in Box 4.C.

Box 4.C Undesirable effects of antipsychotics

Extrapyramidal syndromes
Parkinsonism, akathisia, dystonia, tardive dyskinesia.[31]

Metabolic effects[18,32]
More common with typicals and risperidone
Hyperprolactinemia resulting in amenorrhoea, galactorrhoea, gynaecomastia, sexual dysfunction, osteoporosis.

More common with atypicals, particularly olanzapine, quetiapine and clozapine
Weight gain.
Dyslipidaemia, possibly associated with weight gain.

Type 2 diabetes mellitus, both new onset and exacerbation of pre-existing disease; risk independent of weight gain.

continued

Box 4.C Continued

Cardiovascular effects
QT prolongation: dose-related, affected by presence of other risk factors, highest risk with thioridazine (withdrawn) and ziprasidone.[18,33]

Venous thrombo-embolism; risk possibly highest with atypicals.[34,35]

Stroke and increased risk of death in elderly patients (see Cautions).

Postural hypotension (α-adrenergic antagonism), particularly phenothiazines and clozapine; also seen with quetiapine and risperidone.

Miscellaneous[18]
Reduced seizure threshold (see Cautions).

Antimuscarinic effects; more with phenothiazines and clozapine.

Neuroleptic (antipsychotic) malignant syndrome (see below).

Agranulocytosis is seen in about 1% of patients taking clozapine, generally after 3–6 months.

Neuroleptic (antipsychotic) malignant syndrome

Neuroleptic (antipsychotic) malignant syndrome (NMS) is a potentially life-threatening reaction which occurs in <1% of those prescribed an antipsychotic (Box 4.D).[36,37] This idiosyncratic syndrome is associated with all antipsychotics.[38]

Box 4.D Clinical features of neuroleptic (antipsychotic) malignant syndrome

Essential
Severe muscle rigidity
Pyrexia + sweating

Additional
Muteness → stupor
Tachycardia and elevated/labile blood pressure
Leukocytosis
Raised plasma creatine phosphokinase ± other evidence of muscle injury, e.g. myoglobinuria

Most cases of NMS occur within 2 weeks of starting treatment or a dose increase. It is a hypodopaminergic state; bradykinesia progresses to immobilization, akinesia and stupor, accompanied by lead-pipe rigidity, fever, and autonomic instability.

Symptoms indistinguishable from NMS have been reported in patients with Parkinson's disease when long-term treatment with **levodopa** and **bromocriptine** (a D_2 agonist) has been abruptly discontinued.[39–41] This has led to the suggestion that the syndrome would be better called *acute dopamine depletion syndrome*.[39]

Death occurs in up to 20% of cases, mostly as a result of respiratory failure. The use of a dopamine agonist, e.g. **bromocriptine**, halves the mortality.[42] Subsequent prescription of an antipsychotic carries a 30–50% risk of recurrence.[43]

NMS is self-limiting if the causal antipsychotic drug is discontinued (and an alternative antipsychotic *not* prescribed). Generally it resolves in 1–2 weeks unless caused by a depot antipsychotic, when it takes 4–6 weeks. Antipsychotics are *not* removed by haemodialysis. Specific measures include:

- discontinuation of the causal drug
- prescription of a muscle relaxant, e.g. a benzodiazepine
- in severe cases, prescription of **bromocriptine**.[42]

General supportive measures may need to extend to artificial hydration and nutrition. Complications such as hypoxia, acidosis and renal failure require appropriate acute management.

Use of antipsychotics in palliative care

When long term (>months) use of **olanzapine**, **quetiapine** or phenothiazines is anticipated, consider monitoring weight, glucose and lipids at baseline and 3-monthly thereafter.

Doses are described in individual monographs: **haloperidol** (p.160), **levomepromazine** (p.164), **prochlorperazine** (p.163), **olanzapine** (p.166), **risperidone** (p.168) and **quetiapine** (p.171).

Nausea and vomiting

The D_2 antagonism of all antipsychotics is likely to provide anti-emetic activity in the area postrema (chemoreceptor trigger zone; see p.219). Where specific action at this site is required (e.g. most chemical causes of nausea), a selective dopaminergic agent such as **haloperidol** is used,[44] although studies in palliative care patients are open-label.[45,46] However, most antipsychotics have moderate or high affinity at several receptors, some of which are involved in the transduction of emetic signals.[47] Thus, most antipsychotics are, to a variable extent, broad-spectrum anti-emetics. **Levomepromazine** and **olanzapine** are the most attractive choices (and **haloperidol** is the least) in this respect.[48,49]

Delirium

Delirium is distressing and associated with higher mortality, reduced performance status and increased admission to nursing homes.[50–52] Management guidelines emphasise the importance of treating underlying causes, non-drug management (e.g. orientation strategies, correction of sensory deprivation) and prevention of complications. Because of limited evidence and safety concerns, medication is often advocated only when non-drug measures are insufficient (particularly in patients with dementia; see below).[53]

More recent evidence suggests that antipsychotics (e.g. **haloperidol**, **olanzapine** or **quetiapine**) should be considered alongside non-drug measures in all forms of delirium (agitated, hypo-active and mixed). In 3 RCTs, antipsychotics not only reduced distressing symptoms but shortened the duration of the delirium[54,55] and improved outcomes (e.g. the proportion of patients discharged home).[56] Hypo-active delirium was not excluded and benefit was observed in all symptom domains, not just agitation.[55] Further, early treatment may be important because prophylactic use shortens delirium and hospital stay compared with use after delirium has occurred.[57] It is uncertain whether outcomes improve as a direct consequence of treating delirium and/or because patients are better able to co-operate with other treatments.

Comparative studies with other psychotropics are lacking.[58–60] When antipsychotics alone are insufficient, or when sedation is also required, e.g. for the initial management of a hyperactive, frightened patient, benzodiazepines (see p.132) or **trazodone** (see p.202) can be added. Although benzodiazepines can paradoxically worsen agitation, they are preferred for delirium related to alcohol withdrawal, neuroleptic malignant syndrome or Parkinson's disease. The use of cholinergics has been reported, but **rivastigmine** increased mortality in an RCT.[61] Hallucinations in delirium respond to antipsychotics in hours–days, whereas seemingly identical phenomena in a psychosis may not resolve for 1–2 weeks.

Agitation and challenging behaviours in dementia

Patients with dementia may become agitated for many reasons, including an appropriate response to a distressing situation. Possible precipitants should be treated or modified:

- intercurrent infections
- pain and/or other distressing symptoms
- environmental factors.

When no reversible cause is found and agitation is mild, assurance that such behaviours are often self-limiting may suffice. Training in non-drug management of behavioural disturbances reduces the need for psychotropic medication.[62]

The first-line use of antipsychotics for behavioural disturbance in dementia is inappropriate and actively discouraged.[63–66] In addition to safety concerns (increased risk of stroke and overall mortality, see above), evidence of benefit compared with non-drug measures is limited. A recent large RCT for agitation or psychosis in patients with dementia found both atypicals and typicals to be no better than placebo in all but a few secondary outcomes.[67] Taken together with other studies, the efficacy of antipsychotics in dementia is at best modest, and should be used only where other measures have failed.[68,69]

The use of alternative drugs, i.e. antidepressants, benzodiazepines, anti-epileptics and cholinesterase inhibitors, has been proposed. However, evidence is generally more limited than for antipsychotics, and insufficient to allow clear evidence-based recommendations of one class over another.[69,70] Further, larger studies have not replicated the earlier benefit reported for **trazodone** (see p.202).[69]

Even so, the serious consequences of not treating severe agitation or psychosis in dementia are also recognized.[69] Where drug treatment is required, clinicians should be guided by the individual patient's symptoms and co-morbidities, and their familiarity with the agents available. Options include:

- **haloperidol**
- atypicals, e.g. **olanzapine**, **quetiapine**, **risperidone**
- cholinesterase inhibitors (benefit is marginal, but may be better tolerated).[70]

Whichever drug is selected, use the lowest effective dose for the shortest possible time; attempt dose reduction every 2–3 months; many patients do not deteriorate when medication is withdrawn.[68,70,71]

Intractable hiccup

Chlorpromazine or **haloperidol** are used when more specific treatment, e.g. **simeticone** (an antifoaming agent; see p.3) ± **metoclopramide** (see p.227) for gastric distension, or **baclofen** are ineffective (see Table 1.4, p.21).[72]

Refractory depression

Certain antipsychotics have been used as adjuncts for depression refractory to conventional antidepressants, particularly when switching antidepressants has been unsuccessful. Generally, either **quetiapine** or **olanzapine** is added to an SSRI (see p.180).[13,73,74]

Pain

Dopamine is implicated in pain processing[75] and, in the past, antipsychotics were sometimes used as part of an analgesic cocktail. However, RCTs yield conflicting results.[76] Although no longer used as analgesics themselves, antipsychotics are helpful for treating the undesirable effects of analgesics, particularly nausea and delirium.[77]

Switching antipsychotics

Equivalent doses of typicals have been estimated, predominantly from surveys of psychiatric practice, and provide a starting point if switching from one to another (Table 4.10).[78] However, doses of atypicals are less variable, and thus starting doses are unaffected by the dose of a previous antipsychotic.

Table 4.10 Equivalent doses of typical antipsychotics[78]

Drug	*Dose (mg)*
Chlorpromazine	100
Promazine	100
Perphenazine	8
Trifluoperazine	5
Haloperidol	3

1 Stahl SM (2008) Psychosis and schizophrenia. In: *Essential Psychopharmacology: Neuroscientific Basis and Practical Applications* (3e). Cambridge University Press, USA, pp. 247–325.
2 Boutrel B and Koob GF (2004) What keeps us awake: the neuropharmacology of stimulants and wakefulness-promoting medications. *Sleep*. **27**: 1181–1194.
3 Alves Fda S *et al.* (2008) The revised dopamine hypothesis of schizophrenia: evidence from pharmacological MRI studies with atypical antipsychotic medication. *Psychopharmacology Bulletin*. **41**: 121–132.
4 Jindal RD and Keshavan MS (2008) Classifying antipsychotic agents: need for new terminology. *CNS Drugs*. **22**: 1047–1059.
5 Lal S *et al.* (1993) Levomepromazine receptor binding profile in human brain–implications for treatment-resistant schizophrenia. *Acta Psychiatrica Scandinavica*. **87**: 380–383.
6 NIMH (National Institute of Mental Health) (2006) National Institute of Mental Health's Psychoactive Drug Screening Program. University of North Carolina. Available from: http://pdsp.med.unc.edu/indexR.html
7 Shiloh R *et al.* (2006) Antipsychotic drugs. In: *Atlas of Psychiatric Pharmacotherapy* (2e). Taylor & Francis, London, pp. 90–105.
8 Kapur S and Mamo D (2003) Half a century of antipsychotics and still a central role for dopamine D2 receptors. *Progress in Neuro-psychopharmacology and Biology Psychiatry*. **27**: 1081–1090.
9 Lieberman JA (2004) Dopamine partial agonists: a new class of antipsychotic. *CNS Drugs*. **18**: 251–267.
10 Meltzer HY (2004) What's atypical about atypical antipsychotic drugs? *Current Opinion in Pharmacology*. **4**: 53–57.
11 Rummel-Klage (2006) Antidepressants for the negative symptoms of schizophrenia. *Cochrane Database of Systematic Reviews*. **3**: CD005581.
12 Millan MJ *et al.* (2000) Mirtazapine enhances frontocortical dopaminergic and corticolimbic adrenergic, but not serotonergic, transmission by blockade of alpha2-adrenergic and serotonin2C receptors: a comparison with citalopram. *European Journal of Neuroscience*. **12**: 1079–1095.
13 Shelton RC *et al.* (2010) Therapeutic options for treatment-resistant depression. *CNS Drugs*. **24**: 131–161.
14 Wahlbeck K *et al.* (2000) Clozapine versus typical neuroleptic medication for schizophrenia. *Cochrane Database of Systematic Reviews*. **2**: CD000059.
15 Hunter RH *et al.* (2003) Risperidone versus typical antipsychotic medication for schizophrenia. *Cochrane Database of Systematic Reviews*. **2**: CD000440.
16 Lieberman JA *et al.* (2005) Effectiveness of antipsychotic drugs in patients with chronic schizophrenia. *New England Journal of Medicine*. **353**: 1209–1223.
17 Correll CU *et al.* (2004) Lower risk for tardive dyskinesia associated with second-generation antipsychotics: a systematic review of 1-year studies. *American Journal of Psychiatry*. **161**: 414–425.
18 Haddad PM and Sharma SG (2007) Adverse effects of atypical antipsychotics: differential risk and clinical implications. *CNS Drugs*. **21**: 911–936.
19 Davies A *et al.* (1998) Risperidone versus haloperidol: II. cost-effectiveness. *Clinical Therapeutics*. **20**: 196–213.
20 Eiermann B *et al.* (1997) The involvement of CYP1A2 and CYP3A4 in the metabolism of clozapine. *British Journal of Clinical Pharmacology*. **44**: 439–446.
21 Finn A *et al.* (2005) Bioavailability and metabolism of prochlorperazine administered via the buccal and oral delivery route. *Journal of Clinical Pharmacology*. **45**: 1383–1390.
22 Wooltorton E (2002) Risperidone (Risperdal): increased rate of cerebrovascular events in dementia trials. *Canadian Medical Association Journal*. **167**: 1269–1270.
23 Wooltorton E (2004) Olanzapine (Zyprexa): increased incidence of cerebrovascular events in dementia trials. *Canadian Medical Association Journal*. **170**: 1395.
24 Bullock R (2005) Treatment of behavioural and psychiatric symptoms in dementia: implications of recent safety warnings. *Current Medical Research and Opinion*. **21**: 1–10.
25 Schneider LS *et al.* (2005) Risk of death with atypical antipsychotic drug treatment for dementia: meta-analysis of randomized placebo-controlled trials. *Journal of the American Medical Association*. **294**: 1934–1943.
26 Wang PS *et al.* (2005) Risk of death in elderly users of conventional vs. atypical antipsychotic medications. *New England Journal of Medicine*. **353**: 2335–2341.
27 Gill SS *et al.* (2007) Antipsychotic drug use and mortality in older adults with dementia. *Annals of internal medicine*. **146**: 775–786.
28 Ray WA *et al.* (2009) Atypical antipsychotic drugs and the risk of sudden cardiac death. *New England Journal of Medicine*. **360**: 225–235.
29 Douglas IJ and Smeeth L (2008) Exposure to antipsychotics and risk of stroke: self controlled case series study. *British Medical Journal*. **337**: a1227.
30 Weintraub D and Hurtig HI (2007) Presentation and management of psychosis in Parkinson's disease and dementia with Lewy bodies. *American Journal of Psychiatry*. **164**: 1491–1498.
31 Twycross R and Wilcock A (2008) Drug induced movement disorders. In: *Hospice and Palliative Care Formulary USA* (2e). palliativedrugs.com Nottingham, pp. 547–550.
32 Yood MU *et al.* (2009) The incidence of diabetes in atypical antipsychotic users differs according to agent — results from a multisite epidemiologic study. *Pharmacoepidemiology and Drug Safety*. **18**: 791–799.
33 Twycross R and Wilcock A (2008) Prolongation of the QT interval in palliative care. In: *Hospice and Palliative Care Formulary USA* (2e). palliativedrugs.com, Nottingham, pp. 531–536.
34 Liperoti R *et al.* (2005) Venous thromboembolism among elderly patients treated with atypical and conventional antipsychotic agents. *Archives of Internal Medicine*. **165**: 2677–2682.
35 Parker C *et al.* (2010) Antipsychotic drugs and risk of venous thromboembolism: nested case-control study. *British Medical Journal*. **341**: c4245.
36 Caroff S and Mann S (1993) Neuroleptic malignant syndrome. *Medical Clinics of North America*. **77**: 185–202.
37 Adnet P *et al.* (2000) Neuroleptic malignant syndrome. *British Journal of Anaesthesia*. **85**: 129–135.
38 Isbister GK *et al.* (2002) Comment: neuroleptic malignant syndrome associated with risperidone and fluvoxamine. *Annals of Pharmacotherapy*. **36**: 1293; author reply 1294.
39 Keyser DL and Rodnitzky RL (1991) Neuroleptic malignant syndrome in Parkinson's disease after withdrawal or alteration of dopaminergic therapy. *Archives of Internal Medicine*. **151**: 794–796.
40 Mann S *et al.* (1991) Pathogenesis of neuroleptic malignant syndrome. *Psychiatry Annals*. **21**: 175–180.
41 Ong K *et al.* (2001) Neuroleptic malignant syndrome without neuroleptics. *Singapore Medical Journal*. **42**: 85–88.
42 Sakkas P *et al.* (1991) Pharmacotherapy of neuroleptic malignant syndrome. *Psychiatry Annals*. **21**: 157–164.

43 Wells A *et al.* (1988) Neuroleptic rechallenges after neuroleptic malignant syndrome: case report and literature review. *Drug Intelligence and Clinical Pharmacy.* **22**: 475–479.
44 Buttner M *et al.* (2004) Is low-dose haloperidol a useful antiemetic?: A meta-analysis of published and unpublished randomized trials. *Anesthesiology.* **101**: 1454–1463.
45 Hardy JR *et al.* (2010) The efficacy of haloperidol in the management of nausea and vomiting in patients with cancer. *Journal of Pain and Symptom Management.* **40**: 111–116.
46 Perkins (2009) Haloperidol for the treatment of nausea and vomiting in palliative care patients. *Cochrane Database of Systematic Reviews.*
47 Twycross R and Wilcock A (2008) Antiemetics. In: *Hospice and Palliative Care Formulary USA* (2e), pp. 185–190.
48 Passik SD *et al.* (2004) A phase I trial of olanzapine (Zyprexa) for the prevention of delayed emesis in cancer patients: a Hoosier Oncology Group study. *Cancer Investigation.* **22**: 383–388.
49 Navari RM *et al.* (2005) A phase II trial of olanzapine for the prevention of chemotherapy-induced nausea and vomiting: a Hoosier Oncology Group study. *Supportive Care in Cancer.* **13**: 529–534.
50 Breitbart W *et al.* (2002) The delirium experience: delirium recall and delirium-related distress in hospitalized patients with cancer, their spouses/caregivers, and their nurses. *Psychosomatics.* **43**: 183–194.
51 Marcantonio E *et al.* (2002) Delirium severity and psychomotor types: their relationship with outcomes after hip fracture repair. *Journal of the American Geriatrics Society.* **50**: 850–857.
52 Leslie DL *et al.* (2005) Premature death associated with delirium at 1-year follow-up. *Archives of Internal Medicine.* **165**: 1657–1662.
53 NICE (2010) Clinical Guideline 103. Delirium. Available from: http://guidance.nice.org.uk/CG103
54 Hu (2006) Olanzapine and haloperidol for senile delirium: a randomised controlled observation. *Chinese Journal of Clinical Rehabilitation.* **10**: 188–190.
55 Tahir TA *et al.* (2010) A randomized controlled trial of quetiapine versus placebo in the treatment of delirium. *Journal of Psychosomatic Research.* **69**: 485–490.
56 Devlin JW *et al.* (2010) Efficacy and safety of quetiapine in critically ill patients with delirium: a prospective, multicenter, randomized, double-blind, placebo-controlled pilot study. *Critical Care Medicine.* **38**: 419–427.
57 Kalisvaart KJ *et al.* (2005) Haloperidol prophylaxis for elderly hip-surgery patients at risk for delirium: a randomized placebo-controlled study. *Journal of the American Geriatrics Society.* **53**. 1658–1666.
58 Attard A *et al.* (2008) Delirium and its treatment. *CNS Drugs.* **22**: 631–644.
59 Caraceni A and Simonetti F (2009) Palliating delirium in patients with cancer. *Lancet Oncology.* **10**: 164–172.
60 Fong TG *et al.* (2009) Delirium in elderly adults: diagnosis, prevention and treatment. *Nature Reviews Neurology.* **5**: 210—220.
61 van Eijk MM *et al.* (2010) Effect of rivastigmine as an adjunct to usual care with haloperidol on duration of delirium and mortality in critically ill patients: a multicentre, double-blind, placebo-controlled randomised trial. *Lancet.* **376**: 1829–1837.
62 Fossey J *et al.* (2006) Effect of enhanced psychosocial care on antipsychotic use in nursing home residents with severe dementia: cluster randomised trial. *British Medical Journal.* **332**: 756–761.
63 CSM (Committee on Safety of Medicines) (2004) Antipsychotic drugs and stroke. Available from: www.mhra.gov.uk/Safetyinformation/Safetywarningsalertsandrecalls/Safetywarningsandmessagesformedicines/CON1004298
64 Mowat D *et al.* (2004) CSM warning on atypical psychotics and stroke may be detrimental for dementia. *British Medical Journal.* **328**: 1262.
65 Health Canada (2005) Increased mortality associated with the use of atypical antipsychotic drugs in elderly patients with dementia. Notice to healthcare professionals. Available from: www.hc-sc.gc.ca/dhp-mps/medeff/advisories-avis/prof/_2005/atyp-antipsycho_hpc-cps-eng.php
66 FDA (2008) Alert. Information on antipsychotics (6/16/2008). Available from: www.fda.gov/Drugs
67 Schneider LS *et al.* (2006) Effectiveness of atypical antipsychotic drugs in patients with Alzheimer's disease. *New England Journal of Medicine.* **355**: 1525–1538.
68 Ballard C and Corbett A (2010) Management of neuropsychiatric symptoms in people with dementia. *CNS Drugs.* **24**: 729–739.
69 Jeste DV *et al.* (2008) ACNP White Paper: update on use of antipsychotic drugs in elderly persons with dementia. *Neuropsychopharmacology.* **33**: 957–970.
70 Sink KM *et al.* (2005) Pharmacological treatment of neuropsychiatric symptoms of dementia: a review of the evidence. *Journal of the American Medical Association.* **293**: 596–608.
71 Lee PE *et al.* (2004) Atypical antipsychotic drugs in the treatment of behavioural and psychological symptoms of dementia: systematic review. *British Medical Journal.* **329**: 75.
72 Twycross R *et al.* (2009) *Symptom Management in Advanced Cancer* (4e). palliativedrugs.com, Nottingham, pp. 174–177.
73 NICE (2009) Clinical Guideline 90 and 91. Depression. Available from: www.nice.org.uk
74 Anderson IM *et al.* (2008) Evidence-based guidelines for treating depressive disorders with antidepressants: a revision of the 2000 British Association for Psychopharmacology guidelines. *Journal of Psychopharmacology.* **22**: 343–396.
75 Wood PB (2006) Mesolimbic dopaminergic mechanisms and pain control. *Pain.* **120**: 230–234.
76 Seidel (2008) Antipsychotics for acute and chronic pain in adults. *Cochrane Database of Systematic Reviews.*
77 Coyle N *et al.* (1994) Delirium as a contributing factor to 'crescendo' pain: three case reports. *Journal of Pain and Symptom Management.* **9**: 44–47.
78 Foster P (1989) Neuroleptic equivalence. *Pharmaceutical Journal.* **243**: 431–432.

HALOPERIDOL BNF 4.2.1

Class: Butyrophenone antipsychotic.

Indications: Acute psychotic symptoms, schizophrenia, Gilles de la Tourette's syndrome, †agitation, †delirium, †nausea and vomiting, intractable hiccup.

Pharmacology

Haloperidol is a typical antipsychotic D_2 antagonist. Steady-state plasma concentrations do not vary greatly between patients after injection but they vary considerably after PO administration. The metabolism of haloperidol is not as complex as that of the phenothiazines but, even so, there are many metabolites and some may contribute to its extrapyramidal effects.[1] It is not possible to relate clinical response to plasma haloperidol concentrations. Haloperidol in solution is odourless, colourless and tasteless and can be administered clandestinely in extreme situations.

Compared with **chlorpromazine**, haloperidol has less effect on the cardiovascular system and causes less drowsiness. It has no antimuscarinic properties,[2] but causes *more* extrapyramidal reactions (see Drug-induced movement disorders, p.745). In one study, haloperidol caused akathisia in >50% of schizophrenics.[3] The incidence in palliative care appears to be low, possibly because generally lower doses are used and the duration of treatment is relatively short.

Haloperidol is widely used in palliative care as an anti-emetic and for delirium. By virtue of its D_2 antagonism, it has a profound inhibitory effect on the area postrema (chemoreceptor trigger zone). It is an effective anti-emetic postoperatively and in patients referred to specialist gastro-enterological clinics with multifactorial nausea.[4] Long-standing clinical experience in palliative care indicates that haloperidol is a good anti-emetic for many chemical causes of vomiting,[5] e.g. **morphine**, **digoxin**, renal failure, hypercalcaemia;[6,7] and also after radiotherapy.[8] However, no RCTs have been conducted in palliative care patients.[9] Haloperidol has also been used for obstructive vomiting in relatively small doses, e.g. 2–5mg SC.[10,11] Its benefit in this circumstance is difficult to understand. However, the affinity of haloperidol for D_2-receptors is 10 times that of **domperidone** (see p.229).[12] Thus, haloperidol might have a gastric prokinetic effect.

Bio-availability 45–75% PO.[1]

Onset of action 10–15min SC; >1h PO.

Time to peak plasma concentration 2–6h PO; 10–20min SC.

Plasma halflife 13–35h.

Duration of action up to 24h, sometimes longer.

Cautions

Increased mortality in patients with dementia. Where possible, avoid. Where necessary, use the lowest effective dose for the shortest possible duration; also see stroke risk (p.153) and use for challenging behaviours in dementia (p.156).

Haloperidol can cause potentially fatal prolongation of the QT interval and *torsade de pointes*, particularly if given IV (off-label route) or at higher-than-recommended doses. Caution is required if any formulation of haloperidol is given to patients with an underlying predisposition, e.g. those with cardiac abnormalities, hypothyroidism, familial long QT syndrome, electrolyte imbalance (particularly hypokalaemia or hypomagnesaemia), or taking drugs which prolong the QT interval (see Prolongation of the QT interval in palliative care, p.727). If IV haloperidol is essential, ECG monitoring during administration is recommended.[13,14]

Parkinson's disease; epilepsy (lowered seizure threshold).[15]

Drug interactions

Potentiation of CNS depression caused by other CNS depressants, e.g. anxiolytics, alcohol. Increased risk of extrapyramidal effects and possible neurotoxicity with **lithium**. Plasma concentration of haloperidol is approximately halved by concurrent use of **carbamazepine**.

Undesirable effects

Extrapyramidal effects (see p.745), hypothermia, sedation, hypotension, endocrine effects, blood disorders, altered LFTs, neuroleptic (antipsychotic) malignant syndrome (see p.155).

Dose and use

Haloperidol exacerbates Parkinson's disease: use alternatives where possible (see p.154).

As a general rule, the dose of haloperidol is halved when switching from PO to SC. For CSCI dilute with WFI, or 5% glucose. High concentrations of haloperidol (approaching 2mg/mL after mixing) are incompatible if diluted with 0.9% saline (see p.667).

CSCI compatibility with other drugs: There are 2-drug compatibility data for haloperidol in WFI with **alfentanil**, **clonazepam**, **cyclizine**, **hyoscine *butylbromide***, **hyoscine *hydrobromide***, **midazolam** and **oxycodone**.

Haloperidol is *incompatibile* with **ketorolac**. Concentration-dependent *incompatibility* occurs with **dexamethasone**, **diamorphine**, **hydromorphone** and **morphine sulphate**. For more details and 3-drug compatibility data, see Appendix 3 charts and tables (p.773).

Compatibility charts for mixing drugs in 0.9% saline can be found on www.palliativedrugs.com Syringe Driver Survey Database.

Anti-emetic

For chemical/toxic causes of vomiting, including **morphine**-induced vomiting:

- start with 500microgram–1.5mg PO stat & at bedtime
- typical maintenance dose 1.5–3mg at bedtime (or 500microgram–1.5mg b.d.)
- if necessary, increase the total daily dose progressively to 5–10mg
- if 10mg at bedtime (or 5mg b.d.) is ineffective, review the cause of the vomiting; consider switching to **levomepromazine** (see p.164).

Delirium

If possible, correct underlying causes, and use non-drug measures (e.g. orientation strategies, correction of sensory deprivation).[16] When symptomatic drug treatment is required:

- patient distress mild–moderate and not an immediate danger to self or others:
  - ▹ start with 500microgram stat and q2h p.r.n.
  - ▹ if necessary, increase the dose progressively (e.g. →1mg→1.5mg etc.)[17]
- patient distress severe and/or an immediate danger to self or others:
  - ▹ start with 1.5–3mg stat, possibly combined with a benzodiazepine, and q2h p.r.n.
  - ▹ if necessary, increase the dose further, e.g. 5mg.

The maintenance dose is based on the initial cumulative dose needed to settle the patient; usual maximum ≤5mg/24h. Review daily, particularly if the underlying cause can be resolved. Other strategies include:

- prescribing a more sedating antipsychotic (e.g. **olanzapine** (see p.166), **quetiapine** (see p.171)) *or*
- the concurrent use of **trazadone** (see p.202) or a benzodiazepine (see p.132).

If necessary, seek advice from a psychogeriatrician. Note: for the management of terminal agitation, see p.272.

Behavioural problems in dementia

The management of delirium or psychosis should be distinguished from the long-term treatment of behavioural disturbance in dementia. Antipsychotics are generally not indicated in the latter (see p.156). Training in the non-drug management of behavioural disturbances reduces the need for psychotropic medication; medication is a last resort.[18] When used, dose reduction should be attempted every 2–3 months; many patients do not deteriorate when medication is withdrawn.[19–21]

Intractable hiccup

Haloperidol is generally used only when sequential therapeutic trials of **metoclopramide** (see p.227) ± an anti-foaming agent (see p.3) and **baclofen** (see p.563) have both failed (see Table 1.4, p.21):

- give haloperidol 1.5mg PO t.d.s.
- if no response, consider giving 5mg IV
- maintenance dose 1–3mg at bedtime.[22,23]

Another option is **gabapentin** (see p.251).[24]

Supply

Haloperidol (generic)
Tablets 500microgram, 1.5mg, 5mg, 10mg, 20mg, 28 days @ 5mg at bedtime = £2.
Injection 5mg/mL, 1mL amp = £0.50.

Dozic® (Rosemont)
Oral liquid (sugar-free) 1mg/mL, 28 days @ 5mg at bedtime = £10.

Haldol® (Janssen-Cilag)
Tablets 5mg, 10mg, 28 days @ 5mg at bedtime = £2.
Oral liquid (sugar-free) 2mg/mL, 28 days @ 5mg (2.5mL) at bedtime = £3.
Injection 5mg/mL, 1mL amp = £0.50.

Serenace® (Ivax)
Capsules 500microgram, 28 days @ 5mg at bedtime = £9.
Tablets 1.5mg, 5mg, 10mg, 28 days @ 5mg at bedtime = £3.50.
Oral liquid (sugar-free) 2mg/mL, 28 days @ 5mg (2.5mL) at bedtime = £5.

---

1 Vella-Brincat J and Macleod AD (2004) Haloperidol in palliative care. *Palliative Medicine*. **18**: 195–201.
2 de Leon J (2005) Benztropine equivalents for antimuscarinic medication. *American Journal of Psychiatry*. **162**: 627.
3 Wirshing D *et al.* (1999) Novel antipsychotics: comparison of weight gain liabilities. *Journal of Clinical Psychiatry*. **60**: 358–363.
4 Buttner M *et al.* (2004) Is low-dose haloperidol a useful antiemetic?: A meta-analysis of published and unpublished randomized trials. *Anesthesiology*. **101**: 1454–1463.
5 Hardy JR *et al.* (2010) The efficacy of haloperidol in the management of nausea and vomiting in patients with cancer. *Journal of Pain and Symptom Management*. **40**: 111–116.
6 Bentley A and Boyd K (2001) Use of clinical pictures in the management of nausea and vomiting: a prospective audit. *Palliative Medicine*. **15**: 247–253.
7 Stephenson J and Davies A (2006) An assessment of aetiology-based guidelines for the management of nausea and vomiting in patients with advanced cancer. *Supportive Care in Cancer*. **14**: 348–353.
8 Stoll BA (1962) Radiation sickness. *British Medical Journal*. **2**: 507–510.
9 Perkins P and Dorman S (2009) Haloperidol for the treatment of nausea and vomiting in palliative care patients. *Cochrane Database of Systematic Reviews*. **2**: CD006271.
10 Ventafridda V *et al.* (1990) The management of inoperable gastrointestinal obstruction in terminal cancer patients. *Tumori*. **76**: 389–393.
11 Mercadante S (1995) Bowel obstruction in home-care cancer patients: 4 years experience. *Supportive Care in Cancer*. **3**: 190–193.
12 Sanger G (1993) The pharmacology of anti-emetic agents. In: P Andrews and G Sanger (eds) *Emesis in anti-cancer therapy: mechanisms and treatment*. Chapman and Hall, London, pp. 179–210.
13 FDA (2007) Information for healthcare professionals. Haloperidol (marketed as Haldol, Haldol decanoate and Haldol lactate). Food and Drugs Administration. Available from: www.fda.gov/Drugs/DrugSafety/PostmarketDrugSafetyInformationforPatientsandProviders/DrugSafetyInformationforHeathcareProfessionals/ucm085203.htm
14 Canadian Pharmacists Association (2009) Haloperidol. Compendium of pharmaceuticals and specialities (eCPS). Available from: www.pharmacists.ca/content/products/ecps_english.cfm
15 Hedges D *et al.* (2003) Antipsychotic medication and seizures: a review. *Drugs Today (Barc)*. **39**: 551–557.
16 Twycross R *et al.* (2009) *Symptom Management in Advanced Cancer* (4e). palliativedrugs.com, Nottingham, pp. 207–211.
17 British Geriatrics Society and Royal College of Physicians (2006) The prevention, diagnosis and management of delirium in older people. National Guidelines. Available from: http://bookshop.rcplondon.ac.uk/details.aspx?e = 142
18 Fossey J *et al.* (2006) Effect of enhanced psychosocial care on antipsychotic use in nursing home residents with severe dementia: cluster randomised trial. *British Medical Journal*. **332**: 756–761.
19 Howard R *et al.* (2001) Guidelines for the management of agitation in dementia. *International Journal of Geriatric Psychiatry*. **16**: 714–717.
20 Lee PE *et al.* (2004) Atypical antipsychotic drugs in the treatment of behavioural and psychological symptoms of dementia: systematic review. *British Medical Journal*. **329**: 75.
21 Sink KM *et al.* (2005) Pharmacological treatment of neuropsychiatric symptoms of dementia: a review of the evidence. *Journal of the American Medical Association*. **293**: 596–608.
22 Ives TJ *et al.* (1985) Treatment of intractable hiccups with intramuscular haloperidol. *American Journal of Psychiatry*. **142**: 1368–1369.
23 Scarnati RA (1979) Intractable hiccup (singultus): report of case. *Journal of the American Osteopathic Association*. **79**: 127–129.
24 Twycross R *et al.* (2009) *Symptom Management in Advanced Cancer* (4e). palliativedrugs.com, Nottingham, pp. 174–177.

PROCHLORPERAZINE **BNF 4.2.1**

Class: Phenothiazine antipsychotic, anti-emetic.

Indications: Nausea and vomiting, †vertigo in labyrinthine disorders.

Contra-indications: bone marrow depression.

Pharmacology

Prochlorperazine is a D_2, $5HT_2$, H_1, α_1 and ACh_M antagonist. It has been a popular anti-emetic for many years, particularly for nausea and vomiting caused by chemical stimulation of the chemoreceptor zone. It is too irritant for SC administration, but a buccal formulation is a convenient alternative for patients at home. Although not recommended for motion sickness, prochlorperazine is used for the short-term relief of vertigo in Meniere's disease.

Oral bio-availability is low because of high first-pass hepatic metabolism.[1] Buccal prochlorperazine is about 2.5 times more bio-available and the variance is much less. Prochlorperazine is rapidly metabolized via eight isoforms of cytochrome P450; most extensively by CYP3A4, 2C19 and 2D6.[2,3] The multiple metabolic pathways suggest that clinically important drug interactions are unlikely. Undesirable effects are generally less severe than with **chlorpromazine** but, like all antipsychotics, there is still a risk of extrapyramidal effects.[4]

Bio-availability 6% PO, 14% buccal.[3]

Onset of action 30–40min PO, 10–20min IM, 1h PR.

Time to peak plasma concentration 4h PO, 8h buccal; 4h buccal when given regularly.[3]

Plasma halflife 15–20h.[3]

Duration of action 6–8h PO, PR (possibly longer when taken regularly); 12h buccal, IM.[3,5]

Cautions

Increased mortality in patients with dementia. Where possible, avoid. Where necessary, use the lowest effective dose for the shortest possible duration; also see stroke risk (p.153) and use for challenging behaviours in dementia (p.156).

Epilepsy, hepatic impairment, severe renal impairment.

Drug Interactions

Extrapyramidal effects and neurotoxicity have occurred when given concurrently with **lithium**.[6] Prochlorperazine increases the plasma concentration of **phenytoin** (mechanism unknown); if given concurrently, **phenytoin** levels must be monitored.

Undesirable effects

Very common (>10%): antimuscarinic effects (see p.5).

Frequency not stated: photosensitivity, slate-grey skin pigmentation, extrapyramidal reactions (see p.745), parkinsonism, drowsiness, confusion, paradoxical psychotic behaviour and agitation, seizures, neuroleptic malignant syndrome (see p.155), postural hypotension, blood dyscrasias.

Dose and use

Prochlorperazine is a potent irritant. Avoid direct contact of the oral solution or injection with the skin; do not give by CSCI.

Because of the risk of photosensitivity, patients should be advised to use high-factor (25–30) sun screen cream and a wide-brimmed hat if going outdoors in sunny weather.

Anti-emetic

Recommended maximum 40mg/24h (except for PR route; not UK):

- 3–6mg buccally b.d. *or*
- 5–10mg PO t.d.s.–q.d.s. *or*
- 5–10mg IM q3h–q4h *or*
- 2.5–10mg IV q3h–q4h p.r.n.

- 10mg PR t.d.s.–q.d.s. (not UK).

Labyrinthine disorders

The following regimen is sometimes used:

- start with 5mg PO t.d.s.
- if necessary, increase to 10mg t.d.s.
- reduce gradually to 5mg once daily–b.d. after several weeks.

Supply

Prochlorperazine (generic)
Tablets *(as maleate)* 5mg, 28 days @ 5mg q.d.s. = £3.
Injection *(as mesilate)* 12.5mg/mL, 1mL amp = £0.50.

Stemetil® (Sanofi-Aventis)
Tablets *(as maleate)* 5mg, 28 days @ 5mg q.d.s. = £3.
Oral liquid (syrup) *(as mesilate)* 5mg/5mL, 28 days @ 5mg q.d.s. = £19.
Injection *(as mesilate)* 12.5mg/mL, 1mL amp = £0.50.

Buccastem® (Alliance)
Tablets (buccal) 3mg, 28 days @ 3mg b.d. = £7; *place tablet high between upper lip and gum and leave to dissolve.*

1 Taylor WB and Bateman DN (1987) Preliminary studies of the pharmacokinetics and pharmacodynamics of prochlorperazine in healthy volunteers. *British Journal of Clinical Pharmacology.* **23**: 137–142.
2 Collins JM *et al.* (2004) In-vitro characterization of the metabolism of prochlorperazine. *Clinical Pharmacology and Therapeutics.* **75**: 85.
3 Finn A *et al.* (2005) Bioavailability and metabolism of prochlorperazine administered via the buccal and oral delivery route. *Journal of Clinical Pharmacology.* **45**: 1383–1390.
4 Kawanishi C *et al.* (2007) Unexpectedly high prevalence of akathisia in cancer patients. *Palliative and Supportive Care.* **5**: 351–354.
5 Lacy C *et al.* (eds) (2003) *Lexi-Comp's Drug Information Handbook* (11e). Lexi-Comp and the American Pharmaceutical Association, Hudson, Ohio.
6 Baxter K (2011) Stockley's Drug Interactions (online edition). Pharmaceutical Press, London. Available from: www.medicinescomplete.com

LEVOMEPROMAZINE **BNF 4.2.1**

Class: Phenothiazine antipsychotic, anti-emetic.

Indications: Acute psychotic symptoms, schizophrenia, pain and accompanying distress in the terminally ill, †agitation, †nausea and vomiting.

Pharmacology

Levomepromazine is a D_2, $5HT_{2A}$, α_1- and α_2-adrenergic, H_1 and muscarinic antagonist.[1] It is structurally and functionally similar to **chlorpromazine**, but is more widely used in palliative care, in part because it can be administered SC/CSCI.

The main uses of levomepromazine in palliative care reflect its sedative antipsychotic (i.e. terminal agitation ± delirium) and 'broad spectrum' anti-emetic effects (i.e. nausea and vomiting, see p.219).[2–5] Although traditionally used as a second- or third-line agent in these circumstances, it can be used first-line (unless a prokinetic anti-emetic, e.g. **metoclopramide**, see p.227, is indicated). Doses ⩾25mg/24h tend to cause drowsiness, and also postural hypotension. **Olanzapine** (see p.166) is an alternative broad-spectrum anti-emetic for those unable to tolerate levomepromazine.

Although licensed for pain and accompanying distress in the terminally ill, the evidence on which this is based is relatively limited, involved higher doses (e.g. 25mg by injection) and sedation was common.[6–11] Thus, other adjuvant analgesics which have more supporting evidence and are better tolerated should generally be used in preference. Any such use of levompromazine should be in conjunction with specialist palliative care or pain teams, and will probably be reserved for use alongside other analgesics, e.g. opioids, in patients in severe pain, at the end of life, when sedation is acceptable and when all usual options have been exhausted, or are inappropriate.

Levomepromazine is metabolized by sulphoxidation, N-demethylation and 3- and 7-hydroxylation.[12,13]
Bio-availability 20–40% PO.[14]
Onset of action 30min.
Time to peak plasma concentration 2–3h PO; 30–90min SC.
Plasma halflife 15–30h, sometimes longer.[15]
Duration of action 12–24h.

Cautions

Antipsychotics increase mortality in patients with dementia. Where possible, avoid. Where necessary, use the lowest effective dose for the shortest possible duration; also see stroke risk (p.153) and use for challenging behaviours in dementia (p.156).

Parkinsonism, postural hypotension, antihypertensive medication, epilepsy (lowered seizure threshold), hypothyroidism, myasthenia gravis.

Undesirable effects

Drowsiness, postural hypotension, antimuscarinic effects (see p.5).

Dose and use

When long term (>months) use is anticipated, consider monitoring weight, glucose and lipids at baseline and 3-monthly thereafter.

Levomepromazine is often given by CSCI. To reduce the likelihood of inflammatory reactions at the skin infusion site, dilute to the largest practical volume and consider the use of 0.9% saline as the diluent (see p.667). However, given its long plasma halflife, most patients can be maintained satisfactorily on intermittent injections, 1–3 times/24h.

Terminal agitation ± delirium

Generally given only when a reduced level of consciousness is acceptable:
- 6.25mg SC stat, and q1h p.r.n. together with 12.5–25mg/24h in divided doses SC or by CSCI
- higher starting doses may be required when terminal agitation is severe, e.g. 25–50mg SC stat, together with 50–75mg/24h CSCI
- if necessary, guided by response and frequency of p.r.n. use, progressively increase both p.r.n. and background dose (typically 50–100mg/24h)
- uncommon to need >300mg/24h.[16,17]

Anti-emetic

- start with 6–6.25mg PO/SC stat, at bedtime & p.r.n. (use a 6mg tablet or quarter a 25mg tablet)
- some centres report benefit with even lower starting doses, e.g. 2.5–5mg PO/SC.[18,19]
- if necessary, progressively increase to 12.5–25mg b.d.

Drowsiness generally limits dose titration. In these circumstances consider either switching to **olanzapine** (see p.166) or reducing the dose and combining with an anti-emetic of a different profile of action (e.g. **ondansetron**; see Table 4.19, p.222).

Analgesic

Seek advice from specialist palliative care or pain teams before such use (see Pharmacology):
- stat dose 25mg PO/SC and at bedtime
- titrate dose according to response; usual maximum daily dose 100mg SC/200mg PO.

CSCI compatibility with other drugs: There are 2-drug compatibility data for levomepromazine in 0.9% saline with **diamorphine**, **ketamine** and **oxycodone**.

Incompatibility may occur with **dexamethasone**, **ketorolac**, or **octreotide**. More details, 2 drug and 3-drug compatibility charts can be found on www.palliativedrugs.com Syringe Driver Survey Database.

For compatibility charts for mixing drugs in WFI see Appendix 3 (p.773).

Supply

Nozinan® (Sanofi-Aventis)

Tablets 25mg (scored), 28 days @ 12.5mg at bedtime = £3.50.

Tablets 6mg, 28 days @ 12mg at bedtime = £11. (Unlicensed, available as a named patient supply from United Drugs Group (UDG); see Obtaining unlicensed drugs, p.769.) Cost of a 6mg tablet is £0.19, the equivalent cost of one quarter of a 25mg tablet is £0.06.

Injection 25mg/mL, 1mL amp = £2.

1 Lal S *et al.* (1993) Levomepromazine receptor binding profile in human brain–implications for treatment-resistant schizophrenia. *Acta Psychiatrica Scandinavica.* **87**: 380–383.
2 Kennett A *et al.* (2004) An open study of methotrimeprazine in the management of nausea and vomiting in patients with advanced cancer. *Supportive Care in Cancer.* **13**: 715–721.
3 Eisenchlas JH *et al.* (2005) Low-dose levomepromazine in refractory emesis in advanced cancer patients: an open-label study. *Palliative Medicine.* **19**: 71–75.
4 Twycross RG *et al.* (1997) The use of low dose levomepromazine (methotrimeprazine) in the management of nausea and vomiting. *Progress in Palliative Care.* **5**: 49–53.
5 Higi M *et al.* (1980) Pronounced anti-emetic activity of the antipsychotic drug levomepromazine (methotrimeprazine) in patients receiving cancer chemotherapy. *Journal of Cancer Research and Clinical Oncology.* **97**: 81–86.
6 Bellens J *et al.* (1981) Analgesic treatment with levopromazine (Nozinan) and methadone in patients with acute myocardial infarction. *Ugeskrift nand Laeger.* **143**: 1313–1316.
7 Davidsen O *et al.* (1979) Analgesic treatment with levomepromazine in acute myocardial infarction: A randomized clinical trial. *Acta Medica Scandinavica.* **205**: 191–195.
8 Minuck H (1972) Postoperative analgesia—comparison of methotrimeprazine and meperidine as postoperative analgesic agents. *Canadian Anesthetists Society Journal.* **19**: 87–96.
9 Beaver W *et al.* (1966) A comparison of the analgesic effects of methotrimeprazine and morphine in patients with cancer. *Clinical Pharmacology and Therapeutics.* **5**: 436–446.
10 Bloomfield S *et al.* (1964) Comparative analgesic activity of levomepromazine and morphine in patients with chronic pain. *Canadian Medical Association Journal.* **40**: 1156–1162.
11 Montilla E *et al.* (1963) Analgesic effect of methotrimeprazine and morphine: a clinical comparison. *Archives of Internal Medicine.* **111**: 725–731.
12 Dahl SG and Garle M (1977) Identification of nonpolar methotrimeprazine metabolites in plasma and urine by GLC-mass spectrometry. *Journal of Pharmaceutical Science.* **66**: 190–193.
13 Dahl SG *et al.* (1987) Nuclear magnetic resonance analysis of methotrimeprazine (levomepromazine) hydroxylation in humans. *Journal of Pharmceutical Science.* **76**: 541–544.
14 Bagli M *et al.* (1995) Bioequivalence and absolute bioavailability of oblong and coated levomepromazine tablets in CYP2D6 phenotyped subjects. *International Journal of Clinical Pharmacology and Therapeutics.* **33**: 646–652.
15 Dahl SG *et al.* (1977) Pharmacokinetics and relative bioavailability of levomepromazine after repeated administration of tablets and syrup. *European Journal of Clinical Pharmacology.* **11**: 305–310.
16 Johnson I and Patterson S (1992) Drugs used in combination in the syringe driver: a survey of hospice practice. *Palliative Medicine.* **6**: 125–130.
17 Regnard C and Tempest S (eds) (1998) *A Guide to Symptom Relief in Advanced Disease* (4e). Hochland and Hochland, Manchester.
18 Various authors (2006) The use of s/c levomepromazine as an antiemetic and for terminal agitation. Palliativedrugs.com bulletin board thread. Available from: www.palliativedrugs.com/forum51/read.php?1,10264,10778#msg-10778
19 Zylicz Z (2010) Olanzapine for nausea, insomnia, anorexia, anxiety. Palliativedrugs.com bulletin board thread. Available from: www.palliativedrugs.com/forum51/read.php?1,16506,16536#msg-16536

OLANZAPINE — BNF 4.2.1

Class: Atypical antipsychotic.

Indications: Acute psychotic symptoms, mania and bipolar disorders, schizophrenia, †agitation, †delirium, †nausea and vomiting, †treatment-resistant depression.

Pharmacology

Olanzapine is a potent D_1, D_2, D_3, D_4, $5HT_{2A}$, $5HT_{2C}$, $5HT_3$ and $5HT_6$ antagonist.[1–4] It also binds to other receptors, including α_1-adrenergic, H_1 and muscarinic receptors.[5] Olanzapine is used primarily in schizophrenia and other psychoses.[6] In a non-randomized comparison of olanzapine with **haloperidol** in the treatment of delirium, once daily doses (at bedtime), adjusted according to response, were equally effective, with maximum benefit seen after 1 week.[7] Compared with **haloperidol**, olanzapine causes fewer drug-induced movement disorders, including tardive dyskinesia,[8] but dose-related weight gain is more common (40% vs. 12%).[9] Weight gain is greater than with **risperidone**.[10] It is metabolized in the liver by glucuronidation and, to a lesser extent, oxidation via the cytochrome P450 system (see p.735), primarily via CYP1A2 with a minor contribution via CYP2D6. The major metabolite is the 10-N-glucuronide which does not pass the blood-brain barrier. Elimination of metabolites is both renal (60%) and faecal (30%).[11] Clearance varies 4 times among patients.[2,8]

Not surprisingly, given its receptor site affinities, olanzapine is a potent anti-emetic.[3,4,12] This has been confirmed in Phase 1 and Phase 2 trials in cancer patients receiving either moderately or highly emetogenic chemotherapy.[13,14] Benefit is reported in paraneoplastic sweating.[15]

Bio-availability 60%, sometimes >80% PO.

Onset of action hours–days in delirium; days–weeks in psychoses.

Time to peak plasma concentration 5–8h, not affected by food.

Plasma halflife 34h; 52h in the elderly; shorter in smokers; unchanged in hepatic and renal impairment.

Duration of action 12–48h, situation dependent.

Cautions

Increased mortality in patients with dementia. Where possible, avoid. Where necessary, use the lowest effective dose for the shortest possible duration; also see stroke risk (p.153) and use for challenging behaviours in dementia (p.156).

Injections: fatalities from oversedation or cardiorespiratory depression have occurred after higher than approved doses or *concurrent use with benzodiazepines*. Monitor blood pressure, heart rate, respiratory rate and level of consciousness for at least 4h after IM olanzapine, and do not give parenteral benzodiazepines within 1h of IM olanzapine.

Elderly patients and those with renal or hepatic impairment. Parkinson's disease (exacerbation). Epilepsy (lowers seizure threshold).[16] May cause or adversely affect diabetes mellitus; rare reports of keto-acidosis. Olanzapine potentiates the sedative effects of alcohol and other CNS depressants.

Drug interactions

Omeprazole, **carbamazepine**, **rifampicin** and tobacco exposure stimulate CYP1A2 and decrease the plasma concentration of olanzapine; in contrast, **fluvoxamine**, an inhibitor of CYP1A2, increases the plasma concentration.

Undesirable effects

Common (<10%, >1%): drowsiness, weight gain.

Uncommon (<1%, >0.1%): dry mouth, constipation, orthostatic hypotension,[17–19] agitation, nervousness, dizziness, peripheral oedema.

The incidence and severity of drug-induced movement disorders are significantly less than with **haloperidol**.[8,20] Acute disorders are generally mild and are reversible if the dose is reduced and/or an antimuscarinic antiparkinsonian drug prescribed.

Dose and use

When long term (>months) use is anticipated, consider monitoring weight, glucose and lipids at baseline and 3-monthly thereafter.

Subcutaneous use of parenteral olanzapine is reported without evidence of site reactions.[21]

Psychosis or mania

- Start with 10–15mg at bedtime
- if necessary, increase to 20mg at bedtime.

Agitation and/or delirium

Used as an alternative to **haloperidol**:

- start with 2.5mg PO/SC stat, p.r.n. & at bedtime
- if necessary, increase to 5–10mg at bedtime.[22,23]

Anti-emetic

- start with 1.25–2.5mg PO/SC stat, q2h p.r.n. & at bedtime
- if necessary, increase to 5mg at bedtime, occasionally to 5mg b.d.[3,4]

Orodispersible tablets are placed on the tongue and allowed to dissolve or dispersed in water, orange juice, apple juice, milk or coffee immediately before administration.

Supply

Zyprexa® (Lilly)

Tablets 2.5mg, 5mg, 7.5mg, 10mg, 15mg, 20mg, 28 days @ 5mg at bedtime = £44.

Tablets orodispersible (Velotab®) 5mg, 10mg, 15mg, 20mg, 28 days @ 5mg at bedtime = £48; *place on the tongue and allow to dissolve, or disperse in water, orange juice, apple juice, milk or coffee.*

Injection (powder for reconstitution) 5mg/mL, 10mg vial = £3.50. (Withdrawn from UK market September 2012.)

1 Hale AS (1997) Olanzapine. *British Journal of Hospital Medicine.* **58**: 442–445.
2 Stephenson C and Pilowsky L (1999) Psychopharmacology of olanzapine. A review. *British Journal of Psychiatry Supplement.* **38**: 52–58.
3 Passik SD *et al.* (2002) A pilot exploration of the antiemetic activity of olanzapine for the relief of nausea in patients with advanced cancer and pain. *Journal of Pain and Symptom Management.* **23**: 526–532.
4 Srivastava M *et al.* (2003) Olanzapine as an antiemetic in refractory nausea and vomiting in advanced cancer. *Journal of Pain and Symptom Management.* **25**: 578–582.
5 Raedler T *et al.* (2000) In vivo olanzapine occupancy of muscarinic acetylcholine receptors in patients with schizophrenia. *Neuropsychopharmacology.* **23**: 56–68.
6 Fulton B and Goa K (1997) Olanzapine. A review of phamarcological properties and therapeutic efficacy in the management of schizophrenia and related psychoses. *Drugs.* **53**: 281–297.
7 Sipahimalani A and Masand P (1998) Olanzapine in the treatment of delirium. *Psychosomatics.* **39**: 422–430.
8 Beasley C *et al.* (1997) Efficacy of olanzapine: an overview of pivotal clinical trials. *Journal of Clinical Psychiatry.* **58 (suppl 10)**: 7–12.
9 Eli Lilly Company (2001) *Olanzapine. Clinical and laboratory experience. A comprehensive monograph.* Dextra Court, Basinstoke.
10 Wirshing D *et al.* (1999) Novel antipsychotics: comparison of weight gain liabilities. *Journal of Clinical Psychiatry.* **60**: 358–363.
11 Callaghan J *et al.* (1999) Olanzapine. Pharmacokinetic and pharmacodynamic profile. *Clinical Pharmacokinetics.* **37**: 177–193.
12 Jackson WC and Tavernier L (2003) Olanzapine for intractable nausea in palliative care patients. *Journal of Palliative Medicine.* **6**: 251–255.
13 Passik SD *et al.* (2004) A phase I trial of olanzapine (Zyprexa) for the prevention of delayed emesis in cancer patients: a Hoosier Oncology Group study. *Cancer Investigation.* **22**: 383–388.
14 Navari RM *et al.* (2005) A phase II trial of olanzapine for the prevention of chemotherapy-induced nausea and vomiting: a Hoosier Oncology Group study. *Supportive Care in Cancer.* **13**: 529–534.
15 Zylicz Z and Krajnik M (2003) Flushing and sweating in an advanced breast cancer patient relieved by olanzapine. *Journal of Pain and Symptom Management.* **25**: 494–495.
16 Hedges D *et al.* (2003) Antipsychotic medication and seizures: a review. *Drugs Today (Barc).* **39**: 551–557.
17 Tollefson G *et al.* (1997) Olanzapine versus haloperidol in the treatment of schizophrenia and schizoaffective and schizophreniform disorders: results of an international collaborative trial. *American Journal of Psychiatry.* **154**: 457–465.
18 Conley R and Meltzer H (2000) Adverse events related to olanzapine. *Journal of Clinical Psychiatry.* **61**: 26–29.
19 Worrel J *et al.* (2000) Atypical antipsychotic agents: a critical review. *American Journal of Health-System Pharmacy.* **57**: 238–358.
20 Geddes J *et al.* (2000) Atypical antipsychotics in the treatment of schizophrenia: systematic overview and meta-regression analysis. *British Medical Journal.* **321**: 1371–1376.
21 Elsayem (2010) Subcutaneous olanzapine for hyperactive or mixed delirium in patients with advanced cancer: a preliminary study. *Journal of Pain and Symptom Management.* **40**: 774–782.
22 Passik S and Cooper M (1999) Complicated delirium in a cancer patient successfully treated with olanzapine. *Journal of Pain and Symptom Management.* **17**: 191–223.
23 Meehan K *et al.* (2002) Comparison of rapidly acting intramuscular olanzapine, lorazepam, and placebo: A double-blind, randomized study in acutely agitated patients with dementia. *Neuropsychopharmacology.* **26**: 494–504.

RISPERIDONE — BNF 4.2.1

Class: Atypical antipsychotic.

Indications: Acute psychotic symptoms, mania and bipolar disorders, schizophrenia, †agitation, †delirium.

Pharmacology

Risperidone is a potent D_2 and $5HT_{2A}$ antagonist.[1] It also binds to α_1-adrenergic receptors and with lower affinity to H_1- and α_2-receptors. Unlike **olanzapine**, risperidone does *not* bind to muscarinic receptors. The incidence of drug-induced movement disorders is less than with

haloperidol and phenothiazines but greater than with more sedating atypical antipsychotics (e.g. **olanzapine**, **quetiapine**; see p.154). A retrospective survey reported that >25% of patients developed akathisia or parkinsonism.[2]

In delirium, hallucinations respond to risperidone within hours but generally only after 1–2 weeks in a psychotic illness; this is true of all antipsychotics.

The major metabolite of risperidone is 9-hydroxyrisperidone. This hydroxylation is subject to **debrisoquine**-type genetic CYP2D6-related polymorphism but, because both risperidone and its major metabolite are equally active, the efficacy of risperidone is unaffected.[3] Risperidone is more slowly eliminated in the elderly and in patients with renal impairment. Doses of risperidone should be decreased in patients with hepatic impairment because the mean free fraction of risperidone is increased by up to 35% as a result of decreased levels of albumin and α_1-acid glycoprotein.[4]

Risperidone is as effective as **haloperidol** in treating delirium.[5] Its efficacy as an anti-emetic has not been fully evaluated but, theoretically, it could be better than **haloperidol** because of its antagonism of $5HT_2$-receptors (see **levomepromazine**, p.164). A retrospective review of 20 cancer patients given risperidone 1mg at bedtime for refractory opioid-induced nausea and vomiting reported complete resolution of nausea in half and a partial response in the other half, with cessation of vomiting in two thirds.[6]

Risperidone can cause a weight gain of several kg particularly over the first 2 months; this is generally less than with other atypical antipsychotics but may be more marked if it is given together with **valproate** or **lithium**.[2,7]

Bio-availability 99%.
Time to peak plasma concentration 1–2h, not affected by food.
Onset of action hours–days in delirium; days–weeks in psychoses.
Plasma halflife of active fraction (risperidone +9-hydroxyrisperidone) 24h.
Duration of action 12–48h, situation dependent.

Cautions

Increased mortality in patients with dementia. Where possible, avoid. Where necessary, use the lowest effective dose for the shortest possible duration; also see stroke risk (p.153) and use for challenging behaviours in dementia (p.156).

Elderly patients and those with renal or hepatic impairment.[4] Can cause orthostatic hypotension, particularly initially, because of α-adrenergic receptor antagonism. Parkinson's disease (deterioration). Epilepsy (lowers seizure threshold, although the risk is lower than with more sedating atypical antipsychotics).[8]

Drug interactions

Carbamazepine has been shown to decrease the combined plasma concentration of risperidone and 9-hydroxyrisperidone. A similar effect might be anticipated with other drugs which stimulate metabolizing enzymes in the liver. On initiation of **carbamazepine** or other hepatic enzyme-inducing drugs, the dose of risperidone should be re-evaluated and increased as necessary. Conversely, on discontinuation of such drugs, the dose of risperidone should be re-evaluated and decreased as necessary.

Phenothiazines, TCAs and some β-blockers may increase the plasma concentrations of risperidone but not the combined concentration of risperidone and its active metabolite. **Fluoxetine** may increase the plasma concentration of risperidone but the impact on the combined concentration is less. A dose reduction of risperidone should be considered when **fluoxetine** is added to risperidone therapy. Based on *in vitro* studies, the same interaction may occur with **haloperidol**.

Undesirable effects

Common (<10%, >1%): insomnia, agitation, anxiety, headache, movement disorders (see below), drowsiness, weight gain.

Uncommon (<1%, >0.1%): drowsiness, fatigue, dizziness, impaired concentration, seizures, blurred vision, syncope, dyspepsia, nausea and vomiting, constipation, sexual dysfunction (including priapism and erectile dysfunction), urinary incontinence, rhinitis.

The incidence and severity of drug-induced movement disorders are less than with **haloperidol**.[9–11] Acute disorders are generally mild and are reversible if the dose is reduced and/or an antimuscarinic antiparkinsonian drug prescribed (see Drug-induced movement disorders, p.745).

Dose and use

Despite being commonly given b.d. there is no advantage in dividing the total daily dose, which can conveniently be given at bedtime.[12] Doses above 10mg/24h generally do not provide added benefit and may increase the risk of drug-induced movement disorders.

Psychosis

An atypical antipsychotic should be used preferentially in chronic psychoses:
- start with 1mg b.d.
- if necessary, increase to 2mg b.d. and 3mg b.d. on successive days
- in elderly patients and those with severe hepatic or renal impairment, the starting dose should be halved to 500microgram b.d. (or 1mg once daily) and titration extended over 6 days.[13]

Delirium

- start with 500microgram b.d. & p.r.n.
- if necessary, increase by 500microgram b.d. every other day
- median maintenance dose is 1mg/24h
- uncommon to need >3mg/24h.[5]

Supply

Risperidone (generic)
Tablets 500microgram, 1mg, 2mg, 3mg, 4mg, 6mg, 28 days @ 500microgram b.d. = £3.
Tablets orodispersible 500microgram, 1mg, 2mg, 3mg, 4mg, 28 days @ 500microgram b.d. = £34; *tablets should be placed on the tongue, allowed to dissolve, then swallowed.*
Oral solution 1mg/mL, 28 days @ 500microgram b.d. = £16.

Risperdal® (Janssen-Cilag)
Tablets 500microgram, 1mg, 2mg, 3mg, 4mg, 6mg, 28 days @ 500microgram b.d. = £14.
Tablets orodispersible (Quicklet®) 500microgram, 1mg, 2mg, 3mg, 4mg, 28 days @ 500microgram b.d. = £16.
Oral solution 1mg/mL, 28 days @ 500microgram b.d. = £15; *may be diluted with any non-alcoholic drink except tea.*

1 Green B (2000) Focus on risperidone. *Current Medical Research and Opinion*. **16**: 57–65.
2 Guille C *et al.* (2000) A naturalistic comparison of clozapine, risperidone and olanzapine in the treatment of bipolar disorder. *Journal of Clinical Psychiatry*. **61**: 638–642.
3 Bork J *et al.* (1999) A pilot study on risperidone metabolism: the role of cytochromes P450 2D6 and 3A. *Journal of Clinical Psychiatry*. **60**: 469–476.
4 Snoecke E *et al.* (1995) Influence of age, renal and liver impairment on the pharmacokinetics of risperidone in man. *Psychopharmacology (Berl)*. **122**: 223–229.
5 Sipahimalani A *et al.* (1997) Treatment of delirium with risperidone. *International Journal of Geriatric Psychopharmacology*. **1**: 24–26.
6 Okamoto Y *et al.* (2007) A retrospective chart review of the antiemetic effectiveness of risperidone in refractory opioid-induced nausea and vomiting in advanced cancer patients. *Journal of Pain and Symptom Management*. **34**: 217–222.
7 Wirshing D *et al.* (1999) Risperidone in treatment-refractory schizophrenia. *American Journal of Psychiatry*. **156**: 1374–1379.
8 Hedges D *et al.* (2003) Antipsychotic medication and seizures: a review. *Drugs Today (Barc)*. **39**: 551–557.
9 Geddes J *et al.* (2000) Atypical antipsychotics in the treatment of schizophrenia: systematic overview and meta-regression analysis. *British Medical Journal*. **321**: 1371–1376.
10 Jeste D *et al.* (1999) Lower incidence of tardive dyskinesia with risperidone compared with haloperidol in older patients. *Journal of the American Geriatric Society*. **47**: 716–719.
11 Umbricht D and Kane J (1995) Risperidone: efficacy and safety. *Schizophrenia Bulletin*. **21**: 593–606.
12 Nair N (1998) Therapeutic equivalence of risperidone given once daily and twice daily in patients with schizophrenia. The Risperidone Study. *Journal of Clinical Psychopharmacology*. **18**: 10–110.
13 Luchins D *et al.* (1998) Alteration in the recommended dosing schedule for risperidone. *American Journal of Psychiatry*. **155**: 365–366.

QUETIAPINE **BNF 4.2.1**

Class: Atypical antipsychotic.

Indications: Acute psychotic symptoms, mania and bipolar disorders, schizophrenia, †agitation, †delirium, †treatment-resistant depression, †psychosis in those at risk of parkinsonism.[1]

Pharmacology

Quetiapine is a D_2, D_3, $5HT_{1A}$, $5HT_{2A}$ and $5HT_{2C}$ antagonist. It also binds to other receptors including α_1, α_2-adrenergic, H_1, and muscarinic receptors.[2,3] Quetiapine is used primarily in the treatment of schizophrenia and other psychoses. In off-label use for delirium, the efficacy and tolerability of atypical antipsychotics is comparable to **haloperidol**.[4]

It is rapidly absorbed after oral administration. Although not known precisely, bio-availability is at least 75% (the proportion of radio-labelled quetiapine excreted in urine).[5] Metabolism is predominantly by CYP3A4. The plasma concentration of active metabolites is $\leq$10% that of quetiapine and thus unlikely to contribute significantly to overall activity. Elimination is both renal (75%) and faecal (25%); <1% of quetiapine is excreted unchanged.[5]

Quetiapine and **clozapine** have the lowest risk of extrapyramidal effects of all the atypical antipsychotics (see p.745).[6] The haematological monitoring required for **clozapine** makes quetiapine the drug of choice when an antipsychotic is indicated in someone with Parkinson's disease (see p.154).[1] Quetiapine shares the undesirable metabolic effects, and the increased mortality in patients with dementia, of the other atypicals.[6,7] Compared with **olanzapine** and **risperidone**, it causes more antimuscarinic effects.[3] Like **olanzapine**, it is more sedating than **risperidone**.

Bio-availability $\geq$75%.[5]
Onset of action hours–days in delirium; 1–2 weeks in psychoses.
Time to peak plasma concentration 1.5h.
Plasma halflife 7h (10–14h in the elderly).
Duration of action 12h (although serotoninergic activity may persist for much longer).[5]

Cautions

Increased mortality in patients with dementia. Where possible, avoid. Where necessary, use the lowest effective dose for the shortest possible duration; also see stroke risk (p.153) and use for challenging behaviours in dementia (p.156).

Elderly patients and those with renal or hepatic impairment. Possibly an increased risk of neutropenia. May cause or adversely affect diabetes mellitus. Parkinson's disease (deterioration) but the risk is lower than for other atypicals (see p.154). Epilepsy (lowers seizure threshold).[8,9]

Drug interactions

Plasma quetiapine concentrations can be significantly increased by CYP3A4 inhibitors (e.g. azole antifungals, macrolide antibiotics) and reduced by enzyme inducers (e.g. **carbamazepine**, **phenytoin**).

Undesirable effects

Very common (>10%): drowsiness, dizziness.
Common (<10%, >1%): dry mouth, constipation, leukopenia, tachycardia, orthostatic hypotension, peripheral oedema, altered liver transaminases.

Dose and use

When long term (> months) use is anticipated, consider monitoring weight, glucose and lipids at baseline and 3-monthly thereafter.

Reduce starting dose and rate of titration in the elderly and those with renal or hepatic impairment or Parkinson's disease.

Delirium
- start with 12.5mg b.d.
- if necessary, increase in 12.5–25mg increments
- mean effective dose = 40–100mg/24h.[10–13]

Schizophrenia
- start with 25 mg b.d.
- increase to 50mg b.d. (day 2), 100mg b.d. (day 3), 150mg b.d. (day 4)
- then titrate according to response, up to 750mg/24h
- typical effective dose = 300–450mg/24h.

Bipolar mania
As monotherapy or as adjunct therapy to mood stabilizers:
- start with 50mg b.d.
- increase to 100mg b.d. (day 2), 150mg b.d. (day 3), 200mg b.d. (day 4)
- then titrate according to response, ≤200 mg/24h, up to 800mg/24h
- typical effective dose = 400–800mg/24h.

Supply
Seroquel® (AstraZeneca)
Tablets 25mg, 100mg, 150mg, 200mg, 300mg, 28 days @ 100mg b.d. = £106.

Modified-release
Seroquel XL® (AstraZeneca)
Tablets m/r 50mg, 150mg, 200mg, 300mg, 400mg, 28 days @ 200mg once daily = £53.

1 Weintraub D and Hurtig HI (2007) Presentation and management of psychosis in Parkinson's disease and dementia with Lewy bodies. *American Journal of Psychiatry.* **164**: 1491–1498.
2 NIMH (National Institute of Mental Health) (2006) National Institute of Mental Health's Psychoactive Drug Screening Program. University of North Carolina. Available from: http://pdsp.med.unc.edu/indexR.html
3 Lieberman JA *et al.* (2005) Effectiveness of antipsychotic drugs in patients with chronic schizophrenia. *New England Journal of Medicine.* **353**: 1209–1223.
4 Lonergan E *et al.* (2007) Antipsychotics for delirium. *Cochrane Database of Systematic Reviews.* CD005594.
5 DeVane CL and Nemeroff CB (2001) Clinical pharmacokinetics of quetiapine: an atypical antipsychotic. *Clinical Pharmacokinetics.* **40**: 509–522.
6 Haddad PM and Sharma SG (2007) Adverse effects of atypical antipsychotics: differential risk and clinical implications. *CNS Drugs.* **21**: 911–936.
7 Schneider LS *et al.* (2005) Risk of death with atypical antipsychotic drug treatment for dementia: meta-analysis of randomized placebo-controlled trials. *Journal of the American Medical Association.* **294**: 1934–1943.
8 Yalug I *et al.* (2007) Quetiapine may be associated with new-onset seizures in patients with seizurogenic conditions. *Journal of Neuropsychiatry and Clinical Neurosciences.* **19**: 341–342.
9 Hedges D *et al.* (2003) Antipsychotic medication and seizures: a review. *Drugs Today (Barc).* **39**: 551–557.
10 Tahir TA *et al.* (2010) A randomized controlled trial of quetiapine versus placebo in the treatment of delirium. *Journal of Psychosomatic Research.* **69**: 485–490.
11 Maneeton B *et al.* (2007) An open-label study of quetiapine for delirium. *Journal of the Medical Association of Thailand.* **90**: 2158–2163.
12 Kim KY *et al.* (2003) Treatment of delirium in older adults with quetiapine. *Journal of Geriatric Psychiatry and Neurology.* **16**: 29–31.
13 Lee KU *et al.* (2005) Amisulpride versus quetiapine for the treatment of delirium: a randomized, open prospective study. *International Clinical Psychopharmacology.* **20**: 311–314.

ANTIDEPRESSANTS — BNF 4.3

Indications: Depression, anxiety and panic disorders, stress incontinence and urgency, †neuropathic pain, †agitated delirium, †sweating, †hot flushes, †insomnia, †pruritus, †bladder spasm, †pathological laughing and crying, †drooling.

Pharmacology
Antidepressants enhance transmission of one or more mono-amines. This occurs within hours but beneficial effects are slower to appear because they require normalization of:
- receptor sensitivity *and*
- neuroplasticity.

In depression, mono-amine receptors are upregulated to compensate for a relative mono-amine deficit. Thus antidepressants initially enhance mono-amine transmission against upregulated receptors causing many of the early-onset undesirable effects. As receptor sensitivity returns to normal, these undesirable effects resolve and beneficial effects begin to emerge.

The limbic and prefrontal cortex circuits which regulate mood, attention, energy, appetite and sleep generally adapt structurally and functionally in response to external stimuli (neuroplasticity). This is impaired in depression and restored by antidepressants because mono-amines trigger the release of nerve growth factors (e.g. brain-derived neurotrophic factor).[1] Although these circuits overlap and interact, they do mediate distinct symptoms, and refractory depression may thus respond to a second-line antidepressant which influences a different mono-amine or multiple ones.[2,3]

The analgesic effect of antidepressants is due to enhancement of mono-amine transmission by the descending pain modulation pathway.[4,5] This pathway can induce both analgesia (noradrenergic and serotoninergic activity) and hyperalgesia (serotoninergic activity).[6,7] The latter may explain the inconsistent analgesic effect of SSRIs. Sodium-channel blockade and NMDA-glutamate-receptor antagonism may also contribute to the analgesic efficacy of some antidepressants,[5] including the modest effect of topical **doxepin**.[8,9]

Anxiolytics act on the amygdala's 'fear circuits'. The amygdala is a 'threat sensor' which integrates sensory information with contextual information (e.g. interpretations, memories). If a fear response is required, the amygdala's effector pathway activates the relevant circuits (respiratory and cardiovascular centres, pituitary-adrenal axis, sympathetic autonomic nervous system, and fear-related areas of the cerebral cortex). Antidepressants and benzodiazepines (see p.132) inhibit these 'fear circuits' through $5HT_{1A}$ and $GABA_A$ receptors respectively.[10,11]

The beneficial and undesirable effects of antidepressants vary because of differing:

- mechanisms of action (Figure 4.4)
- mono-amines affected (Box 4.E)
- effects on other receptors (Table 4.11)
- pharmacokinetic profiles (Table 4.12).

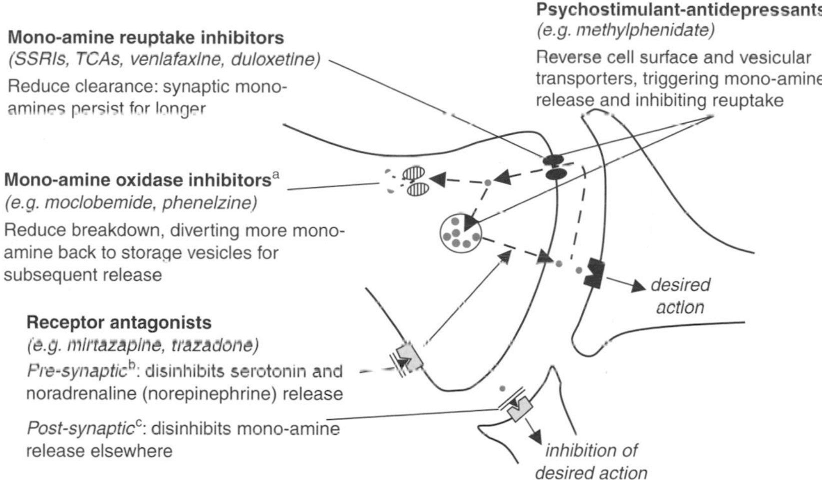

Figure 4.4 Predominant mechanism of action of antidepressants.

a. mono-amine oxidase type A breaks down serotonin, noradrenaline (norepinephrine) and dopamine. Type B breaks down dopamine. Antidepressant-MAOIs are either non-selective (e.g. phenelzine) or type A selective (e.g. moclobemide). Anti-parkinsonian MAOIs (e.g. selegiline) are Type B selective
b. blockade of pre-synaptic α-adrenergic receptors removes inhibition of serotonin and noradrenaline (norepinephrine) release
c. blockade of post-synaptic $5HT_{2A}$ and $5HT_{2C}$-receptors removes inhibition of dopamine and noradrenaline (norepinephrine) release from the post-synaptic neurone (see p.200).

Box 4.E Classification of antidepressants according to principal actions[a]

Mono-amine re-uptake inhibitors (MARIs)

Serotonin and noradrenaline (norepinephrine) (SNRIs[b] or dual inhibitors)

Amitriptyline[c], venlafaxine, duloxetine

Serotonin (selective serotonin re-uptake inhibitors, SSRIs)

Sertraline, citalopram, paroxetine, fluoxetine

Noradrenaline (norepinephrine) (NRIs)

Nortriptyline[c], lofepramine, desipramine[c], reboxetine

Noradrenaline (norepinephrine) and dopamine (NDRIs)

Bupropion

Psychostimulant-antidepressants[d]

Dexamfetamine, methylphenidate, modafinil

Receptor antagonists

Trazodone (α_1, $5HT_2$)

Mirtazapine (central α_2, $5HT_2$, $5HT_3$)

Mono-amine oxidase inhibitors (MAOIs)[e]

Phenelzine, tranylcypromine

a. abbreviated names broadly reflect those found elsewhere;[13] confusion is inevitable because S is used for *Selective*, *Specific*, and *Serotonin*

b. SNRI is sometimes reserved for dual inhibitors without additional receptor binding affinities (e.g. venlafaxine and duloxetine)

c. TCAs differ in their modes of action, and do not comprise a single discrete drug class

d. reverse dopamine re-uptake transporters

e. MAOIs are included for completeness; their use by non-psychiatrists is *not* recommended.

Table 4.11 Transporter and receptor affinities for selected antidepressants[14–16]

	Re-uptake Transporter			*Receptor affinity*					
	5HT	*NAdr*[a]	*DA*	$5HT_{2A}$	$5HT_{2C}$	H_1	α_1	α_2	ACh_M
Amitriptyline	+++	++	−	+++	+++	+++	+++	+	+++
Bupropion	−	+	++	−	−		−	−	−
Citalopram	+++	−	−	−	−	−	−	−	−
Desipramine	+	+++	−	+	−	++	++	−	+
Duloxetine	+++	+++	+	−	−	−	−	−	−
Fluoxetine	+++	−	−	+	+	−	−	−	−
Imipramine	+++	+	−	+	+	+++	++	−	+/+++[b]
Lofepramine	+	+++	−	−		+	+	−	−/++[b]
Methylphenidate	−	−	++	−	−		−	−	−
Mirtazapine	−	−	−	++	++	+++	−	+++	−
Nortriptyline	+	+++	−	+++	+++	+++	++	−	++
Paroxetine	+++	+	−	−	−	−	−	−	+
Reboxetine	−	+++	−	−	−		−	−	
Sertraline	+++	−	+	−	−	−	+	−	−
Trazadone	−	−	−	++	+	−	++	+	−
Venlafaxine	+	+[c]	−	−	−	−	−	−	−

Affinity: +++ high, ++ moderate, + low, − negligible or none; blank = no data.

a. the noradrenaline (norepinephrine) re-uptake transporter also clears dopamine in the prefrontal cortex where dopamine re-uptake transporters are absent. Reduced dopamine in the prefrontal cortex is related to anhedonia and inattention

b. varies with different ACh_m receptor subtypes

c. despite in vitro studies suggesting a relatively low affinity for serotonin and noradrenaline re-uptake transporters, in vivo studies suggest venlafaxine is a dual inhibitor. In vitro assays measure the ability of a drug to displace another compound of known affinity; it may be that venlafaxine binds to a different site on mono-amine re-uptake transporters and so cannot displace the reference compounds.[16]

Table 4.12 Pharmacokinetic details for selected antidepressants (also see individual drug monographs)[17–25]

Drug	*Bio-availability PO (%)*	T_{max} *(h)*	*Plasma halflife (h)*	*Metabolism*
Amitriptyline	45	4	13–36	Multiple pathways[a] (nortriptyline[a])
Bupropion	>87	1.5	21	CYP2B6[a]
Citalopram	80[c]	3	36	Multiple pathways[a]
Desipramine	30–50	4–6	7–77	CYP2D6[a,e]
Duloxetine	90	6	12	CYP1A2, CYP2D6
Fluoxetine	90	4–8	1–4 days 7–15 days[a]	Multiple pathways[a]
Imipramine	45	3	21	Multiple pathways[a] (desipramine[a])
Methylphenidate	30	1–3	2	Non-CYP hepatic carboxylesterase[e]
Mirtazapine	50	2	20–40	CYP1A2, CYP2D6, CYP3A4
Nortriptyline	60	7–8.5	15–39	CYP2D6[a,e]
Paroxetine	50[d]	5	15–20	Multiple pathways
Reboxetine	95	2–4	12	CYP3A4
Sertraline	>44	6–8	26	CYP3A4
Trazadone	65	1	7	CYP2D6, CYP3A4[a]
Venlafaxine	13 45[b]	2.5 4.5–7.5[b]	5 11[a]	CYP2D6, CYP3A4[a]

a. active metabolite(s); listed in table if can be administered separately
b. m/r product
c. tablet product: bio-availability of drops 25% higher
d. increases with multiple dosing
e. significant first pass metabolism.

The clearance of many antidepressants is significantly affected by CYP2D6 metabolizer phenotype, and to a lesser extent by CYP2C19. However, clinical benefit from genotyping has yet to be demonstrated.[12]

St John's wort (hypericum extract) is as effective as **imipramine** and **amitriptyline** in treating mild–moderate depression and causes fewer undesirable effects.[26] However, health professionals should not prescribe or advise its use by patients because of:
- uncertainty about appropriate doses
- variation in the nature of products
- potential serious interactions with other drugs (including oral contraceptives, anticoagulants and anti-epileptics).[27]

Cautions

In patients with a history of mania, antidepressants may precipitate a further episode.

Suicide risk

1 in 1,000 patients attempt suicide in the 6 months after starting antidepressants: one third are successful.[28] In those aged ≤25 years, antidepressants may themselves cause suicidal ideation and non-fatal self harm (NNH 143).[29,30] The risk is greater with SSRIs than TCAs,[31] and is present even when an antidepressant is used for non-depressive illnesses.[30] In adults ≥25 years old, there is a smaller increase in non-fatal self harm (NNH ca. 700), no increase in suicide or suicidal thoughts, and no difference between SSRIs and TCAs.[31–33]

Suicidal ideation should be evaluated when treating depression in all age groups. Consider the safety in overdose of both the antidepressant and concomitant medicines. US and European regulators have re-inforced the need for close follow-up and to encourage changes in mood or behaviour to be reported with all antidepressants.[34,35]

Epilepsy

Antidepressants cause a dose-dependent reduction in seizure threshold. The risk is lowest for SSRIs; and **citalopram** is widely favoured because it lacks significant interactions with anti-epileptic drugs. There are less data and experience with **mirtazapine** and **venlafaxine**. The risk is higher with TCAs, and highest with **clomipramine**, **bupropion** and **maprotiline**.[36] Antidepressants can also cause seizures through hyponatraemia or alterations in anti-epileptic drug levels.

It is hard to quantify the risk of using low-dose TCAs for neuropathic pain in patients with previous seizures because the risk is dose-related and animal studies even suggest a possible anti-epileptic action at low doses.[37]

Epilepsy is associated with both mood disorders and psychosis. Symptoms may occur in between (inter-ictal), during (ictal) or in the days or weeks after (post-ictal) seizures. Optimization of anti-epileptic medication should be considered alongside antidepressant treatment, particularly for ictal and post-ictal symptoms.[38] Further, anti-epileptic drugs can cause (and treat) mood disorders: seek specialist advice when symptoms follow their introduction or titration.[36]

Parkinson's disease

SSRIs can worsen extrapyramidal symptoms because serotonin reduces nigrostriatal dopamine release via inhibitory $5HT_2$ receptors. However, the risk appears small; few RCTs report any worsening.[39] SSRIs are thus still often used in preference to TCAs which can worsen autonomic dysfunction (α blockade) and cognitive impairment (ACh_M blockade).

$5HT_2$ antagonist antidepressants might be expected to avoid serotonin-mediated exacerbations. In small pilot RCTs, Parkinsonian symptoms improved with **nefazodone**[40] but not **mirtazapine**.[41]

Antiparkinsonian D_2 agonists can themselves improve mood. In RCTs evaluating **pramipexole** for motor symptoms, mood and motivation also improved.[42] Further, in an RCT, **pramipexole** was more effective than **sertraline** for depression in patients with Parkinson's disease.[43]

Mono-amine oxidase inhibitors (MAOIs)

Included for general information. MAOIs are *not recommended* in palliative care. They can cause serious adverse events when prescribed concurrently with various other drugs. Seek advice from a psychiatrist if caring for a patient already receiving an MAOI; their previous mental illness is likely to have been difficult to treat and switching or adding other psychotropics is difficult.

MAOIs are potentially dangerous because of the risk of serious dietary and drug interactions. Hypertensive crises are mainly associated with the consumption of tyramine-containing foods (Table 4.13). Typically, the patient experiences severe headache, and may suffer an intracranial haemorrhage. Drug interactions occur with sympathomimetics (e.g. **ephedrine**, **pseudoephedrine**, **dexamfetamine**, **nefopam**), serotoninergics (see below) and **levodopa**.

Toxicity has been reported with serotoninergic opioids (e.g. fentanils, **pethidine**, **tramadol**). However, although the manufacturers of **morphine** and **oxycodone** also advise against concurrent use, their affinity for the serotonin reuptake transporter is negligible,[44] and toxicity has not been reported.[45] Further, insisting on a 2-week washout before treating pain is impracticable.

Table 4.13 Tyramine-containing foods associated with MAOI-related syndrome

Alcohol	Meat (smoked or pickled)
red wine (white wine is safe)	Meat or yeast extracts
beer	Bovril
Broad bean pods	Oxo
Cheese (old)	Marmite
Fava beans	Pickled herring

Drug interactions

MAOIs have numerous clinically significant drug interactions, resulting in hypertensive crises and serotonin toxicity.

Several pharmacodynamic interactions (e.g. serotonin toxicity, bleeding risk, antimuscarinic effects) can be predicted from the mode of action of antidepressants (see Box 4.E and Table 4.11).

In addition, potentially serious interactions may result from induction or inhibition of hepatic metabolism (see p.735). Some antidepressants inhibit cytochrome P450 enzymes:
- CYP1A2 inhibition by **fluvoxamine**: e.g. **tizanidine** levels increased ≤33 times
- CYP2D6 inhibition by **fluoxetine** and **paroxetine**: e.g. TCA levels increased ≤10 times.

The metabolism of others is affected by P450 inhibitors and inducers:
- CYP2D6: most TCAs
- CYP3A4: **mirtazapine**.

Serotonin toxicity ('serotonin syndrome')

Serotonin toxicity results from the ingestion of drug(s) which increase brain serotonin to levels sufficient to cause severe symptoms necessitating hospital admission and medical intervention (see Box 4.F and Box 4.G).[46] It has been characterized as a triad of neuro-excitatory features:
- *autonomic hyperactivity*; sweating, fever, mydriasis, tachycardia, hypertension, tachypnoea, sialorrhoea, diarrhoea
- *neuromuscular hyperactivity*; tremor, clonus, myoclonus, hyperreflexia, and hypertonia (advanced stage)
- *altered mental status*; agitation, hypomania, and delirium (advanced stage).

The onset of toxicity is generally rapid and progressive, typically as a second serotoninergic drug reaches effective blood levels (e.g. after one or two doses). Occasionally, recurrent mild symptoms may occur for weeks before the development of severe toxicity. Clonus (inducible, spontaneous or ocular), agitation, sweating, tremor and hyperreflexia are essential features. Spontaneous clonus, in the presence of a serotoninergic drug, is the most reliable indicator of serotonin toxicity.[47] Neuromuscular signs are initially greater in the lower limbs, then become more generalized as toxicity increases. Other symptoms include shaking, shivering (and chattering of the teeth), and sometimes trismus. It can be distinguished from neuroleptic (antipsychotic) malignant syndrome by its faster onset and pyramidal rather than extrapyramidal neuromuscular findings (Box 4.D, p.155).

Box 4.F Drugs with clinically relevant serotoninergic potency[44,46,48]

Antidepressants

Mono-amine oxidase inhibitors (MAOIs) All types

Selective serotonin re-uptake inhibitors (SSRIs) All

Serotonin and noradrenaline (norepinephrine) re-uptake inhibitors (SNRIs)
Clomipramine and imipramine (but not reported with other TCAs), duloxetine, milnacipran (not UK), venlafaxine

Psychostimulants (serotonin releasers)
Dexamfetamine, methylenedioxymethamfetamine (MDMA, Ecstasy) (but not methylphenidate)

Other drugs

H_1 antihistamines (serotonin re-uptake inhibitors)
Chlorphenamine, brompheniramine (but not other H_1 antihistamines)

Opioids (serotonin re-uptake inhibitors)
Dextromethorphan, dextropropoxyphene, fentanils, methadone, pentazocine, pethidine, tramadol (but not other opioids)

continued

Box 4.F Continued

Miscellaneous
MAOIs
Furazolidone (not UK), linezolid (antibacterials)
Methylene blue
Procarbazine (antineoplastic)
Selegiline (antiparkinsonian)

SNRI
Sibutramine (anorectic)

Different drugs increase serotonin levels to differing degrees. An overdose of the older irreversible MAOI **tranylcypromine** alone will produce hyperpyrexia, and even death,[49] whereas overdoses of reversible MAOIs or SSRIs alone will cause serotoninergic effects but rarely (if ever) life-threatening serotonin toxicity.[50,51] Thus death from serotonin toxicity is generally associated with the combination of two different types of drug which elevate serotonin levels via different mechanisms of action (an MAOI combined with either an SSRI or a serotonin releaser).[50]

Opioids are relatively weak serotonin re-uptake inhibitors and may only cause symptoms in higher doses or susceptible individuals. Fatalities from serotonin toxicity involving opioids have been seen with **dextromethorphan**, **pethidine**, **tramadol**, and possibly **fentanyl**.[44]

Box 4.G Treatment of serotonin toxicity[52]

In severe cases (e.g. rigidity, haemodynamic instability, temperature >38.5°C, deteriorating blood gases) seek urgent advice from a critical care specialist: ventilation and paralysis ± inotropic support may be required.

Discontinue causal medication (toxicity generally resolves within 24h).

Provide supportive care, e.g. IV fluids, oxygen.

Symptomatic measures in mild–moderate cases:
- benzodiazepines for agitation, myoclonus and seizures, e.g. midazolam 5–10mg SC p.r.n.
- $5HT_{2A}$ antagonist[a], e.g.:
  - chlorpromazine 50–100mg IM *or*
  - olanzapine 10mg IM *or*
  - cyproheptadine 12mg PO stat followed by 8mg q6h and 2mg q2h p.r.n. until symptoms resolve; tablets can be crushed and given by enteral feeding tube.

a. prevents deaths from hyperpyrexia in animals and probably in humans. Generally give IM; the PO route is suitable only for mild toxicity and, in the case of overdose, in patients who have *not* received oral activated charcoal.[53,54]

Undesirable effects

A synopsis is contained in Table 4.14; also see individual drug monographs. Overall, discontinuation with SSRIs is marginally less than with TCAs (NNT 33).[55]

GI bleeding and platelet function

SSRIs and SNRIs (e.g. **amitriptyline**, **duloxetine**, **imipramine**, **venlafaxine**) decrease serotonin uptake from the blood by platelets. Because platelets do not synthesize serotonin, the amount of serotonin in platelets is reduced.[59] This adversely affects platelet aggregation.[60] After confounding factors have been controlled for, serotonin re-uptake inhibitors triple the risk of GI bleeding.[61,62] This may be important in already high-risk patients (see p.298). If an antidepressant is indicated in such patients, safer alternatives would include an NRI (e.g. **desipramine** (not UK), **nortriptyline**) or **mirtazapine**.

Table 4.14 Relative frequency and mechanisms of undesirable effects of antidepressants[56–58]

Undesirable effect	*Putative mechanism*	*Relative frequency*													
		SNRI					*NRI*			*SSRI*				*RA*	
		Amitriptyline	*Clomipramine*	*Duloxetine*	*Imipramine*	*Venlafaxine*	*Desipramine*	*Lofepramine*	*Nortriptyline*	*Citalopram*	*Fluoxetine*	*Paroxetine*	*Sertraline*	*Mirtazapine*	*Trazadone*
GI (nausea, diarrhoea)	↑Serotonin (acting on $5HT_3$)	–	+	++	–	++	–	–	–	++	++	++	++	–	–
CNS (agitation, restlessness, anxiety, insomnia)	↑Serotonin (acting on $5HT_2$)	–	+	+	+	+	+	+	+	+	+	+	+	–	–
Weight gain	$5HT_2$ and H_1 antagonism	++	+	–	+	–	–	–	–	–	–	–	–	++	+
Sedation	H_1, ACh_M and α_1-adrenergic antagonism	++	+	–	+	–	+	–	+	–	–	–	–	++	++
Postural hypotension	α_1-adrenergic antagonism	++	++	–	++	–	+	+	+	–	–	–	–	–	++
Sexual dysfunction	↑Serotonin (acting on $5HT_2$)	+	++	++	+	++	+	+	+	++	++	++	++	–	–
Dry mouth, constipation	ACh_M antagonism	++	++	–	++	–	+	+	+	–	–	–	–	–	–
SIADH	↑Serotonin (acting on $5HT_2$); ↑noradrenaline (norepinephrine; acting on α_1)	+	+	+	+	+	+	+	+	++	++	++	++	+	+

Key: ++ = relatively common or strong; + = may occur or moderately strong; – = absent or rare/weak.
Abbreviations: NRI = noradrenaline (norepinephrine) re-uptake inhibitor; SNRI = serotonin and noradrenaline (norepinephrine) re-uptake inhibitor; SSRI = selective serotonin re-uptake inhibitor; RA = receptor antagonist.

Use of antidepressants in palliative care

See individual monographs for doses and titration.

Neuropathic pain

Amitriptyline and **nortriptyline** are commonly used for neuropathic pain.[63] Most RCTs have been of **amitriptyline**, although **nortriptyline** was better tolerated when compared with **amitriptyline**.[64] Their efficacy and tolerability appear comparable to alternatives (e.g. anti-epileptic drugs and other SNRI and NRI antidepressants; see p.281),[65–67] although few have been directly compared.

Bupropion, **duloxetine**, **venlafaxine** and most TCAs are also superior to placebo. SSRIs are modestly effective (3 of 4 RCTs),[68–71] but inferior to **imipramine**.[71] The benefit reported with **mirtazapine**[72] has *not* been confirmed in RCTs.

NICE recommends **duloxetine** as first-line treatment for painful diabetic neuropathy based on a cost-effectiveness model, but no clinical evidence of superiority is provided.[73] Given the comparable efficacy, tolerability and monitoring requirements of cheaper alternatives, this conclusion is clearly questionable.

Alternatives to antidepressants include anti-epileptics (p.237) and opioids (p.281). The efficacy of **amitriptyline** and **nortriptyline** was similar to **gabapentin** in two RCTs, although one found **nortriptyline** to cause more dry mouth, constipation and postural hypotension.[74,75] They are also often used together: **nortriptyline** combined with **gabapentin** was more effective than either drug alone.[76] **Nortriptyline** was as effective as **morphine**.[77]

Other pain syndromes

Antidepressants are of benefit for various other pain syndromes including migraine and tension headache (TCAs),[78] chronic low back pain (TCAs),[79] fibromyalgia (**duloxetine**),[80] and osteo-arthritis (**duloxetine**).[81]

Depression

Treatment is tailored to the severity of symptoms, their functional impact and patient preference (Figure 4.5). First-line treatment is generally with **sertraline** or **citalopram**. They have fewer drug interactions, lower risk in overdose, and are marginally better tolerated than alternatives.[27] Efficacy has been confirmed in palliative populations.[82] Frequent re-evaluation of response, adherence, and alternative and concurrent sources of distress is required throughout.

Methylphenidate, with its rapid onset, may be preferable where prognosis is anticipated to be <2–4 weeks (see p.210). This is shorter than suggested by previous consensus guidance[83] because of the recognition that conventional antidepressants act faster than previously thought.[84] However, trials of psychostimulants are generally of short duration and with outcome measures of uncertain clinical significance. Thus, conventional antidepressants should be used if the patient has a sufficient prognosis for a response to manifest.[83,85,86] Concurrent use with a conventional antidepressant may hasten the response compared with the latter alone, particularly in relation to fatigue.[86] **Modafinil** can be used if **methylphenidate** is poorly tolerated (see p.211).

Although an SNRI or NRI may be considered if depression and neuropathic pain co-exist, slower titration is required to avoid higher rates of discontinuation.[27] They are therefore often treated separately (e.g. with an SSRI plus either **gabapentin** or **nortriptyline**).

Titrating, switching and combining antidepressants

If there is no response after 4 weeks, or only a partial response after 6–8 weeks:

- increase the dose, particularly if there has been a partial response and minimal undesirable effects *or*
- switch antidepressants, particularly if there has been minimal improvement or bothersome undesirable effects *or*
- combine with a second antidepressant or adjuvant psychotropic drug, particularly if a previous switch was unhelpful.[27]

Dose titration is straightforward but, for SSRIs, of uncertain value. A systematic review found dose titration in patients not responding to SSRIs taken for 3–6 weeks no more effective than continuing the dose unaltered.[88] Nonetheless, many guidelines highlight individual variation in effective doses and therefore recommend dose titration if the existing drug is well tolerated.[27,57] There is a dose-response effect with TCAs and **venlafaxine** (225–375mg vs. 75mg).

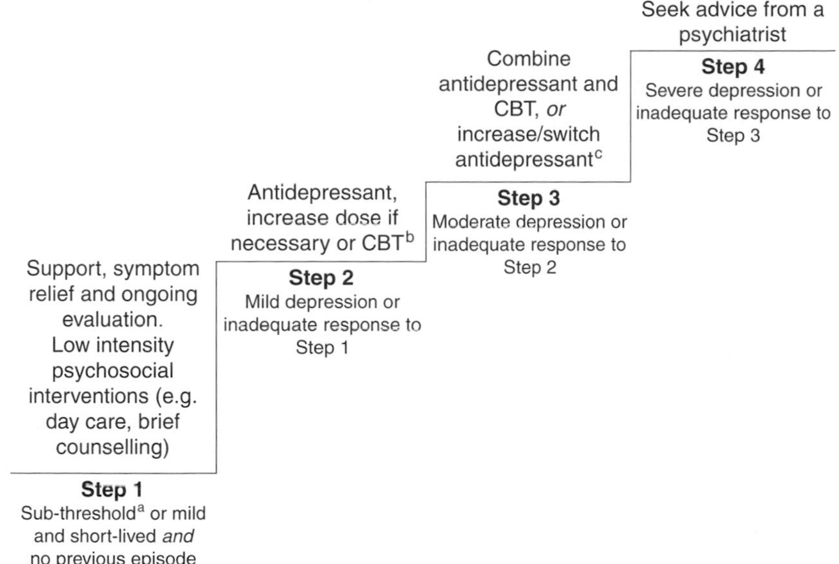

Figure 4.5 Overview of the management of depression.[27,87]

a. sub-threshold symptoms = patients with <5 DSM IV symptoms required for a diagnosis of depression
b. CBT = cognitive-behavioural therapy
c. see p.180 and below, managing an inadequate initial response.

The efficacy of second-line antidepressants appears comparable regardless of mode of action.[57,89,90] Options include an alternative SSRI or **mirtazapine**. One SSRI can be directly substituted for another without cross-tapering or a washout period.[57,90] **Mirtazapine** 15mg can be directly substituted for SSRIs at usual doses (**fluoxetine**, **citalopram** or **paroxetine** 20mg; **sertraline** 50mg).[57,91] Opinion varies on the need to taper higher SSRI doses before switching.[89,91] Switching SSRIs is most effective when the first SSRI is poorly tolerated but benefit is also seen in non-responders,[90] perhaps because of differing additional actions (see p.192). The effect of **mirtazapine** on additional mono-amines is theoretically advantageous (see p.200). **Venlafaxine** has a marginally higher response rate (NNT = 10) compared with switching to a second SSRI[90] but is less well tolerated. Switching to or from TCAs and MAOIs requires additional care.[92]

A partial response to an antidepressant can be increased ('augmented') by adding a second psychotropic drug. This avoids potential loss of the initial improvement but is generally less well tolerated than monotherapy.[27] Options include:

- an antipsychotic (e.g. **quetiapine** or **olanzapine** added to an SSRI)
- **mirtazapine** (added to an SSRI or **venlafaxine**)
- a range of options used only by psychiatrists (e.g. **lithium**, **tri-iodothyronine**).

NICE suggests primary care clinicians seek advice before adding a second drug.[27] Palliative care specialists using some of the above for other indications should be aware of their potential benefit when concurrent depression has only partially responded to an antidepressant.[57,93]

Duration of treatment

Consider stopping treatment 6 months after full remission in those without risk factors for relapse. Risk factors include previous depression and the severity, duration, degree of treatment resistance, and the presence of residual symptoms. Treatment is tapered slowly (see below). Treat those with risk factors for longer: 1 year if full remission but one risk factor; and ≥2 years if ≥2 risk factors.[27,57] In palliative care, the latter is likely to mean lifelong/indefinitely.

Anxiety and panic disorders

The efficacy of cognitive behavioural and drug therapy is comparable.[94] Drug treatment is tailored to the likely duration of use:

- benzodiazepine (see p.132), if prognosis is days to weeks
- SSRI (± a benzodiazepine initially), if prognosis is months.

Although supporting evidence (and licensing) for SSRIs varies for different anxiety disorders,[95] a class effect is plausible. **Citalopram** and **sertraline** are licensed for panic disorder, well tolerated, have fewer drug interactions, and are generally more familiar to prescribers. All SSRIs can initially exacerbate anxiety: start low and consider a concurrent benzodiazepine for the first few weeks.

If response is inadequate, combine with cognitive behavioural therapy (evidence best for panic disorder)[94] or switch to an alternative SSRI or **imipramine** or **clomipramine**.[95,96] Switching is not advocated within 3 months because benefit can take longer to manifest than in depression.[95,96] However, in patients with a short prognosis, consider adding a benzodiazepine to obtain more rapid benefit. **Pregabalin** (see p.254) also acts quickly but is reserved for patients not responding to antidepressants; supporting trials are fewer and mainly confined to generalized anxiety disorder.[95]

Agitated delirium

The benefit reported with **trazodone**[97] remains unconfirmed in clinical trials. Treatment of underlying causes, non-drug management (e.g. orientation strategies, correction of sensory deprivation) and prevention of complications are central to delirium management. Antipsychotics are generally used first-line when medication is needed (see p.156).

Agitation and challenging behaviours in dementia

Evidence for antidepressants is even more limited than for antipsychotics (see p.156), and certainly insufficient to justify routine use.[98,99] Larger studies have not replicated the earlier benefit reported for **trazodone**.[99]

Sweating

Like other antimuscarinics, **amitriptyline** is used for paraneoplastic sweating unresponsive to NSAIDs.[100] However, like all MARIs, it can also cause sweating.[101]

Hot flushes

Venlafaxine is of benefit in hot flushes associated with the menopause, hormone therapy and androgen ablation therapy for prostate cancer (see p.195).

Insomnia

When insomnia co-exists with other indications, sedating antidepressants (e.g. TCAs, **mirtazapine**, **trazodone**) are often selected. **Doxepin** 3–6mg at bedtime PO improves both sleep latency and fragmentation in primary insomnia, although the smallest available UK capsule is 25mg. Benefit is sustained for ⩾12 weeks without rebound insomnia after discontinuation.[102] **Trazodone** is commonly used although evidence is limited.[103]

Pruritus

Two small RCTs suggest benefit within a few days from **sertraline** (cholestatic pruritus)[104] and **paroxetine** (pruritus of mixed cause in cancer patients).[105] Benefit is also reported in pruritus associated with polycythaemia vera.[106] **Mirtazapine** is reported to improve pruritus of mixed cause in advanced disease.[107] Like other H_1 antagonists, **doxepin** can be used for histamine-mediated pruritus and/or for night sedation.

Bladder spasm, stress incontinence and urgency

Antimuscarinic antidepressants (e.g. **amitriptyline**) reduce detrusor contractions associated with urgency, although licensed alternatives have additional direct effects on the detrusor muscle (see p.4).[108] **Duloxetine** has a limited role in stress incontinence.[109]

Pathological laughter and crying

Frequent brief uncontrollable laughter and/or crying, incongruent with external events, can complicate numerous neurological disorders, including Parkinson's disease, cerebral tumours, multiple sclerosis, strokes, MND/ALS, and dementia. It can be socially disabling. Functional

imaging suggests dysregulation of serotoninergic and other mono-aminergic pathways. The differential diagnosis includes:
- seizures: generally complex partial seizures and thus an alteration of consciousness during/after episodes
- depression or other mood disorders: mood alteration is persistent whereas the emotion that may accompany pathological laughter and crying is short-lived.

Validated assessment tools are available to aid diagnosis.[110] First-line treatment is with **citalopram** or **sertraline**. Benefit is often seen within days. Second-line options include **amitriptyline**, **imipramine**, **nortriptyline** and **levodopa**.[111]

Drooling and sialorrhoea

Like other antimuscarinics, **amitriptyline** reduces salivation (p.4).[112]

Stopping antidepressants

Abrupt cessation of antidepressant therapy (particularly an MAOI) after regular administration for >8 weeks may result in a discontinuation reaction (withdrawal syndrome).[113] Discontinuation reactions depend on the class of antidepressant, and are more common with drugs with shorter halflives (Box 4.H). Thus, with SSRIs, they are most common with **paroxetine** and least common with **fluoxetine**.

Box 4.H Antidepressant discontinuation reactions[113]

SSRIs and venlafaxine: *'FINISH'*[114]
Flu-like symptoms (fatigue, lethargy, myalgia, chills)
Insomnia (including vivid dreams)
Nausea
Imbalance (ataxia, vertigo, dizziness)
Sensory disturbances (paraesthesia, sensations of electric shock)
Hyperarousal (restlessness, anxiety, agitation)

TCAs
Flu-like symptoms (fatigue, lethargy, myalgia, chills)
Insomnia (including vivid dreams)
GI disorders (nausea, diarrhoea)
Mood disorders (depression or mania)
Movement disorders (rare: akathisia, parkinsonism)

Trazodone
Flu-like symptoms (fatigue, lethargy, myalgia, chills)
GI disorders (nausea, diarrhoea)
Restlessness
Tremor
Headache

Mirtazapine
Nausea
Dizziness
Hyperarousal (anxiety, agitation)
Headache

MAOIs
Insomnia
Movement disorders (ataxia, athetosis, catatonia, myoclonus)
Mood disorders (lability, depression, agitation, aggression)
Paranoia
Hallucinations
Seizures
Altered speech (pressured, slow)

Discontinuation reactions differ from a depressive relapse or a panic disorder. They generally start abruptly within a few days of stopping the antidepressant (*or reducing its dose*). In contrast, a depressive relapse is uncommon in the first week after stopping an antidepressant, and symptoms tend to build up gradually and persist. Discontinuation reactions generally resolve within 24h of re-instating antidepressant therapy, whereas the response is slower with a depressive relapse.

Ideally, antidepressants taken for $>$8 weeks should be progressively reduced over 4 weeks. If a mild discontinuation reaction is suspected, re-assurance alone may be adequate. If distressing, restart the antidepressant and reduce more gradually.

Some patients experience discontinuation symptoms even during tapering. When this happens, increase the dose and, before continuing with tapering, consider:

- using a liquid formulation and reducing the dose in smaller steps *or*
- switching from **venlafaxine** or a short halflife SSRI to **fluoxetine**.[113]

1 Castren E and Rantamaki T (2010) Role of brain-derived neurotrophic factor in the aetiology of depression: implications for pharmacological treatment. *CNS Drugs*. **24**: 1–7.

2 Belmaker RH and Agam G (2008) Major depressive disorder. *New England Journal of Medicine*. **358**: 55–68.

3 Tran PV *et al.* (2003) Dual monoamine modulation for improved treatment of major depressive disorder. *Journal of Clinical Psychopharmacology*. **23**: 78–86.

4 Sawynok J *et al.* (2001) Antidepressants as analgesics: an overview of central and peripheral mechanisms of action. *Journal of Psychiatry and Neuroscience*. **26**: 21–29.

5 McCleane G (2008) Antidepressants as analgesics. *CNS Drugs*. **22**: 139–156.

6 Heinricher MM *et al.* (2009) Descending control of nociception: Specificity, recruitment and plasticity. *Brain Research Reviews*. **60**: 214–225.

7 Dogrul A *et al.* (2009) Differential mediation of descending pain facilitation and inhibition by spinal 5HT-3 and 5HT-7 receptors. *Brain Research Molecular Brain Research*. **1280**: 52–59.

8 McCleane G (2000) Topical application of doxepin hydrochloride, capsaicin and a combination of both produces analgesia in chronic human neuropathic pain: a randomized, double-blind, placebo-controlled study. *British Journal of Clinical Pharmacology*. **49**: 574–579.

9 McCleane (1999) Topical doxepin hydrochloride reduces neuropathic pain: a randomised, double-blind, placebo-controlled study. *Pain Clinic*. **12**: 47–50.

10 Akimova E *et al.* (2009) The serotonin-1A receptor in anxiety disorders. *Biological Psychiatry*. **66**: 627–635.

11 Maron E and Shlik J (2006) Serotonin function in panic disorder: important, but why? *Neuropsychopharmacology*. **31**: 1–11.

12 Kirchheiner J and Rodriguez-Antona C (2009) Cytochrome P450 2D6 genotyping: potential role in improving treatment outcomes in psychiatric disorders. *CNS Drugs*. **23**: 181–191.

13 Stahl SM (2008) Psychosis and schizophrenia. In: *Essential Psychopharmacology: Neuroscientific Basis and Practical Applications* (3e). Cambridge University Press, USA, pp. 247–325.

14 NIMH (National Institute of Mental Health) (2006) National Institute of Mental Health's Psychoactive Drug Screening Program. University of North Carolina. Available from: http://pdsp.med.unc.edu/indexR.html

15 Stahl SM *et al.* (2004) A Review of the Neuropharmacology of Bupropion, a Dual Norepinephrine and Dopamine Reuptake Inhibitor. *Primary Care Companion Journal of Clinical Psychiatry*. **6**: 159–166.

16 Beique JC *et al.* (1998) Affinities of venlafaxine and various reuptake inhibitors for the serotonin and norepinephrine transporters. *European Journal of Pharmacology*. **349**: 129–132.

17 Wen B *et al.* (2008) Detection of novel reactive metabolites of trazodone: evidence for CYP2D6-mediated bioactivation of m-chlorophenylpiperazine. *Drug Metabolism and Disposition*. **36**: 841–850.

18 Jefferson JW *et al.* (2005) Bupropion for major depressive disorder: Pharmacokinetic and formulation considerations. *Clinical Therapeutics*. **27**: 1685–1695.

19 Hiemke (2000) Pharmacokinetics of selective serotonin reuptake inhibitors. *Pharmacology and Therapeutics*. **85**: 11–28.

20 Fleishaker JC (2000) Clinical pharmacokinetics of reboxetine, a selective norepinephrine reuptake inhibitor for the treatment of patients with depression. *Clinical Pharmacokinetics*. **39**: 413–427.

21 Venkatakrishnan K *et al.* (1998) Five distinct human cytochromes mediate amitriptyline N-demethylation in vitro: dominance of CYP 2C19 and 3A4. *Journal of Clinical Pharmacology*. **38**: 112–121.

22 Richelson E (1997) Pharmacokinetic drug interactions of new antidepressants: A review of the effects on the metabolism of other drugs. *Mayo Clinic Proceedings*. **72**: 835–847.

23 Kaye CM *et al.* (1989) A review of the metabolism and pharmacokinetics of paroxetine in man. *Acta Psychiatr Scand Suppl*. **350**: 60–75.

24 Schulz P *et al.* (1985) Discrepancies between pharmacokinetic studies of amitriptyline. *Clinical Pharmacokinetics*. **10**: 257–268.

25 Abernethyl DR *et al.* (1984) Absolute bioavailability of imipramine: influence of food. *Psychopharmacology (Berl)*. **83**: 104–106.

26 Linde (2008) St John's wort for major depression. *Cochrane Database of Systematic Reviews*.

27 NICE (2009) Clinical Guidleline 90 and 91. Depression. Available from: www.nice.org.uk

28 Simon GE *et al.* (2006) Suicide risk during antidepressant treatment. *American Journal of Psychiatry*. **163**: 41–47.

29 Stone M *et al.* (2009) Risk of suicidality in clinical trials of antidepressants in adults: analysis of proprietary data submitted to US Food and Drug Administration. *British Medical Journal*. **339**: b2880.

30 Bridge JA *et al.* (2007) Clinical response and risk for reported suicidal ideation and suicide attempts in pediatric antidepressant treatment: a meta-analysis of randomized controlled trials. *Journal of the American Medical Association*. **297**: 1683–1696.

31 Martinez C *et al.* (2005) Antidepressant treatment and the risk of fatal and non-fatal self harm in first episode depression: nested case-control study. *British Medical Journal*. **330**: 389.

32 Gunnell D *et al.* (2005) Selective serotonin reuptake inhibitors (SSRIs) and suicide in adults: meta-analysis of drug company data from placebo controlled, randomised controlled trials submitted to the MHRA's safety review. *British Medical Journal*. **330**: 385.

33 Fergusson D *et al.* (2005) Association between suicide attempts and selective serotonin reuptake inhibitors: systematic review of randomised controlled trials. *British Medical Journal.* **330**: 396.

34 Reeves RR and Ladner ME (2010) Antidepressant-induced suicidality: an update. *CNS Neuroscience and Therapeutics.* **16**: 227–234.

35 MHRA (2007) Drug safety update. **1**: 7–8.

36 Harden CL *et al.* (2002) Mood disorders in patients with epilepsy: epidemiology and management. *CNS Drugs.* **16**: 291–302.

37 Dailey JW and Naritoku DK (1996) Antidepressants and seizures: clinical anecdotes overshadow neuroscience. *Biochemical Pharmacology.* **52**: 1323–1329.

38 Blumer D *et al.* (2004) The interictal dysphoric disorder: recognition, pathogenesis, and treatment of the major psychiatric disorder of epilepsy. *Epilepsy and Behaviour.* **5**: 826–840.

39 Skapinakis P *et al.* (2010) Efficacy and acceptability of selective serotonin reuptake inhibitors for the treatment of depression in Parkinson's disease: a systematic review and meta-analysis of randomized controlled trials. *BMC Neurology.* **10**: 49.

40 Avila A *et al.* (2003) Does nefazodone improve both depression and Parkinson disease? A pilot randomized trial. *Journal of Clinical Psychopharmacology.* **23**: 509–513.

41 Zhang (2006) Mirtazapine vs fluoxetine in treatng Parkinson's disease with depression and anxiety. *Medical Journal of Chinese People's Health.*

42 Leentjens AF *et al.* (2009) The effect of pramipexole on mood and motivational symptoms in Parkinson's disease: a meta-analysis of placebo-controlled studies. *Clinical Therapeutics.* **31**: 89–98.

43 Barone P *et al.* (2006) Pramipexole versus sertraline in the treatment of depression in Parkinson's disease: a national multicenter parallel-group randomized study. *Journal of Neurology.* **253**: 601–607.

44 Gillman PK (2005) Monoamine oxidase inhibitors, opioid analgesics and serotonin toxicity. *British Journal of Anaesthesia.* **95**: 434–441.

45 Baxter K (2011) Stockley's Drug Interactions (online edition). Pharmaceutical Press, London. Available from: www.medicinescomplete.com

46 Gillman P (2006) Serotonin toxicity, serotonin syndrome: 2006 update, overview and analysis. Available from: www.psychotropical.com

47 Dunkley EJ *et al.* (2003) The Hunter Serotonin Toxicity Criteria: simple and accurate diagnostic decision rules for serotonin toxicity. *Quarterly Journal of Medicine.* **96**: 635–642.

48 Gillman PK (2006) A review of serotonin toxicity data: implications for the mechanisms of antidepressant drug action. *Biol Psychiatry.* **59**: 1046–1051.

49 Whyte I (2004) Monoamine oxidase inhibitors. In: RC Dart (ed) *Medical Toxicology.* Lippincott Williams & Wilkins, Baltimore, pp. 823–834.

50 Isbister GK *et al.* (2003) Moclobemide poisoning: toxicokinetics and occurrence of serotonin toxicity. *British Journal of Clinical Pharmacology.* **56**: 441–450.

51 Isbister GK *et al.* (2004) Relative toxicity of selective serotonin reuptake inhibitors (SSRIs) in overdose. *Journal of Toxicology and Clinical Toxicology.* **42**: 277–285.

52 Boyer EW and Shannon M (2005) The serotonin syndrome. *New England Journal of Medicine.* **352**: 1112–1120.

53 Gillman PK (1999) The serotonin syndrome and its treatment. *Journal of Psychopharmacology.* **13**: 100–109.

54 Gillman PK (1998) Serotonin syndrome: history and risk. *Fundam Clin Pharmacol.* **12**: 482–491.

55 Anderson IM (2000) Selective serotonin reuptake inhibitors versus tricyclic antidepressants: a meta-analysis of efficacy and tolerability. *Journal of Affective Disorders.* **58**: 19–36.

56 Bhuvaneswar CG *et al.* (2009) Adverse endocrine and metabolic effects of psychotropic drugs: selective clinical review. *CNS Drugs.* **23**: 1003–1021.

57 Anderson IM *et al.* (2008) Evidence based guidelines for treating depressive disorders with antidepressants: a revision of the 2000 British Association for Psychopharmacology guidelines. *Journal of Psychopharmacology.* **22**: 343–396.

58 Jacob S and Spinler SA (2006) Hyponatremia associated with selective serotonin-reuptake inhibitors in older adults. *Annals of Pharmacotherapy.* **40**: 1618–1622.

59 Ross S *et al.* (1980) Inhibition of 5-hydroxytryptamine uptake in human platelets by antidepressant agents in vivo. *Psychopharmacology.* **67**: 1–7.

60 Li N *et al.* (1997) Effects of serotonin on platelet activation in whole blood. *Blood Coagulation Fibrinolysis.* **8**: 517–523.

61 vanWalraven C *et al.* (2001) Inhibition of serotonin reuptake by antidepressants and upper gastrointestinal bleeding in elderly patients: retrospective cohort study. *British Medical Journal.* **323**: 655–657.

62 Paton C and Ferrier IN (2005) SSRIs and gastrointestinal bleeding. *British Medical Journal.* **331**: 529–530.

63 Palliativedrugs.com (2009) Survey Jan-Feb 2009. Available from: www.palliativedrugs.com

64 Watson CP *et al.* (1998) Nortriptyline versus amitriptyline in postherpetic neuralgia: a randomized trial. *Neurology.* **51**: 1166–1171.

65 Saarto T and Wiffen PJ (2007) Antidepressants for neuropathic pain. *Cochrane Database of Systematic Reviews.* CD005454.

66 Dworkin RH *et al.* (2007) Pharmacologic management of neuropathic pain: evidence-based recommendations. *Pain.* **132**: 237–251.

67 Finnerup NB *et al.* (2005) Algorithm for neuropathic pain treatment: an evidence based proposal. *Pain.* **118**: 289–305.

68 Otto M *et al.* (2008) Escitalopram in painful polyneuropathy: a randomized, placebo-controlled, cross-over trial. *Pain.* **139**: 275–283.

69 Sindrup SH *et al.* (1992) The selective serotonin reuptake inhibitor citalopram relieves the symptoms of diabetic neuropathy. *Clinical Pharmacology and Therapeutics.* **52**: 547–552.

70 Max M *et al.* (1992) Effects of desipramine, amitriptyline, and fluoxetine on pain in diabetic neuropathy. *New England Journal of Medicine.* **326**: 1287–1288.

71 Sindrup S *et al.* (1990) The selective serotonin re-uptake inhibitor paroxetine is effective in the treatment of diabetic neuropathy symptoms. *Pain.* **42**: 135–144.

72 Christodoulou C *et al.* (2010) Effectiveness of mirtazapine in the treatment of postherpetic neuralgia. *Journal of Pain and Symptom Management.* **39**: e3–6.

73 NICE (2010) Clinical Guideline 96. Neuropathic pain: the pharmacological management of neuropathic pain in adults in non-specialist settings.

74 Chandra K *et al.* (2006) Gabapentin versus nortriptyline in post-herpetic neuralgia patients: a randomized, double-blind clinical trial–the GONIP Trial. *International Journal of Clinical Pharmacology and Therapeutics.* **44**: 358–363.

75 Morello C *et al.* (1999) Randomized double-blind study comparing the efficacy of gabapentin with amitriptyline on diabetic peripheral neuropathy pain. *Archives of Internal Medicine*. **159**: 1931–1937.
76 Gilron I *et al.* (2009) Nortriptyline and gabapentin, alone and in combination for neuropathic pain: a double-blind, randomised controlled crossover trial. *Lancet*. **374**: 1252–1261.
77 Raja SN *et al.* (2002) Opioids versus antidepressants in postherpetic neuralgia: a randomized, placebo-controlled trial.[see comment]. *Neurology*. **59**: 1015–1021.
78 Jackson JL *et al.* (2010) Tricyclic antidepressants and headaches: systematic review and meta-analysis. *British Medical Journal*. **341**: c5222.
79 Staiger TO *et al.* (2003) Systematic review of antidepressants in the treatment of chronic low back pain. *Spine (Phila Pa 1976)*. **28**: 2540–2545.
80 Lunn (2009) Duloxetine for treating painful neuropathy or chronic pain. *Cochrane Database of Systematic Reviews*. **4**: CD007115.
81 Chappell AS *et al.* (2009) Duloxetine, a centrally acting analgesic, in the treatment of patients with osteoarthritis knee pain: a 13-week, randomized, placebo-controlled trial. *Pain*. **146**: 253–260.
82 Rayner L *et al.* (2011) Antidepressants for the treatment of depression in palliative care: systematic review and meta-analysis. *Palliative Medicine*. **25**: 36–51.
83 Block SD (2000) Assessing and managing depression in the terminally ill patient. ACP-ASIM End-of-Life Care Consensus Panel. American College of Physicians — American Society of Internal Medicine. *Annals of internal medicine*. **132**: 209–218.
84 Tylee A and Walters P (2007) Onset of action of antidepressants. *British Medical Journal*. **334**: 911–912.
85 Candy M *et al.* (2008) Psychostimulants for depression. *Cochrane Database of Systematic Reviews*. **2**: CD006722.
86 Orr K and Taylor D (2007) Psychostimulants in the treatment of depression: a review of the evidence. *CNS Drugs*. **21**: 239–257.
87 Rayner L *et al.* (2011) The development of evidence-based European guidelines on the management of depression in palliative cancer care. *European Journal of Cancer*. **47**: 702–712.
88 Adli M *et al.* (2005) Is dose escalation of antidepressants a rational strategy after a medium-dose treatment has failed? A systematic review. *European Archives of Psychiatry and Clinical Neuroscience*. **255**: 387–400.
89 Rush AJ *et al.* (2009) STAR*D: revising conventional wisdom. *CNS Drugs*. **23**: 627–647.
90 Ruhe HG *et al.* (2006) Switching antidepressants after a first selective serotonin reuptake inhibitor in major depressive disorder: a systematic review. *Journal of Clinical Psychiatry*. **67**: 1836–1855.
91 Fava GA and Mangelli L (2001) Assessment of subclinical symptoms and psychological well-being in depression. *European Archives of Psychiatry and Clinical Neuroscience*. **251 (suppl 2)**: II47–52.
92 Taylor (2007) *The Maundsley Prescribing Guidelines* (9e). Informa Healthcare, London.
93 Shelton RC *et al.* (2010) Therapeutic options for treatment-resistant depression. *CNS Drugs*. **24**: 131–161.
94 Bandelow B *et al.* (2007) Meta-analysis of randomized controlled comparisons of psychopharmacological and psychological treatments for anxiety disorders. *World Journal of Biological Psychiatry*. **8**: 175–187.
95 Baldwin DS *et al.* (2005) Evidence-based guidelines for the pharmacological treatment of anxiety disorders: recommendations from the British Association for Psychopharmacology. *Journal of Psychopharmacology*. **19**: 567–596.
96 NICE (2004) Anxiety: management of anxiety (panic disorder, with or without agoraphobia, and generalised anxiety disorder) in adults in primary,secondary and community care. Clinical guideline 22. Available from: www.nice.org.uk
97 Okamoto Y *et al.* (1999) Trazodone in the treatment of delirium. *Journal of Clinical Psychopharmacology*. **19**: 280–282.
98 Sink KM *et al.* (2005) Pharmacological treatment of neuropsychiatric symptoms of dementia: a review of the evidence. *Journal of the American Medical Association*. **293**: 596–608.
99 Jeste DV *et al.* (2007) ACNP White Paper: Update on Use of Antipsychotic Drugs in Elderly Persons with Dementia. *Neuropsychopharmacology*.
100 Twycross R *et al.* (2009) *Symptom Management in Advanced Cancer* Vol 4. palliativedrugs.com, Nottingham, pp. 331–334.
101 Marcy TR and Britton ML (2005) Antidepressant-induced sweating. *Annals of Pharmacotherapy*. **39**: 748–752.
102 Weber J *et al.* (2010) Low-dose doxepin: in the treatment of insomnia. *CNS Drugs*. **24**: 713–720.
103 Mendelson WB (2005) A review of the evidence for the efficacy and safety of trazodone in insomnia. *Journal of Clinical Psychiatry*. **66**: 469–476.
104 Mayo MJ *et al.* (2007) Sertraline as a first-line treatment for cholestatic pruritus. *Hepatology*. **45**: 666–674.
105 Zylicz Z *et al.* (2003) Paroxetine in the treatment of severe non-dermatological pruritus: a randomized, controlled trial. *Journal of Pain and Symptom Management*. **26**: 1105–1112.
106 Tefferi A and Fonseca R (2002) Selective serotonin reuptake inhibitors are effective in the treatment of polycythemia vera-associated pruritus. *Blood*. **99**: 2627.
107 Zylicz Z *et al.* (eds) (2004) *Pruritus in Advanced Disease*. Oxford University Press, Oxford.
108 Twycross R *et al.* (2009) *Symptom Management in Advanced Cancer* Vol 4. palliativdrugs.com, Nottingham, pp. 289–296.
109 NICE (2006) Urinary incontinence: the management of urinary incontinence in women. In: Clinical guidelines. National Institute for Health and Clinical Excellence. Available from: http://guidance.nice.org.uk/CG40
110 Robinson RG *et al.* (1993) Pathological laughing and crying following stroke: validation of a measurement scale and a double-blind treatment study. *American Journal of Psychiatry*. **150**: 286–293.
111 Wortzel HS *et al.* (2008) Pathological laughing and crying: epidemiology, pathophysiology and treatment. *CNS Drugs*. **22**: 531–545.
112 Twycross R *et al.* (2009) *Symptom Management in Advanced Cancer* Vol 4. palliativedrugs.com, Nottingham, pp. 61–133.
113 Haddad PM (2001) Antidepressant discontinuation syndromes: Clinical relevance, prevention and management. *Drug Safety*. **24**: 183–197.
114 Berber MJ (1998) FINISH: remembering the discontinuation syndrome. Flu-like symptoms, Insomnia, Nausea, Imbalance, Sensory disturbances, and Hyperarousal (anxiety/agitation). *Journal of Clinical Psychiatry*. **59**: 255.

Quick Practice Guide: Depression

Sadness and tears, even if associated with transient suicidal thoughts, do not justify the diagnosis of depression or the prescription of an antidepressant. Often they are part of an adjustment reaction, and improve with time. Other patients are demoralized rather than medically depressed and respond to symptom management and psychosocial support.

Evaluation

1 Screening: about 5–10% of patients with advanced cancer develop a major depression. Cases will be missed unless specific enquiry is made of all patients:
'What has your mood been like lately?... Are you depressed?'
'Have you had serious depression before? Are things like that now?'

2 Assessment interview: if depression is suspected, explore the patient's mood more fully by encouraging the patient to talk further with appropriate prompts. Symptoms suggesting clinical depression include:
- sustained low mood (i.e. most of every day for several weeks) } core symptoms
- sustained loss of pleasure/interest in life (anhedonia) } core symptoms
- diurnal variation (worse in mornings and better in evenings)
- waking significantly earlier than usual (e.g. 1–2h) and feeling 'awful'
- feelings of hopelessness/worthlessness
- excessive guilt
- withdrawal from family and friends
- persistent suicidal thoughts and/or suicidal acts
- requests for euthanasia.

3 Differential diagnosis: the symptoms of depression and cancer, and of depression and sadness overlap. If in doubt whether the patient is suffering from depression, an adjustment reaction or sadness, review after 1–2 weeks of general support and improved symptom management. If still undecided, seek advice from a psychologist/psychiatrist.

4 Medical causes of depression: depression may be the consequence of:
- a medical condition, e.g. hypercalcaemia, cerebral metastases
- a reaction to severe uncontrolled physical symptoms
- drugs, e.g. antineoplastics, benzodiazepines, antipsychotics, corticosteroids, antihypertensives.

Management

5 Correct the correctable: treat medical causes, particularly severe pain and other distressing symptoms.

6 Non-drug treatment:
- explanation and assurance that symptoms can be treated
- depressed patients often benefit from the ambience of a Palliative Care Day Centre
- specific psychological treatments (via a clinical psychologist, etc.)
- other psychosocial professionals, e.g. chaplain and creative therapists, have a therapeutic role, but avoid overwhelming the patient with simultaneous multiple referrals.

7 Drug treatment:
- if the patient is expected to live for >4 weeks, prescribe an antidepressant
- the starting and continuing doses of antidepressants are generally lower in debilitated patients than in the physically fit
- all antidepressants can cause withdrawal symptoms if stopped abruptly; generally withdraw gradually over 4 weeks
- at usual doses, one SSRI can be directly substituted for another without cross-tapering or a washout period. **Mirtazapine** 15mg can be directly substituted for SSRIs (**fluoxetine**, **citalopram** or **paroxetine** 20mg; **sertraline** 50mg)
- taper higher SSRI doses before switching
- switching to or from TCAs and MAOIs requires additional care — seek advice or see reference texts.[92]

continued

PCF preferred antidepressants

First-line
Psychostimulant, e.g. methylphenidate
Particularly if prognosis <2–4 weeks:
- start with 2.5–5mg b.d. (on waking/breakfast time and noon/lunchtime)
- if necessary, increase by daily increments of 2.5mg b.d. to 20mg b.d.
- occasionally higher doses are necessary, e.g. 30mg b.d. or 20mg t.d.s.

SSRI, e.g. sertraline or citalopram
Particularly if prognosis >2–4 weeks, and if associated anxiety:
- no antimuscarinic effects, but may cause an initial increase in anxiety
- if necessary prescribe diazepam at bedtime
- start with sertraline 50mg or citalopram 10mg once daily, increasing the latter to 20mg after 1 week
- if no improvement after 4 weeks, or only a partial improvement after 6–8 weeks, either:
  - ▹ increase dose by sertraline 50mg or citalopram 10mg *or*
  - ▹ switch to a second-line antidepressant
- maximum daily dose sertraline 200mg or citalopram 60mg
- low likelihood of a withdrawal (discontinuation) syndrome.

Second-line
Alternative SSRI, e.g. sertraline or citalopram
Dose as above.

Mirtazapine
Acts on receptors; it is not a MARI. A good choice for patients with anxiety/agitation:
- start with 15mg at bedtime
- if little or no improvement after 2 weeks, increase to 30mg at bedtime
- concurrent H_1-receptor antagonism leads to sedation but this decreases at the higher dose because of noradrenergic effects
- fewer undesirable effects than TCAs.

If no response after 4 weeks, consider third-line options.

Third-line options
- seek advice from a psychiatrist
- dose escalation
- switch antidepressant
- combine an SSRI with mirtazapine, olanzapine or quetiapine.

AMITRIPTYLINE BNF 4.3.1

Class: Serotonin and noradrenaline (norepinephrine) re-uptake inhibitor (SNRI), tricyclic antidepressant (TCA).

Indications: Depression, anxiety and panic disorders, †neuropathic pain, †urgency and urge incontinence, †sweating, †bladder spasm, †pathological laughing and crying, †drooling and sialorrhoea.

Contra-indications: Concurrent administration with an MAOI (see Serotonin toxicity, p.177), recent myocardial infarction, arrhythmias (particularly any degree of heart block), mania, severe hepatic impairment.

Pharmacology

Amitriptyline blocks the presynaptic re-uptake of serotonin and noradrenaline (norepinephrine), and thereby exerts antidepressant and analgesic effects. In addition, it antagonizes muscarinic, $5HT_{2A}$, $5HT_{2C}$, H_1, and α_1-adrenergic receptors.[1] It is these features which account for many of amitriptyline's properties, e.g. antimuscarinic effects (see p.5), drowsiness, and postural hypotension. Sodium channel blockade and NMDA-glutamate-receptor antagonism may also contribute to its analgesic efficacy.[2] Its sedative effect manifests immediately, and improved sleep is often the first benefit of therapy. The analgesic effect may manifest after 3–7 days, whereas the antidepressant effect may not be apparent for ≥2 weeks.

Amitriptyline (and **imipramine** to a lesser extent) has long been regarded as the main reference TCA, the 'gold standard' against which newer antidepressants are evaluated. Although some authorities consider it is still unsurpassed as an antidepressant,[3] meta-analysis shows only a 3% efficacy advantage over SSRIs, and this is more than offset by its disadvantages in terms of undesirable effects.[3,4] Consequently, amitriptyline is generally reserved for severe unresponsive depression.

TCAs are widely used in the management of neuropathic pain and tension headaches (see p.281). The majority of RCTs evaluated amitriptyline, although **nortriptyline** was better tolerated.[5] **Gabapentin** appears better tolerated than TCAs, but is more expensive, a greater tablet burden, and no more effective.[6,7]

A dose-response relationship has been shown for the analgesic effect of amitriptyline,[8] and there appears to be a 'therapeutic window' in some patients.[8] Patients with post-herpetic neuralgia or painful diabetic neuropathy had good relief with amitriptyline 20–100mg (median 50mg). With this dose the pain was reduced from severe to mild. When the dose was increased, the pain became severe again and, when decreased, the pain became mild again. However, some patients appear to benefit from higher doses.

Amitriptyline frequently causes increased appetite and weight gain; this is sometimes desirable in palliative care.

Bio-availability 45%.[9]
Onset of action 2–4 weeks; <1 week in neuropathic pain.[10]
Time to peak plasma concentration 4h PO; 24–48h IM.
Plasma halflife 13–36h; active metabolite nortriptyline 15–39h.
Duration of action 24h, situation dependent.

Cautions

Suicide risk: the possibility of a suicide attempt is inherent in major depression and persists until remission. Antidepressants may themselves cause suicidal ideation, particularly in those aged ≤25 years (see p.175).

Bipolar disorder (can transform into manic phase); epilepsy (lowers seizure threshold); cardiac disease (risk of arrhythmia); hepatic impairment (reduce dose or avoid); urinary hesitancy and narrow-angle glaucoma (antimuscarinic).

Drug interactions

Amitriptyline is metabolized by several hepatic enzymes including CYP2D6. Use with caution in patients thought or known to be 'poor metabolizers' and in patients taking other medications known to be metabolized by CYP2D6, e.g. antipsychotics, **carbamazepine**, **cimetidine**,

clarithromycin, **erythromycin**, **fluconazole**, **fluoxetine**, **gatifloxacin**, **moxifloxacin**, **paroxetine**, **phenytoin**, **quinidine**, **St John's wort**, **sulfamethoxazole**, **tramadol**, **warfarin** (see Cytochrome P450, p.735).

Undesirable effects

Antimuscarinic effects (see p.5), sedation, delirium, postural hypotension, hyponatraemia. The use of amitriptyline in the elderly is associated with a doubling of the incidence of femoral fractures.[11]

Dose and use

Because of the potential for undesirable effects, low doses should be used initially, particularly in the frail elderly.

Amitriptyline can be given as a single dose at bedtime for all indications. If a patient experiences early morning drowsiness, or takes a long time to settle at night, amitriptyline should be taken 2h before bedtime.

Avoid abrupt withdrawal after prolonged use (see Stopping antidepressants, p.183).

A small number of patients are stimulated by amitriptyline and experience insomnia, unpleasant vivid dreams, myoclonus and physical restlessness. In these patients, administer in the morning or change to an SSRI.

Neuropathic pain

- start with 10mg at bedtime
- if tolerated, increase to 25mg after 3–7 days
- if necessary, increase by 25mg every 1–2 weeks
- if successive increases are well tolerated *and bring additional benefit*, increase up to a maximum of 150mg at bedtime (seldom required)
- if helpful but poorly tolerated, consider switching to **nortriptyline**; if dose ≤100mg give the same dose without cross-tapering or a washout period (see p.191)
- if no response, switch to an anti-epileptic (see p.237).

Urgency and urge incontinence, sweating, bladder spasm, drooling and sialorrhoea

Dose as for neuropathic pain. The benefit is from the antimuscarinic action of amitriptyline (and switching to **nortriptyline** would be unhelpful).

Depression, anxiety and panic disorders, †pathological laughing and crying

Amitriptyline is now used less commonly (see pp.180–182). The dose is gradually increased as for neuropathic pain. In depression, 75–100mg at bedtime is generally as effective as higher doses, and better tolerated.[12] However, occasionally 150–225mg/24h may be required.

Supply

Amitriptyline (generic)

Tablets 10mg, 25mg, 50mg, 28 days @ 50mg at bedtime = £1.

Oral solution 25mg/5mL, 50mg/5mL, 28 days @ 50mg at bedtime = £16.

1 NIMH (National Institute of Mental Health) (2006) National Institute of Mental Health's Psychoactive Drug Screening Program. University of North Carolina. Available from: http://pdsp.med.unc.edu/indexR.html
2 McCleane G (2008) Antidepressants as analgesics. *CNS Drugs*. **22**: 139–156.
3 Barbui C and Hotopf M (2001) Amitriptyline v. the rest: still the leading antidepressant after 40 years of randomised controlled trials. *British Journal of Psychiatry*. **178**: 129–144.
4 Thompson C (2001) Amitriptyline: still efficacious, but at what cost? *British Journal of Psychiatry*. **178**: 99–100.
5 Watson CP *et al.* (1998) Nortriptyline versus amitriptyline in postherpetic neuralgia: a randomized trial. *Neurology*. **51**: 1166–1171.
6 Morello C *et al.* (1999) Randomized double-blind study comparing the efficacy of gabapentin with amitriptyline on diabetic peripheral neuropathy pain. *Archives of Internal Medicine*. **159**: 1931–1937.
7 Chandra K *et al.* (2006) Gabapentin versus nortriptyline in post-herpetic neuralgia patients: a randomized, double-blind clinical trial–the GONIP Trial. *International Journal of Clinical Pharmacology and Therapeutics*. **44**: 358–363.
8 Watson C (1984) Therapeutic window for amitriptyline analgesia. *Canadian Medical Association Journal*. **130**: 105–106.
9 Schulz P *et al.* (1985) Discrepancies between pharmacokinetic studies of amitriptyline. *Clinical Pharmacokinetics*. **10**: 257–268.
10 Sindrup SH *et al.* (2005) Antidepressants in the treatment of neuropathic pain. *Basic and Clinical Pharmacology and Toxicology*. **96**: 399–409.
11 Ray WA *et al.* (1987) Psychotropic drug use and the risk of hip fracture. *New England Journal of Medicine*. **316**: 363–369.
12 Furukawa (2009) Low dosage tricyclic antidepressants for depression. *Cochrane Database of Systematic Reviews*.

NORTRIPTYLINE BNF 4.3.1

Class: Noradrenaline (norepinephrine) re-uptake inhibitor (NRI), tricyclic antidepressant (TCA).

Indications: Depression, †neuropathic pain, †pathological laughing and crying.

Contra-indications: Should not be given with an MAOI or within 2 weeks of its cessation (see p.177). Avoid in initial recovery period after an acute myocardial infarction.

Pharmacology

Nortriptyline blocks the presynaptic re-uptake of noradrenaline (norepinephrine), but not of serotonin. In addition, it antagonizes $5HT_{2A}$, $5HT_{2C}$, H_1, and α_1-adrenergic receptors.[1] It is the principal active metabolite of **amitriptyline** (see p.189) but is less antimuscarinic and not so sedating. Nortriptyline undergoes extensive first-pass metabolism to 10-hydroxynortriptyline, which is active.[2]

Overall, nortriptyline is as effective as **amitriptyline**.[3] Although nortriptyline appears to have a therapeutic window at plasma concentrations of 50–150nanogram/mL,[4,5] the dose is generally determined by the clinical response. However, the manufacturer recommends plasma monitoring in patients who are prescribed >100mg/day. Like **amitriptyline**, it generally takes several weeks for the antidepressant effect to manifest. Given the long plasma halflife of nortriptyline, once daily administration is possible, generally at bedtime. However, nortriptyline has both stimulant and sedative properties and, if it disturbs sleep, it should be taken in the morning.

Bio-availability 60%.
Onset of action 2–6 weeks.
Time to peak plasma concentration 7–8.5h.
Plasma halflife 15–39h.
Duration of action variable, possibly several days.

Cautions

Suicide risk: the possibility of a suicide attempt is inherent in major depression and persists until remission. Antidepressants may themselves cause suicidal ideation, particularly in those aged ≤25 years (see p.175).

Bipolar disorder (can transform into manic phase); epilepsy (lowers seizure threshold); cardiac disease (risk of arrhythmia); hepatic impairment (reduce dose or avoid); urinary hesitancy and narrow-angle glaucoma (antimuscarinic).

Drug interactions

Nortriptyline is metabolized by CYP2D6. Use with caution in patients thought or known to be 'poor metabolizers' and in patients taking other medications known to be metabolized by CYP2D6, e.g. antipsychotics, **carbamazepine**, **cimetidine**, **clarithromycin**, **erythromycin**, **fluconazole**, **fluoxetine**, **gatifloxacin**, **moxifloxacin**, **paroxetine**, **phenytoin**, **quinidine**, **St John's wort**, **sulfamethoxazole**, **tramadol**, **warfarin** (see Cytochrome P450, p.735).

Undesirable effects

Very common (>10%): antimuscarinic effects (see p.5), anorexia, nausea, drowsiness, fatigue, weight gain.
Very rare (<0.01%): arrhythmias, AV conduction changes, heart block.

Dose and use

See general advice for **amitriptyline**, p.189.
If stimulation outweighs sedation and sleep is disturbed, administer in the morning. The manufacturer advises monitoring the plasma concentration if the daily dose is ≥100mg.

Avoid abrupt withdrawal after prolonged use (see Stopping antidepressants, p.183).

Depression
- start with 25mg at bedtime
- if necessary, increase the dose by 25mg every 2–4 weeks up to 150mg/day
- if no response with 150mg after 4 weeks, switch to an alternative antidepressant
- if effective, continue on the same dose until the patient has been symptom-free for 6–12 months; after this, discontinue over 2–8 weeks.

†*Neuropathic pain*
- start with 10–25mg at bedtime
- increase by 10mg/day every 3–5 days up to 50mg, or double dose from 25mg to 50mg after 2 weeks[6]
- if successive increases are well tolerated *and result in additional benefit*, increase further to a maximum of 150mg daily (seldom required).

Supply
Allegron® (King)
Tablets 10mg, 25mg, 28 days @ 50mg at bedtime = £13.

1 NIMH (National Institute of Mental Health) (2006) National Institute of Mental Health's Psychoactive Drug Screening Program. University of North Carolina. Available from: http://pdsp.med.unc.edu/indexR.html
2 Nordin C and Bertilsson L (1995) Active hydroxymetabolites of antidepressants. Emphasis on E-10-hydroxy-nortriptyline. *Clinical Pharmacokinetics*. **28**: 26–40.
3 Barbui C and Hotopf M (2001) Amitriptyline v. the rest: still the leading antidepressant after 40 years of randomised controlled trials. *British Journal of Psychiatry*. **178**: 129–144.
4 APA (American Psychiatric Association) (1985) Task Force on the Use of Laboratory Tests in Psychiatry: Tricyclic antidepressants-blood level measurements and clinical outcome. *American Journal of Psychiatry*. **142**: 155–162.
5 Perry PJ (1984) The relationship of free nortriptyline levels to antidepressant response. *Drug Intelligence and Clinical Pharmacy*. **18**: 510.
6 Watson CP *et al*. (1998) Nortriptyline versus amitriptyline in postherpetic neuralgia: a randomized trial. *Neurology*. **51**: 1166–1171.

SELECTIVE SEROTONIN RE-UPTAKE INHIBITORS — BNF 4.3.3

Class: Antidepressant.

Indications: Depression, anxiety and panic disorders, †pruritus, †pathological laughing and crying.

Contra-indications: Concurrent administration with an MAOI (see p.177); mania.

Pharmacology
SSRIs inhibit the serotonin re-uptake transporter. They differ in their propensity for drug interactions, discontinuation reactions and cost (see Supply). They also have varying additional actions that may partly explain why some individuals respond to switching between them (Table 4.15).

In palliative care, **citalopram** or **sertraline** are generally the SSRIs of choice, combining a low risk of drug interactions and discontinuation reactions. They are first-line treatments for depression (see p.180), anxiety and panic disorders (see p.182), and pathological laughter and crying (see p.182).

Two small RCTs suggest benefit in pruritus within a few days from **sertraline** (cholestatic pruritus)[6] and **paroxetine** (pruritus of mixed cause in cancer patients).[7] Benefit is also reported in pruritus associated with polycythaemia vera.[8]

Although SSRIs are modestly effective for neuropathic pain (3 of 4 RCTs),[9–12] they are inferior to **imipramine**.[12] A TCA (e.g. **imipramine**, **amitriptyline**, **nortriptyline**) or an anti-epileptic is preferable (see p.180).

Escitalopram is the *S*-enantiomer of **citalopram**. ***R*-citalopram** does not inhibit the serotonin re-uptake transporter but may hinder the binding of **S-citalopram**. Some fixed-dose comparisons do find a marginally higher response rate with **escitalopram** 10mg vs. **citalopram** 20mg,[13] but titrating **citalopram** might be expected to achieve the same result at lower cost.

For pharmacokinetic details, see Table 4.16.

Table 4.15 Differences between SSRIs[1–5]

Drug	*Additional actions*	*Hepatic enzyme inhibition*					*Discontinuation reaction risk*[a]
		CYP1A2	*CYP2C9*	*CYP2C19*	*CYP2D6*	*CYP3A4*	
Citalopram	H_1 antagonist (*R*-enantiomer)				+		Low
Escitalopram	None				+		Low
Fluoxetine	$5HT_{2C}$ antagonist[b]		++	++	+++	+	Minimal
Fluvoxamine	Sigma-1 agonist[c]	+++		+++		++	Moderate
Paroxetine	Noradrenaline (norepinephrine) re-uptake inhibitor[b]				+++		High
Sertraline	Dopamine re-uptake inhibitor[b]				+		Low

Key: + = weak inhibition; ++ = moderate inhibition; +++ = marked inhibition (also see p.735).
a. approximates to halflife (see Table 4.16)
b. these actions theoretically contribute to their antidepressant effects (see p.172) but the affinity, and overall contribution of these additional actions is much less than the predominant serotonin re-uptake inhibition
c. the action of sigma-1 receptors is poorly defined, but sigma-1 receptor agonists may have antidepressant, pro-seizure, euphoric and/or dysphoric effects.

Table 4.16 Pharmacokinetic details for selected SSRIs[13–15]

Drug	*Bio-availability PO (%)*	T_{max} *(h)*	*Plasma halflife*	*Metabolism*
Citalopram	80[a]	3	36h	Multiple pathways[b]
Escitalopram	80[c]	4	30h	Multiple pathways[b]
Fluoxetine	90	4–8	1–4 days; 1–2 *weeks*[b]	Multiple pathways[b]
Paroxetine	50[d]	5	15–20h	Multiple pathways
Sertraline	>44	6–8	26h	CYP3A4

a. for tablets; bio-availability of drops is nearly 100%
b. active metabolite(s)
c. the bio-availability of tablets and oral solution is comparable
d. increases with multiple dosing.

Cautions

Suicide risk: the possibility of a suicide attempt is inherent in major depression and persists until remission. Antidepressants may themselves cause suicidal ideation, particularly in those aged ≤25 years (see p.175).

Bipolar disorder (can transform into manic phase). Epilepsy (may lower seizure threshold but less than other antidepressants; ***citalopram*** *generally preferred because it lacks significant interactions with anti-epileptics*).

QT prolongation risk factors (see p.727); hepatic impairment (reduce dose or avoid); renal impairment; diabetes mellitus (reduced hypoglycaemic awareness); peptic ulceration or bleeding disorders (SSRIs increase the risk of GI bleeding,[16] particularly in those aged >80 years[17]).

Drug interactions

SSRIs should not be started until 2 weeks after stopping an MAOI.

Additive pharmacodynamic interactions include serotonin toxicity (see p.177), bleeding risk (see p.178), and QT prolongation (particularly **citalopram** and **escitalopram**, see p.727).

Potentially serious interactions with **fluoxetine**, **fluvoxamine** and **paroxetine** result from their inhibition of hepatic metabolism (see Table 4.15 and p.735). **Citalopram**, **escitalopram** and **sertraline** rarely require dose reduction with other enzyme inhibitors (e.g. **cimetidine**, **omeprazole**); consider only if symptoms of toxicity occur.[2,5]

Undesirable effects

Frequencies based on **sertaline** and **citalopram**.

Very common (>10%): somnolence, insomnia, dizziness, headache, dry mouth, nausea, diarrhoea, sweating.

Common (<10%, >1%): agitation, anxiety, nervousness, confusion, tremor, tinnitus, yawning, fatigue, dizziness, paraesthesia, bruxism (teeth grinding), palpitations, altered taste, decreased appetite, vomiting, sexual dysfunction, myalgia, arthralgia, pruritus.

Uncommon (<1%, >0.1%): aggression, depersonalization, hallucinations, mania.

Rare (<0.01%) or unknown incidence: psychosis, hyponatraemia, seizures, movement disorders (e.g. dyskinesia), hepatitis, suicidal ideation (see above), haemorrhage.

The manufacturer reports myocardial infarction as a rare consequence of taking **sertraline**. However, this would be expected in antidepressant RCTs because depression is an independent risk factor for myocardial infarction. Case control studies suggest that SSRIs confer a protective effect,[18] possibly because they impact negatively on platelet aggregation (see p.178). **Sertraline** has been used safely in patients with unstable angina, and after myocardial infarction.[19]

Dose and use

Treatment should not be discontinued abruptly (see p.183).

Sertraline (depression, anxiety and panic)

- if anxiety/panic symptoms are prominent, start with 25mg each morning and increase to 50mg each morning after 1 week
- otherwise, start with 50mg each morning; if necessary, increase to 100mg after 2–4 weeks
- if no response after 4 weeks, or only a partial response after 6–8 weeks, consider further increases to a maximum of 200mg or an alternative (see p.180)
- if effective, continue until the patient has been symptom-free for ⩾6 months (see p.181); after this, discontinue over 2–4 weeks.

Citalopram (depression, anxiety and panic)

- start with 10mg each morning and increase to 20mg each morning after 1 week
- if no response after 4 weeks, or only a partial response after 6–8 weeks, consider further increases to a maximum of 40mg or switch to an alternative (see p.180)
- restrict maximum dose to 20mg in those over 60, hepatic impairment, or with inhibitors of CYP2D6
- if effective, continue until the patient has been symptom-free for ⩾6 months (see p.181); after this, discontinue over 2–4 weeks.

Other indications

- **cholestatic pruritus**
  - ▹ start with **sertraline** 25mg each morning; if necessary, increase in 25mg increments
  - ▹ doses above 100mg rarely give additional relief[6]
- **pathological laughter and crying** often responds to lower doses[20]
  - ▹ start with **citalopram** 5mg each morning; if necessary, increase in 5–10mg increments to a maximum of 40mg each morning *or*
  - ▹ start with **sertraline** 12.5mg each morning; if necessary, increase in 12.5–25mg increments to a maximum of 200mg each morning.

Supply

Citalopram (generic)
Tablets (as *hydrobromide*) 10mg, 20mg, 40mg, 28 days @ 20mg each morning = £1.50.
Oral liquid drops (as hydrochloride) 40mg/mL, 28 days @ 16mg (8 drops) each morning = £13; *16mg as drops is equivalent to 20mg as tablets. Mix with water, orange juice or apple juice before taking.*

Cipramil® (Lundbeck)
Tablets (as *hydrobromide*) 10mg, 20mg, 40mg, 28 days @ 20mg each morning = £9.
Oral liquid drops (as *hydrochloride*) 40mg/mL, 28 days @ 16mg (8 drops) each morning = £8 (note: based on BNF pricing, this is *cheaper* than generic drops); *16mg as drops is equivalent to 20mg as tablets. Mix with water, orange juice or apple juice before taking.*

Sertraline (generic)
Tablets 50mg, 100mg, 28 days @ 50mg each morning = £1.

Lustral® (Pfizer)
Tablets 50mg (scored), 100mg, 28 days @ 50mg each morning = £18.

1 Hashimoto K (2009) Sigma-1 receptors and selective serotonin reuptake inhibitors: clinical implications of their relationship. *Central Nervous System Agents in Medicinal Chemistry.* **9**: 197–204.
2 Rao N (2007) The clinical pharmacokinetics of escitalopram. *Clinical Pharmacokinetics.* **46**: 281–290.
3 Carrasco JL and Sandner C (2005) Clinical effects of pharmacological variations in selective serotonin reuptake inhibitors: an overview. *International Journal of Clinical Practice.* **59**: 1428–1434.
4 Haddad PM (2001) Antidepressant discontinuation syndromes: Clinical relevance, prevention and management. *Drug Safety.* **24**: 183–197.
5 Preskorn SH (1997) Clinically relevant pharmacology of selective serotonin reuptake inhibitors. An overview with emphasis on pharmacokinetics and effects on oxidative drug metabolism. *Clinical Pharmacokinetics.* **32 (suppl 1)**: 1–21.
6 Mayo MJ *et al.* (2007) Sertraline as a first-line treatment for cholestatic pruritus. *Hepatology.* **45**: 666–674.
7 Zylicz Z *et al.* (2003) Paroxetine in the treatment of severe non-dermatological pruritus: a randomized, controlled trial. *Journal of Pain and Symptom Management.* **26**: 1105–1112.
8 Tefferi A and Fonseca R (2002) Selective serotonin reuptake inhibitors are effective in the treatment of polycythemia vera-associated pruritus. *Blood.* **99**: 2627.
9 Otto M *et al.* (2008) Escitalopram in painful polyneuropathy: a randomized, placebo-controlled, cross-over trial. *Pain.* **139**: 275–283.
10 Max M *et al.* (1992) Effects of desipramine, amitriptyline, and fluoxetine on pain in diabetic neuropathy. *New England Journal of Medicine.* **326**: 1287–1288.
11 Sindrup SH *et al.* (1992) The selective serotonin reuptake inhibitor citalopram relieves the symptoms of diabetic neuropathy. *Clinical Pharmacology and Therapeutics.* **52**: 547–552.
12 Sindrup S *et al.* (1990) The selective serotonin re-uptake inhibitor paroxetine is effective in the treatment of diabetic neuropathy symptoms. *Pain.* **42**: 135–144.
13 Garnock-Jones KP and McCormack PL (2010) Escitalopram: a review of its use in the management of major depressive disorder in adults. *CNS Drugs.* **24**: 769–796.
14 Hiemke (2000) Pharmacokinetics of selective serotonin reuptake inhibitors. *Pharmacology and Therapeutics.* **85**: 11–28.
15 Kaye CM *et al.* (1989) A review of the metabolism and pharmacokinetics of paroxetine in man. *Acta Psychiatr Scand Suppl.* **350**: 60–75.
16 Paton C and Ferrier IN (2005) SSRIs and gastrointestinal bleeding. *British Medical Journal.* **331**: 529–530.
17 vanWalraven C *et al.* (2001) Inhibition of serotonin reuptake by antidepressants and upper gastrointestinal bleeding in elderly patients: retrospective cohort study. *British Medical Journal.* **323**: 655–657.
18 Sauer WH *et al.* (2001) Selective serotonin reuptake inhibitors and myocardial infarction. *Circulation.* **104**: 1894–1898.
19 Glassman AH *et al.* (2002) Sertraline treatment of major depression in patients with acute MI or unstable angina. *Journal of the American Medical Association.* **288**: 701–709.
20 Wortzel HS *et al.* (2008) Pathological laughing and crying: epidemiology, pathophysiology and treatment. *CNS Drugs.* **22**: 531–545.

*VENLAFAXINE — BNF 4.3.4

Class: Antidepressant; serotonin and noradrenaline (norepinephrine) re-uptake inhibitor (SNRI).

Indications: Depression, anxiety and panic disorders, †neuropathic pain, †hot flushes.

Contra-indications: Concurrent use with an MAOI or within 2 weeks of previous treatment with an MAOI (see Serotonin toxicity, p.177). Uncontrolled hypertension, high risk for ventricular arrhythmia.[1]

Pharmacology

In vivo studies confirm that venlafaxine inhibits serotonin and noradrenaline (norepinephrine) re-uptake transporters, despite *in vitro* studies suggesting a relatively low affinity.[2] *In vitro* assays measure the ability of a drug to displace another compound of known affinity; it is thus possible that venlafaxine binds to a different site on the transporters and so cannot displace the reference compounds.[3] Inhibition of noradrenaline (norepinephrine) re-uptake increases with higher doses.[4] This also inhibits dopamine re-uptake in the prefrontal cortex (where, in the absence of dopamine re-uptake transporters, dopamine is cleared by noradrenaline (norepinephrine) re-uptake transporters). Venlafaxine has little or no post-synaptic antagonistic effects at muscarinic, α-adrenergic, $5HT_{2A}$, $5HT_{2C}$ or H_1-receptors.

Venlafaxine is generally reserved for the treatment of depression refractory to SSRIs. As a second-line treatment, it is marginally more effective than switching to an alternative SSRI, but less well tolerated (see p.180).[5–7]

Venlafaxine has been shown to have an antinociceptive effect in animals.[8,9] Case reports and case series suggest that venlafaxine relieves several types of chronic pain, e.g. headache, fibromyalgia and neuropathic pain.[10] Benefit in diabetic neuropathy and in a mixed group of patients has been confirmed in RCTs.[11,12] In another RCT (n = 13), benefit appeared to be positively correlated with the plasma concentration of venlafaxine.[13] In an RCT of **imipramine** 75mg daily vs. venlafaxine 112.5mg daily, the two antidepressants were equally effective and both were significantly better than placebo.[14] Dry mouth was more common with **imipramine**, and tiredness more common with venlafaxine.

Venlafaxine is also of benefit in hot flushes associated with the menopause or hormone therapy,[15,16] including androgen ablation therapy for prostate cancer.[17] This is not a specific effect of venlafaxine; SSRIs seem to share this property, e.g. **paroxetine** and **fluoxetine**.[18,19] Venlafaxine is metabolized to a pharmacologically active metabolite, O-desmethylvenlafaxine (ODV), which has a similar pharmacodynamic profile.

Bio-availability 13%; 45% m/r.
Onset of action >2 weeks for depression.
Time to peak plasma concentration about 2.5h; 4.5–7.5h m/r and 6.5–11h ODV m/r.
Plasma halflife 5h; 11h for ODV.
Duration of effect 12–24h, situation dependent.

Cautions

Suicide risk: the possibility of a suicide attempt is inherent in major depression and persists until remission. Antidepressants may themselves cause suicidal ideation, particularly in those aged ≤25 years (see p.175). The risk appears to be greater with venlafaxine than with SSRIs and TCAs, but this may be because patients prescribed venlafaxine (generally not a first-line antidepressant) may already be at greater risk of suicide.[1,20,21]

For patients with risk factors for suicide, the MHRA advises that a maximum of 2 week's supply should be dispensed at a time to reduce the risk from overdose.[1]

Bipolar disorder (can transform into manic phase); epilepsy (lowers seizure threshold); cardiac disease (risk of hypertension and arrhythmia); mild–moderate hepatic impairment (reduce dose); renal impairment (reduce dose); narrow-angle glaucoma (mydriasis reported).

Drug interactions

Concurrent use with drugs which inhibit either CYP2D6 or CYP3A4 may result in higher plasma concentrations (see Cytochrome P450, p.735), and should generally be avoided in order to prevent clinically important interactions in poor metabolizers.[1]

May increase concurrent **haloperidol** plasma concentrations (up to 70% increase in AUC and a possible doubling of the maximum plasma concentration). The dose of **warfarin** may need to be reduced.

Undesirable effects

Very common (>10%): dizziness, dry mouth, insomnia, nervousness, drowsiness, constipation, nausea, abnormal ejaculation/orgasm, asthenia, headache, sweating.
Common (<10%, >1%): agitation, confusion, hypertonia, paraesthesia, tremor, dyspnoea, hypertension, palpitations, postural hypotension, vasodilation, anorexia, diarrhoea, dyspepsia, vomiting, urinary frequency, ecchymosis, decreased libido, impotence, menstrual disorders, arthralgia, myalgia, weight gain/loss, abdominal pain, abnormal dreams, chills, pyrexia, pruritus, rash, abnormal vision/accommodation, mydriasis, tinnitus.
Uncommon (<1%): hallucinations, urinary retention, muscle spasm, hyponatraemia, increased liver enzymes, angioedema, maculopapular eruptions, urticaria.

Dose and use

Because of concerns about its tolerability and safety in overdose, venlafaxine should not be used as a first-line antidepressant.[1,5,22] Specialist supervision required if a dose of ⩾300mg is necessary in severely depressed or hospitalized patients.[1]

Best taken with or after food. If moderate renal or mild–moderate hepatic impairment, reduce the dose by 50% and give once daily.

Monitor blood pressure: consider dose reduction or discontinuation in those who show a sustained increase.[1]

Avoid abrupt withdrawal after prolonged use (see Stopping antidepressants, p.183). If ⩾75mg/day have been taken for > 1 week, taper over at least 1 week; if ⩾150mg/day have been taken for >6 weeks, taper over at least 2 weeks.

Depression

Venlafaxine is reserved for depression refractory to other antidepressants (see p.180)
- generally start with 75mg m/r once daily (the time of day is immaterial, although it should be constant for an individual)
- in frail or elderly patients, start with 37.5mg once daily for 4–7 days
- if necessary, increase the dose progressively in 75mg increments every 2 weeks
- a once daily dose of 225mg is generally sufficient for moderately depressed outpatients
- in severely depressed inpatients, higher once daily doses may be indicated, e.g. ⩽375mg
- if effective, continue until the patient has been symptom-free for ⩾6 months (see p.180); after this, discontinue over 2–4 weeks.

Anxiety and panic

Venlafaxine is reserved for anxiety or panic disorders refractory to other antidepressants (see p.182).
- 75mg m/r once daily.

Neuropathic pain and hot flushes

Venlafaxine is not a first-line treatment for neuropathic pain (see p.180)
- start with 37.5mg m/r once daily
- increase to 75mg m/r once daily after 1 week
- if necessary, increase to 150mg once daily after a further 2 weeks.

Supply

Venlafaxine (generic)
Tablets 37.5mg, 75mg, 28 days @ 75mg b.d. = £5.

Modified-release
Effexor® XL (Wyeth)
Capsules m/r 75mg, 150mg, 28 days @ 150mg once daily = £38.

1 Duff G (2006) Updated prescribing advice for venlafaxine (Efexor/Effexor XL). Letter from the chairman of the Commission on Human Medicines, 31st May 2006. Available from: www.mhra.gov.uk/Safetyinformation/Safetywarningsalertsandrecalls/Safetywarningsandmessagesformedicines/CON2023846
2 Bymaster FP *et al.* (2001) Comparative affinity of duloxetine and venlafaxine for serotonin and norepinephrine transporters in vitro and in vivo, human serotonin receptor subtypes, and other neuronal receptors. *Neuropsychopharmacology.* **25**: 871–880.
3 Beique JC *et al.* (1998) Affinities of venlafaxine and various reuptake inhibitors for the serotonin and norepinephrine transporters. *European Journal of Pharmacology.* **349**: 129–132.
4 Melichar J *et al.* (2001) Venlafaxine occupation at the noradrenaline reuptake site: in-vivo determination in healthy volunteers. *Journal of Psychopharmacology.* **15**: 9–12.
5 NICE (2009) Clinical Guidleline 90 and 91. Depression. Available from: www.nice.org.uk
6 Ruhe HG *et al.* (2006) Switching antidepressants after a first selective serotonin reuptake inhibitor in major depressive disorder: a systematic review. *Journal of Clinical Psychiatry.* **67**: 1836–1855.
7 Anderson IM *et al.* (2008) Evidence-based guidelines for treating depressive disorders with antidepressants: a revision of the 2000 British Association for Psychopharmacology guidelines. *Journal of Psychopharmacology.* **22**: 343–396.
8 Lang E *et al.* (1996) Venlafaxine hydrochloride (Effexor) relieves thermal hyperalgesia in rats with an experimental mononeuropathy. *Pain.* **68**: 151–155.
9 Schreiber S *et al.* (1999) The antinociceptive effect of venlafaxine in mice is mediated through opioid and adrenergic mechanisms. *Neuroscience Letters.* **273**: 85–88.
10 Grothe DR *et al.* (2004) Treatment of pain syndromes with venlafaxine. *Pharmacotherapy.* **24**: 621–629.
11 Kunz N *et al.* (2000) Diabetic neuropathic pain management with venlafaxine XR. In: *CINP* July.
12 Yucel A *et al.* (2005) The effect of venlafaxine on ongoing and experimentally induced pain in neuropathic pain patients: a double blind, placebo controlled study. *European Journal of Pain.* **9**: 407–416.
13 Tasmuth T *et al.* (2002) Venlafaxine in neuropathic pain following treatment of breast cancer. *European Journal of Pain.* **6**: 17–24.
14 Sindrup SH *et al.* (2003) Venlafaxine versus imipramine in painful polyneuropathy: a randomized, controlled trial. *Neurology.* **60**: 1284–1289.
15 Barlow D (2000) Venlafaxine for hot flushes. *Lancet.* **356**: 2025–2026.
16 Loprinzi C *et al.* (2000) Venlafaxine in management of hot flashes in survivors of breast cancer: a randomised controlled trial. *Lancet.* **356**: 2059–2063.
17 Quella S *et al.* (1999) Pilot evaluation of venlafaxine for the treatment of hot flashes in men undergoing androgen ablation therapy for prostate cancer. *Journal of Urology.* **162**: 98–102.
18 Stearns V *et al.* (1997) A pilot trial assessing the efficacy of paroxetine hydrochloride (Paxil) in controlling hot flashes. *Breast Cancer Research Treatment.* **46**: 23–33.
19 Loprinzi C *et al.* (1999) Preliminary data from a randomized evaluation of fluoxetine (Prozac) for treating hot flashes in breast cancer survivors. *Breast Cancer Research Treatment.* **57**: 34.
20 Cipriani A *et al.* (2007) Venlafaxine for major depression. *British Medical Journal.* **334**: 215–216.
21 Rubino A *et al.* (2007) Risk of suicide during treatment with venlafaxine, citalopram, fluoxetine, and dothiepin: retrospective cohort study. *British Medical Journal.* **334**: 242.
22 Buckley NA and McManus PR (2002) Fatal toxicity of serotoninergic and other antidepressant drugs: analysis of United Kingdom mortality data. *British Medical Journal.* **325**: 1332–1333.

DULOXETINE — BNF 4.3.4

Class: Antidepressant, serotonin and noradrenaline (norepinephrine) re-uptake inhibitor (SNRI).

Indications: Depression (Cymbalta®), diabetic neuropathic pain (Cymbalta®), moderate–severe stress incontinence in women (Yentreve®).

Contra-indications: Concurrent use with an MAOI or within 2 weeks of previous treatment with an MAOI (see Serotonin toxicity, p.177). Concurrent use with strong CYP1A2 inhibitors, e.g. **fluvoxamine, ciprofloxacin.**[1] Uncontrolled hypertension, hepatic impairment, end-stage renal failure requiring dialysis or creatinine clearance <30mL/min.

Pharmacology

Like **venlafaxine**, duloxetine inhibits serotonin and noradrenaline (norepinephrine) re-uptake transporters, but lacks the muscarinic, α-adrenergic and H_1-receptor antagonism of **amitriptyline** and other tricyclic SNRIs.[2] Its place relative to other options for depression is unclear. In an RCT, duloxetine was less well tolerated than **venlafaxine.**[3] A meta-analysis found it to be less effective than **escitalopram**, **mirtazapine**, **sertraline** and **venlafaxine.**[4]

Duloxetine is of benefit in painful diabetic neuropathy, fibromyalgia and osteo-arthitic knee pain (NNT 6, 8 and 5.6 respectively for 50% reduction in pain scores).[5,6] Duloxetine has not been directly compared to alternatives. NICE recommends duloxetine as first-line treatment for painful diabetic neuropathy based on a cost-effectiveness model, but no clinical evidence of superiority is provided.[7] Given the comparable efficacy, tolerability and monitoring requirements of cheaper alternatives, this conclusion is clearly questionable.

Duloxetine has a limited role in stress incontinence.[8] Animal studies have shown that serotonin and noradrenaline (norepinephrine) are involved in the central neural control of micturition.[9] Serotonin agonists generally suppress parasympathetic activity and enhance sympathetic and somatic activity in the lower urinary tract, enhancing the bladder's storage capacity. Duloxetine acts through the pudendal motor nucleus in the distal cord and thus stimulates the rhabdosphincter of the urethra. This is also thought to be the mode of action on the urinary tract of peripheral α-adrenergic receptor agents, including those with an indirect action, e.g. **imipramine**. The advantage of duloxetine is that it does not cause postural hypotension or cardiac conduction abnormalities.[10]

The incidence of initial nausea with duloxetine is comparable with that seen with **fluoxetine** and **paroxetine**.[11]

Bio-availability 90%.
Onset of action 2–3 weeks in depression.[12]
Time to peak plasma concentration 6h.
Plasma halflife 12h.
Duration of action >24h, situation dependent.

Cautions

Suicide risk: the possibility of a suicide attempt is inherent in major depression and persists until remission. Antidepressants may themselves cause suicidal ideation, particularly in those aged ≤25 years (see p.175).

Bipolar disorder (can transform into manic phase); epilepsy (lowers seizure threshold); cardiac disease (risk of hypertension and arrhythmia); hepatic impairment (reduce dose); renal impairment (reduce dose); urinary hesitancy and narrow-angle glaucoma (may exacerbate).

Drug interactions

Duloxetine is metabolized by CYP1A2 and CYP2D6, and inhibits these enzymes. Plasma concentration increased by strong CYP1A2 inhibitors, e.g. **fluvoxamine**, **ciprofloxacin** (see Contra-indications) and decreased by up to 50% in smokers.

Duloxetine increases plasma concentrations of **desipramine** (not UK) and possibly other TCAs.[1]

Undesirable effects

Very common (>10%): sexual dysfunction (about 30%), nausea (20%), insomnia (20%), drowsiness (15%), dry mouth (15%), constipation (10%), sweating (10%).
Common (<10%, >1%): lightheadedness, dizziness, blurred vision, headache, altered taste, anorexia, diarrhoea.[13]

Dose and use

The timing of once daily doses is immaterial, although it should be constant for an individual.

Monitor blood pressure: consider dose reduction or discontinuation in those who show a sustained increase.

Avoid abrupt withdrawal after prolonged use (see Stopping antidepressants, p.183).

Diabetic peripheral neuropathy

- start with 60mg once daily
- if necessary, increase to 60mg b.d.
- no dose reduction is required in mild–moderate renal impairment; use is contra-indicated in severe renal impairment (creatinine clearance <30mL/min).

Depression
Duloxetine is less effective and less well tolerated than alternatives (see above). It may have a role in depression with concurrent neuropathic pain.
- 60mg once daily
- no extra benefit likely with higher doses.[14–16]

Stress incontinence in women
Moderate–severe stress incontinence is defined as ⩾14 episodes per week. In physically fit women, management is primarily non-drug, e.g. pelvic floor muscle training (sometimes followed by surgery).[8,17] If prescribing duloxetine:
- start with 20mg b.d.
- if necessary, increase to 40mg b.d. after 2 weeks.

Supply
Cymbalta® (Lilly)
Capsules enclosing e/c pellets 30mg, 60mg, 28 days @ 60mg once daily = £28.

Yentreve® (Lilly)
Capsules enclosing e/c pellets 20mg, 40mg, 28 days @ 20mg b.d. = £31.

1 Baxter K (2011) Stockley's Drug Interactions (online edition). Pharmaceutical Press, London. Available from: www.medicinescomplete.com
2 Bymaster FP *et al.* (2001) Comparative affinity of duloxetine and venlafaxine for serotonin and norepinephrine transporters in vitro and in vivo, human serotonin receptor subtypes, and other neuronal receptors. *Neuropsychopharmacology.* **25**: 871–880.
3 Perahia D *et al.* Comparing duloxetine and venlafaxine in the treatment of major depressive disorder using a global benefit-risk approach. Florida, USA: New Clinical Drug Evaluation Unit; 2005.
4 Cipriani A *et al.* (2009) Comparative efficacy and acceptability of 12 new-generation antidepressants: a multiple-treatments meta-analysis. *Lancet.* **373**: 746–758.
5 Lunn (2009) Duloxetine for treating painful neuropathy or chronic pain. *Cochrane Database of Systematic Reviews.* **4**: CD007115.
6 Chappell AS *et al.* (2009) Duloxetine, a centrally acting analgesic, in the treatment of patients with osteoarthritis knee pain: a 13-week, randomized, placebo-controlled trial. *Pain.* **146**: 253–260.
7 NICE (2009) Clinical Guidleline 90 and 91. Depression. Available from: www.nice.org.uk
8 NICE (2006) Urinary incontinence: the management of urinary incontinence in women. In: Clinical guidelines. National Institute for Health and Clinical Excellence. Available from: http://guidance.nice.org.uk/CG40
9 Norton PA *et al.* (2002) Duloxetine versus placebo in the treatment of stress urinary incontinence. *American Journal of Obstetrics and Gynecology.* **187**: 40–48.
10 Dmochowski RR *et al.* (2003) Duloxetine versus placebo for the treatment of North American women with stress urinary incontinence. *Journal of Urology.* **170**: 1259–1263.
11 Greist J *et al.* (2004) Incidence and duration of antidepressant-induced nausea: duloxetine compared with paroxetine and fluoxetine. *Clinical Therapeutics.* **26**: 1446–1455.
12 Brannan SK *et al.* (2005) Onset of action for duloxetine 60 mg once daily: double-blind, placebo-controlled studies. *Journal of Psychiatric Research.* **39**: 161–172.
13 Goldstein DJ *et al.* (2004) Duloxetine in the treatment of depression: a double-blind placebo-controlled comparison with paroxetine. *Journal of Clinical Psychopharmacology.* **24**: 389–399.
14 Detke MJ *et al.* (2004) Duloxetine in the acute and long-term treatment of major depressive disorder: a placebo- and paroxetine-controlled trial. *European Neuropsychopharmacology.* **14**: 457–470.
15 Mallinckrodt CH *et al.* (2003) Duloxetine: A New Treatment for the Emotional and Physical Symptoms of Depression. *Primary Care Companion Journal of Clinical Psychiatry.* **5**: 19–28.
16 Nemeroff CB *et al.* (2002) Duloxetine for the treatment of major depressive disorder. *Psychopharmacology Bulletin.* **36**: 106–132.
17 DTB (2003) Managing postpartum stress urinary incontinence. *Drug and Therapeutics Bulletin.* **41**: 46–48.

MIRTAZAPINE — BNF 4.3.4

Class: α_2 Adrenergic and $5HT_{2A/C}$ antagonist antidepressant.

Indications: Depression, †anxiety and panic disorders, †pruritus, †serotonin toxicity.

Contra-indications: Should not be given with an MAOI or within 2 weeks of its cessation (see Serotonin toxicity, p.177).

Pharmacology

Mirtazapine antagonises receptors which inhibit mono-amine release:[1,2]

- pre-synaptic α_2-adrenergic antagonism disinhibits serotonin and noradrenaline (norepinephrine) release
- post-synaptic $5HT_{2A}$ and $5HT_{2C}$ antagonism disinhibits noradrenaline (norepinephrine) and dopamine release.

In addition, it antagonizes H_1- and $5HT_3$-receptors. The H_1 antagonistic activity of mirtazapine is responsible for its sedative properties. At lower doses, the antihistaminic effect of mirtazapine predominates, producing sedation. With higher doses, sedation is reduced as noradrenergic neural transmission increases. It has no significant antimuscarinic activity.

The antidepressant effects of mirtazapine are equivalent to TCAs, SSRIs, **venlafaxine** and **trazodone**. A response is sometimes apparent in <1 week. Further, there are fewer relapses compared with **amitriptyline**.[3] Mirtazapine may be combined with an SSRI or **venlafaxine** for refractory depression, particularly if a previous switch of antidepressant monotherapy was unhelpful (see p.180).

Mirtazapine is not associated with cardiovascular toxicity or sexual dysfunction.[3] A blockade of $5HT_2$ leads to appetite stimulation. Its anti-emetic properties may be due to $5HT_2$ and/or $5HT_3$ antagonism.[4,5]

Benefit is reported for neuropathic pain,[6,7] intractable pruritus[8] and serotonin toxicity.[9]

Mirtazapine displays linear pharmacokinetics within the recommended dose range. Food does not affect absorption. Steady-state is reached after 3–4 days of daily administration. Binding to plasma proteins is about 85%. Mirtazapine is extensively metabolized and eliminated via the urine and faeces. Major pathways of biotransformation are demethylation and oxidation, followed by conjugation. Cytochrome P450 enzymes CYP2D6 and CYP1A2 are involved in the formation of the 8-hydroxy metabolite of mirtazapine, whereas CYP3A4 is considered to be responsible for the formation of the N-demethyl and N-oxide metabolites.[10] Clearance in the elderly may be reduced by $\leqslant 40\%$.

The demethyl metabolite is pharmacologically active and appears to have the same pharmacokinetic profile as the parent compound. Overdose produces disorientation, drowsiness, memory impairment and tachycardia.

Bio-availability 50% PO.

Onset of action hours–days (off-label indications); 1–2 weeks (antidepressant).

Time to peak plasma concentration 2h.

Plasma halflife 20–40h; often shorter in men (26h) than women (37h) but can extend up to 65h.

Duration of action variable; up to several days.

Cautions

Suicide risk: the possibility of a suicide attempt is inherent in major depression and persists until remission. Antidepressants may themselves cause suicidal ideation, particularly in those aged $\leqslant 25$ years (see p.175).

Bipolar disorder (can transform into manic phase); epilepsy (seizures occur rarely; risk relative to other antidepressants is uncertain); cardiac disease (manufacturer advises increased monitoring with ischaemic heart disease or risk of arrhythmia); hepatic impairment (reduce dose); renal impairment (reduce dose; clearance of a single oral dose halved when creatinine clearance <10mL/min); diabetes mellitus (may alter glycaemic control); narrow-angle glaucoma (mydriasis reported).

Drug interactions

Clearance doubled by hepatic enzyme inducers (e.g. **carbamazepine**, **phenytoin**); CYP3A4 inhibitors (e.g. **ketoconazole**) increase plasma levels by 40%.

Undesirable effects

Very common (>10%): increase in appetite and weight gain;[11] drowsiness during the first few weeks of treatment. *Dose reduction reduces the likelihood of an antidepressant effect and does not necessarily alleviate drowsiness.*
Uncommon (<1%, >0.1%): hepatic impairment.

Dose and use

Depression, panic and anxiety disorders[3]

- start with 15mg at bedtime
- if necessary, increase the dose by 15mg every 2 weeks up to 45mg
- if no response after 4 weeks on 45mg, switch to an alternative antidepressant
- if effective, continue until the patient has been symptom-free for ≥6 months (see p.180); then discontinue over 2–4 weeks.

Intractable itch

Use as for depression; continue indefinitely.[6,8]

Supply

Mirtazapine (generic)
Tablets 15mg, 30mg, 45mg, 28 days @ 30mg at bedtime = £2.
Tablets orodispersible 15mg, 30mg, 45mg, 28 days @ 30mg at bedtime = £3; *tablets should be placed on the tongue, allowed to disperse, then swallowed.*
Oral solution 15mg/mL, 28 days @ 30mg at bedtime = £40.

Zispin SolTab® (Organon)
Tablets orodispersible 15mg, 30mg, 45mg, 28 days @ 30mg at bedtime = £14; *tablets should be placed on the tongue, allowed to disperse, then swallowed.*

1 Stahl SM (2008) *Essential Psychopharmacology. Neuroscientific basis and practical applications* (3e). Cambridge University Press, Cambridge.
2 Devoto P *et al.* (2004) Mirtazapine-induced corelease of dopamine and noradrenaline from noradrenergic neurons in the medial prefrontal and occipital cortex. *European Journal of Pharmacology.* **487**: 105–111.
3 Croom KF *et al.* (2009) Mirtazapine: a review of its use in major depression and other psychiatric disorders. *CNS Drugs.* **23**: 427–452.
4 Kim SW *et al.* (2008) Effectiveness of mirtazapine for nausea and insomnia in cancer patients with depression. *Psychiatry and Clinical Neurosciences.* **62**: 75–83.
5 Chen CC *et al.* (2008) Premedication with mirtazapine reduces preoperative anxiety and postoperative nausea and vomiting. *Anesthesia and Analgesia.* **106**: 109–113.
6 Brannon G and Stone K (1999) The use of mirtazapine in a patient with chronic pain. *Journal of Pain and Symptom Management.* **18**: 382–385.
7 Ritzenthaler B and Pearson D (2000) Efficacy and tolerability of mirtazapine in neuropathic pain. *Palliative Medicine.* **14**: 346.
8 Krajnik M and Zylicz Z (2001) Understanding pruritus in systemic disease. *Journal of Pain and Symptom Management.* **21**: 151–168.
9 Hoes M and Zeijpveld J (1996) Mirtazapine as treatment for serotonin syndrome. *Pharmacopsychiatry.* **29**: 81.
10 Timmer CJ *et al.* (2000) Clinical pharmacokinetics of mirtazapine. *Clinical Pharmacokinetics.* **38**: 461–474.
11 Abed R and Cooper M (1999) Mirtazapine causing hyperphagia. *British Journal of Psychiatry.* **174**: 181–182.

TRAZODONE — BNF 4.3.1

Class: α-Adrenergic and $5HT_{2A/C}$ antagonist antidepressant; serotonin re-uptake inhibitor.

Indications: Depression, †anxiety and panic disorders, †agitated delirium, †insomnia.

Contra-indications: Should not be given with an MAOI or within 2 weeks of its cessation (see Serotonin toxicity, p.177). Avoid use in the initial recovery period after an acute myocardial infarction.

Pharmacology

Trazodone is an α_1-adenergic, α_2-adrenergic, $5HT_{2A}$- and $5HT_{2C}$-receptor antagonist and, at higher doses, a serotonin re-uptake inhibitor.[1] Its receptor profile accounts for its sedative effect and contributes to its antidepressant action by disinhibiting mono-amine release. It is devoid of antimuscarinic activity. Although generally as effective as other antidepressants,[2] trazodone is not often used to treat depression in palliative care because of unacceptable daytime drowsiness. Thus, when used, it is generally for unlicensed indications.

Food increases its alimentary absorption. Trazodone has an active metabolite, m-chlorophenylpiperazine. Excretion is almost entirely as free or conjugated metabolites. Although trazodone has less effect on cardiac function than TCAs, there are sporadic reports of arrhythmias, ranging from heart block to ventricular tachycardia.[3,4]

Trazodone has been used for behavioural problems in patients with dementia (agitation, restlessness, wandering, physical aggression, inappropriate sexual activity, culturally inappropriate behaviours, hoarding, cursing, shadowing, screaming, sleep disorders).[5,6] However, larger studies have not replicated promising earlier results.[7] Such behaviours occur for many reasons, including an appropriate response to a distressing situation. Possible precipitants should be treated or modified. Medication should only be used as a last resort where non-drug measures have failed (see Antipsychotics, p.156).

Trazodone is sometimes used as a night sedative despite the absence of RCT evidence confirming its efficacy in non-depressed patients. In a dose of 25–50mg at bedtime, it is reported to be effective and well tolerated.[8]

Bio-availability 65%.

Onset of action 30–60min for insomnia or agitation; 1–4 weeks as an antidepressant.

Time to peak plasma concentration 1h if taken fasting; 2h if taken after food.

Plasma halflife 7h; may be doubled in the elderly.

Duration of action variable, situation dependent.

Cautions

Suicide risk: the possibility of a suicide attempt is inherent in major depression and persists until remission. Antidepressants may themselves cause suicidal ideation, particularly in those aged ≤25 years (see p.175).

Bipolar disorder (can transform into manic phase); epilepsy (lowers seizure threshold); cardiac disease (risk of arrhythmia); severe hepatic impairment (increased drowsiness); renal impairment.

Drug interactions

Elimination is delayed if given with inhibitors of CYP3A4, e.g. **ketoconazole** and protease inhibitors, **indinavir** and **ritonavir**. In contrast, inducers of CYP3A4, e.g. **phenytoin**, will accelerate the metabolism of trazodone.

If trazodone is prescribed concurrently, the dose of **warfarin** may need to be increased,[9] but the dose of **digoxin** and **phenytoin** decreased. Trazodone inhibits most of the acute actions of **clonidine** in animals. Thus, although there are no clinical data, the effect of antihypertensive treatment should be monitored if trazodone is prescribed concurrently.

Undesirable effects

Common (<10%, >1%): daytime drowsiness, lethargy, dizziness (orthostatic hypotension), psychomotor impairment.

Uncommon (<1%, >0.1%): nausea, vomiting, sweating.

Rare (<0.1%, >0.01%): increased libido[10,11] and priapism (in 0.01%).[12,13] These have not been reported with low-dose (25–50mg) night sedation.

Dose and use

Depression

- start with 150mg at bedtime (100mg at bedtime in frail elderly patients)
- if necessary, increase dose by 50mg weekly up to 300mg (either as a single night-time dose or in divided doses)
- maximum daily dose 600mg in divided doses (generally inpatients only).

Anxiety

- start with 75mg at bedtime
- if necessary, increase dose gradually up to 300mg daily (as either a single night-time dose or in divided doses).

Insomnia

- start with 25–50mg at bedtime
- if necessary, increase to 100mg
- occasionally may need 150–200mg.

Agitated delirium, and challenging behaviours in those with dementia

Note: Trazodone is not a first-line choice for either indication (see Antipsychotics, p.156).

- start with 25mg t.d.s. or 50–100mg at bedtime
- if necessary, increase the dose
- unlikely to need >300mg/24h.[5,6]

Supply

Trazodone (generic)
Capsules 50mg, 100mg, 28 days @ 100mg at bedtime = £2.50.
Tablets 150mg, 28 days @ 150mg at bedtime = £4.50.

Molipaxin® (Sanofi-Aventis)
Capsules 50mg, 100mg, 28 days @ 100mg at bedtime = £14.
Tablets 150mg, 28 days @ 150mg at bedtime = £16.
Oral solution (sugar-free) 50mg/5mL, 28 days @ 100mg at bedtime = £31.

1 Stahl SM (2008) *Essential Psychopharmacology. Neuroscientific basis and practical applications* (3e). Cambridge University Press, Cambridge.
2 Haria M *et al.* (1994) Trazodone. A review of its pharmacology, therapeutic use in depression and therapeutic potential in other disorders. *Drugs Aging.* **4**: 331–355.
3 Vlay SC and Friedling S (1983) Trazodone exacerbation of VT. *American Heart Journal.* **106**: 604.
4 Johnson BA (1985) Trazodone toxicity. *British Journal of Hospital Medicine.* **33**: 298.
5 Lebert F *et al.* (1994) Behavioral effects of trazodone in Alzheimer's disease. *Journal of Clinical Psychiatry.* **55**: 536–538.
6 Sultzer DL *et al.* (1997) A double-blind comparison of trazodone and haloperidol for treatment of agitation in patients with dementia. *American Journal of Geriatric Psychiatry.* **5**: 60–69.
7 Jeste DV *et al.* (2008) ACNP White Paper: update on use of antipsychotic drugs in elderly persons with dementia. *Neuropsychopharmacology.* **33**: 957–970.
8 Mendelson WB (2005) A review of the evidence for the efficacy and safety of trazodone in insomnia. *Journal of Clinical Psychiatry.* **66**: 469–476.
9 Small NL and Giamonna KA (2000) Interaction between warfarin and trazodone. *Annals of Pharmacotherapy.* **34**: 734–736.
10 Gartrell N (1986) Increased libido in women receiving trazodone. *American Journal of Psychiatry.* **143**: 781–782.
11 Sullivan G (1988) Increased libido in three men treated with trazodone. *Journal of Clinical Psychiatry.* **49**: 202–203.
12 Patel AG *et al.* (1996) Priapism associated with psychotropic drugs. *British Journal of Hospital Medicine.* **55**: 315–319.
13 Pescatori ES *et al.* (1993) Priapism of the clitoris: a case report following trazodone use. *Journal of Urology.* **149**: 1557–1559.

*PSYCHOSTIMULANTS BNF 4.4

Indications: Attention deficit hyperactivity disorder (**methylphenidate**); daytime drowsiness due to narcolepsy (**modafinil**), †obstructive sleep apnoea or chronic shift work-related sleep disorder; †depression particularly when prognosis <2–4 weeks; †opioid-related drowsiness; †fatigue refractory to correction of underlying contributory factors.

Contra-indications: Amphetamines and other psychostimulants should not be prescribed concurrently or <2 weeks of the use of a monoamine oxidase inhibitor (MAOI), including **procarbazine** (an antineoplastic drug and a weak MAOI; see p.176).

Pharmacology

Most psychostimulants act directly or indirectly via dopamine.[1] Dopamine has a central role in reward, motivation, attention and arousal. It is released in response to stimuli and thoughts perceived as relevant, particularly with regard to 'reward' (the mesolimbic and mesocortical systems). These effects are mediated by D_1 and D_2 receptors.[1,2] Psychostimulants (e.g. **cocaine**, **dexamfetamine**, **methylphenidate** and **modafinil**) inhibit or reverse dopamine re-uptake transporters, thus increasing dopamine transmission.[1,3–6] They increase alertness and motivation, and have antidepressant and mood-elevating properties.[1,7]

Other neurotransmitter changes attributed to **modafinil** are likely to represent 'downstream' effects of dopamine elevation.[7,8] **Caffeine** is an adenosine-receptor antagonist; these receptors co-localize with and inhibit D_1 and D_2 receptors. This indirect antidopaminergic effect may explain the sleep-promoting effects of adenosine, which accumulates during wakefulness.[1,9]

Dopaminergic dysfunction in the mesolimbic and mesocortical systems is implicated in several disorders. In attention-deficit hyperactivity disorder, psychostimulants may improve attention by correcting a deficit in dopamine release in response to relevant stimuli.[10] Conversely, in psychoses, dopamine excess ('over-attention') results in hallucinations and delusions, and accounts for the beneficial effects of D_2 antagonists (see p.150).[2] There is also interest in inhibiting dopamine-mediated 'reward' systems in addiction disorders.

Dexamfetamine, **methylphenidate** (see p.210) and **modafinil** (see p.211) have the best evidence base to support use in palliative care.[11] **Methylphenidate** is probably the most widely used.[12,13] **Dexamfetamine** or **methylphenidate** m/r (both generally given once daily) have more risk of insomnia, particularly if taken later in the day.[14]

About half or less of a dose of **dexamfetamine** is excreted renally and largely unchanged; there is thus a theoretical risk of increased toxicity in renal impairment.[12] For selected pharmacokinetic data, see Table 4.17.

Table 4.17 Pharmacokinetic details for selected psychostimulants.[15–18]

	Oral bio-availability (%)	*Time to peak plasma concentration (h)*	*Halflife (h)*	*Metabolism*
Dexamfetamine	No data	2–4	7–17	Multiple routes; ≤50% renally excreted unchanged
Methylphenidate	30[a]	1–3	2	Non-CYP carboxylesterase[b]
Modafinil	≥40	1.5–3	*d*-modafinil 3; *l*-modafinil 10–16	CYP3A4; non-CYP esterase[b]

a. almost completely absorbed but undergoes extensive first-pass hepatic metabolism
b. metabolites are inactive.

Cautions

Psychostimulants may exacerbate cardiovascular disease (e.g. severe hypertension, arrhythmia and angina); psychiatric illness (e.g. anxiety, agitation, psychosis and addiction disorders); epilepsy (possible lowering of seizure threshold); hyperthyroidism and closed-angle glaucoma (not **modafinil**).

Drug interactions

Pharmacodynamic interactions include those with sympathomimetics (e.g. MAOIs, see contra-indications) and antipsychotics (reduced stimulant effect).

Methylphenidate and **modafinil** may increase plasma concentrations of TCAs, **phenytoin** and **warfarin** (check INR at least weekly until stabilized). **Modafinil** may also increase the plasma concentrations of **diazepam**.

Modafinil induces CYP3A4/5 resulting in reduced efficacy of **ciclosporin**, HIV-protease inhibitors, **midazolam**, L-type calcium-channel blockers, statins and hormonal contraception. **Modafinil** also inhibits CYP2C19 and thus may decrease the plasma concentrations of the active metabolites of **clopidogrel**.

Undesirable effects

Undesirable effects have been reported in up to 30% of patients.

Neuropsychiatric: insomnia, agitation and anorexia (generally settle after 2–3 weeks if the drug is continued or resolve after 2–3 days if the drug is discontinued), psychosis, movement disorders.
Cardiovascular: tachyarrhythmias, hypertension and angina (rare).
Other: headache, common and responds to slower dose titration; *very rarely cerebral arteritis occurs with* ***methylphenidate***. Mild rashes are common with **modafinil**; serious skin reactions occur in 1% of children.

Use of psychostimulants in palliative care

Depression

Psychostimulants are used where prognosis is anticipated to be <2–4 weeks. This is shorter than suggested by previous consensus guidance[19] because of the recognition that conventional antidepressants act faster than previously thought.[20] However, trials of psychostimulants are generally of short duration and with outcome measures of uncertain clinical significance. Thus, conventional antidepressants should be used if the patient has a sufficient prognosis for a response to manifest (p.187).[11,19,21] Concurrent use with a conventional antidepressant may hasten the response compared with the latter alone, particularly in relation to fatigue.[21]

Methylphenidate is probably the most commonly used psychostimulant for depression in palliative care. Although undesirable effects are similar for all psychostimulants, some patients may benefit by switching to an alternative (e.g. **modafinil**) if the first choice is ineffective or poorly tolerated.

For doses, see individual monographs (**methylphenidate**, p.210; **modafinil** p.211).

Fatigue

Psychostimulants may be considered for the treatment of fatigue when other approaches are insufficient.[22–24] These include, when feasible, the correction of underlying causal factors (e.g. anaemia, depression and electrolyte disturbance) and modification to the patient's daily routine (e.g. gentle exercise, energy conservation and practical help to aid adjustment to changing circumstances).[23] However, RCTs yield conflicting results and the routine use of psychostimulants for fatigue remains controversial.

In cancer patients, **methylphenidate**[25] and **dexamfetamine**[26] were ineffective for cancer-related fatigue, although results of trials of **dexmethylphenidate** for chemotherapy-related fatigue were conflicting.[27,28] A single-dose study found **modafinil** improved drowsiness, psychomotor speed and attention in patients with advanced cancer.[29] However an RCT found no difference in any predefined outcome measure, although did find benefit in a (non-predefined) subgroup with more severe fatigue.[30] A second trial of **modafinil** in cancer patients is underway.

RCTs examining **modafinil** for fatigue in myotonic dystrophy, Parkinson's disease and traumatic brain injury found little or no effect.[7,31] However, **modafinil** improved HIV related fatigue in 75% of patients (NNT 2.3).[32] Fatigue in multiple sclerosis improved in a small cross-over RCT[33] but not in a larger parallel group study.[34] Benefit was shown in MND/ALS.[35] A lack of clear benefit may relate, in part, to the large placebo response seen in many trials. Further, some have suggested that the b.d. drug regimen may have interfered with sleep and thus exacerbated fatigue in some patients.[36]

Opioid-related drowsiness

Drowsiness is common when opioids are commenced or the dose is increased; it is generally transient. Persistent drowsiness may indicate opioid toxicity; a trial dose reduction should be made and other drug and non-drug approaches considered to provide adequate analgesia (see p.281). However, some patients experience persistent drowsiness despite adjusting the opioid dose. In this circumstance, switching to an alternative opioid may be of benefit (see Opioid dose conversion ratios, p.625).

Psychostimulants are sometimes used for opioid-related drowsiness refractory to these measures. They improve psychomotor performance and allow opioid dose escalation to a higher level than would otherwise be possible.[37] This can be particularly helpful for patients experiencing break-through (episodic) pain.[38–41]

Supply

All products are **CD**.

Dexamfetamine (generic)

Tablets 5mg, 28 days @ 5mg once daily = £16.

---

1 Boutrel B and Koob GF (2004) What keeps us awake: the neuropharmacology of stimulants and wakefulness-promoting medications. *Sleep*. **27**: 1181–1194.

2 Kapur S *et al.* (2005) From dopamine to salience to psychosis–linking biology, pharmacology and phenomenology of psychosis. *Schizophrenia Research*. **79**: 59–68.

3 Volkow ND *et al.* (2009) Effects of modafinil on dopamine and dopamine transporters in the male human brain: clinical implications. *Journal of the American Medical Association*. **301**: 1148–1154.

4 Qu WM *et al.* (2008) Dopaminergic D1 and D2 receptors are essential for the arousal effect of modafinil. *Journal of Neuroscience*. **28**: 8462–8469.

5 Fleckenstein AE *et al.* (2007) New insights into the mechanism of action of amphetamines. *Annual Review of Pharmacology and Toxicology*. **47**: 681–698.

6 Sulzer D *et al.* (2005) Mechanisms of neurotransmitter release by amphetamines: a review. *Progress in Neurobiology*. **75**: 406–433.

7 Kumar R (2008) Approved and investigational uses of modafinil: an evidence-based review. *Drugs*. **68**: 1803–1839.

8 Stahl SM (2008) Disorders of sleep and wakefulness and their treatments. In: *Essential Psychopharmacology: Neuroscientific Basis and Practical Applications* Vol 3. Cambridge University Press, USA, pp. 815–862.

9 Canals M *et al.* (2003) Adenosine A2A-dopamine D2 receptor-receptor heteromerization: qualitative and quantitative assessment by fluorescence and bioluminescence energy transfer. *Journal of Biological Chemistry*. **278**: 46741–46749.

10 Volkow ND *et al.* (2005) Imaging the effects of methylphenidate on brain dopamine: new model on its therapeutic actions for attention-deficit/hyperactivity disorder. *Biological Psychiatry*. **57**: 1410–1415.

11 Candy *et al.* (2008) Psychostimulants for depression. *Cochrane Database of Systematic Reviews*. **2**: CD006722.

12 Dein S and George R (2002) A place for psychostimulants in palliative care? *Journal of Palliative Care*. **18**: 196–199.

13 Masand PS and Tesar GE (1996) Use of stimulants in the medically ill. *Psychiatric Clinics of North America*. **19**: 515–547.

14 Burns MM and Eisendrath SJ (1994) Dextroamphetamine treatment for depression in terminally ill patients. *Psychosomatics*. **35**: 80–83.

15 Challman TD and Lipsky JJ (2000) Methylphenidate: its pharmacology and uses. *Mayo Clinic Proceedings*. **75**: 711–721.

16 de la Torre R *et al.* (2004) Clinical pharmacokinetics of amfetamine and related substances: monitoring in conventional and non-conventional matrices. *Clinical Pharmacokinetics*. **43**: 157–185.

17 Connor DF and Steingard RJ (2004) New formulations of stimulants for attention-deficit hyperactivity disorder: therapeutic potential. *CNS Drugs*. **18**: 1011–1030.

18 Robertson P, Jr. and Hellriegel ET (2003) Clinical pharmacokinetic profile of modafinil. *Clinical Pharmacokinetics*. **42**: 123–137.

19 Block SD (2000) Assessing and managing depression in the terminally ill patient. ACP-ASIM End-of-Life Care Consensus Panel. American College of Physicians — American Society of Internal Medicine. *Annals of Internal Medicine*. **132**: 209–218.

20 Tylee A and Walters P (2007) Onset of action of antidepressants. *British Medical Journal*. **334**. 911–912.

21 Orr K and Taylor D (2007) Psychostimulants in the treatment of depression: a review of the evidence. *CNS Drugs*. **21**: 239–257.

22 NCCN (2008) National comprehensive care network clinical practice guidelines in oncology: cancer related fatigue. Available from: www.nccn.org/professionals/physician_gls/PDF/fatigue.pdf

23 Radbruch L *et al.* (2008) Fatigue in palliative care patients — an EAPC approach. *Palliative Medicine*. **22**: 13–32.

24 Minton O *et al.* (2008) A systematic review and meta-analysis of the pharmacological treatment of cancer-related fatigue. *Journal of the National Cancer Institute*. **100**: 1155–1166.

25 Bruera E *et al.* (2006) Patient-controlled methylphenidate for cancer fatigue: a double-blind, randomized, placebo-controlled trial. *Journal of Clinical Oncology*. **24**: 2073–2078.

26 Auret KA *et al.* (2009) A randomized, double-blind, placebo-controlled trial assessing the impact of dexamphetamine on fatigue in patients with advanced cancer. *Journal of Pain and Symptom Management*. **37**: 613–621.

27 Mar Fan HG *et al.* (2008) A randomised, placebo-controlled, double-blind trial of the effects of d-methylphenidate on fatigue and cognitive dysfunction in women undergoing adjuvant chemotherapy for breast cancer. *Supportive Care in Cancer*. **16**: 577–583.

28 Lower EE *et al.* (2009) Efficacy of dexmethylphenidate for the treatment of fatigue after cancer chemotherapy: a randomized clinical trial. *Journal of Pain and Symptom Management*. **38**: 650–662.

29 Lundorff LE *et al.* (2009) Modafinil for attentional and psychomotor dysfunction in advanced cancer: a double-blind, randomised, cross-over trial. *Palliative Medicine*. **23**: 731–738.

30 Jean-Pierre P *et al.* (2010) A phase 3 randomized, placebo-controlled, double-blind, clinical trial of the effect of modafinil on cancer-related fatigue among 631 patients receiving chemotherapy: a University of Rochester Cancer Center Community Clinical Oncology Program Research base study. *Cancer.* **116**: 3513–3520.
31 Lou JS *et al.* (2009) Using modafinil to treat fatigue in Parkinson disease: a double-blind, placebo-controlled pilot study. *Clinical Neuropharmacology.* **32**: 305–310.
32 Rabkin JG *et al.* (2010) Modafinil treatment for fatigue in HIV/AIDS: a randomized placebo-controlled study. *Journal of Clinical Psychiatry.* **71**: 707–715.
33 Lange R *et al.* (2009) Modafinil effects in multiple sclerosis patients with fatigue. *Journal of Neurology.* **256**: 645–650.
34 Stankoff B *et al.* (2005) Modafinil for fatigue in MS: a randomized placebo-controlled double-blind study. *Neurology.* **64**: 1139–1143.
35 Rabkin JG *et al.* (2009) Modafinil treatment of fatigue in patients with ALS: a placebo-controlled study. *Muscle and Nerve.* **39**: 297–303.
36 Rammohan KW and Lynn DJ (2005) Modafinil for fatigue in MS: a randomized placebo-controlled double-blind study. *Neurology.* **65**: 1995–1997; author reply 1995–1997.
37 Dalal S and Melzack R (1998) Potentiation of opioid analgesia by psychostimulant drugs: a review. *Journal of Pain and Symptom Management.* **16**: 245–253.
38 Bruera E *et al.* (1989) Use of methylphenidate as an adjuvant to narcotic analgesics in patients with advanced cancer. *Journal of Pain and Symptom Management.* **4**: 3–6.
39 Wilwerding M *et al.* (1995) A randomized, crossover evaluation of methylphenidate in cancer patients receiving strong narcotics. *Supportive Care in Cancer.* **3**: 135–138.
40 Bruera E *et al.* (1992) The use of methylphenidate in patients with incident cancer pain receiving regular opiates: a preliminary report. *Pain.* **50**: 75–77.
41 Bruera E *et al.* (1992) Neuropsychological effects of methylphenidate in patients receiving a continuous infusion of narcotics for cancer pain. *Pain.* **48**: 163–166.

Quick Practice Guide: Psychostimulants in depressed patients with a short prognosis

A psychostimulant is the drug of choice for treating depression in patients with a prognosis of <2–4 weeks because they may not live long enough to maximally benefit from a conventional antidepressant. It is often possible to achieve a response in a few days by increasing the dose steadily until benefit or undesirable effects occur. Psychostimulants are not as effective as conventional antidepressants, and these should be considered instead or concurrently in patients with a sufficient prognosis for a response to manifest.

Advantages

Well tolerated and generally effective.
No lag time to effect.
Rapid clearance from the body.
Paradoxically improve appetite in the physically ill.

Disadvantages

Can only be given PO.
May precipitate/exacerbate delirium.
Undesirable effects include restlessness, hallucinations, insomnia, tachycardia, hypertension.
Tolerance may develop.
Withdrawal depression if stopped abruptly after prolonged use.

Drugs

Dexamfetamine

- start with 2.5–5mg each morning
- if necessary, increase progressively every 1–2 days to 20mg each morning.

Methylphenidate

- start with 2.5–5mg b.d. (early morning and noon)
- if necessary, increase progressively every 1–2 days to 20mg b.d.

Dose titration

Check response daily.
Increase dose every 1–2 days by the smallest practical amount until:

- the depression resolves *or*
- unacceptable undesirable effects occur *or*
- the maximum recommended dose is reached.

*METHYLPHENIDATE BNF 4.4

Class: Psychostimulant.

Indications: Attention-deficit hyperactivity disorder; †narcolepsy; †depression where prognosis <2–4 weeks; †opioid-related drowsiness; †fatigue refractory to correction of underlying contributory factors;[1] †hypo-active delirium.[2,3]

Contra-indications: Severe anxiety or agitation, motor tics, hyperthyroidism, severe angina, cardiac arrhythmia, glaucoma.

Pharmacology

Methylphenidate is a CNS stimulant structurally related to **dexamfetamine** but is less potent and has a shorter halflife (2h vs. 10h).[3,4] Both drugs reverse pre-synaptic dopamine re-uptake transporters thus increasing the release, and inhibiting the pre-synaptic re-uptake, of dopamine (see p.205).[5–7] Their action is thus antagonized by antipsychotics.

Methylphenidate is used for depression where prognosis is anticipated to be <2–4 weeks. This is shorter than suggested by previous consensus guidance because of the recognition that conventional antidepressants act faster than previously thought (see p.205).

Methylphenidate may be considered alongside non-drug measures for fatigue unresponsive to the correction of underlying causal factors (e.g. anaemia).[8–10] However, the routine use of psychostimulants for fatigue remains controversial. Methylphenidate also has a limited role in allowing higher doses of opioids without excessive drowsiness in patients with break-through (episodic) pain (see Psychostimulants, p.205).

After almost complete oral absorption, it undergoes extensive first-pass hepatic metabolism via a non-P450 carboxylesterase resulting in an absolute bio-availability of 30%. The effect of food on absorption is unlikely to be significant. Although it is absorbed from the buccal mucosa, this route is not used clinically because of the higher risk of undesirable effects.[11] The major metabolite, ritalinic acid, is inactive and excreted mainly in the urine.[12] Like **dexamfetamine**, little relation exists between plasma levels and behavioural or physiological effects.[13]

Bio-availability 30% (extensive first-pass metabolism).
Onset of action 20–40min.
Time to peak plasma concentration 1–3h.
Plasma halflife 2h.
Duration of action 3–6h.

Cautions

Cardiovascular disease (e.g. severe hypertension, arrhythmia and angina), psychiatric illness (e.g. anxiety, agitation, psychosis and addiction), epilepsy (possible lowering of seizure threshold), hyperthyroidism, closed-angle glaucoma.

Drug interactions

Methylphenidate may inhibit the metabolism of **warfarin**, TCAs and **phenytoin**. Its action is antagonized by antipsychotics.

Undesirable effects

Very common (>10%): nervousness and insomnia (at the beginning of treatment, but can be controlled by reducing the dose).
Common (<10%, >1%): headache, dizziness, dyskinesia, tachycardia, palpitations, arrhythmias, increase in blood pressure, abdominal pain, nausea, vomiting (when starting treatment, but may be alleviated by concurrent food intake), decreased appetite (transient), dry mouth, rash, pruritus, urticaria, fever, arthralgia, scalp hair loss.

Dose and use

Individual dose titration is necessary to maximize benefit and minimize undesirable effects:

- start with 2.5–5mg b.d. (on waking/breakfast time and noon/lunchtime)
- if necessary, increase by *daily* increments of 2.5–5mg b.d.
- usual maximum 20mg b.d. (occasionally, even higher doses are necessary, e.g. 30mg b.d. or 20mg t.d.s.[14]

Supply

All products are **CD**. M/r products are available, but are not appropriate as daytime stimulants in palliative care.

Methylphenidate (generic)
Tablets 5mg, 10mg, 20mg, 28 days @ 10mg b.d. = £13 (note: based on BNF pricing, this is *more expensive* than branded Ritalin® tablets).

Ritalin® (Novartis)
Tablets 10mg, 28 days @ 10mg b.d. = £10 (note: based on BNF pricing, this is *cheaper* than generic tablets).

1 Blockmans D *et al.* (2006) Does methylphenidate reduce the symptoms of chronic fatigue syndrome? *American Journal of Medicine*. **119**: 167 e123–130.
2 Gagnon B *et al.* (2005) Methylphenidate hydrochloride improves cognitive function in patients with advanced cancer and hypoactive delirium: a prospective clinical study. *Journal of Psychiatry and Neuroscience*. **30**: 100–107.
3 Sood A *et al.* (2006) Use of methylphenidate in patients with cancer. *American Journal of Hospice and Palliative Care*. **23**: 35–40.
4 Rozans M *et al.* (2002) Palliative uses of methylphenidate in patients with cancer: a review. *Journal of Clinical Oncology*. **20**: 335–339.
5 Boutrel B and Koob GF (2004) What keeps us awake: the neuropharmacology of stimulants and wakefulness-promoting medications. *Sleep*. **27**: 1181–1194.
6 Sulzer D *et al.* (2005) Mechanisms of neurotransmitter release by amphetamines: a review. *Progress in Neurobiology*. **75**: 406–433.
7 Fleckenstein AE *et al.* (2007) New insights into the mechanism of action of amphetamines. *Annual Review of Pharmacology and Toxicology*. **47**: 681–698.
8 Minton O *et al.* (2008) A systematic review and meta-analysis of the pharmacological treatment of cancer-related fatigue. *Journal of the National Cancer Institute*. **100**: 1155–1166.
9 NCCN-fatigue (2008) National comprehensive care network clinical practice guidelines in oncology: cancer related fatigue. Available from: www.nccn.org/professionals/physician_gls/PDF/fatigue.pdf
10 Radbruch L *et al.* (2008) Fatigue in palliative care patients — an EAPC approach. *Palliative Medicine*. **22**: 13–32.
11 Pleak R (1995) Adverse effects of chewing methylphenidate. *American Journal of Psychiatry*. **152**: 811.
12 Challman TD and Lipsky JJ (2000) Methylphenidate: its pharmacology and uses. *Mayo Clinic Proceedings*. **75**: 711–721.
13 Little K (1993) d-Amphetamine versus methylphenidate effects in depressed inpatients. *Journal of Clinical Psychiatry*. **54**: 349–355.
14 Orr K and Taylor D (2007) Psychostimulants in the treatment of depression: a review of the evidence. *CNS Drugs*. **21**: 239–257.

*MODAFINIL BNF 4.4

Class: Psychostimulant.

Indications: Daytime sleepiness due to narcolepsy, †obstructive sleep apnoea or chronic shift work related sleep disorder, †depression where prognosis <2–4 weeks, †fatigue refractory to correction of underlying contributors.

Contra-indications: Uncontrolled moderate–severe hypertension, arrhythmias.

Pharmacology

Like other psychostimulants, modafinil inhibits the dopamine re-uptake transporter.[1–6] Other changes (e.g. in GABA, glutamate and histamine transmission) appear to be 'downstream' consequences of enhanced dopamine transmission. The effects of modafinil are lost in dopamine-transporter or D_1/D_2-receptor knockout mice and opposed by D_1/D_2 antagonists.[1,2] Positron emission tomography reveals enhanced dopamine transmission in humans.[4]

RCTs of the *adjunctive* use of modafinil in depression found significant improvements in fatigue but not mood. There is less experience than with **methylphenidate** for *monotherapy* and in physically ill patients, although case reports suggest that it may share the mood-elevating properties of other psychostimulants.[7]

An RCT examining modafinil in chemotherapy-related fatigue found no difference in any predefined outcome measure, although it did find benefit in a (non-predefined) subgroup with more severe fatigue.[8] A second trial of **modafinil** in cancer patients is underway.

RCTs for fatigue in myotonic dystrophy, Parkinson's disease and traumatic brain injury found little or no effect.[6,9] However, modafinil improved HIV-related fatigue in 75% of patients (NNT 2.3).[10] Fatigue in multiple sclerosis improved in a small cross-over RCT[11] but not in a larger parallel group study.[12] Benefit was shown in MND/ALS.[13] A lack of clear benefit may relate, in part, to the large placebo response seen in many trials. Further, some have suggested that the b.d. drug regimen may have interfered with sleep and thus exacerbated fatigue in some patients.[14]

Modafinil was previously believed to cause fewer problems with tolerability, tolerance and dependence. However, in direct comparisons with other psychostimulants in patients with prior addiction disorders, few differences were found in subjective 'pleasurable' effects.[6] Its undesirable cardiovascular and psychotropic effects also appear similar. European regulators have recommended withdrawing marketing authorizations for all indications except narcolepsy concerns about because of dermatological and neuropsychiatric effects and abuse potential.[15]

The two enantiomers *d*-modafinil and *l*-modafinil are equipotent, but the latter is cleared more slowly. Its absolute bio-availability is unknown because of the absence of an IV preparation for comparison, but urinary recovery of 40–65% of a dose puts it at ⩾40%. Its absorption is not significantly delayed by food. It is 60% plasma protein-bound. It is inactivated by metabolism to modafinil acid and modafinil sulfone by non-P450 esterases and CYP3A4 respectively. Less than 10% is renally excreted unchanged. Rate of clearance is reduced in the elderly and those with hepatic impairment. The clinical significance of the accumulation of inactive modafinil acid in renal impairment is unclear.[16]

Bio-availability ⩾40%.

Onset of action <5h.[17]

Time to peak plasma concentration 1.5–3h.

Plasma halflife *d*-modafinil 3h; *l*-modafinil10–16h.

Duration of action no data.

Cautions

Cardiovascular disease (e.g. severe hypertension, arrhythmia, angina. Avoid in mitral valve prolapse, cor pulmonale and left ventricular hypertrophy); psychiatric illness (e.g. anxiety, agitation, psychosis, addiction disorders); epilepsy (possible lowering of seizure threshold).

Although rare in adults, serious skin reactions occur in 1% of children; consider alternatives where possible (e.g. **methylphenidate**).

Drug interactions

Modafinil's effects on the cytochrome P450 system are of uncertain clinical significance:[16]

- inhibition of CYP2C19 and 2C9: **phenytoin** (monitor for features of toxicity); **warfarin** (increase INR monitoring for the first 2 months of treatment)
- induction of CYP3A4/5: potential for reduced effect of **ciclosporin**, HIV-protease inhibitors, **midazolam**, calcium-channel blockers, statins and hormonal contraception.

Induction of CYP1A2 and 2B6 also occurs.

Undesirable effects

Very common (>10%): headache.

Common (<10%, >1%): abnormal LFTs, tachycardia, palpitation, dizziness, drowsiness, paraesthesia, blurred vision, abdominal pain, nausea, bowel disturbance, dry mouth, reduced appetite, vasodilation, chest pain, nervousness, insomnia, anxiety, depression, confusion.

Uncommon (<1%, >0.1%): bradycardia, arrhythmia, movement disorders, hostility, suicidal ideation.

Rare (<0.1%): psychosis, mania, angioedema, serious skin reactions (rare in adults but 1% of children): Stevens Johnson syndrome, toxic epidermal necrolysis.

Dose and use

Modafinil is an alternative to **methylphenidate**, particularly where the latter is poorly tolerated. The manufacturer recommends a baseline ECG, and monitoring of BP and heart rate. Dose titration is slower:

- start with 100mg each morning[18]
- if necessary after *1 week*, increase to 200mg each morning
- maximum dose 400mg/24h.

The manufacturer recommends either a single morning dose or divided doses in the morning and at noon. However, the halflife of modafinil raises the possibility of increased sleep disturbance with the latter.

Supply

Provigil® (Cephalon)

Tablets 100mg, 200mg, 28 days @ 200mg each morning = £98.

1 Qu WM *et al.* (2008) Dopaminergic D1 and D2 receptors are essential for the arousal effect of modafinil. *Journal of Neuroscience.* **28**: 8462–8469.
2 Wisor JP *et al.* (2001) Dopaminergic role in stimulant-induced wakefulness. *Journal of Neuroscience.* **21**: 1787–1794.
3 Boutrel B and Koob GF (2004) What keeps us awake: the neuropharmacology of stimulants and wakefulness-promoting medications. *Sleep.* **27**: 1181–1194.
4 Volkow ND *et al.* (2009) Effects of modafinil on dopamine and dopamine transporters in the male human brain: clinical implications. *Journal of the American Medical Association.* **301**: 1148–1154.
5 Lin JS *et al.* (1996) Potential brain neuronal targets for amphetamine-, methylphenidate-, and modafinil-induced wakefulness, evidenced by c-fos immunocytochemistry in the cat. *Proceedings of the National Academy of Sciences of the United States of America.* **93**: 14128–14133.
6 Kumar R (2008) Approved and investigational uses of modafinil: an evidence-based review. *Drugs.* **68**: 1803–1839.
7 Orr K and Taylor D (2007) Psychostimulants in the treatment of depression: a review of the evidence. *CNS Drugs.* **21**: 239–257.
8 Jean-Pierre P *et al.* (2010) A phase 3 randomized, placebo-controlled, double-blind, clinical trial of the effect of modafinil on cancer-related fatigue among 631 patients receiving chemotherapy: a University of Rochester Cancer Center Community Clinical Oncology Program Research base study. *Cancer.* **116**: 3513–3520.
9 Lou JS *et al.* (2009) Using modafinil to treat fatigue in Parkinson disease: a double-blind, placebo-controlled pilot study. *Clinical Neuropharmacology.* **32**: 305–310.
10 Rabkin JG *et al.* (2010) Modafinil treatment for fatigue in HIV/AIDS: a randomized placebo-controlled study. *Journal of Clinical Psychiatry.* **71**: 707–715.
11 Lange R *et al.* (2009) Modafinil effects in multiple sclerosis patients with fatigue. *Journal of Neurology.* **256**: 645–650.
12 Stankoff B *et al.* (2005) Modafinil for fatigue in MS: a randomized placebo-controlled double-blind study. *Neurology.* **64**. 1139–1143.
13 Babkin (2009) Modafinil treatment of fatigue in patients with ALS: a placebo-controlled study. *Muscle Nerve.* **39**: 297–303.
14 Rammohan KW and Lynn DJ (2005) Modafinil for fatigue in MS: a randomized placebo-controlled double-blind study. *Neurology.* **65**: 1995–1997; author reply 1995–1997.
15 EMA (2010) European Medicines Agency recommends stricting the use of modafinil.
16 Robertson P, Jr. and Hellriegel ET (2003) Clinical pharmacokinetic profile of modafinil. *Clinical Pharmacokinetics.* **42**: 123–137.
17 Lundorff LE *et al.* (2009) Modafinil for attentional and psychomotor dysfunction in advanced cancer: a double-blind, randomised, cross-over trial. *Palliative Medicine.* **23**: 731–738.
18 Spathis A *et al.* (2009) Modafinil for the treatment of fatigue in lung cancer: a pilot study. *Palliative Medicine.* **23**: 325–331.

*CANNABINOIDS — BNF 4.6

Indications: refractory spasticity in multiple sclerosis, anti-emesis in chemotherapy, †appetite stimulation in AIDS-related anorexia, †refractory pain in advanced cancer.

Pharmacology

Despite the therapeutic and recreational use of *Cannabis sativa* (marijuana) for thousands of years,[1] currently available cannabinoids are generally poorly tolerated. Their use as anti-emetics has been largely eclipsed by the introduction of $5HT_3$ antagonists (see overleaf), and they are less effective (and/or less well tolerated) than established analgesics in many settings.[2,3] In the future, it is possible that tolerability will improve because of the development of:

- CB_2-selective agonists[4]
- peripherally-acting cannabinoids[5]

- targeting endocannabinoid metabolism or uptake[6]
- combining cannabinoids with different properties, e.g. Δ^9-tetrahydrocannabinol (Δ^9-THC, **dronabinol**) with **cannabidiol** (CBD) (see below).[7]

Cannabinoids may have therapeutic value in other situations including migraine, Parkinson's disease, epilepsy and glaucoma; but the evidence for these claims is either scanty or conflicting.[8] Other possible benefits include an antitumour effect, immunomodulation, mood elevation, and relief of insomnia.[9,10]

Endocannabinoid system

The endocannabinoid system comprises:[11]

- two known receptors
  - ▹ CB_1, expressed by central and peripheral neurones
  - ▹ CB_2, expressed mainly by immune cells
- several endocannabinoids, mainly fatty acids derived from arachidonic acid (a precursor for many other biochemical mediators including prostaglandins)
- enzymes and uptake systems involved in endocannabinoid metabolism, including COX-2.[6]

CB_1, an inhibitory receptor, reduces neuronal excitability and neurotransmitter release by opening potassium channels and blocking N/P-type calcium channels, respectively (see Figure 4.7, p.240).[4] It has an important regulatory role in the synapse. Endocannabinoids are synthesized *de novo* in post-synaptic neurones in response to rising intracellular calcium. They act upon pre-synaptic CB_1-receptors, inhibiting further neurotransmitter release. In this way, they are thought to play an important modulatory role in the release of GABA and glutamate in cortical, limbic, and other areas associated with pain signalling.[11]

CB_2 is implicated in immune regulation. Located on antigen-presenting cells, it influences their cytokine profile and thus that of T-helper cells.[10] This may partly explain its anti-inflammatory and antihyperalgesic effects. Its expression on microglia is upregulated in the dorsal root ganglia and spinal cord following sciatic nerve injury.[4] The antihyperalgesic effects of CB_1 and CB_2 activation are distinct and additive.[12]

Endocannabinoids also act at other receptors, including the capsaicin receptor (TRPV1, involved in pain signalling), and perhaps also G protein-coupled receptors (GPR) 55 and 119.[13]

Most endocannabinoids are fatty acids derived from arachidonic acid, produced *de novo* as required, and then rapidly removed by hydrolysis. Several have been identified, notably anandamide (arachidonylethanolamide) and 2-arachidonyl glycerin (2-AG).[14]

A range of exogenous ligands have been identified, both naturally-occurring cannabinoids from *Cannabis sativa*, e.g. Δ^9-THC (**dronabinol**), CBD, and synthetic substances, e.g. **nabilone** (see p.218).

Cannabinoids as anti-emetics

A systematic review of chemotherapy-induced nausea and vomiting found that cannabinoids had some anti-emetic efficacy in moderate emetogenic settings when compared with placebo, similar to that seen with dopamine antagonists. However, in highly emetogenic settings, cannabinoids were indistinguishable from placebo. Most of these studies were performed before the introduction of specific $5HT_3$ antagonists (see p.234) which have a high therapeutic index. Compared with $5HT_3$ antagonists, the undesirable effects of cannabinoids outweigh their benefits (see below).[15]

Cannabinoids as analgesics

Like opioids, cannabinoids have:

- multiple actions of relevance to nociception, including:
  - ▹ peripheral immunomodulation (antigen-presenting cell CB_2-receptors)
  - ▹ dorsal columns (microglial CB_2-receptors)
  - ▹ disinhibition of antinociceptive neurones of the descending pain modulatory pathway (CB_1-receptors on the pathway's GABAergic 'brake')[4,16,17]
- been used as analgesics for thousands of years.[1]

Further, unlike opioid receptors, CB_1-receptors persist in the spinal cord after peripheral nerve injury.[18,19] However, RCTs have generally found only modest benefit (see p.216 and p.218). A systematic review of cannabinoids as analgesics for mainly postoperative and cancer pain showed that cannabinoids are no more effective than **codeine** 60mg in relieving acute and chronic pain but had more undesirable effects, the most common being drowsiness.[2,8] In the future, it is possible that efficacy/tolerability profile will improve.

Cannabinoids and the respiratory system

Studies of the effects of smoking marijuana cigarettes or inhaling **dronabinol** (not available as a single agent in the UK) have shown a bronchodilator effect together with either an increase in CO_2 sensitivity[20] or a slight respiratory depressant effect.[21,22] However, the potential benefits that could accrue from these actions are overshadowed by the finding that long-term cannabis smoking is associated with a form of chronic bronchitis (although this is not relevant for most patients receiving palliative care). Smoking cannabis appears to increase the overall risk of cancer compared to smoking tobacco alone, particularly of the head and neck and prostate. [23,24]

Undesirable effects

Numerous dose-limiting effects of oral cannabinoids and smoked marijuana have been noted in clinical trials (Box 4.I). Those seen with buccal **cannabis sativa extract** (Sativex®) are comparable. Long-term use of cannabis increases the risk of developing schizophrenia, by a factor of 50.[25,26]

Box 4.I Dose-limiting effects of oral cannabinoids and smoked marijuana reported in clinical trials[8,27]

Physiological	**Psychological**
Ataxia	Drowsiness
Dizziness	Dysphoria
Blurred vision	Abnormal thinking
Dry mouth	Depersonalization
Hypotension	Hallucinations
	Psychosis

The psychotomimetic effects develop 30–90min after oral ingestion, are maximal after 2–4h, and may last up to 12h. Abrupt withdrawal after long-term use of high doses may result in withdrawal phenomena, e.g. anxiety, irritability, insomnia, hot flushes, sweating, rhinorrhoea, diarrhoea, anorexia and hiccup. These are generally mild and the risk is low

1 Mechoulam R (1986) The pharmacohistory of cannabis sativa. In: R Mechoulam (ed) *Cannabinoids as therapeutic agents*. CRC Press, Boca Raton, Fla.

2 Campbell F *et al.* (2001) Are cannabinoids an effective and safe treatment option in the management of pain? A qualitative systematic review. *British Medical Journal*. **323**: 13–16.

3 Frank B *et al.* (2008) Comparison of analgesic effects and patient tolerability of nabilone and dihydrocodeine for chronic neuropathic pain: randomised, crossover, double blind study. *BMJ*. **336**: 199–201.

4 Guindon J and Hohmann AG (2008) Cannabinoid CB2 receptors: a therapeutic target for the treatment of inflammatory and neuropathic pain. *British Journal of Pharmacology*. **153**: 319–334.

5 Yu XH *et al.* (2010) A peripherally restricted cannabinoid receptor agonist produces robust anti-nociceptive effects in rodent models of inflammatory and neuropathic pain. *Pain*. **151**: 337–344.

6 Jhaveri MD *et al.* (2007) Endocannabinoid metabolism and uptake: novel targets for neuropathic and inflammatory pain. *Br J Pharmacol*. **152**: 624–632.

7 Barnes MP (2006) Sativex: clinical efficacy and tolerability in the treatment of symptoms of multiple sclerosis and neuropathic pain. *Expert Opinion on Pharmacotherpy*. **7**: 607–615.

8 Bagshaw SM and Hagan NA (2002) Medical efficacy of cannabinoids and marijuana: a comprehensive review of the literature. *Journal of Palliative Care*. **18 (2)**: 111–122.

9 Walsh D *et al.* (2003) Established and potential therapeutic applications of cannabinoids in oncology. *Supportive Care in Cancer*. **11**: 137–143.

10 Tanasescu R and Constantinescu CS (2010) Cannabinoids and the immune system: an overview. *Immunobiology*. **215**: 588–597.

11 Rea K *et al.* (2007) Supraspinal modulation of pain by cannabinoids: the role of GABA and glutamate. *Br J Pharmacol*. **152**: 633–648.

12 Gutierrez T *et al.* (2007) Activation of peripheral cannabinoid CB1 and CB2 receptors suppresses the maintenance of inflammatory nociception: a comparative analysis. *Br J Pharmacol*. **150**: 153–163.

13 Brown AJ (2007) Novel cannabinoid receptors. *British Journal of Pharmacology*. **152**: 567–575.

14 Mechoulam R *et al.* (1998) Endocannabinoids. *European Journal of Pharmacology*. **359**: 1–18.

15 Davis MP (2008) Oral nabilone capsules in the treatment of chemotherapy-induced nausea and vomiting and pain. *Expert Opinion Investigational Drugs*. **17**: 85–95.

16 Meng ID *et al.* (1998) An analgesia circuit activated by cannabinoids. *Nature*. **395**: 381–383.

17 Welch SP (2009) Interaction of the cannabinoid and opioid systems in the modulation of nociception. *International Reviews on Psychiatry*. **21**: 143–151.
18 Farquhar-Smith WP and Rice AS (2001) Administration of endocannabinoids prevents a referred hyperalgesia associated with inflammation of the urinary bladder. *Anesthesiology*. **94**: 507–513; discussion 506A.
19 Hohmann AG and Herkenham M (1998) Regulation of cannabinoid and mu opioid receptors in rat lumbar spinal cord following neonatal capsaicin treatment. *Neuroscience Letters*. **252**: 13–16.
20 Vachon L *et al.* (1973) Single-dose effect of marihuana smoke. *New England Journal of Medicine*. **288**: 985–989.
21 Bellville J *et al.* (1975) Respiratory effects of delta-9-tetrahydrocannabinol. *Clinical Pharmacology and Therapeutics*. **17**: 541–548.
22 Tashkin D *et al.* (1977) Bronchial effects of aerosolized 9-tetrahydrocannabinol in healthy and asthmatic subjects. *American Review of Respiratory Disease*. **115**: 57–65.
23 Hall W *et al.* (2005) Cannabinoids and cancer: causation, remediation, and palliation. *Lancet Oncology*. **6**: 35–42.
24 Hashibe M *et al.* (2005) Epidemiologic review of marijuana use and cancer risk. *Alcohol*. **35**: 265–275.
25 Zammit S *et al.* (2002) Self reported cannabis use as a risk factor for schizophrenia in Swedish conscripts of 1969: historical cohort study. *British Medical Journal*. **325**: 1199.
26 Fergusson DM *et al.* (2006) Cannabis and psychosis. *British Medical Journal*. **332**: 172–175.
27 Institute of Medicine (1999) *Marijuana and Medicine*. National Academy Press, Washington.

*CANNABIS SATIVA EXTRACT — BNF 4.6

Class: Cannabinoid.

Indications: refractory spasticity in multiple sclerosis; †pain, particularly neuropathic pain and/or painful skeletal muscle spasm.

Contra-indication: History of psychosis; pregnancy, lactation; children.

Pharmacology

Delta-9-tetrahydrocannabinol (Δ^9-THC, dronabinol) and cannabidiol (CBD), present in *Cannabis sativa* extract, are among the best characterized phytocannabinoids. Their actions are distinct. Δ^9-THC is a CB_1 and CB_2 partial agonist; its effects include muscle relaxation, analgesia, anti-emesis, but also psychosis, anxiety and sedation. CBD has a low affinity for CB_1 and CB_2-receptors; it may act by inhibiting the re-uptake or breakdown of the endocannabionoid, anandamide. Although a less potent analgesic and anti-emetic, CBD is non-sedating, anxiolytic and antipsychotic. Further, it reduces Δ^9-THC-induced anxiety in healthy volunteers, perhaps by inhibiting the metabolism of Δ^9-THC to a more psycho-active metabolite, 11-hydroxyTHC.[1–4]

The combined use of Δ^9-THC and CBD (e.g. Sativex®) has been investigated in an attempt to improve the efficacy/tolerability profile of Δ^9-THC alone. Each spray contains Δ^9-THC 2.7mg and CBD 2.5mg. Four RCTs compared Δ^9-THC:CBD with Δ^9-THC alone in patients with pain. Two found modest improvements in tolerability and patient preference,[5,6] one found modest improvements in efficacy, but not tolerability,[7] and one found no difference.[8]

RCTs have compared Δ^9-THC:CBD combinations with placebo for intractable cancer pain and various neuropathic pains. They consistently found a reduction in pain of about 1/10 (NNT for 30% pain reduction 4.5–9). Although modest, these reductions in pain are seen despite cannabinoids being added to optimized conventional analgesia and for difficult pain syndromes. Rates of withdrawal because of undesirable effects varied from 0–14% above that of placebo.[5,7–10] Open-label extension studies found that analgesia was maintained without dose escalation for 1–1.5 years.[9,11]

An RCT of Δ^9-THC alone vs. placebo in patients with multiple sclerosis similarly found only a modest reduction in pain (−0.6/10).[12]

Δ^9-THC and CBD are lipophilic and thus rapidly redistributed to adipose tissue. Δ^9-THC is metabolised by CYP2C9 to 11-hydroxyTHC. CBD is metabolised by multiple routes.[13]

Bio-availability PO (THC) ⩾50%; buccal (no data).
Onset of action 15min.
Time to peak plasma concentration 1–4h (Δ^9-THC and CBD).[13]
Plasma halflife 2–5h (Δ^9-THC); 5–9h (CBD).
Duration of action No data.

Cautions

Severe ischaemic heart disease, arrhythmias or severe heart failure (although healthy volunteer studies found no effect on PR, QTc, QRS intervals, BP or heart rate), epilepsy (cannabinoids can either lower or raise seizure threshold); renal and hepatic impairment (active hepatic metabolites of Δ^9-THC and CBD undergo renal and biliary clearance).

Drug interactions

Sativex® inhibits numerous P450 enzymes, although generally not at typical therapeutic concentrations. Caution is advised when substrates for CYP2C19, 2D6 (e.g. **amitriptyline**) and 3A4 (e.g. **fentanyl, sufentanil**) are used concurrently with Sativex® (see p.735). The metabolism of Sativex® is marginally inhibited by CYP3A4 inhibitors (e.g. **ketoconazole**).

Undesirable effects

Dizziness (30% of patients, dose-dependent).
Cognitive: disorientation, altered mood, dissociation, paranoia.
Physical and psychological dependence.
Cardiovascular: tachycardia, fainting, transient changes in blood pressure.
Buccal: 20% of patients (e.g. irritation, taste alteration, dry mouth).

Dose and use

Direct spray beneath the tongue or inside the cheeks (not towards the pharynx). Vary the site and inspect buccal mucosa regularly for signs of irritation.

Pain

Used for pain relief on a self-titration regimen.

- start with 1 spray up to q4h (maximum 4 sprays in the first 24h)
- titrate up on a daily basis (but more slowly if dizziness occurs)
- median dose required = 5–8 sprays/day. Most patients required ≤12/day.

Spasticity

Reserved for spasticity refractory to other measures (see p.561).

- start with 1 spray at bedtime
- increase over 14 days to 5 sprays in the morning and 7 sprays at bedtime.

Supply

The Home Office is evaluating the CD status of Sativex®. It is currently a **schedule 1 CD** under the Misuse of Drugs Regulations 2001, but prescriptions should be written to comply with the requirements for schedule 2 CDs.

Sativex® (Bayer Healthcare and GW Pharmaceuticals)
Oromucosal spray Cannabis sativa extract (**dronabinol** (Δ^9-THC) 27mg and **cannabidiol** 25mg/mL; about 90 actuations/spray), pack of 3 x 10mL sprays = £375; *the unopened pack should be stored in a refrigerator. Once opened, store at room temperature and use within 6 weeks.*

1 Fusar-Poli P *et al.* (2009) Distinct effects of {delta}9-tetrahydrocannabinol and cannabidiol on neural activation during emotional processing. *Archives of General Psychiatry.* **66**: 95–105.

2 Russo EB and McPartland JM (2003) Cannabis is more than simply delta(9)-tetrahydrocannabinol. *Psychopharmacology (Berl).* **165**: 431–432; author reply 433–434.

3 Zuardi AW *et al.* (1982) Action of cannabidiol on the anxiety and other effects produced by delta 9-THC in normal subjects. *Psychopharmacology (Berl).* **76**: 245–250.

4 Russo E and Guy GW (2006) A tale of two cannabinoids: the therapeutic rationale for combining tetrahydrocannabinol and cannabidiol. *Medical Hypotheses.* **66**: 234–246.

5 Wade DT *et al.* (2003) A preliminary controlled study to determine whether whole-plant cannabis extracts can improve intractable neurogenic symptoms. *Clinical Rehabilitation.* **17**: 21–29.

6 Notcutt W *et al.* (2004) Initial experiences with medicinal extracts of cannabis for chronic pain: results from 34 'N of 1' studies. *Anaesthesia.* **59**: 440–452.

7 Johnson JR *et al.* (2010) Multicenter, double-blind, randomized, placebo-controlled, parallel-group study of the efficacy, safety, and tolerability of THC:CBD extract and THC extract in patients with intractable cancer-related pain. *Journal of Pain and Symptom Management.* **39**: 167–179.
8 Berman JS *et al.* (2004) Efficacy of two cannabis based medicinal extracts for relief of central neuropathic pain from brachial plexus avulsion: results of a randomised controlled trial. *Pain.* **112**: 299–306.
9 Nurmikko TJ *et al.* (2007) Sativex successfully treats neuropathic pain characterised by allodynia: a randomised, double-blind, placebo-controlled clinical trial. *Pain.* **133**: 210–220.
10 Rog DJ *et al.* (2005) Randomized, controlled trial of cannabis-based medicine in central pain in multiple sclerosis. *Neurology.* **65**: 812–819.
11 Wade DT *et al.* (2006) Long-term use of a cannabis-based medicine in the treatment of spasticity and other symptoms in multiple sclerosis. *Multiple Sclerosis.* **12**: 639–645.
12 Svendsen KB *et al.* (2004) Does the cannabinoid dronabinol reduce central pain in multiple sclerosis? Randomised double blind placebo controlled crossover trial. *British Medical Journal.* **329**: 253.
13 Barnes MP (2006) Sativex: clinical efficacy and tolerability in the treatment of symptoms of multiple sclerosis and neuropathic pain. *Expert Opinion on Pharmacotherapy.* **7**: 607–615.

*NABILONE — BNF 4.6

Class: Cannabinoid.

Indications: Chemotherapeutic nausea and vomiting unresponsive to conventional anti-emetics, †breathlessness.

Contra-indication: Severe hepatic impairment.

Pharmacology

Nabilone is the only synthetic cannabinoid licensed for use in the UK. It has significant anti-emetic activity in patients receiving moderately emetogenic chemotherapy.[1,2] Its mechanism of action is not fully understood but there are several points where nabilone could act to block emesis.[3] Nabilone is well absorbed orally. The main metabolite, 9-hydroxynabilone, is pharmacologically active with a plasma halflife up to 5 times longer than that of nabilone itself.[4] Like other cannabinoids, nabilone may cause sedation and, less often, hallucinations and other psychotomimetic effects. Undesirable effects on mental state can last 2–3 days after the last dose. Since the advent of specific $5HT_3$ antagonists, used alone or with **dexamethasone**, there has been little justification for nabilone as an anti-emetic.[1,5]

At a typical anti-emetic dose of 2mg b.d., nabilone has bronchodilator activity in normal subjects and increases the ventilatory response to CO_2.[6] This respiratory stimulation occurs at the time of maximal cortical sedation. Both the bronchodilation and the ventilatory enhancement may be a reflection of a widespread non-specific sympathetic arousal. Thus subjects taking nabilone can feel relaxed and sleepy, and may have demonstrable reduction in PO_2 as a result but, paradoxically, sensitivity to CO_2 is increased. This combination of effects has led to its occasional use in the relief of breathlessness in terminally ill patients.[7] Nabilone should be reserved for patients who:

- are frequently or continuously breathless
- exhibit great anxiety
- would be in danger of slipping into hypercapnic respiratory failure with other conventional respiratory sedatives.

Nabilone and other potentially sedative drugs (e.g. benzodiazepines, opioids, alcohol) have additive CNS depressant events.

Bio-availability 85% PO.
Onset of action 60–90min.
Time to peak plasma concentration 2h.
Plasma halflife 2h; active metabolite 9-hydroxynabilone 5–10h; combined metabolites 35h.
Duration of action 8–12h.

Cautions

Because of possible hypotension and reflex tachycardia, nabilone is unsuitable for patients with atrial fibrillation or in heart failure, and possibly the elderly. History of psychoses.

Undesirable effects

Most frequent: drowsiness, vertigo/dizziness, dysphoria/euphoria, dry mouth, ataxia, visual disturbances, concentration difficulties, sleep disturbance, hypotension, headache, nausea.
Less frequent: confusion, disorientation, hallucinations, psychosis, depression, decreased co-ordination, tremors, tachycardia, decreased appetite and abdominal pain.

Tolerance to CNS effects generally develops after a few days.

Dose and use

Nausea and vomiting

Should be given immediately before, during and for 2 days after each pulse of chemotherapy:

- start with 1mg b.d.
- if necessary, increase to 2mg b.d.
- maximum recommended dose 2mg t.d.s.

Breathlessness

The doses are much lower than for anti emesis:

- start with 100microgram b.d.
- if necessary, increase to 250microgram q.d.s.[8]

Above this dose, most patients with advanced cancer find the sedation unacceptable.

Supply

Unless indicated otherwise, all products are **CD**.

Nabilone
Capsules 250microgram, 30 = £96. (Unlicensed, available as a named patient supply from Creo Pharma; see Obtaining unlicensed drugs, p.769.)
Capsules 1mg, 20 = £126. A lower dose capsule can be prepared by diluting with lactose powder.

1 Gralla R *et al.* (1999) Recommendations for the use of antiemetics: evidence-based, clinical practice guidelines. *Journal of Clinical Oncology.* **17**: 2971–2994.
2 Tramer M *et al.* (2001) Cannabinoids for control of chemotherapy induced nausea and vomiting: quantitative systemic review. *British Medical Journal.* **323**: 16–21.
3 Piomelli D *et al.* (2000) The endocannabinoid system as a target for therapeutic drugs. *Trends in Pharmacological Science.* **21**: 218–224.
4 Rubin A *et al.* (1977) Physiologic disposition of nabilone, a cannabinol derivative, in man. *Clinical Pharmacology and Therapeutics* **22**: 85–91.
5 Davis MP (2008) Oral nabilone capsules in the treatment of chemotherapy-induced nausea and vomiting and pain. *Expert Opinion Investigational Drugs.* **17**: 85–95.
6 McAlpine L and Thomson N (1989) Lidocaine-induced bronchoconstriction in asthmatic patients. Relation to histamine airway responsiveness and effect of preservative. *Chest.* **96**: 1012–1015.
7 Ahmedzai S (1988) Respiratory distress in the terminally ill patient. *Respiratory Disease in Practice.* **5**: 21–29.
8 Ahmedzai S (1997) Palliation of respiratory symptoms. In: D Doyle *et al.* (eds) *Oxford Textbook of Palliative Medicine* (2e). Oxford University Press, Oxford, pp. 583–616.

ANTI-EMETICS — BNF 4.6

The use of anti-emetics in palliative care is currently guided by the probable cause of the nausea and vomiting in relation to the mechanism of action of the drug (Table 4.18; Figure 4.6; Table 4.19),[1–6] largely extrapolated from experimental data and RCTs in postoperative and chemotherapy-related nausea and vomiting. Data from RCTs in palliative care are relatively sparse.[7,8] However, this 'mechanistic approach' is successful in most patients.[2] Other factors to consider include:

- response to anti-emetics already given

- relative merits of alternatives:
  - undesirable effects
  - cost ($5HT_3$ antagonists, **aprepitant** and **octreotide** are expensive)
  - effects on GI motility (i.e. prokinetic (**metoclopramide**, **domperidone**) or antikinetic (antimuscarinics))
  - appropriate route or formulation
- when more than one anti-emetic drug is considered:
  - use combinations with different receptor affinities (e.g. **cyclizine** and **haloperidol**)
  - avoid combinations with antagonistic actions (e.g. **cyclizine** and **metoclopramide**)[9]
  - consider a single broader spectrum drug. **Levomepromazine** (see p.164) and **olanzapine** (see p.166)[10] have affinity at many receptors and may well be as effective as, and easier for patients to handle than, two or more different anti-emetics simultaneously
- adjuvant use of:
  - antisecretory drugs (e.g. **hyoscine *butylbromide***, **glycopyrronium**, **octreotide**)
  - corticosteroids (e.g. **dexamethasone**)
  - benzodiazepines (e.g. **lorazepam**, **midazolam**), particularly with anticipatory nausea[11]
- non-drug treatments.

Generally, the initial choice of an anti-emetic in palliative care lies between three drugs: **metoclopramide** (see p.227), **haloperidol** (see p.159) and **cyclizine** (p.231). These should be prescribed both regularly and as needed (see Quick Practice Guide, p.225).

In bowel obstruction with large-volume vomiting or associated colic, an antisecretory agent (which acts partly by reducing the volume of GI secretions), e.g. **hyoscine *butylbromide*** 60–200mg/24h CSCI, is combined with **cyclizine** 150mg/24h CSCI or **levomepromazine** 6.25–25mg/24h CSCI.

Table 4.18 Classification of drugs used to control nausea and vomiting

Putative site of action	*Class*	*Example*
Central nervous system		
Vomiting centre	Antimuscarinic	Hyoscine *hydrobromide*
	Antihistaminic antimuscarinic[a]	Cyclizine
	Broad-spectrum antipsychotic	Levomepromazine, olanzapine
	NK_1 antagonist	Aprepitant
Area postrema (chemoreceptor trigger zone)	D_2 antagonist	Haloperidol, metoclopramide, domperidone
	$5HT_3$ antagonist	Granisetron, ondansetron
	NK_1 antagonist	Aprepitant
Cerebral cortex	Benzodiazepine	Lorazepam
	Cannabinoid	Nabilone
	Corticosteroid	Dexamethasone
	NK_1 antagonist	Aprepitant
GI tract		
Prokinetic	$5HT_4$ agonist	Metoclopramide
	D_2 antagonist	Metoclopramide, domperidone
	Motilin agonist	Erythromycin
Antisecretory	Antimuscarinic	Hyoscine *butylbromide*, glycopyrronium
	Somatostatin analogue	Octreotide, lanreotide
Vagal $5HT_3$-receptor blockade	$5HT_3$ antagonist	Granisetron, ondansetron, (metoclopramide at high doses)
Anti-inflammatory	Corticosteroid	Dexamethasone

a. antihistamines and phenothiazines both have H_1 antagonistic and antimuscarinic properties (see Table 4.19, p.222).

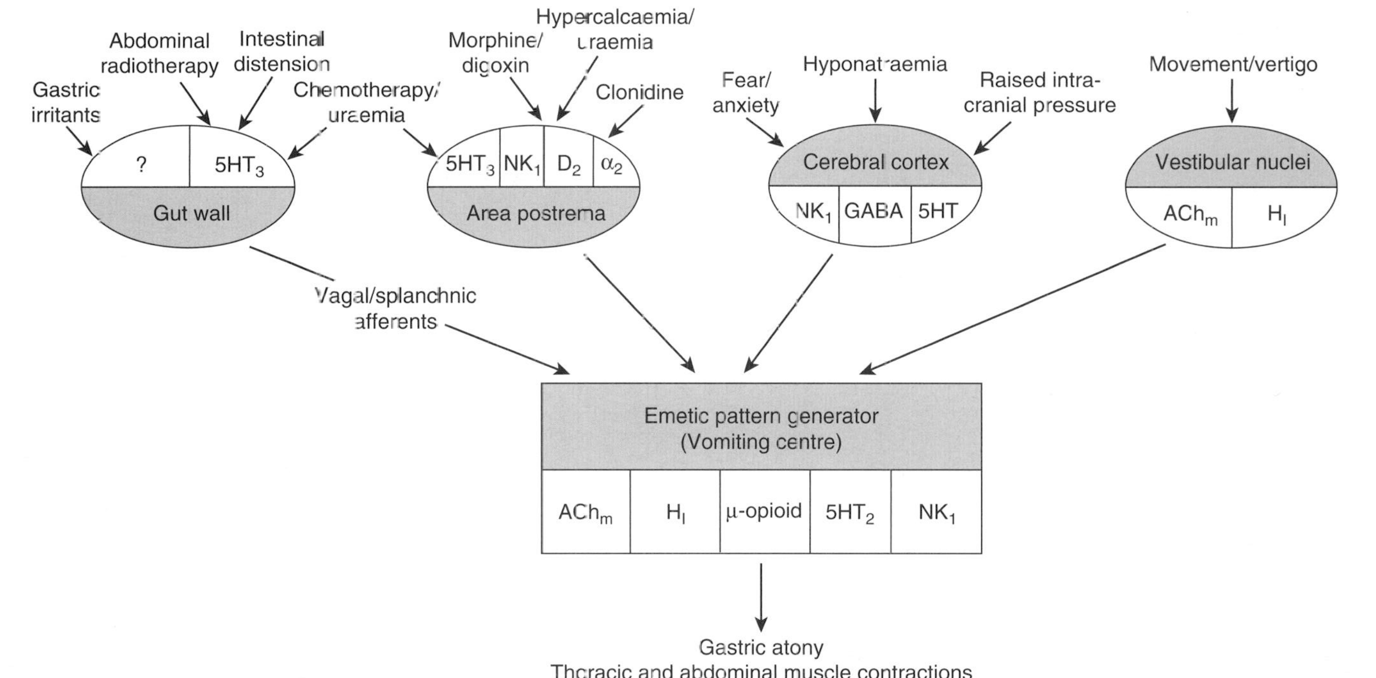

Figure 4.6 Diagram of the neural mechanisms controlling vomiting.

Abbreviations refer to receptor types: AChm = muscarinic cholinergic; α_2 = α_2-adrenergic; D_2 = dopamine type 2; GABA = gamma-aminobutyric acid; 5HT, $5HT_2$, $5HT_3$ = 5-hydroxytriptamine (serotonin) type undefined, type 2, type 3; H_I = histamine type I; NK_1 = neurokinin 1. Anti-emetics act as antagonists at these receptors, whereas the central anti-emetic effects of clonidine and opioids are agonistic.

Table 4.19 Receptor site affinities of selected anti-emetics[4–6,10,11,14,21]

	D_2 antagonist	H_1 antagonist	Muscarinic antagonist	$5HT_2$ antagonist	$5HT_3$ antagonist	NK_1 antagonist	$5HT_4$ agonist	CB_1 agonist	GABAmimetic
Aprepitant	0	0	0	0	0	+++	0	0	0
Chlorpromazine	+++	+++	++	++	0	0	0	0	0
Cyclizine	0	++	++	0	0	0	0	0	0
Domperidone	++[a]	0	0	0	0	0	0	0	0
Haloperidol	+++	0	0	0	+/−	0	0	0	0
Hyoscine *hydrobromide*	0	0	+++	0	0	0	0	0	0
Levomepromazine	++	+++	++	+++	0	0	0	0	0
Lorazepam	0	0	0	0	0	0	0	0	+++
Metoclopramide	++	0	0	0	+	0	++	0	0
Nabilone	0	0	0	0	0	0	0	+++	0
Ondansetron, granisetron	0	0	0	0	+++	0	0	0	0
Olanzapine	++	+	++	++	+	0	0	0	0
Prochlorperazine	+++	++	+	+/++	0	0	0	0	0
Promethazine	+/++	++	++	0	0	0	0	0	0

Pharmacological activity: 0 = none or insignificant; + = slight; ++ = moderate; +++ = marked.
a. domperidone does not normally cross the blood-brain barrier; thus the risk of extrapyramidal effects is negligible (see p.229).

If *nausea* persists, **ondansetron** 16–24mg/24h CSCI is added to **levomepromazine**. If *vomiting* persists, review the patient's oral intake; antisecretory drugs cannot fully alleviate the vomiting of ingested fluid and food. Consider nasogastric aspiration or a trial of **octreotide** (see p.507).

Corticosteroids and **levomepromazine** or **olanzapine** are useful options when first-line anti-emetics fail to relieve nausea and vomiting. **Dexamethasone** is generally added to an existing regimen, whereas **levomepromazine** and **olanzapine** are generally substituted. Sometimes it is necessary to use **dexamethasone** and **levomepromazine** or **olanzapine** concurrently.

$5HT_3$ antagonists were developed primarily to control chemotherapeutic vomiting. In combination with **dexamethasone**, their use is tailored to the risk of nausea and vomiting.[12] If chemotherapy-induced nausea and vomiting persists despite their combined use, options include adding:

- **haloperidol, olanzapine** or **levomepromazine**
- **lorazepam** (particularly if there is anticipatory nausea and vomiting)
- **aprepitant**.[13]

$5HT_3$ antagonists have a definite but limited role in palliative care (see p.234). Drug-induced nausea and vomiting can be problematic. They may be caused by several different mechanisms (Table 4.20), each of which requires a distinct therapeutic response.

Table 4.20 Causes of drug-induced nausea and vomiting

Mechanism	*Drugs*
Gastric irritation	Antibacterials Corticosteroids Iron supplements NSAIDs Tranexamic acid
Gastric stasis	Antimuscarinics Opioids Phenothiazines TCAs
Area postrema stimulation (chemoreceptor trigger zone)	Antibacterials Cytotoxics Digoxin Imidazoles Opioids
$5HT_3$-receptor stimulation	Antibacterials Cytotoxics SSRIs

Aprepitant, a neurokinin 1 (NK_1) antagonist,[14] is approved for the prevention of acute and delayed nausea and vomiting associated with highly emetogenic **cisplatin**-based chemotherapy and moderately emetogenic anthracycline-**cyclophosphamide**-based chemotherapy.[12,15] It is given with **dexamethasone** and a $5HT_3$ antagonist.[16] However, most RCTs examined either its *addition* to sub-optimal regimens (e.g. $5HT_3$ antagonists on day 1 only)[17] or *compared* **aprepitant** to optimal regimens.[18,19] Thus it remains uncertain whether **aprepitant** is beneficial when added to optimally dosed $5HT_3$ antagonists and **dexamethasone**. Postoperatively, **aprepitant** was more effective than **ondansetron** for vomiting but not nausea.[20] A parenteral prodrug, **fosaprepitant**, is available for IV use. Both are expensive. Their place, if any, in the palliative care setting is unclear.

1 Twycross RG and Wilcock A (2001) *Symptom Management in Advanced Cancer* (3e). Radcliffe Medical Press, Oxford, pp. 104–109.
2 Bentley A and Boyd K (2001) Use of clinical pictures in the management of nausea and vomiting: a prospective audit. *Palliative Medicine*. **15**: 247–253.
3 Twycross RG *et al.* (1997) The use of low dose levomepromazine (methotrimeprazine) in the management of nausea and vomiting. *Progress in Palliative Care*. **5**: 49–53.
4 Dollery C (1992) *Therapeutic Drugs: Supplement 1*. Churchill Livingstone, Edinburgh.
5 Dollery C (1991) *Therapeutic Drugs*. Churchill Livingstone, Edinburgh.

6 Peroutka SJ and Snyder SH (1982) Antiemetics: neurotransmitter receptor binding predicts therapeutic actions. *Lancet*. **1**: 658–659.

7 Glare P *et al.* (2004) Systematic review of the efficacy of antiemetics in the treatment of nausea in patients with far-advanced cancer. *Support Care Cancer.* **12**: 432–440.

8 Davis MP *et al.* (2010) A systematic review of the treatment of nausea and/or vomiting in cancer unrelated to chemotherapy or radiation. *Journal of Pain and Symptom Management.* **39**: 756–767.

9 Twycross RG and Back I (1998) Nausea and vomiting in advanced cancer. *European Journal of Palliative Care*. **5**: 39–45.

10 Fleming M and Hawkins C (2005) Use of atypical antipsychotic olanzapine as an anti-emetic. *European Journal of Palliative Care.* **12**: 144–146.

11 Aapro MS *et al.* (2005) Anticipatory nausea and vomiting. *Supportive Care in Cancer.* **13**: 117–121.

12 Hesketh PJ *et al.* (2003) Differential involvement of neurotransmitters through the time course of cisplatin-induced emesis as revealed by therapy with specific receptor antagonists. *European Journal of Cancer.* **39**: 1074–1080.

13 Herrstedt J *et al.* (2009) Chemotherapy-induced nausea and vomiting: ESMO clinical recommendations for prophylaxis. *Annals of Oncology.* **20 Suppl 4**: 156–158.

14 Saito R *et al.* (2003) Roles of substance P and NK(1) receptor in the brainstem in the development of emesis. *Journal of Pharmacology Science.* **91**: 87–94.

15 Navari RM (2004) Role of neurokinin-1 receptor antagonists in chemotherapy-induced emesis: summary of clinical trials. *Cancer Investigation.* **22**: 569–576.

16 Dando TM and Perry CM (2004) Aprepitant: a review of its use in the prevention of chemotherapy-induced nausea and vomiting. *Drugs*. **64**: 777–794.

17 de Wit R *et al.* (2004) The oral NK(1) antagonist, aprepitant, given with standard antiemetics provides protection against nausea and vomiting over multiple cycles of cisplatin-based chemotherapy: a combined analysis of two randomised, placebo-controlled phase III clinical trials. *European Journal of Cancer.* **40**: 403–410.

18 Schmoll HJ *et al.* (2006) Comparison of an aprepitant regimen with a multiple-day ondansetron regimen, both with dexamethasone, for antiemetic efficacy in high-dose cisplatin treatment. *Annals of Oncology.* **17**: 1000–1006.

19 Warr DG *et al.* (2005) Efficacy and tolerability of aprepitant for the prevention of chemotherapy-induced nausea and vomiting in patients with breast cancer after moderately emetogenic chemotherapy. *Journal of Clinical Oncology.* **23**: 2822–2830.

20 Gan TJ *et al.* (2007) A randomized, double-blind comparison of the NK1 antagonist, aprepitant, versus ondansetron for the prevention of postoperative nausea and vomiting. *Anesthesia and Analgesia.* **104**: 1082–1089.

21 Davis M *et al.* (2007) The emerging role of cannabinoid neuromodulators in symptom management. *Supportive Care in Cancer.* **15**: 63–71.

Quick Practice Guide: Management of nausea and vomiting

1 From the patient's history and physical examination, decide what is the most likely cause (or causes) of the nausea and vomiting. Take a blood sample if biochemical derangement is suspected.

2 Correct correctable causes/exacerbating factors, e.g. drugs, severe pain, cough, infection, hypercalcaemia. *(Remember: antibacterial treatment and correction of hypercalcaemia are not always appropriate in a dying patient.)* Anxiety exacerbates nausea and vomiting from any cause and may need specific treatment.

3 Prescribe the most appropriate anti-emetic stat, regularly and p.r.n. (see below). Give by SC injection or CSCI if continuous nausea or frequent vomiting.

Commonly used anti-emetics

Prokinetic anti-emetic (about 50% of prescriptions)
For gastritis, gastric stasis, functional bowel obstruction (peristaltic failure):
metoclopramide 10mg PO stat & q.d.s. or 10mg SC stat & 40–100mg/24h CSCI, & 10mg p.r.n. up to q.d.s.

Anti-emetic acting principally in chemoreceptor trigger zone (about 25% of prescriptions)
For most chemical causes of vomiting, e.g. morphine, hypercalcaemia, renal failure:
haloperidol 1.5–3mg PO stat & at bedtime, or 2.5–5mg SC stat & 2.5–10mg/24h CSCI, & 2.5–5mg p.r.n. up to q.d.s.

Metoclopramide also has a central action.

Antispasmodic and antisecretory anti-emetic
If bowel colic and/or need to reduce GI secretions:
hyoscine *butylbromide* 20mg SC stat, 60–120mg/24h CSCI (occasionally as high as 300mg/24h), & 20mg SC hourly p.r.n.

Anti-emetic acting principally in the vomiting centre
For raised intracranial pressure (in conjunction with dexamethasone), motion sickness and in mechanical bowel obstruction:
cyclizine 50mg PO stat & b.d.–t.d.s. or 50mg SC stat & 150mg/24h CSCI, & 50mg p.r.n. up to b.d.

Broad-spectrum anti-emetic
For mechanical obstruction and when other anti-emetics are unsatisfactory:
levomepromazine 6–12.5mg PO/SC stat, at bedtime & p.r.n. up to q.d.s.

4 Initially, review anti-emetic dose each day; take note of p.r.n. use, and adjust the regular dose accordingly.

5 If little benefit despite upward titration of the dose, reconsider the likely cause(s), and review the route of administration and the choice of anti-emetic.

6 Some patients with nausea and vomiting need more than one anti-emetic.

7 Prokinetics act through a cholinergic system which is competitively antagonized by antimuscarinics; concurrent use is best avoided.

8 A $5HT_3$ antagonist, e.g. granisetron 1–2mg stat & once daily, or ondansetron 8mg stat & b.d.–t.d.s PO/SC should be considered when there is a massive release of 5HT/serotonin from enterochromaffin cells or platelets, e.g. with chemotherapy, abdominal radiation, bowel distension, renal failure. Also consider with chemical causes of nausea and vomiting refractory to haloperidol and levomepromazine.

continued

9 When all else fails, consider adding dexamethasone 8–16mg PO/SC stat & once daily for 7 days, and then review.

10 Continue the anti-emetic(s) unless the cause is self-limiting. Except in mechanical bowel obstruction (see below), consider changing to PO after 3 days of good control with CSCI.

More about bowel obstruction

11 Anti-emetics for inoperable bowel obstruction are best given by CSCI (for typical doses, see above), but levomepromazine can be given as a single SC dose at bedtime:

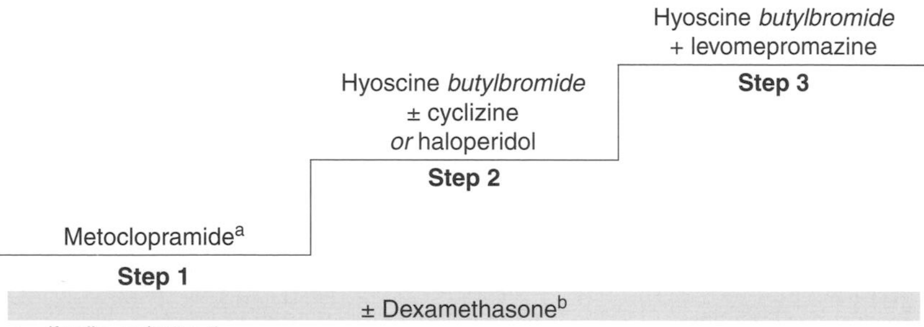

a. if colic, omit step 1

b. the place of dexamethasone in inoperable bowel obstruction is controversial.

12 If levomepromazine is too sedative, consider using olanzapine 1.25–2.5mg SC at bedtime instead; or revert to step 2 but give both cyclizine and haloperidol.

13 If hyoscine butylbromide is inadequate or to obtain more rapid relief, prescribe a somatostatin analogue (= an antisecretory agent without antispasmodic effects), e.g. octreotide 100microgram stat, 250–500microgram/24h CSCI, & 100microgram p.r.n. up to q.d.s.

METOCLOPRAMIDE BNF 4.6

Class: Prokinetic anti-emetic.

Indications: Nausea and vomiting, particularly in GI disorders (e.g. gastric irritation and delayed gastric emptying) and with chemotherapy and radiotherapy, dysmotility dyspepsia, heartburn, migraine, †hiccups.

Contra-indications: Phaeochromocytoma (may induce an acute hypertensive response). GI haemorrhage or perforation. Do not use concurrently with IV $5HT_3$ antagonists (risk of cardiac arrhythmia,[1]) or within <3 days of GI surgery (vigorous contractions may impair healing).

Pharmacology

Metoclopramide is a combined D_2 antagonist and $5HT_4$ agonist. In daily doses above 100mg SC, it manifests $5HT_3$ antagonism. Metoclopramide is therefore a broad-spectrum anti-emetic but its clinical value mainly resides in its prokinetic properties (see Prokinetics, p.19). As a centrally-acting D_2 antagonist, it is second to **haloperidol** (see p.159) and, as a $5HT_3$ antagonist, it is second to the specific $5HT_3$ antagonists (see p.234).

Prokinetics act by triggering a cholinergic system in the wall of the GI tract. Opioids impede this action, and antimuscarinics block it competitively.[2] *Thus, ideally, prokinetics and antimuscarinics should not be given concurrently.* However, if they are, metoclopramide will still exert an antagonistic effect at the dopamine receptors in the area postrema. (**Haloperidol** is generally a better choice in this situation because of the advantage of daily administration, see p.159).

D_2 antagonists block the 'dopamine brake' on gastric emptying induced by stress, anxiety and nausea from any cause. In contrast, $5HT_4$ agonists have a direct excitatory effect which in theory gives them an advantage over the D_2 antagonists particularly for patients with gastric stasis or functional intestinal obstruction. However, when used for dysmotility dyspepsia, metoclopramide and **domperidone** are comparable in standard doses.[3]

Along with other drugs which block central dopamine receptors, there is a risk of developing acute dystonic reactions with facial and skeletal muscle spasms and oculogyric crises (see Drug-induced movement disorders, p.745). These are more common in the young (particularly girls and young women), generally occur within a few days of starting treatment, and subside within 24h of stopping the drug. Thus, when possible, use alternatives in patients aged <20 years.

Bio-availability 50–80% PO.

Onset of action 10–15min IM; 15–60min PO.

Time to peak plasma concentration 1–2.5h PO.

Plasma halflife 2.5–5h.

Duration of action 1–2h (data for single dose and relating to gastric emptying).

Cautions

Epilepsy (lowers seizure threshold); Parkinson's disease or drug-induced parkinsonism; mechanical GI obstruction (but is commonly used in palliative care to restore peristalsis in functional GI obstruction).[4]

Metoclopramide enhances the effects of catecholamines in patients with essential hypertension.[5,6]

Drug interactions

Serious drug interactions: a combination of IV metoclopramide and IV **ondansetron** occasionally causes cardiac arrhythmias.[1] $5HT_3$-receptors influence various aspects of cardiac function, including inotropy, chronotropy and coronary arterial tone,[7] effects which are mediated by both the parasympathetic and the sympathetic nervous systems. Thus, in any given patient, blockade of $5HT_3$-receptors will produce effects dependent on the pre-existing serotoninergic activity in both arms of the autonomic nervous system.

Because antimuscarinics competitively block the final common (cholinergic) pathway through which prokinetics act,[2] concurrent prescription with metoclopramide should be avoided if possible.

Acute dystonic reactions occur in $<5\%$ of patients receiving metoclopramide. The risk is dose-related and greater if also taking other drugs known to cause extrapyramidal effects, e.g. antipsychotics, $5HT_3$ antagonists and antidepressants (see Drug-induced movement disorders, p.745).

Undesirable effects

Extrapyramidal effects, neuroleptic (antipsychotic) malignant syndrome (see p.155). Occasionally drowsiness, restlessness, depression, diarrhoea.

Dose and use

The use of high-dose IV metoclopramide to treat chemotherapy-induced nausea and vomiting is not considered here.[8] In palliative care, metoclopramide is the most commonly used anti-emetic.[9,10] Although it typically has immediate effect, benefit may increase throughout the first week of use.[11] Metoclopramide is also of benefit in dysmotility dyspepsia, delayed gastric emptying, and chronic nausea.[12,13]

Gastric irritation

- 10mg PO q.d.s. or 40–60mg/24h CSCI and 10mg PO/SC p.r.n.; prescribe appropriate gastroprotective drug and, if possible, discontinue causal drug/substance.

Delayed gastric emptying

- as above, consider increasing to 100mg/24h CSCI.

Nausea and vomiting

- as above, but **haloperidol** is generally more convenient if the cause is stimulation of the chemoreceptor trigger zone/area postrema (see p.219).

For nausea and vomiting associated with 5HT release, a selective $5HT_3$ antagonist should be used rather than high-dose metoclopramide (see p.234).

Hiccup

If caused by delayed gastric emptying, gastric distension, or acid reflux:

- 10mg PO t.d.s.–q.d.s. and p.r.n. ± an antifoaming agent (see Table 1.4, p.21)
- if no response to PO treatment, consider 10–20mg IV stat.

Supply

Metoclopramide (generic)
Tablets 10mg, 28 days @ 10mg q.d.s. = £4.
Oral solution 5mg/5mL, 28 days @ 10mg q.d.s. = £49.
Injection 5mg/mL, 2mL amp = £0.50.

Maxolon® (Amdipharm)
Tablets 10mg, 28 days @ 10mg q.d.s. = £7.
Injection 5mg/mL, 2mL amp = £0.50.

Modified-release
Maxolon SR® (Amdipharm)
Capsules enclosing m/r granules 15mg, 28 days @ 15mg b.d. = £7.

---

1 Baguley W *et al.* (1997) Cardiac dysrhythmias associated with the intravenous administration of ondansetron and metoclopramide. *Anesthesia and Analgesia*. **84**: 1380–1381.

2 Schuurkes JAJ *et al.* (1986) Stimulation of gastroduodenal motor activity: dopaminergic and cholinergic modulation. *Drug Development Research*. **8**: 233–241.

3 Barone J (1999) Domperidone: a peripherally acting dopamine$_2$-receptor antagonist. *Annals of Pharmacotherapy*. **33**: 429–440.

4 Twycross R *et al.* (2009) *Symptom Management in Advanced Cancer* (4e). palliativedrugs.com, Nottingham, pp. 108–111.

5 Kuchel O *et al.* (1985) Effect of metoclopramide on plasma catecholamine release in essential hypertension. *Clinical Pharmacology and Therapeutics*. **37**: 372–375.

6 Agabiti-Rosei E (1995) Hypertensive crises in patients with phaeochromocytoma given metoclopramide. *Annals of Pharmacology.* **29**: 381–383.

7 Saxena P and Villalon C (1991) 5-Hydroxytryptamine: a chameleon in the heart. *Trends in Pharmacological Sciences.* **12**: 223–227.

8 Gralla R *et al.* (1999) Recommendations for the use of antiemetics: evidence-based, clinical practice guidelines. *Journal of Clinical Oncology.* **17**: 2971–2994.

9 Twycross RG and Back I (1998) Nausea and vomiting in advanced cancer. *European Journal of Palliative Care.* **5**: 39–45.

10 Ripamonti C *et al.* (2001) Clinical-practice recommendations for the management of bowel obstruction in patients with end-stage cancer. *Supportive Care in Cancer.* **9**: 223–233.

11 Bruera E *et al.* (2004) Dexamethasone in addition to metoclopramide for chronic nausea in patients with advanced cancer: a randomized controlled trial. *Journal of Pain and Symptom Management.* **28**: 381–388.

12 Bruera E *et al.* (1996) Chronic nausea in advanced cancer patients: a retrospective assessment of a metoclopramide-based antiemetic regimen. *Journal of Pain and Symptom Management.* **11**: 147–153.

13 Bruera E *et al.* (2000) A double-blind, crossover study of controlled-release metoclopramide and placebo for the chronic nausea and dyspepsia of advanced cancer. *Journal of Pain and Symptom Management.* **19**: 427–435.

DOMPERIDONE — BNF 4.6

Class: Prokinetic anti-emetic.

Indications: Nausea and vomiting, upper GI dysmotility (due to gastritis and diabetic gastroparesis), gastro-oesophageal reflux, vomiting and hypotension associated with antiparkinsonian drugs.

Contra-indications: Prolactinoma, GI haemorrhage or perforation.

Pharmacology

Domperidone is a D_2 antagonist. It is structurally related to the butyrophenones, but does not normally cross the blood-brain barrier.[1] Domperidone has a dual anti-emetic effect. First, it acts on dopamine receptors in the chemoreceptor trigger zone (CTZ) in the area postrema. (Although situated on the surface of the brain stem, the CTZ is outside the physiological blood-brain barrier.) Second, it acts on D_2-receptors at the gastro-oesophageal and gastroduodenal junctions, and thereby counteracts the gastric 'dopamine brake' associated with nausea from any cause. Domperidone may also inhibit cholinesterase activity.[2] Because negligible amounts of domperidone penetrate the blood-brain barrier, there is negligible risk of extrapyramidal effects (mediated via the basal ganglia). Domperidone is the prokinetic and anti-emetic of choice in Parkinson's disease; it counteracts the emetic effect of **levodopa** and **bromocriptine** without adversely affecting the antiparkinsonian (dopaminergic) effect of these drugs.[3]

Although almost completely absorbed from the GI tract, bio-availability is relatively poor because of extensive first-pass metabolism in the wall of the GI tract and the liver. Bio-availability in healthy volunteers is nearly doubled if taken *after* a meal.[4] Maximal absorption requires an acid environment; H_2 antagonists, PPIs and antacids all reduce absorption, and bio-availability. Under standard conditions, absorption is linear up to a 40mg single dose.

Following absorption, domperidone is metabolized to inactive compounds via the hepatic CYP450 mixed oxidase system, principally CYP3A4 (see Cautions). The plasma halflife is increased by up to 50% in renal failure but the plasma concentrations do not increase (possibly because of an altered volume of distribution). Further, because renal clearance is a minor route of elimination, accumulation is not a concern.[5] Although rectal bio-availability is almost the same as by mouth, the recommended rectal dose is three times the oral dose. This stems from pharmacodynamic studies, and possibly relates to slower absorption from the rectum.

The effect of domperidone on the lower oesophageal sphincter is equivocal.[2] Because domperidone, unlike **metoclopramide**, does not have any $5HT_4$ agonist action, it might be anticipated that domperidone would be less effective in treating gastroparesis. However, the results of a systematic review indicate otherwise (Table 4.21).[6] Domperidone may be effective even when there is no response to **metoclopramide**.[2,7]

Domperidone 20mg q.d.s. causes less frequent and less severe undesirable effects than **metoclopramide** 10mg q.d.s., e.g. less drowsiness and loss of mental acuity.[8] In diabetic patients, the prokinetic effect for solids attenuates after 1–2 months, although the effect on liquid emptying persists.[9,10]

Table 4.21 Comparison of prokinetic drugs[6]

Drug	*Erythromycin*	*Domperidone*	*Metoclopramide*
Mechanism of action			
Motilin agonist	+	−	−
D_2 antagonist	−	+	+
$5HT_4$ agonist	−	−	+
Response to treatment[a]			
Gastric emptying (mean % acceleration)	45	30	20
Symptom relief (mean % improvement)	50	50	40

a. all percentages rounded to nearest 5%.

The usefulness of domperidone is limited by the absence of a parenteral formulation. It was withdrawn in the early 1980s, after several patients died from ventricular arrhythmias when given IV domperidone.[11] Domperidone does not significantly alter the pharmacokinetics or pharmacodynamics of other drugs. Because the prokinetic effect of domperidone is mediated through a cholinergic final common pathway, its prokinetic effect will be impaired by concurrently administered antimuscarinic drugs.[12]

Bio-availability 12–18% PO (fasting), 24% PO (after food).

Onset of action 30min.

Time to peak plasma concentration 0.5–2h PO.

Plasma halflife 7–16h; increasing up to 21h in severe renal impairment.[2]

Duration of action 12–24h (estimate based on halflife).

Cautions

Renal and hepatic impairment; GI haemorrhage or perforation; mechanical GI obstruction.

Drug interactions

The concurrent use of an antimuscarinic drug is likely to reduce the prokinetic effect of domperidone (but will not affect its central anti-emetic effect).

The main metabolic pathway of domperidone is CYP3A4-mediated. The concurrent use of CYP3A4 inhibitors (e.g. **erythromycin**, **ritonavir**, SSRIs, macrolide antibiotics and grapefruit juice) may increase the domperidone plasma concentration, increasing the risk of QT prolongation and thus *torsade de pointes*.[13] The AUC and the peak plasma concentration of domperidone are *trebled* when oral **ketoconazole** is administered concurrently. The QT interval is slightly prolonged (<10msec) by this combination, greater than the increase seen with **ketoconazole** alone. QT prolongation is less likely when domperidone is given alone (Unpublished data on file).

Undesirable effects

Very common (>10%): gynaecomastia, galactorrhoea, amenorrhoea (secondary to increased prolactin secretion), reduced libido, transient colic.[2]

Common (<10%, >1%): pruritus, rash, cramp, headache.[2]

Very rare (<0.01%): extrapyramidal effects (acute dystonias), which resolve rapidly and completely once domperidone is stopped.[14] In two women with polycystic ovaries, hyperoestrogenism may have been a predisposing factor.[2]

Dose and use

The manufacturer recommends giving domperidone t.d.s.–q.d.s. although, given its halflife, b.d. is likely to be satisfactory:

• start with 20mg PO b.d. or 10mg PO q.d.s.

- if necessary, increase to 40mg PO b.d. or 20mg PO q.d.s.
- maximum recommended dose 80mg/24h
- up to 120mg/24h has been used long-term in patients with diabetic gastropathy.[2]

Supply

Domperidone (generic)
Tablets 10mg, 28 days @ 10mg q.d.s. = £2.
Oral suspension 5mg/5mL, 28 days @ 10mg q.d.s. = £67.

Motilium® (Sanofi-Aventis)
Tablets 10mg, 28 days @ 10mg q.d.s. = £10.
Suppositories 30mg, pack of 10 = £3.

1 Barone J (1999) Domperidone: a peripherally acting dopamine$_2$-receptor antagonist. *Annals of Pharmacotherapy*. **33**: 429–440.
2 Prakash A and Wagstaff AJ (1998) Domperidone. A review of its use in diabetic gastropathy. *Drugs*. **56**: 429–445.
3 Langdon N *et al.* (1986) Comparison of levodopa with carbidopa, and levodopa with domperidone in Parkinson's disease. *Clinical Neuropharmacology*. **9**: 440–447.
4 Heykants J *et al.* (1981) On the pharmacokinetics of domperidone in animals and man. IV. The pharmacokinetics of intravenous domperidone and its bioavailability in man following intramuscular, oral and rectal administration. *European Journal of Drug Metabolism and Pharmacokinetics*. **6**: 61–70.
5 Brogden RN *et al.* (1982) Domperidone. A review of its pharmacological activity, pharmacokinetics and therapeutic efficacy in the symptomatic treatment of chronic dyspepsia and as an antiemetic. *Drugs*. **24**: 360–400.
6 Sturm A *et al.* (1999) Prokinetics in patients with gastroparesis: a systematic analysis. *Digestion*. **60**: 422–427.
7 Dumitrascu D and Weinbeck M (2000) Domperidone versus metoclopramide in the treatment of diabetic gastroparesis. *American Journal of Gastroenterology*. **95**: 316–317.
8 Patterson D *et al.* (1999) A double-blind multicenter comparison of domperidone and metoclopramide in the treatment of diabetic patients with symptoms of gastroparesis. *American Journal of Gastroenterology*. **94**: 1230–1234.
9 Horowitz M *et al.* (1985) Acute and chronic effects of domperidone on gastric emptying in diabetic autonomic neuropathy. *Digestive Diseases and Sciences*. **30**: 1–9.
10 Koch KL *et al.* (1989) Gastric emptying and gastric myoelectrical activity in patients with diabetic gastroparesis: effect of long-term domperidone treatment. *American Journal of Gastroenterology*. **84**: 1069–1075.
11 Osborne R *et al.* (1985) Cardiotoxicity of intravenous domperidone. *Lancet*. **2**: 385–385.
12 Schuurkes JAJ *et al.* (1986) Stimulation of gastroduodenal motor activity: dopaminergic and cholinergic modulation. *Drug Development Research*. **8**: 233–241.
13 Health Canada (2007) Domperidone: heart rate and rhythm disorders. *Canadian Adverse Reaction Newsletter*. **17 (January)**: 2.
14 Casteels-Van Daele M *et al.* (1984) Refusal of further cancer chemotherapy due to antiemetic drug. *Lancet*. **1**: 57.

ANTIHISTAMINIC ANTIMUSCARINIC ANTI-EMETICS — BNF 3.4 & 4.6

Indications: Prevention of motion sickness, nausea and vomiting, vertigo and labyrinthine disorders (**cyclizine**, **promethazine**), pruritus, sedation (**promethazine**), anxiety (**hydroxyzine**).

Contra-indications: ***Promethazine:*** intra-arterial or SC injection (is a chemical irritant and may cause local necrosis).

Pharmacology

Antihistaminic antimuscarinic anti-emetics embrace several chemical classes including some phenothiazines (e.g. **promethazine**), piperazines (e.g. **buclizine**, **cyclizine**, **meclozine**, **hydroxyzine**) and mono-ethanolamines (e.g. **diphenhydramine**, **dimenhydrinate**). The piperazines and mono-ethanolamines were first marketed as H_1 antihistamines, and are often classed separately as antihistaminic anti-emetics. They decrease excitability of the inner ear labyrinth and block conduction in the vestibular-cerebellar pathways, as well as acting directly on the vomiting centre in the brain stem. However, there is considerable overlap between their receptor site affinity and that of the antipsychotic phenothiazines (see Table 4.8, p.152).

The piperazines and mono-ethanolamines began to be used for the prevention of motion sickness after a patient with urticaria reported relief from car sickness when taking **dimenhydrinate** (available only in a combination product in the UK).[1] After the Second

World War, studies were conducted in American servicemen crossing the Atlantic Ocean in the General Ballou, a modified freight ship without stabilizers. Although the drugs differ in antihistaminic potency, they were equally effective,[1,2] suggesting that their anti-emetic effect is the result of multiple receptor site activity.

Antihistaminic anti-emetics are effective in many causes of vomiting, including opioid-induced.[3,4] However, in practice **metoclopramide** (see p.227) and **haloperidol** (see p.159) are often used in preference, sometimes because of more specific indications or to avoid drowsiness and antimuscarinic effects. Drowsiness is increased if used with other CNS depressants, e.g. benzodiazepines, barbiturates, antipsychotics, and alcohol. Metabolism is mainly hepatic, and the inactive metabolites are excreted in the urine.

Hydroxyzine is a later addition to this group of drugs, and is principally used as an anxiolytic-sedative and antipruritic. Unlike other anthistaminic drugs, **hydroxyzine** inhibits apomorphine-induced vomiting, suggesting that some of its anti-emetic effect is mediated via the chemoreceptor trigger zone. In postoperative patients, **hydroxyzine** 100mg IM has analgesic activity approaching that of **morphine** 8mg,[5] and **morphine** 5mg and **hydroxyzine** 100mg gave comparable relief to **morphine** 10mg alone.[6] The sedative effect of the combination was not significantly different from **morphine** alone. For pharmacokinetic details, see Table 4.22.

Table 4.22 Pharmacokinetic details

	Cyclizine	*Hydroxyzine*	*Promethazine*
Bio-availability	No data	No data	25% PO
Onset of action	30–60min	15–30min	~20min IM, 3–5min IV
Time to peak plasma concentration	2h PO	~2h	4.5h PO (syrup), 6–9h PR
Plasma halflife	20h	3–7h	7–14h
Duration of effect	4–6h	4–6h	2–6h

Cautions

Hepatic and renal impairment; epilepsy; can precipitate or exacerbate narrow-angle glaucoma; urinary tract obstruction (see Antimuscarinics, p.5). Elderly patients are more susceptible to sedative and central antimuscarinic effects, e.g. postural hypotension, memory impairment, extrapyramidal reactions.

Cyclizine: severe heart failure (antimuscarinic effect → tachycardia).

Hydroxyzine: asthma, COPD, hepatic impairment (restrict to once daily), moderate–severe renal impairment (reduce dose by 50%). When injected IV (not UK), if there is extravasation into the SC tissues, can cause a sterile abscess and tissue induration. Give well diluted as a 15–30min IVI only if strictly necessary.

Undesirable effects

Dry mouth and other antimuscarinic effects (see Antimuscarinics, p.5), drowsiness, headache, fatigue, nervousness, dizziness, thickening of bronchial secretions.

Dose and use

Because of their antimuscarinic properties, the use of this group of drugs tends to be restricted to situations where **metoclopramide** and/or other more specific anti-emetics (e.g. **haloperidol**, $5HT_3$ antagonists) have failed to relieve, e.g. some patients with mechanical bowel obstruction, or as the anti-emetic of choice for raised intracranial pressure.

In the UK, **cyclizine** is generally the antihistaminic antimuscarinic anti-emetic of choice. Depending on circumstances, **cyclizine** is generally given PO or SC:

- 50–100mg PO b.d.–t.d.s. & p.r.n.
- 100–150mg/24h CSCI & 50mg SC p.r.n.
- usual maximum daily dose 200mg PO and CSCI.

Doses of **promethazine** are generally the same as those of **cyclizine**.

For CSCI dilute cyclizine with WFI or 5% glucose; cyclizine (lactate) is *incompatible* with 0.9% saline and will precipitate.

CSCI compatibility with other drugs: There are 2-drug compatibility data for cyclizine in WFI with **haloperidol**, **hyoscine *hydrobromide***, **morphine sulphate**, **and morphine tartrate** (not UK).

Concentration-dependent *incompatibility* occurs with **alfentanil**, **dexamethasone**, **diamorphine** and **oxycodone**. *Incompatbility* has also been reported with **clonazepam**, **hydromorphone**, **hyoscine *butylbromide***, **ketorolac**, **midazolam** and **octreotide**. For more details and 3-drug compatibility data, see Appendix 3 (p.773).

Supply

Oral products

Cyclizine *hydrochloride*
Valoid® (Amdipharm)
Tablets 50mg, 28 days @ 50mg t.d.s. = £6.

Hydroxyzine *hydrochloride*
Atarax® (Alliance)
Tablets 10mg, 25mg, 28 days @ 50mg t.d.s. = £7.

Ucerax® (UCB Pharma)
Tablets 25mg, 28 days @ 50mg t.d.s. = £8. ~~NHS~~
Oral solution (syrup) 10mg/5mL, 28 days @ 50mg t.d.s. = £19.

Promethazine *hydrochloride*
Phenergan® (Sanofi-Aventis)
Tablets 10mg, 25mg, 28 days @ 50mg t.d.s. = £13.
Oral solution 5mg/5mL, 28 days @ 50mg t.d.s. = £112.

Promethazine *teoclate*
Avomine® (Manx)
Tablets 25mg, 28 days @ 50mg t.d.s. = £19.

Injections

Cyclizine *lactate*
Valoid® (Amdipharm)
Injection 50mg/mL, 1mL amp = £0.50.

Promethazine *hydrochloride* (generic)
Injection 25mg/mL, 1mL amp = £0.50, 2mL amp = £1.

Phenergan® (Sanofi-Aventis)
Injection 25mg/mL, 1mL amp = £0.50.

1 Gay L and Carliner P (1949) The prevention and treatment of motion sickness. *Bulletin of John Hopkins Hospital*. **49**: 470–491.
2 Gutner B *et al.* (1952) The effects of potent analgesics upon vestibular function. *Journal of Clinical Investigations*. **31**: 259–266.
3 Dundee J and Jones P (1968) The prevention of analgesic-induced nausea and vomiting by cyclizine. *British Journal of Clinical Practice*. **22**: 379–382.
4 Walder A and Aitkenhead A (1995) A comparison of droperidol and cyclizine in the prevention of postoperative nausea and vomiting associated with patient-controlled analgesia. *Anaesthesia*. **50**: 654–656.
5 Beaver WT and Feise G (1976) Comparison of analgesic effects of morphine sulphate, hydroxyzine and their combination in patients with postoperative pain. In: JJ Bonica and D Albe-Fessard (eds) *Advances in Pain Research and Therapy* Vol 1. Raven Press, New York, pp. 553–557.
6 Hupert C *et al.* (1980) Effect of hydroxyzine on morphine analgesia for the treatment of postoperative pain. *Anesthesia and Analgesia*. **59**: 690–696.

$5HT_3$ ANTAGONISTS BNF 4.6

Indications: Nausea and vomiting after surgery, chemotherapy and radiotherapy, †intractable vomiting due to chemical, abdominal and cerebral causes when usual approaches have failed, †opioid-induced pruritus,[1,2] †uraemic and †cholestatic pruritus.

Contra-indications: Concurrent IV administration with IV **metoclopramide** (risk of arrhythmia: see p.227).

Pharmacology

$5HT_3$ antagonists were developed specifically to control emesis associated with highly emetogenic chemotherapy, e.g. **cisplatin**. They block the amplifying effect of excess 5HT on vagal nerve fibres, and are thus of particular value in situations when excessive amounts of 5HT are released from the body's stores, i.e. from enterochromaffin cells after chemotherapy or radiation-induced damage of the GI mucosa, or because of intestinal distension, or from leaky platelets when there is severe renal impairment.

In an open RCT, **tropisetron** (not UK) was shown to be of benefit in patients with far-advanced cancer and nausea and vomiting of indeterminate cause when given either as a sole agent or with a second anti-emetic, particularly **dexamethasone**.[3] $5HT_3$ antagonists also relieve nausea and vomiting after head injury, brain stem radiotherapy,[4,5] and in multiple sclerosis with brain stem disease;[6] leakage of 5HT from the raphe nucleus probably accounts for the benefit seen in these circumstances. $5HT_3$ antagonists are also effective in nausea and vomiting associated with acute gastro-enteritis.[7] In one patient who experienced persistent nausea after the insertion of an endo-oesophageal tube, a $5HT_3$ antagonist brought about relief after failure with **metoclopramide** and **cyclizine**.[8]

IV **ondansetron** 4–8mg relieves itch induced by spinal opioids in 3–30min.[1,9,10] Although trials have not been conducted with other $5HT_3$ antagonists, it is likely that the benefit shown with **ondansetron** is a class effect.[11] Good results have also been noted in case reports and open studies of both single and multiple doses of IV or PO **ondansetron** in cholestasis[11–14] and uraemia (**ondansetron** 4mg PO b.d. resulted in progressive improvement over 2 weeks).[12] However, two RCTs of **ondansetron** in chronic cholestasis showed either no benefit (IV 8mg stat + tablets 8mg b.d. for 5 days)[15] or minimal benefit (tablets 8mg t.d.s. for 1 week).[16] Similarly, an RCT in uraemic itch showed no benefit with **ondansetron**.[17] For pharmacokinetic details see Table 4.23.

Table 4.23 Pharmacokinetic details of $5HT_3$ antagonists

		Ondansetron	*Granisetron*	*Palonosetron*
Bio-availability	PO	56–71% (60% PR)	60%	n/a
Onset of action	PO IV	<30min <5min	<30min <15min	n/a
Plasma halflife		3–5h (6h PR)	10–11h	40h
Time to peak plasma concentration	PO IM PR	1.5h 10min 6h	No data	n/a n/a n/a
Duration of action		12h	24h	>24h[18]

Cautions

$5HT_3$ antagonists reduce colonic motility and can cause or worsen constipation.
Ondansetron: the dose should be reduced in moderate–severe hepatic impairment.

Drug interactions

Concurrent use of **tropisetron** and **granisetron** can completely block the analgesic effect of **paracetamol**, but **ondansetron** may be safe in this respect (see p.289).

Ondansetron reduces the analgesic effect of **tramadol** (possibly by blocking the action of serotonin at presynaptic 5HT$_3$-receptors on primary afferent nociceptive neurones in the spinal dorsal horn).[19] In postoperative pain, the dose of **tramadol** needed by IV PCA was increased 2–3 times in patients receiving **ondansetron** 1mg/h by CIVI. There was also an increase in vomiting (despite the **ondansetron**).[20] *Note: this is probably a class effect for 5HT$_3$ antagonists.*

Undesirable effects

Very common (>10%): headache.[21]
Common (<10%, >1%): lightheadedness, dizziness, nervousness, tremor, ataxia, asthenia, drowsiness, fever, sensation of warmth or flushing (particularly when given IV), thirst, constipation or diarrhoea.
Uncommon (<1%, >0.1%): **ondansetron**: dystonic reactions, arrhythmia, hypotension, raised LFTs.
Rare (<0.1%, >0.01%): hiccup.
Very rare (<0.01%): **ondansetron**: transient blindness during IV administration (sight generally returns within 20min).

Dose and use

All 5HT$_3$ antagonists are expensive, and it is important not to use them unnecessarily. *In palliative care, first-line use for nausea and vomiting is rarely appropriate.*[22]

When used for intractable nausea and vomiting in advanced cancer, 5HT$_3$ antagonists are often more effective when combined with other anti-emetics.[3] They are typically used in combination with an antipsychotic with affinity for multiple receptors (e.g. **levomepromazine**, **olanzapine**) ± **dexamethasone**.

Generic **ondansetron** is used at some centres as the cheapest option at heavily discounted hospital contract prices. However, **granisetron** needs to be given only once daily (instead of b.d.–t.d.s.). 5HT$_3$ antagonists are equally effective PO and by injection.[23–25] Regimens include:

- **granisetron** 1–2mg PO/SC once daily for 3 days *or*
- **ondansetron** 8mg PO/SC b.d.–t.d.s. (or 16–24mg/24h CSCI) for 3 days
- if clearly of benefit, continue indefinitely unless the cause is self-limiting
- some patients benefit from higher doses, occasionally as high as **granisetron** 9mg daily[26]
- in patients with moderate-severe hepatic impairment, the dose of **ondansetron** should be limited to 8mg daily, whereas no dose reduction is necessary for **granisetron** (in renal impairment, no dose reduction is necessary with either drug).

Note: to control nausea and vomiting caused by severely emetogenic chemotherapy, **granisetron** (or other 5HT$_3$ antagonist) is used with other anti-emetics, typically **dexamethasone** and **metoclopramide**.[27]

For use in pruritus associated with spinally administered opioids or end-stage renal failure, see discussion in Pharmacology section above.

Supply

Granisetron (generic)
Tablets 1mg, 28 days @ 1mg once daily = £143.
Injection 1mg/mL, for dilution and use as an injection or infusion, 1mL amp = £1, 3mL amp = £5.

Kytril® (Roche)
Tablets 1mg, 2mg, 28 days @ 1mg daily = £147.

Ondansetron (generic)
Tablets 4mg, 8mg, 28 days @ 8mg b.d. = £280.
Oral solution 4mg/5mL, 28 days @ 8mg b.d. = £428.
Injection 2mg/mL, 2mL amp = £5, 4mL amp = £11.

Zofran® (GlaxoSmithKline)
Tablets 4mg, 8mg, 28 days @ 8mg b.d. = £403.
Tablets orodispersible (Zofran Melt®) 4mg, 8mg, 28 days @ 8mg b.d. = £403.
Oral solution (sugar-free) 4mg/5mL, 28 days @ 8mg b.d. = £403; *strawberry flavour.*
Injection 2mg/mL, 2mL amp = £6, 4mL amp = £12.
Suppositories 16mg, 1 = £14.

1 Borgeat A and Stimemann H-R (1999) Ondansetron is effective to treat spinal or epidural morphine-induced pruritus. *Anesthesiology.* **90**: 432–436.
2 Kyriakides K *et al.* (1999) Management of opioid-induced pruritus: a role for 5HT antagonists? *British Journal of Anaesthesia.* **82**: 439–441.
3 Mystakidou K *et al.* (1998) Comparison of the efficacy and safety of tropisetron, metoclopramide, and chlorpromazine in the treatment of emesis associated with far advanced cancer. *Cancer.* **83**: 1214–1223.
4 Kleinerman K *et al.* (1993) Use of ondansetron for control of projectile vomiting in patients with neurosurgical trauma: two case reports. *Annals of Pharmacotherapy.* **27**: 566–568.
5 Bodis S *et al.* (1994) The prevention of radiosurgery-induced nausea and vomiting by ondansetron: evidence of a direct effect on the central nervous system chemoreceptor trigger zone. *Surgery and Neurology.* **42**: 249–252.
6 Rice G and Ebers G (1995) Ondansetron for intractable vertigo complicating acute brainstem disorders. *Lancet.* **345**: 1182–1183.
7 Cubeddu L *et al.* (1997) Antiemetic activity of ondansetron in acute gastroenteritis. *Alimentary Pharmacology and Therapeutics.* **11**: 185–191.
8 Fair R (1990) Ondansetron in nausea. *Pharmaceutical Journal.* **245**: 514.
9 Arai L *et al.* (1996) The use of ondansetron to treat pruritus associated with intrathecal morphine in two paediatric patients. *Paediatric Anaesthesia.* **6**: 337–339.
10 Larijani G *et al.* (1996) Treatment of opioid-induced pruritus with ondansetron: report of four patients. *Pharmacotherapy.* **16**: 958–960.
11 Quigley C and Plowman PN (1996) 5HT3 receptor antagonists and pruritus due to cholestasis. *Palliative Medicine.* **10**: 54.
12 Balaskas E *et al.* (1998) Histamine and serotonin in uremic pruritus: effect of ondansetron in CAPD-pruritic patients. *Nephron.* **78**: 395–402.
13 Raderer M *et al.* (1994) Ondansetron for pruritus due to cholestasis. *New England Journal of Medicine.* **330**: 1540.
14 Schworer H and Ramadori G (1993) Improvement of cholestatic pruritus by ondansetron. *Lancet.* **341**: 1277.
15 O'Donohue J *et al.* (1997) Ondansetron in the treatment of pruritus of cholestasis: a randomised controlled trial. *Gastroenterology.* **112**: A1349.
16 Muller C *et al.* (1998) Treatment of pruritus in chronic liver disease with the 5-hydroxytryptamine receptor type 3 antagonist ondansetron: a randomized, placebo-controlled, double-blind cross-over trial. *European Journal of Gastroenterology and Hepatology.* **10**: 865–870.
17 Murphy M *et al.* (2001) A randomised, placebo-controlled, double-blind trial of ondansetron in renal itch. *British Journal of Dermatology.* **145 (suppl 59)**: 20–21.
18 Saito M *et al.* (2009) Palonosetron plus dexamethasone versus granisetron plus dexamethasone for prevention of nausea and vomiting during chemotherapy: a double-blind, double-dummy, randomised, comparative phase III trial. *Lancet Oncology.* **10**: 115–124.
19 De Witte JL *et al.* (2001) The analgesic efficacy of tramadol is impaired by concurrent administration of ondansetron. *Anesthesia and Analgesia.* **92**: 1319–1321.
20 Arcioni R *et al.* (2002) Ondansetron inhibits the analgesic effects of tramadol: a possible 5-HT(3) spinal receptor involvement in acute pain in humans. *Anesthesia and Analgesia.* **94**: 1553–1557.
21 Goodin S and Cunningham R (2002) 5-HT3-receptor antagonists for the treatment of nausea and vomiting: a reappraisal of their side-effect profile. *The Oncologist.* **7**: 424–436.
22 Currow D *et al.* (1997) Use of ondansetron in palliative medicine. *Journal of Pain and Symptom Management.* **13**: 302–307.
23 Perez EA *et al.* (1997) Efficacy and safety of different doses of granisetron for the prophylaxis of cisplatin-induced emesis. *Support Care Cancer.* **5**: 31–37.
24 Perez E *et al.* (1997) Efficacy and safety of oral granisetron versus IV ondansetron in prevention of moderately emetogenic chemotherapy-induced nausea and vomiting. *Proceedings of the American Society of Clinical Oncology.* **16**: 149.
25 Gralla R *et al.* (1997) Can an oral antiemetic regimen be as effective as intravenous treatment against cisplatin: results of a 1054 patient randomized study of oral granisetron versus IV ondansetron. *Proceedings of the American Society of Clinical Oncology.* **16**: 178.
26 Minami M (2003) Granisetron: is there a dose-response effect on nausea and vomiting? *Cancer Chemotherapy and Pharmacology.* **52**: 89–98.
27 Kris MG *et al.* (2006) American Society of Clinical Oncology guideline for antiemetics in oncology: update 2006. *Journal of Clinical Oncology.* **24**: 2932–2947.

ANTI-EPILEPTICS BNF 4.8.1

Indications: (Licensed indications vary; see individual drug monographs for details.) Epilepsy, neuropathic pain, mania, anxiety, †sweats and hot flushes, †refractory hiccup, †terminal agitation, †restless legs syndrome.

Pharmacology

Anti-epileptic drugs are structurally and functionally diverse. The relationship between clinical activity and mode of action is not fully understood. Further, clinically relevant differences exist between anti-epileptics acting in similar ways, and additional actions contribute to the beneficial and/or undesirable effects of some. Choice of drug thus remains partly empirical.[1]

Anti-epileptic drug actions include:

- membrane stabilization:
  - ▹ sodium-channel blockers
- reduced neurotransmitter release:
  - ▹ N/P/Q-type calcium channel blockers ($\alpha 2\delta$ ligands)
  - ▹ SV2A ligands
- increased GABA-mediated inhibition:
  - ▹ GABAmimetics (Table 4.24 and Figure 4.7).

The accumulation of sodium channels at sites of nerve injury is responsible for seizures or neuropathic pain through ectopic action potential generation (see p.257). Membrane stabilizers (e.g. **carbamazepine**, **phenytoin** and **lamotrigine**) reduce the excitability of damaged neurones by blocking such channels.

The $\alpha 2\delta$ ligands, **gabapentin** and **pregabalin**, block N, P and Q-type calcium-channels. This reduces the calcium influx required to trigger neurotransmitter release (see p.249).[10] **Levetiracetam** binds to SV2A, a protein involved in neurotransmitter vesicle release (see p.268).[11]

GABAmimetic anti-epileptics either affect GABA metabolism (synthesis, re-uptake or breakdown, e.g. **vigabatrin, tiagabine**) or act directly on $GABA_A$ receptors (e.g. benzodiazepines, see p.132 and Table 4.24). **Vigabatrin** and **tiagabine** have an effect on all GABA transmission, and this may explain their ability to worsen absence seizures (via thalamic $GABA_B$ receptors), a feature not seen with $GABA_A$-selective anti-epileptics.

The broad spectrum of efficacy of **valproate** is explained by its multiple actions including blockade of T-type calcium channels, implicated in neuropathic pain,[12] the burst firing responsible for absence seizures[1] and perhaps also in regulating pain excitation thresholds in a 'T-rich' subset of peripheral nociceptors.[3] The endocannabinoid system is another important inhibitory neurotransmitter system; cannabinoids have been proposed as potential future anti-epileptics.[13]

Genetic variations in anti-epileptic targets have been identified (e.g. sodium and potassium channels, the $GABA_A$ receptor complex). Some cause inherited epilepsy, but there is no straightforward link between the affected channel/receptor and either the epilepsy type or optimal choice of anti-epileptic.[14,15] A polymorphism in the gene (SCN1A) encoding the sodium channel α-subunit has been linked to **carbamazepine**-resistant epilepsy.[16]

The pharmacokinetics of anti-epileptics are summarized in Table 4.25. Whereas absorption is generally unaffected by increasing age, the volume of distribution may change (reduced albumin, total body water and lean:fat mass ratio) and elimination rates slow (altered metabolism, renal function and volume of distribution).[17,18]

Genetic factors affect both pharmacokinetics and the risk of undesirable effects. Two poor metabolizer CYP2C9 alleles (which occur in 10–20% of Caucasians, 10% of Japanese, and 1–5% of Asians and Africans) reduce the mean effective daily **phenytoin** dose by 20–40%.[15] Human leukocyte antigen (HLA) genes are associated with the risk of Stevens-Johnson syndrome in patients taking **carbamazepine** or **phenytoin** (see p.260).[27,28] The UK MHRA recommends testing HLA B*1502 status before **carbamazepine** is started in people of Han Chinese, Hong Kong Chinese or Thai origin.[17]

Table 4.24 Mechanisms of action of anti-epileptics[1–8]

	Membrane stabilizers		*↓ Neurotransmitter release*		*GABAmimetics*		*↓Thalamic burst firing*
	Na channel blocker	*K channel activator*	*Ca channel blocker (N, P and Q type)*	*↓vesicle release (SV2A)*	*$GABA_A$ receptor modulation*	*Altered GABA synthesis and reuptake*	*Ca channel blocker (T type)*
Benzodiazepines					++		
Carbamazepine	++						
Ethosuximide							++
Gabapentin		+	++				
Lacosamide	++						
Lamotrigine	++		++				
Levetiracetam				++			
Oxcarbazepine	++	+					
Phenobarbital					++		
Phenytoin	++						
Pregabalin			++				
Tiagabine						++[b]	
Topiramate	++				++		
Valproate	+[a]					+[a,b]	+[a]
Vigabatrin						++[b]	
Zonisamide	++		++				++

Key: ++ = predominant action, + = putative or non-predominant action.

a. although many anti-epileptics have more than one mode of action, valproate in particular is thought to have no predominant mode of action, helping to explain its broad spectrum of activity (see p.264)

b. tiagabine and vigabatrin inhibit GABA re-uptake and breakdown (via GABA transaminase) respectively. Valproate affects both synthesis and re-uptake/breakdown of GABA in selected brain regions.

Table 4.25 Pharmacokinetic details of anti-epileptics[18–26]

Drug	*Bio-availability PO (%)*	T_{max} *(h)*	*Plasma binding (%)*	*Plasma halflife (h)*	*Fate*
Carbamazepine	80	4–8	75	8–24	CYP3A4, CYP2C8[h]
Clonazepam	⩾80	1–4	80–90	30–40	CYP3A
Diazepam	⩾80	1–3	95–98	24–48, 48–120[g]	CYP2C19, CYP3A4[h]
Gabapentin	60[a]	1–4	0	6	Excreted unchanged
Lamotrigine	98	1–4	55	15–30, 8–20[d], 30–90[e]	Glucuronidation
Levetiracetam	⩾95	1–2	<10	6–8	Non-hepatic hydrolysis (70% excreted unchanged)
Oxcarbazepine[f]	⩾95	1–3, 3–8[f]	65, 40[f]	1–5, 7–20[f]	Cytosolic keto-reduction to MHD[f], which then undergoes glucuronidation[h]
Phenobarbital	⩾90	2–12	50	72–144	CYP2C9 (25% excreted unchanged)
Phenytoin	90–95	4–8	90	10–70[a]	CYP2C9
Pregabalin	>90	1	0	5–9[b]	Excreted unchanged
Tiagabine	⩾90	1–2	96	4–13, 2–5[d]	CYP3A4
Topiramate	⩾80	1–4	13	20–30, 8–15[d]	Multiple pathways (>60% excreted unchanged)
Valproate	95	1–2[c]	90	9–18, 5–12[d]	Multiple pathways[h] (see p.264)
Vigabatrin	80–90	1–2	0	6	Excreted unchanged
Zonisamide	⩾50	1–4	50	50–70, 25–35[d]	CYP3A4 (15–30% excreted unchanged)

a. dose or plasma concentration dependent
b. >2 days in severe renal impairment and haemodialysis patients
c. 3–5h for e/c tablets, 5–10h for m/r tablets
d. with concurrent enzyme-inducers
e. with concurrent valproate
f. monohydroxycarbazepine, active metabolite of oxcarbazepine (a pro-drug)
g. nordiazepam, active metabolite
h. metabolites biologically active.

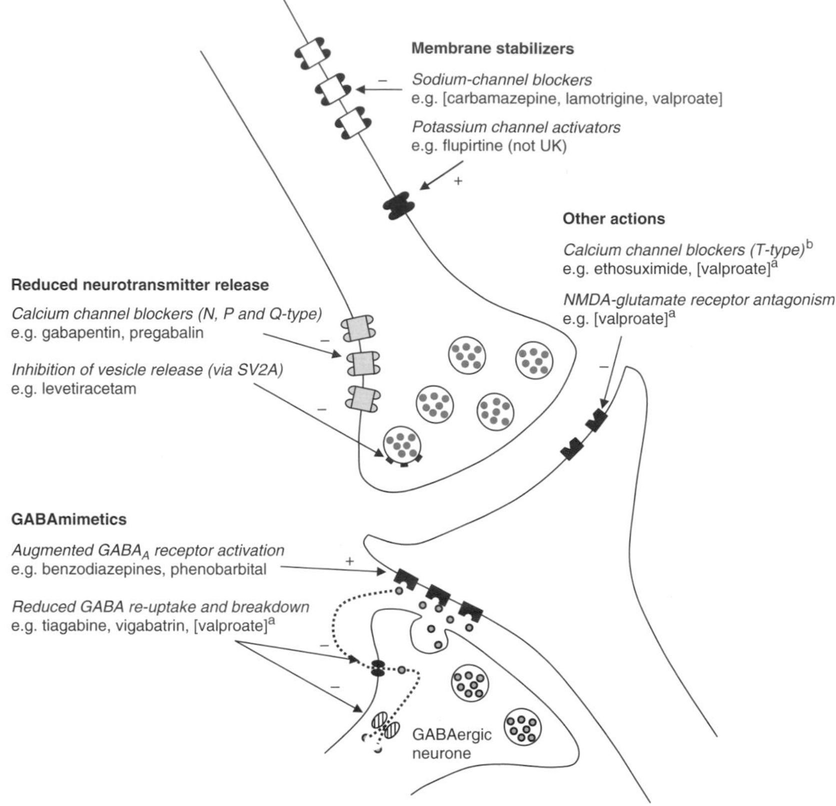

Figure 4.7 Mechanisms of action of anti-epileptics and related drugs.[1–7,9] Squared parentheses indicate a contributory, but not predominant, action of the anti-epileptic.

a. although many anti-epileptics have more than one mode of action, valproate in particular is thought to have no single predominant action (see p.264).

b. T type calcium channels are responsible for thalamic burst firing (implicated in absence seizures); they are also found in some nociceptors, where they may influence firing thresholds (see text).

Cautions

Safety concerns with **vigabatrin** (visual field deficits) and **felbamate** (aplastic anaemia and hepatic failure) limit their use to refractory epilepsy under specialist supervision when all other measures have failed.

Driving

In the UK, patients suffering from epilepsy must notify the DVLA. Generally, a seizure-free period of one year is required before driving can resume (longer for heavy goods vehicles), although this varies (e.g. where a seizure was due to a transient illness).[29] Patients affected by drowsiness should not drive or operate machinery.

Skin rashes and cross-reactive hypersensitivity

In relation to skin rashes, cross-reactive hypersensitivity may occur with various anti-epileptics:[30]

- **carbamazepine**: increased risk if rash occurred with a previous anti-epileptic (particularly **phenytoin, phenobarbital** or **oxcarbazepine**) or TCA; use alternative if possible

- **phenytoin**: increased risk of skin rash if rash has occurred with a previous anti-epileptic (particularly **carbamazepine** or **phenobarbital**); use alternative if possible
- **oxcarbazepine**: 25–30% risk of cross-reactivity if previous reaction to **carbamazepine**
- **zonisamide**: avoid if hypersensitive to sulphonamides
- **lamotrigine**: increased risk of rash if rash has occurred with a previous anti-epileptic, rapidly titrated and/or receiving concurrent **valproate**.

Hepatic impairment

With the exception of **gabapentin**, **pregabalin**, and **vigabatrin**, the manufacturers advise caution with all the anti-epileptics listed in Table 4.25 (i.e. lower initial doses, slower titration and careful monitoring). Specific advice is given for **levetiracetam** (halve the dose in severe hepatic impairment because of probable concurrent renal impairment), **lamotrigine** (see SPC), **oxcarbazepine** (usual dose with mild–moderate impairment, no data with severe impairment), **phenytoin** (monitor plasma concentration), **tiagabine** (reduce dose if mild, avoid if severe), and **zonisamide** (avoid if possible).

Further, previous or concurrent hepatic disease increases the risk of **valproate**- and **carbamazepine**-related hepatic failure. However, no specific information is available about the risks with hepatic metastases. They do not generally affect the hepatic metabolism of drugs unless there is concurrent cirrhosis.[31,32] Increase monitoring or use alternatives.

Renal impairment

With the exception of **phenytoin** and **tiagabine**, the manufacturers advise caution with all the anti-epileptics listed in Table 4.25 (i.e. lower initial doses, slower titration and careful monitoring). Specific advice on dose adjustment is available for **gabapentin** (see Table 4.29, p.253) and **pregabalin** (see Table 4.30, p.256). Further, there are occasional reports of renal failure with **pregabalin** which improved when it was stopped.

Females of child-bearing age

Consider teratogenicity when choosing an anti-epileptic. Enquire about oral contraceptive if using an enzyme-inducing anti-epileptic.

Suicide

Anti-epileptic drugs are associated with suicidal thoughts or behaviour in 1/500 patients from the start of treatment onwards. Monitor for suicidal ideation, and advise patients to get in touch if they experience mood disturbance or suicidal thoughts.[33,34]

Additional cautions with specific anti-epileptics

- atrioventricular block (**carbamazepine** and **oxcarbazepine** may cause complete block)
- previous bone marrow suppression (**carbamazepine**, possible increased risk)
- heart failure (**oxcarbazepine** and **pregabalin**, fluid retention can cause exacerbation; monitor weight and plasma sodium).

Drug interactions

Interactions are described in individual drug monographs:

- **gabapentin** (p.251), **pregabalin** (p.254) and **levetiracetam** (p.268) have no clinically significant pharmacokinetic interactions
- **phenobarbital** (p.270), **carbamazepine** (p.260) and **phenytoin** (p.258) cause numerous interactions through hepatic enzyme induction.

Undesirable effects

Despite their diverse actions and structures, anti-epileptics share many undesirable effects. Their relative incidence is often similar.[35,36]

All anti-epileptics cause psychotropic and CNS depressant effects including drowsiness, ataxia, cognitive impairment, agitation, diplopia and dizziness. Cognitive impairment is worst with **phenobarbital** and least with newer anti-epileptics and **valproate**.[22,37] Anti-epileptics cause suicidal ideation in 1/500 patients (see Cautions).

Most cause haematological derangements. These are often asymptomatic and may not require stopping the drug (see SPCs for advice). Severe derangement (e.g. aplastic anaemia, agranulocytosis) is reported particularly with **felbamate** (limiting use) and **carbamazepine** (monitor blood counts), and with many newer anti-epileptics. Folate deficiency occurs with enzyme-inducers (e.g. **phenytoin**).

Biochemical derangements (particularly of LFTs) are also common but are generally asymptomatic. Albeit rarely, hepatic failure is seen with many anti-epileptics, again particularly with **felbamate** (also limiting its use) and **carbamazepine** (where symptoms of hepatic disease and LFTs should be monitored), as well as with newer anti-epileptics. The incidence compared with **carbamazepine** is unknown. Pancreatitis affects 1:3,000 users of **valproate**.[38] It also occurs with many newer anti-epileptics but the incidence compared with **valproate** is unknown.

Transient rashes are particularly associated with **lamotrigine**, **carbamazepine** and **oxcarbazepine**. Risk factors include rashes with previous anti-epileptics, higher starting doses and rapid titration (and, with **lamotrigine**, childhood and concurrent **valproate**). Severe rashes such as Stevens-Johnson syndrome are reported with all anti-epileptics, but most commonly with **lamotrigine** (affecting 1:1,000 adults). An HLA type is known to predispose specific groups to **carbamazepine**- and **phenytoin**-related Stevens-Johnson syndrome (see above).

Undesirable effects seen with particular anti-epileptics include: urolithiasis (**topiramate** and **zonisamide**); and coarse facies, acne, hirsutism and gingival hypertrophy (**phenytoin**).

Use of anti-epileptics in palliative care

Particularly when prescribing more than one anti-epileptic, it is important to consider:
- pharmacokinetic drug–drug interactions
- seizure type (generalized seizures may be precipitated by **carbamazepine**, **oxcarbazepine**, **gabapentin**, **tiagabine** and **vigabatrin**)
- additive cognitive impairment.

Neuropathic pain

Gabapentin, **pregabalin**, **carbamazepine** and **valproate** are commonly used for central and peripheral neuropathic pain. Their efficacy and tolerability appear comparable to each other and to alternatives (e.g. antidepressants), as judged by NNT and NNH,[39–41] although few have been directly compared.

In some centres **gabapentin** and **pregabalin** are first-line choices for neuropathic pain because this indication is included in their marketing authorizations. Both are beneficial in various non-cancer neuropathic pains. **Pregabalin's** twice daily administration is a possible advantage, but it is more expensive and without evidence of superiority. NICE's recommendations are thus open to question (see p.249) **Gabapentin** is also effective for cancer-related neuropathic pain, although the benefit in an RCT was small (see p.251).[42] **Gabapentin** appeared to act more quickly and with less sedation than **carbamazepine** in relation to neuropathic pain in Guillain-Barre syndrome, but neither was used optimally (dose regimens were fixed).[43]

Valproate is used in some centres as an alternative first choice when a smaller tablet load, oral liquid product or once daily regimen is required, particularly if a TCA cannot be used. Benefit is reported for cancer-related neuropathic pain,[44,45] but the results of RCTs in non-cancer pain are conflicting (see p.264); thus EFNS and IASP guidelines do not recommend its use first line.[41,46] It appears to be well tolerated in both cancer series and RCTs; rates of discontinuation because of adverse events are low (3–5%)[47–50] compared with trials of **gabapentin** (8–19%)[38,40] and **pregabalin** (8–32%)[51–57] in similar populations.

Carbamazepine is a licensed first-line treatment for trigeminal neuralgia. It has long been used off-label for other neuropathic pains despite few supporting RCTs.[58] It requires slow titration and particular care with regard to drug interactions (see p.260). **Phenytoin** is also effective, at least in the short-term.[59] The important role of sodium channels in neuropathic pain (see above) has led to trials of other membrane stabilizers, particularly **oxcarbazepine** and **lamotrigine**, but results are conflicting (see p.257).

Clonazepam is reported to improve both cancer-related and non-cancer neuropathic pain.[60–63] Its concurrent anxiolytic and muscle-relaxant properties have led to its use for selected palliative care patients despite the absence of supporting RCTs.

Alternatives to anti-epileptics include antidepressants (p.172) and opioids (p.345). They are also often used in combination. The efficacy of **gabapentin** was similar to TCAs in two RCTs although, in one, TCAs caused more dry mouth, constipation and postural hypotension.[64,65] Combined use was superior to either treatment alone.[66] **Morphine** was as effective as TCAs,[67] whereas the combination of **morphine** and **gabapentin** was superior to either treatment alone.[68] An open-label trial in cancer pain with a neuropathic component also found this combination to be superior to **morphine** alone.[69]

Combinations of ⩾2 anti-epileptics are used less commonly. Undesirable effects may be increased and alternative options (e.g. antidepressants, opioids, **ketamine** and interventional anaesthesia) are often more appropriate. Where a second anti-epileptic drug is added, the first is generally withdrawn, although examples of combined use are reported. Improvements in efficacy and tolerability have been described in 11 patients with multiple sclerosis whose trigeminal neuralgia had been unsatisfactorily controlled by **carbamazepine** ± **lamotrigine**. The addition of **gabapentin** brought relief in 10 patients. The former were reduced to the minimal effective dose, with improved overall tolerability, but could not be withdrawn completely in any patient, suggesting that both anti-epileptics were contributing to overall relief.[70]

Although generally not used for *nociceptive* pain, **phenytoin**, **lamotrigine**, **gabapentin** and **pregabalin** have an antinociceptive/analgesic effect.[71–74]

Doses are described in individual monographs: †**carbamazepine** (p.260); †**clonazepam** (p.144); **gabapentin** (p.251); †**oxcarbazepine** (p.263); **pregabalin** (p.254) and †**valproate** (p.264).

Epilepsy

Overtreatment with anti-epileptic drugs is common. Seek specialist advice where the diagnosis of seizures or the dose or choice of anti-epileptic drug is in doubt.

Initiating treatment

In palliative care, an anti-epileptic is generally commenced after a first seizure because the persisting underlying cause (e.g. cerebral tumour, multiple sclerosis) makes further seizures probable. In other settings, this risk is lower and an anti-epileptic is often withheld unless a second seizure occurs.[75] Focal lesions cause seizures of partial onset +/− secondary generalization. True generalized convulsive seizures are generally evident within the first two decades of life, and may be exacerbated by some anti-epileptics (see above).

Choice of anti-epileptic is guided by seizure type, potential for drug interactions, co-morbidities, and the simplicity of the regimen (Box 4.J). Because of the risk of teratogenicity with some anti-epileptics, obtain specialist advice when treating women of childbearing age. Enzyme-inducing anti-epileptics can interfere with chemotherapy. **Valproate**, **levetiracetam**, **gabapentin**, **carbamazepine** and **phenytoin** are among the anti-epileptics examined in trials for seizures secondary to cerebral tumours.[76–78]

Box 4.J Anti-epileptics for seizures in palliative care[77,78]

First-line alternatives

Oxcarbazepine

Fewer drug interactions than phenytoin and carbamazepine; effective doses achieved more quickly than with lamotrigine and carbamazepine.

Valproate[a]

Can be titrated rapidly, IV if necessary.

Phenytoin

Can be rapidly titrated, IV if necessary; but numerous drug interactions can occur.

Second-line

Switch to another first-line choice, or prescribe

Levetiracetam

a. despite abnormal in vitro haemostasis, valproate has not been shown to increase neurosurgical bleeding complications,[81,82] but some surgeons advise caution; discuss with surgeons before starting if neurosurgery is planned.

Anti-epileptics are better tolerated if commenced at lower than recommended doses.[79] Doses can be increased if seizures persist. However, less additional benefit is seen when increasing higher doses. In one observational study, 90% of those responding to a first-line anti-epileptic required:

- **valproate** ≤1,500mg/24h
- **lamotrigine** ≤300mg/24h
- **carbamazepine** ≤800mg/24h.[80]

Few patients responded to increases above these doses.[80] In non-responders, a change of anti-epileptic is indicated.

For doses, see individual monographs for **valproate** (p.264), **carbamazepine** (p.260), **oxcarbazepine** (p.263), **gabapentin** (p.251), **pregabalin** (p.254) or **levetiracetam** (p.268), or the manufacturer's SPC.

Switching vs. combining anti-epileptics for epilepsy

If the first choice treatment fails, add a second anti-epileptic (Box 4.J). When the second one is at an adequate or maximally tolerated dose, the first one is slowly withdrawn (see below).[83] Long-term combination therapy is generally avoided unless two trials of monotherapy have proved ineffective because:

- there is an increased likelihood of drug interactions
- toxicity may be enhanced
- evidence of benefit compared with monotherapy is limited.[79,84]

Combinations are guided by the same considerations as those for choosing first- and second-line anti-epileptics. Many successful combinations have been reported,[84,85] but the relative benefits of such combinations have not been established. Studies of older anti-epileptics indicate probable benefit in combining GABAmimetics with sodium channel blockers or possibly with other GABAmimetics, but not in using two sodium channel blockers together.[86] Despite this, combinations of sodium channel blockers are among those used by epileptologists.[84] Combining **valproate** and **lamotrigine** increases the risk of skin reactions.

Do not combine three or more anti-epileptics except on specialist advice; additional benefit is rare.[79]

Prophylaxis in patients with cerebral tumours

Although about 20% of patients diagnosed with cerebral tumours will experience seizures, the risk is not reduced by prophylactic anti-epileptics. Sub-therapeutic levels, a potential explanation in some trials, does not adequately account for this lack of effect. Thus anti-epileptics should not generally be commenced in the absence of a history of seizures.[75,87] Peri-neurosurgical use is an exception, but anti-epileptics should generally be slowly tapered after one week.[87]

Convulsive status epilepticus

Figure 4.8 is modified from NICE guidance.[88] Hypoglycaemia should be excluded in all patients. If alcoholism or severely impaired nutrition is suspected, give thiamine 250mg IV. **Phenobarbital** has been given preference over **phenytoin** because it is more likely to be immediately available in many palliative care units.

Lorazepam is the benzodiazepine of choice in the control of status epilepticus (see p.146)[89] but, if unavailable, **midazolam** 10mg (see p.141) is an alternative. If venous access cannot be obtained give **midazolam** 10mg †buccally or †SC, or **diazepam** 10–20mg PR (see p.139).

Fosphenytoin is a pro-drug of **phenytoin** (1.5mg of the former is equivalent to 1mg of the latter). The dose is expressed as **phenytoin sodium** equivalent (PE). It can be given more rapidly than **phenytoin**. Ideally, heart rate, blood pressure and respiratory function should be monitored during and for 30min after the administration of **fosphenytoin** 15–20mg(PE)/kg (50–100mg(PE)/min). IV **phenytoin sodium** 15mg/kg up to a maximum total dose of 1g (≤50mg/min; dilute 500mg with 50mL 0.9% saline) can be used instead, preferably with ECG monitoring.

Non-convulsive status epilepticus (NCSE)

NCSE is characterised by seizure activity on an EEG but without associated tonic-clonic activity. Presentations include delirium or coma.[90] In one report, NCSE was diagnosed in 5% of patients admitted to a palliative care unit; of these, half responded to treatment with anti-epileptics.[91] Treatment is less urgent than for convulsive status epilepticus (see Box 4.J).

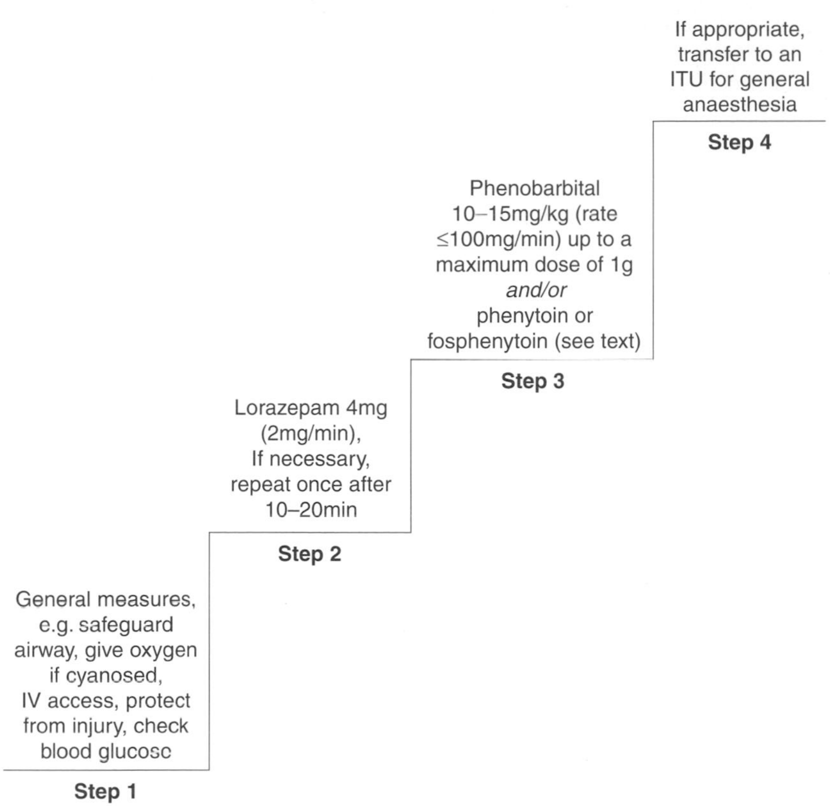

Figure 4.8 Management of status epilepticus in adults. See text for more detail.

Terminal agitation

Phenobarbital is sometimes used in the management of intractable agitation in patients who are imminently dying (see p.270).[92]

Mania

Valproate is generally added only when the response to an antipsychotic and a benzodiazepine is inadequate, but is an alternative first-line therapy particularly when it has been effective previously. **Carbamazepine** and **lamotrigine** can also be used.[93]

Anxiety

Despite benefit in various anxiety disorders,[94] anti-epileptics are not commonly used. In the UK, **pregabalin** (see p.254) is licensed for generalized anxiety disorder. Its efficacy is similar to **lorazepam**, **alprazolam** and **venlafaxine**. It has a faster rate of onset than **venlafaxine**, and causes less nausea. It has a similar rate of onset to **lorazepam** and **alprazolam**, and causes less drowsiness but more dizziness.[95] It is also effective for social phobia.[96] RCTs also show some benefit with **gabapentin**,[97,98] **tiagabine**[99] and **lamotrigine**.[100]

Sweats and hot flushes

Gabapentin is effective for hot flushes associated with breast cancer or the menopause.[101,102] Benefit is also reported in idiopathic sweating in cancer (see p.251).[103]

Refractory hiccup

Gabapentin is reported to be effective for hiccup (see p.251).

Restless legs syndrome

Gabapentin and **clonazepam** are used for restless legs syndrome; alternatives include D_2 agonists (e.g. **ropinirole**) and **levodopa**.[104]

Stopping anti-epileptics

Abrupt cessation of long-term anti-epileptic therapy should be avoided because rebound seizures may be precipitated, even if use is for indications other than epilepsy. If treatment is to be discontinued, particularly barbiturates and benzodiazepines, this is best done *slowly over several months* (Table 4.26). However, both **gabapentin** and **pregabalin** can be stopped progressively over 1–2 weeks.

Table 4.26 Recommended monthly reductions of selected anti-epileptics[105]

Drug[a]	*Reduction*
Carbamazepine	100mg
Clobazam	10mg
Clonazepam	0.5mg
Ethosuximide	250mg
Lamotrigine	25mg
Levetiracetam	1,000mg[b]
Phenobarbital	15mg
Phenytoin	50mg
Topiramate	25mg
Valproate	250mg
Vigabatrin	500mg

a. gabapentin and pregabalin can be stopped progressively over 1–2 weeks
b. data from SPC.

In adults, the risk of relapse of pre-existing epilepsy on stopping treatment is 40–50%.[106] Caution should also be exercised when switching to an alternative anti-epileptic drug. In contrast to switching opioids (see p.354), the first drug should *not* be withdrawn until the new drug has been titrated up to an anticipated effective dose.

For patients who are imminently dying (i.e. death expected within a few days) and who can no longer swallow medication, consider substituting SC **midazolam** or SC **phenobarbital**. However, remember that some anti-epileptics have a long halflife (see Table 4.25) and, in a moribund patient, might continue to be effective for 2–3 days after the last PO dose.

1 Perucca E (2005) An introduction to antiepileptic drugs. *Epilepsia*. **46 (suppl 4)**: 31–37.
2 Lynch BA (2004) The synaptic vesicle protein SV2A is the binding site for the antiepileptic drug levetiracetam. *Proceedings of the National Academy of Sciences of the United States of America*. **101 (26)**: 9861–9866.
3 Jevtovic-Todorovic V *et al.* (2006) The role of peripheral T-type calcium channels in pain transmission. *Cell Calcium*. **40**: 197–203.
4 Kochegarov AA (2003) Pharmacological modulators of voltage-gated calcium channels and their therapeutical application. *Cell Calcium*. **33**: 145–162.
5 Shin HS (2006) T-type Ca2+ channels and absence epilepsy. *Cell Calcium*. **40**: 191–196.
6 Loscher W (2002) Basic pharmacology of valproate: a review after 35 years of clinical use for the treatment of epilepsy. *CNS Drugs*. **16**: 669–694.
7 Lee CH *et al.* (2008) Gabapentin activates ROMK1 channels by a protein kinase A (PKA)-dependent mechanism. *British Journal of Pharmacology*. **154**: 216–225.
8 Sheets PL *et al.* (2008) Differential block of sensory neuronal voltage-gated sodium channels by lacosamide [(2R)-2-(acetylamino)-N-benzyl-3-methoxypropanamide], lidocaine, and carbamazepine. *Journal of Pharmacology and Experimental Therapeutics*. **326**: 89–99.
9 Devulder J (2010) Flupirtine in pain management: pharmacological properties and clinical use. *CNS Drugs*. **24**: 867–881.

10 Taylor CP (2009) Mechanisms of analgesia by gabapentin and pregabalin–calcium channel alpha2-delta [Cavalpha2-delta] ligands. *Pain*. **142**: 13–16.

11 Lynch BA (2004) The synaptic vesicle protein SV2A is the binding site for the antiepileptic drug levetiracetam. *Proceedings of the National Academy of Sciences of the United States of America*. **101 (26)**: 9861–9866.

12 Takahashi T *et al.* (2010) Upregulation of Ca(v)3.2 T-type calcium channels targeted by endogenous hydrogen sulfide contributes to maintenance of neuropathic pain. *Pain*. **150**: 183–191.

13 Bagshaw SM and Hagan NA (2002) Medical efficacy of cannabinoids and marijuana: a comprehensive review of the literature. *Journal of Palliative Care*. **18 (2)**: 111–122.

14 Mann MW and Pons G (2007) Various pharmacogenetic aspects of antiepileptic drug therapy: a review. *CNS Drugs*. **21**: 143–164.

15 Loscher W *et al.* (2009) The clinical impact of pharmacogenetics on the treatment of epilepsy. *Epilepsia*. **50**: 1–23.

16 Abe T *et al.* (2008) Association between SCN1A polymorphism and carbamazepine-resistant epilepsy. *British Journal of Clinical Pharmacology*. **66**: 304–307.

17 MHRA (2008) Drug safety update. 1 (9, April): 5. Available from: www.mhra.gov.uk/Publications/Safetyguidance/DrugSafetyUpdate/CON014505

18 Perucca E (2006) Clinical pharmacokinetics of new-generation antiepileptic drugs at the extremes of age. *Clinical Pharmacokinetics*. **45**: 351–363.

19 Perucca E (1999) The clinical pharmacokinetics of the new antiepileptic drugs. *Epilepsia*. **40 (suppl 9)**: S7–13.

20 Garnett WR (2000) Clinical pharmacology of topiramate: a review. *Epilepsia*. **41 (suppl 1)**: S61–65.

21 Anderson *et al.* (2002) *Handbook of clinical drug data*. (10e). McGraw Hill.

22 Perucca E (2002) Pharmacological and therapeutic properties of valproate: a summary after 35 years of clinical experience. *CNS Drugs*. **16**: 695–714.

23 May TW *et al.* (2003) Clinical pharmacokinetics of oxcarbazepine. *Clinical Pharmacokinetics*. **42**: 1023–1042.

24 Bang LM and Goa KL (2004) Spotlight on oxcarbazepine in epilepsy. *CNS Drugs*. **18**: 57–61.

25 Kwan P and Brodie MJ (2004) Phenobarbital for the treatment of epilepsy in the 21st century: a critical review. *Epilepsia*. **45**: 1141–1149.

26 Patsalos PN and Patsalos PN (2004) Clinical pharmacokinetics of levetiracetam. *Clinical Pharmacokinetics*. **43**: 707–724.

27 Chung WH *et al.* (2004) Medical genetics: a marker for Stevens-Johnson syndrome. *Nature*. **428**: 486.

28 Locharernkul C *et al.* (2008) Carbamazepine and phenytoin induced Stevens-Johnson syndrome is associated with HLA-B*1502 allele in Thai population. *Epilepsia*. **49**: 2087–2091.

29 Carter T (2006) *Fitness to Drive: A Guide for Health Professionals*. Royal Society of Medicine Press, London.

30 Hirsch LJ *et al.* (2008) Cross-sensitivity of skin rashes with antiepileptic drug use. *Neurology*. **71**: 1527–1534.

31 Morgan DJ and McLean AJ (1995) Clinical pharmacokinetic and pharmacodynamic considerations in patients with liver disease. An update. *Clinical Pharmacokinetics*. **29**: 370–391.

32 Ford-Dunn S (2005) Managing patients with cancer and advanced liver disease. *Palliative Medicine*. **19**: 563–565.

33 FDA (2008) Safety information. Antiepileptic drugs. Available from: www.fda.gov/Safety/MedWatch/SafetyInformation/SafetyAlertsforHumanMedicalProducts/ucm074939.htm

34 EMEA (2008) Meeting highlights from the Committee for Medicinal Products for Human Use, 15–18 December 2008. Available from: www.emea.europa.eu/pdfs/human/press/pr/67072408en.pdf

35 Marson AG *et al.* (2007) The SANAD study of effectiveness of valproate, lamotrigine, or topiramate for generalised and unclassifiable epilepsy: an unblinded randomised controlled trial. *Lancet*. **369**: 1016–1026.

36 Marson AG *et al.* (2007) The SANAD study of effectiveness of carbamazepine, gabapentin, lamotrigine, oxcarbazepine, or topiramate for treatment of partial epilepsy: an unblinded randomised controlled trial. *Lancet*. **369**: 1000–1015.

37 Kwan P and Brodie MJ (2001) Neuropsychological effects of epilepsy and antiepileptic drugs. *Lancet*. **357**: 216–222.

38 French JA (2007) First-choice drug for newly diagnosed epilepsy. *Lancet*. **369**: 970–971.

39 Finnerup (2010) The evidence for pharmaceutical treatment of neuropathic pain. *Pain*. **150**: 573–581.

40 Saarto T and Wiffen PJ (2007) Antidepressants for neuropathic pain. *Cochrane Database of Systematic Reviews*. CD005454.

41 Dworkin RH *et al.* (2010) Recommendations for the pharmacological management of neuropathic pain: an overview and literature update. *Mayo Clinic Proceedings*. **85**: S3–14.

42 Caraceni A *et al.* (2004) Gabapentin for neuropathic cancer pain: a randomized controlled trial from the Gabapentin Cancer Pain Study Group. *Journal of Clinical Oncology*. **22**: 2909–2917.

43 Pandey CK *et al.* (2005) The comparative evaluation of gabapentin and carbamazepine for pain management in Guillain-Barre syndrome patients in the intensive care unit. *Anesthesia and Analgesia*. **101**: 220–225.

44 Hardy J *et al.* (2001) A phase II study to establish the efficacy and toxicity of sodium valproate in patients with cancer-related neuropathic pain. *Journal of Pain and Symptom Management*. **21**: 204–209.

45 Snare AJ (1993) Sodium Valproate. Retrospective analysis of neuropathic pain control in patients with advanced cancer. *Journal of Pharmacy Technology*. **9**: 114–117.

46 Attal N *et al.* (2010) EFNS guidelines on the pharmacological treatment of neuropathic pain: 2010 revision. *European Journal of Neurology*. **17**: 1113–e1188.

47 Kochar DK *et al.* (2002) Sodium valproate in the management of painful neuropathy in type 2 diabetes — a randomized placebo controlled study. *Acta Neurologica Scandinavica*. **106**: 248–252.

48 Kochar DK *et al.* (2004) Sodium valproate for painful diabetic neuropathy: a randomized double-blind placebo-controlled study. *Quarterly Journal of Medicine*. **97**: 33–38.

49 Kochar DK *et al.* (2005) Divalproex sodium in the management of post-herpetic neuralgia: a randomized double-blind placebo-controlled study. *Quarterly Journal of Medicine*. **98**: 29–34.

50 Otto M *et al.* (2004) Valproic acid has no effect on pain in polyneuropathy: a randomized, controlled trial. *Neurology*. **62**: 285–288.

51 Richter RW *et al.* (2005) Relief of painful diabetic peripheral neuropathy with pregabalin: a randomized, placebo-controlled trial. *Journal of Pain*. **6**: 253–260.

52 Rosenstock J *et al.* (2004) Pregabalin for the treatment of painful diabetic peripheral neuropathy: a double-blind, placebo-controlled trial. *Pain*. **110**: 628–638.

53 Tolle T *et al.* (2008) Pregabalin for relief of neuropathic pain associated with diabetic neuropathy: a randomized, double-blind study. *European Journal of Pain.* **12**: 203–213.

54 Freynhagen R *et al.* (2005) Efficacy of pregabalin in neuropathic pain evaluated in a 12-week, randomised, double-blind, multicentre, placebo-controlled trial of flexible- and fixed-dose regimens. *Pain.* **115**: 254–263.

55 Sabatowski R *et al.* (2004) Pregabalin reduces pain and improves sleep and mood disturbances in patients with post-herpetic neuralgia: results of a randomised, placebo-controlled clinical trial. *Pain.* **109**: 26–35.

56 van Seventer R *et al.* (2006) Efficacy and tolerability of twice-daily pregabalin for treating pain and related sleep interference in postherpetic neuralgia: a 13-week, randomized trial. *Current Medical Research and Opinion.* **22**: 375–384.

57 Dworkin RH *et al.* (2003) Pregabalin for the treatment of postherpetic neuralgia: a randomized, placebo-controlled trial.[see comment]. *Neurology.* **60**: 1274–1283.

58 Wiffen PJ *et al.* (2005) Carbamazepine for acute and chronic pain. *Cochrane Database of Systematic Reviews.* **3**: CD005451.

59 McCleane G (1999) Intravenous infusion of phenytoin relieves neuropathic pain: a randomized, double-blinded, placebo-controlled, crossover study. *Anesthesia and Analgesia.* **89**: 985–988.

60 Swerdlow M and Cundill J (1981) Anticonvulsant drugs used in the treatment of lancinating pain: a comparison. *Anaesthesia.* **36**: 1129–1132.

61 Bouckoms AJ and Litman RE (1985) Clonazepam in the treatment of neuralgic pain syndrome. *Psychosomatics.* **26**: 933–936.

62 Bartusch S *et al.* (1996) Clonazepam for the treatment of lancinating phantom limb pain. *Clinical Journal of Pain.* **12**: 59–62.

63 Hugel H *et al.* (2003) Clonazepam as an adjuvant analgesic in patients with cancer-related neuropathic pain. *Journal of Pain and Symptom Management.* **26**: 1073–1074.

64 Morello C *et al.* (1999) Randomized double-blind study comparing the efficacy of gabapentin with amitriptyline on diabetic peripheral neuropathy pain. *Archives of Internal Medicine.* **159**: 1931–1937.

65 Chandra K *et al.* (2006) Gabapentin versus nortriptyline in post-herpetic neuralgia patients: a randomized, double-blind clinical trial–the GONIP Trial. *International Journal of Clinical Pharmacology and Therapeutics.* **44**: 358–363.

66 Gilron I *et al.* (2009) Nortriptyline and gabapentin, alone and in combination for neuropathic pain: a double-blind, randomised controlled crossover trial. *Lancet.* **374**: 1252–1261.

67 Raja SN *et al.* (2002) Opioids versus antidepressants in postherpetic neuralgia: a randomized, placebo-controlled trial.[see comment]. *Neurology.* **59**: 1015–1021.

68 Gilron I *et al.* (2005) Morphine, gabapentin, or their combination for neuropathic pain. *New England Journal of Medicine.* **352**: 1324–1334.

69 Keskinbora K *et al.* (2007) Gabapentin and an opioid combination versus opioid alone for the management of neuropathic cancer pain: a randomized open trial. *Journal of Pain and Symptom Management.* **34**: 183–189.

70 Solaro C *et al.* (2000) Low-dose gabapentin combined with either lamotrigine or carbamazepine can be useful therapies for trigeminal neuralgia in multiple sclerosis. *European Neurology.* **44**: 45–48.

71 Webb J and Kamali F (1998) Analgesic effects of lamotrigine and phenytoin on cold-induced pain: a crossover placebo-controlled study in healthy volunteers. *Pain.* **76**: 357–363.

72 Hill CM *et al.* (2001) Pregabalin in patients with postoperative dental pain. *European Journal of Pain.* **5**: 119–124.

73 Ho KY *et al.* (2006) Gabapentin and postoperative pain–a systematic review of randomized controlled trials. *Pain.* **126**: 91–101.

74 Jokela R *et al.* (2008) A randomized controlled trial of perioperative administration of pregabalin for pain after laparoscopic hysterectomy. *Pain.* **134**: 106–112.

75 Miller LC and Drislane FW (2007) Treatment strategies after a single seizure: rationale for immediate versus deferred treatment. *CNS Drugs.* **21**: 89–99.

76 Schaller B (2006) Brain tumor and seizures: pathophysiology and its implications for treatment revisited Epilepsia 2003; 44:1223–1232. *Epilepsia.* **47**: 661; author reply 661.

77 Vecht C (2006) Otimizing therapy of seizures in patients with brain tumours. *Neurology.* **67**: S10–S13.

78 van Breemen MS *et al.* (2007) Epilepsy in patients with brain tumours: epidemiology, mechanisms, and management. *Lancet Neurology.* **6**: 421–430.

79 Perucca E and Kwan P (2005) Overtreatment in epilepsy: how it occurs and how it can be avoided. *CNS Drugs.* **19**: 897–908.

80 Kwan P and Brodie MJ (2001) Effectiveness of first antiepileptic drug. *Epilepsia.* **42**: 1255–1260.

81 Ward MM *et al.* (1996) Preoperative valproate administration does not increase blood loss during temporal lobectomy. *Epilepsia.* **37**: 98–101.

82 Anderson GD *et al.* (1997) Absence of bleeding complications in patients undergoing cortical surgery while receiving valproate treatment. *Journal of Neurosurgery.* **87**: 252–256.

83 NICE (2004) The epilepsies: the diagnosis and management of the epilepsies in adults and children in primary and secondary care. Available from: www.nice.org.uk/nicemedia/pdf/CG020fullguideline.pdf

84 Karceski S *et al.* (2005) Treatment of epilepsy in adults: expert opinion, 2005. *Epilepsy & Behavior.* **7 (suppl 1)**: S1–64.

85 Stephen LJ and Brodie MJ (2002) Seizure freedom with more than one antiepileptic drug. *Seizure.* **11**: 349–351.

86 Deckers CL *et al.* (2000) Selection of antiepileptic drug polytherapy based on mechanisms of action: the evidence reviewed. *Epilepsia.* **41**: 1364–1374.

87 Glantz MJ *et al.* (2000) Practice parameter: anticonvulsant prophylaxis in patients with newly diagnosed brain tumors. Report of the Quality Standards Subcommittee of the American Academy of Neurology. *Neurology.* **54**: 1886–1893.

88 NICE (2010) Clinical Guideline 20. Epilepsy in adults and children: full guideline, appendix C Guidelines for treating status epilepticus in adults and children.

89 Prasad K *et al.* (2005) Anticonvulsant therapy for status epilepticus. *Cochrane Database of Systematic Reviews.* **4**: CD003723.

90 Twycross R *et al.* (2009) *Symptom Management in Advanced Cancer* (4e). palliativedrugs.com, Nottingham, pp. 283–284.

91 Lorenzl S *et al.* (2010) Nonconvulsive status epilepticus in palliative care patients. *Journal of Pain and Symptom Management.* **40**: 460–465.

92 Twycross R *et al.* (2009) *Symptom Management in Advanced Cancer.* palliativedrugs.com, Nottingham, pp. 430–433.

93 NICE (2006) The management of bipolar disorder in adults, children and adolescents, in primary and secondary care. Clinical guideline CG38. Available from: www.nice.guidance.nice.org.uk/CG38

94 Van Ameringen M *et al.* (2004) Antiepileptic drugs in the treatment of anxiety disorders: role in therapy. *Drugs.* **64**: 2199–2220.

95 Frampton JE and Foster RH (2006) Pregabalin: in the treatment of generalised anxiety disorder. *CNS Drugs.* **20**: 685–693; discussion 694–695. [erratum appears in CNS Drugs. 2007;**21**:481].

96 Pande AC *et al.* (2004) Efficacy of the novel anxiolytic pregabalin in social anxiety disorder: a placebo-controlled, multicenter study. *Journal of Clinical Psychopharmacology.* **24**: 141–149.
97 Pande AC *et al.* (1999) Treatment of social phobia with gabapentin: a placebo-controlled study. *Journal of Clinical Psychopharmacology.* **19**: 341–348.
98 Pande AC *et al.* (2000) Placebo-controlled study of gabapentin treatment of panic disorder. *Journal of Clinical Psychopharmacology.* **20**: 467–471.
99 Pollack MH *et al.* (2005) The selective GABA reuptake inhibitor tiagabine for the treatment of generalized anxiety disorder: results of a placebo-controlled study. *Journal of Clinical Psychiatry.* **66**: 1401–1408.
100 Hertzberg MA *et al.* (1999) A preliminary study of lamotrigine for the treatment of posttraumatic stress disorder. *Biological Psychiatry.* **45**: 1226–1229.
101 Pandya KJ *et al.* (2005) Gabapentin for hot flashes in 420 women with breast cancer: a randomised double-blind placebo-controlled trial. *Lancet.* **366**: 818–824.
102 Nelson HD *et al.* (2006) Nonhormonal therapies for menopausal hot flashes: systematic review and meta-analysis. *Journal of the American Medical Association.* **295**: 2057–2071.
103 Porzio G *et al.* (2006) Gabapentin in the treatment of severe sweating experienced by advanced cancer patients. *Supportive Care in Cancer.* **14**: 389–391.
104 Vignatelli L *et al.* (2006) EFNS guidelines on management of restless legs syndrome and periodic limb movement disorder in sleep. *European Journal of Neurology.* **13**: 1049–1065.
105 Chadwick D (1995) The withdrawal of antiepileptic drugs. In: A Hopkins *et al.* (eds) *Epilepsy* (2e). Chapman and Hall, London, pp. 215–220.
106 Hopkins A and Shorvon S (1995) Definitions and epidemiology of epilepsy. In: A Hopkins *et al.* (eds) *Epilepsy* (2e). Chapman and Hall, London, pp. 1–24.

ANTI-EPILEPTIC PRE-SYNAPTIC CALCIUM-CHANNEL BLOCKERS — BNF 4.8.1

Gabapentin and **pregabalin** bind to the $\alpha 2\delta$ type 1 regulatory subunit of pre-synaptic (N, P/Q-type) voltage-gated calcium channels, reducing the calcium influx responsible for triggering neurotransmitter release.[1] Both the spinal dorsal horn and brain stem/forebrain are important sites of action. Calcium channel $\alpha 2\delta$ subunits are upregulated in the spinal dorsal horn by inflammation and neuropathic pain;[2,3] **gabapentin** and **pregabalin** counteract this. Brain stem/forebrain actions influence descending pain inhibitory pathways and pain processing.[1,4,5] Spinal calcium channels are also targeted by **ziconotide**.

Both **gabapentin** and **pregabalin** cause redistribution of calcium channels away from the cell surface, rather than blocking them directly. Effects on sodium and potassium channels have also been shown.[6,7] Despite being GABA analogues, neither **gabapentin** nor **pregabalin** is GABAmimetic.[1] They are unrelated to the L-type calcium-channel blockers, **nifedipine**, **diltiazem** and **verapamil** (Table 4.27). L-type channels are also found on neurones, but the significance of anti-epileptics blocking these neuronal L-type channels (e.g. **carbamazepine**) is unclear.

Table 4.27 Classification of calcium channels

Type	*Location (function)*	*Blocked by*
L-type (Ca_v1.1–1.4)	Cardiovascular and GI tissues (smooth muscle tone, conductivity)	Verapamil, diltiazem, nifedipine (see p.73)
N, P/Q-type (Ca_v2.1–2.2)	Pre-synaptic neurones (calcium influx triggers neurotransmitter release; over-expressed in neuropathic pain)	Gabapentin and pregabalin (N and P/Q-type), ziconotide (N-type)[1]
T-type (Ca_v3.1–3.3)	Thalamic and nociceptive neurones (excitability, threshold setting, pacemaker activity. Thalamic T-type channel dysregulation responsible for absence seizures)	Ethosuximide, valproate (see p.264)[8]
R-type (Ca_v2.3)	Cerebellum (function unknown)	

Table 4.28 Efficacy of gabapentin and pregabalin for neuropathic pain[a]

Pain type	*Gabapentin*			*Pregabalin*[b]		
	Participants	*Studies*[c]	*VAS↓*	*Participants*	*Studies*[c]	*VAS↓*
Painful diabetic neuropathy	225	2	−13	856	5	−12
Post herpetic neuralgia	448	2	−14	513	3	−17
Spinal cord injury	116	2	−17	137	1	−15
Central pain (mixed)				40	1	−24
HIV neuropathy	26	1	−8.5			
Phantom limb pain	86	2	−9.6			
Traumatic nerve injury	240	1	−3.0			

a. mean pain VAS reduction was the most commonly reported outcome measure (11/13 gabapentin RCTs; 10/12 pregabalin RCTs)

b. comparison is hampered by methodological differences (see text). 7/12 pregabalin RCTs compared placebo with ⩾2 fixed dose arms. Only results from highest dose arms are presented (mean VAS reductions are smaller when lower dose arms are included). Enriched recruitment (see text) is likely to result in the presented reductions over-estimating the degree of benefit for pregabalin

c. only 20/25 RCTs considered by NICE are included; 4 did not report mean pain VAS reduction, the other reported results in a mixed pain population.

Gabapentin and **pregabalin** are first-line anti-epileptic drugs for neuropathic pain.[9–11] Their benefit is comparable (Table 4.28), they are free of significant pharmacokinetic drug–drug interactions and neuropathic pain is included in their marketing authorizations. **Pregabalin** is more expensive, without evidence of superiority; but the need to take it only twice daily (rather than thrice) is a practical advantage.

Thus it is surprising that NICE recommended **pregabalin** rather than **gabapentin** for neuropathic pain. The stated reasons for this were:

- a comparison of NNTs for 30% and 50% reductions in pain from separate RCTs
- b.d. vs. t.d.s. administration
- cost-effectiveness.[12]

However, their NNT comparison excluded 10/13 **gabapentin** RCTs and did not take account of enriched enrolment, pain type or important methodological differences. Only 3/13 **gabapentin** RCTs reported NNTs vs. 10/12 **pregabalin** RCTs; and they were less favourable than the remainder (mean pain VAS reduction difference −0.8 vs. −1.2).

Further, enriched enrolment (the exclusion of those not responding to either drug in a previous setting) was more common in **pregabalin** RCTs (4/11 vs. 2/13, 1 not stated). Although the numbers affected are not reported, the mean pain VAS reduction difference is greater in **pregabalin** RCTs using enrichment: −1.3 vs. −1.1 in painful diabetic neuropathy RCTs, and −1.8 *vs.* −1.6 in post-herpetic neuralgia RCTs). Results of enriched **gabapentin** RCTs are not more favourable.

Even if enrichment is disregarded and only higher dose **pregabalin** results included, **gabapentin**'s efficacy is still comparable once pain type is considered (Table 4.28). Further, the combined NNH favours **gabapentin**, 26 (better) vs. 13 (worse) for **pregabalin**. However, this may simply be a reflection of the dose titration regimen in the RCTs, whether flexible or fixed. In summary, NICE provide no direct or indirect clinical evidence of superiority. Given the comparable efficacy, tolerability and monitoring requirements vs. a marked difference in cost, the cost-effectiveness model used in the NICE analysis is questionable.

1 Taylor CP (2009) Mechanisms of analgesia by gabapentin and pregabalin–calcium channel alpha2-delta [Cavalpha2-delta] ligands. *Pain*. **142**: 13–16.

2 Boroujerdi A *et al.* (2008) Injury discharges regulate calcium channel alpha-2-delta-1 subunit upregulation in the dorsal horn that contributes to initiation of neuropathic pain. *Pain*. **139**: 358–366.

3 Lu (2010) Persistent inflammation alters the density and distribution of voltage activated calcium channels in subpopulations of rat cutaneous DRG neurons. *Pain*. **151**: 633–643.

4 Bee LA and Dickenson AH (2008) Descending facilitation from the brainstem determines behavioural and neuronal hypersensitivity following nerve injury and efficacy of pregabalin. *Pain.* **140**: 209–223.
5 Hayashida K *et al.* (2008) Gabapentin acts within the locus coeruleus to alleviate neuropathic pain. *Anesthesiology.* **109**: 1077–1084.
6 Lee CH *et al.* (2008) Gabapentin activates ROMK1 channels by a protein kinase A (PKA)-dependent mechanism. *British Journal of Pharmacology.* **154**: 216–225.
7 Yang RH *et al.* (2009) Gabapentin selectively reduces persistent sodium current in injured type-A dorsal root ganglion neurons. *Pain.* **143**: 48–55.
8 Loscher W (2002) Basic pharmacology of valproate: a review after 35 years of clinical use for the treatment of epilepsy. *CNS Drugs.* **16**: 669–694.
9 Attal N *et al.* (2010) EFNS guidelines on the pharmacological treatment of neuropathic pain: 2010 revision. *European Journal of Neurology.* **17**: 1113–e1188.
10 Dworkin RH *et al.* (2010) Recommendations for the pharmacological management of neuropathic pain: an overview and literature update. *Mayo Clinic Proceedings.* **85**: S3–14.
11 Finnerup (2010) The evidence for pharmaceutical treatment of neuropathic pain. *Pain.* **150**: 573–581.
12 NICE (2010) Clinical Guideline 96. Neuropathic pain: the pharmacological management of neuropathic pain in adults in non-specialist settings.

GABAPENTIN — BNF 4.8.1

Class: Anti-epileptic (pre-synaptic calcium-channel blocker).

Indications: Adjunctive use in epilepsy when conventional treatment is unsatisfactory, neuropathic pain,[1] †intractable itch, †hot flushes,[2,3] †sweating,[4] †refractory hiccup, †restless legs syndrome.

Pharmacology

The mode and site of action of gabapentin is described on p.249. Absorption is by a saturable mechanism and bio-availability is more than halved as the dose increases from 100mg to 1,200mg. Gabapentin is not protein-bound and freely crosses the blood-brain barrier. It is excreted unchanged by the kidneys and accumulates in renal impairment. The halflife increases to 50h when creatinine clearance is <30mL/min, and to over 5 days in anuria. Initial drowsiness or dizziness occurs in 50% of patients and generally resolves over 7–10 days of use.[5] Gabapentin's pharmacokinetic drug interactions are of doubtful clinical significance; **cimetidine** marginally impairs the renal excretion of gabapentin, and antacids containing **aluminum** or **magnesium** reduce gabapentin's bio-availability by 10–20%.

Gabapentin is effective for peripheral and central neuropathic pain.[1] Overall efficacy and tolerability are comparable to those of TCAs and other anti-epileptics,[6–8] but TCAs cause more dry mouth, constipation and postural hypotension.[9,10]

Gabapentin, individually titrated to 300–1,800mg/24h, has been reported to improve cancer-related neuropathic pain when given in addition to opioids.[11,12] This reflects the positive benefit of this combination in non-cancer neuropathic pain.[13] However, in an RCT, although the percentage of patients whose pain reduced by ≥1/3 was significantly higher during the first 5 days in those receiving gabapentin, after 10 days there was no difference; and, again after 10 days, the daily mean global and dysesthesia pain scores differed by <1/10 (mean global pain 4.6 on gabapentin vs. 5.5 on placebo), and there was no significant difference in the scores for stabbing (lancinating) and burning pain.[14] The doses of opioids and other analgesics remained unchanged during the study, although the higher 'as needed' opioid use by the placebo group may have obscured the benefit from gabapentin. Further, the lower doses used compared with non-cancer pain trials (≤1,800mg/24h vs. ≤3,600mg/24h) may also have contributed to the negative results in cancer-related neuropathic pain.[15]

Gabapentin is effective in fibromyalgia[16] and may be of benefit in malignant bone pain,[17] postoperative pain[18] and chronic masticatory myalgia.[19] The use of gabapentin for neuropathic itch is based on extrapolation from neuropathic pain management.[20] Gabapentin is effective for uraemic itch.[21,22] Benefit is also reported for intractable idiopathic itch.[23,24]

Gabapentin has been reported to be of benefit in generalized anxiety disorder,[25] hot flushes associated with breast cancer or the menopause,[2,3] and paraneoplastic sweating.[4] It reduces spasticity and muscle spasm in multiple sclerosis.[26,27] On the other hand, gabapentin occasionally causes myoclonus (a central phenomenon).[28,29] Paradoxically, it has also been used successfully to abolish opioid-related myoclonus.[30]

Gabapentin has been reported to be of benefit in refractory hiccup.[31,32] In one series, 'burst gabapentin' relieved persistent hiccup in patients with a history of brain stem stroke.[33] Patients received 400mg t.d.s. for 3 days, 400mg once daily for 3 days, and then stopped. Only 1/15 patients needed a second treatment.

Gabapentin is also used for restless legs syndrome (alternatives include **clonazepam,** D_2 agonists (e.g. **ropinirole**) and **levodopa**).[34]

Bio-availability PO 100mg, 74%; *but decreases as dose increases*: 300mg, 60%; 600mg, 49%; 1,200mg, 33%.

Onset of action 1–3h.

Time to peak plasma concentration 2–3h PO.

Plasma halflife 5–7h; 2 days or more in moderate–severe renal impairment, 5 days in anuria, 3–4h during haemodialysis.

Duration of action probably 8–12h, much longer in severe renal impairment/failure.

Cautions

Renal impairment; absence seizures (may worsen); psychotic illness (may precipitate psychotic episodes, generally resolving on dose reduction or discontinuation); false positive readings for urinary protein with Ames N-Multistix SG®.

Drug interactions

Aluminium and **magnesium**-containing compounds reduce bio-availability. **Morphine** and **naproxen** may increase gabapentin levels. High doses of gabapentin may decrease **hydrocodone** (not UK) levels; mechanism unknown.

Undesirable effects

Suicidal ideation (1/500; advise patients to report mood or thought disturbance). Possible causal association with acute pancreatitis.

Very common (>10%): drowsiness, dizziness.

Common (<10%, >1%): amnesia, anxiety, fatigue, amblyopia, diplopia, nystagmus, dysarthria, ataxia, tremor, arthralgia, myalgia, peripheral oedema, weight gain, dry mouth, pharyngitis, dyspepsia, diarrhoea.

Uncommon (<1%, >0.1%): leucopenia, impotence, gynaecomastia.[35]

Dose and use

Although the manufacturer advises that gabapentin should be given ⩾2h after aluminium- or magnesium-containing antacids, this is unnecessary in that the effect is relatively small.

Neuropathic pain

- start with 300mg at night
- if necessary, increase by 300mg/24h every 2–3 days, e.g.:
  - ▷ *Day 3* 300mg b.d.
  - ▷ *Day 5* 300mg t.d.s.
  - ▷ *Day 8* 300mg, 300mg, 600mg
  - ▷ *Day 11* 600mg, 300mg, 600mg
  - ▷ *Day 14* 600mg t.d.s.
- in elderly and frail patients, slower titration is advisable, e.g. 100mg at night, increased if necessary by 100mg/24h every 2–3 days
- typical dose 600mg t.d.s.[36]
- maximum recommended dose 1,200mg t.d.s.

The dose of gabapentin should be reduced in adults with renal impairment and those on haemodialysis.[37] Recommendations are shown in Table 4.29. However, although these may be appropriate in physically robust individuals, in palliative care the starting doses should generally be lower.

If required the capsules can be opened and the contents mixed with water, fruit juice, apple sauce, etc.[38]

Table 4.29 Dose adjustments in renal impairment modified from the SPC

Creatinine clearance (mL/min)	*Starting dose*[a]	*Maximum dose*
50–79	200mg t.d.s.	600mg t.d.s.
30–49	100mg t.d.s.	300mg t.d.s.
15–29	300mg alternate days	300mg b.d.[b]
<15	300mg alternate days	300mg at bedtime[b]
After every 4h of haemodialysis	Supplementary single dose of 200–300mg[c]	

a. smaller starting dose is advisable in elderly patients and those receiving other CNS-depressant drugs (see text)
b. the SPC recommends the daily dose be administered in three divided doses, but the prolonged halflife in renal impairment permits b.d. or once daily dosing as indicated
c. for anuric patients on dialysis, no regular dose is required, just a 'supplementary' dose after dialysis.

Hot flushes
- start with a low dose, as for neuropathic pain
- if necessary, increase to 300mg t.d.s.[3]

Hiccup
- in relatively robust patients, consider a 6-day 'burst' of gabapentin', e.g.:
  - ▷ 300–400mg t.d.s. for 3 days
  - ▷ 300–400mg once daily for 3 days
  - ▷ if necessary, re-treat long-term if hiccup recurs after a 'burst'
- in frail elderly patients, proceed slowly as for neuropathic pain:
  - ▷ start with a low dose, e.g. 100mg t.d.s.
  - ▷ if necessary, titrate upwards
  - ▷ if successful, consider reducing/stopping gabapentin
  - ▷ if necessary, re-treat long-term if hiccup recurs after a 'burst'.[33]

Neuropathic pruritus
- as for neuropathic pain.

Stopping gabapentin
To avoid precipitating seizures or pain, gabapentin should be withdrawn gradually over ≥1 week.

Supply
Gabapentin (generic)
Capsules 100mg, 300mg, 400mg, 28 days @ 300mg t.d.s. = £7.
Tablets 600mg, 800mg, 28 days @ 600mg t.d.s. = £21.

Neurontin® (Pfizer)
Capsules 100mg, 300mg, 400mg, 28 days @ 300mg t.d.s. = £36.
Tablets 600mg, 800mg, 28 days @ 600mg t.d.s. = £71.

1 Moore RA *et al.* (2011) Gabapentin for chronic neuropathic pain and fibromyalgia in adults. *Cochrane Database of Systematic Reviews.* **3**: CD007938.
2 Nelson HD *et al.* (2006) Nonhormonal therapies for menopausal hot flashes: systematic review and meta-analysis. *Journal of the American Medical Association.* **295**: 2057–2071.
3 Pandya KJ *et al.* (2005) Gabapentin for hot flashes in 420 women with breast cancer: a randomised double-blind placebo-controlled trial. *Lancet.* **366**: 818–824.
4 Porzio G *et al.* (2006) Gabapentin in the treatment of severe sweating experienced by advanced cancer patients. *Supportive Care in Cancer.* **14**: 389–391.

5 Backonja M and Glanzman RL (2003) Gabapentin dosing for neuropathic pain: evidence from randomized, placebo-controlled clinical trials. *Clinical Therapeutics*. **25**: 81–104.
6 Collins S *et al.* (2000) Antidepressants and anticonvulsants for diabetic neuropathy and postherpetic neuralgia: a quantitative systematic review. *Journal of Pain and Symptom Management*. **20**: 449–458.
7 Wiffen P *et al.* (2000) Anticonvulsant drugs for acute and chronic pain. *Cochrane Database of Systematic Reviews*. **3**: CD001133.
8 Vinik A (2005) Clinical review: Use of antiepileptic drugs in the treatment of chronic painful diabetic neuropathy. *Journal of Clinical Endocrinology and Metabolism*. **90**: 4936–4945.
9 Morello C *et al.* (1999) Randomized double-blind study comparing the efficacy of gabapentin with amitriptyline on diabetic peripheral neuropathy pain. *Archives of Internal Medicine*. **159**: 1931–1937.
10 Chandra K *et al.* (2006) Gabapentin versus nortriptyline in post-herpetic neuralgia patients: a randomized, double-blind clinical trial–the GONIP Trial. *International Journal of Clinical Pharmacology and Therapeutics*. **44**: 358–363.
11 Ross JR *et al.* (2005) Gabapentin is effective in the treatment of cancer-related neuropathic pain: a prospective, open-label study. *Journal of Palliative Medicine*. **8**: 1118–1126.
12 Caraceni A *et al.* (1999) Gabapentin as an adjuvant to opioid analgesia for neuropathic cancer pain. *Journal of Pain and Symptom Management*. **17**: 441–445.
13 Gilron I *et al.* (2005) Morphine, gabapentin, or their combination for neuropathic pain. *New England Journal of Medicine*. **352**: 1324–1334.
14 Caraceni A *et al.* (2004) Gabapentin for neuropathic cancer pain: a randomized controlled trial from the Gabapentin Cancer Pain Study Group. *Journal of Clinical Oncology*. **22**: 2909–2917.
15 Bennett MI (2005) Gabapentin significantly improves analgesia in people receiving opioids for neuropathic cancer pain. *Cancer Treatment Reviews*. **31**: 58–62.
16 Hauser W *et al.* (2009) Treatment of fibromyalgia syndrome with gabapentin and pregabalin–a meta-analysis of randomized controlled trials. *Pain*. **145**: 69–81.
17 Caraceni A *et al.* (2008) Gabapentin for breakthrough pain due to bone metastases. *Palliative Medicine*. **22**: 392–393.
18 Ho KY *et al.* (2006) Gabapentin and postoperative pain–a systematic review of randomized controlled trials. *Pain*. **126**: 91–101.
19 Kimos P *et al.* (2007) Analgesic action of gabapentin on chronic pain in the masticatory muscles: a randomized controlled trial. *Pain*. **127**: 151–160.
20 Zylicz Z *et al.* (eds) (2004) *Pruritus in Advanced Disease*. Oxford University Press, Oxford.
21 Gunal AI *et al.* (2004) Gabapentin therapy for pruritus in haemodialysis patients: a randomized, placebo-controlled, double-blind trial.[see comment]. *Nephrology Dialysis Transplantation*. **19**: 3137–3139.
22 Naini AE *et al.* (2007) Gabapentin: a promising drug for the treatment of uremic pruritus. *Saudi Journal of Kidney Diseases & Transplantation*. **18**: 378–381.
23 Kanitakis J (2006) Brachioradial pruritus: report of a new case responding to gabapentin. *European Journal of Dermatology*. **16**: 311–312.
24 Yesudian PD *et al.* (2005) Efficacy of gabapentin in the management of pruritus of unknown origin. *Archives of Dermatology*. **141**: 1507–1509.
25 Pollack MH *et al.* (1998) Gabapentin as a potential treatment for anxiety disorders. *American Journal of Psychiatry*. **155**: 992–993.
26 Cutter NC *et al.* (2000) Gabapentin effect on spasticity in multiple sclerosis: a placebo-controlled, randomized trial. *Archives of Physical Medicine and Rehabilitation*. **81**: 164–169.
27 Paisley S *et al.* (2002) Clinical effectiveness of oral treatments for spasticity in multiple sclerosis: a systematic review. *Multiple Sclerosis*. **8**: 319–329.
28 Asconape J *et al.* (2000) Myoclonus associated with the use of gabapentin. *Epilepsia*. **41**: 479–481.
29 Scullin P *et al.* (2003) Myoclonic jerks associated with gabapentin. *Palliative Medicine*. **17**: 717–718.
30 Mercadante S *et al.* (2001) Gabapentin for opioid-related myoclonus in cancer patients. *Supportive Care in Cancer*. **9**: 205–206.
31 Jatzko A *et al.* (2007) Alpha-2-delta ligands for singultus (hiccup) treatment: three case reports. *Journal of Pain and Symptom Management*. **33**: 756–760.
32 Alonso-Navarro H *et al.* (2007) Refractory hiccup: successful treatment with gabapentin. *Clinical Neuropharmacology*. **30**: 186–187.
33 Moretti R *et al.* (2004) Gabapentin as a drug therapy of intractable hiccup because of vascular lesion: a three-year follow up. *Neurologist*. **10**: 102–106.
34 Vignatelli L *et al.* (2006) EFNS guidelines on management of restless legs syndrome and periodic limb movement disorder in sleep. *European Journal of Neurology*. **13**: 1049–1065.
35 Zylicz Z (2000) Painful gynecomastia: an unusual toxicity of gabapentin? *Journal of Pain and Symptom Management*. **20**: 2–3.
36 Tremont-Lukats IW *et al.* (2000) Anticonvulsants for neuropathic pain syndromes: mechanisms of action and place in therapy. *Drugs*. **60**: 1029–1052.
37 Dworkin R *et al.* (2003) Advances in neuropathic pain. Diagnosis, mechanisms and treatment recommendations. *Archives of Neurology*. **60**: 1524–1534.
38 Gidal B *et al.* (1998) Gabapentin absorption: effect of mixing with foods of varying macronutrient composition. *Annals of Pharmacotherapy*. **32**: 405–409.

PREGABALIN — BNF 4.8.1

Class: Anti-epileptic (pre-synaptic calcium channel blocker).

Indications: Neuropathic pain, fibromyalgia, adjunctive treatment for partial seizures with or without secondary generalization, generalized anxiety disorder.[1–4]

Pharmacology

The mode and site of action of pregabalin is described on p.249. Pregabalin has a binding affinity 6 times greater than that of **gabapentin**, competitively displacing the latter from the $\alpha2\delta$ subunit.[5] Individual variability in pharmacokinetics is low (<20%). Bio-availability is high and independent of dose. Pregabalin is not protein-bound and undergoes negligible metabolism. More than 90% is excreted unchanged by the kidneys and it thus accumulates in renal impairment.[6] Half of the drug is removed after 4h of haemodialysis. It has no known pharmacokinetic drug interactions (but see Drug interactions below).[7]

Pregabalin has been shown in RCTs to be effective in painful diabetic neuropathy, post-herpetic neuralgia and central pain.[8–16] Response is dose-related; 1/4 of patients on 150mg/24h and up to 1/2 of patients receiving 300–600mg/24h obtain ⩾50% reduction in pain. In relation to pain and sleep, a slower flexible escalation schedule (dose escalation based on a patient's individual response and tolerability, over a period of ⩽4 weeks) ultimately produces similar benefit to a fixed escalation schedule, and is better tolerated. However, the onset of analgesia is delayed with flexible escalation because of the lower daily dose (75mg b.d. compared with 150mg b.d.) during the first week.[13]

In six RCTs, the NNT to achieve ⩾50% pain relief ranged from 3.3–5.6. Patients who had previously failed to respond to **gabapentin** were excluded from three of the trials.[14–16] There are no studies of pregabalin in cancer-related neuropathic pain, nor direct comparisons with **gabapentin** or other neuropathic pain treatments. Although not generally used for other pains, pregabalin is of benefit in post-dental extraction pain,[17] fibromyalgia,[18,19] and postoperative pain.[20]

Pregabalin is as effective as **lorazepam**, **alprazolam** and **venlafaxine** in generalized anxiety disorder. Compared with **venlafaxine**, pregabalin has a faster rate of onset and causes less nausea; it has a similar rate of onset to **lorazapam** and **alprazolam** and causes less drowsiness but more dizziness.[1–4]

Bio-availability ⩾90% PO.

Onset of action 24min post-dental extraction pain; <24h neuropathic pain; 2 days epilepsy.[16,17,21]

Time to peak plasma concentration 1h.

Plasma halflife 5–9h, increasing to >2 days in severe renal impairment (creatinine clearance <15mL/min) and in haemodialysis patients.[6]

Duration of action >12h.

Cautions

Renal impairment (dose adjustment required; renal failure reported which resolved on discontinuation), CHF (exacerbation reported).

Drug interactions

Concurrent use with thiazolidinedione antidiabetic drugs (e.g. **pioglitazone**, **rosiglitazone**) may cause weight gain and peripheral oedema.

Undesirable effects

Suicidal ideation (1/500; advise patients to report mood or thought disturbance).

Very common (>10%): dizziness (about 1/3 of patients), drowsiness (about 1/4); these generally resolve spontaneously after a median of 5–8 weeks.[14–16]

Common (<10%, >1%): confusion, irritability, euphoria, amnesia, reduced attention, blurred vision, diplopia, dysarthria, tremor, ataxia, increased appetite, weight gain, dry mouth, decreased libido, impotence, oedema.

Uncommon (<1%, >0.1%): painful gynaecomastia.[22]

Dose and use for neuropathic pain

- start with 75mg b.d.
- if necessary, at intervals of 3–7 days, increase to 150mg b.d. → 225mg b.d. → 300mg b.d. (maximum recommended dose)
- in debilitated patients, start with 25–50mg b.d.
- if necessary, increase the dose correspondingly cautiously.

The intervals between dose increases are pragmatic rather than pharmacokinetic. In one RCT, the effective doses were:

- 150mg b.d. in about a quarter of patients
- 225mg b.d. in about a third
- 300mg b.d. in another third.[13]

Dose reduction is necessary in renal impairment (Table 4.30). For patients on haemodialysis, the regular dose should be adjusted according to the creatinine clearance and a supplementary single dose given after each dialysis (Table 4.31).

Because epileptic seizures are often sporadic, more time is needed to evaluate the initial response, i.e. a minimum of 1 week.

Table 4.30 Impact of renal impairment on starting and maximum doses (manufacturer's recommendations)

Creatinine clearance (mL/min)	*Starting dose*	*Maximum dose*
>60	75mg b.d.	300mg b.d.
31–60	25mg t.d.s.[a]	150mg b.d.
15–30	25–50mg once daily	150mg once daily
<15	25mg once daily	75mg once daily

a. 37.5mg capsules not available, necessitating t.d.s. regimen.

Table 4.31 Post-haemodialysis supplementary doses

Daily dose	*Supplementary single dose after every 4h of haemodialysis*
25mg	25–50mg
50mg	50–75mg
75mg	100–150mg

Stopping pregabalin

To avoid precipitating pain or seizures, pregabalin should be withdrawn gradually over several weeks.

Supply

Lyrica® (Pfizer)

Capsules 25mg, 50mg, 75mg, 100mg, 150mg, 200mg, 225mg, 300mg, 28 days @ 25mg, 50mg t.d.s. = £97 for both strengths; 28 days @ 75mg, 150mg, 300mg b.d. = £64 for all 3 strengths.

Because of unit costs, the overall daily cost is less if given b.d. rather than t.d.s.

1 Feltner DE *et al.* (2003) A randomized, double-blind, placebo-controlled, fixed-dose, multicenter study of pregabalin in patients with generalized anxiety disorder. *Journal of Clinical Psychopharmacology.* **23**: 240–249.

2 Pande AC *et al.* (2003) Pregabalin in generalized anxiety disorder: a placebo-controlled trial. *American Journal of Psychiatry.* **160**: 533–540.

3 Rickels K *et al.* (2005) Pregabalin for treatment of generalized anxiety disorder: a 4-week, multicenter, double-blind, placebo-controlled trial of pregabalin and alprazolam. *Archives of General Psychiatry.* **62**: 1022–1030.

4 Montgomery SA *et al.* (2006) Efficacy and safety of pregabalin in the treatment of generalized anxiety disorder: a 6-week, multicenter, randomized, double-blind, placebo-controlled comparison of pregabalin and venlafaxine. *Journal of Clinical Psychiatry.* **67**: 771–782.

5 Jones DL and Sorkin LS (1998) Systemic gabapentin and S(+)-3-isobutyl-gamma-aminobutyric acid block secondary hyperalgesia. *Brain Research Reviews.* **810**: 93–99.

6 Randinitis EJ *et al.* (2003) Pharmacokinetics of pregabalin in subjects with various degrees of renal function. *Journal of Clinical Pharmacology.* **43**: 277–283.
7 Ben-Menachem E (2004) Pregabalin pharmacology and its relevance to clinical practice. *Epilepsia.* **45 (suppl 6)**: 13–18.
8 Vranken JH *et al.* (2008) Pregabalin in patients with central neuropathic pain: a randomized, double-blind, placebo-controlled trial of a flexible-dose regimen. *Pain.* **136**: 150–157.
9 Tolle T *et al.* (2008) Pregabalin for relief of neuropathic pain associated with diabetic neuropathy: a randomized, double-blind study. *European Journal of Pain.* **12**: 203–213.
10 van Seventer R *et al.* (2006) Efficacy and tolerability of twice-daily pregabalin for treating pain and related sleep interference in postherpetic neuralgia: a 13-week, randomized trial. *Current Medical Research and Opinion.* **22**: 375–384.
11 Siddall PJ *et al.* (2006) Pregabalin in central neuropathic pain associated with spinal cord injury: a placebo-controlled trial. *Neurology.* **67**: 1792–1800.
12 Richter RW *et al.* (2005) Relief of painful diabetic peripheral neuropathy with pregabalin: a randomized, placebo-controlled trial. *Journal of Pain.* **6**: 253–260.
13 Freynhagen R *et al.* (2005) Efficacy of pregabalin in neuropathic pain evaluated in a 12-week, randomised, double-blind, multicentre, placebo-controlled trial of flexible- and fixed-dose regimens. *Pain.* **115**: 254–263.
14 Sabatowski R *et al.* (2004) Pregabalin reduces pain and improves sleep and mood disturbances in patients with post-herpetic neuralgia: results of a randomised, placebo-controlled clinical trial. *Pain.* **109**: 26–35.
15 Rosenstock J *et al.* (2004) Pregabalin for the treatment of painful diabetic peripheral neuropathy: a double-blind, placebo-controlled trial. *Pain.* **110**: 628–638.
16 Dworkin RH *et al.* (2003) Pregabalin for the treatment of postherpetic neuralgia: a randomized, placebo-controlled trial. *Neurology.* **60**: 1274–1283.
17 Hill CM *et al.* (2001) Pregabalin in patients with postoperative dental pain. *European Journal of Pain.* **5**: 119–124.
18 Crofford LJ *et al.* (2008) Fibromyalgia relapse evaluation and efficacy for durability of meaningful relief (FREEDOM): a 6-month, double-blind, placebo-controlled trial with pregabalin. *Pain.* **136**: 419–431.
19 Hauser W *et al.* (2009) Treatment of fibromyalgia syndrome with gabapentin and pregabalin–a meta-analysis of randomized controlled trials. *Pain.* **145**: 69–81.
20 Jokela R *et al.* (2008) A randomized controlled trial of perioperative administration of pregabalin for pain after laparoscopic hysterectomy. *Pain.* **134**: 106–112.
21 Perucca E *et al.* (2003) Pregabalin demonstrates anticonvulsant activity onset by second day. *Neurology.* **60 (suppl 1)**: A145 [abstract P102. 122].
22 Malaga I and Sanmarti FX (2006) Two cases of painful gynecomastia and lower extremity pain in association with pregabalin therapy. *Epilepsia.* **47**: 1576–1579.

ANTI-EPILEPTIC SODIUM-CHANNEL BLOCKERS (MEMBRANE STABILIZERS) BNF 4.8.1

Membrane stabilizers reduce excitability by blocking sodium channels. Such channels are needed in high densities at sites which initiate action potentials (APs), e.g. sensory nerve endings, but lower densities are sufficient to allow APs to propagate along the remainder of the neurone. Neuronal damage interferes with sodium channel transport resulting in such channels accumulating and creating foci of ectopic AP generation.[1] Depending on the site of injury, these can result in seizures or neuropathic pain. Thus, several classes of drug of benefit in these conditions act through sodium channel blockade:

- some anti-epileptics, e.g. **carbamazepine** (see p.260), **oxcarbazepine** (see p.263), **phenytoin** (Box 4.K), **lamotrigine** and **lacosamide**
- local anaesthetics, e.g. **lidocaine** (see p.61)
- class I anti-arrhythmics, e.g. **flecainide** (see p.65).

All have been shown to have antinociceptive and/or anti-neuropathic pain effects.[2–5] However, the duration of blockade before the drug dissociates from the channel varies. This, and effects on targets other than sodium channels, creates important clinical differences between such drugs.

Carbamazepine is a licensed first-line treatment for trigeminal neuralgia. It has long been used for other neuropathic pains despite few supporting RCTs.[7] It requires slow titration and particular care with regard to drug interactions (see p.260). **Phenytoin** is also effective, at least in the short-term (Box 4.K).[8] **Oxcarbazepine** is reported to improve trigeminal neuralgia and post-herpetic neuralgia unresponsive to **carbamazepine** and **carbamazepine** plus **gabapentin** respectively.[9,10] However, the results of 2 RCTs in painful diabetic neuropathy are conflicting (see p.263).[11,12]

Lamotrigine was effective for neuropathic pain in 3 small RCTs (131 patients in total),[13–15] and was comparable to **amitriptyline** in a comparative cross-over study.[16] However, findings from 6 other RCTs, including 4 larger studies (1,040 patients in total), were equivocal or negative.[17–21] Although **lamotrigine** is advocated by some for the specific pains based on the smaller RCTs (HIV neuropathy and central post-stroke pain),[22,23] the 'negative' studies did include

Box 4.K Phenytoin

Pharmacology

Phenytoin is a sodium channel blocker. It has a narrow therapeutic window. It is about 90% bound to plasma albumin and its effect is limited to the free, unbound portion. This is a greater proportion of the total if the patient is hypo-albuminaemic (cf. hypercalcaemia in the presence of hypo-albuminaemia). Those at risk include the elderly and those with chronic renal impairment; they may develop neurotoxicity even when plasma concentrations are reported as being in the therapeutic range.

Elimination follows zero-order kinetics (i.e. a constant amount is eliminated per unit of time); thus clearance does *not* increase with increasing plasma concentrations of phenytoin. In consequence, a small increase (e.g. 300mg → 350mg) may lead to a big increase in plasma concentration and toxicity.

Phenytoin drug–drug interactions

Phenytoin is a hepatic enzyme inducer with numerous drug interactions (see Table 4.32).

Phenytoin toxicity

Clinical features

Phenytoin toxicity generally manifests as a syndrome of cerebellar, vestibular and ocular effects, including some or all of the following:

- nystagmus:
  - ▹ on lateral gaze only (early sign)
  - ▹ spontaneous (more severe toxicity)
- blurred vision/diplopia
- slurred speech
- ataxia.

These may be accompanied by lethargy and/or delirium. Some patients experience break-through seizures (or an increase in the frequency of seizures) when the free phenytoin plasma concentration increases to toxic levels.

Evaluation

If phenytoin toxicity is suspected, check the plasma phenytoin concentration just before the next dose is due, and the plasma albumin. The normal therapeutic range with a normal plasma albumin is 40–80micromol/L (10–20microgram/mL). However, toxicity can be present despite a level within this range, particularly if hypo-albuminaemic; be prepared to make the diagnosis clinically (e.g. if nystagmus ± other symptoms), and act accordingly.

Management

There is no specific antidote to phenytoin. If the patient has clinical features suggestive of toxicity, reduce the dose of phenytoin to a known previous non-toxic level. If severe, omit a dose and reduce subsequent doses. Generally, symptoms resolve when the plasma phenytoin concentration falls.[6]

Treat break-through seizures with benzodiazepines (see p.244) because other anti-epileptic drugs may exacerbate the toxicity. If the frequency of seizures increases as the phenytoin toxicity resolves, obtain advice from a neurologist.

Supply

Phenytoin (generic)

Tablets phenytoin *sodium* 100mg, 28 days @ 100mg b.d. = £60. (Note: based on BNF prices, this is *more expensive* than branded Epanutin® capsules.)

Injection phenytoin *sodium* 50mg/mL, 5mL amp = £3.50; *contains propylene glycol 40% and alcohol 10% in WFI.*

Epanutin® (Pfizer)

Capsules phenytoin *sodium* 25mg, 50mg, 100mg, 300mg, 28 days @ 100mg b.d. = £2. (Note: based on BNF prices, this is *cheaper* than generic tablets.)

continued

Box 4.K Continued

Tablets chewable (Infatabs®) phenytoin 50mg, 28 days @ 100mg b.d. = £7.

Note: phenytoin *sodium* 55mg is approximately equivalent to phenytoin 50mg; the plasma concentration of phenytoin should be checked after switching from the sodium salt to the free acid form, or *vice versa*.

Oral suspension phenytoin 30mg/5mL, 28 days @ 90mg b.d. = £7.

Injection phenytoin *sodium* 50mg/mL, 5mL amp = £5; *contains propylene glycol 40% and alcohol 10% in WFI.*

Table 4.32 Clinically significant cytochrome P450 interactions with phenytoin resulting in changed drug plasma concentrations

Phenytoin plasma concentration		*Drug plasma concentration*	
increased by	*decreased by*	*increased by phenytoin*	*decreased by phenytoin*
Amiodarone	Antiretrovirals[a]	Phenobarbital	Amiodarone
Antifungal azoles[a]	Benzodiazepines[a]		Antifungal and anthelmintic azoles[a]
Azapropazone	Carbamazepine		Antiretrovirals[a]
Benzodiazepines[a]	Chlorpromazine		Aprepitant
Carbamazepine	Dexamethasone		Benzodiazepines[a]
Celecoxib	Phenobarbital		Calcium-channel blockers[a]
Chlorpromazine	Rifampicin		Carbamazepine
Cimetidine	St John's wort		Clozapine
Dexamethasone	Thioridazine		Corticosteroids
Diltiazem	Valproate		Disopyramide
Ethosuximide	Vigabatrin		Doxycycline
Fluoxetine			Ethosuximide
Fluvoxamine			Fentanyl
Oxcarbazepine			Haloperidol
Phenobarbital			Hormonal contraceptives
Prochlorperazine			Lamotrigine
Stiripentol			Methadone
Thioridazine			Mexiletine
Ticlopidine			Mirtazapine
Topiramate			Primidone
Valproate			Sertindole
			Theophylline
			Tiagabine
			Topiramate
			Tramadol
			Valproate

a. effect not seen with all drug class members.

both peripheral and central neuropathic (spinal cord) pains. Further, slow titration (over ≥6 weeks; see SPC) is essential to reduce the risk of skin reactions. **Lacosamide** is less effective for painful diabetic neuropathy than alternatives: NNT for moderate pain relief 8–11 vs. 1.3 for TCAs, 2.1 for **phenytoin**, 2.3 for **carbamazepine**, and 3.8 for **gabapentin**.[24–28] Thus, important differences exist between sodium channel blockers, and the routine first-line use of newer sodium channel blockers cannot be recommended at present.

Potential future directions in pain management include reduced blood-brain barrier penetration (reducing undesirable central effects by targeting ectopic foci on damaged peripheral neurones)[1] or subtype-selective sodium channel blockers (inherited abnormalities of one subtype, $Na_V1.7$, cause congenital insensitivity to pain while leaving other senses unaffected).[29] The opening of potassium channels also has a membrane-stabilizing effect by hyperpolarizing the cell membrane, and is thought to account for the analgesic effect of **flupirtine** (not UK).[30]

1 Devor M (2006) Sodium channels and mechanisms of neuropathic pain. *Journal of Pain*. **7**: S3–S12.
2 Wiffen PJ *et al.* (2011) Carbamazepine for acute and chronic pain in adults. *Cochrane Database of Systematic Reviews*. **1**: CD005451.
3 Wiffen PJ *et al.* (2010) Anitconvulsant drugs for acute and chronic pain. *Cochrane Database of Systematic Reviews*. **1**: CD001133.
4 von Gunten CF *et al.* (2007) Flecainide for the treatment of chronic neuropathic pain: a Phase II trial. *Palliative Medicine*. **21**: 667–672.
5 Challapalli V *et al.* (2005) Systemic administration of local anesthetic agents to relieve neuropathic pain. *Cochrane Database of Systematic Reviews*. CD003345.
6 Perkin GD (2004) Ch. 24:53. Epilepsy in later childhood and adults. In: DA Warrell *et al.* (eds) *Oxford Textbook of Medicine* (5e). Oxford University Press, Oxford.
7 Wiffen PJ *et al.* (2005) Carbamazepine for acute and chronic pain. *Cochrane Database of Systematic Reviews*. **3**: CD005451.
8 McCleane G (1999) Intravenous infusion of phenytoin relieves neuropathic pain: a randomized, double-blinded, placebo-controlled, crossover study. *Anesthesia and Analgesia*. **89**: 985–988.
9 Criscuolo S *et al.* (2005) Oxcarbazepine monotherapy in postherpetic neuralgia unresponsive to carbamazepine and gabapentin. *Acta Neurologica Scandinavica*. **111**: 229–232.
10 Gomez-Arguelles JM *et al.* (2008) Oxcarbazepine monotherapy in carbamazepine-unresponsive trigeminal neuralgia. *Journal of Clinical Neuroscience*. **15**: 516–519.
11 Dogra S *et al.* (2005) Oxcarbazepine in painful diabetic neuropathy: a randomized, placebo-controlled study. *European Journal of Pain*. **9**: 543–554.
12 Grosskopf J *et al.* (2006) A randomized, placebo-controlled study of oxcarbazepine in painful diabetic neuropathy. *Acta Neurologica Scandinavica*. **114**: 177–180.
13 Simpson DM *et al.* (2000) A placebo-controlled trial of lamotrigine for painful HIV-associated neuropathy. *Neurology*. **54**: 2115–2119.
14 Vestergaard K *et al.* (2001) Lamotrigine for central poststroke pain: a randomized controlled trial. *Neurology*. **56**: 184–190.
15 Eisenberg E *et al.* (2001) Lamotrigine reduces painful diabetic neuropathy: a randomized, controlled study. *Neurology*. **57**: 505–509.
16 Jose VM *et al.* (2007) Randomized double-blind study comparing the efficacy and safety of lamotrigine and amitriptyline in painful diabetic neuropathy. *Diabetic Medicine*. **24**: 377–383.
17 Silver M *et al.* (2007) Double-blind, placebo-controlled trial of lamotrigine in combination with other medications for neuropathic pain. *Journal of Pain and Symptom Management*. **34**: 446–454.
18 Zakrzewska JM *et al.* (1997) Lamotrigine (lamictal) in refractory trigeminal neuralgia: results from a double-blind placebo controlled crossover trial. *Pain*. **73**: 223–230.
19 Finnerup NB *et al.* (2002) Lamotrigine in spinal cord injury pain: a randomized controlled trial. *Pain*. **96**: 375–383.
20 McCleane G (1999) 200 mg daily of lamotrigine has no analgesic effect in neuropathic pain: a randomised, double-blind, placebo controlled trial. *Pain*. **83**: 105–107.
21 Vinik AI *et al.* (2007) Lamotrigine for treatment of pain associated with diabetic neuropathy: results of two randomized, double-blind, placebo-controlled studies. *Pain*. **128**: 169–179.
22 Kumar B *et al.* (2009) Central poststroke pain: a review of pathophysiology and treatment. *Anesthesia and Analgesia*. **108**: 1645–1657.
23 Goodyear-Smith F and Halliwell J (2009) Anticonvulsants for neuropathic pain: gaps in the evidence. *Clinical Journal of Pain*. **25**: 528–536.
24 Wymer JP *et al.* (2009) Efficacy and safety of lacosamide in diabetic neuropathic pain: an 18-week double-blind placebo-controlled trial of fixed-dose regimens. *Clinical Journal of Pain*. **25**: 376–385.
25 Shaibani A *et al.* (2009) Long-term oral lacosamide in painful diabetic neuropathy: a two-year open-label extension trial. *European Journal of Pain*. **13**: 458–463.
26 Saarto T and Wiffen PJ (2007) Antidepressants for neuropathic pain. *Cochrane Database of Systematic Reviews*. CD005454.
27 Rauck RL *et al.* (2007) Lacosamide in painful diabetic peripheral neuropathy: a phase 2 double-blind placebo-controlled study. *Clinical Journal of Pain*. **23**: 150–158.
28 Wiffen PJ *et al.* (2005) Anticonvulsants for acute and chronic pain. *Cochrane Database of Systematic Reviews*. **3**: CD001133.
29 Cummins TR *et al.* (2007) The roles of sodium channels in nociception: Implications for mechanisms of pain. *Pain*. **131**: 243–257.
30 Devulder J (2010) Flupirtine in pain management: pharmacological properties and clinical use. *CNS Drugs*. **24**: 867–881.

CARBAMAZEPINE — BNF 4.8.1

Class: Anti-epileptic (sodium channel blocker).

Indications: Partial seizures ± secondary generalization, trigeminal neuralgia, †neuropathic pain, mania.

Contra-indications: AV block, previous bone marrow depression, concurrent MAOI, hypersensitivity to TCAs (structurally related), porphyria.

Pharmacology

Carbamazepine acts mainly through sodium channel blockade (see p.257). Additional actions of uncertain significance include potassium channel activation, L-type calcium-channel blockade, and antagonism of NMDA-glutamate.[1]

Absorption is affected by formulation; slower rates reduce the incidence of undesirable neurological effects.[2] Carbamazepine is mainly metabolized by CYP3A4 to a pharmacologically active epoxide metabolite; this is subsequently inactivated to several renally excreted metabolites. The halflife decreases over the first 1–2 weeks as a result of hepatic enzyme auto-induction.

Carbamazepine is a first-line drug for trigeminal neuralgia and partial seizures ± secondary generalization. In painful diabetic neuropathy it is superior to placebo (n = 30) and comparable to **nortriptyline** (n = 16).[3] Benefit is also reported for paroxysmal nausea associated with meningeal carcinomatosis[4] and itch associated with haematological malignancy.[5]

A polymorphism in the gene (SCN1A) encoding the sodium channel α-subunit has been linked to carbamazepine-resistant epilepsy.[6] Human leukocyte antigen (HLA) genes, known to influence susceptibility to various infections and auto-immune diseases, are closely associated with the risk of carbamazepine-induced Stevens-Johnson syndrome. In Han Chinese, HLA B*1502 was found in 100% of 44 affected individuals compared with 3% of unaffected carbamazepine-treated individuals.[7] The MHRA recommends testing HLA B*1502 status before carbamazepine is started in people of Han Chinese, Hong Kong Chinese or Thai origin.[8]

Bio-availability ≥85%.

Onset of action generally delayed by the need for slow titration, but anti-epileptic response is sometimes seen as early as 2 days.

Peak plasma concentration 4–8h (normal-release tablets), 12–26h (m/r tablets), 0.5–3h (oral liquid).

Plasma halflife 36h initially, 8–24h after multiple dosing (hepatic auto-induction).

Duration of action No specific data.

Cautions

Agranulocytosis and aplastic anaemia affect about 5 and 2 patients/million/year respectively. Severe hepatic reactions are rare. Mild leukopenia, thrombocytopenia, or cholestatic abnormalities in LFTs should be monitored, and carbamazepine should be discontinued if severe or symptomatic derangement occurs.

Mild skin reactions are common and transient; monitor closely and discontinue carbamazepine if reactions worsen, or if features of Stevens-Johnson syndrome or toxic epidermal necrolysis develop.

Renal, cardiac or hepatic disease; absence seizures (may worsen); previous skin reaction to other anti-epileptic drugs or TCAs.

Drug interactions

Carbamazepine is a hepatic enzyme inducer with numerous drug interactions (see Table 4.33).

Undesirable effects

Very common (>10%): dizziness, ataxia, drowsiness, fatigue, nausea, mild LFT derangement (see above), urticaria, leukopenia.

Common (<10%, >1%): headache, diplopia, blurred vision, oedema, dry mouth, thrombocytopenia, eosinophilia, hyponatraemia, (with suppositories) rectal irritation.

Uncommon (<1%, >0.1%): include suicidal ideation 0.2% (1/500; advise patients to report mood or thought disturbance).

Rare (<0.1%): aseptic meningitis, movement disorders, neuroleptic (antipsychotic) malignant syndrome, arrhythmias and cardiac conduction disorders, pancreatitis, hepatitis, jaundice, renal failure, interstitial nephritis, a delayed-onset multi-organ vasculitic hypersensitivity disorder, severe skin reactions (see above).

Table 4.33 Clinically significant cytochrome P450 interactions with carbamazepine resulting in changed drug plasma concentrations

Carbamazepine[a] plasma concentration		*Drug plasma concentration*	
increased by	*decreased by*	*increased by carbamazepine*	*decreased by carbamazepine*
Antipsychotics[b] Antiretrovirals[b] Azole antifungals[b] Clarithromycin Dextropropoxyphene Diltiazem Erythromycin Fluoxetine Fluvoxamine Haloperidol Isoniazid Lamotrigine Valproate Verapamil	Efavirenz Phenobarbital[c] Phenytoin[c] Valproate[c]	Phenytoin	Antipsychotics[b] Antiretrovirals[b] Azole antifungals[b] Benzodiazepines[b] Calcium-channel blockers[b] Clozapine Corticosteroids[b] Coumarin anticoagulants Ethosuximide Fentanyl Haloperidol Indinavir Lamotrigine Levothyroxine Methadone Oestrogens, progestogens Phenytoin Primidone SSRIs[b] TCAs[b] Tiagabine Topiramate Tramadol Valproate

a. or active metabolite
b. effect not seen with all drug class members
c. increase in active metabolite of carbamazepine.

Dose and use

Starting dose and titration rate will depend on seizure or pain severity. Undesirable effects are minimized by a low starting dose, slow upward titration, and the use of m/r products.

- check:
  - HLA B*1502 status in people of Han Chinese, Hong Kong Chinese or Thai origin[8]
  - baseline FBC, biochemistry, LFTs, and repeat every 2–3 months
- start with 50–100mg PO b.d. (use m/r product for doses ⩾100mg)
- if necessary, increase in 50–100mg increments every 1–2 weeks
- maximum daily dose 2g. In one study, 90% of those responding required ⩽800mg/24h; few patients responded to increases above this dose.[9]

Supply

Note: the BNF advises that the products available in the UK may differ in bio-availability, and that to avoid changes in effectiveness or increased risk of undesirable effects, it is best to avoid switching between formulations.

Carbamazepine (generic)
Tablets 100mg, 200mg, 400mg, 28 days @ 200mg b.d. = £10.

Tegretol® (Novartis)
Tablets 100mg, 200mg, 400mg, 28 days @ 200mg b.d. = £2.50.
Tablets chewable (Chewtabs®) 100mg, 200mg, 28 days @ 200mg b.d. = £6.

Oral liquid (sugar-free) 100mg/5mL, 28 days @ 200mg b.d. = £6.
Suppositories 125mg, pack of 5 = £8; 250mg, pack of 5 = £11.

Modified-release

M/r carbamazepine tablets in the UK are scored to permit splitting into halves.

Carbagen SR® (Generics)
Tablets m/r 200mg, 400mg, 28 days @ 200mg b.d. = £5.

Tegretol Retard® (Novartis)
Tablets m/r 200mg, 400mg, 28 days @ 200mg b.d. = £5.

1 Schmidt D and Elger CE (2004) What is the evidence that oxcarbazepine and carbamazepine are distinctly different antiepileptic drugs? *Epilepsy and Behaviour.* **5**: 627–635.
2 Tothfalusi L *et al.* (2008) Exposure-response analysis reveals that clinically important toxicity difference can exist between bioequivalent carbamazepine tablets. *British Journal of Clinical Pharmacology.* **65**: 110–122.
3 Wiffen PJ *et al.* (2005) Carbamazepine for acute and chronic pain. *Cochrane Database of Systematic Reviews.* **3**: CD005451.
4 Strohscheer I and Borasio GD (2006) Carbamazepine-responsive paroxysmal nausea and vomiting in a patient with meningeal carcinomatosis. *Palliative Medicine.* **20**: 549–550.
5 Korfitis C and Trafalis DT (2008) Carbamazepine can be effective in alleviating tormenting pruritus in patients with hematologic malignancy. *Journal of Pain and Symptom Management.* **35**: 571–572.
6 Abe T *et al.* (2008) Association between SCN1A polymorphism and carbamazepine-resistant epilepsy. *British Journal of Clinical Pharmacology.* **66**: 304–307.
7 Chung WH *et al.* (2004) Medical genetics: a marker for Stevens-Johnson syndrome. *Nature.* **428**: 486.
8 MHRA (2008) Drug safety update. **1 (9):** 5. Available from: www.mhra.gov.uk/Publications/Safetyguidance/DrugSafetyUpdate/CON014506
9 Kwan P and Brodie MJ (2001) Effectiveness of first antiepileptic drug. *Epilepsia.* **42**: 1255–1260.

OXCARBAZEPINE — BNF 4.8.1

Class: Anti-epileptic (sodium channel blocker).

Indications: Monotherapy or adjunctive therapy for partial seizures, †neuropathic pain.

Pharmacology

Oxcarbazepine is structurally related to **carbamazepine**. Both act through sodium channel blockade (see p.257) but differ in tolerability and propensity for drug interactions. Additional actions of uncertain significance include potassium channel activation, N, P and R- type calcium channel blockade and antagonism of NMDA-glutamate receptors.[1]

Oxcarbazepine is a pro-drug which is activated by reduction to its monohydroxy derivative. This is inactivated by glucuronidation and oxidation, and the metabolites are renally excreted.[2] Oxcarbazepine has fewer drug interactions than **carbamazepine** because it is a weaker inducer of hepatic enzymes.

In an RCT, oxcarbazepine was as effective as, but better tolerated than, **carbamazepine**; 14% vs. 25% of patients withdrew because of undesirable effects.[3] Oxcarbazepine is reported to improve trigeminal neuralgia and post-herpetic neuralgia unresponsive to **carbamazepine** and **carbamazepine + gabapentin** respectively.[4,5] However, the results of 2 RCTs in painful diabetic neuropathy are conflicting. A dose of 1,200mg daily was ineffective.[6] Titration to a maximum of 1,800mg daily (mean 1,450mg daily) reduced the mean pain VAS score by 1 (NNT = 6 for > 50% reduction in pain).[7]

Bio-availability ≥95%.
Onset of action pain improved ≤1 week, maximum response ≤4 weeks.[7]
Peak plasma concentration 1–3h.
Plasma halflife 1–5h; 7–20h monohydroxy derivative.
Duration of action no specific data.

Cautions

Previous hypersensitivity to **carbamazepine** (25–30% cross-reactivity), predisposition to hyponatraemia, cardiac insufficiency (fluid retention), abnormal cardiac conduction (arrhythmias and AV block occur rarely).

Drug interactions

Oxcarbazepine can induce CYP3A4 and inhibit CYP2C19 but not often to a clinically significant extent. Oral hormonal contraception may become ineffective. **Lamotrigine** and **phenytoin** may require dose adjustment.

Undesirable effects

Very common (>10%): drowsiness, dizziness, fatigue, headache, diplopia, nausea and vomiting.
Common (<10%, >1%): confusion, agitation, amnesia, altered mood, vertigo, ataxia, tremor, nystagmus, reduced attention, diarrhoea, constipation, abdominal pain, rash, alopecia, acne, asymptomatic hyponatraemia.
Uncommon (<1%, >0.1%): include suicidal ideation 0.2% (1/500; advise patients to report mood or thought disturbance).
Rare (<0.1%): AV block, arrhythmia, pancreatitis, hepatitis, multi-organ hypersensitivity, systemic lupus erythematosus, angioedema, Stevens-Johnson syndrome, toxic epidermal necrolysis, bone marrow depression.

Dose and use

Many palliative care patients have risk factors for hyponatraemia; monitor sodium at baseline, after 2 weeks, then monthly for 3 months. Doses lower than recommended by the manufacturer have been proposed:[2]

- start with 150mg b.d.
- increase the dose to 300mg b.d. after 3 days
- if necessary, increase to 1,200mg b.d. (maximum recommended dose)
- halve the initial dose if creatinine clearance is ≤30mL/min.

Supply

Oxcarbazepine (generic)
Tablets 150mg, 300mg, 600mg, 28 days @ 300mg b.d. = £25.

Trileptal® (Novartis)
Tablets 150mg, 300mg, 600mg, 28 days @ 300mg b.d. = £19.
Oral suspension (sugar-free) 300mg/5mL, 28 days @ 300mg b.d. = £38.

1 Schmidt D and Elger CE (2004) What is the evidence that oxcarbazepine and carbamazepine are distinctly different antiepileptic drugs? *Epilepsy and Behaviour.* **5**: 627–635.
2 May TW *et al.* (2003) Clinical pharmacokinetics of oxcarbazepine. *Clinical Pharmacokinetics.* **42**: 1023–1042.
3 Dam M *et al.* (1989) A double-blind study comparing oxcarbazepine and carbamazepine in patients with newly diagnosed, previously untreated epilepsy. *Epilepsy Research.* **3**: 70–76.
4 Gomez-Arguelles JM *et al.* (2008) Oxcarbazepine monotherapy in carbamazepine-unresponsive trigeminal neuralgia. *Journal of Clinical Neuroscience.* **15**: 516–519.
5 Criscuolo S *et al.* (2005) Oxcarbazepine monotherapy in postherpetic neuralgia unresponsive to carbamazepine and gabapentin. *Acta Neurologica Scandinavica.* **111**: 229–232.
6 Grosskopf J *et al.* (2006) A randomized, placebo-controlled study of oxcarbazepine in painful diabetic neuropathy. *Acta Neurologica Scandinavica.* **114**: 177–180.
7 Dogra S *et al.* (2005) Oxcarbazepine in painful diabetic neuropathy: a randomized, placebo-controlled study. *European Journal of Pain.* **9**: 543–554.

VALPROATE BNF 4.8.1

Class: Anti-epileptic (multimodal action).

Indications: Epilepsy (see SPC for details), †neuropathic pain, †mania associated with bipolar disorder, †migraine prophylaxis.

Contra-indications: active hepatic disease (see text), past or family history of severe hepatic impairment (particularly drug-related), porphyria.

Pharmacology

No single mode of action accounts for the anti-seizure activity of valproate. It is a sodium and T-type calcium channel blocker, an NMDA receptor-channel blocker, it increases potassium conductance and alters GABA, dopamine and serotonin transmission, although the relative significance of these actions is unclear. In contrast to other GABAmimetics, its effect is selective (particularly for the midbrain) and involves several mechanisms (altered synthesis, release, reuptake and degradation).[1] T-type calcium channels are implicated in thalamic burst firing (responsible for absence seizures), neuropathic pain,[2] and perhaps also in regulating pain excitation thresholds in a 'T-rich' subset of peripheral nociceptors.[3]

Valproate is well absorbed orally. It is ≥90% plasma protein-bound, and crosses the blood-brain barrier and neuronal membranes via active transporters. It is metabolized by cytochrome P450-mediated oxidation (10%: CYP2A6, 2B6, 2C9 and 2C19), mitochondrial β-oxidation (40%) and direct microsomal UDP-mediated glucuronidation (50%). Some metabolites are active, but their cerebral concentrations are too low to contribute to valproate's overall effect. Metabolites may be responsible for idiosyncratic hepatic toxicity. CYP enzyme inducers, inhibitors and polymorphisms affect the proportion of cytochrome P450 metabolites, perhaps altering this risk.[4,5]

Valproate remains a first-line treatment for generalized seizures, its efficacy and tolerability comparing favourably to those of newer anti-epileptics.[6,7] Its main safety concerns are idiosyncratic hepatic damage, affecting 1:3,000–1:20,000 people, and teratogenicity.[5,8] However, the incidence of serious idiosyncratic reactions reported with newer anti-epileptics is unknown.

A beneficial effect has been reported for cancer-related neuropathic pain in Australia and Europe respectively.[9,10] However, the results of RCTs in non-cancer pain are less clear, and EFNS and IASP guidelines do not recommend it for first-line use.[11,12] Three RCTs from one group in India found significant benefit in painful diabetic neuropathy (n = 43, n = 57)[13,14] and post-herpetic neuralgia (n = 45).[15] However, a fourth RCT in Europe (n = 37) found no benefit in peripheral neuropathic pain of mixed cause.[16] The discrepancy is difficult to explain. Although conducted in a mixed group, diabetes accounted for ~50% of patients in this fourth RCT; it was a crossover trial (the others were parallel group designs) but no carry-over effect was found; it was shorter (4-week active arm), whereas maximum benefit in the others occurred progressively over 4–12 weeks (although case reports often record a rapid onset of relief). A fifth RCT in central (spinal cord) neuropathic pain found non-significant trends towards benefit of a comparable magnitude to those of the first 3 studies.[17] Its size (n = 20) raises the possibility that it was underpowered. Valproate was well tolerated in all 5 studies, with fewer patients (≤5%) discontinuing because of undesirable effects compared with **gabapentin** (8–19%) and **pregabalin** (8–32%; see p.242).

Bio-availability 95% PO.

Onset of action often within 24h (for neuropathic pain).[9]

Peak plasma concentration 1–2h (3–5h for EC, 5–10h for m/r).

Plasma halflife 9–18h (5–12h with concurrent enzyme inducers).

Duration of action 12–24h.[5]

Cautions

Idiosyncratic, potentially fatal, hepatic failure occurs in 1:3,000–1:20,000 patients, usually within the first 6 months of treatment. Risk factors include age <3 years, pre-existing liver disease and deranged LFTs. Chronic hepatitis was the commonest reported liver disease:[18,19] it is unclear whether hepatic metastases affect the risk. Symptoms (drowsiness, fatigue, vomiting, and increased seizure frequency) may precede altered LFTs,[5] but both are common in palliative care populations. Mildly deranged LFTs do not require discontinuation but should prompt increased monitoring. Valproate should be stopped if co-existent coagulopathy, severely deranged LFTs or rapidly evolving symptoms occur in the absence of an alternative explanation. Treatment with IV **carnitine** has been proposed; seek specialist advice.

Lower initial doses and slower titration may be required in patients with renal impairment. Alternatives may be preferred in women trying to conceive; seek specialist advice. Harmless ketone metabolites, detected by bedside urinalysis, may cause diagnostic confusion in diabetic patients.

Drug Interactions

The clearance of valproate is increased by hepatic enzyme inducers such as **carbamazepine**, **phenytoin**, **phenobarbital** and **rifampicin**.[5] Its clearance is inhibited by **isoniazid**.

Valproate inhibits the metabolism of **carbamazepine**'s active/epoxide metabolite (increasing undesirable effects), **ethosuximide**, **phenytoin**, **phenobarbital**, **lamotrigine** and some antiretrovirals.

Concurrent administration with carbapenem β-lactam antibacterials can decrease the plasma concentration of valproate dramatically by 85–90% through the combined impact on intestinal absorption, distribution and metabolism, with consequential loss of therapeutic effect.[20] Because increasing the dose may not overcome this drug–drug interaction, alternative antibacterials should be considered for patients taking valproate.

Undesirable effects

Hepatic failure (see above) and pancreatitis are the most important idiosyncratic effects. Other rare effects include severe skin reactions (e.g. Stevens-Johnson syndrome) and reversible encephalopathy, parkinsonism, and dementia.

Common problems include gastric intolerance (particularly nausea: reduced by e/c formulations or taking with food), drowsiness and postural tremor (a rarer flapping tremor is seen with hyperammonaemia), although the incidence varies markedly between individual studies. Hyperammonaemia is usually asymptomatic but can cause nausea, ataxia or encephalopathy.

Dose and use

The manufacturer recommends that LFTs, prothrombin time (PT) and FBC be checked before and during the first 6 months of treatment, although this may not improve the early detection of hepatotoxicity.

Epilepsy

- start with valproate 250mg b.d.
- if necessary, increase by 250mg b.d. every 3 days
- maximum recommended dose 2.5g/24h
- 90% of those responding to valproate first-line require ≤1.5g/24h; few patients respond to increases above this dose.[21]

IV valproate is used when the oral route cannot be used. Patients already receiving oral treatment are given the same daily dose in continuous or intermittent (over 3–5 min) infusions. Patients starting valproate are given 500–800mg (max 10mg/kg) followed by continuous or intermittent infusions of up to 2.5g/24h.

Neuropathic pain

- start with valproate 250mg at bedtime
- if necessary, increase by 250mg every 3 days
- response likely at doses lower than those used in epilepsy, e.g. 500–750mg at bedtime
- some patients need 2g/24h.[9,10]

Mania

- start with valproate 250mg t.d.s.
- increase as rapidly as possible to achieve the optimal response, to a maximum of 60mg/kg/24h
- patients receiving >45mg/kg/24h should be carefully monitored
- most patients respond to doses <2g/24h.[22,23]

Migraine prophylaxis

- start with valproate 250mg b.d.[24]
- if necessary, increase progressively to a total daily dose of 1g.[25]

Supply

Note: valproate is the UK generic term for valproic acid and its salts and esters, including sodium valproate. The pharmacokinetics, efficacy, and tolerability of valproic acid and sodium valproate are similar; sodium valproate 579mg is equivalent to valproic acid 500mg,[26] and the manufacturer of valproic acid (Convulex®) advises that it is equipotent with products containing sodium valproate.

Sodium valproate (generic)
Tablets crushable 100mg, 28 days @ 500mg at bedtime = £8.
Tablets e/c 250mg, 500mg, 28 days @ 500mg at bedtime = £3.
Oral solution (sugar-free) 200mg/5mL, 28 days @ 500mg at bedtime = £6.

Epilim® (Sanofi-Aventis)
Tablets crushable 100mg, 28 days @ 500mg at bedtime = £8.
Tablets e/c 250mg, 500mg, 28 days @ 500mg at bedtime = £5.
Oral solution (sugar-free) 200mg/5mL, 28 days @ 500mg at bedtime = £11.
Oral syrup 200mg/5mL, 28 days @ 500mg at bedtime = £9.

Epilim Intravenous® (Sanofi-Aventis)
Injection (powder for reconstitution) 400mg vial = £12; supplied with a 4mL amp of WFI for reconstitution.

Episenta® (Beacon)
Injection 100mg/mL, 3mL amp = £7.

Valproic acid
Convulex® (Pharmacia)
Capsules 150mg, 300mg, 500mg, 28 days @ 500mg at bedtime = £3.50.

Depakote® (Sanofi-Aventis)
Tablets e/c semisodium valproate equivalent to valproic acid 250mg, 500mg, 28 days @ 500mg at bedtime = £8; *semisodium valproate is a mixture of equimolar amounts of valproic acid and sodium valproate.*

Modified-release
Epilim Chrono® (Sanofi-Aventis)
Tablets m/r sodium valproate and valproic acid equivalent to sodium valproate 200mg, 300mg, 500mg, 28 days @ 500mg at bedtime = £8.

Epilim Chronosphere® (Sanofi-Aventis)
Oral granules m/r sodium valproate and valproic acid equivalent to sodium valproate 50mg, 100mg, 250mg, 500mg, 750mg, 1g/sachet, 28 days @ 500mg at bedtime = £28; *the granules may be mixed with soft food or a drink which is cold or at room temperature, and swallowed immediately without chewing.*

Episenta® (Beacon)
Capsules enclosing m/r granules sodium valproate 150mg, 300mg, 28 days @ 300mg at bedtime = £3.50.
Oral granules m/r sodium valproate 500mg, 1g/sachet, 28 days @ 500mg at bedtime = £6.
The granules or contents of the capsules may be mixed with cold food or drink, and swallowed immediately without chewing.

1 Loscher W (2002) Basic pharmacology of valproate: a review after 35 years of clinical use for the treatment of epilepsy. *CNS Drugs*. **16**: 669–694.
2 Takahashi T *et al.* (2010) Upregulation of Ca(v)3.2 T-type calcium channels targeted by endogenous hydrogen sulfide contributes to maintenance of neuropathic pain. *Pain*. **150**: 183–191.
3 Jevtovic-Todorovic V *et al.* (2006) The role of peripheral T-type calcium channels in pain transmission. *Cell Calcium*. **40**: 197–203.
4 Mann MW and Pons G (2007) Various pharmacogenetic aspects of antiepileptic drug therapy: a review. *CNS Drugs*. **21**: 143–164.
5 Perucca E (2002) Pharmacological and therapeutic properties of valproate: a summary after 35 years of clinical experience. *CNS Drugs*. **16**: 695–714.
6 Marson AG *et al.* (2007) The SANAD study of effectiveness of valproate, lamotrigine, or topiramate for generalised and unclassifiable epilepsy: an unblinded randomised controlled trial. *Lancet*. **369**: 1016–1026.
7 Karceski S *et al.* (2005) Treatment of epilepsy in adults: expert opinion. *Epilepsy & Behavior*. **7 (suppl 1)**: S1–64.
8 French JA (2007) First-choice drug for newly diagnosed epilepsy. *Lancet*. **369**: 970–971.
9 Snare AJ (1993) Sodium Valproate. Retrospective analysis of neuropathic pain control in patients with advanced cancer. *Journal of Pharmacy Technology*. **9**: 114–117.
10 Hardy J *et al.* (2001) A phase II study to establish the efficacy and toxicity of sodium valproate in patients with cancer-related neuropathic pain. *Journal of Pain and Symptom Management*. **21**: 204–209.

11 Attal N *et al.* (2010) EFNS guidelines on the pharmacological treatment of neuropathic pain: 2010 revision. *European Journal of Neurology*. **17**: 1113–e1188.
12 Dworkin RH *et al.* (2010) Recommendations for the pharmacological management of neuropathic pain: an overview and literature update. *Mayo Clinic Proceedings*. **85**: S3–14.
13 Kochar DK *et al.* (2002) Sodium valproate in the management of painful neuropathy in type 2 diabetes — a randomized placebo controlled study. *Acta Neurologica Scandinavica*. **106**: 248–252.
14 Kochar DK *et al.* (2004) Sodium valproate for painful diabetic neuropathy: a randomized double-blind placebo-controlled study. *Quarterly Journal of Medicine*. **97**: 33–38.
15 Kochar DK *et al.* (2005) Divalproex sodium in the management of post-herpetic neuralgia: a randomized double-blind placebo-controlled study. *Quarterly Journal of Medicine*. **98**: 29–34.
16 Otto M *et al.* (2004) Valproic acid has no effect on pain in polyneuropathy: a randomized, controlled trial. *Neurology*. **62**: 285–288.
17 Drewes AM *et al.* (1994) Valproate for treatment of chronic central pain after spinal cord injury. A double-blind cross-over study. *Paraplegia*. **32**: 565–569.
18 Konig SA *et al.* (1994) Severe hepatotoxicity during valproate therapy: an update and report of eight new fatalities. *Epilepsia*. **35**: 1005–1015.
19 Koenig SA *et al.* (2006) Valproic acid-induced hepatopathy: nine new fatalities in Germany from 1994 to 2003. *Epilepsia*. **47**: 2027–2031.
20 Mancl EE and Gidal BE (2009) The effect of carbapenem antibiotics on plasma concentrations of valproic acid. *Annals of Pharmacotherapy*. **43**: 2082–2087.
21 Kwan P and Brodie MJ (2001) Effectiveness of first antiepileptic drug. *Epilepsia*. **42**: 1255–1260.
22 Keck PE, Jr. *et al.* (1993) Valproate oral loading in the treatment of acute mania. *Journal of Clinical Psychiatry*. **54**: 305–308.
23 Macritchie K *et al.* (2003) Valproate for acute mood episodes in bipolar disorder. *Cochrane Database of Systematic Reviews*. **1**: CD004052.
24 Kinze S *et al.* (2001) Valproic acid is effective in migraine prophylaxis at low serum levels: a prospective open-label study. *Headache*. **41**: 774–778.
25 Freitag FG (2003) Divalproex in the treatment of migraine. *Psychopharmacol Bull*. **37 (suppl 2)**: 98–115.
26 Fisher (2003) Sodium valproate or valproate semisodium: is there a difference in the treatment of bipolar disorder? *Psychiatric Bulletin*. **27**: 446–448.

LEVETIRACETAM — BNF 4.8.1

Class: Anti-epileptic.

Indications: Mono or adjunctive therapy of partial seizures ± secondary generalization, adjunctive therapy of generalized myoclonic and tonic-clonic seizures, †monotherapy of generalized seizures (see text).

Pharmacology

Levetiracetam binds to synaptic vesicle protein SV2A, and is presumed to interfere with the release of the neurotransmitter stored within the vesicle.[1] Food affects the rate but not the extent of its absorption. It does not bind to plasma proteins. It readily crosses the blood-brain barrier (CSF T_{max} = 3–5h). A third is metabolized predominantly by non-hepatic hydrolysis; the remainder is excreted by the kidneys unchanged. The CSF halflife is 3 times longer than that for plasma.[2]

Levetiracetam is effective for a broad range of seizure types. Its efficacy and tolerability compare favourably to other newer anti-epileptic drugs.[3] It is commonly used second-line (see p.243), or first-line when the seizure type is unclear (also see **valproate**, p.264) or when other anti-epileptics are contra-indicated because of co-morbidities.[4] Levetiracetam is thought *not* to affect the frequency of absences.

Benefit for neuropathic pain, bipolar disorder and hot flushes is reported.[3,5–7] A single-blind RCT found it to be effective for multiple sclerosis-related central neuropathic pain[8] but two double-blind placebo-controlled RCTs found no benefit for post-mastectomy or spinal cord injury pain.[9,10]

Bio-availability ≥95% PO.

Onset of action antiepileptic effect generally evident <3 days of starting treatment.

Peak plasma concentration 1–2h.

Plasma halflife 6–8h.

Duration of action 24h.

Cautions

Dose reduction may be required with renal impairment, look for secondary renal impairment in those with hepatic impairment. Suicidal ideation occurs rarely with all anti-epileptics (p.237).

Drug interactions

Levetiracetam may increase plasma concentrations of **phenytoin**, but reports are conflicting. When given in combination, increased **carbamazepine** toxicity has been reported, even though the plasma concentration was not increased. Although these interactions are probably generally *not* clinically significant, caution should be observed when **carbamazepine** or **phenytoin** are used in combination with levetiracetam.[11]

Valproate increases plasma concentration by a mean of 16%; **carbamazepine**, **oxcarbazepine** and **phenytoin** reduce concentrations ≤30%.[2]

Undesirable effects

Very common (>10%): fatigue, drowsiness.

Common (<10%, >1%): ataxia, hyperkinesis, tremor, dizziness, headache, diplopia, blurred vision, amnesia, abnormal thinking, attention disturbance, behavioural disturbances (emotional lability, irritability, agitation, hostility/aggression, personality disorders), depression, insomnia, anorexia, abdominal pain, diarrhoea, dyspepsia, nausea, vomiting, myalgia, rash, pruritus, thrombocytopenia. Behavioural disturbances occur in 3–4% of patients with epilepsy but only 0.5% of those being treated for other conditions. A history of aggression or psychiatric disturbance is associated with more severe hostility/aggression.[12,13]

Rare (<0.1%): psychosis, suicide, pancreatitis, hepatic failure, bone marrow suppression.

Dose and use

In epilepsy, the PO and IV dose are identical:

- start with 250–500mg PO/IV b.d.
- if starting with 250mg b.d., increase automatically after 2 weeks to 500mg b.d. (the minimum effective dose in most people)
- if necessary, increase by 250–500mg b.d. every 2 weeks
- maximum dose 1.5g b.d.

Renal impairment

For patients with renal impairment, the doses in Table 4.34 should generally be adhered to.

Table 4.34 Dose adjustment for levetiracetam in renal impairment

Creatinine clearance (mL/min/1.73m²)[a]	*Usual Maintenance Dose (mg)*
>80	500–1,500 b.d.
50–79	500–1,000 b.d.
30–49	250–750 b.d.
<30	250–500 b.d.

a. based on the Cockroft-Gault formula adjusted for body surface area (see p.620).

If on dialysis:

- start with 750mg loading dose followed by 500mg–1,000mg *once daily* PO/IV
- give 250–500mg supplementary doses after dialysis.

Hepatic impairment

Dose is unaffected by mild–moderate hepatic impairment. With severe hepatic impairment, creatinine clearance may underestimate the severity of renal impairment. Halve the dose if creatinine clearance <70mL/min.

Discontinuation

Reduce by a maximum of 500mg b.d. every 2–4 weeks to avoid rebound seizures.

Supply

Keppra® (UCB Pharma)

Tablets 250mg, 500mg, 750mg, 1g, 28 days @ 750mg or 1g b.d. = £83 and £94 respectively.

Oral solution (sugar-free) 100mg/mL, 28 days @ 750mg or 1g b.d. = £99 and £133 respectively.
Injection (concentrate for dilution and use as an intravenous infusion) 100mg/mL, 5mL vial = £14.

1 Lynch BA (2004) The synaptic vesicle protein SV2A is the binding site for the antiepileptic drug levetiracetam. *Proceedings of the National Academy of Sciences of the United States of America*. **101 (26)**: 9861–9866.
2 Patsalos PN and Patsalos PN (2004) Clinical pharmacokinetics of levetiracetam. *Clinical Pharmacokinetics*. **43**: 707–724.
3 Zaccara G *et al.* (2006) Comparison of the efficacy and tolerability of new antiepileptic drugs: what can we learn from long-term studies? *Acta Neurologica Scandinavica*. **114**: 157–168.
4 Karceski S *et al.* (2005) Treatment of epilepsy in adults: expert opinion, 2005. *Epilepsy & Behavior*. **7 (suppl 1)**: S1–64.
5 Dunteman ED (2005) Levetiracetam as an adjunctive analgesic in neoplastic plexopathies: case series and commentary. *Journal of Pain and Palliative Care Pharmacotherapy*. **19**: 35–43.
6 Price MJ (2004) Levetiracetam in the treatment of neuropathic pain: three case studies. *Clinical Journal of Pain*. **20**: 33–36.
7 Thompson S *et al.* (2008) Levetiracetam for the treatment of hot flashes: a phase II study. *Supportive Care in Cancer*. **16**: 75–82.
8 Rossi S *et al.* (2009) Effects of levetiracetam on chronic pain in multiple sclerosis: results of a pilot, randomized, placebo-controlled study. *European Journal of Neurology*. **16**: 360–366.
9 Finnerup NB *et al.* (2009) Levetiracetam in spinal cord injury pain: a randomized controlled trial. *Spinal Cord*. **47**: 861–867.
10 Vilholm OJ *et al.* (2008) Effect of levetiracetam on the postmastectomy pain syndrome. *European Journal of Neurology*. **15**: 851–857.
11 Baxter K (ed) (2009) Stockley's Drug Interactions (online edition). Pharmaceutical Press, London. Available from: www.medicinescomplete.com/mc/stockley/current/
12 Dinkelacker V *et al.* (2003) Aggressive behavior of epilepsy patients in the course of levetiracetam add-on therapy: report of 33 mild to severe cases. *Epilepsy Behaviour*. **4**: 537–547.
13 Cramer JA *et al.* (2003) A systematic review of the behavioral effects of levetiracetam in adults with epilepsy, cognitive disorders, or an anxiety disorder during clinical trials. *Epilepsy Behaviour*. **4**: 124–132.

PHENOBARBITAL BNF 4.8.1 & 4.8.2

Class: Anti-epileptic (GABAmimetic).

Indications: Epilepsy (except absence seizures), status epilepticus, †terminal agitation.

Pharmacology

Phenobarbital enhances the post-synaptic inhibitory action of GABA by prolonging the opening of the chloride channel in the GABA receptor-channel complex (see Figure 4.7, p.240).[1] Phenobarbital also inhibits the post-synaptic actions of the excitatory neurotransmitter, glutamate, at non-NMDA-receptor-channels. These actions depress CNS activity, and high doses result in general anaesthesia. There is considerable interindividual variation in the pharmacokinetics of phenobarbital. Peak CNS concentrations occur some 15–20min after peak plasma concentrations. About 25% is excreted unchanged by the kidney; the rest is converted in the liver, mainly to inactive oxidative metabolites via several enzymes including CYP2C9. Phenobarbital is a strong inducer of CYP3A and glucuronidation, thus reducing plasma concentrations of many concurrently administered drugs.[1,2]

Phenobarbital's efficacy in epilepsy is comparable to alternatives but concerns about its cognitive and behavioural effects have led to a decline in its use in developed countries, other than for status epilepticus (see p.244).[1]

Phenobarbital is used at some centres for agitation in the imminently dying which fails to respond to the combined use of **midazolam** and an antipsychotic.[3,4]

Bio-availability >90% PO; no data IM.[2]
Onset of action 5min IV, maximum effect achieved within 30min, onset after SC or IM administration is slightly slower; 2–3 *weeks* PO (= the time to achieve a therapeutic anti-seizure plasma concentration with a once daily dose of 100–200mg).[5]
Time to peak plasma concentration 2–4h IM,[6] 2h PO (some authorities report up to 12h).[5–8]
Plasma halflife 2–6 *days*; 1–3 *days* in children.
Duration of action situation dependent; chronic administration >24h.

Cautions

Elderly, children, debilitated, hepatic impairment, renal impairment, respiratory depression. Avoid sudden withdrawal.

Drug interactions

Phenobarbital induces various enzymes involved in drug metabolism, including CYP1A2, CYP2C9, CYP2C19 and CYP3A4 (manufacturer's data), and thus reduces plasma concentrations of many drugs.[9] Table 4.35 lists selected drugs which have clinically important interactions with phenobarbital.

Table 4.35 Clinically significant cytochrome P450 interactions with phenobarbital resulting in changed drug plasma concentrations[9]

Phenobarbital plasma concentration		*Drug plasma concentration*	
increased by	*decreased by*	*increased by phenobarbital*	*decreased by phenobarbital*
Influenza vaccine	Carbamazepine[a]	Hepatotoxic metabolites of paracetamol (possibly)	Some azole antifungals (itraconazole, ketoconazole)
Felbamate (not UK)	Chlorpromazine	Phenytoin (sometimes)[a]	Some calcium-channel blockers (felodipine, nifedipine, nimodipine, verapamil)
Phenytoin[a]	Folic acid		Carbamazepine[a]
Stiripentol (not UK)	St John's wort		Chlorpromazine
Valproate[a]			Clonazepam
			Corticosteroids (dexamethasone, methylprednisolone, prednisolone)
			Coumarins (oral anticoagulants)
			Ciclosporin
			Disopyramide
			Doxycycline
			Ethosuximide (sometimes)[a]
			IV fentanyl (significance not known for TD)
			Haloperidol
			Lamotrigine
			Methadone
			Metronidazole
			Oral contraceptives
			Paracetamol
			Phenytoin (generally)[a]
			Quinidine (not UK)
			Rifampicin
			TCAs
			Theophylline
			Tiagabine
			Valproate

a. interactions between anti-epileptic drugs are complex and unpredictable; plasma concentrations may be increased, decreased or unchanged.

Undesirable effects

Respiratory depression (high doses), drowsiness, lethargy, ataxia, skin reactions (<3%). Paradoxical excitement, irritability, restlessness/hyperactivity and delirium, particularly in the elderly and children.

Long-term treatment is occasionally complicated by folate-responsive megaloblastic anaemia or by osteomalacia.

Dose and use

Undiluted phenobarbital sodium injection is very alkaline and is formulated in a mixture of propylene glycol and alcohol. If diluted with 10 times its own volume of WFI, it can generally be given safely *on its own* by IV injection or CSCI, but it should *never* be mixed with another drug (see p.670). Local necrosis has been reported after SC injection or IV extravasation (manufacturer's data on file), thus stressing the need to dilute before administration.

However, an alternative formulation (not UK) has been given SC without any problems, thereby highlighting the need to know which product has been used when interpreting reports of SC use.[10]

Epilepsy

Phenobarbital is sometimes used as maintenance anti-epileptic therapy in patients who cannot swallow but for whom a benzodiazepine (e.g. **clonazepam**, **lorazepam** or **midazolam**) is too sedative. Because of the irritant nature of the undiluted injection and the volume after dilution, stat doses are generally given IV, but can be followed by CSCI:

- dilute each 200mg (1mL) ampoule with 10mL of WFI; i.e. total volume 11mL
- give 100mg (i.e. 5.5mL) IV stat
- then 200–400mg/24h CSCI, i.e. total volume 11–22mL.

For use in status epilepticus, see p.244.

Terminal agitation

Phenobarbital is one of several sedative drugs used to treat refractory agitation in the imminently dying (Table 4.36).[11,12] It is generally third-line treatment for patients who fail to respond to **midazolam** 60–120mg/24h together with either **haloperidol** 30mg/24h or **levomepromazine** 200mg/24h.[3]

Because of the irritant nature of the injection (and the volume after dilution), stat doses are generally given IM/IV, but can be followed by CSCI:

- start with loading dose of 200mg (1mL ampoule) as:
  - ▹ *undiluted* IM injection *or*
  - ▹ *diluted* IV bolus given over 2min (1mL ampoule diluted to 10mL with WFI)
- if the patient remains unsettled, give 1 or 2 further doses p.r.n. of 200mg IM/IV 30min apart
- if still unsettled or agitation recurs, give further doses of 200mg IM/IV q1h p.r.n.
- maintain with 800mg/24h CSCI (= total volume 44mL); or more if total initial 'settling' dose was ⩾600mg
- if necessary, increase the dose progressively to 1,600mg/24h, i.e. 800 → 1,200 → 1,600mg (= total volume 88mL)
- occasionally it may be necessary to increase progressively to 3,800mg
- median maximum dose = 1,200–1,600mg/24h (= total volume 66–88mL).[7,13]

Some centres use **propofol** (see p.600) or **dexmedetomidine** (not UK) instead.[14–16]

Table 4.36 Mean, median and range of sedative and antipsychotic doses in final 48h of life (mg/24h)[a,17]

Drug	*Mean dose*	*Median dose*	*Reported range*	*References*
Midazolam	22–70	30–45	3–1,200	18–29
Haloperidol	5	4	5–50	19,21,24
Chlorpromazine	21	50	13–900	19,24,30–33
Levomepromazine	64	100	25–250	19,24,33
Phenobarbital	1,200	800–1,600	200–3,800	13,19,24,30,33,34
Propofol	1,100	500	400–9,600	24,33,35,36

a. mean, median and range may be derived from different studies.

Stopping phenobarbital

Abrupt cessation of long-term anti-epileptic therapy, particularly barbiturates and benzodiazepines, should be avoided because rebound seizures may be precipitated. If it is decided to discontinue anti-epileptic therapy, it should be done *slowly over 6 months or more*. For phenobarbital, the recommended monthly reduction in dose is *15mg*.[37]

In adults the risk of relapse on stopping treatment is 40–50%.[38] Substituting one anti-epileptic drug regimen for another should also be done cautiously, withdrawing the first drug only when the new regimen has been introduced.

Supply

Unless indicated otherwise, all products are **CD**.

Phenobarbital sodium (generic)
Injection 200mg/mL, 1mL amp = £2; *vehicle contains propylene glycol 90%.*

1 Kwan P and Brodie MJ (2004) Phenobarbital for the treatment of epilepsy in the 21st century: a critical review. *Epilepsia*. **45**: 1141–1149.
2 Dollery C (1999) Phenobarbital. In: C Dollery (ed) *Therapeutic Drugs Release 1*. Harcourt Brace Company.
3 de Graeff A and Dean M (2007) Palliative sedation therapy in the last weeks of life: a literature review and recommendations for standards. *Journal of Palliative Medicine*. **10**: 67–85.
4 Twycross R *et al.* (2009) *Symptom Management in Advanced Cancer*. palliativedrugs.com, Nottingham, pp. 430–433.
5 AHFS (2009) AHFS Drug Information (online edition). Available from: www.medicinescomplete.com/mc/ahfs/current/
6 Sweetman S (ed) (2009) Martindale: the Complete Drug Reference (online edition). Available from: www.medicinescomplete.com/mc/martindale/current/
7 Stirling LC *et al.* (1999) The use of phenobarbitone in the management of agitation and seizures at the end of life. *Journal of Pain and Symptom Management*. **17**: 363–368.
8 Holford N (ed) (1998) *Clinical pharmacokinetics: drug data handbook*. (3e). Adis International, Auckland.
9 Baxter K (2011) Stockley's Drug Interactions (online edition). Pharmaceutical Press, London. Available from: www.medicinescomplete.com
10 palliativedrugs.com Bulletin Board (2007) Phenobarbital infusion. Available from: www.palliativedrugs.com/forum-read?&f=1&i=12715&t=12715
11 Truog R *et al.* (1992) Barbiturates in the care of the terminally ill. *New England Journal of Medicine*. **327**: 1672–1682.
12 Greene WR and Davis WH (1991) Titrated intravenous barbiturates in the control of symptoms in patients with terminal cancer. *Southern Medical Journal*. **84**: 332–337.
13 Gillon S *et al.* (2010) Review of phenobarbitone use for deep terminal sedation in a UK hospice. *Palliative Medicine*. **24**: 100–101.
14 Gertler R *et al.* (2001) Dexmedetomidine: a novel sedative-analgesic agent. *Proceedings (Baylor University Medical Center)*. **14**: 13–21.
15 Soares L *et al.* (2002) Dexmedetomidine: a new option for intractable distress in the dying. *Journal of Pain and Symptom Management*. **24**: 6–8.
16 Jackson KC, 3rd *et al.* (2006) Dexmedetomidine: a novel analgesic with palliative medicine potential. *Journal of Pain and Palliative Care Pharmacotherapy*. **20**: 23–27.
17 Wilcock A *et al.* (Unpublished work) Sedation Consensus: Drug selection, dosing and titration.
18 Muller-Busch HC *et al.* (2003) Sedation in palliative care — a critical analysis of 7 years experience. *BMC Palliative Care*. **2**: 2.
19 Morita T *et al.* (2002) Definition of sedation for symptom relief: a systematic literature review and a proposal of operational criteria. *Journal of Pain and Symptom Management*. **24**: 447–453.
20 Chiu TY *et al.* (2001) Sedation for refractory symptoms of terminal cancer patients in Taiwan. *Journal of Pain and Symptom Management*. **21**: 467–472.
21 Fainsinger RL *et al.* (2000) A multicentre international study of sedation for uncontrolled symptoms in terminally ill patients. *Palliative Medicine*. **14**: 257–265.
22 Fainsinger R *et al.* (2000) Sedation for delirium and other symptoms in terminally ill patients in Edmonton. *Journal of Palliative Care*. **16 (2)**: 5–10.
23 Fainsinger RL (1998) Use of sedation by a hospital palliative care support team. *Journal of Palliative Care*. **14**: 51–54.
24 Morita T *et al.* (1996) Sedation for symptom control in Japan: the importance of intermittent use and communication with family members. *Journal of Pain and Symptom Management*. **12**: 32–38.
25 McNamara P *et al.* (1991) Use of midazolam in palliative care. *Palliative Medicine*. **5**: 244–249.
26 Burke A *et al.* (1991) Terminal restlessness — its management and the role of midazolam. *The Medical Journal of Australia*. **155**: 485–487.
27 Bottomley DM and Hanks GW (1990) Subcutaneous midazolam infusion in palliative care. *Journal of Pain and Symptom Management*. **5**: 259–261.
28 Amesbury BDW and Dunphy KP (1989) The use of subcutaneous midazolam in the home care setting. *Palliative Medicine*. **3**: 299–301.
29 de Sousa E and Jepson BA (1988) Midazolam in terminal care. *Lancet*. **1**: 67–68.
30 Roy DJ (1990) Need they sleep before they die? *Journal of Palliative Care*. **6**: 3–4.
31 Cowan J and Walsh D (2001) Terminal sedation in palliative medicine — definition and review of the literature. *Supportive Care in Cancer*. **9**: 403–407.
32 Kohara H *et al.* (2005) Sedation for terminally ill patients with cancer with uncontrollable physical distress. *Journal of Palliative Medicine*. **8**: 20–25.
33 Miccinesi G *et al.* (2006) Continuous deep sedation: physicians' experiences in six European countries. *Journal of Pain and Symptom Management*. **31**: 122–129.
34 Mount B (1996) Morphine drips, terminal sedation, and slow euthanasia: definitions and facts, not anecdotes. *Journal of Palliative Care*. **12**: 31–37.

35 Braun TC *et al.* (2003) Development of a clinical practice guideline for palliative sedation. *Journal of Palliative Medicine*. **6**: 345–350.
36 Cherny NI and Portenoy RK (1994) Sedation in the management of refractory symptoms: guidelines for evaluation and treatment. *Journal of Palliative Care*. **10**: 31–38.
37 Chadwick D (1995) The withdrawal of antiepileptic drugs. In: A Hopkins *et al.* (eds) *Epilepsy* (2e). Chapman and Hall, London, pp. 215–220.
38 Hopkins A and Shorvon S (1995) Definitions and epidemiology of epilepsy. In: A Hopkins *et al.* (eds) *Epilepsy* (2e). Chapman and Hall, London, pp. 1–24.

ORPHENADRINE BNF 4.9.2

Class: Antimuscarinic antiparkinsonian.

Indications: Parkinson's disease, drug-induced parkinsonism, †sialorrhoea (drooling), †extrapyramidal dystonic reactions.

Contra-indications: Glaucoma, prostatic hypertrophy, urinary retention, tardive dyskinesia (see Drug-induced movement disorders, p.745), porphyria.

Pharmacology

Orphenadrine and other antimuscarinic antiparkinsonian drugs are used primarily in Parkinson's disease. They are less effective than **levodopa** in established Parkinson's disease. However, patients with mild symptoms, particularly tremor, may be treated initially with an antimuscarinic drug (alone or with **selegiline**), and **levodopa** added or substituted if symptoms progress. Antimuscarinics exert their antiparkinsonian effect by correcting the relative central cholinergic excess which occurs in parkinsonism as a result of dopamine deficiency. In most patients their effects are only moderate, reducing tremor and rigidity to some extent but without significant action on bradykinesia. They exert a synergistic effect when used with **levodopa** and are also useful in reducing sialorrhoea.

Antimuscarinics reduce the symptoms of drug-induced parkinsonism (mainly antipsychotics) but there is no justification for giving them prophylactically. *Tardive dyskinesia is not improved by the antimuscarinic drugs, and they may make it worse.* No major differences exist between antimuscarinic antiparkinsonian drugs, but orphenadrine sometimes has a mood-elevating effect. Some people tolerate one antimuscarinic better than another. **Procyclidine** may be given parenterally, and is effective emergency treatment for severe acute drug-induced dystonic reactions (see Drug-induced movement disorders, p.745).

Bio-availability readily absorbed PO.
Onset of action 30–60min.
Time to peak plasma concentration 2–4h PO.
Plasma halflife 18h.
Duration of action 12–24h.

Cautions

Hepatic or renal impairment, cardiovascular disease. Avoid abrupt discontinuation. In a psychotic patient receiving a phenothiazine, the addition of orphenadrine to reverse a drug-induced acute dystonia (see Drug-induced movement disorders, p.745) may precipitate a toxic confusional psychosis because of a summation of antimuscarinic effects.

Undesirable effects

Antimuscarinic effects (see p.5). Nervousness, euphoria, insomnia, confusion, hallucinations occasionally.

Dose and use

Parkinsonism

For treatment of previously unrecognized or untreated symptoms in patients with a prognosis of <6 months:

- start with 50mg b.d.–t.d.s.
- if necessary, increase by 50mg every 2–3 days
- normal dose range 150–300mg daily in divided doses
- maximum recommended daily dose 400mg.

Note: **propranolol**, a non-selective β-adrenergic receptor antagonist (β-blocker), is the treatment of choice for akathisia. Antimuscarinic antiparkinsonian drugs are *contra-indicated* in tardive dyskinesia because they may exacerbate the condition (see Drug-induced movement disorders, p.745).

Supply

Orphenadrine (generic)

Tablets 50mg, 28 days @ 50mg t.d.s. = £53. (Note: at BNF prices, this is *more expensive* than branded Disipal® tablets.)

Oral solution 50mg/5mL, 28 days @ 50mg t.d.s. = £20.

Biorphen® (Alliance)

Oral solution (sugar-free) 25mg/5mL, 28 days @ 50mg t.d.s. = £36; *anise flavour.*

Disipal® (Astellas)

Tablets 50mg, 28 days @ 50mg t.d.s. = £3. (Note: at BNF prices, this is *cheaper* than generic tablets.)

5: ANALGESICS

PRINCIPLES OF USE OF ANALGESICS

Analgesics can be divided into three classes:

- non-opioid
- opioid
- adjuvant (Figure 5.1).

The principles governing their use have been summarized in the WHO Method for Relief of Cancer Pain:[1,2]

- 'By the mouth'
- 'By the clock'
- 'By the ladder' (Figure 5.2)
- 'Individual dose titration'
- 'Use adjuvant drugs'
- 'Attention to detail'.

Drugs from different categories are used alone or in combination according to the type of pain and response to treatment (Figure 5.1). Because cancer pain typically has an inflammatory component, it is generally appropriate to optimize treatment with an NSAID (or corticosteroid) and an opioid before introducing adjuvant analgesics.[3] However, with treatment-related pains (e.g. chemotherapy-induced neuropathic pain, chronic postoperative scar pain) and concurrent pains (e.g. post-herpetic neuralgia, muscle spasm pain), an adjuvant may be an appropriate first-line treatment. For example, an antidepressant or an anti-epileptic for non-cancer neuropathic pain, or a benzodiazepine for muscle spasm. Pain management in children is comparable with adults.[4]

Genetic variation involving CYP2D6 (see p.735) has been shown to be important for **codeine** (see p.332), and **tramadol** (see p.340).[5] The clinical significance of polymorphism for other

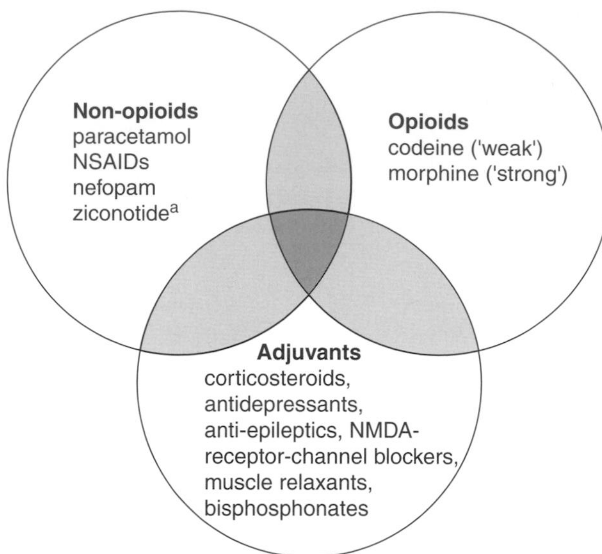

Figure 5.1 Broad-spectrum analgesia; drugs from different categories are used alone or in combination according to the type of pain and response to treatment.

a. ziconotide is an N-type calcium-channel blocker, the first of a new type of non-opioid. Its place in palliative care remains to be determined.[10,11]

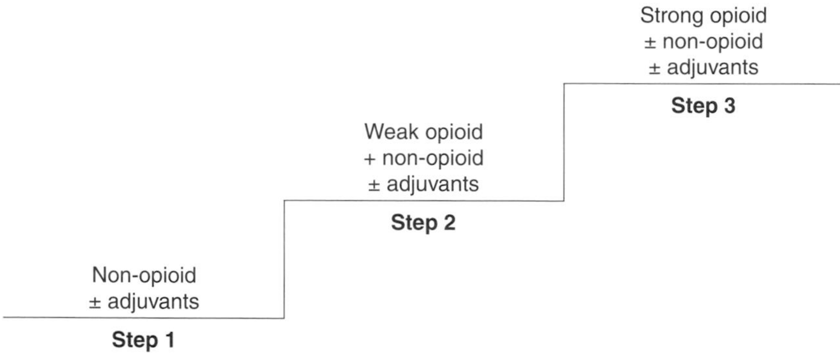

Figure 5.2 The World Health Organization 3-step analgesic ladder.[1]

opioids metabolized by CYP2D6 is unclear (**dextropropoxyphene**, **dihydrocodeine**, **hydrocodone**, **methadone**, **oxycodone**).

Polymorphism is rare for CYP3A4 and of unknown clinical significance.[6] Opioids potentially affected are **buprenorphine** and the fentanils. Dosing differences may be partly attributable to interindividual variation in CYP3A4 activity, which varies up to 10 times.[7] Genetic variations have also been shown for opioid receptors and transporters for **alfentanil**, **morphine** and **pentazocine**.[8]

In relation to the WHO analgesic ladder, there is continuing debate about the need for Step 2.[9] Certainly, there is no absolute pharmacological need for starting with a weak opioid before progressing to a strong opioid. Some paediatric palliative services omitted Step 2 many years ago. However, in most countries, access to a strong opioid remains difficult (e.g. only as a hospital inpatient, and then sparingly by injection) and sometimes impossible. Further, even where strong opioids can be readily prescribed, they are still often stigmatized. Consequently, some patients undoubtedly find a 3-step approach more acceptable.

If Step 2 is omitted, patients will generally start on a lower dose of **morphine** (20–30mg/24h or the equivalent dose of an alternative strong opioid), and be titrated upwards as necessary. Several RCTs indicate that **morphine** 60mg/24h is often too high a starting dose in this circumstance.[9]

Break-through (episodic) pain

Break-through (episodic) pain is a term used to describe a transient exacerbation of pain which occurs either spontaneously or in relation to a specific trigger (predictable or unpredictable) despite relatively stable and adequately controlled background pain.[12] Patients with poorly relieved background pain are excluded because this suggests overall poor pain relief, and is an indication for an increase in regular analgesia. Similarly, pain recurring shortly before the next dose of regular analgesic is due ('end-of-dose-interval pain') is not universally considered true break-through pain. Thus, there are two main types of break-through pain:

- *predictable (incident) pain*, an exacerbation of pain caused by weight-bearing and/or activity (including swallowing, defaecation, coughing, nursing/medical procedures) which may or may not be at the same location as the background (controlled) pain [13]
- *unpredictable (spontaneous) pain*, unrelated to movement or activity, e.g. colic, stabbing pain associated with nerve injury.

Break-through pain is common in both cancer patients (up to 90%) and non-cancer patients (up to 75%) receiving opioid medication for persistent pain.[14,15] It is often a resurgence of the background pain, and thus may be either functional (e.g. tension headache) or pathological, and either nociceptive (associated with tissue distortion or injury) or neuropathic (associated with nerve compression or injury). Patients may experience more than one type of break-through pain, and these may have different causes.

Various strategies reduce the impact of break-through pain (Figure 5.3).[16]

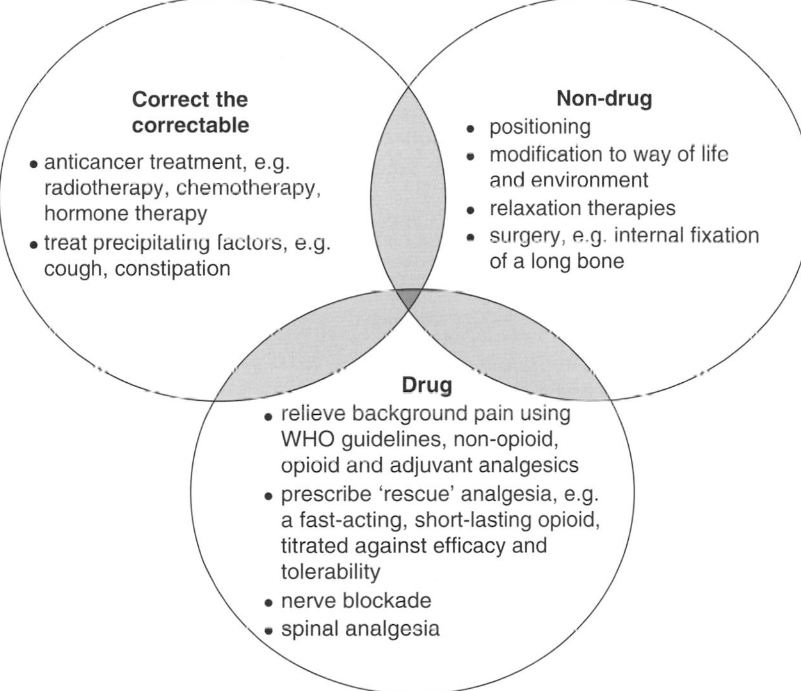

Figure 5.3 A multimodal approach to managing break-through (episodic) pain.

A widespread drug treatment is to give an extra dose of the regular analgesic, e.g. a p.r.n. dose of normal-release morphine for patients taking morphine regularly round-the-clock. A traditional practice, dating from before m/r opioid products were available, was to give an extra dose of the regular q4h dose of oral morphine (i.e. one sixth of the total daily dose). However, many break-through pains are short-lived and this approach effectively doubles the patient's opioid intake for the next 4h.

Increasingly, a more measured approach has been adopted, i.e. many centres recommend that the patient initially takes, as a normal-release formulation, 10% of the total daily regular dose as the p.r.n. dose.[17,18] However, a standard fixed-dose is unlikely to suit all patients and all pains, particularly because the intensity and the impact of break-through pain vary considerably. Thus, when patients are encouraged to optimize their rescue dose, the chosen dose varies from 5–20% of the total daily dose.[19,20]

Generally, break-through pain has a relatively rapid onset and short duration (e.g. 20–30min, ranging from <1min to >3h), whereas oral morphine has a relatively slow onset of action (30min) and long duration of effect (3–6h).[21] This helps to explain why many patients choose *not* to take a rescue dose of PO opioid with every episode of break-through pain, particularly when predictable, mild in intensity, and of relatively short duration.[22,23]

Strategies to circumvent the mismatch between break-through pain duration and drug effect latency include:

- timing a predictable painful activity or procedure to coincide with the peak plasma concentration after a regular or rescue PO dose of morphine (1–2h) or other strong opioid
- using routes of administration, e.g. buccal, intranasal, SL, which permit more rapid absorption of some (lipophilic) opioids, e.g. fentanyl.[24,25]

Experience with transmucosal fentanyl products (see p.400) indicates:[26]

- there is little or no correlation between the dose of the regularly administered strong opioid and the satisfactory rescue dose
- that the rescue dose needs to be individually titrated
- that different products will not be bio-equivalent and cannot be substituted for one another (the formulation and route of administration differ)
- that the cost will be substantially more than PO opioids
- serious adverse events and deaths can occur with inappropriate:
  - ▷ patient selection, e.g. opioid non-tolerant, transient pain (postoperative, migraine)
  - ▷ product use, e.g. exceeding recommended frequency of administration, dose-for-dose substitution of one product with another, i.e. Actiq® for Effentora®.

Other options include SL **alfentanil** (see p.374), and PO/SC **ketamine** (see p.593).

1 WHO (1986) *Cancer Pain Relief*. World Health Organisation, Geneva.
2 WHO (1996) Cancer Pain Relief: *with a guide to opioid availability* (2e). World Health Organisation, Geneva.
3 Twycross R *et al.* (2009) *Symptom Management in Advanced Cancer* (4e). palliativedrugs.com, Nottingham.
4 Zernikow B *et al.* (2006) Paediatric cancer pain management using the WHO analgesic ladder-results of a prospective analysis from 2265 treatment days during a quality improvement study. *European Journal of Pain*. **10**: 587–595.
5 Lotsch J and Geisslinger G (2006) Current evidence for a genetic modulation of the response to analgesics. *Pain*. **121**: 1–5.
6 Pirmohamed M and Park BK (2003) Cytochrome P450 enzyme polymorphisms and adverse drug reactions. *Toxicology*. **192**: 23–32.
7 Haddad A *et al.* (2007) The pharmacological importance of cytochrome CYP3A4 in the palliation of symptoms: review and recommendations for avoiding adverse drug interactions. *Supportive Care in Cancer*. **15**: 251–257.
8 Somogyi AA *et al.* (2007) Pharmacogenetics of opioids. *Clinical Pharmacology & Therapeutics*. **81**: 429–444.
9 Mercadante S (2007) Opioid titration in cancer pain: a critical review. *European Journal of Pain*. **11**: 823–830.
10 Prommer EE (2005) Ziconotide: can we use it in palliative care? *American Journal of Hospice and Palliative Care*. **22**: 369–374.
11 Narayana AK (2005) Elan: ziconotide review focused on off-label uses. *American Journal of Hospice and Palliative Care*. **22**: 408.
12 Davies AN *et al.* (2009) The management of cancer-related breakthrough pain: recommendations of a task group of the Science Committee of the Association for Palliative Medicine of Great Britain and Ireland. *European Journal of Pain*. **13**: 331–338.
13 Douglas I *et al.* (2000) Central issues in the management of temporal variation in cancer pain. In: R Hillier *et al.* (eds) *The Effective Management of Cancer Pain*. Aesculapius Medical Press, London, pp.93–106.
14 Davies A (ed) (2006) *Cancer-related breakthrough pain*. Oxford University Press, Oxford. UK.
15 Portenoy RK *et al.* (2006) Prevalence and characteristics of breakthrough pain in opioid-treated patients with chronic noncancer pain. *Journal of Pain*. **7**: 583–591.
16 Zeppetella G and Ribeiro MD (2002) Episodic pain in patients with advanced cancer. *American Journal of Hospice and Palliative Care*. **19**: 267–276.
17 Davis MP *et al.* (2005) Controversies in pharmacotherapy of pain management. *Lancet Oncology*. **6**: 696–704.
18 Davis MP (2003) Guidelines for breakthrough pain dosing. *American Journal of Hospice and Palliative Care*. **20**: 334.
19 Portenoy K and Hagen N (1990) Breakthrough pain: definition, prevalence and characteristics. *Pain*. **41**: 273–281.
20 Mercadante S *et al.* (2002) Episodic (breakthrough) pain: consensus conference of an expert working group of the EAPC. *Cancer*. **94**: 832–839.
21 Zeppetella G (2008) Opioids for cancer breakthrough pain: a pilot study reporting patient assessment of time to meaningful pain relief. *Journal of Pain and Symptom Management*. **35**: 563–567.

22 Gomez-Batiste X *et al.* (2002) Breakthrough cancer pain: prevalence and characteristics in Catalonia. *Journal of Pain and Symptom Management.* **24**: 45–52.
23 Davies AN *et al.* (2008) The management of cancer-related breakthrough pain: Recommendations of a task group of the Science Committee of the Association for Palliative Medicine of Great Britain and Ireland. *European Journal of Pain.* **13**: 331–338.
24 Davies A *et al.* (2011) Multi-centre European study of breakthrough cancer pain: Pain characteristics and patient perceptions of current and potential management strategies. *European Journal of Pain.* doi: 10.1016/j.ejpain.2010.1012.1004.
25 Zeppetella G and Ribeiro MD (2006) Opioids for the management of breakthrough (episodic) pain in cancer patients. *Cochrane Database of Systematic Reviews.* CD004311.
26 Christie J *et al.* (1998) Dose-titration, multicenter study of oral transmucosal fentanyl citrate for the treatment of breakthrough pain in cancer patients using transdermal fentanyl for persistent pain. *Journal of Clinical Oncology.* **16**: 3238–3248.

ADJUVANT ANALGESICS

Generally speaking, adjuvant analgesics are drugs which:
- are marketed primarily for indications other than pain *and*
- in relation to analgesic efficacy, are often circumstance-specific.

Thus, although *not* classified as analgesics, they may relieve pain resistant to standard analgesics, e.g. NSAIDs and opioids. Adjuvant analgesics include:
- antidepressants
- anti-epileptics
- bisphosphonates
- corticosteroids
- NMDA-receptor-channel blockers
- skeletal muscle relaxants
- smooth muscle relaxants (antispasmodics).

Unfortunately, the term 'adjuvant analgesic' is misleading if taken to mean that they are of benefit only when used together with a standard analgesic. In many situations, adjuvant analgesics *alone* provide pain relief ± a reduction in undesirable effects.

Antidepressants and anti-epileptics

Although opioids have been shown in RCTs to at least partly relieve neuropathic pain,[1,2] an antidepressant and/or an anti-epileptic may be preferable long-term, particularly with non cancer pain.

Comparing drugs used to relieve neuropathic pain

A useful statistic is the NNT, i.e. the *number* of patients *needed* to *treat* in order to achieve a specified benefit (e.g. ⩾50% improvement in one patient) compared with placebo. Thus an NNT of 3 means that 1 in 3 (or 33%) of patients will achieve such a benefit. However, in clinical practice, one hopes to 'capture' the placebo response as well as the pharmacological one. This means that an NNT of 3 in an RCT is likely to become an NNT of 2 in practice (50% of patients achieving a good response).

The opposite of NNT is NNH, i.e. the *number* of patients *needed* to be treated in order to cause a specified *harm* to one patient, e.g. undesirable effects sufficient to cause withdrawal from the trial. This gives a useful measure of comparative drug toxicity.[3]

Use relative to other measures

An antidepressant or an anti-epileptic is often used as a single agent in 'pure' nerve injury pain, e.g. chronic surgical incision pain, painful diabetic neuropathy, and post-herpetic neuralgia.[4–8] However, if the nerve injury pain is caused by an infiltrating cancer, **morphine** and an NSAID should be tried first before *adding* an antidepressant or an anti-epileptic.[9–11]

About 90% of patients with nerve injury pain respond to the use of non-opioids, opioids and adjuvant analgesics.[12] The remainder require spinal analgesia (e.g. **morphine** + **bupivacaine** ± **clonidine**) or a neurolytic procedure to obtain adequate relief. Some patients derive benefit from other non-drug measures, e.g. transcutaneous electrical nerve stimulation (TENS).

Choice of drug

Although few have been directly compared, the efficacy and tolerability of commonly used antidepressants and anti-epileptics appear comparable as judged by NNT and NNH. Expert

Table 5.1 Selected considerations when selecting an adjuvant analgesic for neuropathic pain.[13–17]

Drug	*Supporting evidence*[a]	*Ease of administration*			*Propensity for drug interactions*	*Cautions (also see individual monographs)*			*Approximate typical monthly cost*	*Examples of concurrent indications in palliative care*
		Once daily	*Syrup or dispersible*	*Parenteral*		*Cardiac disease*	*Renal impairment*	*Seizure threshold*		
First line treatments for neuropathic pain										
†Amitriptyline	High	Yes	Yes	No	Moderate	Arrhythmias, CHF, HB, IHD		↓	+ (tablets) ++ (syrup)	Depression, anxiety, bladder spasms, urgency
Duloxetine	Moderate	Yes	No	No	Moderate	Arrhythmias, CHF, HT, IHD	Avoid if GFR < 30	↓	+++	Depression, anxiety, stress incontinence
Gabapentin	High	No	Yes[b]	No	Low		↓Dose		++	Spasticity, seizures
†Nortriptyline	Moderate	Yes	No	No	Moderate	Arrhythmias, CHF, HB, IHD		↓	++	Depression
Pregabalin	High	No	Yes[b]	No	Low	CHF	↓Dose		++++	Anxiety, seizures
†Venlafaxine	High	Yes (m/r)	Yes[e]	No	Moderate	Arrhythmias, CHF, HT, IHD	↓Reduce dose if GFR < 30	↓	+++	Depression, anxiety
Treatments generally reserved for use second line or in specific situations										
Lidocaine 5% plaster[c]	Moderate	Yes	Topical		Low	Limited systemic absorption			++++	
Carbamazepine[d]	Low	No	Yes	No	High	HB	MAC		++	Seizures
†Clonazepam	Very low	Yes	Yes[e]	Yes (SC)	Moderate		↓Dose		+	Spasticity, seizures, anxiety
†Oxcarbazepine	Low	No	Yes	No	Moderate	CCF, HB	↓Dose		++	Seizures
†Valproate	Low	Yes (m/r)	Yes	Yes (IV)	Moderate		↓Dose		++	Seizures

Key: HB = heart block; CHF = congestive heart failure; HT = hypertension; IHD = ischaemic heart disease); MAC = manufacturer advises caution, but no specific dose alteration. Monthly cost; + = ≤£5, ++ = £5–20, +++ = £20–60, ++++ = ≥£60.

a. based on RCTs vs. case reports, methodological quality, consistency within and between studies, and applicability to palliative care population. Although few RCTs have been conducted in palliative care patients, generalizability was considered more likely if benefit demonstrated in ≥2 neuropathic pain types
b. capsules can be opened and sprinkled on food (unlicensed use; see Chapter 22, p.693)
c. licensed for post-herpetic neuralgia only
d. first-line choice (and licensed) for trigeminal neuralgia
e. disperses in 5min (unlicensed use; see Chapter 22, p.693).

guidelines tend to recommend several first-line treatments, depending on individual circumstances (Table 5.1).[13–15] NICE recommends **duloxetine** as first-line treatment for painful diabetic neuropathy and **pregabalin** or **amitriptyline** as first-line treatment for neuropathic pain from other causes. However, using **duloxetine** and **pregabalin** first-line is questionable (see p.249 and p.180 respectively).

Nonetheless, it is important to establish a practical protocol for neuropathic pain management which enables in-depth experience to be gained with 1–2 antidepressants and 1–2 anti-epileptics (Figure 5.4). However, sometimes the choice will be based on a desire to combine the treatment of neuropathic pain with that of another symptom so as to keep a patient's medication as simple as possible.

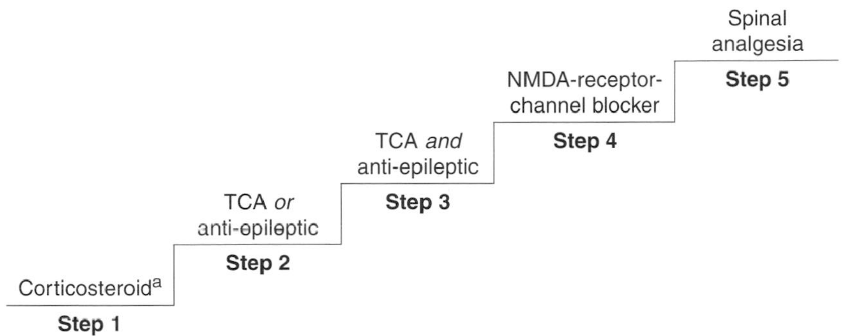

Figure 5.4 Adjuvant analgesics for neuropathic pain. If caused by cancer, use only if the pain does not respond to the combined use of an NSAID and a strong opioid.

a. Corticosteroids are only used for neuropathic pain caused by *an infiltrating cancer.* They are particularly important when neuropathic pain is associated with limb weakness.

Overall, **gabapentin** (p.251) and **amitriptyline** (p.189) are reasonable first-line options. However, alternative TCAs (e.g. **imipramine**, **nortriptyline**) are sometimes advocated on tolerability grounds.[7,15]

The mechanisms by which anti-epileptics relieve pain differ from the antidepressants (Figure 5.5 and Figure 5.6). If combining adjuvant analgesics, the following combinations should be avoided:

- adjuvants with the same action, e.g.:
  - two antidepressants
  - **gabapentin** with **pregabalin**
- an antidepressant with **tramadol** (see Serotonin toxicity, p.177).

Monitoring outcome

Relief is not an 'all or none' phenomenon. Undesirable drug effects are often a limiting therapeutic factor, particularly in frail patients.[18] The crucial first step in many cases is to help the patient obtain a good night's sleep. The second is to reduce pain intensity and allodynia associated with nerve injury pain to a bearable level during the day. Initially there may be marked diurnal variation in relief, with more prolonged periods with less or no pain rather than a decrease in worst pain intensity round the clock.

Patients should be warned that, unlike 'ordinary painkillers', benefit is likely only after several days, although the majority of benefit occurs within the first week.[18] On the other hand, improvement in sleep may well be immediate (particularly with sedative drugs like amitriptyline given at bedtime).

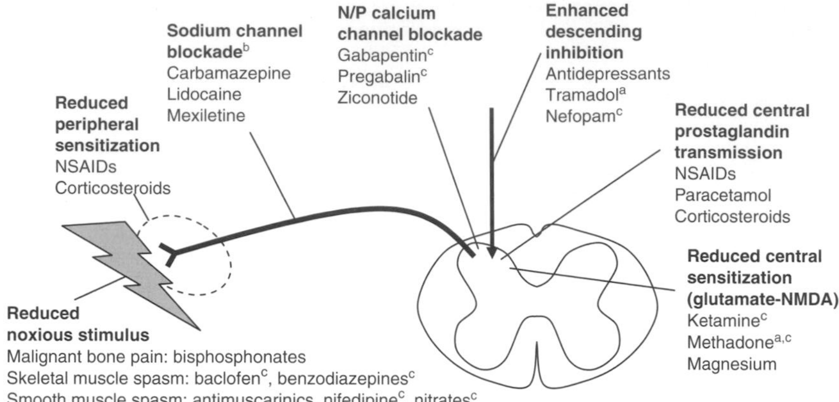

Figure 5.5 Overview of the peripheral and spinal non-opioid sites of action of analgesics.

a. also act as μ-opioid receptor agonists
b. reduces ectopic nerve signal transmission by damaged neurones (see p.257); the higher concentrations of lidocaine used in local/regional anaesthesia completely inhibit nerve signal transmission
c. additional actions (see individual monographs).

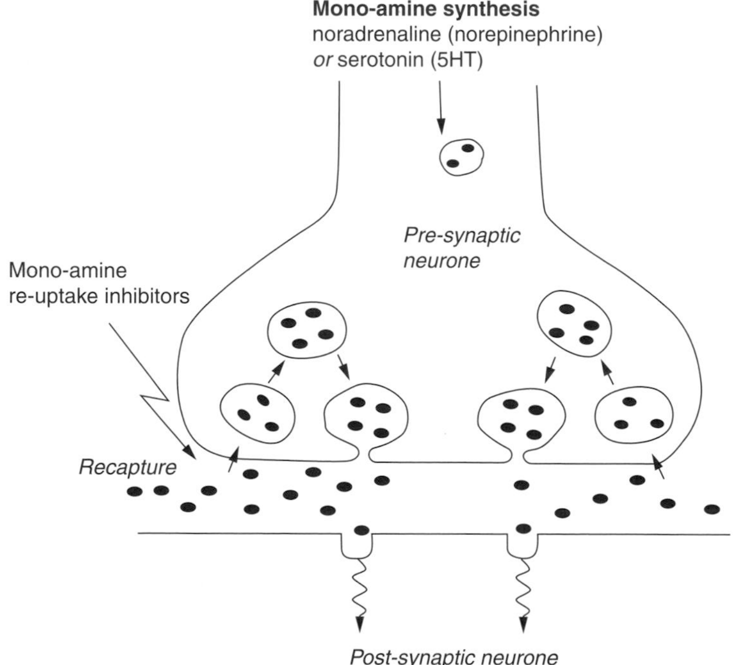

Figure 5.6 Mono-amine re-uptake inhibitors comprise mainly SNRIs, SSRIs, and NRIs (see Box 4.E, p.174), facilitate one or both of the two descending spinal inhibitory pathways by blocking presynaptic re-uptake (one serotoninergic, the other noradrenergic). SNRIs and SSRIs also potentiate opioid analgesia by a serotoninergic mechanism in the brain stem.

It is possible that low-dose combined treatment with an antidepressant and an anti-epileptic may be preferable in patients who do not respond to the introduction of one or other class of drug.[19] Thus, for example, if amitriptyline 50mg at bedtime provides definite but insufficient relief, consider adding an anti-epileptic after, say, 2 weeks rather than continuing to escalate the dose of amitriptyline (see p.189).

Bisphosphonates

Bisphosphonates (see p.469) are osteoclast inhibitors and are used to relieve metastatic bone pain which persists despite analgesics and radiotherapy ± orthopaedic surgery. Although published data relate mainly to breast cancer and myeloma, benefit is also seen with other cancers. About 50% of patients benefit, typically in 1–2 weeks, and this may last for 2–3 months. Benefit may be seen only after a second treatment but, if there is no response after two treatments, nothing is gained by further use.[20] In those who respond, continue to treat p.r.n. for as long as there is benefit.

Corticosteroids

Systemic corticosteroids can be helpful for various types of pain (see Box 7.B, p.483), but are used particularly for pain and weakness associated with:

- nerve root/nerve trunk compression, e.g. **dexamethasone** 4–8mg/24h
- spinal cord compression, e.g. **dexamethasone** 12–16mg/24h.[21,22]

Systemic corticosteroids do not help in pure non-cancer nerve injury pain, e.g. chronic postoperative scar pain, post-herpetic neuralgia. However, in cancer-related nerve injury pain, a 5–7 day trial of **dexamethasone** may be beneficial.

Epidural depot corticosteroids are sometimes used to relieve radicular pain associated with a spinal metastasis (see p.555).

NMDA-receptor-channel blockers

NMDA-receptor-channel blockers are most commonly used when neuropathic pain does not respond well to standard analgesics together with an antidepressant and an anti-epileptic. They have also been used in inflammatory pain, e.g. severe mucositis.[23] NMDA-receptor-channel blockers include:

- **ketamine** (see p.593)[24–26]
- **methadone** (see p.416)[27,28]
- **amantadine**.[29,30]

As with other classes of drugs, NMDA-receptor-channel blockers are not always beneficial. Controlled data show only modest benefit with **amantadine** 200mg IV over 3h, whereas earlier case reports indicated dramatic benefit.[30,31] *PCF does not recommend **amantadine**.*

Skeletal muscle relaxants

These include **baclofen**, **diazepam**, and **tizanidine** (see p.561). Although non-drug treatment is generally preferable for painful skeletal muscle spasm (cramp) and myofascial pain, e.g. physical therapy (local heat, massage, acupuncture),[32] some patients also benefit from relaxation therapy ± **diazepam** (see p.139). Myofascial trigger points often benefit from direct injection of local anaesthetic.[33] *However severe, **morphine** is ineffective for the relief of cramp and trigger point pains.*

Smooth muscle relaxants (antispasmodics)

This is a heterogeneous group of drugs encompassing antimuscarinics, **glyceryl trinitrate** (see p.70), and L-type calcium-channel blockers (e.g. **nifedipine**; see p.73). Antimuscarinics are used to relieve visceral distension pain and colic. In advanced cancer, there is little place for 'weak' antispasmodics, e.g. **dicycloverine**.

Hyoscine *butylbromide* (see p.14) and **glycopyrronium** (see p.11) are quaternary drugs which do not cross the blood-brain barrier, and are widely regarded as the antispasmodics of choice. Although **atropine** and **hyoscine *hydrobromide*** have comparable peripheral effects, they also have central effects, either stimulatory or sedative, and may precipitate delirium (see p.4).

Glyceryl trinitrate and calcium-channel blockers can be used for the same range of indications, but tend to be reserved for painful spasm of the oesophagus, rectum and anus (see p.70).

1 Eisenberg E *et al.* (2006) Efficacy of mu-opioid agonists in the treatment of evoked neuropathic pain: Systematic review of randomized controlled trials. *European Journal of Pain.* **10**: 667–676.
2 Eisenberg E *et al.* (2005) Efficacy and safety of opioid agonists in the treatment of neuropathic pain of nonmalignant origin: systematic review and meta-analysis of randomized controlled trials. *Journal of the American Medical Association.* **293**: 3043–3052.
3 Finnerup NB *et al.* (2005) Algorithm for neuropathic pain treatment: an evidence based proposal. *Pain.* **118**: 289–305.
4 DTB (2000) Drug treatment of neuropathic pain. *Drug and Therapeutics Bulletin.* **38**: 89–93.
5 Collins SL *et al.* (2000) Antidepressants and anticonvulsants for diabetic neuropathy and postherpetic neuralgia: a quantitative systematic review. *Journal of Pain and Symptom Management.* **20**: 449–458.
6 Backonja M (2001) Anticonvulsants and antiarrhythmics in the treatment of neuropathic pain syndromes. In: PT Hansson *et al.* (eds) *Neuropathic pain: pathophysiology and treatment.* IASP, Seattle, pp. 185–201.
7 Sindrup S and Jensen T (2001) Antidepressants in the treatment of neuropathic pain. In: PT Hansson *et al.* (eds) *Neuropathic pain: pathophysiology and treatment.* IASP, Seattle, pp. 169–183.
8 Iskedjian M *et al.* (2009) Anticonvulsants, serotonin-norepinephrine reuptake inhibitors and tricyclic antidepressants in management of neuropathic pain: a meta-analysis and economic evaluation (Technology report number 116). Canadian Agency for Drugs and Technologies in Health, Ottawa. Available from: www.cadth.ca/index.php/en/hta/reports-publications/search/publication/870
9 Dellemijn P *et al.* (1994) Medical therapy of malignant nerve pain. A randomised double-blind explanatory trial with naproxen versus slow-release morphine. *European Journal of Cancer.* **30A**: 1244–1250.
10 Ripamonti C *et al.* (1996) Continuous subcutaneous infusion of ketorolac in cancer neuropathic pain unresponsive to opioid and adjuvant drugs. A case report. *Tumori.* **82**: 413–415.
11 Dellemijn P (1999) Are opioids effective in relieving neuropathic pain? *Pain.* **80**: 453–462.
12 Grond S *et al.* (1999) Assessment and treatment of neuropathic cancer pain following WHO guidelines. *Pain.* **79**: 15–20.
13 Attal N *et al.* (2010) EFNS guidelines on the pharmacological treatment of neuropathic pain: 2010 revision. *European Journal of Neurology.* **17**: 1113–e1188.
14 Finnerup (2010) The evidence for pharmaceutical treatment of neuropathic pain. *Pain.* **150**: 573–581.
15 Dworkin RH *et al.* (2010) Recommendations for the pharmacological management of neuropathic pain: an overview and literature update. *Mayo Clinic Proceedings.* **85**: S3–14.
16 Saarto T and Wiffen PJ (2007) Antidepressants for neuropathic pain. *Cochrane Database of Systematic Reviews.* CD005454.
17 Wiffen PJ *et al.* (2010) Anitconvulsant drugs for acute and chronic pain. *Cochrane Database of Systematic Reviews.* **1**: CD001133.
18 Bennett MI (2010) Effectiveness of antiepileptic or antidepressant drugs when added to opioids for cancer pain: systematic review. *Palliative Medicine.* **25**: 553–559.
19 Gilron I *et al.* (2009) Nortriptyline and gabapentin, alone and in combination for neuropathic pain: a double-blind, randomised controlled crossover trial. *Lancet.* **374**: 1252–1261.
20 Mannix K *et al.* (2000) Using bisphosphonates to control the pain of bone metastases: evidence-based guidelines for palliative care. *Palliative Medicine.* **14**: 455–461.
21 Vecht C *et al.* (1989) Initial bolus of conventional versus high-dose dexamethasone in metastatic spinal cord compression. *Neurology.* **39**: 1255–1257.
22 Loblaw D and Laperriere N (1998) Emergency treatment of malignant extradural spinal cord compression: an evidence-based guideline. *Journal of Clinical Oncology.* **16**: 1613–1624.
23 Jackson K *et al.* (2001) 'Burst' ketamine for refractory cancer pain: an open-label audit of 39 patients. *Journal of Pain and Symptom Management.* **22**: 834–842.
24 Enarson M *et al.* (1999) Clinical experience with oral ketamine. *Journal of Pain and Symptom Management.* **17**: 384–386.
25 Fine P (1999) Low-dose ketamine in the management of opioid nonresponsive terminal cancer. *Journal of Pain and Symptom Management.* **17**: 296–300.
26 Finlay I (1999) Ketamine and its role in cancer pain. *Pain Reviews.* **6**: 303–313.
27 Gannon C (1997) The use of methadone in the care of the dying. *European Journal of Palliative Care.* **4**: 152–158.
28 Morley J and Makin M (1998) The use of methadone in cancer pain poorly responsive to other opioids. *Pain Reviews.* **5**: 51–58.
29 Kornhuber J *et al.* (1995) Therapeutic brain concentration of the NMDA receptor antagonist amantadine. *Neuropharmacology.* **34**: 713–721.
30 Pud D *et al.* (1998) The NMDA receptor antagonist amantadine reduces surgical neuropathic pain in cancer patients: a double blind, randomized, placebo controlled trial. *Pain.* **75**: 349–354.
31 Eisenberg E and Pud D (1998) Can patients with chronic neuropathic pain be cured by acute administration of the NMDA receptor antagonist amantadine? *Pain.* **74**: 337–339.
32 Twycross R *et al.* (2009) *Symptom Management in Advanced Cancer* (4e). palliativedrugs.com, Nottingham.
33 Sola A and Bonica J (1990) Myofascial pain syndromes. In: J Bonica (ed) *The Management of Pain* (2e). Lea and Febiger, Philadelphia, pp. 352–367.

PARACETAMOL BNF 4.7.1

There are increasing reports of unintentional overdose of paracetamol resulting in hepatotoxicity. The dose of paracetamol should always be appropriate for the weight of the patient, and take into account any factors which may increase the risk of hepatotoxicity, e.g. old age, poor nutritional status, fasting/anorexia, concurrent use of enzyme-inducing drugs, chronic alcohol abuse. The maximum recommended dose should not be exceeded.

Class: Non-opioid analgesic.

Indications: Mild–moderate pain, migraine, headache, pyrexia.

Contra-indications: (IV) severe hepatic impairment.

Pharmacology

Paracetamol is a synthetic centrally-acting non-opioid analgesic. Although some studies suggested a peripheral action,[1,2] most evidence points to a purely central effect.[3,4] Like NSAIDs, paracetamol is antipyretic; unlike NSAIDs, it has no discernible peripheral anti-inflammatory effect.

The mode of action of paracetamol in the CNS is still incompletely understood. The suggestion that it blocks the effects of a distinct isoform of cyclo-oxygenase (COX-3)[5] is no longer tenable.[6,7] Rather, by blocking peroxidise regeneration, it prevents the conversion of inactive COX to active oxidized COX. Thus, paracetamol is effective in intact cells (low peroxidase levels), e.g. in the CNS, but essentially ineffective peripherally where the vast amount of released peroxidases associated with tissue damage and/or inflammation overwhelms its inhibitory capacity.[8]

In addition, paracetamol:

- interacts with L-arginine-nitric oxide, opioid and cannabinoid systems[9,10]
- blocks descending serotoninergic inhibitory pain pathways.[11]

It is possible that the analgesic action of paracetamol is dependent on synergy between these mechanisms.[12] There is also evidence suggesting synergy between paracetamol and NSAIDs.[13,14]

The metabolism of paracetamol is age- and dose-dependent. Only 2–5% of a therapeutic dose of paracetamol is excreted unchanged in the urine; the remainder is metabolized mainly by the liver. At therapeutic doses, >80% of paracetamol is metabolized to glucuronide and sulphate conjugates. About 10% is converted by cytochrome P450-dependent hepatic mixed-function oxidase to a highly reactive metabolite N-acetyl-p-benzoquinoneimine (NAPQI; Figure 5.7). In turn, NAPQI is rapidly inactivated by conjugation with glutathione and excreted in the urine after further metabolism.

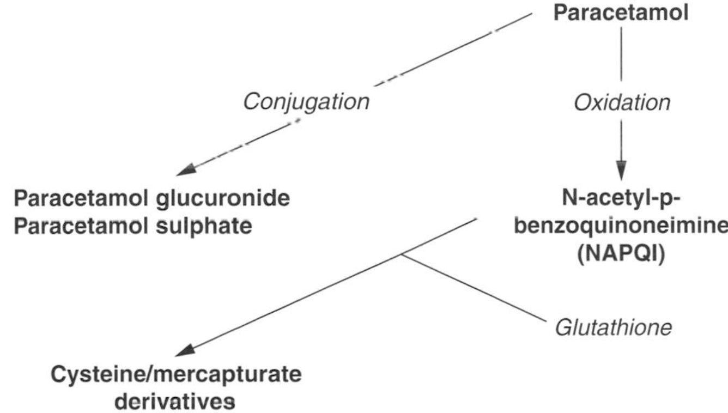

Figure 5.7 Metabolism of paracetamol.

When used *postoperatively* with a strong opioid, paracetamol has been shown to have an 'opioid-sparing' effect and improves overall analgesia.[15] However, the dose reduction may not be large enough to reduce opioid undesirable effects.[16,17] It has also been suggested that, in *cancer* pain, there may be no benefit from adding paracetamol to strong opioids.[18,19] However, the RCTs in question were underpowered,[20] and another RCT showed a small but clinically important additive effect in about one third of patients despite the fact that half were already taking an NSAID or a corticosteroid.[21]

Bearing in mind that, for many patients, paracetamol 1g q.d.s. (a typical dose) is a considerable tablet load, a pragmatic solution might be:

- to limit the long-term use of paracetamol to patients in whom definite benefit is seen within 2 days of starting it
- if already taking paracetamol with definite past benefit and increasing pain necessitates the *addition* of an opioid, to review the need for paracetamol by stopping it after 3–4 days of satisfactory pain relief with both drugs; restart the paracetamol if the pain returns, otherwise do not.

IV use

Single doses of IV paracetamol provide dose-dependent analgesia in doses of ≤2g.[22] In patients undergoing molar dental extraction, compared with 1g, 2g of paracetamol gave 50% more relief for 50% more time (5h vs. 3.2h).[23] Thus, there may be a place for an initial loading dose when prescribing paracetamol.

An IV formulation of paracetamol is available in the UK (see Supply).[24] Because it has low solubility (1g = 100mL), it is given by IV infusion over 15min.

Parenteral **propacetamol**, an inactive pro-drug of paracetamol, is available in many countries, and is used particularly for orthopaedic postoperative pain management.[15] **Propacetamol** 2g yields paracetamol 1g. Because of a significant risk of sensitization, the manufacturer's protocol must be adhered to.

Increased peak plasma concentrations with IV paracetamol lead to earlier and higher concentrations of paracetamol in the CSF, which in turn lead to an earlier onset of action, a longer duration of action, and a greater overall analgesic effect.[25]

Deliberate or unintentional overdose

The main risk associated with paracetamol is overdose, with consequential NAPQI-induced hepatotoxicity. Overdose overwhelms normal metabolism by glucuronidation and sulfonation, shifting more paracetamol into the NAPQI pathway. NAPQI is normally detoxified by conjugation with glutathione but, in overdose, the body's glutathione store becomes exhausted and the accumulation of NAPQI leads to liver parenchymal cell death. Although traditionally overdose is associated with a deliberate suicidal act, reports of unintentional overdose from its analgesic use are increasing.[26,27]

A single overdose of paracetamol below 125mg/kg (7.5g or 15 tablets in a 60kg person) is unlikely to result in liver damage. At twice this dose, the probability of liver damage is around 50%, but the individual may remain well. A dose of 500mg/kg (30g or 60 tablets in a 60kg person) is almost certain to produce life-threatening liver damage. Paracetamol overdose can also lead to acute renal failure, although this is often reversible without the need for dialysis.[28]

Note: acute alcohol intake does not increase the risk of hepatotoxicity. Indeed, because alcohol and paracetamol compete for the same oxidative enzymes, acute alcohol consumption at the time of a paracetamol overdose may be protective. However, because alcohol consumption induces the production of the relevant enzymes, if *chronic* alcohol use suddenly stops, paracetamol will be metabolized more rapidly, and could lead to hepatotoxicity.[29]

Deliberate or unintentional overdose can be treated using a glutathione precursor, e.g. IV **acetylcysteine** or PO **methionine**.[30,31] If given within 15h of the overdose, **acetylcysteine** prevents NAPQI from reacting with liver cell proteins. Further, because it has a protective effect against apoptosis (programmed cell death), **acetylcysteine** can help to a lesser extent if given for ≤3 days after the overdose.

Factors which place a patient at increased risk of hepatotoxicity from paracetamol include:

- old age
- poor nutritional status
- fasting/anorexia

} lower glutathione stores[32]

- concurrent use of enzyme-inducing drugs, e.g. **carbamazepine, phenobarbital, phenytoin, rifampicin, St John's wort**
- chronic alcohol abuse.[33]

For example, a man aged 43 with Crohn's colitis and weighing 30kg died of liver failure after taking 4g/24h for only 4 days.[34] Indeed, there are numerous reports of hepatotoxicity associated with chronic dosing with paracetamol 5–7.5g/24h.[35] Thus, the dose of paracetamol must always be appropriate for the weight and circumstances of the patient, and the maximum recommended dose not exceeded.

Further, an expert advisory committee of the FDA has recommended that:

- the OTC maximum single dose of paracetamol should be lowered to 650mg
- doses of 1g should be limited to prescription only
- combination products including paracetamol should be withdrawn to prevent unintentional overdosing by concurrent use with another paracetamol product.[36]

A final decision about this is awaited. Meanwhile, the FDA has requested manufacturers of combination analgesics to limit paracetamol to 325mg per tablet by 2013.[37]

Bio-availability 60% after 500mg PO, 90% after 1g PO; PR is about two thirds of PO, but is higher with two 500mg suppositories than with one 1g suppository.

Onset of action 15–30min PO; 5–10min IV (pain relief), 30min IV (antipyretic effect).

Time to peak plasma concentration widely variable PO, e.g. 20min in fasting state but 1–2h if delayed gastric emptying;[38] 15min IVI (this is synchronous with the end of a 15min infusion).

Plasma halflife 1.25–3h PO;[38] 2–3h IV.

Duration of action 4–6h PO and IV.

Cautions

Severe hepatic impairment, particularly if associated with alcohol dependence and malnutrition. Chronic paracetamol use increases the risk of renal impairment 2.5 times; and the risk is related to dose and cumulative exposure over a lifetime.[39,40] The risk is higher in diabetics, and in renal impairment associated with systemic vasculitis. In severe renal impairment (creatinine clearance $<$30mL/min), doses should *not* be given more than q.d.s.

Most dispersible paracetamol-containing tablets (alone or combined with a weak opioid) have a Na^+ content of $\geqslant$14mmol/tablet. Thus, a dose of 8 tablets/24h would exceed the recommended maximum daily dietary Na^+ intake of 100mmol (6g of sodium chloride). Dispersible formulations should thus be avoided in patients with hypertension or renal impairment, particularly if already on a salt-restricted diet. In contrast, non-soluble formulations contain negligible Na^+.[41]

The use of paracetamol in pregnancy and early childhood increases the risk of a child developing asthma.[42] However, there is no hard evidence that paracetamol precipitates asthma in established asthmatics.[43,44] Paracetamol can be taken by at least two thirds of patients who are hypersensitive to **aspirin** or other NSAID.[45,46] In people with a history of **aspirin**/NSAID-induced asthma, give a test dose of 250mg (half a tablet) and observe for 2–3h. If no undesirable effects occur, paracetamol can safely be used in standard doses.[44]

Drug interactions

Concurrent use of the $5HT_3$-receptor antagonists **tropisetron** and **granisetron** can completely block the analgesic effect of paracetamol,[12] but **ondansetron** may be safe in this respect.[47]

Concurrent use with **warfarin**: a regular *daily* intake of paracetamol $\geqslant$1300mg for one week may increase the INR to $>$6,[48,49] but a total *weekly* dose of paracetamol of $\leqslant$2g has no effect. The underlying mechanism is not clear, but may relate to interference with the hepatic synthesis of factors II, VII, IX and X. A recent post-mortem series found that concurrent paracetamol increases the risk of a bleed with **warfarin** 2.7 times.[50]

Undesirable effects

Very common (>10%): elevated liver transaminases,[26,51] dyspepsia.

Rare (<0.1%, >0.01%): PO: cholestatic jaundice,[52,53] acute pancreatitis, thrombocytopenia, agranulocytosis, anaphylaxis.[54–56] IV: malaise, hypotension.

Dose and use

In patients already receiving strong opioids ($\pm$ an NSAID), if definite added benefit is not seen within 2 days of starting regular paracetamol, it should be discontinued.[18]

In palliative care, typical PO doses for adults generally range from 500mg–1g q.d.s.[21] Although higher than the licensed maximum daily dose, given the lower bio-availability of PR paracetamol, 1.5g q.d.s. would seem to be a reasonable and safe maximum dose in adults >50kg *without any risk factors for paracetamol-induced hepatotoxicity.*

IV paracetamol is licensed for the short-term treatment of moderate pain (particularly after surgery) and the short-term treatment of fever when administration by other routes is not possible. It is given by infusion over 15min. *The dose depends on body weight:*

- adults and children >50kg, 1g up to q4h, maximum recommended dose 4g/24h
- adults and children >50kg *plus any risk factors for paracetamol-induced hepatotoxicity*, restrict maximum dose to 3g/24h
- adults and children 10–50kg, 15mg/kg up to q4h, maximum recommended dose 60mg/kg/24h.[57]

Supply

Paracetamol (generic)
Tablets 500mg, 28 days @ 1g q.d.s. = £3.
Tablets dispersible 500mg, 28 days @ 1g q.d.s. = £16.
Capsules and ***caplets (capsule-shaped tablets)*** 500mg are available OTC; many patients find these easier to swallow.
Oral suspension 120mg/5mL, 250mg/5mL, 28 days @ 1g q.d.s. = £15.
Suppositories 500mg, 28 days @ 1g q.d.s. = £560.

Perfalgan® (Bristol-Myers Squibb)
Injection (for IV infusion) 10mg/mL, 50mL (500mg) vial = £1.50, 100mL vial (1g) = £1.50.

Oral paracetamol is also available in several combination products with weak opioids.

1 Lim R *et al.* (1964) Site of action of narcotic and non-narcotic analgesics determined by blocking bradykinin-evoked visceral pain. *Archives Internationales de Pharmacodynamie et de Therapie*. **152**: 25–58.
2 Moore U et al. (1992) The efficacy of locally applied aspirin and acetaminophen in postoperative pain after third molar surgery. *Clinical Pharmacology and Therapeutics*. **52**: 292–296.
3 Twycross RG *et al.* (2000) Paracetamol. *Progress in Palliative Care*. **8**: 198–202.
4 Flower RJ and Vane JR (1972) Inhibition of prostaglandin synthetase in brain explains the anti-pyretic activity of paracetamol. *Nature*. **240**: 410–411.
5 Chandrasekharan N *et al.* (2002) COX-3, a cyclooxygenase-1 variant inhibited by acetaminophen and other analgesic/antipyretic drugs: cloning, structure, and expression. *Proceedings of the National Academy of Sciences of the United States of America*. **99**: 13926–13931.
6 Kis B *et al.* (2005) Acetaminophen and the cyclooxygenase-3 puzzle: sorting out facts, fictions, and uncertainties. *Journal of Pharmacology and Experimental Therapeutics*. **315**: 1–7.
7 Li S *et al.* (2008) Acetaminophen: antipyretic or hypothermic in mice? In either case, PGHS-1b (COX-3) is irrelevant. *Prostaglandins and Other Lipid Mediators*. **85**: 89–99.
8 Mattia A and Coluzzi F (2009) What anesthesiologists should know about paracetamol (acetaminophen). *Minerva Anestesiologica*. **75**: 644–653.
9 Bjorkman R *et al.* (1994) Acetaminophen (paracetamol) blocks spinal hyperalgesia induced by NMDA and substance P. *Pain*. **57**: 259–264.
10 Pini L *et al.* (1997) Naloxone-reversible antinociception by paracetamol in the rat. *Journal of Pharmacology and Experimental Therapeutics*. **280**: 934–940.
11 Mallet C *et al.* (2008) Endocannabinoid and serotonergic systems are needed for acetaminophen-induced analgesia. *Pain*. **139**: 190–200.
12 Pickering G *et al.* (2006) Analgesic effect of acetaminophen in humans: first evidence of a central serotonergic mechanism. *Clinical Pharmacology and Therapeutics*. **79**: 371–378.
13 Miranda HF *et al.* (2006) Synergism between paracetamol and nonsteroidal anti-inflammatory drugs in experimental acute pain. *Pain*. **121**: 22–28.
14 Ong CK *et al.* (2010) Combining paracetamol (acetaminophen) with nonsteroidal antiinflammatory drugs: a qualitative systematic review of analgesic efficacy for acute postoperative pain. *Anesthesia and Analgesia*. **110**: 1170–1179.
15 Peduto VA *et al.* (1998) Efficacy of propacetamol in the treatment of postoperative pain. Morphine-sparing effect in orthopedic surgery. Italian Collaborative Group on Propacetamol. *Acta Anaesthesiologica Scandinavica*. **42**: 293–298.
16 Aubrun F *et al.* (2003) Adjunctive analgesia with intravenous propacetamol does not reduce morphine-related adverse effects. *British Journal of Anaesthesia*. **90**: 314–319.
17 Cakan T *et al.* (2008) Intravenous paracetamol improves the quality of postoperative analgesia but does not decrease narcotic requirements. *Journal of Neurosurgical Anesthesiology*. **20**: 169–173.
18 Axelsson B and Christensen S (2003) Is there an additive analgesic effect of paracetamol at step 3? A double-blind randomized controlled study. *Palliative Medicine*. **17**: 724–725.
19 Israel FJ *et al.* (2010) Lack of benefit from paracetamol (acetaminophen) for palliative cancer patients requiring high-dose strong opioids: a randomized, double-blind, placebo-controlled, crossover trial. *Journal of Pain and Symptom Management*. **39**: 548–554.
20 Formby FT (2010) Re: lack of benefit from paracetamol (acetaminophen) for palliative cancer patients. *Journal of Pain and Symptom Management*. **40**: e6; author reply e6–7.

21 Stockler M *et al.* (2004) Acetaminophen (paracetamol) improves pain and well-being in people with advanced cancer already receiving a strong opioid regimen: a randomized, double-blind, placebo-controlled cross-over trial. *Journal of Clinical Oncology.* **22**: 3389–3394.
22 Piguet V *et al.* (1998) Lack of acetaminophen ceiling effect on R-III nociceptive flexion reflex. *European Journal of Clinical Pharmacology.* **53**: 321–324.
23 Juhl GI *et al.* (2006) Analgesic efficacy and safety of intravenous paracetamol (acetaminophen) administered as a 2g starting dose following third molar surgery. *European Journal of Pain.* **10**: 371–377.
24 Flouvat B *et al.* (2004) Bioequivalence study comparing a new paracetamol solution for injection and propacetamol after single intravenous infusion in healthy subjects. *International Journal of Clinical Pharmacology and Therapeutics.* **42**: 50–57.
25 Jarde O and Boccard E (1997) Parenteral versus oral route increases paracetamol efficacy. *Clinical Drug Investigations.* **14**: 474–481.
26 Larson AM *et al.* (2005) Acetaminophen-induced acute liver failure: results of a United States multicenter, prospective study. *Hepatology.* **42**: 1364–1372.
27 MHRA (2010) Intravenous paracetamol (Perfalgan): risk of accidental overdose especially in infants and neonates. *Drug Safety Update.* **3**: 2–3.
28 von Mach MA *et al.* (2005) Experiences of a poison center network with renal insufficiency in acetaminophen overdose: an analysis of 17 cases. *Clinical Toxicology.* **43**: 31–37.
29 Gomez-Moreno G *et al.* (2008) Interaction of paracetamol in chronic alcoholic patients. Importance for odontologists. *Medicina Oral, Patologia Oral Y Cirugia Bucal.* **13**: E235–238.
30 BNF (2011) Emergency treatment of poisoning. In: *British National Formulary (No 60).* British Medical Association and Royal Pharmaceutical Society of Great Britain, London. Current BNF available from: www.bnf.org.
31 Ferner RE *et al.* (2011) Management of paracetamol poisoning. *British Medical Journal.* **342**: 968–972.
32 Horsmans Y *et al.* (1998) Paracetamol-induced liver toxicity after intravenous administration. *Liver.* **18**: 294–295.
33 Zimmerman H and Maddrey W (1995) Acetaminophen (paracetamol) hepatotoxicity with regular intake of alcohol: analysis of instances of therapeutic misadventure. *Hepatology.* **22**: 767–773.
34 Claridge LC *et al.* (2010) Acute liver failure after administration of paracetamol at the maximum recommended daily dose in adults. *British Medical Journal.* **341**: c6764.
35 Krenzelok EP (2009) The FDA Acetaminophen Advisory Committee Meeting — what is the future of acetaminophen in the United States? The perspective of a committee member. *Clinical Toxicology.* **47**: 784–789.
36 Spring S (2009) Food and drug administration. Available from: www.fda.gov/downloads/AdvisoryCommittees/Committees-MeetingMaterials/Drugs/DrugSafetyandRiskManagementAdvisoryCommittee/UCM174697.pdf
37 FDA (2011) Drug Safety Communication. Prescription acetaminophen products to be limited to 325mg per dosage unit; boxed warning will highlight potential for severe liver failure. Available from: www.fda.gov/Drugs/DrugSafety/ucm239821.htm
38 Prescott LF (1996) *Paracetamol (Acetaminophen) A Critical Bibliographic Review.* Taylor & Francis, London.
39 D'Arcy P (1997) Paracetamol. *Adverse Drug Reaction Toxicology Review.* **16**: 9–14.
40 Fored CM *et al.* (2001) Acetaminophen, aspirin, and chronic renal failure. *New England Journal of Medicine.* **345**: 1801–1808.
41 Sullivan L (2006) What is the sodium content of medicines? Available from: www.druginfozone.nhs.uk/Record%20Viewing/viewRecord.aspx?id = 573370
42 Holgate ST (2011) The acetaminophen enigma in asthma. *American Journal of Respiratory Critical Care Medicine.* **183**: 147–148.
43 Shaheen S *et al.* (2000) Frequent paracetamol use and asthma in adults. *Thorax.* **55**: 266–270.
44 Shin G *et al.* (2000) Paracetamol and asthma. *Thorax.* **55**: 882–884.
45 Szczeklik A (1986) Analgesics, allergy and asthma. *Drugs.* **32**: 148–163.
46 Settipane R *et al.* (1995) Prevalence of cross-sensitivity with acetaminophen in aspirin-sensitive asthmatic subjects. *Journal of Allergy and Clinical Immunology.* **96**: 480–485.
47 Jokela R *et al.* (2010) The influence of ondansetron on the analgesic effect of acetaminophen after laparoscopic hysterectomy. *Clinical Pharmacology and Therapeutics.* **87**: 672–678.
48 Bell W (1998) Acetaminophen and warfarin: undesirable synergy. *Journal of the American Medical Association.* **279**: 702–703.
49 Hylek E *et al.* (1998) Acetaminophen and other risk factors for excessive warfarin in anticoagulation. *Journal of the American Medical Association.* **279**: 657–662.
50 Launiainen T *et al.* (2010) Adverse interaction of warfarin and paracetamol: evidence from a post-mortem study. *European Journal of Clinical Pharmacology.* **66**: 97–103.
51 Watkins PB *et al.* (2006) Aminotransferase elevations in healthy adults receiving 4 grams of acetaminophen daily: a randomized controlled trial. *Journal of the American Medical Association.* **296**: 87–93.
52 Waldum H *et al.* (1992) Can NSAIDs cause acute biliary pain and cholestasis? *Journal of Clinical Gastroenterology.* **14**: 328–330.
53 Wong V *et al.* (1993) Paracetamol and acute biliary pain with cholestasis. *Lancet.* **342**: 869.
54 Leung R *et al.* (1992) Paracetamol anaphylaxis. *Clinical and Experimental Allergy.* **22**: 831–833.
55 Mendizabal S and Gomez MD (1998) Paracetamol sensitivity without aspirin intolerance. *Allergy.* **53**. 457–450.
56 Morgan S and Dorman S (2004) Paracetamol (acetaminophen) allergy. *Journal of Pain and Symptom Management.* **27**: 99–101.
57 BNF (2011) Section 4.7.1. In: *British National Formulary (No 60).* British Medical Association and Royal Pharmaceutical Society of Great Britain, London. Current BNF available from www.bnf.org.

NEFOPAM — BNF 4.7.2

Class: Non-opioid analgesic, benzoxazocine.

Indications: Pain (including cancer pain), †hiccup.

Contra-indications: Concurrent use of an MAOI, epilepsy.

Pharmacology

Nefopam is a centrally acting synthetic analgesic. Its dominant mode of action is uncertain. Mono-amine re-uptake inhibition may explain its effect on the descending pain modulatory pathway.[1] However, despite being used for over 30 years, there are no reports of nefopam causing serotonin toxicity either alone or with other drugs which inhibit mono-amine oxidase.[2]

Nefopam also blocks voltage-gated sodium and calcium channels associated with glutamic acid, an excitatory neurotransmitter.[3,4] Its effects are not reversed by **naloxone**. It does not inhibit cyclo-oxygenase (COX) or affect platelet function.[5] Antimuscarinic and sympathomimetic properties may account for some of its undesirable effects.

Nefopam is metabolized in the liver to an active metabolite, desmethylnefopam. This is subsequently renally eliminated.[6] Although excretion of desmethylnefopam is likely to be prolonged in renal impairment, nefopam is commonly used in this situation. Post-operatively, single parenteral doses provided analgesia for ≤5h.[7,8] However, pharmacological effects were seen for ≤12h after oral doses in healthy volunteers,[6] possibly reflecting the longer halflife of desmethylnefopam.

Nefopam is as effective as NSAIDs in cancer pain[9] and osteo-arthritis but less well tolerated.[10] In postoperative pain, IV or IM nefopam 20mg (equivalent to 60mg PO) is:

- comparable with NSAIDs, reducing morphine requirements in the first 24h by 10–15mg[11]
- comparable with ketamine 10mg[12]
- superior to propacetamol 2g.[13]

Although one RCT reported no additional analgesia when nefopam was given postoperatively with an NSAID (in conjunction with a strong opioid),[14] a later RCT reported synergism from such a combination.[15] Nefopam is reported to control refractory hiccup.[16,17]

Bio-availability 36%.
Onset of action < 1h.
Time to peak plasma concentration 1–3h PO, 1.5h IM.
Plasma halflife 4–5h; desmethylnefopam 10–15h.[6]
Duration of action ≤12h PO; ≤5h IV (see text).

Cautions

Hepatic impairment, glaucoma, prostatism.

Drug interactions

Exacerbates the undesirable effects of concurrently administered antimuscarinic or sympathomimetic agents.

Undesirable effects

Most common: nausea and vomiting, drowsiness, hypotension, epigastric pain.[9] In critical care, tachycardia and sweating was reported in ≤30% and ≤20% of patients respectively.[18] Sweating was also common in patients with rheumatoid arthritis.[19] However, in an RCT in cancer patients, tachycardia was noted in only 3%.[9]
Less common: diarrhoea, confusion and hallucinations (particularly in the elderly), tremor, paraesthesia, dizziness, syncope, seizures, palpitations, dry mouth, urinary retention.
Infrequent: blurred vision, insomnia, headache, pink discolouration of the urine.

Dose and use

- start with 60mg PO t.d.s. (30mg PO t.d.s. in the elderly) or 20mg IM q6h
- if necessary, increase to 90mg PO t.d.s.

Supply

Acupan® (Meda)
Tablets 30mg, 28 days @ 60mg t.d.s. = £20.
Injection 10mg/mL, 2mL amp = £2.50. (Unlicensed, available as a named patient supply from IDIS, see Obtaining unlicensed products p.769).

1 Hunskaar S *et al.* (1987) Involvement of central serotonergic pathways in nefopam-induced antinociception. *European Journal of Pharmacology.* **138**: 77–82.
2 Gillman K (2007) *Personal communication.*

3 Novelli A *et al.* (2005) Nefopam inhibits calcium influx, cGMP formation, and NMDA receptor-dependent neurotoxicity following activation of voltage sensitive calcium channels. *Amino Acids.* **28**: 183–191.
4 Verleye M *et al.* (2004) Nefopam blocks voltage-sensitive sodium channels and modulates glutamatergic transmission in rodents. *Brain Research Reviews.* **1013**: 249–255.
5 Dordoni PL *et al.* (1994) Effect of ketorolac, ketoprofen and nefopam on platelet function. *Anaesthesia.* **49**: 1046–1049.
6 Aymard G *et al.* (2003) Comparative pharmacokinetics and pharmacodynamics of intravenous and oral nefopam in healthy volunteers. *Pharmacology and Toxicology.* **92**: 279–286.
7 Beaver WT and Feise GA (1977) A comparison of the analgetic effect of intramuscular nefopam and morphine in patients with postoperative pain. *Journal of Clinical Pharmacology.* **17**: 579–591.
8 Phillips G and Vickers MD (1979) Nefopam in postoperative pain. *British Journal of Anaesthesia.* **51**: 961–965.
9 Minotti V *et al.* (1989) Double-blind evaluation of analgesic efficacy of orally administered diclofenac, nefopam, and acetylsalicylic acid (ASA) plus codeine in chronic cancer pain. *Pain.* **36**: 177–183.
10 Stamp J *et al.* (1989) A comparison of nefopam and flurbiprofen in the treatment of osteoarthrosis. *British Journal of Clinical Practice.* **43**: 24–26.
11 Evans MS *et al.* (2008) Nefopam for the prevention of postoperative pain: quantitative systematic review. *British Journal of Anaesthesia.* **101**: 610–617.
12 Kapfer B *et al.* (2005) Nefopam and ketamine comparably enhance postoperative analgesia. *Anesthesia and Analgesia.* **100**: 169–174.
13 Mimoz O *et al.* (2001) Analgesic efficacy and safety of nefopam vs. propacetamol following hepatic resection. *Anaesthesia.* **56**: 520–525.
14 Moffat AC *et al.* (1990) Postoperative nefopam and diclofenac. Evaluation of their morphine-sparing effect after upper abdominal surgery. *Anaesthesia.* **45**: 302–305.
15 Delage N *et al.* (2005) Median effective dose (ED50) of nefopam and ketoprofen in postoperative patients: a study of interaction using sequential analysis and isobolographic analysis. *Anesthesiology.* **102**: 1211–1216.
16 Bilotta F and Rosa G (2000) Nefopam for severe hiccups. *New England Journal of Medicine.* **343**: 1973–1974.
17 Bilotta F *et al.* (2001) Nefopam for refractory postoperative hiccups. *Anesthesia and Analgesia.* **93**: 1358–1360.
18 Chanques G *et al.* (2010) Analgesic efficacy and haemodynamic effects of nefopam in critically ill patients. *British Journal of Anaesthesia*
19 Emery P and Gibson T (1986) A double-blind study of the simple analgesic nefopam in rheumatoid arthritis. *British Journal of Rheumatology.* **25**: 72–76.

NON-STEROIDAL ANTI-INFLAMMATORY DRUGS (NSAIDS) BNF 10.1.1 & 15.1.4.2

Despite the potential for harm, *PCF* regards NSAIDs as essential analgesics for most patients with cancer pain, and for other pains with an inflammatory component.

Non-steroidal anti-inflammatory drugs (NSAIDs) are essential drugs for cancer pain management,[1,2] and have a major role in postoperative pain.[3,4] However, there is little high level evidence for their usefulness in some forms of chronic non-cancer pain, e.g. low back pain.[5]

NSAIDs prevent or reverse inflammation-induced hyperalgesia, not only locally[6] but also in the CNS.[7,8] NSAIDs are thus of particular benefit for pains associated with inflammation. These include most forms of cancer pain.[2,9,10] The efficacy of NSAIDs in pure neuropathic pain is less well established, but there is some supportive evidence from both animal and human studies.[11] NSAIDs are also antipyretic.[12] It is generally accepted that inhibition of cyclo-oxygenase is the main mechanism of action of NSAIDs.[13]

Quantitatively, the most serious adverse effects of NSAIDs are GI and cardiovascular toxicity. Although quantifying the combined risk is not easy,[14,15] it is important that the dangers are kept in perspective. Based on cohort studies, in patients taking an NSAID for *at least 2 months* the risk of a bleeding ulcer or perforation is of the order of 1 in 500.[16] Further, on average, 1 in 1,200 patients taking NSAIDs for *at least 2 months* will die from gastroduodenal complications.[16]

In relation to selective COX-2 inhibitors (the class of NSAIDs which has caused the most cardiovascular concern), the number of additional thrombotic events (mainly myocardial infarctions) is 3/1,000 patients per year of use.[17] If 1/6–1/3 of these are fatal, this would give a death rate of about 1 in 1,000–2,000 patients *per year of use* from thrombosis. With patients with a short prognosis, the risk may be smaller, although many terminal conditions themselves predispose to thrombosis or other complications.

However, in end-stage disease, the benefit associated with greater physical comfort may far outweigh the potential harm from GI or thrombotic complications. On the other hand, worsening heart failure after an infarct or disability from a stroke can be a high price to pay. Thus, in order to minimize harm as much as possible:

- select the safest drug for each patient (see p.303)[15]

- use the smallest effective dose for the shortest possible time
- prescribe appropriate gastroprotection
- consider whether there are alternative measures which carry less risk.

Cyclo-oxygenase

There are two distinct cyclo-oxygenase (COX) isoforms.[18] COX-1 is mainly 'constitutive', i.e. is part of the body's normal physiological constitution with near constant levels and activity in most tissues, including the CNS. In contrast, COX-2 is 'constitutively' present only in parts of the CNS, renal cortex, stomach, uterus, cartilage, bone and seminal vesicles (Figure 5.8) but is massively 'inducible' within a few hours by inflammation, dehydration or trauma.

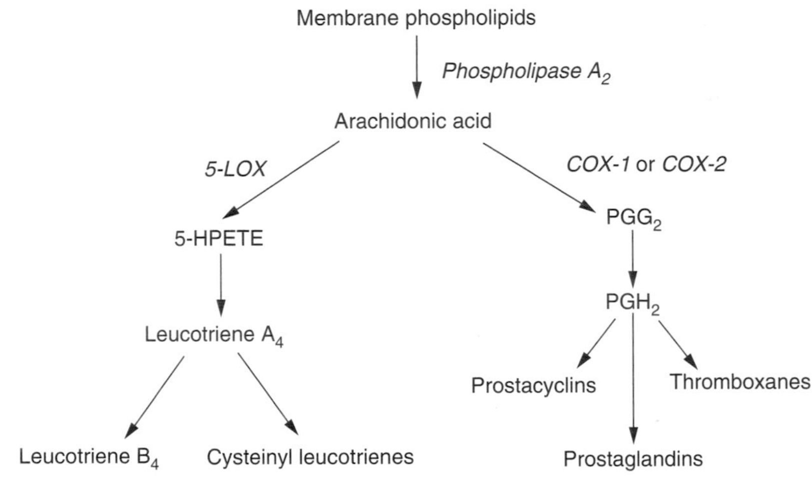

Figure 5.8 Products of arachidonic acid metabolism involved in inflammation.
Key: COX = cyclo-oxygenase; 5-HPETE = hydroperoxyeicosatetrenoic acid; LOX = lipoxygenase; PG = prostaglandin.

COX-1 also plays an essential role in the production of inflammation, producing pro-inflammatory prostaglandins, and is induced at sites of inflammation. COX-1 deficient mice mount a reduced inflammatory response. COX-2 initially produces pro-inflammatory prostaglandins, but later induces anti-inflammatory PGD_2.[19] Both peptic ulcer and bone healing require COX-2.[20,21]

A third isoform, COX-3, has been postulated.[22] However, this is a splice-variant of COX-1, rather than a distinct isoform. It was considered by some to explain both the antipyretic and analgesic effects of **paracetamol**. However, the current consensus is that 'COX-3' is not of physiological importance in humans.[23,24]

Cyclo-oxygenase inhibition

Inflammation is associated with increased prostaglandin (PG) production both in the peripheral tissues and in the CNS.[25] The peripheral free nerve endings responsive to noxious stimuli become hypersensitive in the presence of inflammatory substances. Increased sensitivity of the nerve endings leads to increased transduction, and thus increased pain. Inflammation also leads to the increased production of PGs in the CNS, triggered hormonally, which leads to central sensitization of neurones in the dorsal horn, with further magnification of the noxious stimulus and more severe pain.[26–28] COX-2 plays a key role in central hyperalgesia.[29] There is now some animal evidence that at least some types of inflammatory peripheral hyperalgesia are not prostaglandin-mediated.[29]

By inhibiting the production of COX, NSAIDs block the synthesis of PGs both peripherally in the tissues and in the CNS. The relative peripheral and central contributions to the total analgesic effect depends, *inter alia*, on the NSAID in question, its pharmacokinetic characteristics, and the route of administration.[13]

Spinal COX-2 also inhibits endocannabinoid breakdown. Indeed, some postulate that this mechanism is more important than inhibition of PG synthesis in the reversal of PG-induced spinal hyperexcitability.[30]

Classification

NSAIDs are now generally classified on the basis of their relative ability to inhibit COX-1 and COX-2. However, the degree of COX-2 selectivity varies according to the assay used[31,32] and whether the result is expressed in terms of 50 or 80% inhibition of the enzyme.[33,34] Although 80% inhibition is theoretically a better comparator, most studies use 50% (Table 5.2). Further, the results of *in vitro* assays may not reliably reflect *in vivo* reality.[35] This is certainly the case in relation to **celecoxib**. Despite its relatively modest ranking in (Table 5.2), no significant COX-1 inhibition was seen in volunteers taking 400mg b.d.[36] Dose and inter-patient variation are the main determinants of COX-2 selectivity *in vivo*.[37]

Table 5.2 COX-2 selectivity ratio of IC_{50} COX-1/COX-2 (human whole blood assays)[34]

Drug	*COX-2 selectivity ratio*
Etoricoxib	106
Rofecoxib[a]	35
Valdecoxib[b]	30
Celecoxib	7.6
Nimesulide[c]	7.3
Diclofenac	3.0
Etodolac	2.4
Meloxicam	2.0
Indometacin	0.4
Ibuprofen	0.2
Piroxicam	0.08

a. withdrawn worldwide
b. withdrawn in Europe, the USA and Canada
c. not UK.

Although it is more correct to think of a spectrum of selectivity,[31,33] it is customary to divide NSAIDs into several seemingly disparate categories (Table 5.3). Inevitably, there will be differences of opinion as to where the cut off between categories should come, particularly because selectivity is partly dose-dependent.[31] For example, with **meloxicam** 7.5mg/day, there is 70% COX-2 and 7% COX-1 inhibition but, with 15mg/day, there is 80% COX-2 and 25% COX-1 inhibition.[38] Further, thromboxane B_2 production is reduced 66% by **meloxicam** 15mg/day, the result of COX-1 inhibition.[39]

Table 5.3 Classification of NSAIDs

Preferential COX-1 inhibitors	*Non-selective COX inhibitors*	*Preferential COX-2 inhibitors*	*Selective COX-2 inhibitors*
Flurbiprofen	Aspirin	Diclofenac	Celecoxib
Indometacin	Fenamates	Etodolac	Etoricoxib
Ketoprofen	Ibuprofen	Meloxicam	Parecoxib
Ketorolac	Nabumetone	Nimesulide (not UK)	Valdecoxib
	Naproxen		
	Salicylates		

Additional sites of action

NSAIDs have other sites of actions apart from COX inhibition.[40] It has long been known that the anti-inflammatory properties of an NSAID are not predictive of its analgesic effect, suggesting that other mechanisms must be involved.[41] Other mechanisms have been proposed in relation to the effect of NSAIDs on:

- neutrophils[42–44]
- synthesis and regulation of activity of dorsal horn neurotransmitters and modulators[43]
- modulation of pain transduction through spinal serotoninergic, adrenergic and cholinergic systems[45]
- endocannabinoids[30]
- nitric oxide production[46]
- interleukin release.[40]

NSAIDs also affect brain concentrations of kynurenic acid, an endogenous antagonist which acts on the glycine recognition site of the NMDA-receptor-channel complex.[47] **Diclofenac** (preferential COX-2 inhibitor) and **indometacin** (preferential COX-1 inhibitor) increase brain kynurenic acid concentrations, whereas **meloxicam** and **parecoxib** (preferential and selective COX-2 inhibitors respectively) cause a decrease. It is possible that at least some NSAIDs tonically modulate kynurenic acid metabolism, and thereby impact on central nociceptive mechanisms.

Other laboratory studies have shown that **diclofenac** and **meclofenamic acid** are effective openers of the potassium channels KCNQ2/3, thus facilitating inhibitory M-currents [48] The clinical significance of these findings is unclear.

It is possible that non-selective NSAIDs are intrinsically more broad-spectrum in their central effects than selective COX-2 inhibitors.[49] However, clinically, selective COX-2 inhibitors appear to be equally effective when compared with non-selective NSAIDs in inflammatory, dental and postoperative pain.[50] On the other hand, in dental pain, there is a tendency for weak COX inhibitors to be superior to **aspirin** and for strong inhibitors to be inferior, emphasizing the importance of not adopting too simplistic a view of the mode of action of these drugs (Table 5.4).

Table 5.4 Analgesic efficacy of oral NSAIDs in dental pain compared with aspirin 650mg[41]

Significantly superior	*Not significantly different*	*Significantly inferior*
Azapropazone (3)[a,b]	Diclofenac (1)	Fenbufen (1)
Diflunisal (3)[b]	Etodolac (1)	Nabumetone (1)
Flurbiprofen (1)	Sulindac (1)	Ketoprofen (2)
Ketorolac (3)	Naproxen (3)	Tolmetin (3)[b]

a. numbers indicate capacity to inhibit PG synthesis: 1 = strong; 2 = moderate; 3 = weak
b. no longer available in the UK.

NSAIDs and pyrexia

All NSAIDs are antipyretic.[12,51] Paraneoplastic fever responds to all NSAIDs, not just to naproxen as initially thought.[52] Although the antipyretic effect of NSAIDs tended to wear off after a few months, further benefit was obtained by switching to an alternative NSAID. However, the duration of benefit with second- and third-line drugs was generally shorter.

For guidance on the use of drugs for treating paraneoplastic pyrexia and sweating, see Box 5.A.

Box 5.A Symptomatic drug treatment of paraneoplastic pyrexia and sweating

Begin by prescribing an antipyretic:
- paracetamol 500mg–1g q.d.s. or p.r.n. (generally less toxic than an NSAID)
- NSAID, e.g. ibuprofen 200–400mg t.d.s. or p.r.n. (or the locally preferred alternative).

If the sweating does not respond to an NSAID, prescribe an antimuscarinic drug:
- amitriptyline 25–50mg at bedtime (may cause sedation, dry mouth and other antimuscarinic effects)
- hyoscine *hydrobromide* 1mg/3days TD[53]
- glycopyrronium ≤2mg PO t.d.s.

If an antimuscarinic fails, other options include:
- propranolol 10–20mg b.d.–t.d.s.
- cimetidine 400–800mg b.d.[54]
- olanzapine 5mg b.d.[55]
- thalidomide 100mg at bedtime[56,57]

Thalidomide is generally seen as the last resort even though the response rate appears to be high.[57] This is because it can cause an irreversible painful peripheral neuropathy, and may also cause drowsiness. It is also prohibitively expensive (see p.519).

NSAIDs, platelet function and bleeding time

NSAIDs differ in their effect on platelet function and bleeding time (Table 5.5; also see p.300).

Table 5.5 NSAIDs, platelet function and bleeding time

Drug	*Comment*
Aspirin	Irreversible platelet dysfunction and prolonged bleeding time as a result of acetylation of platelet COX-1
Non-acetylated salicylates e.g. choline magnesium trisalicylate[a], salsalate[a]	No effect on platelet function or bleeding time at recommended doses
Classical NSAIDs (except diclofenac), e.g. flurbiprofen, ibuprofen, ketorolac, naproxen	Reversible platelet dysfunction and prolonged bleeding time
Diclofenac	Reversible inhibition of platelet aggregation in two-third of subjects.[58] IV diclofenac has a measurable effect on bleeding time, but most subjects remain within normal limits
Etodolac	No data
Meloxicam[59] Nabumetone Nimesulide [a,60] Coxibs[38,61]	No effect on platelet function or bleeding time

a. not UK.

Undesirable effects

NSAIDs differ in their propensity to cause a range of undesirable effects. For convenience, these have been categorized as type A and type B. Generally, type A effects are mainly dose-dependent and partly predictable, whereas type B effects are mainly dose-independent and unpredictable (Table 5.6 and Table 5.7).

Table 5.6 Type A ('predictable') reactions to NSAIDs[62]

Organ/system	*Clinical reaction*
Blood	Decreased platelet aggregation, prolonged bleeding time (see Table 5.5)
GI tract	Dyspepsia Peptic ulceration, bleeding, perforation Small bowel stricture Protein-losing enteropathy
Kidney	Salt and water retention
Cardiovascular	Thrombosis, e.g. myocardial infarction, stroke
Lung	Bronchospasm (asthma)

Table 5.7 Type B ('unpredictable') reactions to NSAIDs[62]

Organ/system	*Clinical reaction*	*Most likely NSAIDs*
Immunological	Anaphylaxis	Most NSAIDs
Skin	Morbilliform rash Angioedema	Fenbufen Ibuprofen Azapropazone Piroxicam
Blood	Thrombocytopenia	Diclofenac Ibuprofen Piroxicam
	Haemolytic anaemia	Mefenamic acid Diclofenac
GI tract	Diarrhoea	Fenamates, e.g. mefenamic acid
Kidney	Interstitial nephritis	Fenoprofen[63]
Liver	Reye's syndrome (in children) Hepatotoxicity	Aspirin Diclofenac Sulindac
CNS	Aseptic meningitis	Ibuprofen

NSAIDs and the GI tract

Nabumetone (see p.328) and **celecoxib** (p.312) are the safest by a significant margin; and **diclofenac** (see p.315), low-dose **ibuprofen** (≤1,200mg/24h; see p.320) and **naproxen** (see p.325) are relatively safe. In contrast, the most dangerous NSAIDs are **azapropazone**, **indometacin**, **ketoprofen**, **ketorolac** and **piroxicam**.[64] These latter should not be used routinely in palliative care, although use may be justifiable in specific limited circumstances, e.g. **ketorolac** (see p.323) and **piroxicam** (see p.308).

Stomach and duodenum

The relative risk of gastric ulcer when taking NSAIDs is 5–6.[65] For duodenal ulceration, the relative risk is only 1.1, although a recent population-based nested case-control study suggested it is higher.[66] One patient in 1,200 on NSAIDs for ≥2 months without adequate gastroprotection dies mainly as a result of complicated gastric ulceration (i.e. bleeding or perforation).[16] This translates into 2,000 excess deaths annually in the UK.

Although disputed,[67] it is generally accepted that the incidence of serious gastroduodenal events with the coxibs is reduced by about half.[68–75] How much of the benefit relates to COX-2 selectivity is uncertain; gastroduodenal toxicity depends on several factors (Box 5.B).

Box 5.B Factors intrinsic to NSAIDs which result in low gastroduodenal toxicity[76]

Competitive masking of COX-1 by inactive forms, e.g. R-ibuprofen, R-etodolac.

Weak/no uncoupling of oxidative phosphorylation; Low disruption of phospholipids in protective mucus and mucous membranes } non-acidic compounds, e.g. nabumetone, coxibs.

High protein-binding (less available).

Weak/no inhibition of platelet aggregation, e.g. non-acetylated salicylates, coxibs, meloxicam, and diclofenac sometimes.

The situation may change when dual LOX/COX inhibitors become available. These inhibit lipoxygenase (LOX) as well as COX-1 and COX-2 and appear to have similar GI toxicity to placebo,[77] a positive cardiovascular risk profile, and to reduce cartilage damage in osteo-arthritis.[78]

The nitric oxide NSAIDs (NO-NSAIDs, also known as CINODs, COX-inhibiting NO donors) are another group of novel NSAIDs designed to provide improved GI safety, and lower rather than raise blood-pressure. However, an RCT of one NO-NSAID showed GI safety to be no better than with **naproxen**, although blood pressure was unaffected.[79] Another new concept currently being investigated is linking an NSAID molecule with phosphatidylcholine.[80]

In patients who are *H.pylori* positive, the risk of an NSAID-related ulcer is almost doubled, and the risk of bleeding is increased about 2.5 times.[81] This is because the infection-associated chronic atrophic gastritis, which mainly affects the antrum, makes the extracellular matrix in that part of the stomach wall vulnerable to back-diffusion of acid. Ionized NSAID molecules, circulating in the plasma, are transported passively through leaky capillaries into the inflamed matrix where they become unionized in the acidic environment. In this state, the molecules are lipid-soluble and move freely into the mucosal cells where, at a higher pH, they become ionized again and consequently trapped. The local high concentration of NSAID leads to inhibition of the production of gastroprotective COX-1 in the stomach mucosa. Eradication of *H. pylori* infection (see p.464) corrects the atrophic gastritis and ends the sequence of events initiated by acid back-diffusion. Eradication of *H. pylori* thus renders all COX-1-inhibiting NSAIDs safer to use.[82–86]

However, although *H.pylori* eradication is worthwhile in NSAID-naïve users, surprisingly it is *not* protective in those already taking NSAIDs.[87] Further, when trying to prevent ulcer recurrence in patients on NSAIDs, *H.pylori* eradication is less effective than a PPI.[88]

Risk factors for an NSAID-induced serious gastroduodenal event (i.e. ulceration, bleeding, perforation) are listed in Box 5.C. For example, concurrent administration of a non-selective NSAID and **warfarin** increases the risk of bleeding >10 times, nearly 4 times that of **warfarin** alone, and nearly 4 times the risk when using a coxib plus **warfarin**.[89]

Box 5.C Risk factors for NSAID-related serious GI event[65,90]

Age >65 years (see text).

Peptic ulcer $\pm$ GI bleeding in the last year confirmed by endoscopy, or strong clinical suspicion, e.g. haematemesis, melaena.

Long-term use of maximum recommended doses of an NSAID.

Serious morbidity, e.g. cancer, diabetes mellitus, hypertension, cardiovascular disease, hepatic impairment, renal impairment.

Concurrent use of a corticosteroid, low-dose aspirin, or anticoagulant (warfarin or heparin).

Concurrent use of a serotonin re-uptake inhibitor (see text).

Platelets $<50 \times 10^9$/L.

Acid dyspepsia with an NSAID despite concurrent use of a gastroprotective agent, now or in the past.

Gastric infection with *H. pylori.*

In rheumatoid arthritis, the risk of hospitalization and/or death increases progressively from 50 years.[65] Thus, compared with those under 50, the risk is twice as great in patients aged 50–65 years, 6 times greater in patients aged 65–75, and some 14 times greater in the over 75s. However, in rheumatoid arthritis there may well be concurrent interacting risk factors. Thus, 65 years is widely considered to be the appropriate point for regarding age as a risk factor in other situations.

Antidepressants which inhibit presynaptic serotonin re-uptake, notably SSRIs and **clomipramine**, **amitriptyline** and **venlafaxine**, decrease serotonin uptake from the blood by platelets.[91] Because platelets do not synthesize serotonin, serotonin re-uptake inhibitors decrease the platelet serotonin concentration, and this may adversely affect platelet aggregation. Serotonin re-uptake inhibitors are an independent risk factor for GI bleeding, increasing the risk >6 times, giving an NNH of 106 when combined with an NSAID.[92] Low-dose aspirin in addition to an NSAID and an SSRI reduces the NNH to 28, i.e. is much more dangerous.[93]

Patients with a high risk of serious gastropathy are best treated with an NSAID with a low propensity for causing gastrotoxicity (see p.298). Concurrent prophylaxis with a gastroprotective agent also helps to prevent serious gastric complications.[94–96] There is now evidence that the combination of a coxib and gastroprotection provides the best prophylaxis, and should be recommended in high risk patient.[97,98]However, compliance with guidance about gastroprotection is still low.[99,100]

Misoprostol, PPIs, and *double-dose* H_2-receptor antagonists are all effective at preventing chronic NSAID-related endoscopic gastric and duodenal ulcers.[95] **Misoprostol** 400microgram/24h is less effective than 800microgram and is still associated with diarrhoea. Of all these treatments, only **misoprostol** 800microgram/24h has been definitely shown to reduce the overall incidence of ulcer complications.[95] PPIs reduce the incidence of re-bleeding from endoscopically confirmed peptic ulcers,[101] and may reduce the incidence of ulcer complications.[96]

Small bowel

In the small bowel, NSAIDs can also produce ulceration, bleeding, perforation, stricture (very thin annular strictures that can reduce the bowel lumen to a pinhole) and protein-losing enteropathy. Changes in bowel permeability may be the root cause of NSAID enteropathy,[102] although some have suggested other factors. There is currently no proven treatment for NSAID enteropathy, although there is some suggestion that coxibs and other NSAIDs without an enterohepatic recirculation may be safer (see **nabumetone**, p.328).[103]

Large bowel

In the large bowel, NSAIDs can re-activate Crohn's disease and ulcerative colitis.[104] Although the evidence for this is not strong,[105] NSAIDs should be avoided in these conditions. These and other GI effects are possibly associated with the role of PGs in bowel neuromuscular control[106] and in changes in permeability. NSAIDs can also cause a colitis directly and increase the risk of complications from diverticular disease.[107]

NSAIDs and the cardiovascular system

All NSAIDs raise blood pressure, and this needs to be monitored in patients susceptible to cardiac problems or who are already hypertensive.[108] NSAIDs increase the risk of heart failure;[109] and the use of NSAIDs in heart failure carries a dose-dependent risk of death.[110] Thus, NSAIDs should be generally be avoided in patients with chronic heart failure.[111]

Risk factors for NSAID-related cardiovascular events include age ≥80 years, rheumatoid arthritis, chronic kidney disease, and COPD.[112]

Many NSAIDs increase the likelihood of myocardial infarction.[113] The mechanism is debatable.[114,115] The risk appears to start within a month, increases with continued use, and diminishes but persists for several months after an NSAID is discontinued.[116,117] Likewise, many NSAIDs increase the risk of stroke, and this is probably higher in those who have had a previous stroke.[118]

A recent RCT meta-analysis quantified the risk of **diclofenac**, **ibuprofen**, **naproxen**, and four coxibs (two of which have been withdrawn).[113] A relative risk of ≤1.3 is considered acceptable; generally a higher risk is acceptable only if the potential gains clearly outweigh the risks. Although **diclofenac** carries no excess risk of myocardial infarction, it had one of the highest risks of cardiovascular death (3.98 (1.48–12.70)) and of stroke (2.86 (1.09–8.36)), as well as the highest risk of death from any cause (2.31 (1.00–4.95)).

Ibuprofen increases the risk of myocardial infarction (1.61 (0.50–5.77)), and carries the highest risk for stroke (3.36 (1.00–11.60)). It also increases the risk of death from any cause (2.39 (0.69–8.64)).

Naproxen does *not* increase the risk of myocardial infarction, and its association with cardiovascular death or death from any cause is below the 1.3 threshold. The risk of stroke is higher (1.76 (95% CI 0.91–3.33)).

Celecoxib has acceptable risks for myocardial infarction and stroke, but carries an elevated risk of cardiovascular death (2.07 (0.98–4.55)), suggesting that although fewer myocardial infarcts and strokes occur they are more likely to be fatal. The overall risk of death from any cause with celecoxib was only a little higher than the acceptability threshold (1.50 (0.96–2.54)), and the second best after naproxen.

Etoricoxib appears to carry no increased risk of myocardial infarction, but has the highest risk for cardiovascular death (4.07 (1.23–15.70)), with risks for stroke and death from any cause both being more than doubled.

The thromboprotective effect of aspirin for stroke appears to be compromised in people taking a concurrent NSAID,[119] but possibly less so with the coxibs.[120] However, this combination leads to the loss of the gastroprotective effect of the selective COX-2 inhibitor.[121,122] Thus, ideally, patients on **aspirin** for thromboprotection should *not* take another NSAID of any type. However, if a round-the-clock NSAID is considered essential, stop the **aspirin** and prescribe **naproxen** b.d. because it impairs platelet function and carries no increased risk of myocardial infarction with only a modest increase of risk for stroke.

NSAIDs and the kidneys

All NSAIDs cause an increase in Cl^- resorption from the proximal tubules, and enhance ADH activity, leading to sodium (Na^+) and water retention. Thus NSAIDs antagonize the action of diuretics, and can exacerbate existing hypertension or lead to new onset hypertension.[123] The proximal passive resorption of Na^+ leads to increased resorption of K^+ in the distal tubules; this can result in hyperkalaemia.

NSAIDs can cause acute or acute-on-chronic renal failure.[124,125] Chronic NSAID use increases the risk of chronic renal failure.[126] Sporadic cases of interstitial nephritis ($\pm$ nephrotic syndrome or $\pm$ papillary necrosis) have been reported with most NSAIDs. The renal risks of different NSAIDs, including coxibs, are similar, and thus are not a factor in determining choice.[127] Less than 1% of patients given an NSAID develop renal impairment sufficient to cause discontinuation of therapy.[128]

However, the prevalence in palliative care patients might be higher, because NSAID-induced renal failure is associated with hypovolaemia and conditions of low effective circulating volume. In situations such as hypovolaemia, the plasma concentrations of vasoconstrictor substances such as angiotensin II, noradrenaline (norepinephrine) and vasopressin are increased, e.g. in heart failure, cirrhosis and nephrotic syndrome, persistent vomiting or diarrhoea, third space losses (e.g. ascites) and diuretic use. Normally, this would lead to increased vasodilator prostaglandin secretion in the kidneys to maintain renal perfusion, but the inhibition of renal PG production by NSAIDs prevents this, thereby precipitating renal failure.[125,129] Except in patients expected to die in a few days, dehydrated patients should be rehydrated when starting treatment with an NSAID, or the NSAID should not be used. The acute renal failure due to NSAIDs is generally reversible if the drug is stopped promptly, but not always; it can be fatal.

Patients with multiple myeloma are at particular risk, although this is rare in the absence of Bence-Jones (light chain) proteinuria.[130–132]

NSAIDs and the liver

Patients with hepatic impairment are more susceptible to NSAID-related renal impairment. Hence most SPCs for NSAIDs include active liver disease or significant hepatic impairment as a contra-indication.

In patients with cirrhosis it is difficult to obtain an accurate measure of renal function because the plasma creatinine concentrations tends to be low. This may relate to a reduced muscle mass and reduced conversion of creatine to creatinine.[133] NSAID-related impairment of platelet function may increase the risk of bleeding from oesophageal varices.

Cholestasis may reduce the elimination of NSAIDs excreted in bile (**indometacin**, **sulindac**), and may reduce or delay absorption of fat-soluble NSAIDs, e.g. **ibuprofen**.[134]

Hepatotoxicity is a rare and unpredictable effect seen with most NSAIDs, including COX-2-selective ones. **Diclofenac** and **sulindac** may have the highest risk, and **ibuprofen** the least.[134]

NSAIDs and bronchospasm

Some patients, with or without a history of atopic asthma, give a history of **aspirin**- or NSAID-induced asthma. The prevalence, derived from oral provocation testing studies, is about 20% in the general adult population, and 5% in children.[135] Chronic non-aspirin NSAID users have almost double the risk of developing adult onset asthma.[136]

Genetic polymorphisms in prostanoid receptor genes[137] and leukotriene synthase genes[138] have been described in **aspirin**-induced asthmatics, suggesting that the asthma is caused by an **aspirin**-induced (COX-1 inhibitory) imbalance between bronchodilator PGE_2 and bronchoconstrictor leukotrienes, and is not immunologically mediated (as in atopic asthmatics).[139–141]

Aspirin-induced asthma typically occurs 30min–3h after ingestion of **aspirin**. Half of those affected react to even low-dose **aspirin** (80mg). Cross-sensitivity with other NSAIDs is normal, e.g. **diclofenac** (93%), **ibuprofen** (98%), **naproxen** (100%).[135] A history of allergic-type reactions (asthma, acute rhinitis, nasal polyps, angioedema, urticaria) with **aspirin** or other NSAID calls for extreme caution in prescribing a further NSAID (Table 5.8).

Table 5.8 Use of NSAIDs in asthmatic patients

Patient characteristics	*Recommendations*
Anyone who has ever had an asthmatic reaction to aspirin or other NSAID; or anyone with high risk features of aspirin-induced asthma (severe asthma, nasal polyps, urticaria, or chronic rhinitis)	Avoid all products containing aspirin or other NSAID; use paracetamol instead unless also contra-indicated. Coxibs are almost always safe, but give the first dose under medical supervision
All other asthmatic patients	Any NSAID, including aspirin, may be considered but, if any respiratory reaction occurs, stop the NSAID and manage as above

In contrast, the incidence of cross-sensitivity to **paracetamol** is only 7%, and $<2\%$ of asthmatic patients are sensitive to both **aspirin** and **paracetamol**.[142] Further, reactions to **paracetamol** are generally less severe. Thus, **paracetamol** should always be the initial non-opioid of choice for asthmatic patients.

Bronchospasm has not been observed with **choline salicylate** (available only as a dental gel and ear drops in the UK), **sodium salicylate** (not UK), or **azapropazone**; it is rare with **benzydamine** (available only as a mouthwash and throat spray in the UK).[143]

Coxibs rarely induce asthma, and the cause may well be isolated idiosyncratic allergy and not cross-reactivity with **aspirin** or other NSAID.[144,145]

Management of NSAID-induced asthma is along usual lines, but leukotriene receptor inhibitors, e.g. **montelukast**, have a particular place. Some patients may have been treated by **aspirin** desensitization. Such patients will be on daily **aspirin** and can safely take an NSAID without provoking an attack. It is essential *not* to stop the **aspirin** in such patients or sensitization may return.[145]

NSAIDs and bone healing

Some NSAIDs (**indometacin**, **diclofenac**, **tenoxicam**) delay bone healing in animals, but others (**ibuprofen**, **ketorolac**, **piroxicam**) have not been shown to do this.[146] The clinical impact of this is uncertain, and human data are very limited. However, there is evidence that long-term NSAID use is associated with an increased risk of non-union of fractures.[147] Further, even when used for only 2–5 days, NSAIDs decrease heterotopic (ectopic) bone formation, commonly seen after major hip surgery.[147,148]

Some orthopaedic departments prohibit the use of NSAIDs, including coxibs, for up to 6 weeks postoperatively. There is evidence for impairment in healing with high doses of both non-selective and selective NSAIDs.[146] Thus, when using NSAIDs after fracture or orthopaedic surgery, it would be sensible to use the lowest effective dose for as short a time as necessary. For example, limit the use of an NSAID to ≤10 days, and then discontinue until healing is complete. However, in patients with other risk factors for delayed union or non-union (e.g. smoking, diabetes mellitus, corticosteroids), use **paracetamol** instead.[146] On the other hand, if pain relief is inadequate when using both **paracetamol** and an opioid, an NSAID should be prescribed (instead of the **paracetamol**) despite its potential negative impact.

Contra-indications for NSAIDs

Although the SPCs are not completely consistent in this respect, the following is a general list of contra-indications for NSAIDs:

- hypersensitivity to **aspirin** or other NSAID (urticaria, rhinitis, asthma, angioedema)
- active GI ulceration, bleeding, perforation or inflammation
- severe heart failure
- active liver disease or moderate–severe hepatic impairment
- severe renal impairment (creatinine clearance <30mL/min), deteriorating renal function, hyperkalaemia (>5mmol/L).

These contra-indications are not necessarily absolute. There may well be occasions when 'contra-indication' means 'use with great caution and in the absence of a safer alternative'.

Important NSAID drug–drug interactions

Patients on **warfarin** should have their INR closely monitored during the first week after starting an NSAID; increases of up to 60% have been reported (Table 5.9).[149,150]

Drug interactions are summarized in Table 5.9 and Table 5.10 (also see Cytochrome P450, p.375). Of particular importance is the interaction with **methotrexate** which is 60–80% excreted unchanged by the kidney. *Concurrent administration of* ***methotrexate*** *and an NSAID decreases the excretion of* ***methotrexate*** *and increases its toxicity.*[151] Two deaths have occurred with **aspirin**, three with **ketoprofen** and one with **naproxen**. Fatal or severe renal failure has also developed when intermediate-dose or high-dose **methotrexate** was combined with **ibuprofen** or **indometacin**, and life-threatening neutropenia has been reported with several other NSAIDs.[151,152] Toxicity is related to dose and renal function; it is much less likely with chronic low-dose **methotrexate** in psoriasis or rheumatoid arthritis than with high-dose pulses of cancer chemotherapy, and in patients without pre-existing renal impairment.[151]

Choice of NSAID

In practice, the choice of NSAID will depend on various factors, including availability, efficacy, safety, fashion, cost, and local guidelines. The renal risks of different NSAIDs including coxibs are similar, and thus are not a factor in determining choice.[127]

It is unclear if some cancer patients obtain more benefit from one particular NSAID, as is anecdotally reported in rheumatoid arthritis, or whether apparent differences simply relate to a relative increase in inhibition of PG synthesis.

Although other NSAIDs are sometimes preferred (see p.318 and p.328), current fashion largely favours **diclofenac**, **ibuprofen** and **naproxen**. These all feature in recent large studies in comparison with coxibs. *Because of GI toxicity, all are generally prescribed with gastroprotection*:

- **naproxen** (1g/24h) has a higher risk of GI toxicity but is the drug of choice for patients with cardiovascular risk factors (see p.325)
- **ibuprofen** carries a low risk of GI toxicity at lower doses (≤1,200mg/24h) but a significant risk of stroke or cardiovascular death; it is thus suitable where GI risk matters but needs to be used with caution in patients with cardiovascular problems (see p.320)

Table 5.9 Pharmacokinetic interactions: NSAIDs affecting other drugs[151,153]

Drug affected	*NSAIDs implicated*	*Effect*	*Clinical implications*
Aminoglycosides	All NSAIDs	Reduce renal function in susceptible individuals, thus reducing aminoglycoside clearance and increasing plasma concentration	Monitor plasma concentration and adjust dose
Chlorpropamide and some other sulphonylureas	Aspirin ?other salicylates Fenclofenac	?Inhibits renal tubular excretion, increasing plasma concentration and hypoglycaemic effects	Reduce sulphonylurea dose if necessary
Ciclosporin	Diclofenac Mefenamic acid ?Sulindac	?Inhibit the renal prostacyclin synthesis needed to maintain glomerular filtration and renal blood flow. Increased and decreased ciclosporin plasma concentrations reported; increased risk of renal toxicity	Monitor renal function
Corticosteroids	Indometacin Naproxen	Displace corticosteroids from plasma protein-binding sites, increasing free corticosteroid levels and possibly therapeutic effect	Possible steroid-sparing effect; increased risk of GI bleeding
Digoxin	Most NSAIDs (except ketoprofen, meloxicam, piroxicam)	In heart failure, NSAIDs may precipitate renal failure, reducing digoxin excretion with increased risk of toxicity	In heart failure, avoid NSAIDs if possible; if not, check digoxin and creatinine plasma concentrations and reduce digoxin dose if necessary
Indometacin	Diflunisal	Inhibits glucuronidation, increasing indometacin plasma concentration (by about 50%) and risk of toxicity	Avoid combination
Lithium	All NSAIDs (?except salicylates; sulindac unpredictable)	?Inhibit renal excretion of lithium and increase plasma concentration with increased risk of severe toxicity	Halve dose of lithium and monitor lithium concentration

continued

Table 5.9 Continued

Drug affected	*NSAIDs implicated*	*Effect*	*Clinical implications*
Methotrexate	Salicylates All NSAIDs	Competitively inhibit the tubular excretion of methotrexate. Inhibit PGE_2 synthesis, reducing renal perfusion. Increase methotrexate plasma concentration with risk of severe toxicity	Avoid aspirin and other salicylates during chemotherapy; probably safe between pulses. Use other NSAIDs with caution. Much lower risk with low-dose chronic methotrexate therapy used in psoriasis or rheumatoid arthritis and if no pre-existing renal impairment
Phenytoin	?All NSAIDs	Displace phenytoin from plasma proteins. May inhibit liver enzymes responsible for phenytoin metabolism	Clinical significance uncertain because the excess free phenytoin may be metabolized by the liver. However, phenytoin toxicity can develop even when the plasma concentration is still within the therapeutic range
Probenecid	Aspirin	High dose aspirin and other salicylates antagonize the uricosuric effects of probenecid by blocking the inhibitory effect on tubular reabsorption of uric acid. Aspirin excretion also reduced	Avoid high dose aspirin/salicylates in hyperuricaemia and gout
Valproate	Aspirin ?Other NSAIDS	Displace from plasma proteins, inhibit valproate metabolism and increase plasma concentration	Avoid aspirin. Significance of interaction with other NSAIDs unclear; reduce the dose of valproate if toxicity suspected.
Warfarin	?All NSAIDs	Potentially inhibit metabolism of warfarin and increase INR.	Isolated cases reported with most NSAIDs (including coxibs); check INR and reduce dose of warfarin if necessary
Zidovudine	Ibuprofen ?All NSAIDs	Increased haematological toxicity	Increased risk of bleeding seen in haemophiliacs treated with ibuprofen. Monitor blood count

Table 5.10 Pharmacokinetic interactions: other drugs affecting NSAIDs[151,153]

Drug implicated	*NSAIDs affected*	*Effect*	*Clinical implications*
Antacids	All e/c NSAIDs	Destruction of enteric coating	Administer at different times
Antacids	Aspirin	Decreased absorption and reduced plasma concentration	Use an alternative NSAID
Antacids	?All NSAIDs	Variable. Aluminium-containing antacids can *reduce* rate and/or extent of absorption of fenamates, diflunisal, indometacin and naproxen. Magnesium hydroxide alone can *increase* the absorption of ibuprofen and flurbiprofen but increases endoscopically-detected gastric toxicity of ibuprofen. Sodium bicarbonate *increases* naproxen absorption	Avoid aluminium-containing antacids. Adjust dose of NSAID if necessary
Barbiturates	?All NSAIDs	Increased metabolic clearance of NSAID	May need higher dose of NSAID
Ciclosporin	Diclofenac	Increased plasma concentration of diclofenac	Halve the dose of diclofenac
Colestyramine	Diclofenac Ibuprofen Naproxen ?Other NSAIDs	Anion exchange resin binds NSAIDs in the GI tract, reducing and/or delaying absorption	Separate administration by 4h; may need higher dose of NSAID
Colestyramine	Meloxicam Piroxicam Tenoxicam Sulindac	Binding in GI tract prevents enterohepatic recycling and increases faecal loss, even if NSAID administered IV	Increase NSAID dose if necessary or use alternative NSAID; colestyramine may be used to speed removal of NSAID after overdose
Fluconazole	Flurbiprofen Ibuprofen Celecoxib Parecoxib	Reduced metabolism and increased plasma concentration	Lower doses of flurbiprofen and ibuprofen may be necessary; halve the dose of celecoxib

continued

Table 5.10 Continued

Drug implicated	*NSAIDs affected*	*Effect*	*Clinical implications*
Ketoconazole	Etoricoxib Parecoxib	Reduced metabolism and increased plasma concentration; plasma concentration of active metabolite of parecoxib increased	Reduce dose of coxib if necessary
Metoclopramide	Aspirin	Increased rate of absorption of aspirin in patients with migraine	Can be used therapeutically to speed onset of action of aspirin
Metoclopramide	Ketoprofen ?Other poorly soluble NSAIDs	Reduced absorption, ?because faster gastric transit carries poorly soluble NSAIDs past their absorption site	Take NSAID 1–2h before metoclopramide
Probenecid	?All NSAIDs	Reduced metabolism and renal clearance of NSAIDs and glucuronide metabolite which are hydrolyzed back to parent drug; NSAIDs also reduce the uricosuric effect of probenecid	Increased toxicity seen with indometacin, particularly if renal function impaired. Consider a reduction in the dose of NSAID but could be used therapeutically to increase the response
Rifampicin	Diclofenac Etoricoxib	Plasma concentration reduced because of CYP3A4 induction	Increase NSAID dose if pain returns or consider alternative
Ritonavir	Piroxicam ?Other NSAIDs	Increased plasma concentration with increased risk of toxicity	Manufacturer advises avoid concurrent use
Voriconazole	Diclofenac Ibuprofen	Increased plasma concentration and decreased clearance of NSAID	Lower doses of diclofenac and ibuprofen may be necessary

- **diclofenac** (≤150mg/24h) carries a relatively low GI risk but a higher risk of stroke, cardiovascular death or death from any cause than most other NSAIDs. Its use in patients with cardiovascular risk factors should be discouraged (see p.315).

For gastroprotection, better tolerability in study populations favours the PPIs, although in terms of preventing serious GI events (ulceration, bleeding, perforation) the evidence is more robust for **misoprostol** 800microgram/24h (a large good quality RCT vs. epidemiological studies for PPIs; see p.25).[95] Further, in patients suffering from constipation, **misoprostol** could be a useful 'co-laxative'.

Celecoxib (see p.312) has a low risk of serious GI events and its cardiovascular risk appears to be no greater than non-selective NSAIDs (with the exception of naproxen). It is thus another contender for drug of first choice.

In addition, note:

- **celecoxib** (200mg/24h) + *PPI* is the best choice for patients at very high risk of major GI complications, e.g. recent bleed, and for whom the use of an NSAID is considered essential[95]
- in patients undergoing chemotherapy or with thrombocytopenia from other causes, use an NSAID which has little or no effect on bleeding time, e.g. **celecoxib**, **nabumetone** (see p.297); COX-2 inhibitors (coxibs) are probably safest in this situation because platelets express little or no COX-2
- SC **Ketorolac** + *PPI* is sometimes used in patients with severe nociceptive pain who fail to obtain good relief with other NSAIDs + a strong opioid (see p.323).

Patients with hypertension and with cardiac, hepatic or renal impairment may deteriorate, and should be monitored appropriately. As far as possible, all NSAIDs should be avoided in end-stage heart failure (see p.642).

Route of administration

Except for the relief of biliary and renal colic,[154] NSAIDs should generally be given PO in patients who can swallow. In patients who can no longer reliably take oral medication, SC **diclofenac** 150mg/24h can be given instead. Apart from **ketorolac**,[136,137] there is no evidence of greater efficacy by other routes.[155]

Alternatively, the rectal route can be used:

- **diclofenac** suppositories 50mg b.d.–t.d.s.
- **indometacin** suppositories 100mg up to b.d.

A further option is to switch to **paracetamol** suppositories (see p.287).

Piroxicam given as an orodispersible 20mg tablet (Feldene Melt®) once daily is another option. This dissolves rapidly and completely if placed on the tongue or in the mouth. However, absorption is GI, which means that Feldene Melt® tablets can be used only in patients who can swallow their saliva. However, in someone expected to die within 1–2 days, it is generally possible to discontinue the NSAID without provoking a resurgence of pain.

1 Mercadante S (2001) The use of anti-inflammatory drugs in cancer pain. *Cancer Treatment Reviews*. **27**: 51–61.

2 McNicol E *et al.* (2004) Nonsteroidal anti-inflammatory drugs, alone or combined with opioids, for cancer pain: a systematic review. *Journal of Clinical Oncology*. **22**: 1975–1992.

3 Jirarattanaphochai K and Jung S (2008) Nonsteroidal antiinflammatory drugs for postoperative pain management after lumbar spine surgery: a meta-analysis of randomized controlled trials. *Journal of Neurosurgery Spine*. **9**: 22–31.

4 Derry C *et al.* (2009) Single dose oral ibuprofen for acute postoperative pain in adults. *Cochrane Database of Systematic Reviews*. **3**: CD001548.

5 Roelofs PD *et al.* (2008) Non-steroidal anti-inflammatory drugs for low back pain. *Cochrane Database of Systematic Reviews*. CD000396.

6 Guindon J and Beaulieu P (2006) Antihyperalgesic effects of local injections of anandamide, ibuprofen, rofecoxib and their combinations in a model of neuropathic pain. *Neuropharmacology*. **50**: 814–823.

7 Burian M *et al.* (2003) Peripheral and central antihyperalgesic effects of diclofenac in a model of human inflammatory pain. *Clinical Pharmacology and Therapeutics*. **74**: 113–120.

8 Koppert W *et al.* (2004) The cyclooxygenase isozyme inhibitors parecoxib and paracetamol reduce central hyperalgesia in humans. *Pain*. **108**: 148–153.

9 Shah S and Hardy J (2001) Non-steroidal anti-inflammatory drugs in cancer pain: a review of the literature as relevant to palliative care. *Progress in Palliative Care*. **9**: 3–7.

10 Mercadante S *et al.* (2002) A randomised controlled study on the use of anti-inflammatory drugs in patients with cancer pain on morphine therapy: effects on dose-escalation and a pharmacoeconomic analysis. *European Journal of Cancer*. **38**: 1358–1363.

11 Vo T *et al.* (2009) Non-steroidal anti-inflammatory drugs for neuropathic pain: how do we explain continued widespread use? *Pain*. **143**: 169–171.

12 Simmons DL *et al.* (2000) Nonsteroidal anti-inflammatory drugs, acetaminophen, cyclooxygenase 2, and fever. *Clinical Infectious Diseases*. **31 (suppl 5)**: S211–218.

13 Burian M and Geisslinger G (2005) COX-dependent mechanisms involved in the antinociceptive action of NSAIDs at central and peripheral sites. *Pharmacology and Therepeutics*. **107**: 139–154.

14 Varas-Lorenzo C *et al.* (2007) Quantitative assessment of the gastrointestinal and cardiovascular risk–benefit of celecoxib compared to individual NSAIDs at the population level. *Pharmacoepidemiology and Drug Safety*. **16**: 366–376.

15 Turajane T *et al.* (2009) Gastrointestinal and cardiovascular risk of non-selective NSAIDs and COX-2 inhibitors in elderly patients with knee osteoarthritis. *Journal of the Medical Association of Thailand*. **92 (suppl 6)**: S19–26.

16 Tramer M *et al.* (2000) Quantitative estimation of rare adverse events which follow a biological progression: a new model applied to chronic NSAID use. *Pain*. **85**: 169–182.

17 Kearney PM *et al.* (2006) Do selective cyclo-oxygenase-2 inhibitors and traditional non-steroidal anti-inflammatory drugs increase the risk of atherothrombosis? Meta-analysis of randomised trials. *British Medical Journal*. **332**: 1302–1308.

18 Simmons DL *et al.* (2004) Cyclooxygenase isozymes: the biology of prostaglandin synthesis and inhibition. *Pharmacological Reviews*. **56**: 387–437.

19 Kapoor M *et al.* (2005) Possible anti-inflammatory role of COX-2-derived prostaglandins: implications for inflammation research. *Current Opinion in Investigational Drugs*. **6**: 461–466.

20 Gerstenfeld LC and Einhorn TA (2004) COX inhibitors and their effects on bone healing. *Expert Opinion on Drug Safety*. **3**: 131–136.

21 Peskar BM (2005) Role of cyclooxygenase isoforms in gastric mucosal defense and ulcer healing. *Inflammopharmacology*. **13**: 15–26.

22 Chandrasekharan N *et al.* (2002) COX-3, a cyclooxygenase-1 variant inhibited by acetaminophen and other analgesic/antipyretic drugs: cloning, structure, and expression. *Proceedings of the National Academy of Sciences of the United States of America*. **99**: 13926–13931.

23 Kis B *et al.* (2005) Acetaminophen and the cyclooxygenase-3 puzzle: sorting out facts, fictions, and uncertainties. *Journal of Pharmacology and Experimental Therapeutics*. **315**: 1–7.

24 Qin N *et al.* (2005) Cloning, expression, and functional characterization of human cyclooxygenase-1 splicing variants: evidence for intron 1 retention. *Journal of Pharmacology and Experimental Therapeutics*. **315**: 1298–1305.

25 Schwab JM and Schluesener HJ (2003) Cyclooxygenases and central nervous system inflammation: conceptual neglect of cyclooxygenase 1. *Archives of Neurology*. **60**: 630–632.

26 Baba H *et al.* (2001) Direct activation of rat spinal dorsal horn neurons by prostaglandin E2. *Journal of Neuroscience*. **21**: 1750–1756.

27 Samad T *et al.* (2001) Interleukin-1B-mediated induction of COX-2 in the CNS contributes to inflammatory pain hypersensitivity. *Nature*. **410**: 471–475.

28 Farooqui M *et al.* (2007) COX-2 inhibitor celecoxib prevents chronic morphine-induced promotion of angiogenesis, tumour growth, metastasis and mortality, without compromising analgesia. *British Journal of Cancer*. **97**: 1523–1531.

29 Jain NK *et al.* (2008) COX-2 expression and function in the hyperalgesic response to paw inflammation in mice. *Prostaglandins Leukot Essent Fatty Acids*. **79**: 183–190.

30 Telleria-Diaz A *et al.* (2010) Spinal antinociceptive effects of cyclooxygenase inhibition during inflammation: Involvement of prostaglandins and endocannabinoids. *Pain*. **148**: 26–35.

31 Churchill L *et al.* (1996) Selective inhibition of human cyclo-oxygenase-2 by meloxicam. *Inflammopharmacology*. **4**: 125–135.

32 Brooks P *et al.* (1999) Interpreting the clinical significance of the differential inhibition of cyclooxygenase-1 and cyclooxygenase-2. *Rheumatology*. **38**: 779–788.

33 Warner T *et al.* (1999) Nonsteroidal drug selectivities for cyclo-oxygenase-1 rather than cyclo-oxygenase 2 are associated with human gastrointestinal toxicity: a full in vitro analysis. *Proceedings of the National Academy of Science USA*. **96**: 7563–7568.

34 Riendeau D *et al.* (2001) Etoricoxib (MK-0663). Preclinical profile and comparison with other agents that selectively inhibit cyclooxygenase-2. *Journal of Pharmacology and Experimental Therapeutics*. **296**: 558–566.

35 Blain H *et al.* (2002) Limitation of the in vitro whole blood assay for predicting the COX selectivity of NSAIDs in clinical use. *British Journal of Clinical Pharmacology*. **53**: 255–265.

36 Fries S *et al.* (2006) Marked interindividual variability in the response to selective inhibitors of cyclooxygenase-2. *Gastroenterology*. **130**: 55–64.

37 Capone ML *et al.* (2007) Pharmacodynamic of cyclooxygenase inhibitors in humans. *Prostaglandins Other Lipid Mediat*. **82**: 85–94.

38 vanHecken A *et al.* (2000) Comparative inhibitory activity of rofecoxib, meloxicam, diclofenac, ibuprofen and naproxen on COX-2 versus COX-1 in healthy volunteers. *Journal of Clinical Pharmacology*. **40**: 1109–1120.

39 deMeijer A *et al.* (1999) Meloxicam, 15mg/day, spares platelet function in healthy volunteers. *Clinical Pharmacology and Therapeutics*. **66**: 425–430.

40 Hamza M and Dionne RA (2009) Mechanisms of non-opioid analgesics beyond cyclooxygenase enzyme inhibition. *Current Molecular Pharmacology*. **2**: 1–14.

41 McCormack K and Brune K (1991) Dissociation between the antinociceptive and anti-inflammatory effects of the nonsteroidal anti-inflammatory drugs: a survey of their analgesic efficacy. *Drugs*. **41**: 533–547.

42 Abramson S *et al.* (1991) Non-steroidal anti-inflammatory drugs: effects on a GTP binding protein within the neutrophil plasma membrane. *Biochemical Pharmacology*. **41**: 1567–1573.

43 McCormack K (1994) Nonsteroidal anti-inflammatory drugs and spinal nociceptive processing. *Pain*. **59**: 9–43.

44 Svensson CI and Yaksh TL (2002) The spinal phospholipase-cyclooxygenase-prostanoid cascade in nociceptive processing. *Annual Review of Pharmacology and Toxicology*. **42**: 553–583.

45 Miranda HF *et al.* (2001) An isobolographic analysis of the adrenergic modulation of diclofenac antinociception. *Anesthesia and Analgesia*. **93**: 430–435.

46 Vandivier RW *et al.* (1999) Down-regulation of nitric oxide production by ibuprofen in human volunteers. *Journal of Pharmacology and Experimental Therapeutics*. **289**: 1398–1403.

47 Schwieler L *et al.* (2005) Prostaglandin-mediated control of rat brain kynurenic acid synthesis — opposite actions by COX-1 and COX-2 isoforms. *Journal of Neural Transmission*. **112**: 863–872.

48 Peretz A *et al.* (2005) Meclofenamic acid and diclofenac, novel templates of KCNQ2/Q3 potassium channel openers, depress cortical neuron activity and exhibit anticonvulsant properties. *Molecular Pharmacology*. **67**: 1053–1066.

49 McCormack K and Twycross RG (2001) Are COX-2 selective inhibitors effective analgesics. *Pain Review*. **8**: 13–26.

50 Dougados M *et al.* (2001) Evaluation of the structure-modifying effects of diacerein in hip osteoarthritis: ECHODIAH, a three-year, placebo-controlled trial. Evaluation of the Chondromodulating Effect of Diacerein in OA of the Hip. *Arthritis and Rheumatism*. **44**: 2539–2547.

51 Kathula SK *et al.* (2003) Cyclo-oxygenase II inhibitors in the treatment of neoplastic fever. *Supportive Care in Cancer.* **11**: 258–259.

52 Tsavaris N *et al.* (1990) A randomized trial of the effect of three nonsteroidal anti-inflammatory agents in ameliorating cancer-induced fever. *Journal of Internal Medicine*. **228**: 451–455.

53 Mercadante S (1998) Hyoscine in opioid-induced sweating. *Journal of Pain and Symptom Management.* **15**: 214–215.

54 Pittelkow M and Loprinzi C (2003) Pruritus and sweating in palliative medicine. In: D Doyle *et al.* (eds) *Oxford Textbook of Palliative Medicine* (3e). Oxford University Press, Oxford, pp. 573–587.

55 Zylicz Z and Krajnik M (2003) Flushing and sweating in an advanced breast cancer patient relieved by olanzapine. *Journal of Pain and Symptom Management.* **25**: 494–495.

56 Calder K and Bruera E (2000) Thalidomide for night sweats in patients with advanced cancer. *Palliative Medicine.* **14**: 77–78.

57 Deaner P (2000) The use of thalidomide in the management of severe sweating in patients with advanced malignancy: trial report. *Palliative Medicine.* **14**: 429–431.

58 Ng KF *et al.* (2008) Comprehensive preoperative evaluation of platelet function in total knee arthroplasty patients taking diclofenac. *Journal of Arthroplasty.* **23**: 424–430.

59 Guth B *et al.* (1996) Therapeutic doses of meloxicam do not inhibit platelet aggregation in man. *Rheumatology in Europe*. **25**: Abstract 443.

60 Cullen L *et al.* (1997) Selective suppression of cyclooxygenase-2 during chronic administration of nimesulide in man. In: *Fourth International Congress on essential fatty acids and eicosanoids*; Edinburgh.

61 Clemett D and Goa K (2000) Celecoxib: a review of its use in osteoarthritis, rheumatoid arthritis and acute pain. *Drugs*. **59**: 957–980.

62 Rawlins M (1997) Non-opioid analgesics. In: D Doyle *et al.* (eds) *Oxford Textbook of Palliative Medicine* (2e). Oxford University Press, Oxford, pp. 355–361.

63 Rossert J (2001) Drug-induced acute interstitial nephritis. *Kidney International*. **60**: 804–817.

64 MCA/CSM (2002) Non-steroidal anti-inflammatory drugs (NSAIDS) and gastrointestinal (G) safety. *Current Problems in Pharmacovigilance*. **28**: 5–6.

65 Fries J *et al.* (1991) Nonsteroidal anti-inflammatory drug-associated gastropathy: incidence and risk factor models. *American Journal of Medicine*. **91**: 213–222.

66 Garcia Rodriguez LA and Hernandez-Diaz S (2004) Risk of uncomplicated peptic ulcer among users of aspirin and nonaspirin nonsteroidal antiinflammatory drugs. *American Journal of Epidemiology.* **159**: 23–31.

67 Hippisley-Cox J and Coupland C (2005) Risk of myocardial infarction in patients taking cyclo-oxygenase-2 inhibitors or conventional non-steroidal anti-inflammatory drugs: population based nested case-control analysis. *British Medical Journal.* **330**: 1366.

68 Lanza F *et al.* (1999) Specific inhibition of cyclooxygenase-2 with MK-0966 is associated with less gastroduodenal damage than either aspirin or ibuprofen. *Alimentary Pharmacology and Therapeutics.* **13**: 761–767.

69 Bombardier C *et al.* (2000) Comparison of upper gastrointestinal toxicity of rofecoxib and naproxen in patients with rheumatoid arthritis. *New England Journal of Medicine*. **343**: 1520–1528.

70 Deeks J *et al.* (2002) Efficacy, tolerability, and upper gastrointestinal safety of celecoxib for treatment of osteoarthritis and rheumatoid arthritis; systematic review of randomised controlled trials. *British Medical Journal.* **325**: 619–623.

71 Laine L *et al.* (2002) Upper gastrointestinal event risk with COX-2 inhibitors depended on known risk factors. *Gastroenterology.* **123**: 1006–1012.

72 Mamdani M *et al.* (2002) Observational study of upper gastrointestinal haemorrhage in elderly patients given selective cyclo-oxygenase-2 inhibitors or conventional non-steroidal anti-inflammatory drugs. *British Medical Journal.* **325**: 624–627.

73 Schnitzer TJ *et al.* (2004) Comparison of lumiracoxib with naproxen and ibuprofen in the Therapeutic Arthritis Research and Gastrointestinal Event Trial (TARGET), reduction in ulcer complications: randomised controlled trial. *Lancet*. **364**: 665–674.

74 Watson DJ *et al.* (2004) The upper gastrointestinal safety of rofecoxib vs. NSAIDs: an updated combined analysis. *Current Medical Research Opinion*. **20**: 1539–1548.

75 Ramey DR *et al.* (2005) The incidence of upper gastrointestinal adverse events in clinical trials of etoricoxib vs. non-selective NSAIDs: an updated combined analysis. *Current Medical Research Opinion*. **21**: 715–722.

76 Rainsford K (1999) Profile and mechanisms of gastrointestinal and other side effects of nonsteroidal anti-inflammatory drugs (NsAIDs). *American Journal of Medicine*. **107 (suppl 6A)**: 27s–36s.

77 Kulkarni SK and Singh VP (2008) Licofelone: the answer to unmet needs in osteoarthritis therapy? *Current Rheumatology Reports*. **10**: 43–48.

78 Raynauld JP *et al.* (2009) Protective effects of licofelone, a 5-lipoxygenase and cyclo-oxygenase inhibitor, versus naproxen on cartilage loss in knee osteoarthritis: a first multicentre clinical trial using quantitative MRI. *Annals of the Rheumatic Diseases.* **68**: 938–947.

79 Lohmander LS *et al.* (2005) A randomised, placebo controlled, comparative trial of the gastrointestinal safety and efficacy of AZD3582 versus naproxen in osteoarthritis. *Annals of the Rheumatic Diseases*. **64**: 449–456.

80 Lichtenberger LM *et al.* (2009) Association of phosphatidylcholine and NSAIDs as a novel strategy to reduce gastrointestinal toxicity. *Drugs Today (Barc)*. **45**: 877–890.

81 Papatheodoridis GV *et al.* (2006) Effects of Helicobacter pylori and nonsteroidal anti-inflammatory drugs on peptic ulcer disease: a systematic review. *Clinical Gastroenterology and Hepatology.* **4**: 130–142.

82 McCormack K (1989) Mathematical model for assessing risk of gastrointestinal reactions to NSAIDs. In: K Rainsford (ed) *Azapropazone — over two decades of clinical use*. Kluwer Academic Publishers, Boston, pp. 81–93.

83 Becker JC *et al.* (2004) Current approaches to prevent NSAID-induced gastropathy–COX selectivity and beyond. *British Journal of Clinical Pharmacology.* **58**: 587–600.

84 Sung JJ (2004) Should we eradicate Helicobacter pylori in non-steroidal anti-inflammatory drug users? *Alimentary Pharmacology and Therapeutics*. **20 (suppl 2)**: 65–70.

85 Chang CC *et al.* (2005) Eradication of Helicobacter pylori significantly reduced gastric damage in nonsteroidal anti-inflammatory drug-treated Mongolian gerbils. *World Journal of Gastroenterology.* **11**: 104–108.

86 Di Leo V *et al.* (2005) Effect of Helicobacter pylori and eradication therapy on gastrointestinal permeability. Implications for patients with seronegative spondyloarthritis. *Journal of Rheumatology.* **32**: 295–300.

87 Kiltz U *et al.* (2008) Use of NSAIDs and infection with Helicobacter pylori–what does the rheumatologist need to know? *Rheumatology (Oxford)*. **47**: 1342–1347.

88 Malfertheiner P *et al.* (2007) Current concepts in the management of Helicobacter pylori infection: the Maastricht III Consensus Report. *Gut.* **56**: 772–781.

89 Cheetham TC *et al.* (2009) Gastrointestinal safety of nonsteroidal antiinflammatory drugs and selective cyclooxygenase-2 inhibitors in patients on warfarin. *Annals of Pharmacotherapy.* **43**: 1765–1773.

90 Hawkins C and Hanks G (2000) The gastroduodenal toxicity of nonsteroidal anti-inflammatory drugs. A review of the literature. *Journal of Pain and Symptom Management.* **20**: 140–151.

91 Ross S *et al.* (1980) Inhibition of 5-hydroxytryptamine uptake in human platelets by antidepressant agents in vivo. *Psychopharmacology.* **67**: 1–7.

92 Loke YK *et al.* (2008) Meta-analysis: gastrointestinal bleeding due to interaction between selective serotonin uptake inhibitors and non-steroidal anti-inflammatory drugs. *Alimentary Pharmacology and Therapeutics.* **27**: 31–40.

93 Dall M *et al.* (2009) An association between selective serotonin reuptake inhibitor use and serious upper gastrointestinal bleeding. *Clinical Gastroenterology and Hepatology.* **7**: 1314–1321.

94 Hollander D (1994) Gastrointestinal complications of nonsteroidal anti-inflammatory drugs: prophylactic and therapeutic strategies. *American Journal of Medicine.* **96**: 274–281.

95 Rostom A *et al.* (2002) Prevention of NSAID-induced gastroduodenal ulcers. *Cochrane Database of Systematic Reviews.* **4**: CD002296.

96 Hooper L *et al.* (2004) The effectiveness of five strategies for the prevention of gastrointestinal toxicity induced by non-steroidal anti-inflammatory drugs: systematic review. *British Medical Journal.* **329**: 948.

97 Chan FK *et al.* (2007) Combination of a cyclo-oxygenase-2 inhibitor and a proton-pump inhibitor for prevention of recurrent ulcer bleeding in patients at very high risk: a double-blind, randomised trial. *Lancet.* **369**: 1621–1626.

98 Targownik LE *et al.* (2008) The relative efficacies of gastroprotective strategies in chronic users of nonsteroidal anti-inflammatory drugs. *Gastroenterology.* **134**: 937–944.

99 Helsper CW *et al.* (2009) Trends and determinants of adequate gastroprotection in patients chronically using NSAIDs. *Pharmacoepidemiology and Drug Safety.* **18**: 800–806.

100 Valkhoff VE *et al.* (2010) Time-trends in gastroprotection with nonsteroidal anti-inflammatory drugs (NSAIDs). *Alimentary Pharmacology and Therapeutics.* **31**: 1218–1228.

101 Leontiadis GI *et al.* (2007) Systematic reviews of the clinical effectiveness and cost-effectiveness of proton pump inhibitors in acute upper gastrointestinal bleeding. *Health Technology Assessment.* **11**: iii–iv, 1–164.

102 Bjarnason I and Takeuchi K (2009) Intestinal permeability in the pathogenesis of NSAID-induced enteropathy. *Journal of Gastroenterology.* **44 (suppl 19)**: 23–29.

103 Fortun PJ and Hawkey CJ (2007) Nonsteroidal antiinflammatory drugs and the small intestine. *Current Opinion in Gastroenterology.* **23**: 134–141.

104 Hawkey CJ (2006) NSAIDs, coxibs, and the intestine. *Journal of Cardiovascular Pharmacology.* **47 (suppl 1)**: S72–75.

105 Singh S *et al.* (2009) Do NSAIDs, antibiotics, infections, or stress trigger flares in IBD? *American Journal of Gastroenterology.* **104**: 1298–1313.

106 Fornai M *et al.* (2010) Emerging role of cyclooxygenase isoforms in the control of gastrointestinal neuromuscular functions. *Pharmacology and Therapeutics.* **125**: 62–78.

107 Ballinger A (2008) Adverse effects of nonsteroidal anti-inflammatory drugs on the colon. *Current Gastroenterology Reports.* **10**: 485–489.

108 White WB (2007) Cardiovascular risk, hypertension, and NSAIDs. *Current Pain and Headache Reports.* **11**: 428–435.

109 Huerta C *et al.* (2006) Non-steroidal anti-inflammatory drugs and risk of first hospital admission for heart failure in the general population. *Heart.* **92**: 1610–1615.

110 Gislason GH *et al.* (2009) Increased mortality and cardiovascular morbidity associated with use of nonsteroidal anti-inflammatory drugs in chronic heart failure. *Archives of Internal Medicine.* **169**: 141–149.

111 McGettigan P and Henry D (2006) Cardiovascular risk and inhibition of cyclooxygenase: a systematic review of the observational studies of selective and nonselective inhibitors of cyclooxygenase 2. *Journal of the American Medical Association.* **296**: 1633–1644.

112 Solomon DH *et al.* (2008) Subgroup analyses to determine cardiovascular risk associated with nonsteroidal antiinflammatory drugs and coxibs in specific patient groups. *Arthritis and Rheumatism.* **59**: 1097–1104.

113 Trelle S *et al.* (2011) Cardiovascular safety of non-steroidal anti-inflammatory drugs: network meta-analysis. *British Medical Journal.* **342**: c7086.

114 Joshi GP *et al.* (2007) Cardiovascular thromboembolic adverse effects associated with cyclooxygenase-2 selective inhibitors and nonselective antiinflammatory drugs. *Anesthesia and Analgesia.* **105**: 1793–1804.

115 Dajani EZ and Islam K (2008) Cardiovascular and gastrointestinal toxicity of selective cyclo-oxygenase-2 inhibitors in man. *Journal of Physiology and Pharmacology.* **59 (suppl 2)**: 117–133.

116 García Rodríguez LA *et al.* (2009) Risk of myocardial infarction persisting after discontinuation of non-steroidal anti-inflammatory drugs in the general population. *Journal of Thrombosis and Haemostasis.* **7**: 892–894.

117 Salvo F *et al.* (2009) NSAIDs discontinuation and myocardial infarction. *Journal of Thrombosis and Haemostasis.* **7**: 1600–1601.

118 Cunnington M *et al.* (2008) Risk of ischaemic cardiovascular events from selective cyclooxygenase-2 inhibitors in osteoarthritis. *Pharmacoepidemiology Drug Safety.* **17**: 601–608.

119 Gengo FM *et al.* (2008) Effects of ibuprofen on the magnitude and duration of aspirin's inhibition of platelet aggregation: clinical consequences in stroke prophylaxis. *Journal of Clinical Pharmacology.* **48**: 117–122.

120 Strand V (2007) Are COX-2 inhibitors preferable to non-selective non-steroidal anti-inflammatory drugs in patients with risk of cardiovascular events taking low-dose aspirin? *Lancet.* **370**: 2138–2151.

121 Silverstein FE *et al.* (2000) Gastrointestinal toxicity with celecoxib vs nonsteroidal anti-inflammatory drugs for osteoarthritis and rheumatoid arthritis: the CLASS study: A randomized controlled trial. Celecoxib Long-term Arthritis Safety Study. *Journal of the American Medical Association.* **284**: 1247–1255.

122 Lanas A *et al.* (2006) Risk of upper gastrointestinal ulcer bleeding associated with selective cyclo-oxygenase-2 inhibitors, traditional non-aspirin non-steroidal anti-inflammatory drugs, aspirin and combinations. *Gut.* **55**: 1731–1738.

123 Cheng HF and Harris RC (2004) Cyclooxygenases, the kidney, and hypertension. *Hypertension.* **43**: 525–530.

124 Griffin M *et al.* (2000) Nonsteroidal antiinflammatory drugs and acute renal failure in elderly persons. *American Journal of Epidemiology.* **151**: 488–496.

125 Huerta C *et al.* (2005) Nonsteroidal anti-inflammatory drugs and risk of ARF in the general population. *American Journal of Kidney Disease.* **45**: 531–539.

126 Perneger TV *et al.* (1994) Risk of kidney failure associated with the use of acetaminophen, aspirin, and nonsteroidal antiinflammatory drugs. *New England Journal of Medicine*. **331**: 1675–1679.
127 Schneider V *et al.* (2006) Association of selective and conventional nonsteroidal antiinflammatory drugs with acute renal failure: A population-based, nested case-control analysis. *American Journal of Epidemiology*. **164**: 881–889.
128 Venturini C *et al.* (1998) Nonsteroidal anti-inflammatory drug-induced renal failure: a brief review of the role of cyclooxygenase isoforms. *Current Opinion in Nephrology and Hypertension*. **7**: 79–82.
129 Harirforoosh S and Jamali F (2009) Renal adverse effects of nonsteroidal anti-inflammatory drugs. *Expert Opinion on Drug Safety*. **8**: 669–681.
130 Winearls C (1995) Acute myeloma kidney. *Kidney International*. **48**: 1347–1361.
131 Iggo N *et al.* (1997) The development of cast nephropathy in multiple myeloma. *QJM: monthly journal of the Association of Physicians*. **90**: 653–656.
132 Irish AB *et al.* (1997) Presentation and survival of patients with severe renal failure and myeloma. *QJM: monthly journal of the Association of Physicians*. **90**: 773–780.
133 Delco F *et al.* (2005) Dose adjustment in patients with liver disease. *Drug Safety*. **28**: 529–545.
134 North-Lewis P (ed) (2008) *Drugs and the Liver*. Pharmaceutical Press, London, pp. 178–187.
135 Jenkins C *et al.* (2004) Systematic review of prevalence of aspirin induced asthma and its implications for clinical practice. *British Medical Journal*. **328**: 434.
136 Thomsen SF *et al.* (2009) Regular use of non-steroidal anti-inflammatory drugs increases the risk of adult-onset asthma: a population-based follow-up study. *Clinical Respiratory Journal*. **3**: 82–84.
137 Kim SH *et al.* (2007) Association between polymorphisms in prostanoid receptor genes and aspirin-intolerant asthma. *Pharmacogenet Genomics*. **17**: 295–304.
138 Sanak M and Szczeklik A (2001) Leukotriene C4 synthase polymorphism and aspirin-induced asthma. *Journal of Allergy and Clinical Immunology*. **107**: 561–562.
139 Simon RA (2004) Adverse respiratory reactions to aspirin and nonsteroidal anti-inflammatory drugs. *Current Allergy and Asthma Reports*. **4**: 17–24.
140 Mastalerz L *et al.* (2008) Prostaglandin E2 systemic production in patients with asthma with and without aspirin hypersensitivity. *Thorax*. **63**: 27–34.
141 Taniguchi M *et al.* (2008) Hyperleukotrieneuria in patients with allergic and inflammatory disease. *Allergology International*. **57**: 313–320.
142 Settipane R *et al.* (1995) Prevalence of cross-sensitivity with acetaminophen in aspirin-sensitive asthmatic subjects. *Journal of Allergy and Clinical Immunology*. **96**: 480–485.
143 Dicpinigaitis P (2001) Effect of the cyclooxygenase-2 inhibitor celecoxib on bronchial responsiveness and cough reflex sensitivity in asthmatics. *Pulmonary Pharmacology and Therapeutics*. **14**: 93–97.
144 Kowalski ML and Makowska J (2006) Use of nonsteroidal anti-inflammatory drugs in patients with aspirin hypersensitivity: safety of cyclo-oxygenase-2 inhibitors. *Treatments in Respiratory Medicine*. **5**: 399–406.
145 Stevenson DD (2009) Aspirin sensitivity and desensitization for asthma and sinusitis. *Current Allergy and Asthma Reports*. **9**: 155–163.
146 Boursinos LA *et al.* (2009) Do steroids, conventional non-steroidal anti-inflammatory drugs and selective Cox-2 inhibitors adversely affect fracture healing? *Journal of Musculoskeletal Neuronal Interactions*. **9**: 44–52.
147 Pountos I *et al.* (2008) Pharmacological agents and impairment of fracture healing: what is the evidence? *Injury*. **39**: 384–394.
148 Vuolteenaho K *et al.* (2008) Non-steroidal anti-inflammatory drugs, cyclooxygenase-2 and the bone healing process. *Basic & Clinical Pharmacology and Toxicology*. **102**: 10–14.
149 Brown A *et al.* (2003) An interaction between warfarin and COX-2 inhibitors: two case studies. *The Pharmaceutical Journal*. **271**: 782.
150 Verrico M *et al.* (2003) Adverse drug events involving COX-2 inhibitors. *Annals of Pharmacotherapy*. **37**: 1203–1213.
151 Baxter K (2011) Stockley's Drug Interactions (online edition). Pharmaceutical Press, London. Available from: www.medicinescomplete.com
152 Patrignani P *et al.* (1997) Differential inhibition of human prostaglandin endoperoxide synthase-1 and -2 by nonsteroidal anti-inflammatory drugs. *Journal of Physiology and Pharmacology*. **48**: 623–631.
153 Tonkin A and Wing L (1988) Interactions of nonsteroidal anti-inflammatory drugs. In: P Brooks (ed) *Bailliere's Clinical Rheumatology Anti-rheumatic drugs* Vol 2. Bailliere Tindall, London, pp. 455–483.
154 Lundstam SOA *et al.* (1982) Prostaglandin-synthetase inhibition with diclofenac sodium in treatment of renal colic: comparison with use of a narcotic analgesic. *Lancet*. **1**: 1096–1097.
155 Tramer M *et al.* (1998) Comparing analgesic efficacy of non-steroidal anti-inflammatory drugs given by different routes in acute and chronic pain: a qualitative systematic review. *Acta Anaesthesiologica Scandinavica*. **42**: 71–79.

CELECOXIB — BNF 10.1.1

Class: Non-opioid analgesic, NSAID, selective COX-2 inhibitor.

Indications: Pain and inflammation in osteoarthritis, rheumatoid arthritis, and ankylosing spondylitis, †acute pain, †cancer pain.

Contra-indications: Hypersensitivity to **aspirin** or other NSAID (urticaria, rhinitis, asthma, angioedema), *hypersensitivity to sulphonamides*, active GI ulceration, severe heart failure, severe hepatic impairment, severe renal impairment (creatinine clearance <30 mL/min), deteriorating renal function, hyperkalaemia, inflammatory bowel disease.

Pharmacology

No significant COX-1 inhibition was observed in healthy volunteers on 400mg b.d.[1] Thus, despite its modest selectivity when tested *in vitro*,[2,3] celecoxib is correctly classified as a selective COX-2 inhibitor.[4]

Celecoxib is less lipophilic and is less bio-available than other coxibs. A high volume of distribution suggests widespread tissue binding. Non-COX-2 inhibitory properties may account for some of its activity; celecoxib inhibits endoplasmic reticulum Ca^{2+} ATPase[5] and inhibits phosphodiesterase-5 activity.[6] The capacity to interact with non-COX-2 targets may be enhanced by accumulation of celecoxib within cells.[7]

Celecoxib is as effective as non-selective NSAIDs in treating pain in rheumatoid arthritis[8,9] and osteoarthritis.[10,11] It is effective in postoperative pain[12] and dysmenorrhoea,[13] but not in renal colic.[14]. There is a lack of data relating to cancer pain. Unlike opioids, celecoxib failed to control pain in mice with bone tumours.[15,16]

In RCTs, discontinuation rates for adverse events were *not* significantly higher than placebo. Celecoxib produces significantly fewer GI symptoms and serious adverse events than non-selective NSAIDs.[11,17,18] The lower risk of peptic ulceration and bleeding is also borne out in extended studies, mostly ≥12 weeks.[18] Translated into clinical terms, compared with a non-selective NSAID, one less patient in 28 taking celecoxib will have a serious GI events (ulceration, bleeding, perforation), and one less in 17 will have a fall in haematocrit of 5% or more.

Celecoxib has no effect on platelet function in healthy volunteers.[19] Further, unlike **etoricoxib**, celecoxib does not cause new onset hypertension.[20,21] Company data suggest that a raised creatinine is equally likely with celecoxib as with other NSAIDs or placebo.[18]

A recent meta-analysis of RCTs showed that celecoxib causes no appreciable increase in myocardial infarction or stroke, but doubles the risk of cardiovascular death, with a more modest increase in the risk of death from any cause.[22] This suggests that, although it leads to fewer cardiovascular events, those which occur are more often fatal. However, the risk is low, and is in the mid-range of NSAIDs for cardiovascular death. The risk for all-type adverse cardiovascular events is dose and dose frequency related: it is highest with 400mg b.d., less with 200mg b.d, and least with 400mg once daily.[23]

Coxibs have been shown to have an anti-cancer effect in several situations.[24,25] The adjuvant use of celecoxib in chemotherapy is being investigated.[26–28] In mice, chronic administration of morphine stimulates angiogenesis, tumour growth, and metastasis and leads to earlier mortality; these effects are neutralized by the co-administration of celecoxib without compromising analgesia.[29] The relevance of these findings to clinical practice remains to be elucidated.

All things considered, the relative GI safety of celecoxib (compared with most non-selective NSAIDs) makes it a preferred NSAID (see p.303).

Bio-availability Not known in humans; 22–40% in dogs.[30]

Onset of action 60min.[31]

Time to peak plasma concentration 3h; high fat meals may delay peak by 1–2 hours; aluminium- and magnesium-containing antacids reduce peak concentration.

Plasma halflife 11h, celecoxib is eliminated almost entirely by hepatic excretion.

Duration of action 5h in single-dose post-dental extraction pain;[31] but given that recommended frequency of administration is once daily–b.d., presumably longer when given regularly.

Cautions

To minimize the potential for serious undesirable effects, use the lowest effective dose for the shortest treatment duration possible. Because they cause sodium and fluid retention, all NSAIDs can decrease the effect of diuretics, ACE inhibitors and antihypertensives. Use with caution in established ischaemic heart disease, peripheral arterial disease, cerebrovascular disease.

Drug interactions

Celecoxib may increase **lithium** levels leading to toxicity. **Fluconazole** significantly increases the plasma level and AUC of celecoxib.[32]

Because an increase in INR is occasionally seen when celecoxib and **warfarin** are taken concurrently, if celecoxib is prescribed for a patient already taking **warfarin**, monitor the INR weekly for 3–4 weeks and adjust the dose of **warfarin** if necessary.[32]

Undesirable effects

Also see NSAIDs, p.293.

Common (<10%, >1%): abdominal pain, diarrhoea, dyspepsia, flatulence (but all comparable to or less than other NSAIDs), pharyngitis, rhinitis, allergy, pruritus, insomnia, dizziness, hypertonia, rash, flu-like symptoms, peripheral oedema, fluid retention.

Dose and use

- start with 100mg b.d. or 200mg once daily
- if necessary, increase to 200mg b.d.

Supply

Celebrex® (Pharmacia)

Capsules 100mg, 200mg, 28 days @ 200mg daily = £20.

1 Fries S *et al.* (2006) Marked interindividual variability in the response to selective inhibitors of cyclooxygenase-2. *Gastroenterology.* **130**: 55–64.

2 Warner TD and Mitchell JA (2008) COX-2 selectivity alone does not define the cardiovascular risks associated with non-steroidal anti-inflammatory drugs. *Lancet.* **371**: 270–273.

3 Riendeau D *et al.* (2001) Etoricoxib (MK-0663): Preclinical profile and comparison with other agents that selectively inhibit cyclooxygenase-2. *Journal of Pharmacology and Experimental Therapeutics.* **296**: 558–566.

4 Schwartz JI *et al.* (2008) Comparative inhibitory activity of etoricoxib, celecoxib, and diclofenac on COX-2 versus COX-1 in healthy subjects. *Journal of Clinical Pharmacology.* **48**: 745–754.

5 Alloza I *et al.* (2006) Celecoxib inhibits interleukin-12 alphabeta and beta2 folding and secretion by a novel COX2-independent mechanism involving chaperones of the endoplasmic reticulum. *Molecular Pharmacology.* **69**: 1579–1587.

6 Klein T *et al.* (2007) Celecoxib dilates guinea-pig coronaries and rat aortic rings and amplifies NO/cGMP signaling by PDE5 inhibition. *Cardiovascular Research.* **75**: 390–397.

7 Maier TJ *et al.* (2009) Cellular membranes function as a storage compartment for celecoxib. *Journal of Molecular Medicine.* **87**: 981–993.

8 Emery P *et al.* (1999) Celecoxib versus diclofenac in long-term management of rheumatoid arthritis: randomised double-blind comparison. *Lancet.* **354**: 2106–2111.

9 Simon LS *et al.* (1999) Anti-inflammatory and upper gastrointestinal effects of celecoxib in rheumatoid arthritis: a randomized controlled trial. *Journal of the American Medical Association.* **282**: 1921–1928.

10 Bensen WG *et al.* (1999) Treatment of osteoarthritis with celecoxib, a cyclooxygenase-2 inhibitor: a randomized controlled trial. *Mayo Clinic Proceedings.* **74**: 1095–1105.

11 Chen YF *et al.* (2008) Cyclooxygenase-2 selective non-steroidal anti-inflammatory drugs (etodolac, meloxicam, celecoxib, rofecoxib, etoricoxib, valdecoxib and lumiracoxib) for osteoarthritis and rheumatoid arthritis: a systematic review and economic evaluation. *Health Technology Assessment.* **12**: 1–278, iii.

12 Derry S (2008) Single dose oral celecoxib for acute postoperative pain in adults. *Cochrane Database of Systematic Reviews.* **4**: CD004233.

13 Daniels S *et al.* (2009) Celecoxib in the treatment of primary dysmenorrhea: results from two randomized, double-blind, active- and placebo-controlled, crossover studies. *Clinical Therapeutics.* **31**: 1192–1208.

14 Phillips E *et al.* (2009) Celecoxib in the management of acute renal colic: a randomized controlled clinical trial. *Urology.* **74**: 994–999.

15 Saito O *et al.* (2005) Analgesic effects of nonsteroidal antiinflammatory drugs, acetaminophen, and morphine in a mouse model of bone cancer pain. *Journal of Anesthesia.* **19**: 218–224.

16 Mouedden ME and Meert TF (2007) Pharmacological evaluation of opioid and non-opioid analgesics in a murine bone cancer model of pain. *Pharmacology, Biochemistry, and Behavior.* **86**: 458–467.

17 Niculescu L *et al.* (2009) Pooled analysis of GI tolerability of 21 randomized controlled trials of celecoxib and nonselective NSAIDs. *Current Medical Research Opinion.* **25**: 729–740.

18 Moore RA *et al.* (2005) Tolerability and adverse events in clinical trials of celecoxib in osteoarthritis and rheumatoid arthritis: systematic review and meta-analysis of information from company clinical trial reports. *Arthritis Research and Therapy.* **7**: R644–665.

19 Leese PT *et al.* (2000) Effects of celecoxib, a novel cyclooxygenase-2 inhibitor, on platelet function in healthy adults: a randomized, controlled trial. *Journal of Clinical Pharmacology.* **40**: 124–132.

20 Chan CC *et al.* (2009) Do COX-2 inhibitors raise blood pressure more than nonselective NSAIDs and placebo? An updated meta-analysis. *Journal of Hypertension.* **27**: 2332–2341.

21 Solomon DH *et al.* (2004) Relationship between COX-2 specific inhibitors and hypertension. *Hypertension.* **44**: 140–145.

22 Trelle S *et al.* (2011) Cardiovascular safety of non-steroidal anti-inflammatory drugs: network meta-analysis. *British Medical Journal.* **342**: c7086.

23 Solomon SD *et al.* (2008) Cardiovascular risk of celecoxib in 6 randomized placebo-controlled trials: the cross trial safety analysis. *Circulation.* **117**: 2104–2113.

24 Zhou R *et al.* (2010) Effect of celecoxib on proliferation, apoptosis, and survivin expression in human glioma cell line U251. *Chinese Journal of Cancer.* **29**: 294–299.

25 Fujimura T *et al.* (2007) Cyclooxygenase-2 (COX-2) in carcinogenesis and selective COX-2 inhibitors for chemoprevention in gastrointestinal cancers. *Journal of Gastrointestinal Cancer.* **38**: 78–82.

26 Lipton A *et al.* (2010) Phase II trial of gemcitabine, irinotecan, and celecoxib in patients with advanced pancreatic cancer. *Journal of Clinical Gastroenterology.* **44**: 286–288.

27 Debucquoy A *et al.* (2009) Double blind randomized phase II study with radiation+5-fluorouracil+/-celecoxib for resectable rectal cancer. *Radiotherapy and Oncology.* **93**: 273–278.
28 Schonthal AH *et al.* (2008) Celecoxib analogs that lack COX-2 inhibitory function: preclinical development of novel anticancer drugs. *Expert Opinion on Investigational Drugs.* **17**: 197–208.
29 Farooqui M *et al.* (2007) COX-2 inhibitor celecoxib prevents chronic morphine-induced promotion of angiogenesis, tumour growth, metastasis and mortality, without compromising analgesia. *British Journal of Cancer.* **97**: 1523–1531.
30 Paulson S *et al.* (2001) Pharmacokinetics of celecoxib after oral administration in dogs and humans: effects of food and site absorption. *Journal of Pharmacology and Experimental Therapeutics.* **297**: 638–645.
31 Malmstrom K *et al.* (1999) Comparison of rofecoxib and celecoxib, two cyclooxygenase-2 inhibitors, in postoperative dental pain: a randomised, placebo- and active-comparator-controlled clinical trial. *Clinical Therapeutics.* **21**: 1653–1663.
32 Baxter K (2011) Stockley's Drug Interactions (online edition). Pharmaceutical Press, London. Available from: www.medicinescomplete.com

DICLOFENAC SODIUM — BNF 10.1.1

Class: Non-opioid analgesic, NSAID, preferential COX-2 inhibitor.

Indications: Pain and inflammation in arthritic conditions and other musculoskeletal disorders, postoperative pain, †dysmenorrhoea, acute gout, †cancer pain, †neoplastic fever.

Contra-indications: Hypersensitivity to **aspirin** or other NSAID (urticaria, rhinitis, asthma, angioedema), active GI ulceration, cerebrovascular bleeding or other bleeding disorders, severe heart failure, active liver disease or severe hepatic impairment, severe renal impairment (creatinine clearance <30mL/min), deteriorating renal function, hyperkalaemia, systemic lupus erythematosus.
BNF advises not using IV diclofenac if plasma creatinine >160micromol/L.

Pharmacology

Diclofenac is a preferential COX-2 inhibitor (see Tables 5.2 and 5.3, p.295).[1–3] The analgesic effect of diclofenac has been shown in animals to be both peripheral and central.[4–6] In addition to inhibiting COX, diclofenac:
- activates the nitric oxide-cGMP nociceptive pathway[7]
- impacts on central nociception by increasing brain concentrations of kynurenic acid, an endogenous antagonist on the glycine recognition site of the NMDA-receptor-channel complex[8]
- facilitates inhibitory M-currents by opening potassium channels KCNQ2/3.[9,10]

It is possible that diclofenac is intrinsically more broad-spectrum in its central effects than other NSAIDs.[11]

It is a potent reversible inhibitor of platelet aggregation *in vitro*, but typical PO doses have no effect on bleeding time.[12] In contrast, IV diclofenac has a measurable effect on bleeding time, but most subjects remain within normal limits. However, with invasive procedures, bleeding time is a poor predictor of blood loss.[13] Using indicators which best correlate with peri-operative blood loss, diclofenac causes platelet dysfunction in about two thirds of healthy volunteers.[14]

About 10–15% of patients experience undesirable effects (mainly gastric intolerance).[15] These are generally mild and transient; diclofenac needs to be withdrawn in only 2%.[12] Age[16] and renal or hepatic impairment do not have any significant effect on plasma concentrations of diclofenac, although metabolite concentrations increase in severe renal impairment. The principal metabolite, hydroxydiclofenac, possesses little anti-inflammatory effect.

When used for >6 months in patients with osteo-arthritis and rheumatoid arthritis, diclofenac caused no more gastrotoxicity than **celecoxib**.[17,18] Over 18 months and with most patients also taking a PPI, diclofenac caused more upper GI ulceration than **etoricoxib**; but the frequency of *complicated* upper GI events (serious bleeding, perforation, obstruction) was similar.[19]

Despite some disagreement,[20,21] there is now a broad consensus that diclofenac carries a higher cardiovascular risk than non-selective NSAIDs.[22–24] This was confirmed by a recent meta-analysis which showed that, although not associated with an increased risk of myocardial infarction, it carries the second highest risk of stroke and cardiovascular death out of the seven NSAIDs reviewed, and the highest risk of death from any cause.[25]

Numerous observational (case-control or cohort) studies confirm that, in previously healthy individuals (including those with no risk factors,[26]) diclofenac carries a higher risk than non-selective COX-inhibitors,[27] and that the risk increases with increasing duration of use.[28] For those who have had a previous myocardial infarction, there is an increased risk of death or re-infarction.[29]

Severe local necrosis has been described anecdotally after IM and SC use.[30] Diclofenac is available as the *sodium* and *potassium* salts; diclofenac *potassium* is absorbed more quickly and peak plasma concentration is reached sooner.

Bio-availability 50% PO (both normal-release and m/r products); suppositories about 33%.

Onset of action 20–30min.

Time to peak plasma concentration diclofenac *sodium:* 2.5h e/c (fasting), 6h e/c (taken with food), ⩾4h m/r, 1h suppositories; diclofenac *potassium* PO 20–60min (not significantly affected by food).

Plasma halflife 1–2h.

Duration of action 8h.

Cautions

To minimize the potential for serious undesirable effects, use the lowest effective dose for the shortest treatment duration possible. Because they cause sodium and fluid retention, all NSAIDs can decrease the effect of diuretics, ACE inhibitors and antihypertensives.

The thromboprotective effect of **aspirin** for stroke is compromised in people taking a concurrent NSAID.[31,32] Thus, ideally, people on **aspirin** for thromboprotection should *not* take another NSAID of any type. However, if an NSAID is considered essential, stop the **aspirin** and prescribe **naproxen** b.d. (see p.300)

Drug interactions

Diclofenac is a substrate of CYP1A2, 3A4, 2B6, 2C8/9, 2C19 and 2D6, and inhibits CYP1A2, 2C8/9 and 2E1. It can increase the plasma concentrations of **digoxin**, **lithium**, **methotrexate**, and sulfonylureas (see Table 5.9, p.304 and Table 5.10, p.306).

Because an increase in INR is occasionally seen when diclofenac and **warfarin** are taken concurrently, if diclofenac is prescribed for a patient already taking **warfarin**, monitor the INR weekly for 3–4 weeks and adjust the dose of **warfarin** if necessary.[33]

Undesirable effects

Also see NSAIDs, p.293.

Common (<10%, >1%): headache, dizziness, oedema, indigestion, abdominal discomfort, nausea, constipation or diarrhoea, pruritus, rash, ecchymosis.

Dose and use

Typical regimens of diclofenac sodium are:

- 50mg PO b.d.–t.d.s.
- m/r 75mg PO b.d. or 100mg once daily
- 50mg PR b.d.–t.d.s.

Diclofenac *potassium* is also available (see Supply). It is theoretically a better alternative in patients already troubled by Na^+ and water retention. However, it is much more expensive.

Some patients obtain greater benefit from 200mg/24h with no immediately apparent increase in undesirable effects, e.g. m/r 100mg b.d. However, doses > 150mg/day are unlicensed and are associated with an increased cardiovascular risk (see Pharmacology).

Diclofenac is available as an injection and is used primarily to relieve biliary and renal colic (75mg IM p.r.n.).[34,35] If given by CSCI, it must be given via a separate syringe driver (or other delivery device) because it is incompatible with other drugs. A typical regimen is 75mg SC/IM stat and 150mg/day CSCI.

Supply

Diclofenac *sodium* (generic)
Tablets e/c 25mg, 50mg, 28 days @ 50mg t.d.s. = £1.50.
Suppositories 100mg, 10 = £4.50.

Voltarol® (Novartis)
Tablets e/c 25mg, 50mg, 28 days @ 50mg t.d.s. = £4.50.
Tablets dispersible 50mg, 28 days @ 50mg t.d.s. = £25.
Injection 25mg/mL, 3mL amp = £1.
Suppositories 12.5mg, 25mg, 50mg, 100mg; 50mg × 10 = £2; 100mg × 10 = £3.

Diclofenac *potassium* (generic)
Tablets 50mg, 28 days @50mg t.d.s. = £5.

Voltarol® Rapide (Novartis)
Tablets 25mg, 50mg, 28 days @ 50mg t.d.s. = £19.

Modified-release
Diclomax SR® (Galen)
Capsules m/r 75mg, 28 days @ 75mg b.d. = £11.

Diclomax Retard® (Galen)
Capsules m/r 100mg, 28 days @ 100mg once daily = £8.

Motifen® 75mg (Daiichi Sankyo)
Capsules e/c 75mg, 28 days @ 75mg b.d. = £8.

Voltarol® 75mg SR (Novartis)
Tablets m/r 75mg, 28 days @ 75mg b.d. = £13.
Voltarol® Retard (Novartis)
Tablets m/r 100mg, 28 days @ 100mg once daily = £10.

With **misoprostol**
Arthrotec® 50 (Pharmacia)
Tablets e/c diclofenac *sodium* 50mg + **misoprostol** 200microgram, 28 days @ 1 t.d.s. = £17.

Arthrotec® 75 (Pfizer)
Tablets EC diclofenac *sodium* 75mg + **misoprostol** 200microgram, 28 days @ 1 b.d. = £15.

Topical
Voltarol Emulgel® (Novartis)
Gel containing diclofenac *diethylammonium* 1.16% (equivalent to diclofenac sodium 1%), 100g = £7.
Voltarol Gel Patch® (Novartis)
Topical patch containing diclofenac *epolamine* (equivalent to 140mg diclofenac sodium per patch) Adults aged >15 years 1 patch for up to 3 days; 10 patches = £14.

1 John V (1979) The pharmacokinetics and metabolism of diclofenac sodium (Voltarol) in animals and man. *Rheumatology and Rehabilitation* **(suppl 2)**: 22–37.
2 Patrignani P *et al.* (1997) Differential inhibition of human prostaglandin endoperoxide synthase-1 and -2 by nonsteroidal anti-inflammatory drugs. *Journal of Physiology and Pharmacology.* **48**: 623–631.
3 Schwartz JI *et al.* (2008) Comparative inhibitory activity of etoricoxib, celecoxib, and diclofenac on COX-2 versus COX-1 in healthy subjects. *Journal of Clinical Pharmacology.* **48**: 745–754.
4 McCormack K (1994) Nonsteroidal anti-inflammatory drugs and spinal nociceptive processing. *Pain.* **59**: 9–43.
5 Svensson CI and Yaksh TL (2002) The spinal phospholipase-cyclooxygenase-prostanoid cascade in nociceptive processing. *Annual Review of Pharmacology and Toxicology.* **42**: 553–583.
6 Ortiz MI *et al.* (2008) Additive interaction between peripheral and central mechanisms involved in the antinociceptive effect of diclofenac in the formalin test in rats. *Pharmacology, Biochemistry and Behavior.* **91**: 32–37.
7 Ortiz MI *et al.* (2003) The NO-cGMP-K+ channel pathway participates in the antinociceptive effect of diclofenac, but not of indomethacin. *Pharmacology, Biochemistry and Behavior.* **76**: 187–195.
8 Schwieler L *et al.* (2005) Prostaglandin-mediated control of rat brain kynurenic acid synthesis — opposite actions by COX-1 and COX-2 isoforms. *Journal of Neural Transmission.* **112**: 863–872.
9 Peretz A *et al.* (2005) Meclofenamic acid and diclofenac, novel templates of KCNQ2/Q3 potassium channel openers, depress cortical neuron activity and exhibit anticonvulsant properties. *Molecular Pharmacology.* **67**: 1053–1066.
10 Gan TJ (2010) Diclofenac: an update on its mechanism of action and safety profile. *Current Medical Research Opinion.* **26**: 1715–1731.
11 McCormack K and Twycross RG (2001) Are COX-2 selective inhibitors effective analgesics. *Pain Review.* **8**: 13–26.
12 Todd P and Sorkin E (1988) Diclofenac sodium: a reappraisal of its pharmacodynamic and pharmacokinetic properties, and therapeutic efficacy. *Drugs.* **35**: 244–285.

13 Peterson P *et al.* (1998) The preoperative bleeding time test lacks clinical benefit: College of American Pathologists' and American Society of Clinical Pathologists' position article. *Archives of Surgery.* **133**: 134–139.
14 Ng KF *et al.* (2008) Comprehensive preoperative evaluation of platelet function in total knee arthroplasty patients taking diclofenac. *Journal of Arthroplasty.* **23**: 424–430.
15 Medsafe (2010) New Zealand Medicines and Medical Devices Safety Authority. Available from: www.medsafe.govt.nz/profs/datasheet/d/diclaxtab.htm
16 Willis JV and Kendall MJ (1978) Pharmacokinetic studies on diclofenac sodium in young and old volunteers. *Scandinavian Journal of Rheumatology.* (**suppl**): 36–41.
17 Bombardier C (2002) An evidence-based evaluation of the gastrointestinal safety of coxibs. *American Journal of Cardiology.* **89 (suppl 6)**: 3d–9d.
18 Juni P *et al.* (2002) Risk of myocardial infarction associated with selective COX-2 inhibitors: questions remain. *Archives of Internal Medicine.* **162**: 2639–2640.
19 Laine L *et al.* (2007) Assessment of upper gastrointestinal safety of etoricoxib and diclofenac in patients with osteoarthritis and rheumatoid arthritis in the Multinational Etoricoxib and Diclofenac Arthritis Long-term (MEDAL) programme: a randomised comparison. *Lancet.* **369**: 465–473.
20 Helin-Salmivaara A *et al.* (2006) NSAID use and the risk of hospitalization for first myocardial infarction in the general population: a nationwide case-control study from Finland. *European Heart Journal.* **27**: 1657–1663.
21 Gudbjornsson B *et al.* (2010) Rofecoxib, but not celecoxib, increases the risk of thromboembolic cardiovascular events in young adults-a nationwide registry-based study. *European Journal of Clinical Pharmacology.* **66**: 619–625.
22 Kearney PM *et al.* (2006) Do selective cyclo-oxygenase-2 inhibitors and traditional non-steroidal anti-inflammatory drugs increase the risk of atherothrombosis? Meta-analysis of randomised trials. *British Medical Journal.* **332**: 1302–1308.
23 Krotz F and Struthmann L (2010) A Review on the risk of myocardial infarction associated with the NSAID diclofenac. *Cardiovascascular and Hematological Disorders Drug Targets.* **10**: 53–65.
24 Fosbol EL *et al.* (2010) Cardiovascular safety of non-steroidal anti-inflammatory drugs among healthy individuals. *Expert Opinion on Drug Safety.* **9**: 893–903.
25 Trelle S *et al.* (2011) Cardiovascular safety of non-steroidal anti-inflammatory drugs: network meta-analysis. *British Medical Journal.* **342**: c7086.
26 Jick H *et al.* (2006) Nonsteroidal antiinflammatory drugs and acute myocardial infarction in patients with no major risk factors. *Pharmacotherapy.* **26**: 1379–1387.
27 Fosbol EL *et al.* (2009) Risk of myocardial infarction and death associated with the use of nonsteroidal anti-inflammatory drugs (NSAIDs) among healthy individuals: a nationwide cohort study. *Clinical Pharmacology and Therapeutics.* **85**: 190–197.
28 Jick SS *et al.* (2007) Diclofenac and acute myocardial infarction in patients with no major risk factors. *British Journal of Clinical Pharmacology.* **64**: 662–667.
29 Gislason GH *et al.* (2006) Risk of death or reinfarction associated with the use of selective cyclooxygenase-2 inhibitors and nonselective nonsteroidal antiinflammatory drugs after acute myocardial infarction. *Circulation.* **113**: 2906–2913.
30 Kirkpatrick G (2003) SC diclofenac. In: *Bulletin board discussion.* Palliativedrugs.com. Available from: www.palliativedrugs.org/forum/read.php?f=1&i=3710&t=3710
31 Gengo FM *et al.* (2008) Effects of ibuprofen on the magnitude and duration of aspirin's inhibition of platelet aggregation: clinical consequences in stroke prophylaxis. *Journal of Clinical Pharmacology.* **48**: 117–122.
32 Gladding PA *et al.* (2008) The antiplatelet effect of six non-steroidal anti-inflammatory drugs and their pharmacodynamic interaction with aspirin in healthy volunteers. *American Journal of Cardiology.* **101**: 1060–1063.
33 Baxter K (2011) Stockley's Drug Interactions (online edition). Pharmaceutical Press, London. Available from: www.medicinescomplete.com
34 Lundstam SOA *et al.* (1982) Prostaglandin-synthetase inhibition with diclofenac sodium in treatment of renal colic: comparison with use of a narcotic analgesic. *Lancet.* **1**: 1096–1097.
35 Thompson JF *et al.* (1989) Rectal diclofenac compared with pethidine injection in acute renal colic. *British Medical Journal.* **299**: 1140–1141.

FLURBIPROFEN — BNF 10.1.1

Class: Non-opioid analgesic, NSAID, preferential COX-1 inhibitor.

Indications: Pain and inflammation in arthritic conditions, musculoskeletal disorders and trauma, dental pain, dysmenorrhoea, migraine, postoperative analgesia, sore throat (lozenges, see p.574), †cancer pain, †neoplastic fever, †detrusor instability.[1]

Contra-indications: Hypersensitivity to **aspirin** or other NSAID (urticaria, rhinitis, asthma, angioedema), active GI ulceration, cerebrovascular bleeding or other bleeding disorders, severe heart failure, active liver disease or severe hepatic impairment, severe renal impairment (creatinine clearance <30mL/min), deteriorating renal function, hyperkalaemia, systemic lupus erythematosus.

Pharmacology

Flurbiprofen is a propionic acid derivative and a highly potent COX inhibitor. It inhibits both COX-1 and COX-2 but, along with **indometacin**, **ketoprofen** and **ketorolac**, has higher COX-1 selectivity than many NSAIDs.[2] The molar potency for 50% inhibition of PGE_2 synthesis *in* *vitro* is >5,000 times that of **aspirin**, 250 times that of **ibuprofen**, and 125 times that of **naproxen**.[3] In animals, mg for mg, it is 8–20 times more potent than **aspirin**. Flurbiprofen is excreted in the urine both as unchanged drug and several hydroxylated metabolites.

Flurbiprofen has been used for many years by some palliative care services as the NSAID of choice (without routine gastroprotection). It is convenient to use and apparently highly effective. However, flurbiprofen does not feature in any of the recent surveys and meta-analyses, and it is in danger of becoming a forgotten drug even though there are no specific adverse data to justify its exclusion.

In addition to its analgesic use, flurbiprofen has been used to relieve frequency caused by instability of the detrusor muscle of the bladder. Animal studies show that PGs are produced by the detrusor (bladder muscle) and that they increase tone and bladder contractile activity. In humans, frequency, urgency, and urge incontinence are all significantly decreased by flurbiprofen 50mg t.d.s.[1]

Bio-availability (85% PO.
Onset of action 30–60min.
Time to peak plasma concentration 1–2h PO; 4–6h m/r.
Plasma halflife 3–6h.
Duration of action 8–16h.[4]

Cautions

To minimize the potential for serious undesirable effects, use the lowest effective dose for the shortest treatment duration possible. Because they cause sodium and fluid retention, all NSAIDs can decrease the effect of diuretics, ACE inhibitors and antihypertensives.

The thromboprotective effect of **aspirin** for stroke is compromised in people taking a concurrent NSAID.[5,6] Thus, ideally, people on **aspirin** for thromboprotection should *not* take another NSAID of any type. However, if an NSAID is considered essential, stop the **aspirin** and prescribe **naproxen** b.d. (see p.300)

Drug interactions

Flurbiprofen is a substrate of, and also inhibits, CYP2C8/9. It can increase the plasma concentrations of **digoxin**, **lithium** and **methotrexate** (see Table 5.9, p.304 and Table 5.10, p.306).

Because an increase in INR is occasionally seen when flurbiprofen and **warfarin** are taken concurrently, if flurbiprofen is prescribed for a patient already taking **warfarin**, monitor the INR weekly for 3–4 weeks and adjust the dose of **warfarin** if necessary.[7]

Undesirable effects

Also see NSAIDs, p.293.
Common (<10%, >1%): headache, dizziness, oedema, indigestion, abdominal discomfort, nausea, constipation or diarrhoea, pruritus, rash, ecchymosis.

Dose and use

For cancer pain:
- start with 100mg b.d.
- if necessary, increase to 100mg t.d.s.
- in very elderly or debilitated, start with 50mg b.d.; if necessary, increase to normal adult dose (see above).

Supply

Flurbiprofen (generic)
Tablets 50mg, 100mg, 28 days @ 100mg b.d. = £16.

Froben® (Abbott)
Tablets 50mg, 100mg, 28 days @ 100mg b.d. = £10.

1 Cardozo L *et al.* (1980) Evaluation of flurbiprofen in detrusor instability. *British Medical Journal*. **280**: 281–282.
2 Uzan A (2005) The unexpected side effects of new nonsteroidal anti-inflammatory drugs. *Expert Opinion on Emerging Drugs*. **10**: 687–688.
3 Crook D *et al.* (1976) Effect of aspirin-like drug therapy. Prostaglandin synthetase activity from human rheumatoid synovial microsomes. *Annals of the Rheumatic Diseases*. **35**: 327–332.
4 Kowanko I *et al.* (1981) Circadian variations in the signs and symptoms of rheumatoid arthritis and in the therapeutic effectiveness of flurbiprofen at different times of day. *British Journal of Clinical Pharmacology*. **11**: 477–484.
5 Gengo FM *et al.* (2008) Effects of ibuprofen on the magnitude and duration of aspirin's inhibition of platelet aggregation: clinical consequences in stroke prophylaxis. *Journal of Clinical Pharmacology*. **48**: 117–122.
6 Gladding PA *et al.* (2008) The antiplatelet effect of six non-steroidal anti-inflammatory drugs and their pharmacodynamic interaction with aspirin in healthy volunteers. *American Journal of Cardiology*. **101**: 1060–1063.
7 Baxter K (2011) Stockley's Drug Interactions (online edition). Pharmaceutical Press, London. Available from: www.medicines-complete.com

IBUPROFEN — BNF 10.1.1

Class: Non-opioid analgesic, NSAID, non-selective COX inhibitor.

Indications: Pain and inflammation in arthritic conditions and other musculoskeletal disorders, postoperative pain, dental pain, dysmenorrhoea, headache, migraine, fever, †cancer pain.

Contra-indications: Hypersensitivity to **aspirin** or other NSAID (urticaria, rhinitis, asthma, angioedema), active GI ulceration, cerebrovascular bleeding or other bleeding disorders, severe heart failure, active liver disease or severe hepatic impairment, severe renal impairment (creatinine clearance <30mL/min), deteriorating renal function, hyperkalaemia, systemic lupus erythematosus.

Pharmacology

Ibuprofen is a non-selective COX inhibitor (see Tables 5.2 and 5.3, p.295). Like **flurbiprofen** and **naproxen**, it is a propionic acid derivative. The analgesic effect of ibuprofen is mediated by several non-COX mechanisms in addition to COX inhibition (see p.296).[1] Doses of 2,400mg/day are well tolerated by most patients. Ibuprofen is three times more potent than **aspirin**, i.e. 200mg is equivalent to 600mg of **aspirin**. Higher doses of ibuprofen have a greater analgesic effect than standard doses of **aspirin**.

Ibuprofen is a chiral NSAID, i.e. it is a mixture of roughly equal amounts of S and R enantiomers, mirror-image molecules which rotate polarized light in opposite directions.[2,3] The anti-inflammatory activity resides mostly in the S enantiomer, but about half the R enantiomer is converted to the S form in the GI tract and liver.[1] Thus, the clinical effects of the racemic mixture depend on absorption rate.[4]

Ibuprofen shares this property of enantiomeric inversion with similar NSAIDs, e.g. **ketoprofen**. This has led to the production of **dexibuprofen** and **dexketoprofen** (both licensed in the UK) which are pure S enantiomers and thus theoretically more potent mg for mg. The enantiomers are metabolized via CYP450. Age also affects the S enantiomer free drug concentrations and clearance; the S enantiomer reaches higher levels and persists for longer in the elderly.[5]

Inversion takes time, and the time frame for single doses in acute situations is too short for inversion to play an important part.[6] Even so, a single dose of ibuprofen for acute postoperative pain is highly effective, with an NNT of around 2.5 for 200–400mg PO.[7]

In arthritis, ibuprofen is concentrated at sites of inflammation, e.g. the joint synovium.[8] At low doses (200–400mg) it is as effective as **paracetamol** 1g, and efficacy increases as the dose increases.[9]

Although a non-selective COX inhibitor, *low dose* ibuprofen (i.e. ≤1,200mg/24h) has a low propensity for causing serious GI events (ulceration, bleeding, perforation),[10] and, in consequence, is available OTC. However, at doses >1,800mg/24h, ibuprofen is no safer than other non-selective NSAIDs;[11] and even at low doses it causes significantly more ulcers than **celecoxib**.[12] Further, a small RCT found that ibuprofen 2,400mg/24h+ **misoprostol** 800mg/24h is no safer than **nabumetone** alone.[13] Concern has been expressed about the possibility that OTC ibuprofen may occasionally cause small bowel damage.[14]

However, although the GI risk of low-dose ibuprofen is low, the cardiovascular risk is higher. In a recent meta-analysis the risk of stroke was increased >3 times compared with placebo (the highest risk of seven NSAIDs), and the risk of cardiovascular death was increased nearly two and half times, inferior only to the risk with **etoricoxib** and **diclofenac**.[15] The risk was seen with both low and high dose ibuprofen, is higher with long-term use and in association with coronary artery disease.

Ibuprofen is safe in overdose; only 10 deaths attributable to ibuprofen alone have been reported, e.g. involving overdoses of 36g and 105g.[16–19] It is certainly safer than two other commonly used antipyretic analgesics, **paracetamol** and **aspirin**.[1]

Ibuprofen can be used topically (as a locally prepared preparation), particularly for sprains, strains and arthritis.[20] Although application to the skin produces plasma concentrations which are only 5% of those obtained with oral administration, the underlying muscle and fascial concentrations are 25 times greater.[21,22] An RCT showed that patients with sprains and bruises treated with TD ibuprofen did significantly better in relation to speed of resolution, relief of pain, reduction in swelling and return of function.[23]

A Health Technology Assessment found that topical and PO ibuprofen were equally effective for chronic knee pain in patients aged ≥50 years, although those with more severe or widespread pain preferred PO treatment.[24] The incidence of major undesirable effects were similar, but topical treatment led to fewer minor undesirable effects and less treatment discontinuation. Based on the cost per quality-adjusted life-year, topical ibuprofen was more cost-effective over the first year, whereas PO treatment was more cost-effective over 2 years.[24] Systemic undesirable effects with topical ibuprofen for acute pain are uncommon, and even local effects were not significantly different from placebo.[25]

Bio-availability 90% PO.
Onset of action 20–30min.
Time to peak plasma concentration 1–2h.
Plasma halflife 2–3h.[1]
Duration of action 4–6h.

Cautions

To minimize the potential for serious undesirable effects, use the lowest effective dose for the shortest treatment duration possible. Because they cause sodium and fluid retention, all NSAIDs can decrease the effect of diuretics, ACE inhibitors and antihypertensives.

The thromboprotective effect of **aspirin** for stroke is compromised in people taking a concurrent NSAID.[26,27] Thus, ideally, people on **aspirin** for thromboprotection should *not* take another NSAID of any type. However, if an NSAID is considered essential, stop the **aspirin** and prescribe **naproxen** b.d. (see p.300)

Drug interactions

Ibuprofen is a substrate of CYP2C8/9 and 2C19, and inhibits CYP2C8/9. It can increase plasma concentrations of **digoxin**, **lithium** and **methotrexate** (see Table 5.9, p.304 and Table 5.10, p.306). Its plasma concentration may be reduced by analgesic doses of **aspirin**.

Because an increase in INR is occasionally seen when ibuprofen and **warfarin** are taken concurrently, if ibuprofen is prescribed for a patient already taking **warfarin**, monitor the INR weekly for 3–4 weeks, and adjust the dose of **warfarin** if necessary.[28]

Undesirable effects

Also see NSAIDs, p.293.
Common (<10%, >1%): headache, dizziness, oedema, indigestion, abdominal discomfort, nausea, constipation or diarrhoea, pruritus, rash, ecchymosis.

Dose and use

- start with 400mg t.d.s.
- if necessary, increase to 600–800mg t.d.s.

Supply

Ibuprofen tablets and capsules 200mg and 400mg, and ibuprofen suspension and gel are available OTC.

Ibuprofen (generic)
Tablets 200mg, 400mg, 600mg, 28 days @ 400mg t.d.s. = £2.
Oral suspension 100mg/5mL, 120mL bottle, 28 Days @400mg t.d.s. = £30.

Brufen® (Abbott)
Tablets 200mg, 400mg, 600mg, 28 days @ 400mg t.d.s. = £7.
Oral syrup 100mg/5mL, 28 days @ 400mg t.d.s. = £30.
Granules 600mg/sachet, 28 days @ 600mg b.d. = £18 *(contains 9mmol Na^+/sachet).*

Modified-release
Brufen Retard® (Abbott)
Tablets m/r 800mg, 28 days @1,600mg once daily. = £6.

Fenbid® (Goldshield)
Capsules enclosing m/r pellets 300mg, 28 days @ 600mg b.d. = £9.

Topical (generic)
Gel 5%, 100g = £6.

Fenbid® Forte Gel (Goldshield)
Gel 10%, 100g = £6.

Ibugel® Forte (Dermal)
Gel 10%, 100g = £6.

1 Rainsford KD (2009) Ibuprofen: pharmacology, efficacy and safety. *Inflammopharmacology*. **17**: 275–342.
2 Rudy AC *et al.* (1991) Stereoselective metabolism of ibuprofen in humans: administration of R-, S- and racemic ibuprofen. *Journal of Pharmacology and Experimental Therapeutics*. **259**: 1133–1139.
3 Jamali F *et al.* (1992) Human pharmacokinetics of ibuprofen enantiomers following different doses and formulations: intestinal chiral inversion. *Journal of Pharmaceutical Sciences*. **81**: 221–225.
4 Ding G *et al.* (2007) Effect of absorption rate on pharmacokinetics of ibuprofen in relation to chiral inversion in humans. *Journal of Pharmacy and Pharmacology*. **59**: 1509–1513.
5 Tan SC *et al.* (2003) Influence of age on the enantiomeric disposition of ibuprofen in healthy volunteers. *British Journal of Clinical Pharmacology*. **55**: 579–587.
6 Evans AM (2001) Comparative pharmacology of S(+)-ibuprofen and (RS)-ibuprofen. *Clinical Rheumatology*. **20 (suppl 1)**: S9–14.
7 Derry C *et al.* (2009) Single dose oral ibuprofen for acute postoperative pain in adults. *Cochrane Database of Systematic Reviews*. **3**: CD001548.
8 Glass RC and Swannell AJ (1978) Concentrations of ibuprofen in serum and synovial fluid from patients with arthritis [proceedings]. *British Journal of Clinical Pharmacology*. **6**: 453P–454P.
9 McQuay HJ and Moore RA (2007) Dose-response in direct comparisons of different doses of aspirin, ibuprofen and paracetamol (acetaminophen) in analgesic studies. *British Journal of Clinical Pharmacology*. **63**: 271–278.
10 Masso Gonzalez EL *et al.* (2010) Variability among nonsteroidal antiinflammatory drugs in risk of upper gastrointestinal bleeding. *Arthritis and Rheumatism*. **62**: 1592–1601.
11 Henry D and McGettigan P (2003) Epidemiology overview of gastrointestinal and renal toxicity of NSAIDs. *International Journal of Clinical Practice Supplement*. 43–49.
12 Scheiman JM *et al.* (2004) A randomized, controlled comparison of ibuprofen at the maximal over-the-counter dose compared with prescription-dose celecoxib on upper gastrointestinal mucosal injury. *Clinical Gastroenterology and Hepatology*. **2**: 290–295.
13 Roth SH *et al.* (1993) A controlled study comparing the effects of nabumetone, ibuprofen, and ibuprofen plus misoprostol on the upper gastrointestinal tract mucosa. *Archives of Internal Medicine*. **153**: 2565–2571.
14 Sidhu R *et al.* (2010) Undisclosed use of nonsteroidal anti-inflammatory drugs may underlie small-bowel injury observed by capsule endoscopy. *Clinical Gastroenterology and Hepatology*. **8**: 992–995.
15 Trelle S *et al.* (2011) Cardiovascular safety of non-steroidal anti-inflammatory drugs: network meta-analysis. *British Medical Journal*. **342**: c7086.
16 Wood DM *et al.* (2006) Fatality after deliberate ingestion of sustained-release ibuprofen: a case report. *Critical Care*. **10**: R44.
17 Krenova M and Pelclova D (2005) Fatal poisoning with ibuprofen. *Clinical Toxicology*. **43**: 537.
18 Volans G et al. (2003) Ibuprofen overdose. *International Journal of Clinical Practice Supplement*. 54–60.
19 Holubek W *et al.* (2007) A report of two deaths from massive ibuprofen ingestion. *Journal of Medical Toxicology*. **3**: 52–55.
20 Chlud K and Wagener H (1987) Percutaneous nonsteroidal anti-inflammatory drug (NSAID) therapy with particular reference to pharmacokinetic factors. *EULAR Bulletin*. **2**: 40–43.
21 Mondino A *et al.* (1983) Kinetic studies of ibuprofen on humans. Comparative study for the determination of blood concentrations and metabolites following local and oral administration. *Medizinische Welt*. **34**: 1052–1054.
22 Kageyama T (1987) A double blind placebo controlled multicenter study of piroxicam 0.5% gel in osteoarthritis of the knee. *European Journal of Rheumatology and Inflammation*. **8**: 114–115.
23 Peters H *et al.* (1987) Percutaneous kinetics of ibuprofen (German). *Aktuelle Rheumatologie*. **12**: 208–211.

24 Underwood M *et al.* (2008) Topical or oral ibuprofen for chronic knee pain in older people. The TOIB study. Available from: www.hta.ac.uk/project/1302.asp
25 Massey T *et al.* (2010) Topical NSAIDS for acute pain in adults. *Cochrane Database of Systematic Reviews.* **6**: CD007402.
26 Gengo FM *et al.* (2008) Effects of ibuprofen on the magnitude and duration of aspirin's inhibition of platelet aggregation: clinical consequences in stroke prophylaxis. *Journal of Clinical Pharmacology.* **48**: 117–122.
27 Gladding PA *et al.* (2008) The antiplatelet effect of six non-steroidal anti-inflammatory drugs and their pharmacodynamic interaction with aspirin in healthy volunteers. *American Journal of Cardiology.* **101**: 1060–1063.
28 Baxter K (ed) (2010) Stockley's Drug Interactions (online edition). The Pharmaceutical Press, London. Available from: www.medicinescomplete.com

*KETOROLAC TROMETAMOL — BNF 15.1.4.2

Class: Non-opioid analgesic, NSAID, preferential COX-1 inhibitor.

Indications: Short-term management of moderate–severe acute postoperative pain, †intractable nociceptive cancer pain.

Contra-indications: Hypersensitivity to **aspirin** or other NSAID (urticaria, rhinitis, asthma, angioedema), history of or active GI ulceration, cerebrovascular bleeding or other bleeding disorders, severe heart failure, severe hepatic impairment, renal impairment (creatinine >160micromol/L), deteriorating renal function, hyperkalaemia, systemic lupus erythematosus. Concurrent prescription with **warfarin**, **heparin**, **aspirin**, other NSAID, **pentoxifylline**, **lithium** and **probenecid**.

Pharmacology

Ketorolac is a cyclic propionate structurally related to the acetate NSAIDs, **tolmetin** and **indometacin**.[1,2] It inhibits both COX-1 and COX-2 but, along with **flurbiprofen**, **indometacin** and **ketoprofen**, has higher COX-1 selectivity than many NSAIDs.[3]

Ketorolac trometamol is more water-soluble than the parent substance. Over 99% of the oral dose is absorbed and about 75% of a dose is excreted in the urine within 7h, and over 90% within 2 days, over half as unmodified ketorolac.[4] The rest is excreted in the faeces. The analgesic and anti-inflammatory activity of ketorolac resides mainly in the S-enantiomer, which is cleared more rapidly than the less active R-enantiomer. The analgesic effect is far greater than the antipyretic and anti-inflammatory properties. In animal studies, ketorolac is about 350 times more potent than **aspirin** as an analgesic but only 20 times more potent as an antipyretic.[5] As an anti-inflammatory ketorolac is about half as potent as **indometacin** and twice as potent as **naproxen**. Like most NSAIDs, ketorolac inhibits platelet aggregation.

Of all the NSAIDs, ketorolac (PO or parenteral) appears to carry the highest risk for upper GI bleeding or perforation. A meta-analysis calculated a 15 times increase in risk with ketorolac, which is three times the risk of non-specific NSAIDs generally. [6] A retrospective case-crossover study of 38,000 people with strokes found PO ketorolac to be associated with only a modest increase in the risk of stroke (odds ratio 1.9) but after parenteral use, the risk of ischaemic or haemorrhagic stroke was increased 4–6 times respectively.[7]

Other postoperative studies indicate that, compared with opioids, the short-term use of ketorolac is associated with only a small increased risk of GI and operative site bleeding.[8,9] The risk is largely related to old age and increases significantly if treatment is continued for >1 week.[8,10] Thus, approval for ketorolac is restricted to short-term postoperative use.[11,12] In some countries, approval has been withdrawn, e.g. France and Germany. Ketorolac has been used in emergency departments for post-traumatic pain.[9] However, high dose ketorolac after spinal surgery is associated with an increased rate of bony non-union.[13]

Studies submitted to the FDA to obtain marketing authorization in the USA related to acute pain.[14] Data on management of chronic pain are scanty and of low quality. In palliative care, ketorolac has been used for extended periods but always with a gastroprotective drug.[5,15–17]

In a week-long RCT in cancer pain, PO ketorolac 10mg q.d.s. was no better than **paracetamol** 600mg + **codeine** 60mg q.d.s.[18] It was also found to be no better than PO **diclofenac**.[19] However, anecdotal clinical experience suggests that parenteral ketorolac may be effective in some patients, notably with bone pain, who fail to obtain relief with NSAIDs PO.[5,15–17]

Bio-availability 100% PO.
Onset of action 30min PO, 10–30min IM/IV.
Time to peak plasma concentration 44 min PO, 35min IM, 1.1min IV.
Plasma halflife 5h; 7h in the elderly;[20] 6–19h with renal impairment.[10]
Duration of action 6h PO, 4–6h IM.

Cautions

To minimize the potential for serious undesirable effects, use the lowest effective dose for the shortest treatment duration possible. In the elderly and those with renal impairment, the maximum daily dose should be reduced (see below). Because they cause sodium and fluid retention, all NSAIDs can decrease the effect of diuretics, ACE inhibitors and antihypertensives. **Warfarin**, **heparin**, **aspirin** and **pentoxifylline** may increase the bleeding tendency.

Drug interactions

Ketorolac can increase the plasma concentrations of **lithium** and **methotrexate**. **Probenecid** increases ketorolac levels and halflife.

Undesirable effects

Also see NSAIDs, p.293.
Very common (>10%): headache, dyspepsia, nausea, abdominal pain.
Common (<10%, >1%): dizziness, drowsiness, tinnitus, oedema, hypertension, anaemia, stomatitis, vomiting, bloating, flatulence, GI ulceration, diarrhoea, constipation, abnormal renal function, pruritus, purpura, rash, bleeding and pain at injection site (less with CSCI).

Dose and use

Moderate–severe acute pain

Approved in the UK for a maximum of 2 days IM/IV or 7 days PO for postoperative pain only.
For adults <65 years, with normal renal function and weighing >50kg:
- 10–30mg IM/IV q6h–q4h *or* 10mg PO q6h–q4h
- maximum recommended daily dose 90mg IM/IV, 40mg PO (the latter is less than the parenteral dose possibly because it is generally given when postoperative analgesic requirements are diminishing).

For those aged >65 years, those with renal impairment, and those weighing <50kg:
- maximum recommended daily dose 60mg IM/IV
- 10mg PO q8h–q6h.

Cancer pain

Ketorolac is used at some centres when a parenteral NSAID is needed for a few weeks to help relieve metastatic bone pain while arranging and awaiting benefit from more definitive therapy, e.g. radiotherapy. However, ketorolac has been used for up to 6 months without causing serious GI events.[17]

Ketorolac can be given by intermittent injections 15–30mg SC t.d.s. but these are uncomfortable; it is better given by CSCI:
- start with 60mg/24h by CSCI; also the recommended maximum dose in people over 65 and those <50kg
- if necessary, increase by 15mg/24h to 90mg/24h
- prescribe a gastroprotective drug concurrently, preferably either **misoprostol** 200microgram t.d.s.–q.d.s.,[15] or a PPI once daily.

CSCI: because ketorolac is irritant, dilute to the largest volume possible, and consider the use of 0.9% saline as the diluent (see p.667).

CSCI compatibility with other drugs: Ketorolac is alkaline in solution and there is a high risk of *incompatibility* when mixed with acidic drugs. There are 2-drug compatibility data for ketorolac in 0.9% saline with **diamorphine** and **oxycodone**.[21]

Incompatibility has been reported with **cyclizine**, **glycopyrronium**, **haloperidol**, **hydromorphone**, **hydroxyzine**, **levomepromazine**, **midazolam**, **morphine**, **pethidine**, and **promethazine** (see, p.669).

For more details, 2-drug and 3-drug compatibility charts can be found on www.palliativedrugs.com Syringe Driver Survey Database (SDSD).

For compatibility charts for mixing drugs in WFI see Appendix 3, p.773.

Supply

Ketorolac trometamol (generic)
Injection 30mg/mL, 1mL amp = £1, *vehicle contains alcohol.*

Toradol® (Roche)
Tablets 10mg, 7 days @ 10mg q.d.s = £8.
Injection 10mg/mL, 30mg/mL, both 1mL amp = £1 *vehicle contains alcohol.*

1 Buckley MM-T and Brogden R (1990) Ketorolac: a review of its pharmacodynamic and pharmacokinetic properties, and therapeutic potential. *Drugs.* **39**: 86–109.
2 Gillis J and Brogden R (1997) Ketorolac: A reappraisal of its pharmacodynamic and pharmacokinetic properties and therapeutic use in pain management. *Drugs.* **53**: 139–188.
3 Uzan A (2005) The unexpected side effects of new nonsteroidal anti-inflammatory drugs. *Expert Opinion on Emerging Drugs.* **10**: 687–688.
4 Litvak K and McEvoy G (1990) Ketorolac: an injectable nonnarcotic analgesic. *Clinical Pharmacy.* **9**: 921–935.
5 Blackwell N *et al.* (1993) Subcutaneous ketorolac — a new development in pain control. *Palliative Medicine.* **7**: 63–65.
6 Masso Gonzalez EL *et al.* (2010) Variability among nonsteroidal antiinflammatory drugs in risk of upper gastrointestinal bleeding. *Arthritis and Rheumatism.* **62**: 1592–1601.
7 Chang CH *et al.* (2010) Increased risk of stroke associated with nonsteroidal anti-inflammatory drugs: a nationwide case-crossover study. *Stroke.* **41**: 1884–1890.
8 Strom B *et al.* (1996) Parenteral ketorolac and risk of gastrointestinal and operative site bleeding. A postmarketing surveillance study. *Journal of the American Medical Assocation.* **275**: 376–382.
9 Rainer T *et al.* (2000) Cost effectiveness analysis of intravenous ketorolac and morphine for treating pain after limb injury: double blind randomised controlled trial. *British Medical Journal.* **321**: 1247–1251.
10 Reinhart D (2000) Minimising the adverse effects of ketorolac. *Drug Safety.* **22**: 487–497.
11 Choo V and Lewis S (1993) Ketorolac doses reduced. *Lancet.* **342**: 109.
12 Lewis S (1994) Ketorolac in Europe. *Lancet.* **343**: 784.
13 Li Q *et al.* (2010) High-Dose Ketorolac Affects Adult Spinal Fusion: A Meta-Analysis of the Effect of Perioperative Nonsteroidal Anti-Inflammatory Drugs on Spinal Fusion. *Spine (Phila Pa 1976).*
14 Ridgway D (2004) Analgesics for acute pain: Meeting the United States Food and Drug Administration's requirements for proof of efficacy. *Clinical Journal of Pain.* **20**: 123–132.
15 Myers K and Trotman I (1994) Use of ketorolac by continuous subcutaneous infusion for the control of cancer-related pain. *Postgraduate Medical Journal.* **70**: 359–362.
16 Middleton RK *et al.* (1996) Ketorolac continuous infusion: a case report and review of the literature. *Journal of Pain and Symptom Management.* **12**: 190–194.
17 Hughes A *et al.* (1997) Ketorolac: continuous subcutaneous infusion for cancer pain. *Journal of Pain and Symptom Management.* **13**: 315–317.
18 Carlson RW *et al.* (1990) A multiinstitutional evaluation of the analgesic efficacy and safety of ketorolac tromethamine, acetaminophen plus codeine, and placebo in cancer pain. *Pharmacotherapy.* **10**: 211–216.
19 Pannuti F *et al.* (1999) A double-blind evaluation of the analgesic efficacy and toxicity of oral ketorolac and diclofenac in cancer pain. The TD/10 recordati Protocol Study Group. *Tumori.* **85**: 96–100.
20 Greenwald R (1992) Ketorolac: an innovative nonsteroidal analgesic. *Drugs of Today.* **28**: 41–61.
21 Dickman A et al. (2005) *The Syringe Driver: Continuous Subcutaneous Infusions in Palliative Care* (2e). Oxford University Press, Oxford.

NAPROXEN — BNF 10.1.1

Class: Non-opioid analgesic, NSAID, non-selective COX inhibitor.

Indications: Pain and inflammation in arthritic conditions and other musculoskeletal disorders, dysmenorrhoea, acute gout †cancer pain, †fever.

Contra-indications: Hypersensitivity to **aspirin** or other NSAID (urticaria, rhinitis, asthma, angioedema), active GI ulceration, cerebrovascular bleeding or other bleeding disorders, severe heart failure, active liver disease or severe hepatic impairment, severe renal impairment (creatinine clearance <30mL/min), deteriorating renal function, hyperkalaemia, systemic lupus erythematosus.

Pharmacology

Naproxen is a non-selective COX inhibitor. Like **flurbiprofen** and **ibuprofen**, it is a propionic acid derivative. Absorption is not affected by food or antacids. A steady-state is achieved after 4–5 days of b.d. administration. Excretion is almost entirely urinary, mainly as conjugated naproxen, with some unchanged drug. Plasma concentrations do not increase with doses >500mg b.d. because of rapid urinary excretion.[1]

The GI risk with naproxen has been reported as both moderate (just over twice the risk of low-dose ibuprofen)[2] and low (next safest after low dose **ibuprofen**).[3] The differing estimates may be accounted for by differences in risk factors in the populations surveyed.[4] As with all NSAIDs, concurrent administration with an SSRI is associated with an increased risk of GI bleeding. A combination product with **misoprostol** is available but the total daily dose of **misoprostol** is half that needed for optimal protection.

Attempts are being made to improve naproxen's GI safety by linking it with an NO-donating moiety to produce naproxicinod, or by combining it with phosphatidylcholine (see p.298) to produce naproxen-PC.[5] However, in an RCT in nearly 1,000 volunteers, naproxicinod was no better than naproxen.[6]

Naproxen is *not* associated with an increase in myocardial infarction.[7] It may carry no increased risk even in people with known[8] and severe cardiovascular disease.[9–11] It carries only a moderate risk of stroke, no additional risk of cardiac death, and a negligible increase in risk of death from any cause.[7]

The underlying reasons for the apparent cardiovascular safety of naproxen are unclear. However, on current evidence, it is the safest NSAID to use in patients with cardiovascular risk factors (with **celecoxib** as second choice). As with all NSAIDs, naproxen should be avoided in cardiac failure.[12]

Although generally given b.d., a single dose of naproxen 500mg at bedtime was equal in efficacy to 250mg b.d. in patients with osteo-arthritis[13,14] and with rheumatoid arthritis.[15]

Naproxen *sodium* 275mg is equivalent to 250mg naproxen. Naproxen *sodium* is more rapidly absorbed, resulting in plasma concentrations about 1.5–2 times higher than those of naproxen over the first hour, and better analgesia from 4h onwards.[16] However, it is approximately 3 times more expensive than naproxen base.

Bio-availability 95% PO.
Onset of action 20–30min.
Time to peak plasma concentration 1.5–5h depending on dose and formulation.[17,18]
Plasma halflife 12–15h.
Duration of action 6–8h single dose; >12h multiple doses.

Cautions

To minimize the potential for serious undesirable effects, use the lowest effective dose for the shortest treatment duration possible. Because they cause sodium and fluid retention, all NSAIDs can decrease the effect of diuretics, ACE inhibitors and antihypertensives.

Naproxen carries a similar risk of inducing acute renal failure as other NSAIDs.[19] Because of their Na^+ content (see Supply), naproxen *sodium* products should be used with caution in patients on a salt-restricted diet.

The thromboprotective effect of **aspirin** for stroke is compromised in people taking a concurrent NSAID.[20,21] Thus, ideally, people on **aspirin** for thromboprotection should *not* take another NSAID of any type. However, if an NSAID is considered essential, prescribe naproxen b.d., and stop the **aspirin** (see p.300). As stated above, naproxen does *not* increase thrombotic risk, and it impairs platelet function round-the-clock if given regularly.

Drug interactions

Naproxen is a substrate of CYP1A2 and CYP2C8/9. It can increase plasma concentrations of **methotrexate** (possibly partly through an effect on tubular transporter systems[22] and **lithium**, and slightly increase **warfarin** levels (see Table 5.9, p.304–7). Naproxen plasma concentrations are increased by **probenecid**.

Although studies have not shown any increase in INR when naproxen and **warfarin** are taken concurrently, if naproxen is prescribed for a patient already taking **warfarin**, it is still advisable to monitor the INR weekly for 3–4 weeks, and adjust the dose of **warfarin** if necessary.[23]

Undesirable effects

Also see NSAIDs, p.293.

Very common (>10%): headache.

Common (<10%, >1%): headache, dizziness, oedema, indigestion, abdominal discomfort, nausea, constipation or diarrhoea, pruritus, rash, ecchymosis.

Dose and use

Naproxen is the NSAID of choice at some centres:

- typically 250–500mg b.d.
- can be taken as a single daily dose, either each morning or each evening with food
- occasionally, with careful monitoring, it may be worth titrating up to a total daily dose of 1.5g (e.g. 500mg t.d.s.); this is higher than the manufacturer's recommended maximum daily doses of 1–1.25g (depending on indication) and should normally be done for only a limited period. This is comparable to doses used for severe rheumatoid arthritis.

Supply

Naproxen (generic)
Tablets 250mg, 500mg, 28 days @ 500mg b.d. = £3.50.
Tablets e/c 250mg, 375mg, 500mg, 28 days @ 500mg b.d. = £5.

Naprosyn® (Roche)
Tablets 250mg, 500mg, 28 days @ 500mg b.d. = £9.
Tablets e/c 250mg, 375mg, 500mg, 28 days @ 500mg b.d. = £9.

Naproxen *sodium*
Synflex® (Roche)
Tablets containing naproxen sodium 275mg equivalent to 250mg naproxen, 28 days @ 550mg b.d. = £13 (each tablet contains 25mg of sodium).

1 Simon L and Mills J (1980) Nonsteroidal anti-inflammatory drugs. Part 2. *New England Journal of Medicine*. **302**: 1237–1243.
2 Henry D *et al.* (1996) Variability in risk of gastrointestinal complications with individual non-steroidal anti-inflammatory drugs: results of a collaborative meta-analysis. *British Medical Journal*. **312**: 1563–1566.
3 MCA/CSM (2002) Non-steroidal anti-inflammatory drugs (NSAIDS) and gastrointestinal (G) safety. *Current Problems in Pharmacovigilance*. **28**: 5–6.
4 Rahme E *et al.* (2009) Discrepancy among observational studies: example of naproxen-associated adverse events. *Open Rheumatology Journal*. **3**: 1–8.
5 Lichtenberger LM *et al.* (2009) Naproxen-PC: a GI safe and highly effective anti-inflammatory. *Inflammopharmacology*. **17**: 1–5.
6 Lohmander LS *et al.* (2005) A randomised, placebo controlled, comparative trial of the gastrointestinal safety and efficacy of AZD3582 versus naproxen in osteoarthritis. *Annals of the Rheumatic Diseases*. **64**: 449–456.
7 Trelle S *et al.* (2011) Cardiovascular safety of non-steroidal anti-inflammatory drugs: network meta-analysis. *British Medical Journal*. **342**: c7086.
8 Roumie CL *et al.* (2008) Nonaspirin NSAIDs, cyclooxygenase 2 inhibitors, and the risk for stroke. *Stroke*. **39**: 2037–2045.
9 Duff G (2006) Safety of selective and non-selective NSAIDs. In: *Letter to health professionals from the Chairman of the Commission on Human Medicines*, 24th October 2006. Available from: www.mhra.gov.uk/SafetyInformation/Safetywarningsalertsandrecalls/Safetywarningsandmessagesformedicines/CON2025040
10 Patrignani P *et al.* (2008) NSAIDs and cardiovascular disease. *Heart*. **94**: 395–397.
11 Ray W *et al.* (2009) Cardiovascular risks of nonsteroidal anti-inflammatory drugs in patients after hospitalization for serious coronary heart disease. *Circulation Cardiovascular Quality and Outcomes*. **2**: 155–163.
12 Gislason GH *et al.* (2009) Increased mortality and cardiovascular morbidity associated with use of nonsteroidal anti-inflammatory drugs in chronic heart failure. *Archives of Internal Medicine*. **169**: 141–149.
13 Brooks P *et al.* (1982) Evaluation of a single daily dose of naproxen in osteoarthritis. *Rheumatology and Rehabilitation*. **21**: 242–246.
14 Mendelsohn s (1991) Clinical efficacy and tolerability of naproxen in osteoarthritis patients using twice-daily and once-daily regimens. *Clinical Therapy*. **13 (suppl A)**: 8–15.
15 Graziano F (1991) Once-daily or twice-daily administration of naproxen in patients with rheumatoid arthritis. *Clinical Therapy*. **13 (suppl A)**: 20–25.
16 Sevelius H *et al.* (1980) Bioavailability of naproxen sodium and its relationship to clinical analgesic effects. *British Journal of Clinical Pharmacology*. **10**: 259–263.
17 Kelly J *et al.* (1989) Pharmacokinetic properties and clinical efficacy of once-daily sustained-release naproxen. *European Journal of Clinical Pharmacology*. **36**: 383–388.
18 Davies N and Anderson K (1997) Clinical pharmacokinetics of naproxen. *Clinical Pharmacokinetics*. **32**: 268–293.
19 Schneider V *et al.* (2006) Association of selective and conventional nonsteroidal antiinflammatory drugs with acute renal failure: A population-based, nested case-control analysis. *American Journal of Epidemiology*. **164**: 881–889.
20 Gengo FM *et al.* (2008) Effects of ibuprofen on the magnitude and duration of aspirin's inhibition of platelet aggregation: clinical consequences in stroke prophylaxis. *Journal of Clinical Pharmacology*. **48**: 117–122.

21 Gladding PA *et al.* (2008) The antiplatelet effect of six non-steroidal anti-inflammatory drugs and their pharmacodynamic interaction with aspirin in healthy volunteers. *American Journal of Cardiology.* **101**: 1060–1063.

22 El-Sheikh AA *et al.* (2007) Interaction of nonsteroidal anti-inflammatory drugs with multidrug resistance protein (MRP) 2/ABCC2- and MRP4/ABCC4-mediated methotrexate transport. *Journal of Pharmacology and Experimental Therapeutics.* **320**: 229–235.

23 Baxter K (ed) (2010) Stockley's Drug Interactions (online edition). The Pharmaceutical Press, London. Available from: www.medicinescomplete.com

NABUMETONE — BNF 10.1.1

Class: Non-opioid analgesic, NSAID, non-selective COX-2 inhibitor.

Indications: Pain in osteo-arthritis and rheumatoid arthritis, †cancer pain.

Contra-indications: Hypersensitivity to **aspirin** or other NSAID (urticaria, rhinitis, asthma, angioedema), active GI ulceration, severe heart failure, active liver disease or severe hepatic impairment, severe renal impairment (creatinine clearance <30mL/min), deteriorating renal function, hyperkalaemia.

Pharmacology

Worldwide, nabumetone is one of the most commonly prescribed NSAIDs.[1] It is a unique NSAID in that it is both a pro-drug and non-acidic; this may explain its low risk for GI toxicity (see below).

Absorption is mainly unaffected by food, and is increased if taken with milk.[1] It undergoes rapid and extensive first-pass metabolism in the liver to mainly 6-methoxy-2-naphthylacetic acid (6-MNA), which is further metabolized by O-methylation and conjugation to inactive compounds.[2] Less than 1% is excreted as 6-MNA. Steady-state plasma concentrations of 6-MNA are not altered in patients with renal impairment even though the renal excretion of 6-MNA is reduced.[1] This could relate to non-linear protein-binding, changes in apparent volume of distribution[3] or increased excretion by other routes.

Although early studies suggested that nabumetone is COX-2 selective, later studies using whole blood assay indicate that it is non-selective.[4–6] Nabumetone has no effect on platelet aggregation in clinical studies.[1,5,7–9] In most patients, once daily administration is satisfactory.

A systematic review of single-dose nabumetone in postoperative pain failed to find any study showing significant benefit.[10] However, when given in a regular dose of 1g/24h in rheumatoid and osteo-arthritis and after acute soft tissue injury, nabumetome is as effective as other NSAIDs.[11–13]

In patients with osteo-arthritis, nabumetone is significantly less gastrotoxic than **diclofenac** and **piroxicam**; the incidence of serious GI events (ulceration, bleeding, perforation) over 6 months is 1.1% vs. 4.3%, and no hospitalizations vs. 1.4%.[14] Nabumetone produced fewer endoscopic ulcers over 12 weeks than **ibuprofen**, and was comparable to **ibuprofen** 2,400mg/24h + **misoprostol** 800microgram/24h.[15] It is less gastrotoxic than **naproxen** (endosopic monitoring for 5 years).[16] This persistent low level of ulcer formation is unique to nabumetone; most NSAIDs have a high level of risk when started, which then diminishes but continues significantly above the baseline even at 5 years.

Meta-analysis of 13 studies, incorporating some 50,000 patients, showed that serious GI events were 10–36 times less likely than with the comparator NSAIDs. However, it should be noted that the confidence intervals for this were extremely wide, approximately 5–760.[17] Hospitalization for NSAID-related events was also less frequent (odds ratio 3.7, 95% CI 1–11).[17] A more recent review of the GI tolerability of nabumetone is also available.[18]

Over some 30 years on the ARAMIS database (for patients with rheumatoid arthritis; www.aramis.stanford.edu), nabumetone has had the least hospitalizations for serious GI events of all the NSAIDs.[19] In practice this means that, except when there is very high risk of gastrotoxicity, a gastroprotective drug need *not* be prescribed with nabumetone. Nabumetone's decreased propensity for causing gastroduodenal toxicity is probably related to the following features:

- it is non-acidic and thus does not damage phosphatidylcholine in the mucous layer and is not subject to acid-trapping (see p.298)

- because it is non-acidic, it has only a weak uncoupling effect on oxidative phosphorylation, and thus causes little disruption of the tight junctions which control mucosal permeability to acid
- it is a pro-drug activated in the liver, and thus causes little direct damage to the stomach and duodenum[20]
- there is no enterohepatic recirculation of the active metabolite.

Nabumetone's cardiovascular risk appears comparable to other NSAIDs.[21,22] In patients with treated hypertension, compared with **ibuprofen**, fewer on nabumetone had a significant increase in blood pressure (17% vs. 6%).[23]

Nabumetone is the NSAID of choice at one major UK palliative care service. It is convenient to use, and the higher cost (vs. **diclofenac**, **ibuprofen** and **naproxen**) is largely offset by generally *not* needing to prescribe concurrent gastroprotection (e.g. a PPI or **misoprostol**). However, nabumetone does not feature in any of the recent major trials and meta-analyses, and thus is in danger of being overlooked despite its favourable risk profile.

Bio-availability *of 6-MNA* 38% (increased by administration with milk).[1,24]
Onset of action 1–2h.
Time to peak plasma concentration *for 6-MNA* 3–6h.[2]
Plasma halflife *of 6-MNA* about 24h.
Duration of action >24h.

Cautions

As with all NSAIDs, use the lowest effective dose for the shortest treatment duration possible to minimize the potential for serious undesirable effects. Because they cause sodium and fluid retention, all NSAIDs can decrease the effect of diuretics, ACE inhibitors and antihypertensives.

In patients with systemic lupus erythematosus (SLE) and other auto-immune disorders, there is probably an increased risk of aseptic meningitis.

Drug interactions

6-MNA is highly protein-bound and may displace other highly bound drugs from plasma proteins, e.g. **phenytoin**, sulfonylureas.

Although nabumetone does not generally alter platelet aggregation or affect the INR in anticoagulated patients, there is an isolated report of haemarthrosis and raised INR in a patient taking **warfarin** concurrently.[25] Thus, if nabumetone is prescribed to a patient already taking **warfarin**, monitor the INR weekly for 3–4 weeks and adjust the dose of **warfarin** if necessary.[26]

Undesirable effects

Also see NSAIDs, p.293.
Very common (>10%): dyspepsia, abdominal pain, diarrhoea (dose-dependent).[27]
Common (<10%, >1%): headache, nausea.

Dose and use

- start with 1g each evening
- if necessary, increase to 500mg each morning and 1g each evening
- if necessary, increase further to 1g b.d.
- in very elderly (80+ years) frail patients, start with 500mg, and limit to 1g once daily.

Dose reduction is not necessary in patients with mild–moderate renal impairment.[1]

Supply

Nabumetone (generic)
Tablets 500mg, 28 days @ 1g daily = £6.

Relifex® (Meda)
Tablets 500mg, 28 days @ 1g daily = £6.
Suspension 500mg in 5mL, 28 days @ 1g daily = £22.

1 Hedner T *et al.* (2004) Nabumetone: Therapeutic use and safety profile in the management of osteoarthritis and rheumatoid arthritis. *Drugs*. **64**: 2315–2343; discussion 2344–2345.
2 Davies NM (1997) Clinical pharmacokinetics of nabumetone. The dawn of selective cyclo-oxygenase-2 inhibition? *Clinical Pharmacokinetics*. **33**: 404–416.
3 Brier ME *et al.* (1995) Population pharmacokinetics of the active metabolite of nabumetone in renal dysfunction. *Clinical Pharmacology and Therapeutics*. **57**: 622–627.
4 Patrignani P *et al.* (1994) Biochemical and pharmacological characterization of the cyclooxygenase activity of human blood prostaglandin endoperoxide synthases. *Journal of Pharmacology and Experimental Therapeutics*. **271**: 1705–1712.
5 Cipollone F *et al.* (1995) Effects of nabumetone on prostanoid biosynthesis in humans. *Clinical Pharmacology and Therapeutics*. **58**: 335–341.
6 van Kraaij DJ *et al.* (2002) A comparison of the effects of nabumetone vs meloxicam on serum thromboxane B2 and platelet function in healthy volunteers. *British Journal of Clinical Pharmacology*. **53**: 644–647.
7 Hilleman DE *et al.* (1993) Nonsteroidal antiinflammatory drug use in patients receiving warfarin: emphasis on nabumetone. *American Journal of Medicine*. **95 (suppl)**: 30S–34S.
8 Knijff-Dutmer EA *et al.* (1999) Effects of nabumetone compared with naproxen on platelet aggregation in patients with rheumatoid arthritis. *Annals of Rheumatic Diseases*. **58**: 257–259.
9 Jennings MB *et al.* (2009) A double-blind study of the effect of hemostasis of nabumetone (Relafen) compared to placebo. *Journal of Foot and Ankle Surgery*. **39**: 168–173.
10 Moore RA *et al.* (2009) Single dose oral nabumetone for acute postoperative pain in adults. *Cochrane Database of Systematic Reviews*. **4**: CD007548.
11 Friedel HA *et al.* (1993) Nabumetone. A reappraisal of its pharmacology and therapeutic use in rheumatic diseases. *Drugs*. **45**: 131–156.
12 Lister BJ *et al.* (1993) Efficacy of nabumetone versus diclofenac, naproxen, ibuprofen, and piroxicam in osteoarthritis and rheumatoid arthritis. *American Journal of Medicine*. **95 (suppl)**: 2S–9S.
13 Morgan GJ *et al.* (1993) Efficacy and safety of nabumetone versus diclofenac, naproxen, ibuprofen, and piroxicam in the elderly. *American Journal of Medicine*. **95 (suppl)**: 19S–27S.
14 Scott DL and Palmer RH (2000) Safety and efficacy of nabumetone in osteoarthritis: emphasis on gastrointestinal safety. *Alimentary Pharmacology and Therapeutics*. **14**: 443–452.
15 Roth SH *et al.* (1993) A controlled study comparing the effects of nabumetone, ibuprofen, and ibuprofen plus misoprostol on the upper gastrointestinal tract mucosa. *Archives of Internal Medicine*. **153**: 2565–2571.
16 Roth SH *et al.* (1994) A longterm endoscopic evaluation of patients with arthritis treated with nabumetone vs naproxen. *Journal of Rheumatology*. **21**: 1118–1123.
17 Huang JQ *et al.* (1999) Gastrointestinal safety profile of nabumetone: a meta-analysis. *American Journal of Medicine*. **107 (suppl)**: 55S–61S; discussion 61S–64S.
18 Bannwarth B (2008) Safety of the nonselective NSAID nabumetone: focus on gastrointestinal tolerability. *Drug Safety*. **31**: 485–503.
19 Ashworth NL *et al.* (2004) A population based historical cohort study of the mortality associated with nabumetone, Arthrotec, diclofenac, and naproxen. *Journal of Rheumatology*. **31**: 951–956.
20 Jeremy JY *et al.* (1990) The effect of nabumetone and its principal active metabolite on in vitro human gastric mucosal prostanoid synthesis and platelet function. *British Journal of Rheumatology*. **29**: 116–119.
21 Helin-Salmivaara A *et al.* (2006) NSAID use and the risk of hospitalization for first myocardial infarction in the general population: a nationwide case-control study from Finland. *European Heart Journal*. **27**: 1657–1663.
22 Huang WF *et al.* (2006) Cardiovascular events associated with the use of four nonselective NSAIDs (etodolac, nabumetone, ibuprofen, or naproxen) versus a cyclooxygenase-2 inhibitor (celecoxib): a population-based analysis in Taiwanese adults. *Clinical Therapeutics*. **28**: 1827–1836.
23 Palmer R *et al.* (2003) Effects of nabumetone, celecoxib, and ibuprofen on blood pressure control in hypertensive patients on angiotensin converting enzyme inhibitors. *American Journal of Hypertension*. **16**: 135–139.
24 Dollery C (1999) *Therapeutic Drugs*. (2e). Churchill Livingstone, Edinburgh.
25 Dennis VC *et al.* (2000) Potentiation of oral anticoagulation and hemarthrosis associated with nabumetone. *Pharmacotherapy*. **20**: 234–239.
26 Baxter K (2011) Stockley's Drug Interactions (online edition). Pharmaceutical Press, London. Available from: www.medicinescomplete.com
27 Willkens RF (1990) An overview of the long-term safety experience of nabumetone. *Drugs*. **40 (suppl) 5**: 34–37.

WEAK OPIOIDS — BNF 4.7.1 & 4.7.2

There is no pharmacological need for Step 2 of the WHO Analgesic Ladder. Low doses of **morphine**, or an alternative strong opioid, can be used instead.[1,2] Moving directly from Step 1 to Step 3 is now the preferred option at some centres. However, from an international perspective, Step 2 remains a practical necessity because of the highly restricted availability (or even non-availability) in many countries of oral **morphine**, and other strong opioids.

Codeine is the archetypical weak opioid (and **morphine** the archetypical strong opioid).[3] However, the division of opioids into 'weak' and 'strong' is to a certain extent arbitrary. In reality, opioids manifest a range of strengths which is not fully reflected in two discrete categories.

By IM injection, weak opioids can all provide analgesia equivalent, or almost equivalent, to **morphine** 10mg but most weak opioids are not marketed as injections. High-dose **codeine** (or alternative) is comparable to low-dose **morphine** (or alternative), and vice versa.

Weak opioids are said to have a 'ceiling' effect for analgesia. This is an oversimplification; although mixed agonist-antagonists (e.g. **pentazocine**) have a true ceiling effect, the maximum effective dose of weak opioid agonists is arbitrary. At higher doses, there are progressively more undesirable effects, e.g. nausea and vomiting, which outweigh any additional analgesic effect.

The amount of **dextropropoxyphene** in **co-proxamol** tablets was originally chosen so that only a small minority of patients would experience nausea and vomiting with two tablets. This adds a further constraint because the upper dose limit in practice is likely to be determined by the number of tablets which patients will readily accept (possibly only 2–3 of any one preparation). Further, with some compound preparations, the dose of the non-opioid (e.g. **paracetamol**) will be an additional dose-limiting factor.

There is little to choose between the weak opioids in terms of efficacy (Table 5.11)[4] but, at present, there is no consensus about which is the weak opioid of choice. The following should be noted:

- **codeine** has little or no analgesic effect until metabolized to **morphine** mainly via CYP2D6; it is thus essentially ineffective in slow metabolizers (see p.332)
- **dihydrocodeine**, like **codeine**, is a substrate for CYP2D6 and its partial metabolism is limited in slow metabolizers and is blocked by CYP2D6 inhibitors.[5] However, unlike **codeine**, there is no evidence that such inhibition reduces its analgesic effect, i.e. **dihydrocodeine** is an active substance, not a pro-drug like **codeine**[6–8]
- **tramadol** use has increased in the UK in recent years (as the use of **dextropropoxyphene** has decreased). It is less constipating than **dihydrocodeine** and **codeine**,[9–11] but causes more vomiting, dizziness and anorexia.[12] Further, if used with another drug which affects serotonin metabolism or availability, it can lead to serotonin toxicity, particularly in the elderly (see p.177). It also lowers seizure threshold, and has a much reduced analgesic effect unless metabolized to O-desmethyltramadol (M1) via CYP2D6; it is thus practically ineffective in slow metabolizers (see p.340)
- **dextropropoxyphene** has effectively been withdrawn in the UK, throughout Europe,[13] and the USA.[14] This is because of its relatively common use in intentional overdose, and its potential fatal toxicity in accidental overdose (see p.337)[15,16] Anecdotal evidence suggests that it is less constipating than **codeine**
- **pentazocine** should *not* be used, it often causes psychotomimetic effects (dysphoria, depersonalization, frightening dreams, hallucinations).[17]

Table 5.11 Weak opioids

Drug	*Bio-availability (%)*	*Time to peak plasma concentration (h)*	*Plasma halflife (h)*	*Duration of analgesia (h)*[a]	*Approximate potency ratio with codeine*
Codeine	40 (12–84)	1–2	2.5–3.5	4–6	1
Dextropropoxyphene	40	2–2.5	6–12[b]	6–8	2/3[c]
Dihydrocodeine	20	1.6–1.8	3.5–4.5	3–4	4/3
Tramadol	75[d]	2	6[e]	4–6	1[f]

a. when used in typical doses for mild–moderate pain
b. increased >50% in elderly
c. for single dose; given its halflife, potency ratio for multiple doses (t.d.s.–q.d.s.) of dextropropoxyphene likely to be greater
d. multiple doses >90%
e. active metabolite (M1) 7.4h; both figures double in cirrhosis and severe renal failure
f. estimated on basis of potency ratio with morphine.

Whichever weak opioid is preferred locally, the following general rules should be observed:

- a weak opioid should be added to, not substituted for, a non-opioid analgesic
- it is generally inappropriate to switch from one weak opioid to another weak opioid

- if a weak opioid is inadequate when given regularly, change to **morphine** (or an alternative strong opioid).

As with all opioids, patients must be monitored for undesirable effects, particularly nausea and vomiting, and constipation. Depending on individual circumstances, an anti-emetic should be prescribed for regular or p.r.n. use, (see p.225) and, routinely, a laxative prescribed (see p.38).

1 Maltoni M *et al.* (2005) A validation study of the WHO analgesic ladder: a two-step vs three-step strategy. *Supportive Care in Cancer.* **13**: 888–894.
2 Marinangeli F *et al.* (2004) Use of strong opioids in advanced cancer pain: a randomized trial. *Journal of Pain and Symptom Management.* **27**: 409–416.
3 WHO (1986) *Cancer Pain Relief.* World Health Organisation, Geneva.
4 Moore RA and McQuay HJ (1997) Single-patient data meta-analysis of 3453 postoperative patients: oral tramadol versus placebo, codeine and combination analgesics. *Pain.* **69**: 287–294.
5 Fromm M *et al.* (1995) Dihydrocodeine: A new opioid substrate for the polymorphic CYP2D6 in humans. *Clinical Pharmacology and Therapeutics.* **58**: 374–382.
6 Wilder-Smith CH *et al.* (1998) The visceral and somatic antinociceptive effects of dihydrocodeine and its metabolite, dihydromorphine. A cross-over study with extensive and quinidine-induced poor metabolizers. *British Journal of Clinical Pharmacology.* **45**: 575–581.
7 Webb JA *et al.* (2001) Contribution of dihydrocodeine and dihydromorphine to analgesia following dihydrocodeine administration in man: a PK-PD modelling analysis. *British Journal of Clinical Pharmacology.* **52**: 35–43.
8 Schmidt H *et al.* (2003) The role of active metabolites in dihydrocodeine effects. *International Journal of Clinical Pharmacology and Therapeutics.* **41**: 95–106.
9 Wilder-Smith CH and Bettiga A (1997) The analgesic tramadol has minimal effect on gastrointestinal motor function. *British Journal of Clinical Pharmacology.* **43**: 71–75.
10 Wilder-Smith CH *et al.* (1999) Effect of tramadol and morphine on pain and gastrointestinal motor function in patients with chronic pancreatitis. *Digestive Diseases and Sciences.* **44**: 1107–1116.
11 Wilder-Smith C *et al.* (2001) Treatment of severe pain from osteoarthritis with slow-release tramadol or dihydrocodeine in combination with NSAID's: a randomised study comparing analgesia, antinociception and gastrointestinal effects. *Pain.* **91**: 23–31.
12 Rodriguez RF *et al.* (2007) Incidence of weak opioids adverse events in the management of cancer pain: a double-blind comparative trial. *Journal of Palliative Medicine.* **10**: 56–60.
13 European Medicines Agency (2009) Press Release. European Medicines Agency recommends withdrawal of dextropropoxyphene-containing medicines. Available from: www.emea.europa.eu/pdfs/human/press/pr/40106209en.pdf
14 FDA (2010) FDA recommends against the continued use of propoxyphene. In: FDA drug safety communication (issued 19th November 2010). Available from: www.fda.gov/Drugs/DrugSafety/ucm234338.htm
15 Hawton K *et al.* (2003) Co-proxamol and suicide: a study of national mortality statistics and local non-fatal self poisonings. *British Medical Journal.* **326**: 1006–1008.
16 Hawton K *et al.* (2009) Effect of withdrawal of co-proxamol on prescribing and deaths from drug poisoning in England and Wales: time series analysis. *British Medical Journal.* **338**: b2270.
17 Woods A *et al.* (1974) Medicines evaluation and monitoring group: central nervous system effects of pentazocine. *British Medical Journal.* **1**: 305–307.

CODEINE PHOSPHATE BNF 1.4.2, 3.9.1, 4.7.1 & 4.7.2

Class: Opioid analgesic.

Indications: Mild–moderate pain, cough, diarrhoea.

Contra-indications: None absolute if titrated carefully to effect.

Pharmacology

Codeine (methylmorphine) is an opium alkaloid, about one tenth as potent as **morphine**. An increasing analgesic response has been reported with IM doses up to 360mg.[1] However, in practice, codeine is generally used PO in doses of 15–60mg, often in combination with a non-opioid. Although widely prescribed, there is a lack of RCT data on the efficacy and tolerability of fixed-dose **paracetamol**-codeine combinations in cancer pain. Codeine is metabolized mainly by conjugation to codeine-6-glucuronide, but also by O-demethylation to **morphine** (via CYP2D6) and by N-demethylation (via CYP3A3/4).

It is unclear how much of the analgesic effect of codeine is a direct one.[2] Codeine is at least partly a pro-drug, with typically ≤10% of codeine biotransformed to **morphine**.[3,4] When the biotransformation to **morphine** is blocked by CYP2D6 inhibitors (e.g. **fluoxetine**, **paroxetine**, **quinidine**), codeine lacks significant analgesic activity. The major metabolite (80%) is codeine-6-glucuronide, and this may also contribute to codeine's analgesic effect.[5,6]

However, because of genetic polymorphism, there is wide interindividual variation in the production of **morphine** (Table 5.12), which results in a wide range of responses to codeine.[7–10] Compared to the general population (rapid metabolizers), slow metabolizers produce little or no **morphine**, and obtain little or no pain relief from codeine. At the other extreme, ultra-rapid metabolizers produce greater than usual amounts of **morphine**, which can lead to life-threatening opioid intoxication.[11–13]

Table 5.12 Prevalence of CYP2D6 polymorphisms affecting codeine metabolism[14,15]

Ethnic group	*Slow metabolizers*[a]	*Ultra-rapid metabolizers*
Caucasians	5–10%	1–7%
Asians	≤1%	?
Africans	0–34%	9–30%

a. lesser degrees of reduced enzyme activity may be present in up to 50%.[15]

Although slow metabolizers obtain little or no analgesic effect from codeine,[16] in a single dose RCT in healthy volunteers, the incidence of undesirable effects was comparable in both slow and rapid metabolizers.[10]

Like **morphine**, codeine is antitussive and also slows GI transit.[17] Given that opioids can cause pruritus, it is noteworthy that a patient with primary biliary cirrhosis obtained relief with regular oral codeine (also see Opioid antagonists, p.429).[18] Because of constipation, codeine was stopped and the pruritus returned. When codeine was restarted, together with a laxative, the patient again obtained relief.

Bio-availability 40% (12–84%) PO.[3]

Onset of action 30–60min for analgesia; 1–2h for antitussive effect.

Time to peak plasma concentration 1–2h.

Plasma halflife 2.5–3.5h.[3]

Duration of action 4–6h.

Cautions

Driving ability may be impaired by a dose of 50mg.[19,20] Like **morphine** and **dihydrocodeine**, codeine is more toxic in renal failure. This is because of accumulation of **morphine** and of other active metabolites of both codeine and **morphine** (see p.362).

Undesirable effects

Codeine can produce the whole range of opioid undesirable effects, with constipation occurring invariably (see p.349). Data detailing the frequency of other undesirable effects are not readily available.

Dose and use

It is bad practice to prescribe codeine to patients already taking ***morphine*** *or any other strong opioid; if a greater effect is needed, the dose of* ***morphine*** *(or other strong opioid) should be increased.*

Pain relief

Codeine is often given in a combination product with a non-opioid. The codeine content of these products is generally 15mg, 30mg or 60mg (lower strengths, e.g. 8mg, are present in some OTC **paracetamol**-codeine products). Thus patients with inadequate relief may benefit by changing to a higher strength product. When given alone, the dose is generally 30–60mg q4h. Higher doses can be given but equivalent analgesic doses of **morphine** (one tenth of the dose of codeine) may be less constipating.

Cough
Codeine is effective as an antitussive by any route. The dose is tailored to the patient's need, e.g. 15–30mg p.r.n., up to q4h. Administration as an oral liquid or syrup is *not* necessary.

Diarrhoea
To control diarrhoea, a dose of 30–60mg is used both p.r.n. and regularly up to q4h. However, **loperamide** may be preferable (see p.32).

As with all opioids, patients must be monitored for undesirable effects, particularly nausea and vomiting, and constipation (see Box 5.G, p.349). Depending on individual circumstances, an anti-emetic should be prescribed for regular or p.r.n. use, (see p.225) and, routinely, a laxative prescribed (see p.38).

Supply
Codeine phosphate (generic)
Tablets 15mg, 30mg, 60mg, 28 days @ 30mg q.d.s. = £6.
Oral syrup 25mg/5mL, 28 days @ 25mg q.d.s. = £5.
Injections **CD** are available but are not recommended.

Codeine linctus BP
Oral solution 15mg/5mL, 28 days @ 30mg q.d.s. = £8.
Diabetic oral solution 15mg/5mL, 28 days @ 30mg q.d.s. = £8.

With **aspirin**
Co-codaprin (generic)
Tablets dispersible codeine phosphate 8mg, **aspirin** 400mg, 28 days @ 2 q.d.s. = £74.

With **paracetamol**
Co-codamol 8/500 (generic)
Capsules codeine phosphate 8mg, **paracetamol** 500mg, 28 days @ 2 q.d.s. = £19.
Tablets codeine phosphate 8mg, **paracetamol** 500mg, 28 days @ 2 q.d.s. = £9.
Tablets dispersible codeine phosphate 8mg, **paracetamol** 500mg, 28 days @ 2 q.d.s. = £12.

Co-codamol 15/500
Codipar® (Goldshield)
Caplets (capsule-shaped tablets) codeine phosphate 15mg, **paracetamol** 500mg, 28 days @ 2 q.d.s. = £18.

Co-codamol 30/500 (generic)
Capsules codeine phosphate 30mg, **paracetamol** 500mg, 28 days @ 2 q.d.s. = £15.
Tablets codeine phosphate 30mg, **paracetamol** 500mg, 28 days @ 2 q.d.s. = £10.
Tablets effervescent codeine phosphate 30mg, **paracetamol** 500mg, 28 days @ 2 q.d.s. = £22; *contain* Na^+ *13.6mmol/tablet, avoid in renal impairment.*

This is not a complete list; see BNF for more information.

1 Beaver W (1966) Mild analgesics: a review of their clinical pharmacology (Part II). *American Journal of Medical Science.* **251**: 576–599.
2 Quiding H *et al.* (1993) Analgesic effect and plasma concentrations of codeine and morphine after two dose levels of codeine following oral surgery. *European Journal of Clinical Pharmacology.* **44**: 319–323.
3 Persson K *et al.* (1992) The postoperative pharmacokinetics of codeine. *European Journal of Clinical Pharmacology.* **42**: 663–666.
4 Findlay JWA *et al.* (1978) Plasma codeine and morphine concentrations after therapeutic oral doses of codeine-containing analgesics. *Clinical Pharmacology and Therapeutics.* **24**: 60–68.
5 Lotsch J *et al.* (2006) Evidence for morphine-independent central nervous opioid effects after administration of codeine: contribution of other codeine metabolites. *Clinical Pharmacology and Therapeutics.* **79**: 35–48.
6 Vree TB *et al.* (2000) Codeine analgesia is due to codeine-6-glucuronide, not morphine. *International Journal of Clinical Practice.* **54**: 395–398.
7 Sindrup SH and Brosen K (1995) The pharmacogenetics of codeine hypoalgesia. *Pharmacogenetics.* **5**: 335–346.
8 Caraco Y *et al.* (1996) Pharmacogenetic determination of the effects of codeine and prediction of drug interactions. *Journal of Pharmacology and Experimental Therapeutics.* **278**: 1165–1174.
9 Lurcott G (1999) The effects of the genetic absence and inhibition of CYP2D6 on the metabolism of codeine and its derivatives, hydrocodone and oxycodone. *Anesthesia Progress.* **45**: 154–156.

10 Eckhardt K *et al.* (1998) Same incidence of adverse drug events after codeine administration irrespective of the genetically determined differences in morphine formation. *Pain.* **76**: 27–33.
11 Gasche Y *et al.* (2004) Codeine intoxication associated with ultrarapid CYP2D6 metabolism. *New England Journal of Medicine.* **351**: 2827–2831.
12 Koren G *et al.* (2006) Pharmacogenetics of morphine poisoning in a breastfed neonate of a codeine-prescribed mother. *Lancet.* **368**: 704.
13 Kirchheiner J *et al.* (2007) Pharmacokinetics of codeine and its metabolite morphine in ultra-rapid metabolizers due to CYP2D6 duplication. *Pharmacogenomics Journal.* **7**: 257–265.
14 Smith HS (2009) Opioid metabolism. *Mayo Clinic Proceedings.* **84**: 613–624.
15 Williams DG *et al.* (2002) Pharmacogenetics of codeine metabolism in an urban population of children and its implications for analgesic reliability. *British Journal of Anaesthesia.* **89**: 839–845.
16 Lotsch J *et al.* (2004) Genetic predictors of the clinical response to opioid analgesics: clinical utility and future perspectives. *Clinical Pharmacokinetics.* **43**: 983–1013.
17 Anonymous (1989) Drugs in the management of acute diarrhoea in infants and young children. *Bulletin of the World Health Organization.* **67**: 94–96.
18 Zylicz Z and Krajnik M (1999) Codeine for pruritus in primary biliary cirrhosis. *Lancet.* **353**: 813.
19 Linnoila M and Hakkinen S (1974) Effects of diazepam and codeine, alone and in combination with alcohol, on simulated driving. *Clinical Pharmacology and Therapeutics.* **15**: 368–373.
20 Linnoila M and Mattila MJ (1973) Proceedings: Drug interaction on driving skills as evaluated by laboratory tests and by a driving simulator. *Pharmakopsychiatric Neuropsychopharmakologie.* **6**: 127–132.

DIHYDROCODEINE — BNF 4.7.1 & 4.7.2

Class: Opioid analgesic.

Indications: Moderate–severe pain.

Contra-indications: None absolute if titrated carefully to effect.

Pharmacology

Dihydrocodeine is a semisynthetic analogue of **codeine**. It relieves pain and cough,[1–3] and causes constipation.[4] Like **codeine**, dihydrocodeine is a substrate for CYP2D6 and its partial metabolism to dihydromorphine is limited in slow metabolizers and is blocked by CYP2D6 inhibitors such as **fluoxetine**, **paroxetine** and **quinidine**.[5] However, unlike **codeine**, there is no evidence that such inhibition reduces the analgesic effect of dihydrocodeine.[6] In other words, dihydrocodeine is an active substance, not a pro-drug like **codeine**.[7,8]

By injection 60mg provides significantly more analgesia than 30mg and is comparable to **morphine** 10mg.[9,10] Dihydrocodeine is about twice as potent as **codeine** by injection but, because its oral bio-availability is low, the two drugs are essentially equipotent by mouth.[11]

Bio-availability 20% PO.
Onset of action 30min.
Time to peak plasma concentration 1.7h.
Plasma halflife 3.5–4.5h.
Duration of action 4h.

Cautions

May impair the ability to perform skilled tasks, e.g. driving. Prolonged erections have occurred when **sildenafil** was taken concurrently with dihydrocodeine, possibly because abnormally high concentrations of cyclic guanosine monophosphate were produced in peripheral nerve endings.[12]

Like **morphine** and **codeine**, dihydrocodeine is more toxic in renal failure, probably because of accumulation of an active glucuronide (also see p.618).[13]

Undesirable effects

Common (<10%, >1%): sedation, dizziness, disturbed dreams, headache, vertigo, nausea and vomiting, constipation, pruritus, rash.
Uncommon (<1%): hallucinations, paralytic ileus, urinary retention.

Dose and use

As a single agent analgesic:

- start with 30mg q6h–q4h
- if necessary, increase to 60mg q6h–q4h.

The higher dose is associated with a significant increase in undesirable effects.[14]

Supply

Dihydrocodeine (generic)
Tablets 30mg, 28 days @ 30mg q.d.s. = £6.
Oral solution 10mg/5mL, 28 days @ 30mg q.d.s. = £34.
***Injection* CD** 50mg/mL, 1mL amp = £3.

DF118 Forte® (Martindale)
Tablets 40mg, 28 days @ 40mg t.d.s. = £10.

Modified-release
DHC Continus® (Napp)
Tablets m/r 60mg, 90mg, 120mg, 28 days @ 60mg b.d. = £5.

With **paracetamol**
Co-dydramol 10/500 (generic)
Tablets dihydrocodeine tartrate 10mg, **paracetamol** 500mg, 28 days @ 2 q.d.s. = £9.

Remedeine® (Napp)
Tablets dihydrocodeine tartrate 20mg, **paracetamol** 500mg, 28 days @ 2 q.d.s. = £21.
Tablets Forte dihydrocodeine tartrate 30mg, **paracetamol** 500mg, 28 days @ 2 q.d.s. = £26.

---

1 Keats AS *et al.* (1957) Studies of analgesic drugs: dihydrocodeine. *Journal of Pharmacology and Experimental Therapeutics*. **120**: 354–360.
2 Weiss B (1959) Dihydrocodeine. A pharmacologic review. *American Journal of Pharmacy*. **August**: 286–301.
3 Luporini G *et al.* (1998) Efficacy and safety of levodropropizine and dihydrocodeine on nonproductive cough in primary and metastatic lung cancer. *European Respiratory Journal*. **12**: 97–101.
4 Freye E *et al.* (2001) Dose-related effects of controlled release dihydrocodeine on oro-cecal transit and pupillary light reflex. A study in human volunteers. *Arzneimittelforschung*. **51**: 60–66.
5 Fromm M *et al.* (1995) Dihydrocodeine: A new opioid substrate for the polymorphic CYP2D6 in humans. *Clinical Pharmacology and Therapeutics*. **58**: 374–382.
6 Wilder-Smith CH *et al.* (1998) The visceral and somatic antinociceptive effects of dihydrocodeine and its metabolite, dihydromorphine. A cross-over study with extensive and quinidine-induced poor metabolizers. *British Journal of Clinical Pharmacology*. **45**: 575–581.
7 Webb JA *et al.* (2001) Contribution of dihydrocodeine and dihydromorphine to analgesia following dihydrocodeine administration in man: a PK-PD modelling analysis. *British Journal of Clinical Pharmacology*. **52**: 35–43.
8 Schmidt H *et al.* (2003) The role of active metabolites in dihydrocodeine effects. *International Journal of Clinical Pharmacology and Therapeutics*. **41**: 95–106.
9 Seed JC *et al.* (1958) A comparison of the analgesic and respiratory effects of dihydrocodeine and morphine in main. *Archives Internationales de Pharmacodynamie et de Therapie*. **116**: 293–339.
10 Palmer RN *et al.* (1966) Incidence of unwanted effects of dihydrocodeine bitartrate in healthy volunteers. *Lancet*. **2**: 620–621.
11 Anonymous (1991) Dihydrocodeine (tartrate). In: C Dollery (ed) *Therapeutic Drugs*. Churchill Livingstone, Edinburgh, pp. 133–136.
12 Goldmeier D and Lamba H (2002) Prolonged erections produced by dihydrocodeine and sildenafil. *British Medical Journal*. **324**: 1555.
13 Barnes J *et al.* (1985) Dihydrocodeine in renal failure: further evidence for an important role in the kidney in the handling of opioid drugs. *British Medical Journal*. **290**: 740–742.
14 McQuay H *et al.* (1993) A multiple dose comparison of ibuprofen and dihydrocodeine after third molar surgery. *British Journal of Oral and Maxillofacial Surgery*. **31**: 95–100.

DEXTROPROPOXYPHENE BNF 4.7.1

Class: Opioid analgesic.

Indications: Mild–moderate pain.

Withdrawal of licence

In 2007, the MHRA withdrew the licence for **co-proxamol**, the only dextropropoxyphene-containing product in the UK. The EMEA has also withdrawn the marketing authorization for all dextropropoxyphene-containing medicines throughout the EU. This was primarily because of its use in intentional overdose and its potentially fatal toxicity in accidental overdose through its effects on cardiac conduction and respiration, particularly when taken with alcohol.[1,2] It was stated that there is no good evidence that **co-proxamol** is superior to **paracetamol** alone in relieving mild–moderate acute and chronic musculoskeletal pain.[3] However, although this may be true for single doses, it is *not* true for chronic regular use (see below).

In 2010, the FDA withdrew the drug from the market in the USA after new data showed that, even at normal therapeutic doses, dextropropoxyphene can cause potentially serious prolongation of the PR and QT intervals, and widened QRS complexes.[4,5]

In the UK, there is provision for prescribers to supply **co-proxamol** on a named-patient basis if there is an identified clinical need, e.g. if alternatives prove ineffective.[3,6]

Pharmacology

Dextropropoxyphene is a synthetic derivative of **methadone**. It is a μ-opioid receptor agonist with affinity similar to that of **codeine**. However, whereas **codeine** is mainly a pro-drug (see p.332), dextropropoxyphene is an active substance. It is also a weak NMDA-receptor-channel blocker[7] but this is unlikely to be clinically relevant. Dextropropoxyphene undergoes extensive dose-dependent first-pass hepatic metabolism; systemic availability increases with increasing doses.[8] The principal metabolite, nordextropropoxyphene, is also analgesic but crosses the blood-brain barrier to a lesser extent.

In *single-dose* RCTs in patients with postoperative pain, arthritis and musculoskeletal pain, no added benefit is seen when dextropropoxyphene combined with **paracetamol** is compared with **paracetamol** alone.[9] Such reports have led to doubts about the efficacy of dextropropoxyphene. However, dextropropoxyphene *hydrochloride* 65mg has been shown to have a definite analgesic effect in several placebo-controlled trials,[10] and a dose-response curve has been established (Figure 5.9).[11,12] *Placebos do not have a dose-response curve.*

Because of the long halflife of both dextropropoxyphene and nordextropropoxyphene in elderly patients, it takes about 1 week to achieve a steady-state when dextropropoxyphene is taken regularly t.d.s.–q.d.s., and plasma concentrations are some 5 and 7 times greater than after a single dose.[13,14] Thus, rather like **methadone** (see p.416), the effect of multiple doses cannot be estimated from single-dose studies.[15,16] Further, whereas the NNT in single-dose studies for a 50% reduction in moderate or severe postoperative pain for dextropropoxyphene *hydrochloride* 65mg is 8, for 130mg the NNT is only 3. Because of accumulation when given regularly round-the-clock, the latter is likely to more closely reflect the response with multiple doses of 65mg.

The relative potency of a *single* dose of dextropropoxyphene is 1/2–2/3 that of **codeine**.[8] However, because of accumulation with multiple doses, when given regularly t.d.s.–q.d.s., it is reasonable to assume that it is approximately as potent as **codeine** and **dihydrocodeine**, i.e. is about one tenth as potent as PO **morphine** on a weight-for-weight basis. Dextropropoxyphene causes less nausea and vomiting, drowsiness and dry mouth than low-dose **morphine**, particularly during initial treatment.[17] Anecdotally, it is said to cause less constipation than **codeine**.

Bio-availability 40% PO.

Onset of action 20–30min.

Time to peak plasma concentation 2–2.5h.

Plasma halflife 6–12h, nordextropropoxyphene 30–36h; increasing in the elderly to 36h, nordextropropoxyphene to >50h.[13]

Duration of action single dose 4–6h; longer in the elderly and when taken regularly.

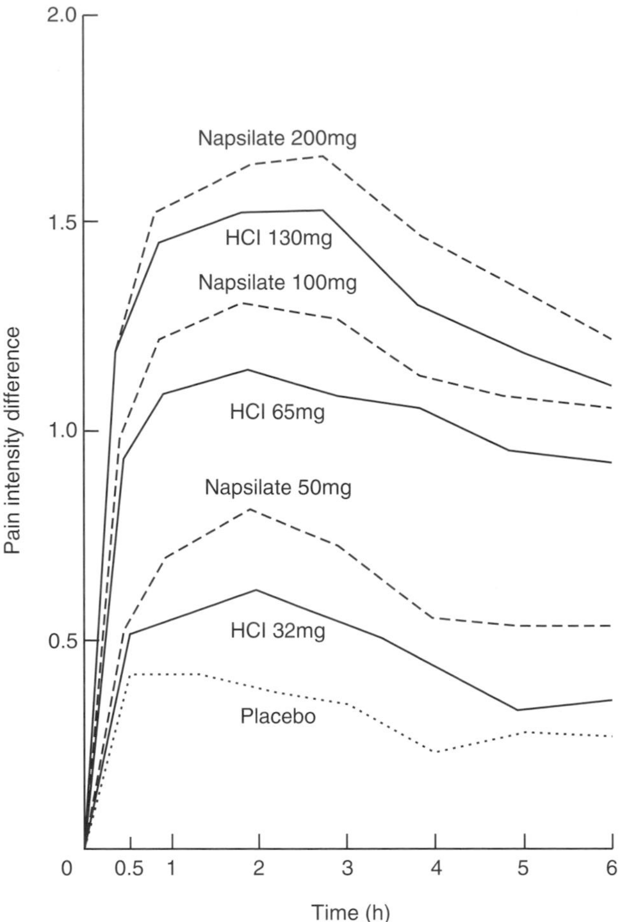

Figure 5.9 Incremental pain relief with increasing doses of dextropropoxyphene *hydrochloride* and dextropropoxphene *napsilate*[11]

Cautions

Even at normal therapeutic doses, dextropropoxyphene can cause potentially serious prolongation of the PR and QT intervals, and widened QRS complexes.[4,5]

May impair the ability to perform skilled tasks, e.g. driving. In elderly patients prescribed a standard dose regimen, because of increased plasma halflife, accumulation leading to drowsiness, delirium and respiratory depression is possible after 7–10 days.

Hepatic or renal impairment. Dextropropoxyphene may enhance the effect of **warfarin**, **carbamazepine**[18] and CNS depressants, including alcohol. Dextropropoxyphene prolongs the plasma halflife of **alprazolam** by 50% (12h→18h) but it has no effect on the metabolism of **lorazepam** and a clinically unimportant effect on **diazepam**.[19]

Avoid the concurrent use of **co-proxamol** with other **paracetamol**-containing medicines.

Undesirable effects

More frequent: dizziness, drowsiness, nausea and vomiting.

Less frequent: headache, weakness, euphoria/dysphoria, hallucinations, minor visual disturbances, constipation, abdominal pain, rashes.

Dextropropoxyphene (as a single agent) has also been associated with abnormal LFTs and, more rarely, with reversible jaundice (both hepatocellular and cholestatic). Dextropropoxyphene *napsilate* has been associated with hypoglycaemia.

Subacute painful myopathy has occurred after chronic ingestion of larger-than-recommended doses; doses exceeding 720mg/24h have caused toxic psychoses and seizures.

Dose and use

Worldwide, where available, dextropropoxyphene is marketed as either the *hydrochloride* salt or as *napsilate*. Dextropropoxyphene *napsilate* 100mg is equivalent to dextropropoxyphene *hydrochloride* 65mg, the difference relating to the different molecular weights of the two salts.

In the UK, dextropropoxyphene is available only in combination tablets with **paracetamol** as **co-proxamol**, an unlicensed product. The traditional maximum recommended dose is 2 tablets q.d.s., i.e. 8 tablets/24h. This is an artificial limit; clinically, the dose need be limited only to the total daily dose of **paracetamol** (12 tablets contain 4g).

Co-proxamol (or a comparable combination tablet) is used by palliative care services in some countries, e.g. India, as the Step 2 analgesic of choice.

As with all opioids, patients must be monitored for undesirable effects, particularly nausea and vomiting, and constipation. Depending on individual circumstances, an anti-emetic should be prescribed for regular or p.r.n. use, (see p.225) and a laxative prescribed (see p.38).

Overdose

The advice in Box 5.D is adapted from information on the MHRA website.

Box 5.D Co-proxamol overdose

For an adult, a fatal single dose of co-proxamol may be as little as 10–20 tablets (dextropropoxyphene 325–650mg, paracetamol 3.25 6.5g), particularly if combined with CNS depressants such as alcohol, anxiolytic-sedatives and/or antipsychotic drugs.

Symptoms

Early features reflect the dextropropoxyphene (opioid) content, and include coma, respiratory depression, seizures, and cardiac arrest. These may occur <30min after ingestion, particularly if alcohol has also been ingested.

Cardiac arrhythmias including ventricular tachycardia may occur up to 12h after ingestion, particularly if features of CNS depression are also present.

In less severe cases, pallor, nausea and vomiting may persist for about 24h. Psychotic reactions may occur.

Late features (after 1–3 days) reflect paracetamol-induced hepatocellular damage, and include nausea and vomiting, right subcostal pain and tenderness, followed by jaundice. Loin pain, haematuria and proteinuria after the first 24h strongly suggest the development of renal tubular necrosis and the risk of acute renal failure.

Abnormalities of glucose metabolism and metabolic acidosis may occur. In severe poisoning, hepatic failure may progress to encephalopathy, coma and death.

Management

This should include general symptomatic and supportive measures. Naloxone will reduce the respiratory depression and should be given IV if coma or respiratory depression is present. Consider gastric lavage and/or activated charcoal if the patient presents <1h after ingestion of a potentially toxic amount.

continued

Box 5.D Continued

The ECG should be monitored and hypoxia, electrolyte abnormalities and acid-base disturbance should be corrected.

The need for N-acetylcysteine as treatment for paracetamol intoxication should be determined by measuring the plasma paracetamol concentration at least 4h after ingestion. N-acetylcysteine should be started immediately if it is thought that more than either 150mg/kg body weight or 12g in an adult has been ingested >8h earlier. If risk of liver damage is confirmed by measurement of plasma paracetamol concentration, continue administration of the antidote.

Hepatic and renal failure should be managed conventionally.

Supply

Co-proxamol (generic)

Tablets dextropropoxyphene *hydrochloride* 32.5mg + **paracetamol** 325mg, 28 days @ 2 q.d.s. = £48 (unlicensed, available as a named patient supply from Clinigen; see Appendix 1, Obtaining unlicensed products, p.769).

1 Hawton K *et al.* (2003) Co-proxamol and suicide: a study of national mortality statistics and local non-fatal self poisonings. *British Medical Journal.* **326**: 1006–1008.

2 Hawton K *et al.* (2009) Effect of withdrawal of co-proxamol on prescribing and deaths from drug poisoning in England and Wales: time series analysis. *British Medical Journal.* **338**: b2270.

3 Anonymous (2006) The withdrawal of co-proxamol: alternative analgesics for mild to moderate pain. *MeReC Bulletin.* **16**: 13–16.

4 FDA (2010) FDA recommends against the continued use of propoxyphene,. In: *FDA drug safety communication (issued 19th November 2010).* Available from: www.fda.gov/Drugs/DrugSafety/ucm234338.htm

5 MHRA (2011) (Dextro)propoxyphene new studies confirm cardiac risks. *Drug Safety Update.* **4 (6)**: H1.

6 CHM (2006) Withdrawal of co-proxamol (Distalgesic, Cosalgesic, Dolgesic). *Current Problems in Pharmacovigilance.* **31 (May)**: 11.

7 Ebert B *et al.* (1998) Dextropropoxyphene acts as a noncompetitive N-methyl D-aspartate antagonist. *Journal of Pain and Symptom Management.* **15**: 269–274.

8 Perrier D and Gibaldi M (1972) Influence of first-pass effect on the systemic availability of propoxyphene. *The Journal of Clinical Pharmacology.* **Nov/Dec**: 449–452.

9 Li-Wan-Po A and Zhang W (1997) Systematic overview of co-proxamol to assess analgesic effects of addition of dextropropoxyphene to paracetamol. *British Medical Journal.* **315**: 1565–1571.

10 Collins S *et al.* (1998) Single-dose dextroproxpoxphene in post-operative pain: a quantitative systematic review. *European Journal of Clinical Pharmacology.* **54**: 107–112.

11 Beaver WT (1984) Analgesic efficacy of dextropropoxyphene and dextropropoxyphene-containing combinations: a review. *Human Toxicology.* **3 (suppl)**: 191s–220s.

12 Collins SL *et al.* (1998) Single-dose dextropropoxyphene in post-operative pain: a quantitative systematic review. *European Journal of Clinical Pharmacology.* **54**: 107–112.

13 Crome P *et al.* (1984) Pharmacokinetics of dextropropoxyphene and nordextropropoxyphene in elderly hospital patients after single and multiple doses of distalgesic. Preliminary analysis of results. *Human Toxicology.* **3 (suppl)**: 41s–48s.

14 Twycross RG (1984) Plasma concentrations of dextropropoxyphene and norpropoxyphene. *Human Toxicology.* **3 (suppl)**: 58s–59s.

15 Sykes JV *et al.* (1996) Coproxamol revisited. *Lancet.* **348**: 408.

16 Hanks GW and Forbes K (1998) Co-proxamol is effective in chronic pain. *British Medical Journal.* **316**: 1980.

17 Mercadante S *et al.* (1998) Dextropropoxyphene versus morphine in opioid-naive cancer patients with pain. *Journal of Pain and Symptom Management.* **15**: 76–81.

18 Bergendal L *et al.* (1997) The clinical relevance of the interaction between carbamazepine and dextropropoxyphene in elderly patients in Gothenburg, Sweden. *European Journal of Clinical Pharmacology.* **53**: 203–206.

19 Abernethy D *et al.* (1985) Interaction of propoxyphene with diazepam, alprazolam and lorazepam. *British Journal of Clinical Pharmacology.* **19**: 51–57.

TRAMADOL — BNF 4.7.2

Class: Opioid analgesic.

Indications: Moderate–severe pain.

Contra-indications: Use of MAOIs concurrently or within 14 days, severe renal impairment (creatinine clearance <10mL/min), uncontrolled epilepsy.

Pharmacology

Tramadol is a synthetic centrally-acting analgesic with both non-opioid and opioid properties.[1,2] It is a racemic mixture which stimulates neuronal serotonin release and inhibits the presynaptic re-uptake of both serotonin (mainly mediated via (+) enantiomer) and noradrenaline (norepinephrine; mainly mediated via (−) enantiomer). The agonist effect at the μ-opioid receptor is mediated mainly via the main metabolite (M1).[3,4]

A comparison of opioid receptor site affinities and mono-amine re-uptake inhibition indicates that the analgesic effect of tramadol is the result of synergism between these two mechanisms (Table 5.13 and Table 5.14).[2] In animal models, tramadol also has an anti-inflammatory effect which is independent of PG inhibition.[5]

Although **naloxone** can only partially reverse the effects of tramadol,[3,6] in a series of 11 patients with a tramadol overdose, seven had a good response to **naloxone**, and only one had no response.[7]

Tramadol is converted in the liver mainly via CYP2D6 to O-desmethyltramadol (M1). This is an active metabolite which, in animals, is 6 times more potent than tramadol.[8] Further biotransformation results in many inactive metabolites which are excreted by the kidneys.

Slow metabolizers, who comprise 7–10% of the Caucasian population in Europe, lack CYP2D6.[9,10] Slow metabolizers have a decreased response to tramadol.[11–13]

Tramadol has a negligible antihyperalgesic effect.[14] However, in a short-term experimental pain study in volunteers, when combined with **paracetamol** (a non-opioid with known antihyperalgesic properties), the combination manifested greater analgesia and greater antihyperalgesia, even when the dose of both drugs was halved.[14]

In placebo-controlled trials, tramadol significantly improves neuropathic pain (e.g. diabetic neuropathy, post-herpetic neuralgia, polyneuropathy), with an NNT of 3.8.[15] This is comparable with several anti-epileptics, but not as good as the TCAs (NNT = 2.3, see p.281) Further, **oxycodone** has an NNT of 2.5 in post-herpetic neuralgia[16] and, in an RCT of cancer and non-cancer patients with and without neuropathic pain, tramadol was indistinguishable from **morphine**.[17]

Tramadol is as effective as **codeine** as a cough suppressant.[18] Tramadol causes less constipation and respiratory depression than equi-analgesic doses of **morphine**,[19–21] but more vomiting, dizziness and anorexia than **codeine** and **dihydrocodeine**.[22] In contrast to **morphine**, tramadol reduces the basal pressure in the Sphincter of Oddi (for less than 20min after IM administration) and does not increase the pressure in the common bile duct.[23] Its dependence liability is also considerably less,[21] and it is not a controlled drug in the UK. As with other opioids, physical dependence develops with chronic use.[25]

By injection, tramadol is generally regarded as one tenth as potent as **morphine** (e.g. tramadol 100mg is equivalent to **morphine** 10mg).[26] In fact, various pre- and postoperative studies give a range of potency ratios, from 1:11–1:19,[27,28] suggesting that the figure of 1:10 is more of a 'convenient to remember' ratio than a scientifically precise one. Some of the postoperative studies also suggest that, to produce adequate analgesia, tramadol needs to be administered more frequently than **morphine** over the first few hours (by IV PCA), after which doses become less frequent. The need for the equivalent of a loading dose with tramadol may reflect its different mode of action from **morphine**. A delayed maximum effect has also been reported in an RCT of oral tramadol and **morphine**.[17]

By mouth compared with **morphine**, RCTs indicate a potency ratio of 1:5 and 1:4 respectively (i.e. tramadol 100mg PO = **morphine** 20–25mg).[29,30] However, extensive clinical experience has led many physicians to regard the potency ratio for PO tramadol and PO **morphine** to be 1:10 (i.e. tramadol 100mg PO = **morphine** 10mg PO), i.e. the same as by injection.[31,32]

Bio-availability 65–75% PO; 90% with multiple doses;[33] 77% PR.[34,35]
Onset of action 30min–1h.
Time to peak plasma concentration 2h; 4–8h m/r.
Plasma halflife 6h; active metabolite 7.4h; these more than double in cirrhosis and severe renal failure.
Duration of action 4–9h.

Table 5.13 Opioid receptor affinities: K_i (micromol) values[a,3]

	μ	δ	κ
Morphine	0.0003	0.09	0.6
Dextropropoxyphene	0.03	0.38	1.2
Codeine	0.2	5	6
Tramadol	2	58	43

a. the lower the K_i value, the greater the receptor affinity.

Table 5.14 Inhibition of mono-amine uptake: K_i (micromol) values[a,3]

	Norepinephrine	*Serotonin*
Imipramine	0.0066	0.021
Tramadol	0.78	0.99
Codeine, Dextropropoxyphene, Morphine	IA[b]	IA[b]

a. the lower the Ki value, the greater the receptor affinity
b. IA = inactive at 10micromol.

Cautions

Epilepsy, head trauma or raised intracranial pressure. In severe hepatic impairment or severe renal impairment (creatinine clearance <30mL/min), halve the dose, e.g. by reducing frequency from q.d.s. to q12h.

Tramadol has been associated with seizures, notably when the total daily dose exceeds 400mg or when tramadol is used concurrently with other medications which lower the seizure threshold, e.g. TCAs, SSRIs, antipsychotics, and other opioids.[7,36,37] Seizures have also been reported in patients after rapid IV injection of tramadol. Treat with standard measures, i.e. IV benzodiazepines (see p.132). Resolution generally occurs in <1 day.[7] Fatalities resulting from tramadol-induced seizures are rare.[8]

Serotonin toxicity has occasionally occurred when tramadol has been taken concurrently with a second drug which also interferes with presynaptic serotonin re-uptake (see p.177). Caution is necessary in patients with a history of substance abuse because of the risk of tramadol-dependence in such individuals.[31]

The FDA has warned of an increased risk of suicide in emotionally unstable patients taking tramadol, particularly if they are also taking antidepressants or tranquillizers. As with other opioids, an overdose of tramadol can lead to central nervous system depression, respiratory depression and death.[38]

Drug interactions

The analgesic effect of tramadol is reduced by **ondansetron** (possibly by blocking the action of serotonin at presynaptic $5HT_3$-receptors on primary afferent nociceptive neurones in the spinal dorsal horn).[39] In postoperative pain, the dose of tramadol needed by IV PCA was 2–3 times greater in patients also receiving **ondansetron** 1mg/h by CIVI. There was also an increase in vomiting (despite the **ondansetron**).[40] This is probably a class effect for $5HT_3$ antagonists.

Carbamazepine decreases the effect of tramadol. CYP2D6 inhibitors, e.g. **fluoxetine**, **paroxetine**, **quinidine**, and **ritonavir** inhibit the conversion of tramadol to its active metabolite and may thus decrease analgesia.[41,42] Tramadol occasionally prolongs the INR of patients taking **warfarin**.[43] Monitor the INR closely for 3–4 weeks if tramadol is prescribed for a patient already taking **warfarin**, and adjust the dose if necessary.[41]

Undesirable effects

Very common (>10%): dizziness, nausea, vomiting.
Common (<10%, >1%): headache, drowsiness, fatigue, sweating, dry mouth, constipation.
Rare (<0.1%): seizures (dose-dependent, see Cautions above)
Also see Strong opioids, p.345.

Dose and use

With cancer pain, most patients will already be taking a non-opioid:

- start with 50mg q.d.s. *or* 200mg m/r once daily
- in severe renal impairment (creatinine clearance 10–30mL/min) or severe hepatic impairment, *halve* the starting dose to 50mg q12h *or* 100mg m/r once daily; likewise in very frail patients[1]
- if necessary, increase the dose in stages to a maximum recommended total daily dose of 400mg (less in those with severe renal or hepatic impairment and in very frail patients)
- higher doses have been given, e.g. 600mg/24h, and sometimes more[31,32,44]
- for break-through (episodic) pain when taking m/r tramadol, consider normal-release tramadol or normal-release **morphine** (see p.362).

As with all opioids, patients must be monitored for undesirable effects, particularly nausea and vomiting, and constipation (see Box 5.G, p.349). Depending on individual circumstances, an anti-emetic should be prescribed for regular or p.r.n. use, (see p.225) and, routinely, a laxative prescribed (see p.38).

If tramadol becomes inadequate, the patient will generally be switched to a strong opioid. It has been suggested that the dose of tramadol should be tapered over several days, rather than being stopped abruptly.[2] However, this is not necessary when switching to **morphine** (or other strong opioid); an abrupt switch from tramadol does *not* result in an antidepressant type discontinuation/withdrawal syndrome.[45]

Supply

Tramadol (generic)
Capsules 50mg, 28 days @ 100mg q.d.s. = £6.
Injection 50mg/mL, 2mL amp = £1.

Zamadol® (Meda)
Capsules 50mg, 28 days @ 100mg q.d.s. = £18.
Injection 50mg/mL, 2mL amp = £1.

Zamadol Melt® (Meda)
Orodispersible tablets 50mg, 28 days @ 100mg q.d.s. = £26.

Modified-release
Maxitram® SR (Chiesi)
Capsules m/r 50mg, 100mg, 150mg, 200mg, 28 days @ 200mg b.d. = £23.

Zamadol® SR (Meda)
Capsules m/r 50mg, 100mg, 150mg, 200mg, 28 days @ 200mg b.d. = £28.

Zamadol® 24hr (Meda)
Tablets m/r 150mg, 200mg, 300mg, 400mg, 28 days @ 400mg once daily = £28.

With **paracetamol**
Tramacet® (Grünenthal)
Tablets tramadol hydrochloride 37.5mg, **paracetamol** 325mg, 28 days @ 2 q.d.s. = £36.
Tablets soluble tramadol hydrochloride 37.5mg, **paracetamol** 325mg, 28 days @ 2 q.d.s. = £36.

This is not a complete list; see BNF for more information.

1 Grond S and Sablotzki A (2004) Clinical pharmacology of tramadol. *Clinical Pharmacokinetics*. **43**: 879–923.
2 Dickman A (2007) Tramadol: a review of this atypical opioid. *European Journal of Palliative Care*. **14**: 181–185.
3 Raffa RB *et al*. (1992) Opioid and nonopioid components independently contribute to the mechanism of action of tramadol, an 'atypical' opioid analgesic. *Journal of Pharmacology and Therapeutics*. **260**: 275–285.

4 Raffa RB *et al.* (1993) Complementary and synergistic antinociceptive interaction between enantiomers of tramadol. *Journal of Pharmacology and Experimental Therapeutics.* **267**: 331–340.
5 Buccellati C *et al.* (2000) Tramadol anti-inflammatory activity is not related to a direct inhibitory action on prostaglandin endoperoxide synthases. *European Journal of Pain.* **4**: 413–415.
6 Shipton EA (2000) Tramadol — present and future. *Anaesthesia and Intensive Care.* **28**: 363–374.
7 Marquardt KA *et al.* (2005) Tramadol exposures reported to statewide poison control system. *Annals of Pharmacotherapy.* **39**: 1039–1044.
8 Close BR (2005) Tramadol: does it have a role in emergency medicine? *Emergency Medicine Australasia.* **17**: 73–83.
9 Sachse C *et al.* (1997) Cytochrome P450 2D6 variants in a Caucasian population: allele frequencies and phenotypic consequences. *American Journal of Human Genetics.* **60**: 284–295.
10 Zanger UM *et al.* (2004) Cytochrome P450 2D6: overview and update on pharmacology, genetics, biochemistry. *Naunyn Schmiedebergs Arch Pharmacol.* **369**: 23–37.
11 Stamer UM *et al.* (2003) Impact of CYP2D6 genotype on postoperative tramadol analgesia. *Pain.* **105**: 231–238.
12 Poulsen L *et al.* (1996) The hypoalgesic effect of tramadol in relation to CYP2D6. *Clinical Pharmacology and Therapeutics.* **60**: 636–644.
13 Collart L *et al.* (1993) [Duality of the analgesic effect of tramadol in humans]. *Schweizerische Medizinische Wochenschrift.* **123**: 2241–2243.
14 Filitz J *et al.* (2008) Supra-additive effects of tramadol and acetaminophen in a human pain model. *Pain.* **136**: 262–270.
15 Duehmke RM (2006) tramadol for neuropathic pain. *Cochrane Database of Systematic Reviews.* **3**: CD003726.
16 Watson C and Babul N (1998) Efficacy of oxycodone in neuropathic pain: a randomized trial in postherpetic neuralgia. *Neurology.* **50**: 1837–1841.
17 Leppert W (2001) Analgesic efficacy and side effects of oral tramadol and morphine administered orally in the treatment of cancer pain. *Nowotwory.* **51**: 257–266.
18 Szekely SM and Vickers MD (1992) A comparison of the effects of codeine and tramadol on laryngeal reactivity. *European Journal of Anaesthesiology.* **9**: 111–120.
19 Wilder-Smith C and Bettiga A (1997) The analgesic tramadol has minimal effect on gastrointestinal motor function. *British Journal of Clinical Pharmacology.* **43**: 71–75.
20 Wilder-Smith CH *et al.* (1999) Effect of tramadol and morphine on pain and gastrointestinal motor function in patients with chronic pancreatitis. *Digestive Diseases and Sciences.* **44**: 1107–1116.
21 Houmes R *et al.* (1992) Efficacy and safety of tramadol versus morphine for moderate and severe postoperative pain with special regard to respiratory depression. *Anesthesia and Analgesia.* **74**: 510–514.
22 Rodriguez RF *et al.* (2007) Incidence of weak opioids adverse events in the management of cancer pain: a double-blind comparative trial. *Journal of Palliative Medicine.* **10**: 56–60.
23 Wu SD *et al.* (2004) Effects of narcotic analgesic drugs on human Oddi's sphincter motility. *World Journal of Gastroenterology.* **10**: 2901–2904.
24 Preston K *et al.* (1991) Abuse potential and pharmacological comparison of tramadol and morphine. *Drug and Alcohol Dependency.* **27**: 7–18.
25 Soyka M *et al.* (2004) Tramadol use and dependence in chronic noncancer pain patients. *Pharmacopsychiatry.* **37**: 191–192.
26 Vickers M *et al.* (1992) Tramadol: pain relief by an opioid without depression of respiration. *Anaesthesia.* **47**: 291–296.
27 Naguib M *et al.* (1998) Perioperative antinociceptive effects of tramadol. A prospective, randomized, double-blind comparison with morphine. *Canadian Journal of Anaesthesia.* **45**: 1168–1175.
28 Pang WW *et al.* (1999) Comparison of patient-controlled analgesia (PCA) with tramadol or morphine. *Canadian Journal of Anaesthesia.* **46**: 1030–1035.
29 Wilder-Smith CH *et al.* (1994) Oral tramadol, a mu-opioid agonist and monoamine reuptake-blocker, and morphine for strong cancer-related pain. *Annals of Oncology.* **5**: 141–146.
30 Tawfik MO *et al.* (1990) Tramadol hydrochloride in the relief of cancer pain: a double blind comparison against sustained release morphine. *Pain.* **(suppl 5)**: S377.
31 Leppert W and Luczak J (2005) The role of tramadol in cancer pain treatment–a review. *Supportive Care in Cancer.* **13**: 5–17.
32 Grond S *et al.* (1999) High-dose tramadol in comparison to low-dose morphine for cancer pain relief. *Journal of Pain and Symptom Management.* **18**: 174–179.
33 Gibson T (1996) Pharmacokinetics, efficacy, and safety of analgesia with a focus on tramadol HCl. *American Journal of Medicine.* **101 (suppl 1A)**: 47s–53s.
34 Mercadante S *et al.* (2005) Randomized double-blind, double-dummy crossover clinical trial of oral tramadol versus rectal tramadol administration in opioid-naive cancer patients with pain. *Supportive Care in Cancer.* **13**: 702–707.
35 Lintz W *et al.* (1998) Pharmacokinetics of tramadol and bioavailability of enteral tramadol formulations. 3rd Communication: suppositories. *Arzneimittelforschung.* **48**: 889–899.
36 Boyd IW (2005) Tramadol and seizures. *Medical Journal of Australia.* **182**: 595–596.
37 Spiller HA *et al.* (1997) Prospective multicenter evaluation of tramadol exposure. *Journal of Toxicology and Clinical Toxicology.* **35**: 361–364.
38 FDA (2010) Safety alerts for human medical products Ultram (tramadol hydrochloride), Ultracet (tramadol hydrochloride/acetaminophen). Available from: www.fda.gov/Safety/MedWatch/SafetyInformation/SafetyAlertsforHumanMedicalProducts/ucm213264.htm (accessed 10th Aug 2010)
39 De Witte JL *et al.* (2001) The analgesic efficacy of tramadol is impaired by concurrent administration of ondansetron. *Anesthesia and Analgesia.* **92**: 1319–1321.
40 Arcioni R *et al.* (2002) Ondansetron inhibits the analgesic effects of tramadol: a possible 5-HT(3) spinal receptor involvement in acute pain in humans. *Anesthesia and Analgesia.* **94**: 1553–1557.
41 Baxter K (2011) Stockley's Drug Interactions (online edition). Pharmaceutical Press, London. Available from: www.medicinescomplete.com
42 Laugesen S *et al.* (2005) Paroxetine, a cytochrome P450 2D6 inhibitor, diminishes the stereoselective O-demethylation and reduces the hypoalgesic effect of tramadol. *Clinical Pharmacology and Therapeutics.* **77**: 312–323.
43 Sabbe JR *et al.* (1998) Tramadol-warfarin interaction. *Pharmacotherapy.* **18**: 871–873.
44 Osipova N *et al.* (1991) Analgesic effect of tramadol in cancer patients with chronic pain: A comparison with prolonged-action morphine sulfate. *Current Therapeutic Research.* **50**: 812–815.
45 Leppert W (2008) *Personal communication.*

STRONG OPIOIDS

Strong opioids are essential drugs in palliative care; their use should be dictated by therapeutic need and response, not by brevity of prognosis.[1,2]

Contra-indications: Provided the dose of an opioid is carefully titrated against the patient's pain, there are generally no absolute contra-indications to the use of strong opioids in palliative care. However, there are circumstances, e.g. renal impairment, when it may be better to avoid the use of certain opioids and/or positively choose certain other ones (see p.355; also see Guidance about prescribing in palliative care, p.605).

Chemical classes

Opioids can be divided into four chemical classes (Table 5.15). Knowledge of the different chemical classes is of value when dealing with cases of intolerance (i.e. unacceptable undesirable effects) to a particular opioid, e.g. cutaneous histamine release causing a rash and pruritus. However, in many situations switching from one phenanthrene to another phenanthrene is satisfactory, e.g. neurotoxicity (see p.352).

Table 5.15 Chemical classification of opioids

Phenanthrenes	*Benzomorphans*	*Phenylpiperidines*	*Diphenylheptanes*
Codeine	Diphenoxylate	Fentanils	Dextropropoxyphene
Dextromethorphan	Loperamide	Pethidine[a]	Methadone
Dihydrocodeine	Pentazocine[a]		
Hydrocodone			
Tramadol			
Morphine			
Diamorphine			
Buprenorphine			
Hydromorphone			
Oxycodone			
Oxymorphone			
Tapentadol			

a. *not* recommended for use in palliative care.

Opioid receptors

There are four opioid receptors (μ, κ, δ, and ORL-1) distributed in varying densities throughout the body, particularly in nervous tissue. Their naturally-occurring ligands are peptides, and together they contribute to various physiological functions including the modulation of pain, hormones and the immune system (Table 5.16).[3,4]

In nervous tissue, the peptides function as neural transmitters. Like other peptides, they are synthesized as large inactive precursors in the neuronal cell body, and are then cleaved while being transported to the nerve terminals. The active fragment is released into the synapse and binds to one or more receptors.

Opioid receptors are found both pre- and post-synaptically, with the former predominating. Generally, opioid receptor agonists lead to an inhibitory effect. Pre-synaptic receptor activation controls the release of several neurotransmitters. Endogenous peptides are rapidly degraded, and have a relatively short duration of action. In contrast, exogenous opioids such as **morphine** have a prolonged effect. They produce analgesia primarily by interacting with μ-opioid receptors in the CNS.

In the presence of local inflammation, opioids also have a peripheral analgesic action because inflammation activates otherwise dormant opioid receptors in the peripheral nerve terminals.

Undesirable effects relate to both central and peripheral receptors, mainly in the CNS and GI tract.

Table 5.16 Opioid receptors, ligands,[9,10] and effects[a]

Receptors	*Mu* (μ)	*Delta* (δ)	*Kappa* (κ)	*ORL-1*
Endogenous opioid	β-Endorphin Endormorphins	Enkephalins	Dynorphins	Nociceptin
Exogenous agonist	Morphine Buprenorphine[b] Codeine Dextropropoxphene Dihydrocodeine Fentanils Hydromorphone Methadone Oxycodone Pethidine Tapentadol Tramadol	DSTBULET Methadone (?)	U50488H Oxycodone (?)	Buprenorphine
Antagonists	Naloxone Naltrexone	Buprenorphine Naloxone	Buprenorphine Naloxone	
Effector mechanism	G protein opens K^+ channel	G protein opens K^+ channel	G protein closes Ca^{++} channel	G protein opens K^+ channel
Effects[c]	*Hyperpolarization of neurons, inhibition of neurotransmitter release*			
	Analgesia Euphoria Nausea Constipation Cough suppression Dependence Respiratory depression Miosis	Similar to μ but less marked	Analgesia Aversion Diuresis	Mixed analgesia (spinal) and anti-opioid (brain)

a. also see individual drug monographs
b. partial agonist
c. not an exhaustive list; other roles include hormone and immune system.

All clinically important opioid analgesics act as agonists at the μ-opioid receptor (Table 5.16), and some may also have significant effects on δ-opioid receptors (e.g. **methadone**, see p.416) and κ-opioid receptors (e.g. **oxycodone**, see p.424). Some opioids are mixed agonist-antagonists (e.g. **buprenorphine** is a partial μ *agonist*, an opioid-receptor-like (ORL-1) *agonist*, and a κ and δ *antagonist*.)[5–8]

Some opioids also possess non-opioid activity. Thus, **methadone** blocks the pre-synaptic re-uptake of serotonin and the NMDA-receptor-channel (see p.416), **tapentadol** blocks re-uptake of noradrenaline (norepinephrine; see below), and **tramadol** (a weak opioid) blocks re-uptake of both serotonin and noradrenaline (see p.340).

Clinical use

Morphine is the strong opioid of choice for cancer pain management (see p.362).[11–13] Other strong opioids are used mainly when:

- **morphine** is not readily available
- the TD route is preferable
- the patient has unacceptable undesirable effects with **morphine**.[14]

Differences in receptor affinity (Table 5.16) may partly explain why some patients report better pain relief after switching opioids (see p.354). Similarly, the pattern and severity of undesirable effects may be altered, e.g. when switching from **morphine** to **oxycodone** (see p.424) or TD **fentanyl** (see p.390).

Both **methadone** (see p.416) and **tapentadol** have opioid and non-opioid effects which, in the case of **tapentadol**, are analgesically synergistic (Box 5.E). The potential role of **tapentadol** in palliative care is currently uncertain, although studies in cancer pain are underway.

Box 5.E Tapentadol

Tapentadol is a centrally-acting analgesic which is both a μ agonist and an inhibitor of synaptic re-uptake of noradrenaline (norepinephrine).[15–17] It is authorized for use in both moderate–severe acute and severe chronic pain.

Tapentadol is relatively expensive, comparable in cost to m/r oxycodone. Thus, at present, its use is best restricted to patients who fail to get satisfactory analgesia from, for example, morphine ± an NSAID.

By mouth, it is some 5 times *less* potent than oxycodone (i.e. tapentadol 50mg is approximately equivalent to oxycodone 10mg). By extrapolation, this suggests that it is about 3 times *less* potent than morphine (i.e. tapentadol 50mg is approximately equivalent to morphine 15–20mg).

RCTs have been conducted in both acute (e.g. postoperative orthopaedic)[18] and chronic pain (e.g. osteo-arthritis, low back pain, diabetic neuropathy).[19,20] These have shown tapentadol to be superior to placebo and/or non-inferior to oxycodone. An RCT in cancer pain is underway.

Tapentadol is mainly metabolized in the liver by glucuronidation, independent of CYP450, thus reducing the likelihood of pharmacokinetic drug–drug interactions. It has no active metabolites.

Undesirable GI effects are significantly less than with oxycodone (less nausea, vomiting, constipation). In chronic pain studies, withdrawals were about 40% for tapentadol vs. 60% for oxycodone.[20]

Switching from another μ agonist (e.g. morphine, oxycodone) to tapentadol may cause low-grade opioid withdrawal, and p.r.n. doses of the original opioid should be used to counter this (e.g. give a normal-release formulation at 1/4–1/2 of the original dose).

The absence of an impact on serotonin re-uptake means that there should be no risk of tapentadol precipitating serotonin toxicity.

Strong opioids are not the panacea for cancer pain; effective analgesia generally requires the use of both a strong opioid and a non-opioid. Further, even combined use does not guarantee success, particularly with neuropathic pain or if the psychosocial dimension of suffering is ignored. Other reasons for poor relief include:

- underdosing (failure to titrate the dose upwards or dose at the correct interval)
- poor patient adherence (patient not taking medication)
- poor alimentary absorption, e.g. because of vomiting.

Pentazocine should *not* be used; it is a weak opioid by mouth,[21,22] and often causes psychotomimetic effects (dysphoria, depersonalization, frightening dreams, hallucinations).[23] **Pethidine** also should *not* be used (Box 5.F).

Box 5.F Pethidine

The use of pethidine is actively discouraged in palliative care.

Pethidine is a synthetic μ agonist. In typical doses PO it is little more than a weak opioid (see Table 5.18, p.355). It has a relatively short duration of action (2–3h) and is thus a bad choice for round-the-clock analgesia.

Pethidine has a toxic metabolite, norpethidine, which accumulates when pethidine is given regularly. Particularly in renal impairment, norpethidine causes tremors, multifocal myoclonus, agitation, and occasionally seizures.[24]

Pethidine:

- is not antitussive
- is less constipating than morphine but causes more vomiting
- causes less smooth muscle spasm (e.g. sphincter of Oddi)
- is antimuscarinic (anticholinergic)
- does not cause constriction of the pupils.[25]

Drug-drug interaction with:

phenobarbital } increase production of norpethidine.
chlorpromazine }
MAOIs

Serotonin toxicity

Pethidine must not be given concurrently with an MAOI because of the risk of serotonin toxicity (see p.177).[26–28]

Overdose and effect of naloxone

Overdose is a mixed picture of CNS depression (pethidine) and excitation (norpethidine), with both stupor and seizures.

Naloxone will reverse the pethidine-induced stupor but not the stimulant effects of norpethidine. Seizures should be treated with a benzodiazepine (see p.132).

Undesirable effects

Strong opioids tend to cause the same undesirable effects (Box 5.G), although to a varying degree. Strategies are necessary to deal with the undesirable effects of **morphine** and other strong opioids, particularly nausea and vomiting (see p.225), and constipation (see p.38).[29]

Respiratory depression

Pain is a physiological antagonist to the central depressant effects of opioids.

When appropriately titrated against the patient's pain, strong opioids do not cause clinically important respiratory depression in patients in pain.[30–32] Strong opioids also relieve moderate-severe breathlessness at rest at doses which do not cause respiratory depression (see p.368).

Box 5.G Undesirable effects of opioids when used for analgesia

Common initial
Nausea and vomiting[a]
Drowsiness
Lightheadedness/unsteadiness
Delirium (acute confusional state)

Common ongoing
Constipation
Nausea and vomiting[a]
Dry mouth

Possible ongoing
Suppression of hypothalamic-pituitary axis
Suppression of immune system

Less common
Neurotoxicity:
- hyperalgesia
- allodynia
- myoclonus
- cognitive failure/delirium
- hallucinations

Sweating
Urinary retention
Postural hypotension
Spasm of the sphincter of Oddi
Pruritus

Rare
Respiratory depression
Psychological dependence

a. generally, opioid-related nausea and vomiting is transient and improves after 5–7 days; if persistent despite an anti-emetic (see p.225), consider other possible causes before switching to another opioid (see p.354).

Naloxone, a specific opioid antagonist, is rarely needed in palliative care (see p.435). In contrast to postoperative patients, cancer patients with pain:

- have generally been receiving a weak opioid for some time, i.e. are not opioid-naïve
- take medication PO (slower absorption, lower peak concentration)
- titrate the dose upwards step by step (less likelihood of an excessive dose being given).

The relationship of the therapeutic dose to the lethal dose of a strong opioid (the therapeutic ratio) is greater than commonly supposed. For example, patients who take a double dose of **morphine** at bedtime are no more likely to die during the night than those who do not.[33]

The *belief* that the lethal dose of **morphine** is the weight of the patient in kg given as mg of **morphine** is *false*, and, in any case, is irrelevant to palliative care practice. Patients receiving an individually titrated dose of PO **morphine** on a regular basis to relieve pain are not the same physiologically as people without pain who receive *de novo* **morphine** 40–80mg by injection.

Tolerance and dependence

Generally, tolerance to strong opioids is not a practical problem.[34,35] Psychological dependence (addiction) to **morphine** is rare in patients.[32,36,37] Caution in this respect should be reserved for patients with a present or past history of substance abuse (Box 5.H); but even then strong opioids should be used when there is clinical need.[38,39] Physical dependence does not prevent a reduction in the dose if the patient's pain ameliorates, e.g. as a result of radiotherapy or nerve block.[40]

Opioid-induced pruritus

Pruritus occurs in about 1% of those who receive an opioid agonist systemically but in ≤80% of patients who receive spinal opioids. The incidence depends on which opioid is used and whether the patient is opioid-naïve.[42,43] After spinal injection, pruritus spreads rostrally through the thorax from the level of the injection and is characteristically maximal in the face and, in some patients, limited just to the nose.[44]

Except in cases of true allergy, pruritus induced by clinical doses of opioids administered spinally or systemically is *not* caused by histamine release from mast cells in the skin. *In vitro* studies indicate that the dose of **morphine** or **methadone** needed to release histamine from mast cells is some 10,000 times greater than the dose needed for μ agonist effects.[45] Thus, a central opioid receptor-mediated mechanism is the likely cause for generalized pruritus associated with spinal or systemic opioids.[44,46] This explains why the pruritus can respond to **naloxone** but not to an antihistamine (see p.688).

Box 5.H Example of a contract for controlled substance prescriptions with addicts[a]

Controlled substance medications (narcotics, tranquillizers and barbiturates) are very useful, but have high potential for misuse and are therefore closely controlled by the local, state, and federal government. They are intended to relieve pain, to improve function and/or ability to work, not simply to feel good. Because my physician is prescribing such medication for me to help manage my condition, I agree to the following conditions

1 I am responsible for my controlled substance medications. If the prescription of medication is lost, misplaced, or stolen, or if I use it up sooner than prescribed, I understand that it will not be replaced.

2 I will not request or accept controlled substance medication from any other physicians or individual while I am receiving such medication from Dr.________________. Besides being illegal to do so, it may endanger my health. The only exception is if it is prescribed while I am admitted in a hospital.

3 Refills of controlled substance medication:
- Will be made only during Dr.__________________ regular office hours, in person, once each month during a scheduled office visit. Refills will not be made at night, on holidays, or weekends.
- Will not be made if I "run out early". I am responsible for taking the medication in the dose prescribed and for keeping track of the amount remaining.
- Will not be made as an "emergency", such as on Friday afternoon because I suddenly realize I will "run out tomorrow". I will call at least seventy-two hours ahead if I need assistance with a controlled substance medication prescription.

4 I will bring in the containers of all medications prescribed by Dr. ________________ each time I see him even if there is no medication remaining. These will be in the original containers from the pharmacy for each medication.

5 I understand that if I violate any of the above conditions, my controlled substances prescription and/or treatment with Dr.________________ may be ended immediately. If the violation involves obtaining controlled substances from another individual, as described above, I may also be reported to my physician, medical facilities, and other authorities.

6 I understand that the main treatment goal is to improve my ability to function and/or work. In consideration of that goal and the fact that I am being given potent medication to help me reach that goal, I agree to help myself by the following better health habits: exercise, weight control, and the non-use of tobacco and alcohol. I understand that only through following a healthier life-style can I hope to have the most successful outcome to my treatment.

I have been fully informed by Dr._____________ and his staff regarding psychological dependence (addiction) of a controlled substance, which I understand is rare. I know that some persons may develop a tolerance, which is the need to increase the dose of the medication to achieve the same effect of pain control, and I do know that I will become physically dependent on the medication. This will occur if I am on the medication for several weeks, and, when I stop the medication, I must do so slowly and under medical supervision or I may have withdrawal symptoms.

I have read this contract and it has been explained to my by Dr.________________ and/or his staff. In addition, I fully understand the consequences of violating said contract.

____________________	_______	_________________	_______
Patient's Signature	Date	Witness	Date

a. reproduced with permission from Hansen 1999.[41] ©Southern Medical Association.

Other neurotransmitter systems interact with the opioid system in relation to the mediation of pruritus, notably the serotonin system, and this possibly explains why **ondansetron**, a specific $5HT_3$-receptor antagonist, relieves pruritus caused by spinal **morphine** (see p.688).

Opioid-induced pruritus is uncommon in palliative care; few patients receive spinal opioids and those who do are not opioid-naïve. Further, such patients almost always receive **bupivacaine** concurrently, and this tends to restrict pruritus to just the face.

When pruritus is induced by a systemic opioid, options include a trial of a H_1-antihistamine, switching the opioid and **ondansetron** (see Table 5.30, p.432).

Opioid-related serotonin toxicity

Serotonin toxicity results from the ingestion of drug(s) which increase brain serotonin above a critical level (see p.177).[47] Toxicity manifests as a triad of neuro-excitatory features:

- *autonomic hyperactivity*; sweating, fever, mydriasis, tachycardia, hypertension, tachypnea, sialorrhoea, diarrhoea
- *neuromuscular hyperactivity*; tremor, clonus, myoclonus, hyperreflexia, and pyramidal rigidity (advanced stage)
- *altered mental status*; agitation, hypomania, and delirium (advanced stage).

Clonus (inducible, spontaneous or ocular), agitation, sweating, tremor and hyperreflexia are essential features. Spontaneous clonus, in the presence of a serotoninergic drug, is the most reliable indicator of serotonin toxicity.[48]

Opioids are relatively weak serotonin re-uptake inhibitors and only cause symptoms in higher doses or susceptible individuals, or when used concurrently with a second drug with serotoninergic potency, notably an MAOI but also with many other antidepressants and some psychostimulants (see Box 4.F, p.177).

Fatalities from serotonin toxicity have occurred with **dextromethorphan**, **pethidine** (see Box 5.F, p.348), **tramadol**, and possibly **fentanyl**.[49] Non-fatal serotonin toxicity has also been observed with other **fentanils**, **dextropropoxyphene**, **methadone**, and **pentazocine**. It has *not* been observed with other opioids, and the 'blanket' warning against the concurrent use of an MAOI and other opioids is misplaced (Box 5.I).

Box 5.I A misleading report about morphine and MAOIs[50]

A patient who regularly took an MAOI and trifluoperazine 20mg/24h was given pre-operative promethazine 50mg IM and morphine 1mg IV followed by two doses of morphine 2.5mg IV. About 3min later she became unresponsive and hypotensive (systolic pressure 40mmHg); responding within 2min to IV naloxone.

Although repeatedly referenced as such, this was *not* MAOI-related serotonin toxicity; it was a hypotensive response to IV morphine in someone chronically taking trifluoperazine, an α antagonist.

The onset of toxicity is generally rapid and progressive, typically as the second drug reaches effective blood levels (one or two doses). Occasionally, recurrent mild symptoms may occur for weeks before the development of severe toxicity. The patient is often alert or agitated, with tremor (sometimes severe), myoclonus and hyperreflexia. Ankle clonus is generally demonstrable or, in severe toxicity, occurs spontaneously. Neuromuscular signs are initially greater in the lower limbs, then become more generalized as toxicity increases. Other symptoms include shaking, shivering (often including chattering of the teeth), and sometimes trismus. Pyramidal rigidity is a late development in severe cases, and can impair respiration. Rigidity, a fever of $>38.5°C$ or deteriorating blood gases indicate life-threatening toxicity.

Opioids and hypothalamic-pituitary function

Chronic administration of opioids can interfere with hypothalamic-pituitary function:

- inhibition of hypothalamic gonadotrophin-releasing hormone from the hypothalamus:
  - ▹ ↓ luteinizing hormone (LH) release from the pituitary → ↓ production of testosterone (testes) or oestrogen (ovaries)
  - ▹ ↓ follicle-stimulating hormone (FSH) release from the pituitary → ↓ production of sperm or ovarian follicles
  - ▹ associated with loss of libido, impotence, irregular menses or amenorrhoea, subfertility and other consequences of hypogonadism, e.g. reduced muscle mass, osteoporosis
- inhibition of adrenocorticotrophic hormone (ACTH) from the pituitary:
  - ▹ ↓ cortisol production and release (adrenals)
  - ▹ associated with symptoms such as fatigue, weight loss, anorexia, vomiting, diarrhoea, abdominal pain, hypoglycaemia, hypotension
- inhibition of growth hormone from the pituitary:
  - ▹ associated with decreased exercise tolerance, decreased mood and general wellbeing, reduced bone remodelling activity, altered body fat distribution (increased central adiposity), hyperlipidaemia and increased predisposition to atherogenesis.[51]

In patients with chronic non-cancer pain, hormone suppression is evident after 1 week of opioid administration and appears dose-related; in one study, abnormally low levels of sex hormones were found in three quarters of men receiving opioids by mouth equivalent to <150mg **morphine**/24h, and in all receiving >150mg/24h.[52]

IT **morphine** (mean doses 5–12mg/24h) produced hypogonadism in most subjects, both men and women.[53–55] In one study, one third of patients also developed hypocortisolism ± growth hormone deficiency, leading to an Addisonian crisis in one patient.[53] Thus, in patients due to receive long-term IT opioids, it is recommended to measure sex hormone levels at baseline, and annually thereafter (see Table 21.5, p.686).

However, when any patient receiving long-term opioids for non-cancer pain has symptoms suggestive of hypothalamic dysfunction, it may be necessary to refer to an endocrinologist for investigation and possible replacement hormone therapy.[53]

Compared with **morphine** and other opioids, **buprenorphine** appears less likely to suppress the gonadal axis or testosterone levels (see p.381).

Opioids and immune function

Opioids modulate immune cell function directly and indirectly via activation of the hypothalamic-pituitary-adrenal axis (HPA) and the autonomic nervous system. Lymphocytes and mononuclear phagocytes express μ-, κ- and δ-opioid receptors, which when activated trigger cellular apoptosis. Immune function is suppressed by the opioid-induced release of glucocorticoids and catecholamines (e.g. adrenaline (epinephrine), noradrenaline (norepinephrine) and dopamine) from the adrenal medulla and the release of catecholamines from sympathetic nerve fibres which innervate lymphoid tissue (e.g. lymph nodes, spleen).[56] Thus, **morphine** depresses natural killer cell activity, T-lymphocyte proliferation, monocyte/macrophage function and cytokine function (e.g. interleukin (IL)-2, interferon (IFN)-γ), potentially reducing host resistance to bacterial, fungal and viral infections.[57–59] Further, partly through its effects on the immune system, **morphine** can influence cancer cell growth and metastasis. However, it is unclear if the overall effect is beneficial or deleterious.[60]

Compared with **morphine** (and **diamorphine**), other opioids are less immunosuppressive and **buprenorphine**, **hydromorphone**, **methadone**, **oxycodone**, **oxymorphone** and **tramadol** have little or no effect.[61–64]

The clinical implications of these effects are uncertain.[60,64,65] However, they may help to explain the increased susceptibility to infection seen in opioid abusers.[66] On the other hand, because pain is immunosuppressive, opioid analgesia may improve immune function in patients with pain.[67]

Opioid-induced hyperalgesia

Opioid-induced hyperalgesia (OIH) appears important in both acute and chronic pain. Although poorly understood, it appears to result from sustained sensitization of the nervous system in which the excitatory amino acid neurotransmitter system and the NMDA-receptor-channel complex play important roles.[68,69] Possible causes include:

- opioid-induced activation of glial cells, which play a role in inflammation, pain signal transmission, pain hypersensitivity and opioid tolerance[70–72]
- alteration in the G protein coupling of opioid receptors, i.e. G_s rather than $G_{i/o}$; the G_s variant has an excitatory rather than an inhibitory effect[73]
- in the case of **morphine**, accumulation of M3G.[74]

Genetic make-up probably plays an important part in its development.

Clinical features

In surgical pain, OIH may contribute to exaggerated levels of pain in the immediate postoperative period and the development of a chronic pain state. In patients with cancer, OIH may manifest in various ways:

- rapidly developing tolerance to opioids
- short-lived benefit from increased doses
- a change of pain pattern (Table 5.17).

Table 5.17 Opioid-induced hyperalgesia.[75]

What the patient says	*What the doctor finds*
Increased sensitivity to pain stimulus (hyperalgesia)	Any dose of any opioid, but particularly with high-dose morphine or hydromorphone, and in renal failure
Worsening pain despite increasing doses of opioids	Pain elicited from ordinary non-painful stimuli, e.g. stroking skin with cotton (allodynia)
Pain which becomes more diffuse, extending beyond the distribution of the pre-existing pain	Presence of other manifestations of opioid-induced neural hyperexcitability: myoclonus, seizures, delirium

The extreme upper end of the spectrum may be those patients who manifest evidence of severe neural hyperexcitability (myoclonus, allodynia, and/or hyperalgesia), particularly when taking high doses of **morphine** or an alternative strong opioid. This may be accompanied by sedation and delirium (when it is often described as opioid neurotoxicity). However, OIH:

- is *not* limited to very high doses, or to any one opioid
- is probably under-diagnosed
- is more common than generally thought.

Severe pain which does not respond to increasing doses of opioids, or is complicated by severe undesirable effects, should raise the *possibility* of OIH.[75]

Evaluation

A diagnosis of OIH is generally made on the basis of a high level of clinical suspicion, probability, and pattern recognition. OIH must be differentiated from increased pain caused by disease progression or the development of opioid tolerance, both of which may be managed by increasing the opioid dose.

Management

Management is based largely on theoretical grounds and clinical observation.

Prophylaxis

Use a multimodal approach to analgesia, e.g.:

- an NSAID may help to reduce the production of excitatory amino acid neurotransmitters which activate the pronociceptive and anti-opioid systems
- **gabapentin** may block calcium channels which may contribute to hyperalgesia in nerve pain.

Treatment

- progressively and rapidly reduce the dose of the causal opioid to about 25% of the peak dose
- switch to an opioid with less risk of OIH, i.e. **fentanyl** (highest) → **morphine** → **methadone** → **buprenorphine** (lowest)[76]
- (rarely) if occurring at very low doses (< 10mg/24h), discontinue the opioid completely

- use a multimodal approach to analgesia, i.e. use non-opioids, e.g. **paracetamol** or an NSAID, and adjuvant analgesics, e.g. **gabapentin**
- start oral or parenteral **ketamine** (an NMDA-receptor-channel blocker).[77]

Note that when switching from **morphine** because of severe neural hyperexcitability, a lower than expected dose of the alternative opioid is likely to be needed unless the dose of **morphine** has been much reduced (as suggested above).[78,79] If these steps do not lead to a resolution of the OIH:

- consider spinal, regional or local analgesia (with local anaesthetics), and tail off systemic opioids completely
- check for hypomagnesaemia because this can aggravate OIH.[80,81]
- consider treatment with ultralow doses of an opioid antagonist.[82–84]

Opioid switching ('rotation')

It is crucial to appreciate that conversion ratios are *never* more than an approximate guide. Thus, careful monitoring during conversion is necessary to avoid both underdosing and excessive dosing.

Generally, switching from **morphine** (or other strong opioid) to an alternative is undertaken in an attempt to improve analgesia and/or reduce undesirable effects. Before switching, it is worth considering if other options may be more appropriate, e.g. the use of adjuvant analgesics or modifying the management of the undesirable effects.

Switching, is necessary in about 20% of patients according to one prospective survey.[85] Changes from **morphine** to TD **fentanyl** (or vice versa) are included in this figure. Higher figures have been published elsewhere, e.g. 44%.[86] The lower figure better reflects clinical experience in the UK.[87] Examples of when switching may be appropriate include:

- poor adherence (→ TD **fentanyl**)
- poor response to **morphine** plus an NSAID (→ **methadone**)[88]
- intolerable undesirable effects, e.g. *intractable* constipation (→ TD **fentanyl**)
- significant decline in the patient's renal function (**morphine** → **methadone**, TD **fentanyl** or **hydromorphone**)
- opioid-induced hyperalgesia or other manifestations of neurotoxicity, e.g. cognitive failure/ delirium, hallucinations, myoclonus, allodynia.

In cases of neurotoxicity, **hydromorphone**, **oxycodone** and **methadone** have all been substituted successfully for **morphine**.[89–91] Similarly, in the presence of inadequate pain relief and intolerable undesirable effects, TD **buprenorphine** has been substituted successfully for TD **fentanyl**, and vice versa.[92]

When converting from **morphine** to an alternative strong opioid, or vice versa, the initial dose depends on the relative potency of the two drugs (Table 5.18). (Also see Opioid dose conversion ratios, p.625). However, potency and thus conversion ratios are *never* more than an approximate guide because of:[94–97]

- wide interindividual variation in opioid pharmacokinetics; influencing factors include age, ethnicity, renal or hepatic impairment
- other variables including dose and duration of opioid treatment, direction of switch in opioid, nutritional status and concurrent medications
- their method of derivation, e.g. single dose rather than chronic dose studies, using typical doses.

Thus, careful monitoring during conversion is necessary to avoid both underdosing and excessive dosing.

Providing explicit guidance on switching opioids is difficult because the reasons for switching are varied, as are the patient's circumstances. One guideline, based on expert consensus, recommends routinely reducing the calculated equivalent dose of the new opioid by 25–50%[98] Various patient factors are then taken into account to modify the reduction, which potentially could see it removed (e.g. young patient, no undesirable effects, in severe pain, switching at low dose) or increased further (e.g. older patient, delirious, in moderate pain, switching at high dose).

Certainly, a dose reduction of at least 50% would seem prudent when switching at high doses (e.g. **morphine** or equivalent doses of ≥1g/24h), in elderly or frail patients, because of intolerable undesirable effects (e.g. delirium), or when there has been a recent rapid escalation of

Table 5.18 Approximate PO opioid potency ratios (morphine = 1)[a]

Analgesic	*Potency ratio with morphine*	*Duration of action (h)*[b]
Codeine Dihydrocodeine Dextropropoxyphene	1/10	3–6
Tramadol	1/10	4–6
Pethidine	1/8	2–4
Hydrocodone (not UK)	2/3	4–8
Papaveretum	2/3[c]	3–5
Oxycodone	1.5 (2)[d]	3–4
Methadone	5–10[e]	8–12
Hydromorphone	4–5 (5–7.5)[d]	4–5
Buprenorphine (SL)	80	6–8
Buprenorphine (TD)	100 (75–115)[d]	Formulation dependent
Fentanyl (TD)	100 (150)[d]	72

a. multiply dose of opioid by its potency ratio to determine the equivalent dose of morphine sulphate/hydrochloride; conversely, divide morphine dose by the appropriate potency ratio to determine the equivalent dose of another opioid
b. dependent in part on severity of pain and on dose; often longer lasting in very elderly and those with renal impairment
c. papaveretum (strong opium) is standardized to contain 50% morphine base; potency expressed in relation to morphine sulphate
d. the numbers in parenthesis are the manufacturers' preferred ratios; for explanation of divergence, (see individual drug monographs)
e. a single 5mg dose of methadone is equivalent to morphine 7.5mg, but a variable long plasma halflife and broad-spectrum receptor affinity result in a much higher than expected potency ratio when administered regularly, sometimes much higher than the range given above (see p.416).[78,93]

the first opioid (possibly due to opioid-induced hyperalgesia).[99] In such circumstances, p.r.n. doses can be relied on to make up any deficit while re-titrating to a satisfactory dose of the new opioid.

A separate strategy is necessary for **methadone** (see p.416).

Combining opioids

It is generally considered to be bad practice to prescribe two or more opioids for simultaneous use. Thus, for example, regular **morphine** is best backed up by p.r.n **morphine** for break-through (episodic) pain. However, there are circumstances when the p.r.n. opioid differs from the regular opioid, for example TD **fentanyl** backed up by p.r.n. **morphine** (see p.398). Also, someone with good pain relief from a regular weak opioid may have a supply of **morphine** for back-up use in case of severe break-through (episodic) pain.

However, there are reports of two strong opioids being used successfully in combination, i.e. providing better pain relief at relatively lower doses and reduced undesirable effects.[100–102] For example, in one, regular **oxycodone** plus p.r.n. **morphine** was more beneficial than regular **morphine** plus p.r.n. **morphine**.[100] In another, patients on regular morphine benefited from the addition of a second regular opioid in low dose (either **methadone** or TD **fentanyl**).[101] Nonetheless, the quality of this evidence is low or very low[103] and despite such reports, patients should *not* normally have two opioids prescribed concurrently on a regular basis.[104,105]

Opioids in renal impairment and end-stage renal failure

In renal impairment and end-stage renal failure, regardless of the opioid used, extra caution is *always* required whether or not the patient is on dialysis. This is particularly necessary in patients with rapidly deteriorating renal function or when acutely unwell, e.g. because of sepsis.

Clear written instructions regarding analgesic drug regimens should routinely be provided together with close monitoring. Patients and their carers should be educated about the early symptoms of opioid toxicity and the actions required should they occur.

Table 5.19 Opioid analgesia and severe renal impairment or renal failure[106,110–112]

Opioid[a]	*Main metabolite(s)*	*Active metabolite(s)*[b]	*Effect of renal impairment*	*Removed by dialysis*[c]	*Comment*
Recommended for chronic use					
Alfentanil	Noralfentanil	No	No accumulation. Possible increase in unbound fraction but clinical significance unknown	No	When used as a rescue analgesic, its short duration of action may necessitate frequent p.r.n. use
Buprenorphine	Norbuprenorphine	Yes[d]	Possible accumulation of metabolites but clinical significance unknown	No	Less experience of its use in this setting compared with fentanyl
Fentanyl	Norfentanyl	No	Possible accumulation of parent drug but clinical significance unknown	No[e]	
Methadone	Methadol, EDDP, EMDP[f]	No	No accumulation	No	Use requires caution; unpredictable accumulation and toxicity even in the absence of renal impairment (see p.416)
Use cautiously					
Hydromorphone	Hydromorphone-3-glucuronide (H3G)	Yes	Accumulation of H3G can occur to a clinically significant degree	Yes	H3G has no analgesic effect but may cause neurotoxicity. Generally, no additional dose required with dialysis
Tramadol	O-desmethyltramadol (M1)	Yes	Accumulation of parent drug and metabolites can occur to a clinically significant degree	Yes	Generally, no additional dose required with dialysis

continued

Table 5.19 Continued

Opioid[a]	*Main metabolite(s)*	*Active metabolite(s)*[b]	*Effect of renal impairment*	*Removed by dialysis*[c]	*Comment*
Not recommended for chronic use					
Codeine	Codeine-6-glucuronide, morphine-3-glucuronide (M3G), morphine-6-glucuronide (M6G)	Yes	Accumulation of M3G and M6G can occur to a clinically significant degree	Yes	
Morphine	M3G, M6G	Yes	Accumulation of M3G and M6G can occur to a clinically significant degree	Yes	M6G more active than morphine. Human studies suggest M3G has no analgesic effect but may cause neurotoxicity
Oxycodone	Noroxycodone, oxymorphone	Yes	Accumulation of oxycodone and metabolites can occur to a clinically significant degree	Yes	

a. close monitoring of the patient is required whichever opioid is used
b. in sufficient quantities with the potential to produce a clinical effect
c. the removal of the parent drug or metabolites when patients are undergoing regular dialysis depends on several factors, and evidence is limited and contradictory. If loss of analgesia occurs either prior to or soon after dialysis, consider giving an additional dose of the opioid
d. norbuprenorphine has similar receptor binding to buprenorphine but does not readily cross the blood-brain barrier
e. certain dialysis membranes may remove fentanyl, e.g. cellulose triacetate 190
f. EDDP = 1,5,-dimethyl-2-ethyl-3,3-diphenylpyrroline, EMDP = 2-ethyl-5-methyl-3,3-diphenylpyrrolidine.

Opioids differ in their potential to cause toxicity when renal function is impaired. However, the evidence base from clinical studies is limited,[106] and stratification of risk is based on the presence of active metabolites, risk of accumulation, and expert opinion.

The pharmacokinetics and pharmacodynamics of opioids are altered by renal impairment (see p.618). Accumulation of an opioid or active metabolite will lead to a prolonged duration of action and increased toxicity. Changes in plasma protein concentrations or alterations in the blood-brain barrier also increase the potential for toxicity with any opioid. Thus in renal impairment, when possible optimize the use of adjuvant analgesics before introducing an opioid, e.g. in neuropathic pain (see p.281). If an opioid is necessary, it is important to:

- start at lower than usual doses
- consider increasing the intervals between doses
- monitor closely for toxicity, both immediate and delayed.

(Also see Principles of dose adjustment in renal impairment, p.618.)

Weak and strong opioids with active metabolites (e.g. **codeine**, **hydromorphone**, **morphine**, **oxycodone**, **tramadol**) can be used with caution in patients with *mild–moderate* renal impairment. However, in *severe* renal impairment (and in renal *failure*), it is generally

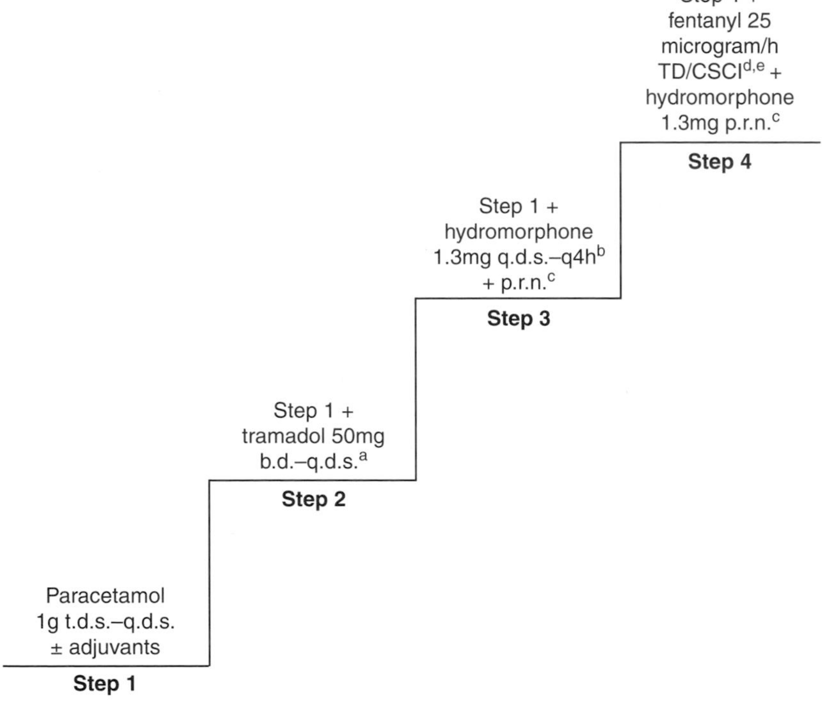

Figure 5.10 Example of an analgesic ladder for patients with severe renal impairment or failure; doses PO unless stated otherwise.

a. equivalent to about morphine 10–20mg/24h PO; the maximum dose of tramadol is limited to 100mg/24h in patients not on dialysis and 200mg/24h in those on dialysis
b. equivalent to about morphine 20–30mg/24h PO; start with q.d.s and increase if necessary and if tolerated to q4h. Fentanyl TD/CSCI 12microgram/h is an alternative to q4h hydromorphone and is preferred in patients *not* on dialysis
c. equivalent to about morphine 5mg PO
d. equivalent to about morphine 60mg/24h PO; use when unacceptable pain relief in step 3 despite frequent p.r.n. use, i.e. 4–6/24h
e. CSCI alfentanil can be substituted for CSCI fentanyl: it is about one quarter as potent as fentanyl (see p.374).

preferable to use a strong opioid which has no active metabolite and is not removed by dialysis (Table 5.19). On the other hand, expert opinion (with a limited objective evidence base) suggests that **tramadol** and **hydromorphone** can still be used with caution in this setting, e.g. by reducing the upper dose limit (Figure 5.10).[106–109]

Fentanyl can be administered continuously TD or CSCI.[106,109,113] There is also an increasing range of SL, buccal and nasal **fentanyl** products suitable for p.r.n. use, although these are licensed only for break-through (episodic) cancer pain (see p.400).

Buprenorphine, like **fentanyl**, is not removed by haemodialysis and it could become a popular choice in patients with renal impairment.[112,114,115] It does have an active metabolite (norbuprenorphine) with similar opioid receptor-binding affinities to **buprenorphine**, but this does not usually cross the blood-brain barrier and thus has little, if any, central effect (see p.381).[116,117] However, renal impairment increases the permeability of the blood-brain barrier and more experience is required with **buprenorphine** in this setting.[106]

Ketamine may also have a role to play in some patients with renal impairment (see p.593).[118]

At the end of life, UK guidelines for analgesia in patients with severe renal impairment or failure (GFR <30mL/min) also opt for **fentanyl** as the preferred strong opioid.[119] Experience with this approach is increasing. However, in some centres or settings, the cautious use of a familiar opioid may still be preferred over switching to an unfamiliar (albeit 'renally safer') one.

1 Portenoy RK *et al.* (2006) Opioid use and survival at the end of life: a survey of a hospice population. *Journal of Pain and Symptom Management.* **32**: 532–540.
2 Ballantyne JC (2007) Regulation of opioid prescribing. *British Medical Journal.* **334**: 811–812.
3 Mika J (2008) The opioid systems and the role of glial cells in the effects of opioids. *Advances in Palliative Medicine.* **7**: 185–196.
4 Sauriyal DS *et al.* (2011) Extending pharmacological spectrum of opioids beyond analgesia: Multifunctional aspects in different pathophysiological states. *Neuropeptides e-pub ahead of print.*
5 Rothman R (1995) Buprenorphine: a review of the binding literature. In: A Cowan and J Lewis (eds) *Buprenorphine: combatting drug abuse with a unique opioid.* Wiley-Liss, New York, pp. 19–29.
6 Zaki P *et al.* (2000) Ligand-induced changes in surface mu-opioid receptor number: relationship to G protein activation? *Journal of Pharmacology and Experimental Therapeutics.* **292**: 1127–1134.
7 Lutfy K *et al.* (2003) Buprenorphine-induced antinociception is mediated by mu-opioid receptors and compromised by concomitant activation of opioid receptor-like receptors. *Journal of Neuroscience.* **23**: 10331–10337.
8 Lewis JW and Husbands SM (2004) The orvinols and related opioids–high affinity ligands with diverse efficacy profiles. *Current Pharmaceutical Design.* **10**: 717–732.
9 Hill RG (1992) Multiple opioid receptors and their ligands. *Frontiers of Pain.* **4**: 1–4.
10 Corbett AD *et al.* (1993) Selectivity of ligands for opioid receptors. In: A Herz (ed) *Opioids.* Springer-Verlag, London, pp. 657–672.
11 WHO (1986) *Cancer Pain Relief.* World Health Organisation, Geneva.
12 Hanks G *et al.* (2001) Morphine and alternative opioids in cancer pain: the EAPC recommendations. *British Journal of Cancer.* **84**: 587–593.
13 Quigley C (2005) The role of opioids in cancer pain. *British Medical Journal.* **331**: 825–829.
14 Cherny N (1996) Opioid analgesics: comparative features and prescribing guidelines. *Drugs.* **51**: 713–737.
15 Tzschentke TM *et al.* (2009) Tapentadol hydrochloride: a next-generation, centrally acting analgesic with two mechanisms of action in a single molecule. *Drugs Today (Barc).* **45**: 483–496.
16 Schroder W *et al.* (2010) Differential contribution of opioid and noradrenergic mechanisms of tapentadol in rat models of nociceptive and neuropathic pain. *European Journal of Pain.* **14**: 814–821.
17 Kress HG (2010) Tapentadol and its two mechanisms of action: is there a new pharmacological class of centrally-acting analgesics on the horizon? *European Journal of Pain.* **14**: 781–783.
18 Frampton JE (2010) Tapentadol immediate release: a review of its use in the treatment of moderate to severe acute pain. *Drugs.* **70**: 1719–1743.
19 Schwartz S *et al.* (2011) Safety and efficacy of tapentadol ER in patients with painful diabetic peripheral neuropathy: results of a randomized-withdrawal, placebo-controlled trial. *Current Medical Research Opinion.* **27**. 151–162.
20 Lange B *et al.* (2010) Efficacy and safety of tapentadol prolonged release for chronic osteoarthritis pain and low back pain. *Advances in Therapy.* **27**: 381–399.
21 Hoskin P and Hanks G (1991) Opioid agonist-antagonist drugs in acute and chronic pain states. *Drugs.* **41**: 326–344.
22 Twycross RG (1994) Pentazocine. In: *Pain Relief in Advanced Cancer.* Churchill Livingstone, Edinburgh, pp. 247–248.
23 Woods A *et al.* (1974) Medicines evaluation and monitoring group: central nervous system effects of pentazocine. *British Medical Journal.* **1**: 305–307.
24 Plummer JL *et al.* (2001) Norpethidine toxicity. *Pain Reviews.* **8**: 159–170.
25 Sweetman SC (ed) (2005) *Martindale: The Complete Drug Reference* (34e). Pharmaceutical Press, London, pp. 80–82.
26 Shee JC (1960) Dangerous potentiation of pethidine by iproniazid, and its treatment. *British Medical Journal.* **ii**: 507–509.
27 Taylor D (1962) Alarming reaction to pethidine in patients on phenelzine. *Lancet.* **2**: 401–402.
28 Rogers KJ and Thornton JA (1969) The interaction between monoamine oxidase inhibitors and narcotic analgesics in mice. *British Journal of Pharmacology.* **36**: 470–480.
29 Cherny N *et al.* (2001) Strategies to manage the adverse effects of oral morphine: an evidence-based report. *Journal of Clinical Oncology.* **19**: 2542–2554.
30 Borgbjerg FM *et al.* (1996) Experimental pain stimulates respiration and attenuates morphine-induced respiratory depression: a controlled study in human volunteers. *Pain.* **64**: 123–128.
31 Estfan B *et al.* (2007) Respiratory function during parenteral opioid titration for cancer pain. *Palliative Medicine.* **21**: 81–86.
32 Sykes NP (2007) Morphine kills the pain, not the patient. *Lancet.* **369**: 1325–1326.

33 Regnard CFB and Badger C (1987) Opioids, sleep and the time of death. *Palliative Medicine*. **1**: 107–110.
34 Collin E *et al.* (1993) Is disease progression the major factor in morphine 'tolerance' in cancer pain treatment? *Pain*. **55**: 319–326.
35 Portenoy RK (1994) Tolerance to opioid analgesics: clinical aspects. *Cancer Surveys*. **21**: 49–65.
36 Passik S and Portenoy R (1998) Substance abuse issues in palliative care. In: A Berger (ed) *Principles and Practice of Supportive Oncology*. Lippincott-Raven, Philadelphia, pp. 513–529.
37 Joranson D *et al.* (2000) Trends in medical use and abuse of opioid analgesics. *Journal of the American Medical Association*. **283**: 1710–1714.
38 Passik S *et al.* (1998) Substance abuse issues in cancer patients. Part 1: prevalence and diagnosis. *Oncology*. **12**: 517–521.
39 Passik S *et al.* (1998) Substance abuse issues in cancer patients. Part 2: evaluation and treatment. *Oncology*. **12**: 729–734.
40 Twycross RG and Wald SJ (1976) Longterm use of diamorphine in advanced cancer. In: JJ Bonica and D Albe-Fessard (eds) *Advances in Pain Research and Therapy* Vol 1. Raven Press, New York, pp. 653–661.
41 Hansen H (1999) Treatment of chronic pain with antiepileptic drugs. *Southern Medical Journal*. **92**: 642–649.
42 Woodham M (1988) Pruritus with sublingual buprenorphine. *Anaesthesia*. **43**: 806–807.
43 Katcher J and Walsh D (1999) Opioid-induced itching: morphine sulfate and hydromorphone hydrochloride. *Journal of Pain and Symptom Management*. **17**: 70–72.
44 Ballantyne J *et al.* (1988) Itching after epidural and spinal opiates. *Pain*. **33**: 149–160.
45 Barke K and Hough L (1993) Opiates, mast cells and histamine release. *Life Sciences*. **53**: 1391–1399.
46 Reisine T and Pasternak G (1996) Opioid analgesics and antagonists. In: J Hardman *et al.* (eds) *Goodman and Gilman's The Pharmacological Basis of Therapeutics* (9e). McGraw-Hill, London, pp. 521–555.
47 Gillman P (2006) Serotonin toxicity, serotonin syndrome: 2006 update, overview and analysis. Available from: www.psychotropical.com
48 Dunkley EJ *et al.* (2003) The Hunter Serotonin Toxicity Criteria: simple and accurate diagnostic decision rules for serotonin toxicity. *Quarterly Journal of Medicine*. **96**: 635–642.
49 Gillman PK (2005) Monoamine oxidase inhibitors, opioid analgesics and serotonin toxicity. *British Journal of Anaesthesia*. **95**: 434–441.
50 Barry B (1979) Adverse effects of MAO inhibitors with narcotics reversed with naloxone. *Anaesthesia and Intensive Care*. **7**: 194.
51 The Society for Endocrinology and the Royal College of Physicians (2002) Health Technology Appraisal of Human Growth Hormone Replacement in Adults. In: *National Institute for Clinical Excellence*. Available from: www.endocrinology.org/SFE/GHAppraisal.pdf
52 Daniell HW (2002) Hypogonadism in men consuming sustained-action oral opioids. *The Journal of Pain*. **3**: 377–384.
53 Abs R *et al.* (2000) Endocrine consequences of long-term intrathecal administration of opioids. *Journal of Clinical Endocrinology and Metabolism*. **85**: 2215–2222.
54 Finch PM *et al.* (2000) Hypogonadism in patients treated with intrathecal morphine. *Clinical Journal of Pain*. **16**: 251–254.
55 Roberts LJ *et al.* (2002) Sex hormone suppression by intrathecal opioids: a prospective study. *Clinical Journal of Pain*. **18**: 144–148.
56 Vallejo R *et al.* (2004) Opioid therapy and immunosuppression: a review. *American Journal of Therapeutics*. **11**: 354–365.
57 Sacerdote P *et al.* (1997) Antinociceptive and immunosuppressive effects of opiate drugs: a structure-related activity study. *British Journal of Pharmacology*. **121**: 834–840.
58 Risdahl JM *et al.* (1998) Opiates and infection. *Journal of Neuroimmunology*. **83**: 4–18.
59 McCarthy L *et al.* (2001) Opioids, opioid receptors, and the immune response. *Drug and Alcohol Dependence*. **62**: 111–123.
60 Afsharimani B *et al.* (2011) Morphine and tumor growth and metastasis. *Cancer Metastasis Reviews*. **30**: 225–238.
61 Sacerdote P *et al.* (2000) The effects of tramadol and morphine on immune responses and pain after surgery in cancer patients. *Anesthesia and Analgesia*. **90**: 1411–1414.
62 Budd K and Shipton E (2004) Acute pain and the immune system and opioimmunosuppression. *Acute Pain*. **6**: 123–135.
63 Budd K and Raffa R (eds) (2005) *Buprenorphine — the unique opioid analgesic*. Georg Thieme Verlag, Stuttgart, Germany, p.134.
64 Sacerdote P *et al.* (2008) Buprenorphine and methadone maintenance treatment of heroin addicts preserves immune function. *Brain, Behavior, and Immunity*. **22**: 606–613.
65 Rittner HL *et al.* (2010) The clinical (ir)relevance of opioid-induced immune suppression. *Current Opinion in Anaesthesiology*. **23**: 588–592.
66 Alonzo NC and Bayer BM (2002) Opioids, immunology, and host defenses of intravenous drug abusers. *Infectious Disease Clinics of North America*. **16**: 553–569.
67 Page GG (2005) Immunologic effects of opioids in the presence or absence of pain. *Journal of Pain and Symptom Management*. **29**: S25–31.
68 Simonnet G (2008) Preemptive antihyperalgesia to improve preemptive analgesia. *Anesthesiology*. **108**: 352–354.
69 Bekhit MH (2010) Opioid-induced hyperalgesia and tolerance. *American Journal of Therapeutics*. **17**: 498–510.
70 Ren K and Dubner R (2008) Neuron-glia crosstalk gets serious: role in pain hypersensitivity. *Current Opinion in Anaesthesiology*. **21**: 570–579.
71 Romero-Sandoval EA *et al.* (2008) Neuroimmune interactions and pain: focus on glial-modulating targets. *Current Opinion in Investigational Drugs*. **9**: 726–734.
72 Milligan ED and Watkins LR (2009) Pathological and protective roles of glia in chronic pain. *Nature Reviews Neurosciene*. **10**: 23–36.
73 Crain S and Shen K (2000) Antagonists of excitatory opioid receptor functions enhance morphine's analgesic potency and attenuate opioid tolerance/dependence liability. *Pain*. **84**: 121–131.
74 Bartlett S *et al.* (1994) Pharmacology of morphine and morphine-3-glucuronide at opioid, excitatory amino acid, GABA and glycine binding sites. *Pharmacology and Toxicology*. **75**: 73–81.
75 Zylicz Z and Twycross R (2008) Opioid-induced hyperalgesia may be more frequent than previously thought. *Journal of Clinical Oncology*. **26**: 1564; author reply 1565.
76 Filitz J *et al.* (2008) Supra-additive effects of tramadol and acetaminophen in a human pain model. *Pain*. **136**: 262–270.
77 Walker SM and Cousins MJ (1997) Reduction in hyperalgesia and intrathecal morphine requirements by low-dose ketamine infusion. *Journal of Pain and Symptom Management*. **14**: 129–133.
78 Bruera E *et al.* (1996) Opioid rotation in patients with cancer pain. *Cancer*. **78**: 852–857.
79 Lawlor P *et al.* (1998) Dose ratio between morphine and methadone in patients with cancer pain. *Cancer*. **82**: 1167–1173.
80 Dubray C *et al.* (1997) Magnesium deficiency induces an hyperalgesia reversed by the NMDA receptor antagonist MK801. *Neuroreport*. **8**: 1383–1386.

81 Begon S *et al.* (2002) Magnesium increases morphine analgesic effect in different experimental models of pain. *Anesthesiology.* **96**: 627–632.
82 Gan T *et al.* (1997) Opioid-sparing effects of a low-dose infusion of naloxone in patient-administered morphine sulfate. *Anesthesiology.* **87**: 1075–1081.
83 Chindalore VL *et al.* (2005) Adding ultralow-dose naltrexone to oxycodone enhances and prolongs analgesia: a randomized, controlled trial of Oxytrex. *Journal of Pain.* **6**: 392–399.
84 Rauck RL *et al.* (2006) A randomized, double-blind, placebo-controlled study of intrathecal ziconotide in adults with severe chronic pain. *Journal of Pain and Symptom Management.* **31**: 393–406.
85 Sarhill N *et al.* (2001) Parenteral opioid rotation in advanced cancer: A prospective study. Abstracts of the MASCC/ISOO 13th International Symposium Supportive Care in Cancer, Copenhagen, Denmark, June 14–16. *Supportive Care Cancer.* **9**: 307.
86 Cherny NJ *et al.* (1995) Opioid pharmacotherapy in the management of cancer pain: a survey of strategies used by pain physicians for the selection of analgesic drugs and routes of administration. *Cancer.* **76**: 1283–1293.
87 Twycross RG Unpublished work.
88 Morley J and Makin M (1998) The use of methadone in cancer pain poorly responsive to other opioids. *Pain Reviews.* **5**: 51–58.
89 Sjogren P *et al.* (1994) Disappearance of morphine-induced hyperalgesia after discontinuing or substituting morphine with other opioid agonists. *Pain.* **59**: 313–316.
90 Hagen N and Swanson R (1997) Strychnine-like multifocal myoclonus and seizures in extremely high-dose opioid administration: treatment strategies. *Journal of Pain and Symptom Management.* **14**: 51–58.
91 Ashby M *et al.* (1999) Opioid substitution to reduce adverse effects in cancer pain management. *Medical Journal of Australia.* **170**: 68–71.
92 Aurilio C *et al.* (2009) Opioids switching with transdermal systems in chronic cancer pain. *Journal of Experimental and Clinical Cancer Research.* **28**: 61.
93 Nixon AJ (2005) Methadone for cancer pain: a case report. *American Journal of Hospice and Palliative Care.* **22**: 337.
94 Anderson R *et al.* (2001) Accuracy in equianalgesic dosing: conversion dilemmas. *Journal of Pain and Symptom Management.* **21**: 397–406.
95 Pasternak G (2001) Incomplete cross tolerance and multiple mu opioid peptide receptors. *Trends in Pharmacological Sciences.* **22**: 67–70.
96 Pereira J *et al.* (2001) Equianalgesic dose ratios for opioids: a critical review and proposals for long-term dosing. *Journal of Pain and Symptom Management.* **22**: 672–687.
97 Knotkova H *et al.* (2009) Opioid rotation: the science and the limitations of the equianalgesic dose table. *Journal of Pain and Symptom Management.* **38**: 426–439.
98 Fine PG and Portenoy RK (2009) Establishing "best practices" for opioid rotation: conclusions of an expert panel. *Journal of Pain and Symptom Management.* **38**: 418–425.
99 Twycross R *et al.* (2009) *Symptom Management in Advanced Cancer* (4e). palliativedrugs.com, Nottingham.
100 Lauretti GR *et al.* (2003) Comparison of sustained-release morphine with sustained-release oxycodone in advanced cancer patients. *British Journal of Cancer.* **89**: 2027–2030.
101 Mercadante S *et al.* (2004) Addition of a second opioid may improve opioid response in cancer pain: preliminary data. *Supportive Care Cancer.* **12**: 762–766.
102 Kotlinska-Lemieszek A (2010) Rotation, partial rotation (semi-switch), combining opioids, and titration. Does "opioid plus opioid" strategy make a step forward on our way to improving the outcome of pain treatment? *Journal of Pain and Symptom Management.* **40**: e10–12.
103 Fallon MT and Laird BJA (2011) A systematic review of comination strong opioid therapy in cancer pain (in press). *Palliative Medicine.*
104 Davis MP *et al.* (2005) Look before leaping: combined opioids may not be the rave. *Supportive Care in Cancer.* **13**: 769–774.
105 Strasser F (2005) Promoting science in a pragmatic world: not (yet) time for partial opioid rotation. *Supportive Care in Cancer.* **13**: 765–768.
106 King S *et al.* (2011) A systematic review of the use of opioid medication for those with moderate to severe cancer pain and renal impairment: an EPCRC opioid guidleines project. *Palliative Medicine.* **In press**.
107 Clemens KE and Klaschik E (2009) Morphine and hydromorphone in palliative care patients with renal impairment. *Anasthesiologie und Intensivmedizin.* **50**: 70–76.
108 Lee MA *et al.* (2001) Retrospective study of the use of hydromorphone in palliative care patients with normal and abnormal urea and creatinine. *Palliative Medicine.* **15**: 26–34.
109 Ferro CJ *et al.* (2004) Management of pain in renal failure. In: EJ Chambers *et al.* (eds) *Supportive Care for the Renal Patient.* Oxford University Press, Oxford, UK, pp. 105–153.
110 Dean M (2004) Opioids in renal failure and dialysis patients. *Journal of Pain and Symptom Management.* **28**: 497–504.
111 Davison SN *et al.* (2010) Management of pain in renal failure. In: EJ Chambers *et al.* (eds) *Supportive Care for the Renal Patient* (2e). Oxford University Press, Oxford, pp. 139–188.
112 Niscola P *et al.* (2010) The use of major analgesics in patients with renal dysfunction. *Current Drug Targets.* **11**: 752–758.
113 Douglas C *et al.* (2009) Symptom management for the adult patient dying with advanced chronic kidney disease: a review of the literature and development of evidence-based guidelines by a United Kingdom Expert Consensus Group. *Palliative Medicine.* **23**: 103–110.
114 Murtagh FE *et al.* (2007) The use of opioid analgesia in end-stage renal disease patients managed without dialysis: recommendations for practice. *Journal of Pain and Palliative Care Pharmacotherapy.* **21**: 5–16.
115 Boger RH (2006) Renal impairment: a challenge for opioid treatment? The role of buprenorphine. *Palliative Medicine.* **20 (suppl 1)**: s17–23.
116 Hand CW *et al.* (1990) Buprenorphine disposition in patients with renal impairment: single and continuous dosing, with special reference to metabolites. *British Journal of Anaesthesia.* **64**: 276–282.
117 Elkader A and Sproule B (2005) Buprenorphine: clinical pharmacokinetics in the treatment of opioid dependence. *Clinical Pharmacokinetics.* **44**: 661–680.
118 Murphy EJ (2005) Acute pain management pharmacology for the patient with concurrent renal or hepatic disease. *Anaesthesia and Intensive Care.* **33**: 311–322.
119 Marie Curie Palliative Care Institute (2008) Liverpool Care Pathway for the Dying Patient (LPC), National LCP Renal Project Group Guidelines for LCP Drug Presribing in Advanced Chronic Kidney Disease. Available from: www.mcpcil.org.uk/about_the_institute/news/june_2008/06_june_2008

MORPHINE BNF 4.7.2

Class: Opioid analgesic.

Indications: Severe or †moderate pain, diarrhoea, †cough, †dyspnoea.

Contra-indications: None absolute if titrated carefully against a patient's pain (also see Strong opioids, p.345).

Pharmacology

Morphine is the main pharmacologically active constituent of opium. Its effects are mediated by specific opioid receptors both within the CNS and peripherally. Under normal circumstances, its main peripheral action is on smooth muscle. However, in the presence of inflammation, normally silent peripheral receptors become activated.[1,2] The liver is the principal site of morphine metabolism.[3] Metabolism also occurs in other organs,[4] including the CNS.[5] Glucuronidation is rarely impaired except in severe hepatic impairment,[6] and morphine is well tolerated in patients with mild–moderate hepatic impairment.[7] However, with impairment severe enough to prolong the prothrombin time, the plasma halflife of morphine may be increased[4] and the dose of morphine may need to be reduced or given less often, e.g. q6h or even q8h (see p.615).

The major metabolites of morphine are morphine-3-glucuronide (M3G; 55–80%) and morphine-6-glucuronide (M6G; 10–15%) which are excreted by the kidneys.[8] M6G binds to opioid receptors and contributes substantially to the effects of morphine, both desirable (e.g. analgesia) and undesirable (e.g. nausea and vomiting, sedation and respiratory depression).[9–11] In renal failure, the plasma halflife of M6G increases from 2.5h up to 7.5h, and is likely to lead to accumulation and enhanced toxicity unless the frequency of administration and/or the dose of morphine is reduced (see p.355). M3G will also accumulate, but the significance of this is unclear; it binds poorly to opioid receptors and is considered devoid of an analgesic effect. Although animal studies suggest a neuro-excitatory effect, this has not been clearly demonstrated in humans.[12]

Morphine is administered by a range of routes. Systemic absorption from topical application to ulcers or inflamed surfaces varies with the amount and concentration of the gel used; bio-availability ranges from negligible (with 0.06–0.125% gel) to almost the same as SC (0.125–0.5% gel applied to large ulcers).[13–16]

Bio-availability 35% PO, ranging from 15–64%; 25% PR.

Peak effect ≤60min PO (normal-release tablets); 20min IV; 30–60min IM; 50–90min SC.

Time to peak plasma concentration 15–60min PO (normal-release tablets), 1–6h m/r (product dependent); 10–20min IM; 15min SC; 45–60min PR.

Plasma halflife 1.5–4.5h PO; 1.5h IV.

Duration of action 3–6h; 12–24h m/r (product dependent).

Undesirable effects

See Table 5.20 and Strong opioids, p.345.

Dose and use

Morphine should generally be given with a non-opioid, when the non-opioid ± a weak opioid does not provide adequate analgesia (see p.277).

PO

Morphine is available as normal-release tablets and solutions, and m/r tablets, capsules and suspensions. Most m/r products are administered b.d., some once daily. Because the pharmacokinetic profiles of m/r products differ,[18–20] it is best to keep individual patients on the same brand.

Patients can be started on either an ordinary (normal-release) or an m/r formulation (Box 5.J).[21,22] An observational study supports a starting dose of 5mg q4h as generally safe for opioid-naïve patients, and 10mg q4h for those being switched from a regular weak opioid.[23] However, slight variation exists between guidelines, e.g. in the recommended starting dose.[24] It is important to recognize that guidelines are just guidelines; and for each patient, when deciding the starting dose, it is necessary to consider the individual circumstances, e.g. severity of the pain, current analgesia, presence of renal impairment, increasing age or frailty. In every case, the patient must be monitored closely, and the dose titrated as necessary.

Table 5.20 Potential intolerable effects of morphine

Type	*Effects*	*Initial action*	*Comment*
For general undesirable effects of opioid analgesics, see Box 5.G, p.349.			
Gastric stasis	Epigastric fullness, flatulence, anorexia, hiccup, persistent nausea	Prescribe a prokinetic, e.g. metoclopramide 10–20mg t.d.s.–q.d.s. (see p.227)	If the problem persists, change to an alternative opioid, with less impact on the GI tract
Sedation	Intolerable persistent sedation	Reduce dose of morphine; consider a psychostimulant, e.g. methylphenidate 5mg b.d., (see p.210)	Sedation may be caused by other factors; stimulant rarely appropriate
Cognitive failure	Agitated delirium with hallucinations	Prescribe an antipsychotic, e.g. haloperidol 1mg stat & q2h p.r.n. (see p.159); reduce dose of morphine and, if no improvement, switch to an alternative opioid	Some patients develop intractable delirium with one opioid but not with an alternative opioid
Myoclonus	Multifocal twitching ± jerking of limbs	Prescribe a benzodiazepine, e.g. diazepam/midazolam 5mg or lorazepam 500microgram stat & q1h p.r.n.; reduce morphine but increase again if pain recurs	Uncommon with typical oral doses; more common with high dose IV and spinal morphine
Neurotoxicity	Abdominal muscle spasms, symmetrical jerking of legs; whole-body allodynia, hyperalgesia (manifests as excruciating pain)	Prescribe a benzodiazepine, e.g. diazepam/midazolam 5mg or lorazepam 500microgram stat & q1h p.r.n.; reduce dose of morphine; consider changing to an alternative opioid	A rare syndrome in patients receiving intrathecal or high dose IV morphine; occasionally seen with typical oral and SC doses
Vestibular stimulation	Movement-induced nausea and vomiting	Prescribe an antihistaminic antimuscarinic anti-emetic, e.g. cyclizine 25–50mg q8h–q6h (see p.231)	If intractable, try levomepromazine or switch to an alternative opioid
Pruritus	Whole-body itch with systemic morphine; localized to upper body or face/nose with spinal morphine	With systemic opioids, prescribe PO H_1-antihistamine (e.g. chlorphenamine 4–8mg stat; if beneficial continue with 4mg t.d.s. or p.r.n. for 2–3 days). Possibly switch opioids, e.g. morphine → oxycodone. For spinal opioids, see Box 21.C, p.688.	Pruritus after systemic opioids is uncommon. Sometimes caused by cutaneous histamine release and self-limiting but most are chronic and antihistamine-resistant. Centrally-acting opioid antagonists relieve the pruritus but also antagonize analgesia[17]
Histamine release	Bronchoconstriction → breathlessness	Treat as for anaphylaxis (see p.751); change to a chemically distinct opioid immediately, e.g. methadone	Rare

Box 5.J Starting a patient on PO morphine

The starting dose of morphine is calculated to give a greater analgesic effect than the medication already in use:

- if the patient was previously receiving a weak opioid regularly (e.g. codeine 240mg/24h or equivalent), give 10mg q4h or m/r 20–30mg q12h, but less if suspected a poor codeine metabolizer (see p.332)
- if changing from an alternative strong opioid (e.g. fentanyl, methadone) a much higher dose of morphine may be needed
- if the patient is frail and elderly, or opioid-naïve, a lower dose helps to reduce initial drowsiness, confusion and unsteadiness, e.g. 5mg q4h
- because of accumulation of an active metabolite, a lower and/or less frequent regular dose may suffice in mild–moderate renal impairment, e.g. 5–10mg q8h–q6h (but the use of a 'renally safer' opioid is generally advisable with moderate–severe renal impairment, see p.355).

When adjusting the dose of morphine, p.r.n. use should be taken into account; increments should not exceed 33–50% every 24h.

As with all opioids, patients must be monitored for undesirable effects, particularly nausea and vomiting, and constipation (see Box 5.G, p.349). Depending on individual circumstances, an anti-emetic should be prescribed for regular or p.r.n. use (see p.225) and, routinely, a laxative prescribed (see p.38).

Upward titration of the dose of morphine stops when either the pain is relieved or unacceptable undesirable effects occur. In the latter case, it is generally necessary to consider alternative measures. The aim is to have the patient free of pain and mentally alert after the initial drowsiness has cleared.

Because of poor absorption, m/r morphine may not be satisfactory in patients troubled by frequent vomiting or those with diarrhoea or an ileostomy.

Scheme 1: ordinary (normal-release) morphine tablets or solution

- morphine given q4h 'by the clock' with p.r.n. doses 1/10–1/6 of the 24h dose
- after 1–2 days, recalculate q4h dose by dividing the total used in previous 24h (regular + p.r.n. use) by 6
- continue q4h and p.r.n. doses
- increase the regular dose until there is adequate relief throughout each 4h period, taking p.r.n. use into account
- a double dose at bedtime obviates the need to wake the patient for a dose during the night
- >90% of patients achieve satisfactory pain relief within 5 days.

Scheme 2: ordinary (normal-release) morphine and modified-release (m/r) morphine

- begin as for Scheme 1
- when the q4h dose is stable, replace with m/r morphine q12h, or once daily if a 24h product is prescribed
- the q12h dose will be three times the previous q4h dose; a q24h dose will be six times the previous q4h dose, rounded to a convenient number of tablets or capsules
- continue to provide ordinary morphine tablets or solution for p.r.n. use; give 1/10–1/6 of the 24h dose.

Scheme 3: m/r morphine and ordinary (normal-release) morphine

- generally start with m/r morphine 20–30mg q12h, or 10mg q12h in frail elderly patients
- use ordinary morphine tablets or solution for p.r.n. medication; give 1/10–1/6 of the 24h dose
- if necessary, increase the dose of m/r morphine every 2–3 days until there is adequate relief throughout each 12h period, guided by p.r.n. use.

Traditionally, to make things easier for patients, morphine q4h has been given on waking, 1000h, 1400h, 1800h with a double dose at bedtime. Despite contrary results in a non-blinded study,[25] RCT evidence has shown that this approach results in less pain through the night, better sleep, and no increase in early morning pain.[26]

When adjusting the dose of morphine, p.r.n. use should be taken into account; increments should not exceed 33–50% every 24h.[27] Two-thirds of patients never need >30mg q4h (or m/r morphine 100mg q12h); the rest need up to 200mg q4h (or m/r morphine 600mg q12h), and occasionally more.[28] Instructions must be clear: extra p.r.n. morphine does not mean that the next regular dose is omitted.

P.r.n. doses of morphine for break-through pain are typically 1/10–1/6 of the regular 24h dose but, as with the regular dose, there is need to consider individual variation. In practice, satisfactory p.r.n. doses vary from 1/20 (5%) to 1/5 (20%) of the 24h dose.[29]

As a general rule, the p.r.n. dose should be increased when the regular dose is increased. A p.r.n. dose is generally permitted every q2–4h as required (up to q1h when pain severe, or in the last days of life). However, frequent use of p.r.n. doses, i.e. ⩾2 a day, should prompt a review of pain management. The time to peak plasma concentration is significantly shorter with a solution of morphine compared with a normal-release tablet (median 1h vs. 2h),[30] suggesting that morphine solution is the better option for p.r.n. use (also see p.400).

An anti-emetic, e.g. haloperidol 1.5mg stat and at bedtime, should be supplied for p.r.n. use during the first week or prescribed regularly if the patient has had nausea with a weak opioid. Warn patients about the possibility of initial drowsiness. A laxative should be prescribed routinely unless there is a definite reason for not doing so, e.g. the patient has an ileostomy (see Guidelines: Opioid-induced constipation, p.38). *Constipation may be more difficult to manage than the pain.* Laxative suppositories and enemas continue to be necessary in about one third of patients.[31]

SC/CSCI

In the UK, if the PO route becomes an unreliable means of administering regular morphine, e.g. because of difficulty swallowing or vomiting, generally the CSCI route is used (see p.665).

The oral to SC potency ratio of morphine is between 1:2 and 1:3 (i.e. the SC dose is 2–3 times more potent than a PO dose) and, correspondingly, the SC dose is 1/2–1/3 of the oral dose. The same ratio holds true for IM and IV injections.[6,32] In practice, most centres divide the PO dose by 2, and re-titrate as necessary, e.g.:

- patient taking m/r morphine 30mg b.d. PO = 60mg/24h PO
- 60mg/24h divided by 2 = 30mg/24h CSCI
- the p.r.n. dose is 1/10–1/6 of the 24h dose, i.e. 3–5mg SC.

For CSCI dilute with WFI, 0.9% saline or 5% glucose.

CSCI compatibility with other drugs: There are 2-drug compatibility data for morphine sulphate in WFI with **clonazepam**, **cyclizine**, **glycopyrronium**, **hyoscine *butylbromide***, **hyoscine *hydrobromide***, **ketamine**, **levomepromazine**, **metoclopramide**, and **octreotide**.

Morphine sulphate is *incompatible* with **ketorolac** and may be *incompatible* with higher concentrations of **haloperidol** or **midazolam**. For more details and 3-drug compatibility data, see Appendix 3 charts A3.1 (p.776) and A3.5 (p.784).

Compatibility charts in 0.9% saline can be found on www.palliativedrugs.com Syringe Driver Survey Database.

IV/CIVI

IV morphine is widely used for the rapid relief of severe pain caused by acute trauma or medical emergencies. In opioid-naïve patients:

- give a prophylactic anti-emetic IV, e.g. metoclopramide 10mg
- give morphine 5–10mg (2.5–5mg in the elderly) IV over 5–10min
- when insufficient, give additional morphine at a rate not exceeding 1–2mg/min until satisfactory relief obtained; monitor for undesirable effects, e.g. excessive sedation, respiratory depression
- the dose can be repeated q2–4h as required.

Although uncommon in UK, CIVI morphine and/or p.r.n. IV morphine are used in palliative care units in Europe and North America.[33,34] Generally, this is in the context of the first few days of an inpatient admission for pain control.

When subsequently switching from IV to PO, a potency ratio of between 2:1 and 3:1 appears to hold true (i.e. the PO dose should be 2–3 greater than the IV dose). In a recent observational study, about 80% of patients achieved a satisfactory 24h PO dose at 3 times the previous 24h IV dose, rounded down to convenient strength m/r tablets.[35]

Rapid IV/SC titration of morphine dose for severe cancer pain

Although rapid IV/SC titration of morphine is generally *not* necessary, it can be useful in patients with severe acute pain, whether already taking opioids ('opioid-tolerant') or 'opioid-naïve'.[36,37] Further, because of difficulties in relation to follow-up, rapid IV titration is the norm at some centres in India for new patients presenting with pain of ⩾5/10.

Two IV methods are included here; the first with 10min and the second with 1min intervals between each IV bolus.(Box 5.K and Box 5.L).[37–41] In India, a single cumulative IV dose is given, followed immediately by PO medication (Box 5.K). About 80% of patients obtain relief with 10mg or less.[38,39] At the Cleveland Clinic (USA), patients are maintained on CIVI for several days before conversion to PO medication (Box 5.L). Although these methods have been used safely in many patients, **naloxone** should be readily available (see p.435).

IV patient-controlled analgesia (PCA) can also be used but is more costly, requires inpatient admission and may take > 10h to achieve relief.[42,43] Some centres use a more rapidly acting strong opioid, e.g. IV **fentanyl**, with subsequent doses given after pauses of only 5–10min.[44]

Note: patients who have required a rapid escalation in opioid requirements must be monitored closely. The underlying cause may be transient, e.g. haemorrhage into a liver metastasis, and a subsequent reduction in dose will be necessary.

Alternative routes

Buccal morphine

Morphine is slowly absorbed through the buccal mucosa.[45] However, most of a morphine solution given sublingually or into the gingival gutter will be swallowed and absorbed from the GI tract. Nonetheless, in the past, this route was successfully used in moribund patients.

Rectal morphine

Morphine is absorbed from suppositories.[46] From the lower and middle rectum, it will enter the systemic circulation bypassing the liver. From the upper rectum, it will undergo hepatic first-pass metabolism after it enters the portal circulation. However, there are extensive anastomoses between the rectal veins which make it impossible to predict how much will enter the portal circulation.[47,48] Despite the uncertainty, in practice the same dose is given PR as PO and titrated as necessary.

Although not licensed for this route and not generaly recommended, m/r morphine tablets have been used PR to provide analgesia in moribund patients, generally while organizing a more reliable delivery method.[49]

Spinal morphine

In the UK, <5% of cancer patients needing morphine receive it spinally, i.e. ED or IT. This route of administration (see p.681) is normally undertaken by an anaesthetist. Particularly with neuropathic pain, morphine is generally combined with a local anaesthetic (e.g. **bupivacaine**), and sometimes with **clonidine**.

Topical morphine

Nociceptive afferent nerve fibres contain peripheral opioid receptors which are silent except in the presence of local inflammation.[1,2,14,50] This property is exploited in joint surgery where morphine is given intra-articularly at the end of the operation.[51] Topical morphine has also been used successfully to relieve otherwise intractable pain associated with cutaneous ulceration, often decubitus ulcers.[52–55] It is often given as a 0.1% (1mg/mL) gel, using IntraSite®. If prepared under sterile conditions, morphine sulphate is stable for at least 28 days when mixed with IntraSite® gel at a concentration of 0.125% (1.25mg/mL). This preparation can be made by thoroughly mixing 1mL of morphine sulphate 10mg/mL injection with an 8g sachet of IntraSite® gel.[56]

Higher concentrations, namely 0.3–0.5%, have been used when managing pain associated with:

- vaginal inflammation associated with a fistula
- rectal ulceration.[53]

Box 5.K Rapid titration of morphine dose in 'opioid-naïve' patients (Institute of Palliative Medicine, India)[38,39]

Prerequisites
Pain ⩾5/10 on a numerical scale.
Probability of a partial or complete response to morphine.[a]

Method
Obtain venous access with a butterfly cannula.
Give metoclopramide 10mg IV routinely.
Dilute the contents of 15mg morphine ampoule in a 10mL syringe.[b]
Inject 1.5mg (1mL) every 10min until the patient is pain-free or complains of undue sedation.[c]
If patients experience nausea, give additional metoclopramide 5mg IV.

Results
Dose required (with approximate percentages):

- 1.5–4.5mg (40%)
- 6–9mg (40%)
- 10.5–15mg (15%)
- >15mg (5%).

Complete relief in 80%; none in 1%.
Drop outs 2%.
Undesirable effects: sedation 32%; other 3%.

Ongoing treatment
Prescribe a dose of oral morphine q4h similar to the IV dose, rounded to nearest 5mg, e.g. needed morphine 3–6mg IV → 5mg PO; the minimum dose is 5mg. Advise about p.r.n. doses and, if >2/24h needed, to increase the dose the next day. In practice, 20% of patients need a dose increase within 3 days.

a. most patients will already be taking an NSAID
b. ampoule strengths varies from country to country; use local standard
c. if ampoule = 10mg/mL (diluted to 10mg in 10mL), a bolus dose of 2mg would be reasonable.

Box 5.L Rapid titration of morphine dose in both 'opioid-tolerant' and 'opioid-naïve' patients (based on practice at Cleveland Clinic, Ohio, USA)[36,40,41]

Sequence	*IV*	*SC*
Dose	1mg/min up to 10mg	2mg q5min up to 10mg
Pause	5min	10min
Dose	1mg/min up to 10mg	2mg q5min up to 10mg
Pause	5min	10min
Dose	1mg/min up to 10mg[a]	2mg q5min up to 10mg[a]

Maintenance IV/SC dose
Regard cumulative effective dose as the equivalent of a q4h dose, and prescribe accordingly.

Example
Cumulative effective IV dose = 9mg.
If giving intermittent injections, dose = 9mg q4h, rounded to 10mg.
If CIVI, total daily IV dose = 9mg x 6 = 54mg/24h.
Round this up or down to convenient number of ampoules, i.e. 50mg or 60mg.
P.r.n. dose = 5–10mg q1h.

a. review cause if relief inadequate after a total of 30mg.

The amount of gel applied varies according to the size and the site of the ulcer, but is typically 5–10mL applied b.d.–t.d.s. The topical morphine is kept in place with either a non-absorbable pad or dressing, e.g. Opsite® or Tegaderm®, or gauze coated with petroleum jelly. Other opioids, e.g. **diamorphine**, **methadone**, and other carriers, e.g. Stomahesive® paste, **medronidazole** gel have also been used.[57]

A 0.2% (2mg/mL) morphine solution without alcohol, (15mL used to rinse the mouth for 2min, q3h) has also been used for cancer treatment-related mucositis. It provides better pain relief than a placebo mouthwash, or one containing **co-magaldrox** + **lidocaine** + **diphenhydramine.**[58,59] Significant relief occurs after about 30min, and lasts about 3.5h.[60]

Morphine for breathlessness

Generally, opioids are more beneficial in patients who are breathless at rest than in those who are breathless only on exertion. Even with maximal exertion, breathlessness generally recovers within a few minutes, much quicker than the time it takes to locate, administer and obtain benefit from an opioid. Thus, non-drug measures are of primary importance in this circumstance.[61]

A systematic review supports the use of opioids by the oral and parenteral but *not* the nebulized route, and the latter should not be used outside of a clinical trial.[62–68]

Morphine and other opioids reduce the ventilatory response to hypercapnia, hypoxia and exercise, decreasing respiratory effort and breathlessness.[61] Improvements are seen at doses that *do not* cause respiratory depression.[69–74] In opioid-naïve patients:

- start with small doses of morphine, e.g. 2.5–5mg PO p.r.n.; larger doses can be poorly tolerated
- if ⩾2 doses/24h are needed, prescribe morphine regularly and titrate the dose according to response, duration of effect and undesirable effects
- relatively small doses may suffice, e.g. 20–60mg/24h.[65,66,69–73,75–78]

In patients already taking morphine for pain and with:

- severe breathlessness (i.e. ⩾7/10), a dose that is 100% or more of the q4h analgesic dose may be needed
- moderate breathlessness (i.e. 4–6/10), a dose equivalent to 50–100% of the q4h analgesic dose may suffice
- mild breathlessness (i.e. ⩽3/10), a dose equivalent to 25–50% of the q4h analgesic dose may suffice.

However, as with pain, individual titration is required for optimal benefit. In some patients, morphine by CSCI is better tolerated and provides greater relief, possibly by avoiding the peaks (with undesirable effects) and troughs (with loss of effect) of oral medication. If using an alternative opioid to morphine, adopt the same approach as above.

Opioids are also used in patients with severe COPD who have distressing breathlessness despite usual treatments. A low-dose and slow titration is generally advocated, e.g.:

- start with morphine 1mg PO b.d., increasing to 1–2.5mg q4h over one week
- thereafter, increase dose by 25% each week until satisfactory relief obtained
- when a stable dose is found, consider switching to a m/r formulation.[79]

For severe breathlessness in the last days of life:

- patients often fear suffocating to death and a positive approach to the patient, their family and colleagues about the relief of terminal breathlessness is important
- no patient should die with distressing breathlessness
- failure to relieve terminal breathlessness is a failure to utilize drug treatment correctly.

Because of the distress, inability to sleep and exhaustion, patients and their carers generally accept that drug-related drowsiness may need to be the price paid for greater comfort. However, unless there is overwhelming distress, sedation is not the primary aim of treatment and some patients become mentally brighter when their breathlessness is reduced.

Even so, because increasing drowsiness also generally reflects the deteriorating clinical condition, it is important to stress the gravity of the situation and the aim of treatment to the relatives. Drug treatment typically comprises:[80]

- parenteral administration of an opioid and a sedative-anxiolytic, e.g. morphine and **midazolam** or **lorazepam** by CSCI and p.r.n.
- **haloperidol** or **levomepromazine** if the patient develops an agitated delirium (may be aggravated by a benzodiazepine).

Supply

Unless indicated otherwise, all products are **CD**.

Morphine solution is available in two strengths, 2mg/mL and a high potency concentrate of 20mg/mL supplied with a calibrated syringe. *Deaths have occurred from accidental overdose with the concentrated solution*, mostly when doses prescribed in *mg* were administered as *mL*, resulting in *20 times* the prescribed dose being given.[81]

Normal-release oral products
Sevredol® (Napp)
Tablets 10mg, 20mg, 50mg; 10mg and 100mg dose = £0.10 and £1 respectively.

Oramorph® (Boehringer Ingelheim)
Oral solution 2mg/mL (**PoM**, not **CD**); 10mg dose = £0.07 (contains alcohol)
Concentrated oral solution 20mg/mL, 100mg dose = £0.80.

Oral solution 2mg/mL without alcohol (**PoM** not **CD**), 100mL = £235 (Unlicensed, available as a special order from Martindale Pharmaceuticals; see Obtaining unlicensed products, p.769.)

Modified-release oral products

Because the pharmacokinetic profiles of m/r products differ, and to minimize the risk of mistakes (e.g. mixing up normal-release and m/r products), it is best to keep individual patients on the same m/r brand, and to label with both the generic and proprietary names.

Morphgesic® SR (Amdipharm)
Tablets m/r 10mg, 30mg, 60mg, 100mg, 28 days @ 30mg q12h = £9.

MST Continus® (Napp)
Tablets m/r 5mg, 10mg, 15mg, 30mg, 60mg, 100mg, 200mg, 28 days @ 30mg q12h = £12.
Oral suspension (sachet of m/r granules to mix with water) 20mg, 30mg, 60mg, 100mg, 200mg/sachet, 28 days @ 30mg q12h = £48.

MXL® (Napp)
Capsules containing m/r granules 30mg, 60mg, 90mg, 120mg, 150mg, 200mg, 28 days @ 60mg once daily = £15. *May be swallowed whole or opened and the granules sprinkled on soft food.*

Zomorph® (Archimedes)
Capsules m/r 10mg, 30mg, 60mg, 100mg, 200mg, 28 days @ 30mg q12h = £8.

Normal-release rectal products
Morphine *hydrochloride* or *sulphate* (generic)
Suppositories 10mg, 15mg, 20mg, 30mg; 10mg dose = £1; *the required salt should be specified on the prescription.*

Parenteral products
Morphine *sulphate* (generic)
Injection 10, 15, 20 and 30mg/mL, 1mL and 2mL amp = £1.
Infusion 1mg/mL 50mL vial = £5, 2mg/mL 50mL vial = £6.

Minijet® Morphine Sulphate (UCB Pharma)
Injection 1mg/mL, 10mL disposable syringe = £15.

1 Krajnik M *et al.* (1998) Opioids affect inflammation and the immune system. *Pain Reviews.* **5**: 147–154.
2 Smith HS (2008) Peripherally-acting opioids. *Pain Physician.* **11**: S121–132.
3 Hasselstrom J *et al.* (1986) The metabolism and bioavailability of morphine in patients with severe liver cirrhosis. *British Journal of Clinical Pharmacology.* **29**: 289–297.
4 Mazoit J-X *et al.* (1987) Pharmacokinetics of unchanged morphine in normal and cirrhotic subjects. *Anesthesia and Analgesia.* **66**: 293–298.
5 Sandouk P *et al.* (1991) Presence of morphine metabolites in human cerebrospinal fluid after intracerebroventricular administration of morphine. *European Journal of Drug Metabolism and Pharmacology.* **16**: 166–171.
6 Max MB et al. (1992) *Principles of Analgesic Use in the Treatment of Acute Pain and Cancer Pain* (3e). American Pain Society, Skokie, Illinois, p.12.
7 Regnard CFB and Twycross RG (1984) Metabolism of narcotics (letter). *British Medical Journal.* **288**: 860.

8 McQuay HJ *et al.* (1990) Oral morphine in cancer pain: influences on morphine and metabolite concentration. *Clinical Pharmacology and Therapeutics.* **48**: 236–244.
9 Osborne RJ *et al.* (1986) Morphine intoxication in renal failure: the role of morphine-6-glucuronide. *British Medical Journal.* **292**: 1548–1549.
10 Thompson P *et al.* (1992) Mophine-6-glucuronide: a metabolite of morphine with greater emetic potency than morphine in the ferret. *British Journal of Pharmacology.* **106**: 3–8.
11 Buetler TM *et al.* (2000) Analgesic action of i.v. morphine-6-glucuronide in healthy volunteers. *British Journal of Anaesthesia.* **84**: 97–99.
12 Gretton S and Riley J (2008) Morphine metabolites: a review of their clinical effects. *European Journal of Palliative Care.* **15**: 110–114.
13 Westerling D *et al.* (1994) Transdermal administration of morphine to healthy subjects. *British Journal of Clinical Pharmacology.* **37**: 571–576.
14 Ribeiro MD *et al.* (2004) The bioavailability of morphine applied topically to cutaneous ulcers. *Journal of Pain and Symptom Management.* **27**: 434–439.
15 Watterson G *et al.* (2004) Peripheral opioids in inflammatory pain. *Archives of Disease in Childhood.* **89**: 679–681.
16 Jansen M (2006) Morphine gel. Palliativedrugs.com bulletin board message. Available from: www.palliativedrugs.com/forum/read.php?f = 1&i = 9271&t = 9189
17 Twycross RG *et al.* (2003) Itch: scratching more than the surface. *Quarterly Journal of Medicine.* **96**: 7–26.
18 Bloomfield S *et al.* (1993) Analgesic efficacy and potency of two oral controlled-release morphine preparations. *Clinical Pharmacology and Therapeutics.* **53**: 469–478.
19 Gourlay G *et al.* (1993) A comparison of Kapanol (a new sustained-release morphine formulation), MST Continus and morphine solution in cancer patients: pharmacokinetic aspects. In: *The Seventh World Congress on Pain*; Seattle. IASP Press.
20 West R and Maccarrone C (1993) Single dose pharmacokinetics of a new oral sustained-release morphine formulation, Kapanol capsules. In: *The Seventh World Congress on Pain*; Seattle. IASP Press.
21 Mercadante S (2007) Opioid titration in cancer pain: a critical review. *European Journal of Pain.* **11**: 823–830.
22 De Conno F *et al.* (2008) The MERITO Study: a multicentre trial of the analgesic effect and tolerability of normal-release oral morphine during 'titration phase' in patients with cancer pain. *Palliative Medicine.* **22**: 214–221.
23 Ripamonti CI *et al.* (2009) Normal-release oral morphine starting dose in cancer patients with pain. *Clinical Journal of Pain.* **25**: 386–390.
24 Taubert M *et al.* (2010) Re: Update on cancer pain guidelines. *Journal of Pain and Symptom Management.* **24**: 1–5.
25 Todd J *et al.* (2002) An assessment of the efficacy and tolerability of a 'double dose' of normal-release morphine sulphate at bedtime. *Palliative Medicine.* **16**: 507–512.
26 Dale O *et al.* (2009) A double-blind, randomized, crossover comparison between single-dose and double-dose immediate-release oral morphine at bedtime in cancer patients. *Journal of Pain and Symptom Management.* **37**: 68–76.
27 Carver AC and Foley KM (2001) Symptom assessment and management. *Neurologic Clinics.* **19**: 921–947.
28 Schug SA *et al.* (1992) A long-term survey of morphine in cancer pain patients. *Journal of Pain and Symptom Management.* **7**: 259–266.
29 Donnelly S *et al.* (2002) Morphine in cancer pain management: a practical guide. *Supportive Care in Cancer.* **10**: 13–35.
30 Sawe J *et al.* (1983) Steady-state kinetics and analgesic effect of oral morphine in cancer patients. *European Journal of Clinical Pharmacology.* **24**: 537–542.
31 Twycross RG and Harcourt JMV (1991) The use of laxatives at a palliative care centre. *Palliative Medicine.* **5**: 27–33.
32 Hanks G *et al.* (2001) Morphine and alternative opioids in cancer pain: the EAPC recommendations. *British Journal of Cancer.* **84**: 587–593.
33 Mercadante S *et al.* (2008) Intravenous morphine for breakthrough (episodic-) pain in an acute palliative care unit: a confirmatory study. *Journal of Pain and Symptom Management.* **35**: 307–313.
34 Mercadante S (2010) Intravenous morphine for management of cancer pain. *Lancet Oncology.* **11**: 484–489.
35 Lasheen W *et al.* (2010) The intravenous to oral relative milligram potency ratio of morphine during chronic dosing in cancer pain. *Palliative Medicine.* **24**: 9–16.
36 Hagen N *et al.* (1997) Cancer pain emergencies: a protocol for management. *Journal of Pain and Symptom Management.* **14**: 45–50.
37 Davis MP *et al.* (2004) Opioid dose titration for severe cancer pain: a systematic evidence-based review. *Journal of Palliative Medicine.* **7**: 462–468.
38 Kumar K *et al.* (2000) Intravenous morphine for emergency treatment of cancer pain. *Palliative Medicine.* **14**: 183–188.
39 Harris JT *et al.* (2003) Intravenous morphine for rapid control of severe cancer pain. *Palliative Medicine.* **17**: 248–256.
40 Davis MP (2004) Acute pain in advanced cancer: an opioid dosing strategy and illustration. *American Journal of Hospice and Palliative Care.* **21**: 47–50.
41 Davis MP (2005) Rapid opioid titration in severe cancer pain. *European Journal of Palliative Care.* **12**: 11–14.
42 Radbruch L *et al.* (1999) Intravenous titration with morphine for severe cancer pain: report of 28 cases. *Clinical Journal of Pain.* **15**: 173–178.
43 Schiessl C *et al.* (2010) Rhythmic pattern of PCA opioid demand in adults with cancer pain. *European Journal of Pain.* **14**: 372–379.
44 Soares LG *et al.* (2003) Intravenous fentanyl for cancer pain: a "fast titration" protocol for the emergency room. *Journal of Pain and Symptom Management.* **26**: 876–881.
45 Coluzzi P (1998) Sublingual morphine: efficacy reviewed. *Journal of Pain and Symptom Management.* **16**: 184–192.
46 deBoer AG *et al.* (1982) Rectal drug administration: clinical pharmacokinetic considerations. *Clinical Pharmacokinetics.* **7**: 285–311.
47 Johnson AG and Lux G (1988) *Progress in the Treatment of Gastrointestinal Motility Disorder. The role of cisapride.* Excerpta Medica, Amsterdam.
48 Ripamonti C and Bruera E (1991) Rectal, buccal and sublingual narcotics for the management of cancer pain. *Journal of Palliative Care.* **7 (1)**: 30–35.
49 Wilkinson T *et al.* (1992) Pharmacokinetics and efficacy of rectal versus oral sustained-release morphine in cancer patients. *Cancer Chemotherapy and Pharmacology.* **31**: 251–254.
50 Krajnik M and Zylicz Z (1997) Topical opioids — fact or fiction? *Progress in Palliative Care.* **5**: 101–106.
51 Likar R *et al.* (1999) Dose-dependency of intra-articular morphine analgesia. *British Journal of Anaesthesia.* **83**: 241–244.

52 Back NI and Finlay I (1995) Analgesic effect of topical opioids on painful skin ulcers. *Journal of Pain and Symptom Management*. **10**: 493.
53 Krajnik M *et al.* (1999) Potential uses of topical opioids in palliative care — report of 6 cases. *Pain*. **80**: 121–125.
54 Twillman R *et al.* (1999) Treatment of painful skin ulcers with topical opioids. *Journal of Pain and Symptom Management*. **17**: 288–292.
55 Zeppetella G *et al.* (2003) Analgesic efficacy of morphine applied topically to painful ulcers. *Journal of Pain and Symptom Management*. **25**: 555–558.
56 Zeppetella G and Ribeiro MD (2005) Morphine in intrasite gel applied topically to painful ulcers. *Journal of Pain and Symptom Management*. **29**: 118–119.
57 Le Bon B *et al.* (2009) Effectiveness of topical administration of opiods inpalliative care a systematic review. *Journal of Pain and Symptom Management*. **37**: 913–917.
58 Cerchietti LC *et al.* (2002) Effect of topical morphine for mucositis-associated pain following concomitant chemoradiotherapy for head and neck carcinoma. *Cancer*. **95**: 2230–2236.
59 Vayne-Bossert P *et al.* (2010) Effect of topical morphine (mouthwash) on oral pain due to chemotherapy — and/or radiotherapy-induced mucositis: a randomized double-blinded study. *Journal of Palliative Medicine*. **13**: 125–128.
60 Cerchietti LC *et al.* (2003) Potential utility of the peripheral analgesic properties of morphine in stomatitis-related pain: a pilot study. *Pain*. **105**: 265–273.
61 Twycross R *et al.* (2009) *Symptom Management in Advanced Cancer* (4e). palliativedrugs.com, pp. 145–158.
62 Davis C (1999) Nebulized opioids should not be prescribed outside a clinical trial. *American Journal of Hospice and Palliative Care*. **16**: 543.
63 Jennings A *et al.* (2002) A systematic review of the use of opioids in the management of dyspnoea. *Thorax*. **57**: 939–944.
64 Foral PA *et al.* (2004) Nebulized opioids use in COPD. *Chest*. **125**: 691–694.
65 Brown SJ *et al.* (2005) Nebulized morphine for relief of dyspnea due to chronic lung disease. *Annals of Pharmacotherapy*. **39**: 1088–1092.
66 Bruera E *et al.* (2005) Nebulized versus subcutaneous morphine for patients with cancer dyspnea: a preliminary study. *Journal of Pain and Symptom Management*. **29**: 613–618.
67 Bruera E *et al.* (2006) Can we really say that nebulized morphine works? (authors response). *Journal of Pain and Symptom Management*. **32**: 102–103.
68 Lasheen W *et al.* (2006) Can we really say that nebulized morphine works? *Journal of Pain and Symptom Management*. **32**: 101–102; author reply 102–103.
69 Bruera E *et al.* (1990) Effects of morphine on the dyspnea of terminal cancer patients. *Journal of Pain and Symptom Management*. **5**: 341–344.
70 Bruera E *et al.* (1993) Subcutaneous morphine for dyspnoea in cancer patients. *Annals of internal medicine*. **119**: 906–907.
71 Mazzocato C *et al.* (1999) The effects of morphine on dyspnoea and ventilatory function in elderly patients with advanced cancer: A randomized double-blind controlled trial. *Annals of Oncology*. **10**: 1511–1514.
72 Abernethy AP *et al.* (2003) Randomised, double blind, placebo controlled crossover trial of sustained release morphine for the management of refractory dyspnoea. *British Medical Journal*. **327**: 523–528.
73 Allen S *et al.* (2005) Low dose diamorphine reduces breathlessness without causing a fall in oxygen saturation in elderly patients with end-stage idiopathic pulmonary fibrosis. *Palliative Medicine*. **19**: 128–130.
74 Clemens KE *et al.* (2008) Is there a higher risk of respiratory depression in opioid-naive palliative care patients during symptomatic therapy of dyspnea with strong opioids? *Journal of Palliative Medicine*. **11**: 204–216.
75 Cohen M *et al.* (1991) Continuous intravenous infusion of morphine for severe dyspnoea. *Southern Medical Journal*. **84**: 229–234.
76 Boyd K and Kelly M (1997) Oral morphine as symptomatic treatment of dyspnoea in patients with advanced cancer. *Palliative Medicine*. **11**: 277–281.
77 Poole PJ *et al.* (1998) The effect of sustained-release morphine on breathlessness and quality of life in severe chronic obstructive pulmonary disease. *American Journal of Respiratory and Critical Care Medicine*. **157**: 1877–1880.
78 Allard P *et al.* (1999) How effective are supplementary doses of opioids for dyspnea in terminally ill cancer patients? A randomized continuous sequential clinical trial. *Journal of Pain and Symptom Management*. **17**: 256–265.
79 Rocker G *et al.* (2009) Palliation of dyspnoea in advanced COPD: revisiting a role for opioids. *Thorax*. **64**: 910–915.
80 Navigante AH *et al.* (2006) Midazolam as adjunct therapy to morphine in the alleviation of severe dyspnea perception in patients with advanced cancer. *Journal of Pain and Symptom Management*. **31**: 38–47
81 FDA (2011) Medwatch safety alert. Morphine sulfate oral solution 100mg per 5mL (20mg/mL): medication use error — reports of accidental overdose. Available from: www.fda.gov/Safety/MedWatch/SafetyInformation/SafetyAlertsforHumanMedicalProducts/ucm239559.htm?sms_ss = email&at_xt = 4d372d1d29c3a5e2%2C0

DIAMORPHINE — BNF 4.7.2

Class: Strong opioid analgesic (available only in the UK).

Indications: As for **morphine**; used in the UK instead of parenteral **morphine** because of its greater solubility, particularly when large doses are necessary.

Contra-indications: None absolute if titrated carefully against a patient's pain (also see Strong opioids, p.345).

Pharmacology

Diamorphine (di-acetylmorphine, heroin) is generally considered to be a pro-drug without intrinsic activity.[1] *In vivo*, it is rapidly de-acetylated (plasma halflife 3min) to an active metabolite, 6-mono-acetylmorphine (6-MAM) (plasma halflife 20min), and then to **morphine** itself.[2]

IM diamorphine is more than twice as potent as **morphine**.[3–5] The greater potency of parenteral diamorphine could be because 6-MAM is more potent than **morphine**[6] or because diamorphine and 6-MAM cross the blood-brain barrier more readily than **morphine**. However, by mouth the two opioids are almost equipotent.[7]

Diamorphine IM acts more quickly than **morphine**,[5,8] but **morphine** acts more quickly IV.[9] This paradox is not easily explained, but it could relate to differences in plasma protein-binding (diamorphine 40%, **morphine** 20%).

In terms of analgesic efficacy and effect on mood, diamorphine has no clinical advantage over **morphine** by oral or SC/IM routes.[3,4,7] Diamorphine hydrochloride is much more water-soluble than **morphine** sulphate/hydrochloride and, in the UK, is the strong opioid of choice for parenteral use when high doses are needed (Table 5.21).

Table 5.21 Solubility of selected opioids[10]

Preparation	*Amount of water needed to dissolve 1g at 25°C (mL)*
Morphine	5,000
Morphine hydrochloride	24
Morphine sulphate	21
Diamorphine hydrochloride	1.6[a]
Hydromorphone	3

a. 1g of diamorphine hydrochloride dissolved in 1.6mL has a volume of 2.4mL.

Like **morphine**, diamorphine can be given by many different routes, including spinally. Diamorphine can also be given intranasally using a nasal dosing device, a route used mainly in children.[11] It can be used for the same range of indications as **morphine**, including bladder spasms (intravesical administration)[12,13] and painful decubitus ulcers (topically in Intrasite® gel).[14–16]

Bio-availability (as 6-MAM) no data.

Onset of action 5–10min SC.

Time to peak plasma concentration 1.5–2h PO as 6-MAM and **morphine**.

Plasma halflife 3min IV; metabolized to active metabolites.

Duration of action 4h.

Stability

Diamorphine hydrochloride is stable indefinitely when stored as a powder[17] but de-acetylates when in solution, first to 6-mono-acetylmorphine (6-MAM) and then to **morphine**. The rate of de-acetylation is situation dependent. Thus, *in vivo*, diamorphine is converted to 6-MAM in minutes. In contrast, the stability of diamorphine hydrochloride in simple aqueous solution is relatively long. Further, because 6-MAM is the primary active agent, there is no loss of potency until 6-MAM is degraded to **morphine**.[6]

In one study, after 3 months in simple aqueous solution, 30% of the diamorphine had degraded to 6-MAM, but it was only at 12 months that a trace of **morphine** became detectable.[18] A second study looked at the effect of ambient temperature and of mixing the diamorphine with other drugs.[19,20] At 22°C, the loss of 10% of diamorphine to 6-MAM took 8 weeks but, at 37°C, only 2 weeks. When mixed with **prochlorperazine** or **chlorpromazine** and kept at 22°C, the 'shelf life' was 2 weeks, i.e. the same as the aqueous solution at 37°C.[19,20] Based on these data, it is reasonable to conclude that diamorphine in solution in a syringe, even for several days with other drugs, remains a mixture of diamorphine and 6-MAM, and is not simply a solution of **morphine** by another name.

Undesirable effects

See Strong opioids, p.345.

Dose and use

In the UK, diamorphine has been used for all the same indications as **morphine**, and by the same range of routes, including topically and spinally (see p.362). Intranasal sprays (not commercially available) are used for children in many Emergency Departments in England and Wales.[11,21,22]

Although in the past diamorphine was often administered PO instead of **morphine**, it is now generally reserved for parenteral use (see p.665). The following are practical clinical conversion ratios:

- PO **morphine** to SC diamorphine, give one third of the PO dose
- PO diamorphine to SC diamorphine, give one half of the PO dose.

For CSCI dilute with WFI, concentration-dependent *incompatibility* occurs with 0.9% saline (see p.667).

CSCI compatibility with other drugs: There are 2-drug compatibility data for diamorphine in WFI with **clonazepam, dexamethasone, glycopyrronium, hyoscine *butylbromide*, hyoscine *hydrobromide*, ketorolac, levomepromazine, metoclopramide, midazolam, octreotide,** and **ondansetron**.

Concentration-dependent *incompatibility* occurs with **cyclizine** or **haloperidol** at higher concentrations. For more details and 3-drug compatibility data, see Appendix 3 charts A3.1 (p.776) and A3.3 (p.780).

Compatibility charts for mixing drugs in 0.9% saline can be found on www.palliativedrugs.com Syringe Driver Survey Database.

Supply

Diamorphine hydrochloride is available for medicinal use only in the UK. Because diamorphine ampoules cost about 3 times more than **morphine** ampoules, many palliative care units in the UK now use **morphine** as their standard parenteral strong opioid, unless the need for high doses makes diamorphine more convenient because of its greater solubility.[23]

Unless indicated otherwise, all preparations are **CD**.

Diamorphine (generic)

Tablets 10mg, 10mg dose = £0.16.

Injection (powder for reconstitution) 5mg amp = £2.50; 10mg amp = £3.50; 30mg amp = £4; 100mg amp = £9; 500mg amp = £42.

1 Inturrisi CE *et al.* (1984) The pharmacokinetics of heroin in patients with chronic pain. *New England Journal of Medicine.* **310**: 1213–1217.

2 Barrett DA *et al.* (1992) The effect of temperature and pH on the deacetylation of diamorphine in aqueous solution and in human plasma. *Journal of Pharmacy and Pharmacology.* **44**: 606–608.

3 Kaiko RF *et al.* (1981) Analgesic and mood effects of heroin and morphine in cancer patients with postoperative pain. *New England Journal of Medicine.* **304**: 1501–1505.

4 Beaver WT *et al.* (1981) Comparison of the analgesic effect of intramuscular heroin and morphine in patients with cancer pain. *Clinical Pharmacology and Therapeutics.* **29**: 232.

5 Reichle CW *et al.* (1962) Comparative analgesic potency of heroin and morphine in postoperative patients. *Journal of Pharmacology and Experimental Therapeutics.* **136**: 43–46.

6 Wright CI and Barbour FA (1935) The respiratory effects of morphine, codeine and related substances. *Journal of Pharmacology and Experimental Therapeutics.* **54**: 25–33.

7 Twycross RG (1977) Choice of strong analgesic in terminal cancer: diamorphine or morphine? *Pain.* **3**: 93–104.

8 Dundee JW *et al.* (1966) Studies of drugs given before anaesthesia XI: diamorphine (heroin) and morphine. *British Journal of Anaesthesia.* **38**: 610–619.

9 Morrison L *et al.* (1991) Comparison of speed of onset of analgesic effect of diamorphine and morphine. *British Journal of Anaesthesia.* **66**: 656–659.

10 Hanks GW and Hoskin PJ (1987) Opioid analgesics in the management of pain in patients with cancer: a review. *Palliative Medicine.* **1**: 1–25.

11 Kendall J *et al.* (2001) Multicentre randomised controlled trial of nasal diamorphine for analgesia in children and teenagers with clinical fractures. *British Medical Journal.* **322**: 261–265.

12 McCoubrie R and Jeffrey D (2003) Intravesical diamorphine for bladder spasm. *Journal of Pain and Symptom Management.* **25**: 1–3.

13 Duckett J (1997) Intravesical morphine analgesia after bladder surgery. *Journal of Urology.* **157**: 1407–1409.

14 Abbas SQ (2004) Diamorphine-Intrasite dressings for painful pressure ulcers. *Journal of Pain and Symptom Management.* **28**: 532–534.

15 Zeppetella G and Ribeiro MD (2003) Pharmacotherapy of cancer-related episodic pain. *Expert Opinion in Pharmacotherapy.* **4**: 493–502.

16 Flock P (2003) Pilot study to determine the effectiveness of diamorphine gel to control pressure ulcer pain. *Journal of Pain and Symptom Management.* **25**: 547–554.

17 Lerner M and Mills A (1963) Some modern aspects of heroin analysis. *Bulletin on Narcotics.* **15**: 37–42.

18 Rizzotti G (1935) Contributo allo studio delle alterazioni delle soluzioni acquose di eroina. *Archives Internationales de Pharmacodynamie et de Therapie*. **52**: 87–96.
19 Twycross RG and Gilhooley RA (1973) Euporiant elixirs. *British Medical Journal*. **4**: 552.
20 Twycross RG (1974) Diamorphine and cocaine elixir BPC. *Pharmaceutical Journal*. **212**: 153 & 159.
21 Shelley K and Paech MJ (2008) The clinical applications of intranasal opioids. *Current Drug Delivery*. **5**: 55–58.
22 Hadley G *et al.* (2010) A survey of intranasal medication use in the paediatric emergency setting in England and Wales. *Emergency Medical Journal*. **27**: 553–554.
23 Palliativedrugs.com (2010) Diamorphine: essential opioid or time to say goodbye? Available from: www.palliativedrugs.com/download/100223_diamorphine_essential_opioid.pdf

*ALFENTANIL BNF 4.7.2

Class: Opioid analgesic.

Indications: Intra-operative analgesia, analgesia and procedure-related pain in mechanically ventilated patients on intensive care units, †an alternative in cases of intolerance to other strong opioids, particularly in renal failure,[1] †procedure-related pain in non-ventilated patients,[2,3] †break-through (episodic) pain.[4,5]

Contra-indications: Do not administer concurrently with MAOIs or within two weeks of their discontinuation. Generally no absolute if titrated carefully against a patient's pain (also see Strong opioids, p.345).

Pharmacology

Alfentanil is a synthetic lipophilic opioid in the same class as **fentanyl** and **sufentanil** (not UK). Compared with these, it has a more rapid onset of action and time to peak effect, and a shorter duration of action (Table 5.22). Its potency is approximately one quarter that of **fentanyl**[6] (and 10–20 times more than parenteral **morphine**).

Alfentanil is less lipophilic than **fentanyl** and is 90% bound to mainly α_1-acid glycoprotein.[7] However, because most of the unbound alfentanil is unionized, it rapidly enters the CNS. It is metabolized in the liver by CYP3A4 to inactive metabolites that are excreted in the urine. Alfentanil can accumulate with chronic administration, particularly when clearance is reduced, e.g. in the elderly and the obese, and when there is hepatic impairment.[8] In consequence, if switching from an alfentanil infusion to another opioid, it is safer to use conservative dose estimates. It has been suggested that analgesic tolerance occurs rapidly with alfentanil,[9] but this has been refuted.[10] Certainly, tolerance does not seem to be a problem in palliative care.[11,12]

Although dose reductions may be necessary in patients with severe hepatic impairment, this is not necessary in renal failure. Consequently, alfentanil is used at some centres as the parenteral opioid of choice in end-stage renal failure (see p.355).[13] Alfentanil is available in a more concentrated form (500microgram/mL) than **fentanyl** (50microgram/mL), reducing the dose volume and facilitating its administration by CSCI or SL (see p.665). For similar reasons, in countries where alfentanil is not available, **sufentanil** is used instead (Table 5.22 and Box 5.M).[14]

Alfentanil has been used successfully by short-term PCA or CSCI for dressing changes in burns or trauma patients.[2,3] It can be used SL and nasally for episodic pain, including severe intractable angina in inoperable coronary artery disease.[4,15,16] In the UK, a spray bottle containing alfentanil 5mg in 5mL is manufactured from alfentanil powder, delivering 140microgram/0.14mL spray. Details and instructions for use can be downloaded from palliativedrugs.com.[5] In an audit of patients already on regular strong opioids, about three quarters benefited from SL alfentanil in doses of 560–1,680microgram (4–12 sprays; titrated as necessary). Pain relief was seen within 10min.

Spinal administration of lipophilic opioids remains controversial because of the rapid clearance into the systemic circulation (see Chapter 21, Spinal analgesia).[17,18]

Table 5.22 Pharmacokinetics of single IV doses of fentanils[19–21]

	Alfentanil	*Sufentanil*	*Fentanyl*
Onset of action (min)	0.75[a]	1	1.5
Time to peak effect (min)	1.5	2.5	4.5
Plasma halflife (min)	95	165	220
Duration of action (min)	30[a]	60	60

a. onset slower if given IM (<5min), and duration of action longer (60min).

Box 5.M Sufentanil (not UK)

A lipophilic opioid with a strong affinity for the μ-opioid receptor. Time to onset of action and to peak effect is mid-way between that of alfentanil and fentanyl (see Table 5.22).[20]

Sufentanil is about 7.5–10 times more potent than fentanyl,[22 23] and this allows a smaller volume to be given. Divide the dose of fentanyl by 10 to obtain an easy-to-calculate starting dose.

Example
Fentanyl 1,000microgram/24h CSCI (i.e. 20mL of 50microgram/mL)
→ sufentanil 100microgram/24h CSCI (i.e. 2mL of 50microgram/mL).

Sufentanil can be administered SC, IV or spinally.[24] By CSCI, it is compatible with other commonly prescribed drugs.[25]

Also given by intranasal or SL routes as pre-operative sedation and for rescue analgesia for episodic cancer pain (see Table 5.22).[26]

Accumulates in fat tissue when given continuously;[27] monitor carefully when switching to another opioid.

Is not dependent on renal function for elimination, and is thus useful in renal impairment.

Cautions

Alfentanil levels are increased by inhibitors of CYP3A4 (see Table 5.23 and Cytochrome P450, p.735). Thus, it may be necessary to adjust the dose of alfentanil if any of these drugs are prescribed concurrently.[28]

Table 5.23 Clinically significant cytochrome P450 interactions with alfentanil resulting in changed drug plasma concentrations

Alfentanil plasma concentration	
Increased by	*Decreased by*
Cimetidine	Rifampicin
Diltiazem	
Erythromycin	
Fluconazole, itraconazole, ketoconazole, voriconazole	
Protease inhibitors	
Troleandomycin	

Undesirable effects

See Strong opioids, p.349.

Dose and use

Procedure-related pain (see Quick Practice Guide, p.379)

- 250–500microgram SL (from ampoule for injection) or SC/IV.

As an alternative to morphine

Used mostly for patients in renal failure in whom there is evidence of **morphine** neurotoxicity (see p.352). Given the shorter duration of action of alfentanil, it is difficult to give a single precise dose conversion ratio. However, the following are safe practical conversion ratios:

- PO **morphine** to CSCI alfentanil, give one thirtieth of the 24h dose, e.g. **morphine** 60mg/24h PO = alfentanil 2mg/24h CSCI
- CSCI **morphine** to CSCI alfentanil, give one fifteenth of the 24h dose, e.g. **morphine** 30mg/24h = alfentanil 2mg/24h
- CSCI **diamorphine** to CSCI alfentanil, give one tenth of the 24h dose, e.g. **diamorphine** 30mg/24h = alfentanil 3mg/24h.

Conventionally, SC p.r.n. doses of alfentanil are 1/6–1/10 of the total 24h CSCI dose. Because of the short duration of action of alfentanil (about 30min), even with an optimally titrated p.r.n. dose, frequent dosing may be required; the CSCI dose of alfentanil should be reviewed at least daily, and titrated accordingly. For CSCI dilute with WFI, 0.9% saline or 5% glucose.

CSCI compatibility with other drugs: There are 2-drug compatibility data for alfentanil in WFI with **clonazepam, dexamethasone, glycopyrronium, haloperidol, hyoscine *butylbromide*, levomepromazine, metoclopramide, midazolam, octreotide,** and **ondansetron**.

Concententration-dependent *incompatibility* occurs with **cyclizine**. For more details, and 3-drug compatibility data, see Appendix 3 charts A3.1 (p.776) and A3.2 (p.778).

Compatibility charts for mixing drugs in 0.9% saline can be found on *www.palliativedrugs.com* Syringe Driver Survey Database.

An alternative dosing schedule

The recommendations above may well be too conservative for some patients. It is important to review sooner rather than later, and increase the dose if necessary. At one centre, a conversion ratio for **diamorphine** to alfentanil of one sixth has been used for many years without clinical evidence of respiratory depression.[29]

At this centre, p.r.n. **diamorphine/morphine** is given to supplement CSCI alfentanil, giving the same p.r.n. dose as used before the switch to alfentanil. When the switch has been prompted by opioid neurotoxicity, a recurrence has not been observed with 1–2 p.r.n. doses/24h of **diamorphine/morphine**.

Break-through (episodic) cancer pain, SL administration

Given the variability in the intensity of break-through pains, p.r.n. recommendations are best expressed as a range of doses rather than a single fixed dose. There is a poor relationship between the effective SL p.r.n. dose and regular CSCI dose. Individual dose titration is necessary, e.g. starting with 1/10–1/6 of the daily alfentanil dose, and titrating upwards if necessary. Retaining even 2mL in the mouth (sublingually or buccally) for 5–10min is difficult. Thus, the smaller the volume, the easier it is for the patient (see Table 5.24).

As with all opioids, patients must be monitored for undesirable effects, particularly nausea and vomiting, and constipation (see p.348). Depending on individual circumstances, an anti-emetic should be prescribed for regular or p.r.n. use, (see p.225) and, routinely, a laxative prescribed (see p.38).

Supply

Unless indicated otherwise, all preparations are **CD**.

The high-strength intensive care injection is used at some centres when the CSCI/CIVI dose is >5mg/24h. However, to avoid the risk of the high-strength injection being administered by mistake, in many hospitals its availability is restricted to the Intensive Care Unit.

Table 5.24 Equivalent volumes of parenteral formulations of alfentanil, sufentanil and fentanyl for SL use[a]

Alfentanil (500microgram/mL)		*Sufentanil (50microgram/mL)*		*Fentanyl (50microgram/mL)*	
Dose (microgram)	*Volume (mL)*	*Dose (microgram)*	*Volume (mL)*	*Dose (microgram)*	*Volume (mL)*
100	0.2	2.5	N/A	25	0.5
200	0.4	5	0.1	50	1
300	0.6	7.5	0.15	75	1.5
400	0.8	10	0.2	100	2
500	1	12.5	0.25	125	N/O[b]
600	1.2	15	0.3	150	N/O
800	1.6	20	0.4	200	N/O
1,000	2	25	0.5	250	N/O
2,000	N/O[b]	50	1	500	N/O
3,000	N/O	75	1.5	750	N/O
4,000	N/O	100	2	1,000	N/O

a. this is *not* a true dose conversion chart. Alfentanil, sufentanil and fentanyl have differing properties and, although bio-availability and onset of effect are broadly similar, duration of effect differs (fentanyl > sufentanil > alfentanil). As always with analgesics, individual patient dose titration is required

b. N/O = not optimal, because > 2mL.

Alfentanil (generic)

Nasal spray (with attachment for buccal/SL use) 5mg/5mL, 5mL bottle = £12; minimum order value = £25. (Unlicensed, available as a special order from the pharmacy manufacturing unit, Torbay hospital, see Obtaining unlicensed products, p.769). *Telephone number for enquiries: 01803 664707; orders must be faxed to the manufacturing unit on 01803 664354. The solution is stable for 1 year unopened and for 28 days after opening.*

Injection 500microgram/mL, 2mL amp = £0.50, 10mL amp = £3.

Intensive care injection (for dilution and use as a continuous infusion) 5mg/mL, 1mL amp = £2.50.

Rapifen® (Janssen Cilag)

Injection 500microgram/mL, 2mL amp = £0.50, 10mL amp = £3.

Intensive care injection (for dilution and use as a CIVI) 5mg/mL, 1mL amp = £2.50.

1 Kirkham SR and Pugh R (1995) Opioid analgesia in uraemic patients. *Lancet.* **345**: 1185.

2 Sim KM *et al.* (1996) Use of patient-controlled analgesia with alfentanil for burns dressing procedures: a preliminary report of five patients. *Burns.* **22**: 238–241.

3 Gallagher G *et al.* (2001) Target-controlled alfentanil analgesia for dressing change following extensive reconstructive surgery for trauma. *Journal of Pain and Symptom Management.* **21**: 1–2.

4 Duncan A (2002) The use of fentanyl and alfentanil sprays for episodic pain. *Palliative Medicine.* **16**: 550.

5 Palliativedrugs.com (2003) Hot Topics: alternatives to sublingual fentanyl. In: *August Newsletter.* Available from: www.palliativedrugs.com

6 Larijani G and Goldberg M (1987) Alfentanil hydrochloride: a new short acting narcotic analgesic for surgical procedures. *Clinical Pharmacy.* **6**: 275–282.

7 Bernards C (1999) Clinical implications of physicochemical properties of opioids. In: C Stein (ed) *Opioids in Pain Control: basic and clinical aspects.* Cambridge University Press, Cambridge, pp. 166–187.

8 Bodenham A and Park GR (1988) Alfentanil infusions in patients requiring intensive care. *Clinical Pharmacokinetics.* **15**: 216–226.

9 Kissin I *et al.* (2000) Acute tolerance to continuously infused alfentanil: the role of cholecystokinin and N-methyl-D-aspartate-nitric oxide systems. *Anesthesia and Analgesia.* **91**: 110–116.

10 Schraag S *et al.* (1999) Lack of rapid development of opioid tolerance during alfentanil and remifentanil infusions for postoperative pain. *Anesthesia and Analgesia.* **89**: 753–757.

11 Hill HF *et al.* (1992) Patient-controlled analgesia infusions: alfentanil versus morphine. *Pain.* **49**: 301–310.

12 Urch CE *et al.* (2004) A retrospective review of the use of alfentanil in a hospital palliative care setting. *Palliative Medicine.* **18**: 516–519.

13 Chambers EJ *et al.* (eds) (2004) *Supportive Care for the Renal Patient.* Oxford University Press, Oxford, pp. 122, 262–265.

14 Gardner-Nix J (2001) Oral transmucosal fentanyl and sufentanil for incident pain. *Journal of Pain and Symptom Management.* **22**: 627–630.

15 Osborn H and Jefferson M (2010) Intranasal alfentanil for severe intractable angina in inoperable coronary artery disease. *Palliative Medicine.* **24**: 94–95.

16 Brenchley J and Ramlakhan S (2006) Intranasal alfentanil for acute pain in children. *Emergency Medical Journal.* **23**: 488.

17 Burm A *et al.* (1994) Pharmacokinetics of alfentanil after epidural administration. Investigation of systemic absorption kinetics with a stable isotope method. *Anesthesiology.* **81**: 308–315.
18 Ummenhofer W *et al.* (2000) Comparative spinal distribution and clearance kinetics of intrathecally administered morphine, fentanyl, alfentanil, and sufentanil. *Anesthesiology.* **92**: 739–953.
19 Willens JS and Myslinski NR (1993) Pharmacodynamics, pharmacokinetics, and clinical uses of fentanyl, sufentanil, and alfentanil. *Heart Lung*. **22**: 239–251.
20 Scholz J *et al.* (1996) Clinical pharmacokinetics of alfentanil, fentanyl and sufentanil. An update. *Clinical Pharmacokinetics*. **31**: 275–292.
21 Hall T and Hardy J (2005) The lipophilic opioids: fentanyl, alfentanil, sufentanil and remifentanil. In: M Davis *et al.* (eds) *Opioids in Cancer Pain*. Oxford University Press, Oxford.
22 Reynolds L *et al.* (2004) Relative analgesic potency of fentanyl and sufentanil during intermediate-term infusions in patients after long-term opioid treatment for chronic pain. *Pain.* **110**: 182–188.
23 Scott JC *et al.* (1991) Electroencephalographic quantitation of opioid effect: comparative pharmacodynamics of fentanyl and sufentanil. *Anesthesiology.* **74**: 34–42.
24 Waara-Wolleat KL *et al.* (2006) A review of intrathecal fentanyl and sufentanil for the treatment of chronic pain. *Pain Medicine*. **7**: 251–259.
25 White C *et al.* (2008) Subcutaneous sufentanil for palliative care patients in a hospital setting. *Palliative Medicine*. **22**: 89–90.
26 Good P *et al.* (2009) Intranasal sufentanil for cancer-associated breakthrough pain. *Palliative Medicine*. **23**: 54–58.
27 Alazia M *et al.* (1992) Pharmacokinetics of long term sufentanil infusion (72 hours) used for sedation in ICU patients. *Anesthesiology.* **77**: A364 (abstract).
28 Saari TI *et al.* (2006) Voriconazole, but not terbinafine, markedly reduces alfentanil clearance and prolongs its half-life. *Clinical Pharmacology and Therapeutics*. **80**: 502–508.
29 Kirkham S (2010) *Personal communication.*

Quick Practice Guide: Management of procedure-related pain

1 Palliative care patients may experience pain while undergoing procedures, e.g.:
- position change
- investigation, e.g. MRI
- wound dressing change
- venous cannulation
- urethral catheterization
- removing impacted faeces
- insertion of nasogastric tube
- insertion/removal of central line
- insertion/removal of spinal line
- drainage of chest/abdomen
- treatment, e.g. radiotherapy.

2 The goal is adequate pain relief without undesirable effects. What is appropriate depends on the anticipated pain severity, procedure duration, current opioid use, and the patient's past personal experience. Thus, severe procedure-related pain may necessitate parenteral analgesia and sedation as first-line therapy.

3 Always include non-drug approaches:
- discuss past experiences of procedure-related pain, identify what was helpful or unhelpful, and clarify present concerns
- explain the procedure thoroughly before starting
- assure that you will stop immediately if requested
- as far as possible, choose the most comfortable position for the patient
- distract and relax, e.g. through talking, music, hypnosis and other relaxation techniques.

4 Use a local anaesthetic for:
- venous cannulation; use EMLA® cream if needle phobic or if requested (wait 60min)
- urethral catheterization; use lidocaine gel (wait 5min)
- chest aspiration; use lidocaine for tissue infiltration (wait 5min).

5 If available, consider nitrous oxide-oxygen (Entonox®) inhalation if the procedure is short and the patient is able to use the mask or mouthpiece effectively.

6 Give analgesia from the appropriate step of the ladder. (General anaesthetic approaches are beyond the scope of these guidelines.)

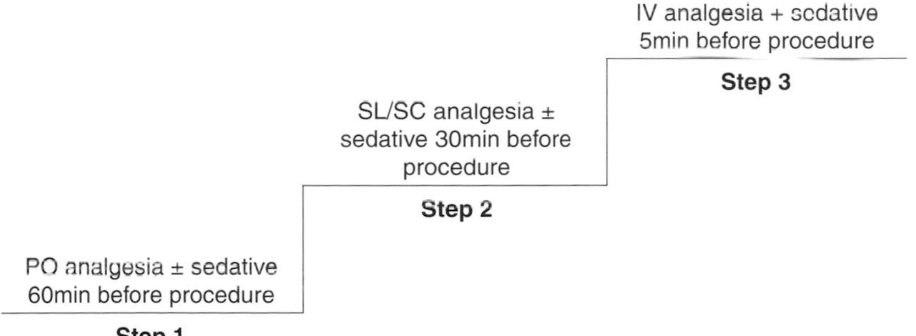

7 If pain relief inadequate, give a repeat dose and wait again; if still inadequate, move to the next step.

8 When a sedative or sedative analgesic is used, practitioners must be competent in airway management. Monitor the patient to ensure that the airway remains patent, and intervene if the patient becomes cyanosed because of severely depressed respiration.

continued

Examples of analgesia for procedure-related pain

Step 1: If anticipating mild–moderate pain
Give 60min before the procedure:
PO morphine, give the patient's usual rescue dose for break-through (episodic) pain.
If necessary, combine with:
- PO diazepam 5mg *or*
- SL lorazepam 500microgram–1mg *or*
- an alternative sedative.

Step 2: If anticipating moderate–severe pain
Give 30min before procedure:
SC morphine, give 50% of the patient's usual PO morphine rescue dose.
If necessary, combine with:
- SL/SC midazolam 2.5–5mg *or*
- SL lorazepam 500microgram–1mg *or*
- an alternative sedative.

Step 3: If anticipating severe–excruciating pain
Give 5min before procedure:
IV morphine, give 50% of the patient's usual PO morphine rescue dose *or*
IV ketamine 0.5–1mg/kg (typically 25–50mg). Combine with:
- IV midazolam 2.5–5mg *or*
- an alternative sedative.

Note: there is a risk of marked sedation when ketamine and a sedative such as midazolam are combined in this way; use only if competent in airway management.

Alternatives to SC/IV morphine
- fentanyl 50–100microgram or more transmucosally using a licensed product (see p.400)
- alfentanil 250–500microgram SL (*from ampoule for injection or spray*) or SC/IV
- fentanyl 50–100microgram SL (*from ampoule for injection*) or SC/IV
- sufentanil 12.5–25microgram SL (*from ampoule for injection*) or SC/IV.

9 An opioid antagonist (naloxone) and a benzodiazepine antagonist (flumazenil) should be available in case of need. To prevent the complete reversal of any background regular opioid analgesic therapy, use naloxone 20–100microgram IV, repeated every 2min until the respiratory rate and cyanosis have improved. The initial dose of flumazenil is 200microgram IV over 15 seconds. If the desired level of consciousness is not obtained after 1 minute, further 100microgram doses can be given at 1 minute intervals p.r.n. up to a maximum total dose of 1mg.

10 If the procedure is to be repeated, give analgesia based on previous experience, e.g. drugs used and the patient's comments.

BUPRENORPHINE BNF 4.7.2

Buprenorphine is experiencing a renaissance in the management of chronic cancer and non-cancer pain and opioid dependence (high-dose SL formulation ± **naloxone**).[1–6] Compared to **morphine** and other opioids, buprenorphine appears to cause less hyperalgesia (see p.352) and tolerance, and adversely affects the immune and endocrine systems to a lesser extent. However, clinical trials are needed to find out whether such differences represent real clinical advantages.

Class: Opioid analgesic.

Indications: ***SL and injection*** moderate–severe pain, premedication and peri-operative analgesia, †intolerance to other strong opioids.
SL high-dose tablet withdrawal and maintenance therapy for opioid addicts (also available as a combined formulation with naloxone, to prevent parenteral misuse).
TD moderate (BuTrans®) or severe (Transtec®) non-cancer pain; moderate–severe cancer pain (Transtec®), †intolerance to other strong opioids.

Contra-indications: None absolute if titrated carefully against a patient's pain (also see Strong opioids, p.345). TD buprenorphine should not be used for acute (transient, intermittent or short-term) pain, e.g. postoperative, or when there is need for rapid dose titration for severe uncontrolled pain.

Pharmacology

Buprenorphine is a partial μ-opioid receptor and opioid-receptor-like (ORL-1) *agonist* and a κ- and δ-opioid receptor *antagonist*.[7–9] It has high affinity at the μ-, κ- and δ-opioid receptors, but affinity at the ORL-1 receptor is 500-fold less. It associates and dissociates slowly from receptors.[10] Subjective and physiological effects are generally similar to **morphine** (μ-opioid receptor agonist).

A study in volunteers suggests that buprenorphine may have an antihyperalgesic effect as well as an analgesic effect.[11,12] Animal studies and case reports also suggest that buprenorphine may be of particular benefit in neuropathic pain.[2,13] However, controlled studies are required to determine what place, if any, buprenorphine should have in the clinical management of neuropathic pain.[6,14–16] As with other opioids, ultra-low doses of opioid antagonists potentiate the analgesic effect of buprenorphine (see p.435).[17]

Antagonist effects at the κ-opioid receptor may limit spinal analgesia, sedation and psychotomimetic effects.[18] In animal studies, buprenorphine shows a ceiling effect or a bell-shaped dose-response curve for analgesic (>1mg/kg) and respiratory effects (0.1mg/kg). This is thought to be due to its partial agonist effect at the μ-opioid receptor. An agonist effect at the pronociceptive supraspinal ORL-1 receptor may also contribute.[19] In humans, a ceiling effect has been shown for respiratory depression (~200microgram/70kg IV)[20,21] and other effects, e.g. euphoria (4–8mg SL),[22,23] but not for analgesia.[21] Total daily doses as high as 16–24mg SL provide effective analgesia.[24,25] Thus, the ceiling dose for analgesia in humans is much higher than the 'maximum' TD dose recommended by the UK manufacturers, namely 3.36mg/day (70microgram/h patches x 2).

Studies of buprenorphine TD or SL up to 1.6mg/day have confirmed it is possible to use **morphine** (or other μ-opioid receptor agonist) for break-through (episodic) pain[26] and to switch either way between buprenorphine and **morphine** (or other μ-opioid receptor agonist) without loss of analgesia.[27,28]

Buprenorphine has either no effect or a smaller effect than **morphine** on pressure within the biliary and pancreatic ducts.[29,30] Buprenorphine does slow intestinal transit, but possibly less so than **morphine**.[31,32] Constipation may be less severe.[33]

Compared with **morphine** and other opioids, buprenorphine appears less likely to suppress the gonadal axis or testosterone levels (see p.352).[34] This may relate to its κ-opioid receptor *antagonist* effect.[35] Because hypogonadism is associated with reduced sexual desire and function, mood disturbance, fatigue and other physiological effects, e.g. muscle wasting, osteoporosis, this may become an important consideration in patients requiring long-term opioid therapy.[36–38]

Compared with **morphine** and other opioids, buprenorphine has little or no immunosuppressive effect (see p.352).[2,39–41]

Compared with **methadone**, buprenorphine has less effect on the QT interval (see p.418).[42,43]

In an anecdotal report, 2 out of 5 patients with cholestatic pruritus responded to treatment with buprenorphine.[44,45] However, there are insufficient data at present to recommend its use in this circumstance.

TD buprenorphine

Buprenorphine is highly lipid-soluble making it suitable for TD delivery. It is available in the UK as two formulations delivering either 5, 10 or 20microgram/h over 7 days (BuTrans®) or 35, 52.5 or 70microgram/h over 4 days (Transtec®)[46] and, like other strong opioids, is an alternative to both weak opioids and **morphine**.[47] Buprenorphine is evenly distributed in a drug-in-adhesive matrix. Its release is controlled by the physical characteristics of the matrix and is proportional to the surface area of the patch. Absorption of the buprenorphine through the skin and into the systemic circulation is influenced by the stratum corneum and blood flow. Thus, if the skin is warm and vasodilated, the rate of absorption increases.

There are few practical differences in the use of the buprenorphine or **fentanyl** matrix patches, and similar safety considerations apply, e.g. not to expose the patch to external sources of heat. Compared with **fentanyl**, TD buprenorphine (as Transtec®) adheres better. However, after patch removal, it is associated with more persistent erythema (± localized pruritus), and sometimes a more definite dermatitis.[48] This is generally caused by the adhesive, but occasionally buprenorphine itself causes a contact dermatitis ± more widespread skin rash.[49]

Retrospective analysis suggests that, compared with TD **fentanyl**, patients receiving TD buprenorphine (as Transtec®) have a slower rate of dose increase and longer periods of dose stability.[50] This requires confirmation in an RCT. Indeed, a systematic review has highlighted a relative lack of high quality studies of TD buprenorphine.[51]

SL opioid-maintenance therapy in addicts

Studies in addicts indicate that buprenorphine 16mg SL leads to 80% of the μ-opioid receptors in the brain being occupied which is sufficient to antagonize the subjective and respiratory depressant effects of **hydromorphone**, a μ-opioid receptor agonist.[10,52] This has implications for the management of acute pain in these patients, e.g. postoperative or traumatic pain (see p.655).

Respiratory depression

Significant respiratory depression is rarely seen with clinically recommended doses. A lower risk of respiratory depression may also explain why buprenorphine (mainly SL ± **naloxone**) appears to have a better safety profile than **methadone**.[53] However, serious or fatal respiratory depression has occurred in addicts misusing buprenorphine, generally in high-dose IV and in combination with benzodiazepines or other CNS depressants, e.g. alcohol.[54] Because buprenorphine has very strong receptor affinity (reflected in its high relative potency with **morphine**), **naloxone** in standard doses does not reverse the effects of buprenorphine and higher doses must be used (Box 5.N).[2,55–58] The non-specific respiratory stimulant **doxapram** can also be used, 1–1.5mg/kg IV over 30sec, repeated if necessary at hourly intervals or 1.5–4mg/min CIVI.[55,58–60]

Box 5.N Reversal of buprenorphine-induced respiratory depression

1 Discontinue buprenorphine (stop CSCI/CIVI, remove TD patch).
2 Give oxygen by mask.
3 Give IV naloxone *2mg* stat over 90sec.
4 Commence naloxone *4mg/h* by CIVI.
5 Continue CIVI until the patient's condition is satisfactory (probably <90min).
6 Monitor the patient frequently for the next 24h, and restart CIVI if respiratory depression recurs.
7 If the patient's condition remains satisfactory, restart buprenorphine at a reduced dose, e.g. half the previous dose.

Potency ratio

Buprenorphine has a longer duration of action than **morphine**. In postoperative single-dose studies, buprenorphine provided analgesia for 6–7h compared with 4–5h with **morphine**.[61] This is reflected in the recommended dose frequency (q8h–q6h vs. q4h for **morphine**). However, the longer duration of action of buprenorphine almost certainly means that potency ratios based on *single-dose* studies will *underestimate* the potency of buprenorphine. Thus, the following ratios should be *not* be regarded as 'cast iron'. They merely provide a rough guide for use when switching route or opioids (see Opioid dose conversion ratios, p.625):

- SL buprenorphine is about half as potent as IV/IM/SC buprenorphine; thus, in round figures, 2mg SL is equivalent to 1mg by injection[62,63]
- SL buprenorphine is about 80 times more potent than PO **morphine**;[27] thus, in round figures, 1mg SL buprenorphine is equivalent to 80mg PO **morphine**
- IV/IM/SC buprenorphine is 30–40 times more potent than IV/IM/SC **morphine**;[64] thus, in round figures, 300microgram IV buprenorphine is equivalent to 10mg IV **morphine**
- TD buprenorphine is 70–115 times more potent than PO **morphine**.[65–67]

The lower limit of the last ratio is based on a small prospective study and the upper limit on a large retrospective chart review. As a convenient compromise, *PCF* favours a potency ratio of 100:1.

A TD buprenorphine:PO **morphine** potency ratio of 100:1 also means that TD buprenorphine and TD **fentanyl** can be considered essentially equipotent (see Table 15.2, p.628). However, a TD **fentanyl**:TD buprenorphine potency ratio of 1.4:1 is suggested by others,[28,67] making TD **fentanyl** 25 and 50microgram/h patches equivalent to buprenorphine 35 and 70microgram/h patches respectively. Even so, when switching opioids because of possible opioid-induced hyperalgesia, it is prudent to reduce the calculated equivalent dose of the new opioid by 25–50% (see Switching opioids, p.354).

Switching opioids

As with any opioid switch, patients changing from another opioid to buprenorphine may experience opioid-withdrawal symptoms. These manifest with symptoms like gastric flu and last for a few days. With TD and lower doses of SL buprenorphine, p.r.n. doses of the previous opioid will relieve troublesome symptoms.

However, in addiction medicine, when switching generally involves high-dose SL buprenorphine, the practice is to discontinue the first opioid, await the development of withdrawal symptoms and only then commence buprenorphine. In this way, opioid withdrawal will not be precipitated by buprenorphine (because of its greater affinity for the μ-opioid receptor) but, rather, once withdrawal symptoms are present, they should be relieved by it.

Pharmacokinetics

The bio-availability of PO buprenorphine is low (15%); it undergoes extensive first-pass metabolism in the GI mucosa and liver, where it is almost completely converted by CYP3A4 to norbuprenorphine. Norbuprenorphine has similar opioid receptor-binding affinities to buprenorphine but does not readily cross the blood-brain barrier and has little, if any, central effect.[60] Both buprenorphine and norbuprenorphine undergo glucuronidation to inactive metabolites.[69]

The bio-availability of SL buprenorphine is about 50%; it is rapidly absorbed into the oral mucosa (2–3min), followed by a slower absorption into the systemic circulation (t_{max} 30min–3.5h after a single dose; 1–2h with repeat dosing).[68] This, together with a duration of action of 6–8h, suggests that SL buprenorphine is *not* ideal for the treatment of breakthrough (episodic) pain. Nonetheless, onset of analgesia in 10–20min is reported for SL buprenorphine,[31] and it has been successfully used as a rescue analgesic in patients receiving higher dose TD buprenorphine (i.e. Transtec®).[70] After parenteral and SL administration, 70% of buprenorphine is excreted unchanged in the faeces and some enterohepatic recirculation is likely; whereas norbuprenorphine is mainly excreted in the urine.[71] Vomiting is more common with SL administration than IM or TD.

Buprenorphine has a large volume of distribution and is highly protein-bound (96%; α- and β-globulins).[68] It is generally safe to use in patients with renal impairment as buprenorphine does not accumulate; it is not removed by haemodialysis and thus analgesia is unaffected (see p.355).[72,73] Although accumulation of norbuprenorphine can occur, this may be of little clinical relevance given its lack of central effect.[68,72] Smaller starting doses and careful titration are advisable in patients with severe but not mild–moderate hepatic impairment. Buprenorphine crosses the placenta and enters breast milk. The incidence, severity and duration of the neonatal abstinence syndrome appears to be less than with **methadone**.[74,75]

The bio-availability of IV buprenorphine is by definition 100%, and that of SC essentially the same. Bio-availability is irrelevant in relation to TD patches; the stated delivery rates reflect the mean amount of drug delivered to patients throughout the patch's recommended duration of use. Inevitably, there will be interindividual variation in the amount delivered. Extrapolating from data relating to TD fentanyl, the absorption of TD buprenorphine could also be impaired in patients with cachexia, possibly because of a loss of skin hydration.[76] Pharmacokinetic data are summarized in Table 5.25.

Table 5.25 Pharmacokinetic details for buprenorphine

	IV	*TD (Transtec®)*	*TD (BuTrans®)*	*SL*
Onset of action	5–15min[61]	21h for 35microgram/h patch; 11h for 70microgram/h patch	18–24h	10–20min[31]
Time to peak plasma concentration	5min	60h	3 days	30min–3.5h single dose; 1–2h multiple doses[18,68]
Plasma halflife	3–16h[68]	25–36h[a]	13–35h[a]	24–69h[68]
Duration of action	6–8h	4 days	7 days	6–8h

a. the halflife after a patch has been removed and not replaced.

Cautions

Hepatic impairment. The combination of high-dose buprenorphine SL with antiretrovirals, particularly **delavirdine** and **ritonavir** increases the QT interval, but the clinical significance of this is uncertain.[77]

Drug interactions

A single case report describes respiratory depression when IM **ketorolac** was added to ED buprenorphine.[78] Buprenorphine is mainly a substrate of CYP3A4 and accordingly the manufacturers and others suggest caution with CYP3A4 inhibitors, or avoiding their concurrent use (e.g. **cimetidine**, **clarithromycin**, **erythromycin**, **troleandomycin**, **ketoconazole**, **indinavir**, **ritonavir** and **saquinavir**) which theoretically could lead to an increase in buprenorphine levels.

Conversely, CYP3A4 inducers (e.g. **carbamazepine**, **phenobarbital**, **phenytoin** and **rifampin**) could reduce buprenorphine levels.[79] Studies have confirmed that **ketoconazole** approximately doubles buprenorphine levels in patients receiving high-dose buprenorphine (8–16mg/day) SL but not 5–20microgram/h TD.[80,81] Thus, halving of the dose of buprenorphine is recommended in patients receiving high-dose buprenorphine SL if used with **ketoconazole** or other CYP3A4 inhibitors.

Undesirable effects

Also see Strong opioids, p.345.

Very common (>10%): nausea; erythema and pruritus at the patch application site.

Common (<10%, >1%): asthenia, drowsiness, dizziness, headache, oedema, vomiting, constipation, sweating.

Dose and use

In Europe, the TD patches are the commonest formulation of buprenorphine used in chronic cancer and non-cancer pain. Compared to the SL and parenteral routes, the TD patches permit smaller initial doses of buprenorphine to be delivered more consistently (without large peaks and troughs) and are thus better tolerated.[82]

TD

In the UK, TD buprenorphine patches are available in two formulations: 7-day patches; 5, 10 and 20microgram/h (BuTrans®) and 4-day patches, 35, 52.5, 70microgram/h (Transtec®) (see Quick Practice Guide, p.388). For patients who have not already been taking an opioid, the lowest patch strength should be prescribed, i.e. 5microgram/h (equivalent to **morphine** 12mg/24h PO). General advice and recommended starting doses are detailed in the manufacturer's SPC.

SL

The tablet should not be chewed or swallowed as this will reduce efficacy:

- manufacturer's recommended starting dose 200microgram (equivalent to approximately **morphine** 15mg PO) q8h; this may be too much for some patients
- use with a sip of water if mouth is dry
- use an appropriate dose of a strong opioid as a rescue analgesic. Note. SL buprenorphine is *not* an ideal rescue analgesic but, if used, allow one tenth of the total daily dose, rounded to a convenient tablet size, q3h p.r.n.; some limit this to a maximum of four doses per 24h
- titrate the dose every 4–5 days, based on p.r.n. use
- typical dose 800–1,200microgram/day, given as 200–400microgram q8h–q6h
- doses of 2–16mg/day have been reported in chronic pain patients switched from other opioids.[24]

SC/IM/IV

- manufacturer's recommended starting dose 300microgram (equivalent to approximately **morphine** 10mg SC/IM/IV) q8h; this may be too much for some patients
- if necessary, titrate to 600microgram q8h–q6h
- for patients receiving CSCI/CIVI buprenorphine, p.r.n. injections about one tenth of the total daily dose can be used for break-through (episodic) pain.

Supply

Unless indicated otherwise, all preparations are **CD**.

Temgesic® (RB Pharmaceuticals)
Tablets SL 200microgram, 400microgram, 28 days @ 200microgram t.d.s. = £9.
Injection 300microgram/mL, 1mL amp = £0.50.

Subutex® (RB Pharmaceuticals)
Tablets SL 400microgram, 2mg, 8mg, 28 days @ 4mg b.d. = £103.

With **naloxone**
Suboxone® (RB Pharmaceuticals)
Tablets SL buprenorphine 2mg, **naloxone** 500microgram, pack of 28 = £26.
Tablets SL buprenorphine 8mg, **naloxone** 2mg, pack of 28 = £78.

Transdermal products
BuTrans® (Napp)
Patches (for 7 days) 5microgram/h, 1 = £4.50; 10microgram/h, 1 = £8; 20microgram/h, 1 = £14.

Transtec® (Napp)
Patches (for 4 days) 35microgram/h, 1 = £4; 52.5microgram/h, 1 = £6; 70microgram/h, 1 = £8.

1 Resnick RB (2003) Food and Drug Administration approval of buprenorphine-naloxone for office treatment of addiction. *Annals of internal medicine*. **138**: 360.

2 Budd K and Raffa R (eds) (2005) *Buprenorphine — the unique opioid analgesic*. Georg Thieme Verlag, Stuttgart, Germany, p.134.

3 Griessinger N *et al.* (2005) Transdermal buprenorphine in clinical practice–a post-marketing surveillance study in 13,179 patients. *Current Medical Research and Opinion*. **21**: 1147–1156.

4 Gowing L *et al.* (2006) Buprenorphine for the management of opioid withdrawal. *Cochrane Database Systematic Reviews*. CD002025.

5 Landau CJ *et al.* (2007) Buprenorphine transdermal delivery system in adults with persistent noncancer-related pain syndromes who require opioid therapy: a multicenter, 5-week run-in and randomized, double-blind maintenance-of-analgesia study. *Clinical Therapeutics*. **29**: 2179–2193.

6 Kress HG (2009) Clinical update on the pharmacology, efficacy and safety of transdermal buprenorphine. *European Journal of Pain*. **13**: 219–230.

7 Rothman R (1995) Buprenorphine: a review of the binding literature. In: A Cowan and J Lewis (eds) *Buprenorphine: combatting drug abuse with a unique opioid.* Wiley-Liss, New York, pp. 19–29.
8 Zaki P *et al.* (2000) Ligand-induced changes in surface mu-opioid receptor number: relationship to G protein activation? *Journal of Pharmacology and Experimental Therapeutics.* **292**: 1127–1134.
9 Lewis JW and Husbands SM (2004) The orvinols and related opioids–high affinity ligands with diverse efficacy profiles. *Current Pharmaceutical Design.* **10**: 717–732.
10 Greenwald M *et al.* (2007) Buprenorphine duration of action: mu-opioid receptor availability and pharmacokinetic and behavioral indices. *Biological Psychiatry.* **61**: 101–110.
11 Koppert W *et al.* (2005) Different profiles of buprenorphine-induced analgesia and antihyperalgesia in a human pain model. *Pain.* **118**: 15–22.
12 Simonnet G (2005) Opioids: from analgesia to anti-hyperalgesia? *Pain.* **118**: 8–9.
13 Hans G (2007) Buprenorphine–a review of its role in neuropathic pain. *Journal of Opioid Management.* **3**: 195–206.
14 Sanchez-Blazquez P and Garzon J (1988) Pertussis toxin differentially reduces the efficacy of opioids to produce supraspinal analgesia in the mouse. *European Journal of Pharmacology.* **152**: 357–361.
15 Likar R and Sittl R (2005) Transdermal buprenorphine for treating nociceptive and neuropathic pain: four case studies. *Anesthesia and Analgesia.* **100**: 781–785.
16 Penza P *et al.* (2008) Short- and intermediate-term efficacy of buprenorphine TDS in chronic painful neuropathies. *Journal of the Peripheral Nervous System.* **13**: 283–288.
17 Hay JL *et al.* (2010) Potentiation of buprenorphine antinociception with ultra-low dose naltrexone in healthy subjects. *European Journal of Pain.* DOI:10.1016/j.ejpain.2010.1007.1009.
18 Johnson RE *et al.* (2005) Buprenorphine: considerations for pain management. *Journal of Pain and Symptom Management.* **29**: 297–326.
19 Lutfy K *et al.* (2003) Buprenorphine-induced antinociception is mediated by mu-opioid receptors and compromised by concomitant activation of opioid receptor-like receptors. *Journal of Neuroscience.* **23**: 10331–10337.
20 Dahan A *et al.* (2005) Comparison of the respiratory effects of intravenous buprenorphine and fentanyl in humans and rats. *British Journal Anaesthesia.* **94**: 825–834.
21 Dahan A *et al.* (2006) Buprenorphine induces ceiling in respiratory depression but not in analgesia. *British Journal of Anaesthesia.* **96**: 627–632.
22 Budd K (2002) *Buprenorphine: a review. Evidence Based Medicine in Practice.* Hayward Medical Communications, Newmarket.
23 Walsh S *et al.* (1994) Clinical pharmacology of buprenorphine: ceiling effects at high doses. *Clinical Pharmacology and Therapeutics.* **55**: 569–580.
24 Malinoff HL *et al.* (2005) Sublingual buprenorphine is effective in the treatment of chronic pain syndrome. *American Journal of Therapeutics.* **12**: 379–384.
25 Heit HA and Gourlay DL (2008) Buprenorphine: new tricks with an old molecule for pain management. *Clinical Journal of Pain.* **24**: 93–97.
26 Mercadante S *et al.* (2006) Safety and effectiveness of intravenous morphine for episodic breakthrough pain in patients receiving transdermal buprenorphine. *Journal of Pain and Symptom Management.* **32**: 175–179.
27 Atkinson R *et al.* (1990) The efficacy in sequential use of buprenorphine and morphine in advanced cancer pain. In: D Doyle (ed) *Opioids in the treatment of cancer pain.* Royal Society of Medicine Services, London, pp. 81–87.
28 Mercadante S *et al.* (2007) Switching from transdermal drugs: an observational "N of 1" study of fentanyl and buprenorphine. *Journal of Pain and Symptom Management.* **34**: 532–538.
29 Pausawasdi S *et al.* (1984) The effect of buprenorphine and morphine on intraluminal pressure of the common bile duct. *Journal of the Medical Association of Thailand.* **67**: 329–333.
30 Staritz M *et al.* (1986) Effect of modern analgesic drugs (tramadol, pentazocine, and buprenorphine) on the bile duct sphincter in man. *Gut.* **27**: 567–569.
31 Robbie DS (1979) A trial of sublingual buprenorphine in cancer pain. *British Journal of Clinical Pharmacology.* **7 (suppl 3)**: S315–S317.
32 Bach V *et al.* (1991) Buprenorphine and sustained release morphine–effect and side-effects in chronic use. *The Pain Clinic.* **4**: 87–93.
33 Pace MC *et al.* (2007) Buprenorphine in long-term control of chronic pain in cancer patients. *Frontiers in Bioscience.* **12**: 1291–1299.
34 Hallinan R *et al.* (2009) Hypogonadism in men receiving methadone and buprenorphine maintenance treatment. *International Journal of Andrology.* **32**: 131–139.
35 Bliesener N *et al.* (2005) Plasma testosterone and sexual function in men receiving buprenorphine maintenance for opioid dependence. *Journal of Clinical Endocrinology and Metabolism.* **90**: 203–206.
36 Daniell HW (2002) Hypogonadism in men consuming sustained-action oral opioids. *The Journal of Pain.* **3**: 377–384.
37 Rajagopal A *et al.* (2004) Symptomatic hypogonadism in male survivors of cancer with chronic exposure to opioids. *Cancer.* **100**: 851–858.
38 Hallinan R *et al.* (2008) Erectile dysfunction in men receiving methadone and buprenorphine maintenance treatment. *Journal of Sexual Medicine.* **5**: 684–692.
39 Sacerdote P *et al.* (2000) The effects of tramadol and morphine on immune responses and pain after surgery in cancer patients. *Anesthesia and Analgesia.* **90**: 1411–1414.
40 Budd K and Shipton E (2004) Acute pain and the immune system and opioimmunosuppression. *Acute Pain.* **6**: 123–135.
41 Sacerdote P *et al.* (2008) Buprenorphine and methadone maintenance treatment of heroin addicts preserves immune function. *Brain, Behavior, and Immunity.* **22**: 606–613.
42 Wedam EF *et al.* (2007) QT-interval effects of methadone, levomethadyl, and buprenorphine in a randomized trial. *Archives of Internal Medicine.* **167**: 2469–2475.
43 Esses JL *et al.* (2008) Successful transition to buprenorphine in a patient with methadone-induced torsades de pointes. *Journal of Interventional Cardiac Electrophysiology.* **23**: 117–119.
44 Juby L *et al.* (1994) Buprenorphine and hepatic pruritus. *British Journal of Clinical Practice.* **48**: 331.
45 Reddy L *et al.* (2007) Transdermal buprenorphine may be effective in the treatment of pruritus in primary biliary cirrhosis. *Journal of Pain and Symptom Management.* **34**: 455–456.
46 Likar R *et al.* (2007) Transdermal buprenorphine patches applied in a 4-day regimen versus a 3-day regimen: a single-site, Phase III, randomized, open-label, crossover comparison. *Clinical Therapeutics.* **29**: 1591–1606.
47 Davis MP (2005) Buprenorphine in cancer pain. *Supportive Care in Cancer.* **13**: 878–887.

48 Schmid-Grendelmeier P *et al.* (2006) A comparison of the skin irritation potential of transdermal fentanyl versus transdermal buprenorphine in middle-aged to elderly healthy volunteers. *Current Medical Research Opinion.* **22**: 501–509.
49 Vander Hulst K *et al.* (2008) Allergic contact dermatitis from transdermal buprenorphine. *Contact Dermatitis.* **59**: 366–369.
50 Sittl R *et al.* (2006) Patterns of dosage changes with transdermal buprenorphine and transdermal fentanyl for the treatment of noncancer and cancer pain: a retrospective data analysis in Germany. *Clinical Therapeutics.* **28**: 1144–1154.
51 Deandrea S *et al.* (2009) Managing severe cancer pain: the role of transdermal buprenorphine: a systematic review. *Therapeutics and Clinical Risk Management.* **5**: 707–718.
52 Greenwald MK *et al.* (2003) Effects of buprenorphine maintenance dose on mu-opioid receptor availability, plasma concentrations, and antagonist blockade in heroin-dependent volunteers. *Neuropsychopharmacology.* **28**: 2000–2009.
53 Dasgupta N *et al.* (2010) Post-marketing surveillance of methadone and buprenorphine in the United States. *Pain Medicine.* **11**: 1078–1091.
54 Kintz P (2001) Deaths involving buprenorphine: a compendium of French cases. *Forensic Science International.* **121**: 65–69.
55 Knape J (1986) Early respiratory depression resistant to naloxone following epidural buprenorphine. *Anesthesiology.* **64**: 382–384.
56 van Dorp E *et al.* (2006) Naloxone reversal of buprenorphine-induced respiratory depression. *Anesthesiology.* **105**: 51–57.
57 Sarton E *et al.* (2008) Naloxone reversal of opioid-induced respiratory depression with special emphasis on the partial agonist/antagonist buprenorphine. *Advances in Experimental Medicine and Biology.* **605**: 486–491.
58 Gal T (1989) Naloxone reversal of buprenorphine-induced respiratory depression. *Clinical Pharmacology and Therapeutics.* **45**: 66–71.
59 Orwin JM (1977) The effect of doxapram on buprenorphine induced respiratory depression. *Acta anaesthesiologica Belgica.* **28**: 93–106.
60 BNF (2011) Section 3.5.1 Respiratory stimulants. In: *British National Formulary* (No. 61). British Medical Association and Royal Pharmaceutical Society of Great Britain, London. Current BNF available from: www.bnf.org.
61 Heel RC *et al.* (1979) Buprenorphine: a review of its pharmacological properties and therapeutic efficiency. *Drugs.* **17**: 81–110.
62 Ellis R *et al.* (1982) Pain relief after abdominal surgery-a comparison of i.m. morphine, sublingual buprenorphine and self-administered i.v. pethidine. *British Journal of Anaesthesia.* **54**: 421–428.
63 Bullingham RE *et al.* (1984) Mandatory sublingual buprenorphine for postoperative pain. *Anaesthesia.* **39**: 329–334.
64 Cuschieri RJ *et al.* (1984) Comparison of morphine and sublingual buprenorphine following abdominal surgery. *British Journal of Anaesthesia.* **56**: 855–859.
65 Sittl R *et al.* (2005) Equipotent doses of transdermal fentanyl and transdermal buprenorphine in patients with cancer and noncancer pain: results of a retrospective cohort study. *Clinical Therapeutics.* **27**: 225–237.
66 Likar R *et al.* (2008) Challenging the equipotency calculation for transdermal buprenorphine: four case studies. *International Journal of Clinical Practice.* **62**: 152–156.
67 Mercadante S *et al.* (2009) Equipotent doses to switch from high doses of opioids to transdermal buprenorphine. *Supportive Care in Cancer.* **17**: 715–718.
68 Elkader A and Sproule B (2005) Buprenorphine: clinical pharmacokinetics in the treatment of opioid dependence. *Clinical Pharmacokinetics.* **44**: 661–680.
69 McQuay H and Moore R (1995) Buprenorphine kinetics in humans. In: A Cowan and J Lewis (eds) *Buprenorphine: combatting drug abuse with a unique opioid.* Wiley-Liss, New York, pp. 137–147.
70 Poulain P *et al.* (2008) Efficacy and safety of transdermal buprenorphine: a randomized, placebo-controlled trial in 289 patients with severe cancer pain. *Journal of Pain and Symptom Management.* **36**: 117–125.
71 Cone EJ *et al.* (1984) The metabolism and excretion of buprenorphine in humans. *Drug Metabolism and Disposition.* **12**: 577–581.
72 Hand CW *et al.* (1990) Buprenorphine disposition in patients with renal impairment: single and continuous dosing, with special reference to metabolites. *British Journal of Anaesthesia.* **64**: 276–282.
73 Filitz J *et al.* (2006) Effect of intermittent hemodialysis on buprenorphine and norbuprenorphine plasma concentrations in chronic pain patients treated with transdermal buprenorphine. *European Journal of Pain.* **10**: 743–748.
74 Fischer G (2000) Treatment of opioid dependence in pregnant women. *Addiction.* **95**: 1141–1144.
75 Lacroix I *et al.* (2004) Buprenorphine in pregnant opioid-dependent women: first results of a prospective study. *Addiction.* **99**: 209–214.
76 Heiskanen T *et al.* (2009) Transdermal fentanyl in cachectic cancer patients. *Pain.* **144**: 218–222.
77 Baker JR *et al.* (2006) Effect of buprenorphine and antiretroviral agents on the QT interval in opioid-dependent patients. *Annals of Pharmacotherpy.* **40**: 392–396.
78 Jain PN and Shah SC (1993) Respiratory depression following combination of epidural buprenorphine and intramuscular ketorolac. *Anaesthesia.* **48**: 898–899.
79 Genelex Corporation (2006) GeneMedRx Database. (Subscription required). Available from: www.genelex.com
80 Schering-Plough Limited (2006) *Data on file.*
81 Noveck R *et al.* (2005) Lack of effect of CYP3A4 inhibitor ketoconazole on transdermally administered buprenorphine (abstract). In: *Annual Meeting of the American Society for Clinical Pharmacology and Therapeutics* 2–5 March; Orlando.
82 James IG *et al.* (2010) A randomized, double-blind, double-dummy comparison of the efficacy and tolerability of low-dose transdermal buprenorphine (BuTrans seven-day patches) with buprenorphine sublingual tablets (Temgesic) in patients with osteoarthritis pain. *Journal of Pain and Symptom Management.* **40**: 266–278.

Quick Practice Guide: Use of transdermal buprenorphine

1 Indications for using transdermal (TD) buprenorphine instead of morphine include:
- intolerable undesirable effects with morphine, e.g. nausea and vomiting, constipation, hallucinations, dysphagia
- renal failure (no centrally active metabolites)
- 'tablet phobia' or poor compliance with oral medication
- high risk of tablet misuse/diversion (although the patch can still be abused).

2 TD buprenorphine is contra-indicated in patients with acute (short-term) pain and in those who need rapid dose titration for severe uncontrolled pain.

3 TD buprenorphine patches are available in two formulations:
- 7-day patches; 5, 10 and 20microgram/h (BuTrans®)
- 4-day patches, 35, 52.5, 70microgram/h (Transtec®).

The maximum *licensed* dose is two 70microgram/h patches.

Use the Table below to decide a safe starting dose for TD buprenorphine and an appropriate rescue dose of morphine. These recommendations are based on a PO morphine:TD buprenorphine dose conversion ratio of 100:1 derived from published data, which is in keeping with the manufacturer's dose ratio range of 75–115:1 (see SPC). It is an approximation, and inevitably there will be individual variation. If switching to buprenorphine because of possible opioid-induced hyperalgesia, reduce the calculated equivalent dose by 25–50%.

4 Patients not previously receiving opioids should start on 5 or 10microgram/h patches; patients with unrelieved pain despite maximum dose of a Step 2 analgesic should commence on 20 or 35microgram/h patches, according to circumstances.

5 For patients taking a dose of morphine that is not the exact equivalent of a buprenorphine patch, it will be necessary to opt for a patch which is either slightly more or slightly less than the morphine dose. Thus, if the patient still has pain, round up to a higher patch strength; if pain-free and frail, round down.

Comparative doses based on dose conversion ratio 100:1

PO Morphine[a]		*SC/IV Morphine*[a]		*TD Buprenorphine*	
mg/24h	*p.r.n. mg*[b]	*mg/24h*[c]	*p.r.n. mg*[b]	*microgram/h*	*microgram/24h*
				BuTrans®	
12	2[d]	6	1	5	120
24	5[d]	12	2.5	10	240
48	10	24	5	20	480
				Transtec®	
84	15	42	7.5	35	840
126	20	63	10	52.5	1,260
168	30	84	15	70[e]	1,680

a. an alternative strong opioid can be used, calculated using the appropriate conversion factor. Note. SL buprenorphine is *not* an ideal rescue medication but some centres use an initial dose of 200microgram SL q3h, up to 4 doses per 24h, for patients receiving any strength of Transtec®

b. using traditional one sixth of total daily dose as p.r.n. dose and rounded to a convenient dose; give up to q1h; some centres opt for one tenth of total daily dose

c. assuming potency ratio of morphine SC/IV to PO of 2:1

d. at these doses, p.r.n. codeine/dihydrocodeine (30–60mg) or tramadol (50mg) may suffice

e. for combinations of patches, add the p.r.n. doses together, e.g. 70 + 52.5microgram/h patches = 15 + 10mg morphine SC/IV = 25mg morphine SC/IV, but can round up to 30mg or down to 20mg for convenience.

continued

6 The date of application and/or the date for renewal should be written in a consistent manner on the patch. Apply to dry, non-inflamed, non-irradiated, hairless skin on the upper trunk or arm. Body hair may be clipped with scissors but not shaved. If the skin is washed beforehand, use only water; do not use soap and do not apply oils, cream or ointment to the area. Press patch firmly in place for at least 30 seconds. Micropore® or Tegaderm® can be used to ensure adherence. Careful removal of the patch helps to minimize local skin irritation.

7 Systemic analgesic concentrations are generally reached within 12–24h but levels continue to rise for 32–54h. If converting from:
- 4-hourly PO morphine, give regular doses for the first 12h after applying the patch
- 12-hourly m/r morphine, apply the patch and the final m/r dose at the same time
- 24-hourly m/r morphine, apply the patch 12h after the final m/r dose
- CSCI/CIVI opioids, continue the infusion for about 12h after applying the patch.

8 Steady-state plasma concentrations of buprenorphine are reached after 9 days (1–2 days with patch strength of ≤20microgram/h); the patient should use p.r.n. doses liberally, particularly during the first 24h, either the previously used weak opioid, or morphine/other strong opioid, or buprenorphine (see Table above).

9 After 72h, if a patient continues to need 2 or more rescue doses of analgesic/day, the next strength patch should be used.

10 Patients could experience opioid-withdrawal symptoms when changed from another opioid (particularly large doses) to TD buprenorphine. These manifest with symptoms like gastric flu and last for a few days; p.r.n. doses of the previous opioid will relieve troublesome symptoms.

11 Buprenorphine is less constipating than morphine; halve the dose of laxatives when starting buprenorphine and re-titrate.

12 Buprenorphine may cause nausea and vomiting; if necessary, prescribe an anti-emetic, e.g. haloperidol 1.5mg stat & at bedtime.

13 In febrile patients, the rate of absorption of buprenorphine increases, and may cause toxicity, e.g. drowsiness. Absorption is also enhanced by an external heat source over the patch, e.g. electric blanket or hot-water bottle; patients should be warned about this. Patients may swim or shower with a patch but should not soak in a hot bath.

14 Remove and replace patches once (7-day patch) or twice (4-day patch) a week. The 4 day patch can be replaced on fixed days in the week, i.e. after 3 and 4 days alternatively. Change the position of the new patches so as to rest the underlying skin for at least 9 days.

15 A reservoir of buprenorphine cumulates in the body, particularly in adipose tissue, and significant plasma levels persist for at least 24h after discontinuing TD buprenorphine.

16 TD buprenorphine is unsatisfactory in <5% of patients.

17 In moribund patients, continue TD buprenorphine and give additional SC morphine p.r.n. (see Table above). If >2 p.r.n. doses are required/24h, give morphine by CSCI, starting with a dose equal to the sum of the p.r.n. doses over the preceding 24h. If necessary, adjust the p.r.n. dose taking into account the total opioid dose (i.e. TD buprenorphine + CSCI morphine).

18 Used patches still contain buprenorphine; after removal, fold the patch with the adhesive side inwards, and then discard in a sharps container (hospital) or dustbin (home), and wash hands. Ultimately, any unused patches should be returned to a pharmacy.

FENTANYL BNF 4.7.2 & 15.1.4.3

For transmucosal fentanyl for cancer-related breakthrough (episodic) pain or procedure-related pain, see p.400.

Class: Strong opioid analgesic.

Indications: ***TD*** severe chronic (persistent, long-term) pain, including cancer, †AIDS,[1] †intolerance to other strong opioids.[2] ***Injection*** severe pain, premedication and peri-operative analgesia, analgesic/respiratory depressant in patients requiring assisted ventilation, neurolepta-nalgesia (i.e. in combination with an antipsychotic/neuroleptic), †intolerance to other strong opioids.

Contra-indications: TD fentanyl should not be used for acute (transient, intermittent or short-term) pain, e.g. postoperative, or when there is need for rapid dose titration for severe uncontrolled pain. In the UK, TD fentanyl is licensed for first-line use in adults (see Dose and use). However, in Canada and the USA, TD fentanyl is contra-indicated in opioid-naïve patients because of reports of unintentional overdoses, with serious (sometimes fatal) consequences.[3]

Pharmacology

Fentanyl (*like* **morphine**) is a strong μ-opioid receptor agonist. It has a relatively low molecular weight and (*unlike* **morphine**) is lipophilic. This makes it suitable for TD and transmucosal administration (see p.400).

Fentanyl is sequestrated in body fats, including epidural fat and the white matter of the CNS.[4,5] Thus, by any route (including spinally), after systemic redistribution, fentanyl acts supraspinally mainly in the thalamus (white matter). Any effect in the dorsal horn (grey matter) is probably minimal.[4] This may account for the clinical observation that patients with poor pain relief despite using very high doses (e.g. 600microgram/h TD) sometimes obtain good relief with relatively smaller doses of **morphine**, e.g. 10–20mg SC.[6]

The lipophilic nature of fentanyl also provides one explanation for the difference in undesirable effects profile compared with **morphine** (Figure 5.11).[7] Thus, when converting from PO or parenteral **morphine** to TD or parenteral fentanyl, there is a massive decrease in opioid molecules outside the CNS with, in consequence, less constipation. This also explains why peripherally-mediated withdrawal symptoms are also sometimes seen.

TD fentanyl is used in the management of chronic severe pain,[8–10] particularly in cancer.[11–18] Steady-state plasma concentrations of fentanyl are generally achieved after 36–48h[1] but, according to manufacturer data[19] this is sometimes achieved only after 9–12 days.

Elimination of fentanyl mainly involves biotransformation in the liver by CYP3A4 to inactive norfentanyl which is excreted in the urine. Less than 7% is excreted unchanged. The SPCs generally advise caution in the use of fentanyl in patients with moderate-severe liver or renal impairment, but this is based on limited data which suggest reduced clearance of fentanyl via, for example, alterations in metabolic clearance and plasma protein-binding. Nonetheless, fentanyl is a reasonable option for patients with renal impairment or failure (see p.355).

If effective analgesia does not last for 3 days, the correct response is to increase the patch strength. Even so, a small percentage of patients do best if the patch is changed every 2 days.[18,20]

Matrix and reservoir patches are now available from several manufacturers. All the SPCs contain dose conversion recommendations from PO morphine which, although broadly similar, do vary. The original manufacturer recommends a dose conversion ratio for **morphine** and fentanyl of 150:1. However, several RCTs support a smaller ratio, ranging between 70–125:1. Consequently, *PCF* has opted for a ratio of 100:1.[21]

PCF also favours a TD **buprenorphine**:PO **morphine** potency ratio of 100:1 and this means that TD **buprenorphine** and TD fentanyl can be considered essentially equipotent (see Buprenorphine, p.381). However, a TD fentanyl:TD **buprenorphine** potency ratio of 1.4:1 is suggested by others,[22,23] which would make TD fentanyl 25 and 50microgram/h patches equivalent to **buprenorphine** 35 and 70microgram/h patches respectively. Even so, when switching opioids because of possible opioid-induced hyperalgesia, it is prudent to reduce the calculated equivalent dose of the new opioid by 25–50% (see, p.354).

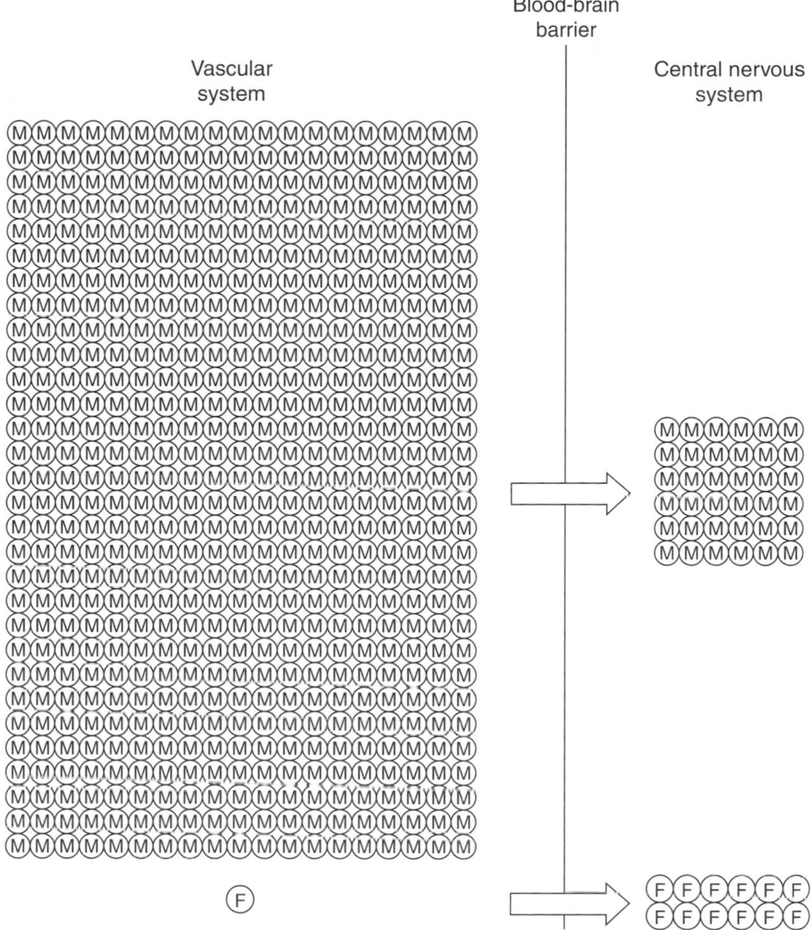

Figure 5.11 Distribution of equipotent doses of morphine and fentanyl in the vascular and central nervous systems based on animal data.[7] For clinical relevance, see p.390

Because fentanyl is less constipating than **morphine**,[11,20,24–26] when converting from **morphine** to fentanyl, the dose of laxative should be halved and subsequently adjusted according to need. Some patients experience withdrawal symptoms (e.g. diarrhoea, colic, nausea, sweating, restlessness) when changed from PO **morphine** to TD fentanyl despite satisfactory pain relief. This is probably related to differences between the two opioids in relation to their relative impact on peripheral and central μ-opioid receptors (see Figure 5.11). Such symptoms are easily treatable by using rescue doses of **morphine** until they resolve after a few days. Like **buprenorphine**, fentanyl appears to have little effect on the sphincter of Oddi.[27]

At one PCU, it was noted that patients admitted on fentanyl TD were receiving relatively higher equivalent opioid doses than other patients.[28] The reasons for this are not clear but may include a failure to appreciate the potency of fentanyl, and the induction of opioid-induced hyperalgesia by inappropriately high doses. It is noteworthy that fentanyl TD was successfully reduced or discontinued in 60% of patients.[28]

Pharmacokinetic data are summarized in Table 5.26. Bio-availability is irrelevant in relation to TD patches; the stated delivery rates reflect the mean amount of drug delivered to patients throughout the patch's recommended duration of use. Inevitably, there will be interindividual variation in the amount delivered, e.g. for the 100microgram/h patch, the mean (±SD) delivery is 97 (±15) microgram/h,[29] and the amount of unused fentanyl in the patch after 3 days can vary from 30–85% of the original contents.[30]

Table 5.26 Pharmacokinetic data for fentanyl

	TD	*SC/IM*	*IV*
Onset of action	3–23h[33]	7–15min IM	No formal data, but likely <5min
Time to peak plasma concentration	24–72h	Median 15min, range 10–30min [34]	No formal data, but likely <5min
Plasma halflife	13–22h[a,35]	Median 10h, range 6–16h[34]	3–14h
Duration of action	72h; for some patients, 48h[36]	1–2h IM	30–60min

a. the halflife after a patch has been removed and not replaced.

In cachectic patients, plasma concentrations of fentanyl are reduced by 1/3–1/2.[31] The reason for this is unclear; it appears not to relate to loss of subcutaneous adipose tissue,[32] but loss of skin hydration is one possibility.[31]

Cautions

The reservoir patches should not be cut because damage to the rate-controlling membrane can lead to a rapid release of fentanyl and overdose. Although cutting matrix patches is theoretically safer, some strongly discourage it because of similar concerns.[37] However, cutting has become unnecessary with the introduction of a 12microgram/h patch.

After reports of serious adverse events (overdoses and deaths), regulatory authorities in Canada and the USA have issued safety warnings about the use of TD fentanyl.[3,38] Factors contributing to adverse drug events include:

- lack of appreciation that fentanyl is a strong opioid analgesic
- inappropriate use for short-term, intermittent or postoperative pain in patients who had not previously been receiving a strong opioid
- lack of patient education regarding directions for safe use, storage and disposal
- lack of awareness of the signs of an overdose and when to seek attention
- lack of awareness that the rate of absorption of fentanyl may be increased if the skin under the patch becomes vasodilated, e.g. in febrile patients, or by an external heat source, e.g. electric blanket, heat lamps, saunas, hot tubs
- lack of awareness of drug interactions which can increase fentanyl levels.

Deaths continue to occur from incorrect use.[39] Additional errors include the failure to remove old patches, and the dispensing and application of higher strength patches than prescribed.

Patients with COPD or other medical conditions which predispose to respiratory depression (e.g. myasthenia gravis) or who are susceptible to the intracranial effects of hypercapnia (e.g. those with raised intracranial pressure). Caution is also needed if bradyarrhythmia, elderly, cachectic, debilitated, moderate–severe hepatic or renal impairment, hypovolaemic, hypotensive, and if a history or high risk of abuse or diversion. Muscle rigidity can occur (generally transiently following IV injection).

Although fentanyl analgesia is generally unaffected by haemodialysis,[40] there are rare reports of pain recurring in patients on TD fentanyl during and after haemodialysis.[41] This probably relates only to certain dialysis membranes (see p.355) and may reflect loss of fentanyl through membrane adsorption rather than loss into the dialysate solution.[40]

Addicts misuse TD fentanyl in various ways, e.g. heating the patch, applying buccally, chewing, ingesting, inhaling, IV injection of patch contents, sometimes with fatal consequences.[42,43]

Drug interactions

Fentanyl is metabolized by CYP3A4. Thus, fentanyl plasma concentrations may be increased by CYP3A4 inhibitors such as azole antifungals (e.g. **fluconazole**, **ketoconzole**, **itraconazole**), macrolide antibiotics (e.g. **erythromycin**, **clarithromycin**), protease inhibitors (e.g. **ritonavir**, **nelfinavir**), **aprepitant**, **cimetidine**, **diltiazem** and **verapamil**.[44]

In contrast, concentrations are decreased by potent CYP3A4 inducers (e.g. **carbamazepine**, **phenytoin**, **phenobarbitone**, **rifampicin**) and this may lead to a loss of analgesia.[44–48]

Fentanyl is best avoided in patients who have used a MAOI within the past 2 weeks. Although they have been used safely together, serotonin toxicity (sometimes fatal) has occurred (also see p.177).[44]

Undesirable effects

Also see Strong opioids, p.345.

Very common (>10%): drowsiness, dizziness, headache, insomnia, nausea, vomiting, constipation; muscle rigidity (including the thoracic muscles) when given IV.

Common (<10%, >1%): abdominal pain, anorexia, anxiety, diarrhoea, dry mouth, dyspepsia, visual disturbance, palpitations, sweating, vasodilatation.

Topical effects: Occasional skin irritation, hypersensitivity.

Dose and use

TD fentanyl

The use of TD fentanyl patches is summarized in the Quick Practice Guide (See p.398). These and the comments in this section are based on a dose conversion ratio with PO **morphine** of 1:100. Prescribers using the manufacturer's preferred ratio of 1:150 should follow the dose conversion guidelines in the SPC (see Box 15.B, p.630).

Under no circumstances should a *reservoir* patch be cut in an attempt to reduce the dose. Leakage from the cut reservoir could result in either the patient receiving minimal or no fentanyl, or, alternatively, an overdose from the rapid absorption of fentanyl through the surrounding skin.

Two different TD formulations are currently available:

- *reservoir* patch (e.g. Fentalis®, Tilofyl®) the fentanyl is contained within a reservoir, and the release of fentanyl is controlled by a rate-limiting membrane
- *matrix* patch (e.g. Durogesic DTrans®, Matrifen®) the fentanyl is evenly distributed throughout a drug-in-adhesive matrix, and the release of fentanyl is controlled by the physical characteristics of the matrix.)

Absorption of the fentanyl through the skin and into the systemic circulation is influenced by both the condition of the skin and cutaneous blood flow. Thus, if the skin is warm and vasodilated, the rate of absorption will be increased.

Bio-equivalence has been demonstrated between two different makes of *matrix* patches, and between the *matrix* and *reservoir* patches. Thus, patients can be switched from one to the other with no loss of efficacy or increase in undesirable effects.[19,49–51]

The matrix patch is thinner (because there is no reservoir), and smaller (for equal strengths, the matrix patch is more than one-third smaller). Consequently, to avoid confusing the patients and carers, it is generally better if one formulation is prescribed consistently for any one individual.

In North America, the manufacturer stresses that TD fentanyl should be commenced *only* in patients who have been receiving strong opioids in a dose at least equivalent to a 25microgram/h patch for ≥1 week, such as:

- **morphine** 60mg/day PO
- **oxycodone** 30mg/day PO
- **hydromorphone** 8mg/day PO.

However, in the UK, TD fentanyl is licensed for use as a *first-line strong opioid* in adults and has been used satisfactorily in, for example, patients with severe dysphagia, renal failure or who are living in social circumstances where there is a high risk of diversion and tablet misuse. (Note: misuse of TD fentanyl can also occur; see Cautions).

TD fentanyl is also used in *totally opioid-naïve patients* at centres which skip Step 2 of the WHO analgesic ladder.[52–54] Licensed starting doses for TD fentanyl as a *first-line strong opioid* in the UK are 12microgram/h and 25microgram/h, depending on the individual product, equivalent to **morphine** 30mg and 60mg PO respectively. Thus, the 12microgram/h dose will be a safer starting dose for *totally opioid-naïve* patients and for some *strong* (but not weak) *opioid-naïve* patients, e.g. frail patients using low doses of weak opioid with moderate pain. Undesirable effects, e.g. nausea and vomiting, are more frequent in *strong* opioid-naïve patients and, in separate studies, resulted in one-sixth and one-third of patients discontinuing TD fentanyl 12microgram/h and 25microgram/h respectively.[55,56]

Although not recommended by the manufacturer, when using the 25microgram/h patch to initiate TD treatment, some practitioners cover part of the underside of the patch (*reservoir*) or cut patches (*matrix*) so as to decrease the initial dose. These practices have become unnecessary since the introduction of the 12microgram/h patch.

It should be noted that, unless patients have been taking several rescue doses per day of **morphine** (or other strong opioid) for break-through (episodic) pain, escalating in one step from 25 to 50microgram/h (a dose increase of 100%) can cause a marked (but temporary) increase in undesirable effects.[57]

It is important to give adequate rescue doses of **morphine** (see Quick Practice Guide, p.398) or other strong opioid. Adjusting the patch strength on a daily basis is not recommended.[58] With inpatients, the use of a fentanyl patch chart is recommended (Box 5.O).

SC/IM/IV

- start with a stat dose of 50–200microgram, and subsequently 50microgram p.r.n.
- reduce the dose in the elderly and debilitated
- traditionally p.r.n. dosing intervals are q1h, but more frequent dosing with close monitoring may be required in severe acute pain
- give IV by slow injection; this reduces the risk of muscular rigidity.

CIVI

Fentanyl CIVI is used in some (generally non-UK) centres for initial control of cancer pain. When an effective stable dose is found, the route is switched to TD over 6h:

- start by applying patch(es) which deliver the same dose/h as the CIVI (rounded for convenience)
- after 3h, halve the fentanyl CIVI dose
- after a further 3h, discontinue the CIVI.[59]

Supply

Unless indicated otherwise, all preparations are **CD**.

Fentanyl (generic)
Reservoir patches (for 3 days) 12microgram/h, 1 = £3.50, 25microgram/h, 1 = £5; 50microgram/h, 1 = £9; 75microgram/h, 1 = £13; 100microgram/h, 1 = £16.
Generic products include Tilofyl®, Fentalis.

Matrix patches (for 3 days) 12microgram/h, 1 = £3.50; 25microgram/h, 1 = £5; 50microgram/h, 1 = £9; 75microgram/h, 1 = £13; 100microgram/h, 1 = £16.
Generic products include Matrifen®, Mezolar®, Osmanil®, Victanyl®

Durogesic DTrans® (Janssen-Cilag)
Matrix patches (for 3 days) 12microgram/h, 1 = £3.50; 25microgram/h, 1 = £5; 50microgram/h, 1 = £9; 75microgram/h, 1 = £13; 100microgram/h, 1 = £16.

Fentanyl citrate (generic)
Injection 50microgram/mL, 2mL amp = £0.50, 10mL amp = £0.50.

Sublimaze® (Janssen-Cilag)
Injection 50microgram/mL, 10mL amp = £1.50.

Box 5.O Fentanyl patch chart: example of a nursing record

Fentanyl Patch Chart

Patient's name: Hospital No:
Date of birth:

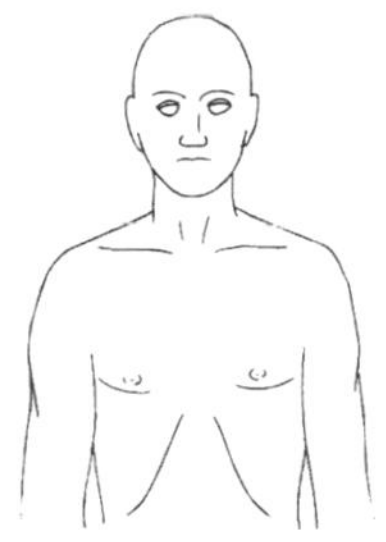

Generally apply to dry, flat, non-hairy skin on the trunk or upper arm.

Press firmly in place with the hand for 30 seconds to ensure good contact.

Mark the patch with the date and time it was applied, and record the site of application on the chart.

Rotate sites.

General Information

- Fentanyl patches need to be prescribed on the inpatient medicine chart; sign the administration box as usual, and also complete this chart.
- A nurse should check that each patch is still in place twice daily, e.g. 10am and 10pm, and sign below.
- Comments should be made about any problems, stating the action taken, e.g. *patch lifted, secured with Tegaderm.*
- Fentanyl patches are normally replaced every 72 hours.
- When removed, fold patches in half with the adhesive side inwards and discard in the sharps bin. A second nurse should witness this and countersign below.

Date & time patch applied	Strength (microgram/h) No. of patches Site	Signature	12 hourly observation				Comments Removal & discarding Date & Time Signatures
			10am	Sig	10pm	Sig	
23/02/11 1000h	25 × 1 Left arm	*S Thorp*			23/2 ✓	*AS*	
			24/2 ✓	*ST*	24/2 ✓	*MB*	
			25/2 ✓	*ST*	25/2 ✓	*MB*	
			26/2 ✓	*AS*			26/2/11 1000h *A Smith S Thorp*

1 Newshan G and Lefkowitz M (2001) Transdermal fentanyl for chronic pain in AIDS: a pilot study. *Journal of Pain and Symptom Management.* **21**: 69–77.
2 Morita T *et al.* (2005) Opioid rotation from morphine to fentanyl in delirious cancer patients: an open-label trial. *Journal of Pain and Symptom Management.* **30**: 96–103.
3 Health Canada (2008) Fentanyl transdermal patch and fatal adverse reactions. *Canadian Adverse Reaction Newsletter.* **18(3)**: 1–2.
4 Bernards C (1999) Clinical implications of physicochemical properties of opioids. In: C Stein (ed) *Opioids in Pain Control: basic and clinical aspects.* Cambridge University Press, Cambridge, pp. 166–187.
5 Ummenhofer W *et al.* (2000) Comparative spinal distribution and clearance kinetics of intrathecally administered morphine, fentanyl, alfentanil, and sufentanil. *Anesthesiology.* **92**: 739–953.
6 Zylicz Z (2001) *Personal communication.*
7 Herz A and Teschemacher H-J (1971) Activities and sites of antinociceptive action of morphine-like analgesics and kinetics of distribution following intravenous, intracerebral and intraventricular application. *Advances in Drug Research.* **6**: 79–119.
8 Simpson R *et al.* (1997) Transdermal fentanyl as treatment for chronic low back pain. *Journal of Pain and Symptom Management.* **14**: 218–224.
9 Milligan K and Campbell C (1999) Transdermal fentanyl in patients with chronic, nonmalignant pain: a case study series. *Advances in Therapy.* **16**: 73–77.
10 Allan L *et al.* (2001) Randomised crossover trial of transdermal fentanyl and sustained release oral morphine for treating chronic non-cancer pain. *British Medical Journal.* **322**: 1154–1158.
11 Ahmedzai S and Brooks D (1997) Transdermal fentanyl versus sustained-release oral morphine in cancer pain: preference, efficacy and quality of life. *Journal of Pain and Symptom Management.* **13**: 254–261.
12 Wong J-N *et al.* (1997) Comparison of oral controlled-release morphine with transdermal fentanyl in terminal cancer pain. *Acta Anaesthesiologica Singapore.* **35**: 25–32.
13 Yeo W *et al.* (1997) Transdermal fentanyl for severe cancer-related pain. *Palliative Medicine.* **11**: 233–239.
14 Kongsgaard U and Poulain P (1998) Transdermal fentanyl for pain control in adults with chronic cancer pain. *European Journal of Pain.* **2**: 53–62.
15 Payne R *et al.* (1998) Quality of life and cancer pain: satisfaction and side effects with transdermal fentanyl versus oral morphine. *Journal of Clinical Oncology.* **16**: 1588–1593.
16 Sloan P *et al.* (1998) A clinical evaluation of transdermal therapeutic system fentanyl for the treatment of cancer pain. *Journal of Pain and Symptom Management.* **16**: 102–111.
17 Nugent M *et al.* (2001) Long-term observations of patients receiving transdermal fentanyl after a randomized trial. *Journal of Pain and Symptom Management.* **21**: 385–391.
18 Radbruch L *et al.* (2001) Transdermal fentanyl for the management of cancer pain: a survey of 1005 patients. *Palliative Medicine.* **15**: 309–321.
19 Janssen-Cilag Ltd *Data on file.*
20 Donner B *et al.* (1998) Long-term treatment of cancer pain with transdermal fentanyl. *Journal of Pain and Symptom Management.* **15**: 168–175.
21 Donner B *et al.* (1996) Direct conversion from oral morphine to transdermal fentanyl: a multicenter study in patients with cancer pain. *Pain.* **64**: 527–534.
22 Mercadante S *et al.* (2007) Switching from transdermal drugs: an observational "N of 1" study of fentanyl and buprenorphine. *Journal of Pain and Symptom Management.* **34**: 532–538.
23 Mercadante S *et al.* (2009) Equipotent doses to switch from high doses of opioids to transdermal buprenorphine. *Supportive Care in Cancer.* **17**: 715–718.
24 Grond S *et al.* (1997) Transdermal fentanyl in the long-term treatment of cancer pain: a prospective study of 50 patients with advanced cancer of the gastrointestinal tract or the head and neck region. *Pain.* **69**: 191–198.
25 Megens A *et al.* (1998) Comparison of the analgesic and intestinal effects of fentanyl and morphine in rats. *Journal of Pain and Symptom Management.* **15**: 253–258.
26 Tassinari D *et al.* (2008) Adverse effects of transdermal opiates treating moderate-severe cancer pain in comparison to long-acting morphine: a meta-analysis and systematic review of the literature. *Journal of Palliative Medicine.* **11**: 492–501.
27 Koo HC *et al.* (2010) Effect of transdermal fentanyl patches on the motility of the sphincter of oddi. *Gut and Liver.* **4**: 368–372.
28 Botterman J and Criel N (2011) Inappropriate use of high doses of transdermal fentanyl at admission to a palliative care unit. *Palliative Medicine.* **25**: 111–116.
29 Van Nimmen NF *et al.* (2010) Fentanyl transdermal absorption linked to pharmacokinetic characteristics in patients undergoing palliative care. *Journal of Clinical Pharmacology.* **50**: 667–678.
30 Marquardt KA *et al.* (1995) Fentanyl remaining in a transdermal system following three days of continuous use. *Annals of Pharmacotherpy.* **29**: 969–971.
31 Heiskanen T *et al.* (2009) Transdermal fentanyl in cachectic cancer patients. *Pain.* **144**: 218–222.
32 Hadgraft J and Lane ME (2005) Skin permeation: the years of enlightenment.[see comment]. *International Journal of Pharmaceutics.* **305**: 2–12.
33 Gourlay GK *et al.* (1989) The transdermal administration of fentanyl in the treatment of post-operative pain: pharmacokinetics and pharmacodynamic effects. *Pain.* **37**: 193–202.
34 Capper SJ *et al.* (2010) Pharmacokinetics of fentanyl after subcutaneous administration in volunteers. *European Journal of Anaesthesiology.* **27**: 241–246.
35 Portenoy RK *et al.* (1993) Transdermal fentanyl for cancer pain. *Anesthesiology.* **78**: 36–43.
36 Smith J and Ellershaw J (1999) Improvement in pain control by change of fentanyl patch after 48 hours compared with 72 hours. *Poster EAPC Congress, Geneva.* PO1/1376.
37 Anonymous (2007) Safe use of fentanyl (Duragesic) patches. *Pharmacist's Letter/Prescriber's Letter.* **23**: 1–5.
38 FDA (2007) Fentanyl transdermal system (marketed as Duragesic) Information. Available from: www.fda.gov/Drugs/DrugSafety/PostmarketDrugSafetyInformationforPatientsandProviders/ucm114961.htm
39 Jumbelic MI (2010) Deaths with transdermal fentanyl patches. *American Journal of Forensic Medicine and Pathology.* **31**: 18–21.
40 Dean M (2004) Opioids in renal failure and dialysis patients. *Journal of Pain and Symptom Management.* **28**: 497–504.
41 Hardy JR *et al.* (2007) Opioids in patients on renal dialysis. *Journal of Pain and Symptom Management.* **33**: 1–2.
42 Prosser JM *et al.* (2010) Complications of oral exposure to fentanyl transdermal delivery system patches. *Journal of Medical Toxicology.* **6**: 443–447.
43 Carson HJ *et al.* (2010) A fatality involving an unusual route of fentanyl delivery: Chewing and aspirating the transdermal patch. *Legal Medicine (Tokyo).* **12**: 157–159.

44 Baxter K (2011) Stockley's Drug Interactions (online edition). Pharmaceutical Press, London. Available from: www.medicinescomplete.com

45 Kharasch ED *et al.* (2004) Influence of hepatic and intestinal cytochrome P4503A activity on the acute disposition and effects of oral transmucosal fentanyl citrate. *Anesthesiology.* **101**: 729–737.

46 Takane H *et al.* (2005) Rifampin reduces the analgesic effect of transdermal fentanyl. *Annals of Pharmacotherpy.* **39**: 2139–2140.

47 Sasson M and Shvartzman P (2006) Fentanyl patch sufficient analgesia for only one day. *Journal of Pain and Symptom Management.* **31**: 389–391.

48 Morii H *et al.* (2007) Failure of pain control using transdermal fentanyl during rifampicin treatment. *Journal of Pain and Symptom Management.* **33**: 5–6.

49 Freynhagen R *et al.* (2005) Switching from reservoir to matrix systems for the transdermal delivery of fentanyl: a prospective, multicenter pilot study in outpatients with chronic pain. *Journal of Pain and Symptom Management.* **30**: 289–297.

50 Marier JF *et al.* (2006) Pharmacokinetics, tolerability, and performance of a novel matrix transdermal delivery system of fentanyl relative to the commercially available reservoir formulation in healthy subjects. *Journal of Clinical Pharmacology.* **46**: 642–653.

51 Kress HG *et al.* (2010) Transdermal fentanyl matrix patches Matrifen and Durogesic DTrans are bioequivalent. *European Journal of Pharmceutics and Biopharmaceutics.* **75**: 225–231.

52 Vielvoye-Kerkmeer A *et al.* (2000) Transdermal fentanyl in opioid-naive cancer pain patients: an open trial using transdermal fentanyl for the treatment of chronic cancer pain in opioid-naive patients and a group using codeine. *Journal of Pain and Symptom Management.* **19**: 185–192.

53 van Seventer R *et al.* (2003) Comparison of TTS-fentanyl with sustained-release oral morphine in the treatment of patients not using opioids for mild-to-moderate pain. *Current Medical Research Opinion.* **19**: 457–469.

54 Tawfik MO *et al.* (2004) Use of transdermal fentanyl without prior opioid stabilization in patients with cancer pain. *Curr Med Res Opin.* **20**: 259–267.

55 Mercadante S *et al.* (2010) Low doses of transdermal fentanyl in opioid-naive patients with cancer pain. *Current Medical Research Opinion.* **26**: 2765–2768.

56 Chang JT *et al.* (2010) Transdermal fentanyl for pain caused by radiotherapy in head and neck cancer patients treated in an outpatient setting: a multicenter trial in Taiwan. *Japanese Journal of Clinical Oncology.* **40**: 307–312.

57 Mercadante S *et al.* (2001) Clinical problems with transdermal fentanyl titration from 25 to 50mcg/h. *Journal of Pain and Symptom Management.* **21**: 448–449.

58 Korte W *et al.* (1996) Day-to-day titration to initiate transdermal fentanyl in patients with cancer pain: short and long term experiences in a prospective study of 39 patients. *Journal of Pain and Symptom Management.* **11**: 139–146.

59 Nomura M *et al.* (2011) Six- versus 12-h conversion method from intravenous to transdermal fentanyl in chronic cancer pain: a randomized study. *Supportive Care in Cancer.* **19**: 691–695.

Quick Practice Guide: Use of transdermal fentanyl patches

These recommendations use a dose conversion ratio for PO morphine to TD fentanyl of 100:1 and, as such, differ from those in UK SPCs. It is an approximation, and inevitably there will be individual variation.
Note: pain not relieved by morphine will generally not be relieved by fentanyl. If in doubt, seek specialist advice before prescribing TD fentanyl.

1 Indications for using TD fentanyl instead of morphine include:
- intolerable undesirable effects with morphine, e.g. nausea and vomiting, constipation, hallucinations, dysphagia
- renal failure (fentanyl has no active metabolite)
- 'tablet phobia' or poor compliance with oral medication
- high risk of tablet misuse/diversion.

2 TD fentanyl is contra-indicated in patients with acute (short-term) pain and in those who need rapid dose titration for severe uncontrolled pain. TD fentanyl is most appropriate for patients already on a stable dose of morphine (or other opioid analgesic) for ⩾1 week.

3 TD fentanyl patches are available in five strengths: 12, 25, 50, 75 and 100microgram/h for 3 days.

4 Use the table below to decide a safe starting dose for TD fentanyl, and an appropriate rescue dose. Patients taking a weak opioid should start on 12microgram/h.

5 For patients taking a dose of morphine that is not the exact equivalent of a fentanyl patch, it will be necessary to opt for a patch which is either slightly more or slightly less than the morphine dose. Thus, if the patient still has pain, round up to a higher patch strength; if pain-free and frail, round down. However, if switching because of possible opioid-induced hyperalgesia, reduce the calculated equivalent dose by 25–50%.

Comparative doses of PO morphine and TD fentanyl (based on dose ratio 100:1)

PO Morphine		*SC/IV Morphine*		*TD Fentanyl*	
mg/24h	*p.r.n mg*[a]	*mg/24h*[b]	*p.r.n mg*[a]	*microgram/h*	*mg/24h*
30	5	15	2.5	12	0.3
60	10	30	5	25	0.6
120	20	60	10	50	1.2
180	30	90	15	75	1.8
240	40	120	20	100[c]	2.4

a. using traditional 1/6 of total daily dose as p.r.n. dose
b. assuming potency ratio of morphine SC/IV to PO of 2:1
c. for combinations of patches, add the p.r.n. doses together, e.g. 100 + 75microgram/h patches = 20 + 15mg morphine SC/IV = 35mg morphine SC/IV, but can round up to 40mg or down to 30mg for convenience.

6 The date of application and/or the date for renewal should be written on the patch. Apply to dry, non-inflamed, non-irradiated, hairless skin on the upper trunk or arm. Body hair may be clipped with scissors but not shaved. If the skin is washed beforehand, use only water; do not use soap and do not apply oils, cream or ointment to the area. Press patch firmly in place for at least 30 seconds. Micropore® or Tegaderm® can be used to ensure adherence. Careful removal of the patch helps to minimize local skin irritation.

7 Effective systemic analgesic concentrations are generally reached in <12h. When converting from:
- 4-hourly PO morphine, give regular doses for the first 12h after applying the patch
- 12-hourly m/r morphine, apply the patch and the final m/r dose at the same time
- 24-hourly m/r morphine, apply the patch 12h after the final m/r dose

- CSCI/CIVI morphine, continue the infusion unchanged for 8–12h after applying the patch
- CSCI/CIVI fentanyl, continue the infusion unchanged for 3h after applying the patch, then halve the dose for the next 3h, then discontinue.

8 Steady-state plasma concentrations of fentanyl are generally achieved in 36–48h; the patient should use p.r.n. doses liberally during the first 3 days, particularly the first 24h. Safe rescue doses of PO morphine are given in the table above.

9 After 48h, if a patient still needs 2 or more rescue doses of morphine/day, the strength of the next patch to be applied should be increased by 12–25microgram/h. (Note: with the manufacturer's recommended starting doses, about 50% of patients need to increase the patch strength after the first 3 days.)

10 About 10% of patients experience opioid withdrawal symptoms when changed from morphine to TD fentanyl. These manifest with symptoms like gastric flu and last for a few days; p.r.n. doses of morphine will relieve troublesome symptoms.

11 Fentanyl is less constipating than morphine; halve the dose of laxatives when starting fentanyl and re-titrate.

12 Fentanyl may cause nausea and vomiting; if necessary, prescribe an anti-emetic, e.g. haloperidol 1.5mg stat & at bedtime.

13 In febrile patients, the rate of absorption of fentanyl increases, and may cause toxicity, e.g. drowsiness. Absorption is also enhanced by an external heat source over the patch, e.g. electric blanket or hot-water bottle; patients should be warned about this. Patients may shower with a patch but should not soak in a hot bath.

14 Remove patches after 72h; change the position of the new patches so as to rest the underlying skin for 3–6 days.

15 A reservoir of fentanyl accumulates in the body, and significant blood concentrations persist for at least 24h after discontinuing TD fentanyl.

16 TD fentanyl is unsatisfactory in <5% of patients. However, discontinuation is more common when TD fentanyl is used in strong opioid-naïve patients.

17 Additional or alternative analgesic approaches should be considered when the dose exceeds 300microgram/h.

18 In moribund patients, continue TD fentanyl and give additional SC morphine p.r.n. (see Table). If >2 p.r.n. doses are required/24h, give morphine by CSCI, starting with a dose equal to the sum of the p.r.n. doses over the preceding 24h. If necessary, adjust the p.r.n. dose taking into account the total opioid dose (i.e. TD fentanyl + CSCI morphine).

19 Used patches still contain fentanyl; after removal, fold the patch with the adhesive side inwards and discard in a sharps container (hospital) or dustbin (home), and wash hands. Ultimately, any unused patches should be returned to a pharmacy.

FENTANYL (TRANSMUCOSAL) BNF 4.7.2

This is a rapidly changing area, with several transmucosal fentanyl products available and more expected. Relative to PO opioids, the licensed products are expensive (about £4–12/episode). They are more effective than placebo, but direct comparison with PO morphine, or each other, is limited. Careful patient selection, training, titration and monitoring are required to ensure optimum use. They are *not* interchangeable.

Medicine advisory boards (Scottish Medicines Consortium, All Wales Medicines Strategy Group) have recommended restricting their use to patients unsuitable for other short-acting opioids, e.g. PO morphine.

Class: Strong opioid analgesic.

Indications: Break-through (episodic) pain in patients on regular strong opioids. The use of fentanyl injection SL or nasally is off-label.

Contra-indications: Use in strong opioid-naïve patients, acute non-cancer pain (e.g. postoperative pain, migraine), severe obstructive airways disease. *Instanyl®*: previous facial radiotherapy, recurrent epistaxis.

Pharmacology

Fentanyl (*like* **morphine**) is a strong μ-opioid receptor agonist. It has a relatively low molecular weight and (*unlike* **morphine**) is lipophilic. This makes it suitable for TD (see p.390) and transmucosal administration. Several formulations are licensed for the treatment of break-through (episodic) cancer pain, with others on the way, e.g. a buccal soluble film.[1]

Break-through cancer pain generally has a relatively rapid onset and short duration, e.g. 20–30min, but ranging from 1min to 2–3h (see p.279).[2] By comparison, strong opioids such as **morphine**, on average, take about 30–40min to achieve meaningful pain relief and have a long duration of effect (3–6h).[3] Thus, transmucosal fentanyl products aim to provide rapid onset pain relief which better matches the characteristics of break-through pain. Available products include:

- lozenge on a stick (Actiq®)
- SL (Abstral®) or buccal/SL (Effentora®) tablet
- nasal spray (Instanyl®, Pecfent®).

Formulations range from an aqueous solution of fentanyl (Instanyl®) to combinations with bio-adhesive substances, e.g. croscarmellose (Abstral®), pectin (Pecfent®). Thus, the pharmacokinetic characteristics of the products vary and they are *not* interchangeable (Table 5.27). Fentanyl is readily absorbed transmucosally and these modifications tend to *slow* the rate of absorption. Various justifications are given (e.g. to aid mucosal adherence, to attenuate the peak plasma concentration) but the fact that a novel delivery system can be patented (although not fentanyl itself) is also relevant.

With the buccal/SL products, the amount of fentanyl absorbed directly across the mucosa or swallowed varies with formulation and route of administration. About two thirds of any swallowed fentanyl will be eliminated by intestinal or hepatic first-pass metabolism. Nonetheless, significant amounts of swallowed fentanyl are absorbed, e.g. about 25% and 15% of the systemically available Actiq® and Effentora® respectively is via GI absorption.[9,12] The effects of the GI absorption on the plasma concentration of fentanyl include producing a 'double peak', maintaining high levels for longer (e.g. >2h) and contributing to the wide range in T_{max}.[6]

The rate and degree of absorption of fentanyl from the nasal cavity is dependent on mucosal perfusion. Vasoconstrictive nasal decongestants, e.g. **oxymetazoline**, double the time to maximum plasma concentration and halve the maximum plasma concentration of a dose of nasal fentanyl. Thus, the concurrent use of vasoconstrictive nasal decongestants with Instanyl® or Pecfent® should be avoided.

Once absorbed, fentanyl is rapidly distributed to the best perfused tissues, i.e. brain, heart, lungs, and then to fat, muscle and other tissues. Subsequently, fentanyl is redistributed between the deep tissue compartment and plasma. Up to 85% of fentanyl is protein bound, mainly to α_1-acid glycoprotein, but also albumin and lipoproteins. This pattern of rapid distribution, followed

Table 5.27 Selected characteristics and pharmacokinetic data for transmucosal fentanyl products[a,b]

	Abstral	*Actiq*	*Effentora*[c]	*Instanyl*	*Pecfent*
Formulation	SL tablet	Buccal lozenge	Buccal/SL tablet	Nasal spray	Nasal spray
Dose range and presentation	100, 200, 300, 400, 600, 800microgram Different shapes and colour coded packs of 10 or 30	200, 400, 600, 800, 1,200, 1,600microgram On a stick, marked with dose, in colour coded cartons, in pack of 3 or 30	100, 200, 400, 600, 800microgram 100 smaller in size; embossed 1, 2, etc., in pack of 4 or 28	50, 100, 200microgram/spray (100microL) 1 dose repeated once after 10min p.r.n.; colour coded and in 10 and 20 dose bottles	100, 200, 400 and 800microgram; given as 1 or 2 doses of 100 or 400microgram/spray (100microL); colour coded and in 8 dose bottles
Maximum dose/episode	800microgram	1,600microgram	800microgram	400microgram	800microgram
Maximum frequency of use	Maximum 4 episodes/24h, ideally ≥4h apart (see Dose and use)	Maximum 4 episodes/24h, ideally ≥4h apart (see Dose and use)	Maximum 4 episodes/24h, ≥4h apart	Maximum 4 episodes/24h, ≥4h apart	Maximum 4 episodes/24h, ≥4h apart
Approximate cost/tablet or spray	£5	£6	£5	£6; over 1/2 require 2 doses, thus average cost ≥£9	£3.80; about 1/2 require 200 or 800microgram dose, thus average cost = £5.70
Time to dissolution	<2min	Applied over 15min	Buccal 14–25min; SL quicker	N/A	N/A
Onset of action[d]	10min	15min	10min	5min	10min
Time to peak plasma concentration, median (range)	30–60min (10–90) Longer with higher strengths, but 600 and 800microgram not examined in patients	Across dose range 90min (30–480)[4,5]	Pooled data 53min (20–240)[6]	Across dose range 12–15min (6–90min)[7]	Across dose range 15–21min (5–180min)[5]

continued

Table 5.27 Continued

	Abstral	*Actiq*	*Effentora*[c]	*Instanyl*	*Pecfent*
Plasma halflife	Mean 5–6h, but 600 and 800microgram not examined in patients	Median 18h (7–49) 800microgram[4]	Median 12h (2–44), pooled data[6]	Median 19h (8–30); 200microgram, 2 doses 10min apart[8]	Mean 15–25h
Duration of action	⩾1h	⩾1h (⩽3.5h reported with higher doses)[9]	⩾2h	⩾1h	⩾1h
Bio-availability	70% (estimated)	50% (25% transmucosal, 25% PO)[9]	65% (50% transmucosal, 15% PO)	90%	No data
Comments		Requires continual movement around the mouth; less effective if finished < 15min as more is swallowed	Absorption not affected by mild (grade 1) mucositis[10]	Non-preserved solution, pH 6.6, osmolality ~0.9% saline	Preserved solution containing pectin, adjusted for pH and osmolality. C_{max} is about 1/3 of that of Instanyl. Audible click denotes dose administered; visual priming guide and dose counter, end-of-use lock

a. the source (i.e. healthy volunteers vs. patients) and quality (e.g. small number of subjects, whole dose range not studied, use of massage over buccal tablet) of the data varies widely
b. data based on venous blood sampling; with arterial sampling, a higher maximum concentration is achieved about 15min quicker[11]
c. pharmacokinetics are similar for either buccal or SL placement
d. earliest *statistically significant* difference between fentanyl product and placebo in mean pain intensity difference; a *clinically meaningful* difference has been variably defined and generally takes longer (see text).

by a slower redistribution explains why fentanyl has a relatively short duration of action despite a long halflife.

Elimination of fentanyl mainly involves biotransformation in the liver by CYP3A4 to inactive norfentanyl which is excreted in the urine. Less than 7% is excreted unchanged. The SPCs of all of the transmucosal fentanyl products advise caution in their use in patients with moderate–severe hepatic or renal impairment but this is based on limited data which suggests a reduced clearance of fentanyl, e.g. via alterations in metabolic clearance and plasma protein binding.

Pharmacokinetic studies of repeat/chronic dosing of the transmucosal products are limited. Repeating a dose of Pecfent® after an interval of 1 or 2h significantly increases the maximum plasma concentration, but not when given 4h apart.[5] Accumulation of fentanyl can occur with regular use; when Effentora® 400microgram is given q6h, steady state is reached after about 5 days, and the maximum plasma concentration becomes double that of the initial dose.[13] Thus, even when an effective and tolerable dose is identified through titration, with subsequent regular use, accumulation, and undesirable effects could occur.

Generally, patients recruited to the development studies for the fentanyl transmucosal products were relatively young (mean age 55–60 years), had a good performance status (ECOG PS 0–2), no clinically relevant renal or hepatic impairment and were taking reasonable doses of regular opioids (mean morphine equivalent dose of 190–280mg PO/24h). Thus, additional caution is required when giving these products to patients outside of this group, particularly those who are elderly. A sober critique of the published papers is also required for various reasons, including:

- they are studies sponsored by the manufacturer and lack impartiality
- although similar methods of evaluation are used across studies, the criteria used to define a response vary, making direct comparison difficult (see below)
- some approaches undertaken in the studies do not reflect recommended clinical practice, e.g.:
  - only single doses of Abstral® were used for titration and maintenance in the study on which its safety data is based, with the effective dose confirmed over several consecutive episodes; by comparison, in the SPC, a second dose is permitted during titration and intermediate doses suggested, with no mention of confirmation of the effective dose[14]
  - Effentora® tablet remnants were 'massaged' after 10–15min in the pharmacokinetic and efficacy studies, potentially artificially enhancing absorption and efficacy data[15]
  - patients who had already used Instanyl® were enrolled into an efficacy study, artificially enhancing the proportion achieving successful titration (>90% vs. more usual 60–70%)[8]
  - in some instances the regulatory authorities expressed concerns about the amount and/or the quality of the data, e.g. Abstral® pharmacokinetic data, Instanyl® safety reporting.[8,16]

For speed of onset of analgesia, generally what is promoted is the earliest *statistically significant* difference in pain intensity between the fentanyl product and placebo (generally 5–15min). Although some patients report a reduction in pain intensity which is considered *clinically meaningful* by this time, this generally takes longer for most products. Reliable comparison of the different products is difficult because how a clinically meaningful change is defined and calculated varies, e.g. reduction in pain intensity score from baseline of ≥2/10 or 30–33%, by episode (at least one or all) or by patient. Further, applying different criteria to the same data can produce different times, e.g. for Pecfent®, half of the patients experience a reduction in pain intensity score of ≥2 by 15min, but a ≥33% reduction takes 30min.[5,17] (Note: it has been suggested that a ≥50% improvement in pain intensity is required to be of *substantial* clinical importance.[18]

However, for half of the episodes, an improvement in pain intensity of at least moderate clinical importance appears by about 10min (Instanyl®[19]), 15min (Pecfent®[17]) or 30min (Abstral®,[20] Actiq®,[21] Effentora®[22]). Even so, in up to a quarter of episodes, a second rescue analgesic is needed after 20–30min (product-dependent) because of an inadequate response. Careful explanation is required to ensure that both rescue analgesics are used correctly.

Comparative data either between products or with PO analgesia is limited. When compared to PO **morphine**, Actiq® and Pecfent® have generally performed statistically significantly better, but the absolute differences in outcomes are relatively small, making their clinical relevance uncertain (Box 5.P).

Box 5.P Active comparator studies of transmucosal fentanyl products

Actiq® vs. PO morphine tablets[21]

Actiq®, titrated to an effective dose, has been compared with morphine *tablets* (previously identified effective dose, encapsulated to maintain blinding) in a double-blind, double-dummy, multiple cross-over study. For the primary and secondary outcomes, Actiq® was statistically superior to PO morphine tablets. However, the differences were small and their clinical relevance uncertain.

For example, for Actiq® vs. PO morphine tablets, the proportion of episodes after 15min with clinical meaningful pain relief (defined as a ≥33% reduction in pain intensity) was 42 vs. 32%. Nonetheless, >90% of patients chose to continue with Actiq®.[21]

Pecfent® vs. PO morphine tablets[23,24]

Pecfent®, titrated to an effective dose, has been compared with encapsulated morphine *tablets* (one sixth of the total daily dose, or previously identified effective dose) in a double-blind, double-dummy, multiple cross-over study. For the primary and most secondary outcomes, Pecfent® was statistically superior to PO morphine tablets. However, the differences were small and their clinical relevance uncertain.

For example, for Pecfent® vs. PO morphine tablets:

- mean (SD) pain intensity difference at 15min (primary outcome) was 3.0 (0.2) vs. 2.7 (0.2)
- percentage of episodes with clinical meaningful pain relief (defined as a ≥2 reduction in pain intensity) was 25 vs. 23% (5min); 52 vs. 45% (10min) and 76 vs. 69% (15min).

Instanyl® vs. Actiq®[8,25]

Instanyl® and Actiq® (both titrated to an effective dose) have been compared in an open label RCT. The primary outcome was time to meaningful pain relief, measured by stop-watch. The fastest time to meaningful pain relief was significantly more likely with Instanyl® than Actiq®, with a median difference of 5min (11 vs. 16min respectively). A second dose of Instanyl® or Actiq® was required in about 60% and 30% of episodes respectively. For Instanyl® this was permitted 10min after the first dose, and for Actiq® 15min after fully consuming the first dose, i.e. at least 30min after starting the first dose. Usual rescue analgesia was required in 5–8% of episodes. Patients found the administration of Instanyl® easier and overall preferred Instanyl® (75%) to Actiq® (25%).

Indeed, PO **morphine** performs relatively well, particularly when considered that, unlike the fentanyl product, the **morphine** dose will not have been optimized in a titration phase, and is also given in tablet form. To fully determine the relative advantage of the transmucosal products over PO **morphine** in relation to speed of onset of action, **morphine** *solution* is the more appropriate comparator than *tablets*, because it is absorbed and acts more quickly. For example, studies have reported a median (range) T_{max} of 60min (20–90) vs. 125min (40–240) and mean time to meaningful pain relief of about 15min vs. 30min for **morphine** solution vs. tablets respectively.[26,27]

The lack of more extensive comparison between the transmucosal products limits the evidence to determine which are best to use. However, the practical aspects of using some of the products have been compared in a patient satisfaction survey.[28] Following instruction, 30 patients were asked to use a single *placebo* version of Abstral®, Effentora® and Instanyl® and to rate factors such as ease of access from packaging, ease of administration and palatability; they also rated their current rescue analgesic (generally PO **morphine** or **oxycodone**) similarly. They were asked to indicate if they would be prepared to use the transmucosal product and, if so, which they felt was the best and why. Several themes emerged:

- *ease of access:* the fentanyl products were generally more difficult to access than usual rescue analgesia, particularly the child-proof container for Instanyl®
- *ease of use:* Abstral® and the usual rescue analgesia were joint best
- *palatability:* Abstral® was rated best
- *patients willing to use:* Abstral® (90%) vs. Effentora® and Instanyl® (about 60% each); three patients would not use any (did not like the product or could not open the packaging)

- *which is best and why?*:
  - ▹ Abstral® (~70%); easy to access and use, dissolved quickly
  - ▹ Instanyl® (~20%); quick to use (once you get into package), route familiar
  - ▹ Effentora® (~10%); liked sensation in the mouth
  - ▹ one could not choose between Abstral® and Effentora®.

The use of placebos means that overall satisfaction with the products could not be compared. Nonetheless, taking these practical issues and other factors into account, *PCF* suggests the following in patients with cancer taking regular strong opioids and experiencing break-through pain:

- use PO strong opioids first-line and titrate accordingly (include a trial of a PO solution if tablets not adequate); only when inadequate with regards to speed of onset of action or prolonged undesirable effects should the transmucosal products be considered
- a patient's circumstances should be considered carefully to ensure they fulfil the necessary requirements for use of a transmucosal product, e.g. current opioid dose, ability to access, use, store and dispose of the product reliably etc. (see Dose and use)
- decide which route and product is the most appropriate, i.e.:
  - ▹ *nasal:* generally works quicker and shorter lasting (less PO absorption) than the SL/buccal route; Pecfent® works slightly slower than Instanyl®, but has a safer, accountable delivery system, and is cheaper
  - ▹ *SL/buccal:* there is little to choose from in terms of efficacy and cost; Abstral® dissolves quickest, making it more convenient to use than Actiq® or Effentora®.

There may be other more specific reasons which guide choice of route, e.g. patient preference, presence of severe dry mouth or mucositis (use nasal), or frequent nose bleeds (use SL/buccal).

As a cheaper alternative to the licensed transmucosal fentanyl products, some palliative care services use the parenteral formulation of various fentanils for SL administration, e.g. fentanyl (50microgram/mL), **sufentanil** (50microgram/mL, not UK) and **alfentanil** (500microgram/mL and 5mg/mL).[29–31] Onset of analgesic effect may be broadly similar (5–10min) but duration of effect is likely to differ (fentanyl > **sufentanil** > **alfentanil**) (see Alfentanil, p.374). Several small doses can be given until pain relief is obtained. Using a 1mL graduated oral syringe:

- start with fentanyl 25–50microgram (0.5–1mL of 50microgram/mL)
- if necessary, increase to 50–100microgram; many patients do not need more than this
- doses > 100microgram are impractical because 2mL is the maximum volume that can be reliably kept in the mouth for transmucosal absorption.[30]

Drawing up the correct amount of the parenteral formulation into a syringe is inconvenient, but this can be overcome by the use of a spray bottle.[31,32]

The 50microgram/mL fentanyl solution has also been administered as a nasal spray. In adults this approach is limited by the large dose volume. However, it has provided effective analgesia in children 1–16 years old presenting to the emergency department with acute moderate–severe pain.[33–35] A 1mL syringe attached to a mucosal atomizer device permits the appropriate amount of fentanyl to be converted into a spray. The initial dose is 1.5microgram/kg, with some centres permitting a second dose of 0.5microgram/kg after 10min if required.[35]

Cautions

All companies provide additional information for prescribers, pharmacists and patients; these include check-lists to ensure proper patient selection and education around use, signs of opioid overdose, safe storage and disposal. Store out of reach of children (accidental deaths have occurred).

In 2007, after reports of serious overdoses and deaths in the USA, the FDA issued a safety warning about the use of Fentora® (Effentora®). Factors which contributed to the adverse drug events included improper:

- patient selection, e.g. non-opioid tolerant, acute (non-cancer) pain
- dosing, e.g. wrong dose prescribed, exceeding recommended maximum use
- product substitution, e.g. like for like swap from Actiq® to Fentora®.

Thus, these products need to be used correctly, specifically:

- do *not* use in opioid naïve (non-tolerant) patients, including those who only take strong opioids p.r.n.
- they are contra-indicated in the management of acute or postoperative pain, including headache/migraine

- they are not interchangeable; do *not* convert patients on a microgram per microgram basis from one to another; it is necessary to titrate the new formulation
- when dispensing, do *not* substitute one product for another.

Use with caution in patients with COPD or other medical conditions predisposing them to respiratory depression (e.g. myasthenia gravis) or susceptible to the intracranial effects of hypercapnia (e.g. those with raised intracranial pressure). Also if bradyarrhythmia, elderly, cachectic, debilitated, moderate–severe hepatic or renal impairment, hypovolaemia, hypotension; and if a history or high risk of abuse or diversion.

Mouth wounds, mucositis (may enhance absorption); nasal vasoconstrictive decongestants (reduce the effect), other nasal medications (the SPC for Instanyl® recommends avoiding because of lack of data, whereas that for Pecfent® advises avoiding within 15min of a dose), epistaxis.

Actiq® contains 2g of sugars; inform diabetic patients, also risk of tooth decay (uncommon).

Drug interactions

Fentanyl is metabolized by CYP3A4. Thus, fentanyl plasma concentrations may be increased by CYP3A4 inhibitors such as azole antifungals (e.g. **fluconazole**, **ketoconzole**, **itraconazole**), macrolide antibiotics (e.g. **erythromycin**, **clarithromycin**), protease inhibitors (e.g. **ritonavir**, **nelfinavir**), **aprepitant**, **cimetidine**, **diltiazem** and **verapamil**.[36]

In contrast, concentrations are decreased by potent CYP3A4 inducers (e.g. **carbamazepine**, **phenytoin**, **phenobarbitone**, **rifampicin**) and this may lead to a loss of analgesia.[36–40]

Fentanyl is best avoided in patients who have used a MAOI within the past 2 weeks. Although they have been used safely together, serotonin toxicity (sometimes fatal) has occurred.[36]

Undesirable effects

Also see Strong opioids, p.34. Except Actiq®, all products are marked with a black triangle, and undesirable effects should be reported using the Yellow card scheme (www.yellowcard.mhra.gov.uk).

Very common (>10%): drowsiness, dizziness, headache, confusion, nausea, vomiting, sweating.

Topical effects: less common and formulation-dependent, but include: oral and nasal discomfort, inflammation or ulceration, rhinorrhoea, epistaxis, sore throat, dysguesia, dental caries with Actiq® (uncommon).

Dose and use

For TD and SC routes of administration, see p.390.

Prescribers of transmucosal fentanyl products should:

- be experienced in the management of opioid-therapy in cancer patients
- limit use to opioid-tolerant patients who can adhere to the instructions regarding indication, administration, storage and returns
- provide ongoing supervision
- keep in mind the potential for fentanyl to be misused
- understand that the formulations are *not* bio-equivalent and thus *not* interchangeable; when switching products, de novo titration is required.

Transmucosal fentanyl products should be used only in adults on a regular strong opioid for chronic cancer pain for ⩾1 week:

- **morphine** 60mg/24h PO
- fentanyl 25microgram/h TD (50microgram/h required in some studies)
- **hydromorphone** 8mg/24h PO
- **oxycodone** 30mg/24h PO
- an equivalent dose of another opioid.

Individual titration is required because a successful dose cannot be predicted from the maintenance dose of opioid.[41,42] Careful monitoring is required during initial or subsequent titration; the complexity of the titration schedules varies between products (Box 5.Q, Box 5.R, Box 5.S, Box 5.T, Box 5.U). Even so, transmucosal fentanyl products are unsatisfactory in about 1/4–1/3 of patients, either because they fail to provide relief at the highest practical dose or cause unacceptable undesirable effects.

The optimal dose found during successful titration (Box 5.Q, Box 5.R, Box 5.S, Box 5.T, Box 5.U), can be used to treat up to 4 break-through pain episodes/24h. Except for Abstral® and

Actiq®, the SPC of all products specify that these should be ⩾4h apart, which includes after the use of a second rescue analgesic. However, applying this rule across all products would be reasonable because more frequent dosing than q4h appears to increase the maximum plasma concentration achieved with the subsequent dose of fentanyl.[5] Thus, an alternative p.r.n. analgesic, e.g. **morphine** PO, will be required to treat any additional, more frequent episodes. Further, in about 5–25% of episodes, the transmucosal products fail to provide adequate relief and an alternate analgesic is required.[43,44]

Box 5.Q Abstral® dose and use

Follow the manufacturer's guidance on administration, titration, storage and disposal in the SPC, Prescribers guide, Dose titration guide, and Patient Information Leaflet. A hospital/ hospice referral pad for GPs is also available.

Abstral® is a SL tablet, placed in the deepest part under the tongue. The tablets must not be chewed or sucked and patients should not eat or drink until they have dissolved. Those with a dry mouth may moisten it with water beforehand. The tablet generally dissolves quickly (<5min), with the particles produced adhering to the oral mucosa from which the fentanyl is subsequently absorbed.

Evaluate each dose after 15–30min and if successful, i.e. a *single* dose provides adequate analgesia with little or no undesirable effects, this is the maintenance dose. If unsuccessful, during titration, a further dose can be given and subsequently a higher dose used for the next episode:

- start with 100microgram, if unsuccessful, give an additional 100microgram dose
- for the next episode give 200microgram, if unsuccessful, give an additional 100microgram tablet
- for the next episode give 300microgram, if unsuccessful, give an additional 100microgram tablet
- for the next episode give 400microgram, if unsuccessful, give an additional 200microgram tablet
- for the next episode give 600microgram, if unsuccessful, give an additional 200microgram tablet
- for the next episode give 800microgram, the maximum dose.

The SPC suggests that intermediate doses of 500 and 700microgram can be considered if there is adequate analgesia but undesirable effects at either the 600 or 800microgam doses respectively. However, in practice, such doses are rarely used. It requires the use of a 100microgram tablet plus a 400 or 600microgram tablet, and doubles the cost of treating an episode (£10).

Note: in the efficacy and safety study, only single doses of Abstral® were used for titration and maintenance, with the effective dose confirmed over several consecutive episodes.[14]

More than two thirds of patients find an effective and tolerable dose. However, because of inadequate relief after 30min, an alternative rescue analgesic is needed in about 10% of episodes.[14]

A maximum of 4 break-through pain episodes/24h can be treated. In studies, this had to be ⩾2h apart (each pain episode was limited to treatment with a single dose);[14,39] ⩾4h apart is the ideal (see text). Regular daily use of break-through medication (traditionally ⩾2/24h) should prompt a review and possible increase in the dose of the regular strong opioid. Subsequently, if a single dose of Abstral® fails to provide consistent relief, the dose should be further titrated as above.

Abstral® is generally well tolerated and remains effective. Use of a median dose of 600microgram treating a mean of 3 episodes/day for 5–6 months showed that:

- opioid-related undesirable effects (e.g. nausea) are common but not a major cause of discontinuation
- application site irritation rarely occurred
- about 75% of patients were satisfied or very satisfied with its use.[14,45]

Box 5.R Actiq® dose and use

Follow the manufacturer's guidance on administration, titration, storage and disposal in the SPC, Patients and caregivers guide and Patient Information Leaflet.

Actiq® is a 'lozenge on a stick' containing fentanyl in a hard sweet matrix. In order to achieve maximum mucosal exposure to the fentanyl, the lozenge should be placed between the cheek and the gum and moved constantly up and down, and changed at intervals from one cheek to the other. It should not be chewed. The lozenge should be consumed completely over 15min; quicker than this and more fentanyl is swallowed. Patients with xerostomia (dry mouth) may find it hard to consume it in this time period.[46] If necessary, moisten the mouth with water beforehand. Initially, prescribe 6 doses of one strength at a time:

- start with fentanyl 200microgram and consume over 15min; drinking or eating is not permitted during administration
- wait 15min; if there is inadequate analgesia, use a second 200microgram lozenge
- not more than two lozenges should be used for any one episode of pain
- continue with 200microgram for a further 2 episodes of pain, allowing a second lozenge when necessary
- if on review, the break-through (episodic) pain is not controlled satisfactorily with a single 200microgram dose, increase to 400microgram
- wait 15min; use a second 400microgram lozenge if necessary
- continue this upwards titration through the available dose strengths until a *single* dose provides adequate analgesia with little or no undesirable effects; this is the maintenance dose
- the maximum dose is 1,600microgram.

The lozenge should be removed from the mouth once the pain is relieved; partly consumed lozenges should be dissolved under hot running water and the handle discarded in a waste container out of reach of children.

About three quarters of patients find an effective and tolerable dose. An alternative rescue analgesic is required in 5–15% of episodes (permitted if inadequate response 15min after Actiq® dose fully completed).

A maximum of 4 break-through pain episodes/24h can be treated. In studies, this generally had to be ⩾2h apart (each pain episode was limited to treatment with a single dose);[21] ⩾4h apart is the ideal (see text). Regular daily use of break-through medication (traditionally ⩾2/24h) should prompt a review and possible increase in the dose of the regular strong opioid. Subsequently, if a single dose of Actiq® fails to provide consistent relief, the dose should be further titrated as detailed above.

Actiq® is generally well tolerated and remains effective. Follow up over a mean of about 3 months showed that:

- opioid-related undesirable effects are common (e.g. nausea) but not a major cause of discontinuation
- a single dose is effective in 85–90% of episodes
- about 1/2–3/4 of patients require a dose adjustment; mostly upwards, but sometimes downwards
- patient ratings of global medication performance remain the same (generally 'very good').[47,48]

Box 5.S Effentora® dose and use

Follow the manufacturer's guidance on administration, titration, storage and disposal in the SPC, Patients and caregivers guide and Patient Information Leaflet.

Effentora® is a tablet which can be placed either buccally (between the cheek and gum near a molar tooth) or SL. Absorption is similar from both sites, but it dissolves quicker SL.[49] A dry mouth should be moistened with water beforehand. Mild mucositis (grade 1) does not affect absorption,[10] but avoid use in more severe grades because the impact on absorption has not been examined.

The tablets must not be chewed or sucked and patients should not eat or drink until they have dissolved. The time to dissolution is generally 15–25min but can be longer. However, any tablet remnants should be swallowed after 30min with a glass of water.

Evaluate each dose after 30min and, if successful, this is the maintenance dose. If unsuccessful, during the titration phase, a further dose can be given and subsequently a higher dose used for the next episode. Titration packs, each containing 4 tablets, are available; prescribing 1 pack of 100microgram and 3 packs of 200microgram is sufficient to escalate through the dose range over 5 break-through episodes:

- start with 100microgram, if unsuccessful, give an additional 100microgram dose
- for the next episode give 200microgram (2 x 100microgram tablets), if unsuccessful, give an additional 200microgram tablet
- for the next episode give 400microgram (2 x 200microgram tablets), if unsuccessful, give an additional 200microgram tablet
- for the next episode give 600microgram (3 x 200microgram tablets), if unsuccessful, give an additional 200microgram tablet
- for the next episode give the maximum dose of 800microgram (4 x 200microgram tablets).

About two thirds of patients find an effective and tolerable dose. Subsequently only a *single* dose of the appropriate strength tablet is used per episode, which can be prescribed in 28 tablet packs. An alternative rescue analgesic is required in about 10–25% of episodes.

A maximum of 4 break-through pain episodes/24h can be treated, with at least 4h between doses (including any other rescue analgesic used). Regular daily use of break-through medication (traditionally ⩾2/24h) should prompt a review and possible increase in the dose of the regular strong opioid. Subsequently, if a single dose of Effentora® fails to provide consistent relief, the dose may require further titration as above.

Effentora® is generally well tolerated and remains effective. Follow up over a mean of 6 months showed that:

- opioid-related undesirable effects are common (e.g. nausea) but not a major cause of discontinuation
- application site problems (e.g. pain, irritation, ulceration) are seen in 6% and lead to discontinuation in <2%
- 70% of patients continue on the same dose
- patient ratings of global medication performance remain the same (generally 'good').[50]

Although only licensed for break-through cancer pain, data exist for the use of Effentora® in:

- opioid-tolerant patients with non-cancer break-through pain, e.g. degenerative back pain, complex regional pain syndrome[51–54]
- opioid-naïve patients with severe pain attending emergency departments with possible or definite fractures or dislocations (single dose of 100microgram).[55]

However, such use is controversial, and concerns exist around safety and the potential for misuse.[54,56,57]

Box 5.T Instanyl® dose and use

Follow the guidance on priming, administration, storage and disposal in the manufacturer's SPC, Physician and Pharmacist guides, Patient brochure/Information Leaflet.

Instanyl® is a nasal spray. Not all patients feel the spray and they should be warned not to repeat the dose because of this. There is no dose counter.

Evaluate each dose after 10min and if successful, this is the maintenance dose; if unsuccessful, a maximum of one further dose can be given.

Evaluate each dose strength over several (i.e. 3–4) episodes; increase to the next higher strength if there is frequent need for a second dose:

- start with 50microgram in one nostril, if unsuccessful give an additional 50microgram in the other nostril
- if unsuccessful over several episodes, give 100microgram in one nostril, if necessary give an additional 100microgram in the other nostril
- if unsuccessful over several episodes, give 200microgram in one nostril, if necessary give an additional 200microgram in the other nostril; this is the *maximum* dose.

About 2/3–3/4 of patients find an effective and tolerable dose. Although the aim is to use only one dose per episode, >50% require a second dose. An alternative rescue analgesic is required in about 15% of episodes; this is given after waiting ≥10min after a dose of Instanyl®.

A maximum of 4 break-through pain episodes/24h can be treated, with at least 4h between doses (including any other rescue analgesic used). Regular daily use of break-through medication (traditionally ≥2/24h) should prompt a review and possible increase in the dose of the regular strong opioid. The dose of Instanyl® may subsequently need to be re-titrated.

Instanyl® is generally well tolerated; opioid-related undesirable effects are common (e.g. nausea) but not a major cause of discontinuation.

The bottles should be stored upright in the child-resistant container for safety; if not used for >1 week, they need to be primed again by spraying a single dose in the air.

Box 5.U Pecfent® dose and use

Follow the guidance on priming, administration, storage and disposal in the manufacturer's SPC, Physician and Pharmacist guides, Patient brochure/Information Leaflet.

Pecfent® is a nasal spray. Not all patients feel the spray, but there is an audible click when the dose is administered, and the dose counter advances by one. Advise patients not to blow their nose for 1h after administration:

- start with 100microgram in one nostril
- if unsuccessful, for the next episode, give 200microgram (100microgram in each nostril)
- if unsuccessful, for the next episode, prescribe higher concentration formulation and give 400microgram in one nostril
- if unsuccessful, for the next episode, increase to the maximum dose of 800microgram (400microgram in each nostril).

Evaluate each dose after 30min and, if ineffective, an alternative rescue analgesic can be given.

If any of the above doses are successful, this should be confirmed in the next episode. About three quarters of patients find an effective and tolerable dose; an alternative rescue analgesic is needed in about 5–10% of episodes. Subsequently, if a previously effective dose fails to provide relief over several episodes, consider titration to a higher dose.

A maximum of 4 break-through pain episodes/24h can be treated, with at least 4h between doses (including any other rescue analgesic used). Regular daily use of break-through medication (traditionally ≥2/24h) should prompt a review and a possible increase in the dose of the regular strong opioid. The dose of Pecfent® may subsequently need to be re-titrated.

Pecfent® is generally well tolerated and remains effective. Follow up over a mean of 4 months showed that:

- <3% of patients dropped out because of drug-related undesirable effects
- 90% continued on the same dose
- 90% were satisfied or very satisfied with its use.[17,44]

The bottles should be kept in the child-resistant container for safety, and disposed of 2 weeks after priming or if >5 days have elapsed since last use.

Supply

All preparations are fentanyl citrate and **CD**.

Buccal products
Abstral® (ProStrakan)
Tablet sublingual 100microgram, 200microgram, 300microgram, 400microgram, 600microgram, 800microgram. 1 tablet = £5 regardless of strength

Actiq® (Flynn)
Lozenge buccal with oromucosal applicator 200microgram, 400microgram, 600microgram, 800microgram, 1,200microgram and 1,600microgram, 1 lozenge = £6 regardless of strength.

Effentora® (Cephalon)
Tablet buccal 100microgram, 200microgram, 400microgram, 600microgram, 800microgram. 1 tablet = £5 regardless of strength.

Nasal spray
Instanyl® (Nycomed)
Nasal spray 50micrograms/metered dose spray, 100microgram/metered dose spray, 200microgram/metered dose spray, 1 spray = £6 regardless of strength.

Pecfent® (Archimedes)
Nasal spray 100microgram/metered dose spray, 400microgram/metered dose spray, 1 spray = £3.80 regardless of strength; the dose required may consist of 1 or 2 sprays.

Fentanyl citrate (generic)
Injection 50microgram/mL, 2mL amp = £0.50, 10mL amp = £0.50.

Sublimaze® (Janssen-Cilag)
Injection 50microgram/mL, 2mL amp = £0.50, 10mL amp = £1.50

---

1 Rauck R *et al.* (2010) Fentanyl buccal soluble film (FBSF) for breakthrough pain in patients with cancer: a randomized, double-blind, placebo-controlled study. *Annals of Oncology.* **21**: 1308–1314.
2 Gomez-Batiste X *et al.* (2002) Breakthrough cancer pain: prevalence and characteristics in Catalonia. *Journal of Pain and Symptom Management.* **24**: 45–52.
3 Zeppetella G (2008) Opioids for cancer breakthrough pain: a pilot study reporting patient assessment of time to meaningful pain relief. *Journal of Pain and Symptom Management.* **35**: 563–567.
4 Darwish M *et al.* (2007) Absolute and relative bioavailability of fentanyl buccal tablet and oral transmucosal fentanyl citrate. *Journal of Clinical Pharmacology.* **47**: 343–350.
5 European Medicines Agency (2010) Assessment report for Pecfent. Procedure No. EMA/H/C/001164.
6 European Medicines Agency (2008) Effentora: EPAR — Scientific discussion.
7 Kaasa S *et al.* (2010) Pharmacokinetics of intranasal fentanyl spray in patients with cancer and breakthrough pain. *Journal of Opioid Management.* **6**: 17–26.
8 European Medicines Agency (2009) Assessment report for Instanyl. Procedure No. EMEA/H/C/959. London.
9 Lichtor J *et al.* (1999) The relative potency of oral transmucosal fentanyl citrate compared with intravenous morphine in the treatment of moderate to severe postoperative pain. *Anesthesia and Analgesia.* **89**: 732–738.
10 Darwish M *et al.* (2007) Absorption of fentanyl from fentanyl buccal tablet in cancer patients with or without oral mucositis: a pilot study. *Clinical Drug Investigation.* **27**: 605–611.
11 Darwish M *et al.* (2006) Comparison of equivalent doses of fentanyl buccal tablets and arteriovenous differences in fentanyl pharmacokinetics. *Clinical Pharmacokinetics.* **45**: 843–850.
12 Darwish M *et al.* (2007) Absorption of fentanyl from fentanyl buccal tablet in cancer patients with or without oral mucositis: a pilot study. *Clinical Drug Investigation.* **27**: 605–611.
13 Darwish M *et al.* (2007) Single-dose and steady-state pharmacokinetics of fentanyl buccal tablet in healthy volunteers. *Journal of Clinical Pharmacology.* **47**: 56–63.
14 Rauck RL *et al.* (2009) Efficacy and long-term tolerability of sublingual fentanyl orally disintegrating tablet in the treatment of breakthrough cancer pain. *Current Medical Research Opinion.* **25**: 2877–2885.
15 Slatkin NE *et al.* (2007) Fentanyl buccal tablet for relief of breakthrough pain in opioid-tolerant patients with cancer-related chronic pain. *Journal of Supportive Oncology.* **5**: 327–334.
16 European Medicines Agency (2008) Committee for medicinal products for human use (CHMP). Opinion following article 29(4) referral for Rapinyl.
17 Portenoy RK *et al.* (2010) A multicenter, placebo-controlled, double-blind, multiple-crossover study of Fentanyl Pectin Nasal Spray (FPNS) in the treatment of breakthrough cancer pain. *Pain.* **151**: 617–624.
18 Dworkin RH *et al.* (2008) Interpreting the clinical importance of treatment outcomes in chronic pain clinical trials: IMMPACT recommendations. *Journal of Pain.* **9**: 105–121.
19 Kress HG *et al.* (2009) Efficacy and tolerability of intranasal fentanyl spray 50 to 200 microg for breakthrough pain in patients with cancer: a phase III, multinational, randomized, double-blind, placebo-controlled, crossover trial with a 10-month, open-label extension treatment period. *Clinical Therapeutics.* **31**: 1177–1191.

20 Prostraken (2010) *Personal communication.*
21 Coluzzi P *et al.* (2001) Breakthrough cancer pain: a randomized trial comparing oral transmucosal fentanyl citrate (OTFC) and morphine sulfate immediate release (MSIR). *Pain.* **91**: 123–130.
22 Zeppetella G *et al.* (2010) Consistent and clinically relevant effects with fentanyl buccal tablet in the treatment of patients receiving maintenance opioid therapy and experiencing cancer-related breakthrough pain. *Pain Practice.* **10**: 287–293.
23 Fallon M *et al.* (2010) Efficacy, safety and patient acceptability of fentanyl pectin nasal spray compared with immediate-release morphine sulphate tablets in the treatment of breakthrough cancer pain: A multicentre, double-blind, double-dummy, multiple cross-over study. Poster presentation at the European Association for Palliative Care Research Congress, Glasgow.
24 Davies A *et al.* (2011) Consistency of efficacy, patient acceptability, and nasal tolerability of fentanyl pectin nasal spray compared with immediate-release morphine sulfate in breakthrough cancer pain. *Journal of Pain and Symptom Management.* **41**: 358–366.
25 Mercadante S *et al.* (2009) A comparison of intranasal fentanyl spray with oral transmucosal fentanyl citrate for the treatment of breakthrough cancer pain: an open label, randomised, crossover trial. *Current Medical Research Opinion.* **25**: 2805–2815.
26 Sawe J *et al.* (1983) Steady-state kinetics and analgesic effect of oral morphine in cancer patients. *European Journal of Clinical Pharmacology.* **24**: 537–542.
27 Freye E *et al.* (2007) Effervescent morphine results in faster relief of breakthrough pain in patients compared to immediate release morphine sulfate tablet. *Pain Practice.* **7**: 324–331.
28 Wilcock A (2011) *Personal communication.*
29 Gardner-Nix J (2001) Oral transmucosal fentanyl and sufentanil for incident pain. *Journal of Pain and Symptom Management.* **22**: 627–630.
30 Zeppetella G (2001) Sublingual fentanyl citrate for cancer-related breakthrough pain: a pilot study. *Palliative Medicine.* **15**: 323–328.
31 Palliativedrugs.com (2003) Hot Topics: alternatives to sublingual fentanyl. In: *August Newsletter.* Available from: www.palliativedrugs.com
32 Duncan A (2002) The use of fentanyl and alfentanil sprays for episodic pain. *Palliative Medicine.* **16**: 550.
33 Younge P *et al.* (1999) A prospective randomized pilot comparison of instranasal fentanyl and intramuscular morphine for analgesia in children presenting to the emergency department with clinical fractures. *Emergency Medical Journal.* **11**: 90–94.
34 Finn M and Harris D (2010) Intranasal fentanyl for analgesia in the paediatric emergency department. *Emergency Medical Journal.* **27**: 300–301.
35 Cole J *et al.* (2009) Intranasal fentanyl in 1–3-year-olds: a prospective study of the effectiveness of intranasal fentanyl as acute analgesia. *Emergency Medicine Australasia.* **21**: 395–400.
36 Baxter K (ed) (2010) Stockley's Drug Interactions (online edition). The Pharmaceutical Press, London. Available from: www.medicinescomplete.com
37 Kharasch ED *et al.* (2004) Influence of hepatic and intestinal cytochrome P4503A activity on the acute disposition and effects of oral transmucosal fentanyl citrate. *Anesthesiology.* **101**: 729–737.
38 Takane H *et al.* (2005) Rifampin reduces the analgesic effect of transdermal fentanyl. *Annals of Pharmacotherpy.* **39**: 2139–2140.
39 Sasson M and Shvartzman P (2006) Fentanyl patch sufficient analgesia for only one day. *Journal of Pain and Symptom Management.* **31**: 389–391.
40 Morii H *et al.* (2007) Failure of pain control using transdermal fentanyl during rifampicin treatment. *Journal of Pain and Symptom Management.* **33**: 5–6.
41 Christie J *et al.* (1998) Dose-titration, multicenter study of oral transmucosal fentanyl citrate for the treatment of breakthrough pain in cancer patients using transdermal fentanyl for persistent pain. *Journal of Clinical Oncology.* **16**: 3238–3248.
42 Portenoy R *et al.* (1999) Oral transmucosal fentanyl citrate (OTFC) for the treatment of breakthrough pain in cancer patients: a controlled use titration study. *Pain.* **79**. 303–312.
43 Portenoy RK *et al.* (2006) A randomized, placebo-controlled study of fentanyl buccal tablet for breakthrough pain in opioid-treated patients with cancer. *Clinical Journal of Pain.* **22**: 805–811.
44 Portenoy RK *et al.* (2010) Long-term safety, tolerability, and consistency of effect of fentanyl pectin nasal spray for breakthrough cancer pain in opioid-tolerant patients. *Journal of Opioid Management.* **6**: 319–328.
45 Nalamachu S *et al.* (2011) Long-term effectiveness and tolerability of sublingual fentanyl orally disintegrating tablet for the treatment of breakthrough cancer pain. *Current Medical Research Opinion.* **27**: 519–530.
46 Davies AN and Vriens J (2005) Oral transmucosal fentanyl citrate and xerostomia. *Journal of Pain and Symptom Management.* **30**: 496–497.
47 Payne R *et al.* (2001) Long-term safety of oral transmucosal fentanyl citrate for breakthrough cancer pain. *Journal of Pain and Symptom Management.* **22**: 575–583.
48 Hanks GW *et al.* (2004) Oral transmucosal fentanyl citrate in the management of breakthrough pain in cancer: an open, multicentre, dose-titration and long term use study. *Palliative Medicine.* **18**: 698–704.
49 Darwish M *et al.* (2008) Bioequivalence following buccal and sublingual placement of fentanyl buccal tablet 400 microg in healthy subjects. *Clinical Drug Investigation.* **28**: 1–7.
50 Weinstein SM *et al.* (2009) Fentanyl buccal tablet for the treatment of breakthrough pain in opioid-tolerant patients with chronic cancer pain: A long-term, open-label safety study. *Cancer.* **115**: 2571–2579.
51 Portenoy RK *et al.* (2007) Fentanyl buccal tablet (FBT) for relief of breakthrough pain in opioid-treated patients with chronic low back pain: a randomized, placebo-controlled study. *Current Medical Research Opinion.* **23**: 223–233.
52 Simpson DM *et al.* (2007) Fentanyl buccal tablet for the relief of breakthrough pain in opioid-tolerant adult patients with chronic neuropathic pain: a multicenter, randomized, double-blind, placebo-controlled study. *Clinical Therapy.* **29**: 588–601.
53 Farrar JT *et al.* (2010) A novel 12-week study, with three randomized, double-blind placebo-controlled periods to evaluate fentanyl buccal tablets for the relief of breakthrough pain in opioid-tolerant patients with noncancer-related chronic pain. *Pain Medicine.* **11**: 1313–1327.
54 Fine PG *et al.* (2010) Long-term safety and tolerability of fentanyl buccal tablet for the treatment of breakthrough pain in opioid-tolerant patients with chronic pain: an 18-month study. *Journal of Pain and Symptom Management.* **40**: 747–760.
55 Shear ML *et al.* (2010) Transbuccal fentanyl for rapid relief of orthopedic pain in the ED. *American Journal of Emergency Medicine.* **28**: 847–852.
56 Markman JD (2008) Not so fast: the reformulation of fentanyl and breakthrough chronic non-cancer pain. *Pain.* **136**: 227–229.
57 Passik SD *et al.* (2010) Aberrant Drug-Related Behavior Observed During Clinical Studies Involving Patients Taking Chronic Opioid Therapy for Persistent Pain and Fentanyl Buccal Tablet for Breakthrough Pain (in press). *Journal of Pain and Symptom Management.*

HYDROMORPHONE BNF 4.7.2

Class: Opioid analgesic.

Indications: Severe pain in cancer; †an alternative in cases of intolerance to other strong opioids.

Contra-indications: None absolute if titrated carefully against a patient's pain. (Also see Cautions below, and Strong opioids, p.345).

Pharmacology

Hydromorphone is an analogue of **morphine** with similar pharmacokinetic and pharmacodynamic properties.[1–3] Thus, hydromorphone and **morphine** are comparable in terms of analgesic efficacy, undesirable effects, and patient preference.[4,5] Like **morphine**, hydromorphone is an antitussive.

According to the UK manufacturer, hydromorphone PO and SC/IM is about 7.5 times more potent than **morphine**,[6,7] and this accounts for the choice of capsule content (1.3mg and 2.6mg; stated to be equivalent to **morphine** 10mg and 20mg PO respectively). However, others suggest that when switching from **morphine** to hydromorphone, the conversion ratio is approximately 5:1 (i.e. the hydromorphone dose should be one fifth of the **morphine** dose)[8,9] and when switching from hydromorphone to **morphine** a ratio of 1:4 should be used (i.e. the **morphine** dose should be 4 times the hydromorphone dose).[10,11] (Also see Switching opioids, p.354 and Opioid dose conversion ratios, p.625).

PO hydromorphone is absorbed mainly in the small intestine. As with **morphine**, bio-availability is subject to wide inter-individual variation.[11,12] Hydromorphone is metabolized in the liver by 6-ketoreduction with subsequent glucuronidation. The main metabolite is hydromorphone-3-glucuronide (H3G). All the metabolites are renally excreted and can accumulate in renal impairment.

H3G has no analgesic activity but is estimated to be about 2.5 times more potent than morphine-3-glucuronide as a neuro-excitant.[13] In animal studies, dose-dependent allodynia, myoclonus, and seizures are seen.[14]

Bio-availability 37–62% PO.[11]
Onset of action <5min IV;[15] 15min SC/IM; 30min PO.[16]
Time to peak plasma concentration 1h PO.
Plasma halflife 2.5h early phase, with a prolonged late phase.
Duration of action 4–5h normal-release; 12–24h m/r (product-dependent).[17–19]

Cautions

In 2005, the FDA warned that the concurrent ingestion of alcohol could hasten the release of hydromorphone from one m/r product resulting in 'dose dumping', i.e. a rapid rise in plasma concentrations. In 2011, the EMEA reported the results of a review of the interaction between alcohol and opioid m/r mechanisms, and concluded that the risk is minor for most m/r products except those using polymethylmethacrylate-triethylcitrate (none in the UK).[20]

Little is known about the impact of hepatic and renal impairment.[21,22] The SPC for hydromorphone lists hepatic impairment as a contra-indication, although there are no pharmacokinetic data to support this contention. Despite the probability of accumulation of H3G and other glucuronide metabolites, hydromorphone is used at some centres as a preferred strong opioid in severe renal impairment (see p.355).

An osmotic-release oral delivery system (OROS®) for once daily administration has been developed, but as yet is unlicensed in the UK and Ireland. This 'extended-release' hydromorphone displays dose-dependent linear pharmacokinetics which are not significantly affected by food or alcohol.[23]

Undesirable effects

Also see Strong opioids, p.345.

Dose and use

As with all opioids, patients must be monitored for undesirable effects, particularly nausea and vomiting, and constipation (see p.348). Depending on individual circumstances, an anti-emetic should be prescribed for regular or p.r.n. use (see p.225) and, routinely, a laxative prescribed (see p.38).

PO hydromorphone is used in the same way as PO **morphine**, generally q4h as normal-release capsules or q12h as m/r capsules; both formulations can be swallowed whole or, if necessary, opened and the contents sprinkled on a small amount of soft food, e.g. yoghurt. Note:

- the m/r granules should not be crushed or chewed because this could lead to a rapid release of an overdose
- when converting hydromorphone from PO to SC, use half the PO dose
- if given by CSCI, high potency ampoules can be used (unlicensed in the UK)
- for CSCI dilute with WFI, 0.9% saline or 5% glucose.

CSCI compatibility with other drugs: Although most data are for dilution in 0.9% saline, there are 2-drug compatibility data for hydromorphone in WFI with **levomepromazine** and **metoclopramide**.

Concentration-dependent *incompatibility* may occur with **cyclizine**, **dexamethasone**, **haloperidol** and **ketorolac**. For more details and 3-drug compatibility data, see Appendix 3 charts A3.1 (p.776) and A3.4 (p.782).

Compatibility charts in 0.9% saline can be found on www.palliativedrugs.com Syringe Driver Survey Database.

In the UK, hydromorphone is unlikely to be used primarily as an antitussive but theoretically could be (see Antitussives, p.128).

Supply

Unless indicated otherwise, all products are **CD**.

Palladone® (Napp)
Capsules 1.3mg, 2.6mg, 1.3mg dose = £0.16.

Modified-release
Palladone® SR (Napp)
Capsules enclosing m/r granules 2mg, 4mg, 8mg, 16mg, 24mg, 28 days @ 2mg, 8mg or 24mg 12h = £21, £56 and £160 respectively.

Injectable formulation
Hydromorphone hydrochloride
Injection 10mg/mL, 1mL amp = £6; 20mg/mL, 1mL amp = £7; high-potency 50mg/mL, 1mL amp = £9. (Unlicensed, available as a special order from Martindale Products; See Obtaining unlicensed products, p.769).

1 Sarhill N *et al.* (2001) Hydromorphone: pharmacology and clinical applications in cancer patients. *Supportive Care in Cancer.* **9**: 84–96.
2 Murray A and Hagen NA (2005) Hydromorphone. *Journal of Pain and Symptom Management.* **29 (suppl 5)**: s57–s66.
3 Quigley C and Glare P (2009) Hydromorphone. In: M Davis *et al.* (eds) *Opioids in Cancer Pain* (2e). Oxford University Press, Oxford, pp. 245–252.
4 Quigley C (2002) Hydromorphone for acute and chronic pain. *Cochrane Database of Systematic Reviews.* **1**: CD003447.
5 Hong D *et al.* (2008) The side effects of morphine and hydromorphone patient-controlled analgesia. *Anesthesia and Analgesia* **107**: 1384–1389.
6 McDonald C and Miller A (1997) A comparative potency study of a controlled release tablet formulation of hydromorphone with controlled release morphine in patients with cancer pain. *European Journal of Palliative Care Abstracts of the Fifth Congress.*

7 Moriarty M *et al.* (1999) A randomised crossover comparison of controlled release hydromorphone tablets with controlled release morphine tablets in patients with cancer pain. *Journal of Clinical Research.* **2**: 1–8.
8 Wallace MS and Thipphawong J (2007) Clinical Trial Results with OROS((R)) Hydromorphone. *Journal of Pain and Symptom Management.* **33**: S25–32.
9 Palangio M *et al.* (2002) Dose conversion and titration with a novel, once-daily, OROS osmotic technology, extended-release hydromorphone formulation in the treatment of chronic malignant or nonmalignant pain. *Journal of Pain and Symptom Management.* **23**: 355–368.
10 Anderson R *et al.* (2001) Accuracy in equianalgesic dosing: conversion dilemmas. *Journal of Pain and Symptom Management.* **21**: 397–406.
11 Pereira J *et al.* (2001) Equianalgesic dose ratios for opioids: a critical review and proposals for long-term dosing. *Journal of Pain and Symptom Management.* **22**: 672–687.
12 Vallner J *et al.* (1981) Pharmacokinetics and bioavailability of hydromorphone following intravenous and oral administration to human subjects. *Journal of Clinical Pharmacology.* **21**: 152–156.
13 Wright AW *et al.* (2001) Hydromorphone-3-glucuronide: a more potent neuro-excitant than its structural analogue, morphine-3-glucuronide. *Life Sciences.* **69**: 409–420.
14 Babul N and Darke AC (1992) Putative role of hydromorphone metabolites in myoclonus. *Pain.* **51**: 260–261.
15 Coda B *et al.* (1997) Hydromorphone analgesia after intravenous bolus administration. *Pain.* **71**: 41–48.
16 Benedetti CB and Butler SH (1990) Systemic analgesics. In: Bonica J.J (ed) *The Management of Pain.* Lea and Febiger, Philedelphia.
17 Bruera E *et al.* (1996) A randomized, double-blind, double-dummy, crossover trial comparing the safety and efficacy of oral sustained-release hydromorphone with immediate-release hydromorphone in patients with cancer pain. Canadian Palliative Care Clinical Trials Group. *Journal of Clinical Oncology.* **14**: 1713–1717.
18 Hagen N *et al.* (1995) Steady-state pharmacokinetics of hydromorphone and hydromorphone-3-glucuronide in cancer patients after immediate and controlled-release hydromorphone. *Journal of Clinical Pharmacology.* **35**: 37–44.
19 Hays H *et al.* (1994) Comparative clinical efficacy and safety of immediate release and controlled release hydromorphone for chronic severe cancer pain. *Cancer.* **74**: 1808–1816.
20 European Medicines Agency (2010) Concludes review of modified-release oral opioids of the WHO level III. Available from: www.ema.europa.eu/ema/index.jsp?curl = pages/medicines/human/public_health_alerts/2010/09/human_pha_detail_000008.jsp&murl = menus/medicines/medicines.jsp&mid = WC0b01ac058001d126
21 Niscola P *et al.* (2010) The use of major analgesics in patients with renal dysfunction. *Current Drug Targets.* **11**: 752–758.
22 Lee MA *et al.* (2001) Retrospective study of the use of hydromorphone in palliative care patients with normal and abnormal urea and creatinine. *Palliative Medicine.* **15**: 26–34.
23 Gardner-Nix J and Mercadante S (2010) The role of OROS hydromorphone in the management of cancer pain. *Pain Practice.* **10**: 72–77.

*METHADONE — BNF 4.7.2

Class: Opioid analgesic.

Methadone should be used as a strong opioid analgesic only by those fully conversant with its pharmacology. It is generally best reserved for patients who fail to respond well to **morphine** or another μ-opioid receptor agonist. Important facts about methadone include:
- a widely variable plasma halflife
- dosing which is more complicated than for other strong opioids
- metabolism which is modified to a clinically important extent by other drugs which may be used in palliative care
- an association with a potentially fatal cardiac arrhythmia (see Cautions below and Prolongation of the QT interval in palliative care, p.727).

In addition, because methadone is used to treat opioid addiction, there is a social stigma attached to its use.

Indications: Moderate–severe pain, †cough, †an alternative in cases of intolerance to other strong opioids, †**morphine** poorly-responsive pain, †pain relief in severe renal impairment.[1,2] Also treatment of opioid addiction.

Contra-indications: None absolute if titrated carefully against a patient's pain (also see Strong opioids, p.345).

Pharmacology

Methadone is a synthetic strong opioid with mixed properties.[3,4] Thus, it is a μ-opioid receptor agonist, possibly a δ-opioid receptor agonist,[5] an NMDA-receptor-channel blocker,[6,7] and a presynaptic blocker of serotonin re-uptake.[8] Methadone is a racemic mixture; L-methadone is responsible for most of the analgesic effect, whereas D-methadone is antitussive. Methadone is a non-acidic and lipophilic drug which is absorbed well from all routes of administration.

Partly because of its lipid-solubility methadone has a high volume of distribution with only about 1% of the drug in the blood.[9] Methadone accumulates in tissues when given repeatedly, creating an extensive reservoir.[10] Protein-binding (principally to a glycoprotein) is 60–90%;[11] this is double that of **morphine**. Both volume of distribution and protein-binding contribute to the long plasma halflife, and accumulation is a potential problem. Methadone is metabolized mainly in the liver to several inactive metabolites.[12] About half of the drug and its metabolites are excreted by the intestines and half by the kidneys, most of the latter unchanged.[13] Renal and hepatic impairment do not affect methadone clearance.[14,15] Even so, in renal and hepatic failure (see p.605), it is generally best to reduce the starting dose, e.g. by at least 50%, and titrate according to response.

In single doses, methadone PO is about one half as potent as IM,[16] and IM a single dose of methadone is marginally more potent than **morphine**. With repeated doses, methadone is several times more potent and longer-acting; analgesia lasts 8–12h and sometimes more.[17,18] There is no single potency ratio between methadone and **morphine**. When patients with inadequate pain relief or undesirable effects with **morphine** are switched, the eventual 24h dose of methadone *is typically 5–10 times smaller than the previous dose of* ***morphine****, but sometimes 20–30 times smaller, and occasionally even smaller.*[19–22] The potency ratio tends to increase as the dose of **morphine** increases, i.e. proportionately less methadone is required as the **morphine** dose increases.[21,22]

When considering the use of methadone, the difficulty of a subsequent switch from methadone to another opioid should also be borne in mind. For such switches, the typical potency ratio of 5–10:1 appears to hold (i.e. typically the PO morphine equivalent dose will be 5–10 times greater than the PO methadone dose) with a wide range again reported, e.g. 1–75:1.[21,23] Thus, it is prudent to use conservative dose calculations and monitor the patient closely.

Methadone is used in several different settings. A systematic review of methadone for cancer pain identified eight RCTs but, because different methods were used, meta-analysis was not possible.[24] First-line, methadone provides similar analgesia to **morphine** but more undesirable effects. In an RCT, 20% of patients allocated to methadone 7.5mg b.d. discontinued treatment compared with 5% of those who received **morphine** 15mg b.d. Half of the withdrawals occurred in the first week, and most were because of sedation or nausea. For patients remaining in the study, there was no difference in efficacy or undesirable effects.[18] This suggests that a smaller starting dose of methadone (e.g. 2.5–5mg b.d., or even 1–2mg b.d.) would have been more appropriate.[25,26]

Second-line, patients who experience inadequate analgesia with **morphine**, with or without unacceptable undesirable effects such as nausea, vomiting, hallucinations or sedation, can obtain good relief with relatively low-dose methadone with few undesirable effects.[27–29] Patients who experience more specific neurotoxicity with **morphine**, e.g. hyperalgesia, allodynia and/or myoclonus ± sedation and delirium, generally also benefit by switching to methadone. However, switching to other opioids also helps.[30–33] Thus, when switching from **morphine**, it would seem sensible to choose an opioid which is easier and safer to use than methadone, e.g. **oxycodone**, **hydromorphone**, **fentanyl**.

Methadone is an alternative strong opioid for patients with severe renal impairment at risk of excessive drowsiness ± delirium with **morphine** because of accumulation of morphine-6-glucuronide.[2] Methadone is poorly removed by haemodialysis.[34] However, for moribund patients, **alfentanil** or **fentanyl** are probably better choices (see p.355). Methadone can also be used as a strong opioid analgesic in former opioid addicts who are being maintained on methadone.[35]

Methadone has been successfully used for cancer break-through (episodic) pain, either PO or SL (maximum volume of 1mL held for 2min); the average time to meaningful pain relief is 30min and 10min respectively.[36,37]

Bio-availability 80% (range 40–100%) PO.

Onset of action <30min PO, 15min IM.

Time to peak plasma concentration 4h PO; 1h IM.

Plasma halflife highly variable, mean 20–35h (range 5–130h);[38] longer in older patients; acidifying the urine results in a shorter halflife (20h) and raising the pH with sodium bicarbonate a longer halflife (>40h).[39]

Duration of action 4–5h PO and 3–5h IM single dose; 8–12h repeated doses.

Cautions

In 2006, after a review of deaths and life-threatening adverse events (e.g. respiratory depression, cardiac arrhythmia) associated with unintentional overdose, drug interactions, and prolongation of the QT interval, the FDA in the USA issued a safety warning about the use of methadone. This highlighted the need for:
- physicians to be fully aware of the pharmacology of methadone
- close monitoring of the patient when starting methadone, particularly when switching from a high dose of another opioid
- slow dose titration, and close monitoring of the patient when changing the dose of methadone
- warning the patient not to exceed the prescribed dose.

Because methadone generally has a long plasma halflife, accumulation to a variable extent should be anticipated, particularly in the elderly. Drowsiness and respiratory depression may develop after several days/weeks on a steady dose. *PCF* recommends p.r.n. dose titration to minimize the risk of this occurring (see below).[40]

QT interval prolongation and, rarely, a serious ventricular arrhythmia (*torsade de pointes*) have been observed during treatment with methadone. Generally, the latter is associated with, but not limited to, higher dose treatment (>200mg/24h) (see Prolongation of the QT interval in palliative care, p.727).[41] The SPC recommends that methadone is administered with caution to patients at risk of developing QT prolongation, e.g. those with:
- a history of cardiac conduction abnormalities
- a family history of sudden death
- advanced heart disease or ischaemic heart disease
- liver disease
- electrolyte abnormalities
- concurrent treatment with drugs which:
  - ▷ may cause electrolyte abnormalities
  - ▷ have a potential to prolong QT
  - ▷ inhibit cytochrome P450 3A4.

Note: the IV formulation of methadone in the USA (but *not* the UK), contains a preservative chlorobutanol, which has an additive QT prolonging effect.[42]

The risk this rare but potentially fatal cardiac complication poses must be considered in the context of the patient's circumstances. A commonsense approach should prevail, and ECG monitoring will be largely irrelevant in the last days of life. On the other hand, for a patient with a prognosis of several months or longer, it may be appropriate to identify any risk factors for QT prolongation and consider ECG ± electrolyte monitoring (see p.727).

Even so, research is needed to establish the magnitude of the risk of *torsade de pointes* with methadone, and the overall value of monitoring in the palliative care setting.[41]

Drug interactions

Methadone is metabolized by several cytochrome P450 iso-enzymes, mainly CYP3A4 and CYP2B6, with CYP2D6, CYP2C9, CYP2C19, and CYP1A2 also involved to varying degrees. Clinically relevant and well-established CYP-related drug-drug interactions are listed in Table 5.28. Note particularly that **carbamazepine**, **phenobarbital**, **phenytoin**, **rifampicin** and **St John's wort** increase the metabolism of methadone, and may reverse previously satisfactory pain relief, or even precipitate withdrawal symptoms.[43,44]

Symptomatic bradycardia has been reported in a patient on **thalidomide** given methadone.[45]

Undesirable effects

As for all strong opioids (see p.345). Methadone may occasionally cause neurotoxicity, e.g. myoclonus,[46] or more florid opioid-induced hyperalgesia.[47,48] Local erythema and induration when given by CSCI.[49]

Table 5.28 Cytochrome P450 interactions with methadone resulting in changed drug plasma concentrations[43]

Methadone increased by	*Methadone decreased by*	*Increased by methadone*	*Decreased by methadone*
SSRIs Cimetidine Ciprofloxacin Diazepam (high-dose) Fluconazole Voriconazole	Carbamazepine Phenobarbital Phenytoin Rifampicin St John's wort Antiretrovirals, e.g. abacavir, amprenavir, efavirenz, lopinavir, nelfinavir, nevirapine, ritonavir, tipranavir	Desipramine Zidovudine (AZT)	Amprenavir

Dose and use

As with all opioids, monitor for undesirable effects, particularly nausea and vomiting, and constipation (see p.348). Depending on individual circumstances, an anti-emetic should be prescribed for regular or p.r.n. use (see p.225) and a laxative prescribed routinely (see p.38).

Because of the wide interindividual variation in the pharmacokinetics of methadone, dose titration is different from **morphine**. Several methods exist for switching from **morphine** to methadone, but none has been shown to be definitely superior.[21] However, all require practitioners to be experienced in the use of methadone and close observation of the patient, generally as an inpatient.[2,19,27–29,50–54] Some have reported carefully controlled outpatient regimens, but pain relief can take weeks rather than days to achieve.[51,54]

With methadone, the implication of its large volume of distribution must be considered. During the first few days, while the body tissues become saturated, a greater daily dose of methadone will be required for satisfactory analgesia than subsequently; once saturation is complete, a smaller daily dose of methadone will then be sufficient. Continuing on the initial daily dose is likely to result in sedation after a few days, and possibly respiratory depression and even death.[55,56]

PCF favours a 'stop and go' approach, i.e. the abrupt cessation of the **morphine** and introduction of methadone p.r.n. (see Quick Practice Guide, p.422). These guidelines are an evolution from earlier ones, incorporating feedback to www.palliativedrugs.com from clinicians.[2,19,57] A single loading dose aids tissue saturation and helps to reduce the number of p.r.n. doses required in the first 48h.[19] The recommendations may be overcautious but are safer, particularly in the elderly and for those switching from large doses of **morphine**.

Several other methods for switching from **morphine** or from another strong opioid have been published.[53,58–62 63] Regardless of the method used, the importance of close supervision cannot be overemphasized. Caution is also required when there has been rapid dose escalation of the pre-switch opioid; in these circumstances it is probably safer to calculate the initial dose of methadone using the pre-escalation dose.[64] Maintenance doses vary considerably, but most are $<$80mg/24h.[52] *Subsequent switching from methadone to other opioids can be difficult. In one series 12/13 patients experienced increased pain ± dysphoria.*[65]

Methadone SC (generally doses $>$25mg) or CSCI can cause marked local inflammation necessitating site rotation, and possibly other measures (see Quick Practice Guide, p.422).[66,67] When switching from methadone PO to SC, a safe conversion is to halve the methadone PO dose. However, for some patients, particularly those receiving a small dose of methadone ($<$80mg/24h), a 1:1 conversion ratio may be more appropriate and subsequent upwards dose titration may be required.[67] Methadone can also be given SL, PR, IV, CIVI ± PCA.[59,68–70] It has also been used as a topical analgesic for mouth ulcers (as a mouthwash),[71] and for open wounds and ulcers (in powder form mixed with Stomahesive®).[72]

Supply

Unless indicated otherwise, all preparations are **CD**.

Methadone (generic)

Tablets 5mg, 28 days @ 30mg b.d. = £19.

Oral solution 1mg/mL and 5mg/mL, 28 days @ 30mg b.d. = £38 and £25 respectively.

Injection 10mg/mL, 1mL amp = £1, 2mL amp = £2, 3.5mL amp = £2.50, 5mL amp = £2.50; 25mg/mL, 2mL amp = £2; 50mg/mL, 1mL amp = £2.

Methadose® (Rosemont)

Oral concentrate 10mg/mL; 20mg/mL, 28 days @ 30mg b.d. = £13. (The oral concentrate should be dispensed only after dilution to the required strength using Methadose® Diluent.)

1 Gannon C (1997) The use of methadone in the care of the dying. *European Journal of Palliative Care*. **4**: 152–158.
2 Morley J and Makin M (1998) The use of methadone in cancer pain poorly responsive to other opioids. *Pain Reviews*. **5**: 51–58.
3 Watanabe S (2001) Methadone the renaissance. *Journal of Palliative Care*. **17 (2)**: 117–120.
4 Davis MP and Walsh D (2001) Methadone for relief of cancer pain: a review of pharmacokinetics, pharmacodynamics, drug interactions and protocols of administration. *Supportive Care in Cancer*. **9**: 73–83.
5 Raynor K *et al.* (1994) Pharmacological characterization of the cloned kappa-, delta-, and mu-opioid receptors. *Molecular Pharmacology*. **45**: 330–334.
6 Ebert B *et al.* (1995) Ketobemidone, methadone and pethidine are non-competitive N-methyl-D-aspartate (NMDA) antagonists in the rat cortex and spinal cord. *Neuroscience Letter*. **187**: 165–168.
7 Gorman A *et al.* (1997) The d- and l- isomers of methadone bind to the non-competitive site on the N-methyl-D-aspartate (NMDA) receptor in rat forebrain and spinal cord. *Neuroscience Letters*. **223**: 5–8.
8 Codd E *et al.* (1995) Serotonin and norepinephrine uptake inhibiting activity of centrally acting analgesics: structural determinants and role in antinociception. *Journal of Pharmacology and Experimental Therapeutics*. **274**: 1263–1270.
9 Ferrari A *et al.* (2004) Methadone-metabolism, pharmacokinetics and interactions. *Pharmacological Research*. **50**: 551–559.
10 Robinson AE and Williams FM (1971) The distribution of methadone in man. *Journal of Pharmacy and Pharmacology*. **23**: 353–358.
11 Eap CB *et al.* (1990) Binding of D-methadone, L-methadone and DL-methadone to proteins in plasma of healthy volunteers: role of variants of X1-acid glycoprotein. *Clinical Pharmacology and Therapeutics*. **47**: 338–346.
12 Fainsinger R *et al.* (1993) Methadone in the management of cancer pain: clinical review. *Pain*. **52**: 137–147.
13 Inturrisi CE and Verebely K (1972) The levels of methadone in the plasma in methadone maintenance. *Clinical Pharmacology and Therapeutics*. **13**: 633–637.
14 Kreek MJ *et al.* (1980) Methadone use in patients with chronic renal disease. *Drug Alcohol Dependence*. **5**: 197–205.
15 Novick DM *et al.* (1981) Methadone disposition in patients with chronic liver disease. *Clinical Pharmacology and Therapeutics*. **30**: 353–362.
16 Beaver WT *et al.* (1967) A clinical comparison of the analgesic effects of methadone and morphine administered intramuscularly, and of orally and parenterally administered methadone. *Clinical Pharmacology and Therapeutics*. **8**: 415–426.
17 Sawe J *et al.* (1981) Patient-controlled dose regimen of methadone for chronic cancer pain. *British Medical Journal*. **282**: 771–773.
18 Bruera E *et al.* (2004) Methadone versus morphine as a first-line strong opioid for cancer pain: a randomized, double-blind study. *Journal of Clinical Oncology*. **22**: 185–192.
19 Cornish CJ and Keen JC (2003) An alternative low-dose ad libitum schedule for conversion of other opioids to methadone. *Palliative Medicine*. **17**: 643–644.
20 Nixon AJ (2005) Methadone for cancer pain: a case report. *American Journal of Hospice and Palliative Care*. **22**: 337.
21 Weschules DJ and Bain KT (2008) A systematic review of opioid conversion ratios used with methadone for the treatment of pain. *Pain Medicine*. **9**: 595–612.
22 Benitez-Rosario MA *et al.* (2009) Morphine-methadone opioid rotation in cancer patients: analysis of dose ratio predicting factors. *Journal of Pain and Symptom Management*. **37**: 1061–1068.
23 Walker PW *et al.* (2008) Switching from methadone to a different opioid: what is the equianalgesic dose ratio? *Journal of Palliative Medicine*. **11**: 1103–1108.
24 Nicholson AB (2007) Methadone for cancer pain. *Cochrane Database of Systematic Reviews*. **4**: CD003971.
25 Mercadante S *et al.* (2008) Sustained-release oral morphine versus transdermal fentanyl and oral methadone in cancer pain management. *European Journal of Pain*. **12**: 1040–1046.
26 Gallagher R (2009) Methadone: an effective, safe drug of first choice for pain management in frail older adults. *Pain Medicine*. **10**: 319–326.
27 Tse DM *et al.* (2003) An ad libitum schedule for conversion of morphine to methadone in advanced cancer patients: an open uncontrolled prospective study in a Chinese population. *Palliative Medicine*. **17**: 206–211.
28 Mercadante S *et al.* (2001) Switching from morphine to methadone to improve analgesia and tolerability in cancer patients: a prospective study. *Journal of Clinical Oncology*. **19**: 2898–2904.
29 Mercadante S *et al.* (1999) Rapid switching from morphine to methadone in cancer patients with poor response to morphine. *Journal of Clinical Oncology*. **17**: 3307–3312.
30 Sjogren P *et al.* (1994) Disappearance of morphine-induced hyperalgesia after discontinuing or substituting morphine with other opioid agonists. *Pain*. **59**: 313–316.
31 Hagen N and Swanson R (1997) Strychnine-like multifocal myoclonus and seizures in extremely high-dose opioid administration: treatment strategies. *Journal of Pain and Symptom Management*. **14**: 51–58.
32 Ashby M *et al.* (1999) Opioid substitution to reduce adverse effects in cancer pain management. *Medical Journal of Australia*. **170**: 68–71.
33 Morita T *et al.* (2005) Opioid rotation from morphine to fentanyl in delirious cancer patients: an open-label trial. *Journal of Pain and Symptom Management*. **30**: 96–103.
34 Furlan V *et al.* (1999) Methadone is poorly removed by haemodialysis. *Nephrology, Dialysis, Transplantation*. **14**: 254–255.

35 Manfredi P *et al.* (2001) Methadone analgesia in cancer pain patients on chronic methadone maintenance therapy. *Journal of Pain and Symptom Management.* **21**: 169–174.
36 Fisher K *et al.* (2004) Characterization of the early pharmacodynamic profile of oral methadone for cancer-related breakthrough pain: a pilot study. *Journal of Pain and Symptom Management.* **28**: 619–625.
37 Hagen NA *et al.* (2010) A formal feasibility study of sublingual methadone for breakthrough cancer pain. *Palliative Medicine.* **24**: 696–706.
38 Lugo RA *et al.* (2005) Pharmacokinetics of methadone. *Journal of Pain and Palliative Care Pharmacotherapy.* **19**: 13–24.
39 Nilsson MI *et al.* (1982) Pharmacokinetics of methadone during maintenance treatment: adaptive changes during the induction phase. *European Journal of Clinical Pharmarcology.* **22**: 343–349.
40 Hendra T *et al.* (1996) Fatal methadone overdose. *British Medical Journal.* **313**: 481–482.
41 Wilcock A and Beattie JM (2009) Prolonged QT interval and methadone: implications for palliative care. *Current Opinion in Supportive and Palliative Care.* **3**: 252–257.
42 Kornick CA *et al.* (2003) QTc interval prolongation associated with intravenous methadone. *Pain.* **105**: 499–506.
43 Baxter K (2011) Stockley's Drug Interactions (online edition). Pharmaceutical Press, London. Available from: www.medicinescomplete.com
44 Kreek MJ *et al.* (1976) Rifampin-induced methadone withdrawal. *New England Journal of Medicine.* **294**: 1104–1106.
45 Buchanan D (2010) Sinus bradycardia related to methadone in a patient with myeloma receiving thalidomide therapy. *Palliative Medicine.* **24**: 742–743.
46 Sarhill N *et al.* (2001) Methadone-induced myoclonus in advanced cancer. *American Journal of Hospice and Palliative Care.* **18 (1)**: 51–53.
47 Davis MP *et al.* (2007) When opioids cause pain. *Journal of Clinical Oncology.* **25**: 4497–4498.
48 El Osta B *et al.* (2007) Intractable pain: intoxication or undermedication? *Journal of Palliative Medicine.* **10**: 811–814.
49 Bruera E *et al.* (1991) Local toxicity with subcutaneous methadone. Experience of two centers. *Pain.* **45**: 141–143.
50 Ripamonti C *et al.* (1997) An update on the clinical use of methadone cancer pain. *Pain.* **70**: 109–115.
51 Hagen N and Wasylenko E (1999) Methadone: outpatient titration and monitoring strategies in cancer patients. *Journal of Pain and Symptom Management.* **18**: 369–375.
52 Scholes C *et al.* (1999) Methadone titration in opioid-resistant cancer pain. *European Journal of Cancer Care.* **8**: 26–29.
53 Nauck F *et al.* (2001) A German model for methadone conversion. *American Journal of Hospice and Palliative Care.* **18 (3)**: 200–202.
54 Soares LG (2005) Methadone for cancer pain: what have we learned from clinical studies? *American Journal of Hospice and Palliative Care.* **22**: 223–227.
55 Twycross RG (1977) A comparison of diamorphine with cocaine and methadone. *British Journal of Clinical Pharmacology.* **4**: 691–692.
56 Lipman AG (2005) Methadone: effective analgesia, confusion, and risk. *Journal of Pain and Palliative Care Pharmacotherapy.* **19 (2)**: 3–5.
57 Palliativedrugs.com (2005) Hot Topics: new draft methadone monograph. In: *September Newsletter.* Available from: www.palliativedrugs.com
58 Mercadante S *et al.* (2001) Switching from morphine to methadone to improve analgesia and tolerability in cancer patients: a prospective study. *Journal of Clinical Oncology.* **19**: 2898–2904.
59 Santiago-Palma J *et al.* (2001) Intravenous methadone in the management of chronic cancer pain: safe and effective starting doses when substituting methadone for fentanyl. *Cancer.* **92**: 1919–1925.
60 Blackburn D *et al.* (2002) Methadone: an alternative conversion regime. *European Journal of Palliative Care.* **9**: 93–96.
61 Benitez-Rosario MA *et al.* (2004) Opioid switching from transdermal fentanyl to oral methadone in patients with cancer pain. *Cancer.* **101**: 2866–2873.
62 Blackburn D (2005) Methadone: the analgesic. *European Journal of Palliative Care.* **12**: 188–191.
63 Bruera E *et al.* (1996) Opioid rotation in patients with cancer pain. *Cancer.* **78**: 852–857.
64 Zimmermann C *et al.* (2005) Rotation to methadone after opioid dose escalation: How should individualization of dosing occur? *Journal of Pain and Palliative Care Pharmacotherapy.* **19 (2)**: 25–31.
65 Moryl N *et al.* (2002) Pitfalls of opioid rotation: substituting another opioid for methadone in patients with cancer pain. *Pain.* **96**: 325–328.
66 Mathew P and Storey P (1999) Subcutaneous methadone in terminally ill patients: manageable local toxicity. *Journal of Pain and Symptom Management.* **18**: 49–52.
67 Centeno C and Vara F (2005) Intermittent subcutaneous methadone administration in the management of cancer pain. *Journal of Pain and Palliative Care Pharmacotherapy.* **19**: 7–12.
68 Fitzgibbon D and Ready L (1997) Intravenous high-dose methadone administered by patient controlled analgesia and continuous infusion for the treatment of cancer pain refractory to high-dose morphine. *Pain.* **73**: 259–261.
69 Davis M and Walsh D (2001) Methadone for relief of cancer pain: a review of pharmacokinetics, pharmacodynamics, drug interactions and protocols of administration. *Supportive Care in Cancer.* **9**: 73–83.
70 Manfredi PL and Houde RW (2003) Prescribing methadone, a unique analgesic. *Journal of Supportive Oncology.* **1**: 216–220.
71 Gallagher R (2004) Methadone mouthwash for the management of oral ulcer pain. *Journal of Pain and Symptom Management.* **27**: 390–391.
72 Gallagher RE *et al.* (2005) Analgesic effects of topical methadone: a report of four cases. *Clinical Journal of Pain.* **21**: 190–192.

Quick Practice Guide: Use of methadone for cancer pain

Methadone has both opioid and non-opioid properties, and a long variable halflife (range 5–130h vs. 2.5h for morphine). Thus there is no single potency ratio for methadone and other opioids. When switching from morphine, the eventual 24h dose of methadone is typically 5–10 times smaller than the dose of morphine, sometimes 20–30 times smaller, and occasionally even smaller. Inevitable accumulation is the reason for the week-long intervals between dose adjustments. *Switching must be closely supervised by specialists*, generally as an inpatient.

Indications for use

- neuropathic or mixed nociceptive-neuropathic pain not responding to an NSAID + morphine + adjuvant analgesics, e.g. an antidepressant ± an anti-epileptic
- neurotoxicity with morphine at any dose (e.g. myoclonus, allodynia, hyperalgesia) which does not respond to a reduction in morphine dose and switching to another easier-to-use opioid (e.g. fentanyl, hydromorphone, oxycodone) is not possible
- the strong opioid of choice, instead of morphine
- end-stage renal failure.

Dose titration

1 When prescribing PO methadone as first-line strong opioid:
   - start with methadone 5mg (1–2.5mg in the elderly) q12h regularly and q3h p.r.n.
   - if necessary, titrate the regular dose upwards once a week, guided by p.r.n. use
   - continue with 5mg p.r.n., or 1–2.5mg in the elderly
   - with doses ⩾30mg q12h, increase the p.r.n. dose to 1/6–1/10 of the q24h dose, rounded to a convenient tablet size or volume.

2 If the patient is already receiving morphine, use the following method.

PO morphine to PO methadone

Morphine is stopped abruptly when methadone is started.
If switching from:
- normal-release morphine, give the first dose of methadone ⩾2h (pain present) or 4h (pain-free) after last dose of morphine
- m/r morphine, give the first dose of methadone ⩾6h (pain present) or 12h (pain-free) after the last dose of a 12h preparation, or ⩾12h (pain present) or 24h (pain-free) after the last dose of a 24h preparation.

Give a single loading dose of PO methadone one tenth of the previous total 24h PO morphine dose, up to a maximum of 30mg.

Give q3h p.r.n. doses of methadone one third of the loading dose (i.e. 1/30 of the previous total 24h PO morphine dose), rounded to a convenient tablet size or volume, up to a maximum of 30mg per dose.

Example 1: Morphine 300mg/24h PO = loading dose of methadone 30mg PO, and 10mg q3h p.r.n.

Example 2: Morphine 1,200mg/24h PO = loading dose of methadone 120mg PO, and 40mg q3h p.r.n.; however, both are limited to the maximum of 30mg.

For patients in severe pain who need more analgesia in <3h, see point 6 below.

On Day 6, the amount of methadone taken over the previous 2 days is noted and divided by 4 to give a regular q12h dose, with 1/6–1/10 of the 24h dose q3h p.r.n., e.g. *methadone 80mg PO in previous 48h → 20mg q12h and 5mg PO q3h p.r.n.*

If ⩾2 doses/day of p.r.n. methadone continue to be needed, the dose of regular methadone should be increased once a week, guided by p.r.n. use.

3 If using another strong opioid, calculate the morphine equivalent daily dose and then follow the guidelines for morphine.

4 If converting from PO methadone to SC/IV methadone, or from another CSCI/CIVI opioid, see the respective boxes below.

5 If there has been recent rapid escalation of the pre-switch opioid dose, calculate the initial dose of methadone using the pre-escalation dose of the opioid.

6 For patients in severe pain and who need more analgesia in <3h, options include:
- taking the previously used opioid q1h p.r.n. (50–100% of the p.r.n. dose used before switching)
- if neurotoxicity with the pre-switch opioid, use an appropriate dose of an alternative strong opioid
- ketamine.

7 The switch to methadone is successful (i.e. improved pain relief and/or reduced toxicity) in about 75% of patients.

8 If a patient:
- becomes oversedated, reduce the dose generally by 33–50% (some centres monitor the level of consciousness and respirations q4h for 24h)
- develops opioid abstinence symptoms, give p.r.n. doses of the previous opioid to control these.

PO methadone to SC/IV or CSCI/CIVI methadone

To convert PO methadone to SC/IV methadone, halve the PO dose, e.g. methadone 10mg/24h PO = 5mg/24h SC/IV. This is a safe conversion ratio; for some patients the SC/IV dose = PO dose.

Because of its long halflife, methadone (10mg/mL) can be given SC q12h–q8h. If SC injection is painful or causes local inflammation, give by CSCI/CIVI instead.

If CSCI methadone causes a skin reaction:
- administer as a more dilute solution in a 20–30mL syringe
- change the site daily
- consider applying hydrocortisone cream 1% topically around the needle entry site (under an occlusive dressing)
- consider adding dexamethasone 1mg to the diluted combination of drugs (compatibility data permitting).

For additional rescue doses of methadone SC/IV, give 1/6–1/10 of the 24h SC/IV dose q3h p.r.n., e.g. methadone 20mg CIVI/24h = 2mg q3h p.r.n. SC/IV.

If ≥2 p.r.n doses/day continue to be needed, the 24h SC/IV dose should be increased once a week, guided by p.r.n. use.

For patients in severe pain who need more analgesia in <3h, see point 6 above.

Other CSCI/CIVI opioids to CSCI/CIVI methadone

The safest approach is to follow the method for PO switching, using bolus injections of SC/IV methadone instead of PO doses.

Convert the opioid 24h CSCI/CIVI dose to its PO equivalent and determine the PO methadone dose (Dose titration, point 2).

The SC/IV dose of methadone is half the PO dose; the maximum initial dose of SC/IV methadone will be 15mg. This is a safe conversion ratio; for some patients the SC/IV dose = PO dose.

OXYCODONE BNF 4.7.2

Class: Opioid analgesic.

Indications: Moderate–severe cancer and non-cancer pain, †an alternative in cases of intolerance to other strong opioids.

Contra-indications: None absolute if titrated carefully against a patient's pain (also see Strong opioids, p.345). Do not use in severe renal impairment (creatinine clearance <30mL/min).

Pharmacology

Oxycodone is a strong opioid with similar properties to **morphine**.[1–5] However, its opioid receptor site affinities remain a matter of controversy.[6,7] Studies with selective opioid antagonists suggest that oxycodone and **morphine** produce analgesia through different populations of opioid receptors.[8] Thus, in rats, naloxonazine (a selective μ-opioid receptor antagonist) completely blocks **morphine**-induced antinociception but does not attenuate the effect of oxycodone.[9] In contrast, norbinaltorphimine (a selective κ-opioid receptor antagonist) completely blocks oxycodone-induced antinociception but does not attenuate the effect of **morphine**. On the other hand, in other studies (rats, mice, and humans), oxycodone showed definite μ-opioid receptor activity.[10–12] However, some of this activity could have been mediated by active metabolites, e.g. **oxymorphone**.[12] Although synergy between **morphine** and oxycodone has been shown in rats,[13] no synergy is seen in humans.[14]

Oxycodone is metabolized principally to noroxycodone via CYP3A4, and 10% to **oxymorphone** via CYP2D6[15,16] Parenteral **oxymorphone** is 10 times more potent than parenteral **morphine**.[17] However, after blocking CYP2D6 with **quinidine**, the non-analgesic effects of oxycodone in volunteers are unchanged.[16] Further, postoperatively, no differences are found between CYP2D6 rapid or slow metabolizers in the dose requirements or analgesic efficacy of oxycodone.[18] Thus it is unlikely that, in most people, **oxymorphone** contributes significantly to the analgesic effect of oxycodone. However, CYP2D6 ultra-rapid metabolizers may be at risk of undesirable CNS effects even with low-dose oxycodone.[19] This may relate to an enhanced production of **oxymorphone** (also see Cytochrome P450, p.735).

By mouth, oxycodone has a mean bio-availability of 75%, whereas **morphine**'s is about half this (see p.362). This partly explains why PO oxycodone is more potent than PO **morphine** (i.e. *fewer* mg of oxycodone are needed than **morphine** to have a comparable analgesic effect).[20–25] The PO potency ratio for oxycodone to **morphine** is about 1.5:1, and thus the dose of oxycodone by mouth is about two thirds that of **morphine** (i.e. oxycodone 10mg is equivalent to **morphine** 15mg). Hence, the recommendation by the manufacturer to halve the dose of PO **morphine** when converting to PO oxycodone, although reasonable in terms of caution and safety, almost certainly exaggerates the actual potency of oxycodone.

Parenterally, when bio-availability is comparable, the situation is different. Despite a short-term (2h) postoperative PCA study which suggested that **morphine** is less potent parenterally than oxycodone (i.e. *more* mg of **morphine** will be needed, as with PO administration),[26] earlier single-dose studies and two more recent longer PCA studies (1–2 days) suggest that by injection **morphine** is more potent than oxycodone, in the region of 4:3. Thus, *fewer* mg of **morphine** will be needed, e.g. **morphine** 10mg is approximately equivalent to oxycodone 13mg.[17,25,27] However, given the modest difference in potency, together with the constraints of ampoule size, it is reasonable in clinical practice to use a parenteral potency ratio of 1:1 when converting from oxycodone injections to **morphine** injections (or vice versa), i.e. regard IV/SC oxycodone 10mg as equivalent to IV/SC **morphine** 10mg.

About 20% of oxycodone is excreted unchanged in the urine. In mild–moderate hepatic impairment, oxycodone and noroxycodone concentrations increase (but the **oxymorphone** concentration decreases) and the elimination halflife increases by about 2h. In renal impairment the clearance of oxycodone, noroxycodone and conjugated **oxymorphone** are reduced. Oxycodone plasma concentration increases by 50% and the halflife lengthens by 1h.[24,28] The clearance of oxycodone also reduces with increasing age, partly because of the associated renal impairment.[29]

Bio-availability 75% PO, ranging from 60–87%.[30,31]

Onset of action 20–30min PO.

Time to peak plasma concentration 1–1.5h; 3h m/r.

Plasma halflife 3.5h; 4.5h in renal failure.
Duration of action 4–6h; 12h m/r.

Cautions

M/r preparations should be swallowed whole; crushing or chewing them may lead to a rapid release of an overdose of oxycodone.

Interactions

Inhibitors of CYP3A4 (e.g. **ketoconazole**, **voriconazole**, **erythromycin**, **telithromycin** and **ritonavir**) can inhibit oxycodone metabolism, and may enhance its effects.[32–35] However, inhibition of CYP2D6 (e.g. with **quinidine**) appears to have no detectable clinical impact.[36] **Rifampicin**, an enzyme inducer has been reported to decrease plasma concentrations of oxycodone.[33,37]

Undesirable effects

Also see Strong opioids, p.345. Essentially the same as **morphine**.

Various studies have suggested possible differences in the undesirable effect profiles of oxycodone and **morphine**.[38] However, a systematic review comparing efficacy and tolerability of oxycodone versus other opioids found no difference in the undesirable effect profile between oxycodone and either **morphine** or **hydromorphone**.[39]

Dose and use

Because oxycodone is more expensive, it should generally be reserved for patients who cannot tolerate **morphine**. In Scotland, oxycodone injections are restricted to cancer patients who cannot tolerate **diamorphine** or **morphine** injections.

A combination product of oxycodone with **naloxone** is available (Targinact® Box 5.V).

> Note: remains of m/r tablets (Oxycontin®) and Targinact® may appear in the patient's faeces ('ghost tablets'), but these are inert residues, and do not affect the efficacy of the products.

Oral

Normal-release oxycodone is generally given q4h but, in some patients, q6h is satisfactory.[49] M/r tablets are biphasic in their release of oxycodone, i.e. there is an initial fast release which leads to the early onset of analgesia and a slow release which provides a prolonged duration of action. For strong opioid-naïve patients:

- start with 5mg q6h–q4h for normal-release capsules and liquid formulations
- start with 10mg b.d. for m/r tablets
- titrate the dose to optimize analgesia.

For patients transferring from PO **morphine**:

- start with a dose conversion ratio of 1.5:1 (e.g. replace **morphine** 15mg by oxycodone 10mg)
- titrate the dose to optimize analgesia.

> Note: this recommendation differs from the manufacturer's dose conversion ratio of 2:1 (see Pharmacology above; also see Table 15.1 p.627).

The manufacturer recommends that the initial dose is reduced in patients with mild hepatic impairment or mild–moderate renal impairment, i.e. start with 2.5mg q6h for oral solution or 5mg b.d. for m/r tablets. This will generally include most elderly/frail patients.

Injection

Oxycodone injection may be given IV or SC as a bolus or by infusion. For CSCI, dilute with WFI, 0.9% saline or 5% glucose.

For opioid-naïve patients:

- start with 7.5mg/day
- if necessary, titrate the dose upwards, guided by p.r.n. use.

Box 5.V Oxycodone combined with naloxone (Targinact®)

Targinact® is marketed as a range of tablets containing m/r formulations of oxycodone and naloxone in a fixed-dose ratio of 2:1, i.e. oxycodone 5mg/naloxone 2.5mg; 10mg/5mg; 20mg/10mg and 40mg/20mg. The primary reason for the addition of naloxone is to antagonize the constipating effect of oxycodone. The desire to develop a formulation which deters misuse (e.g. by crushing and injecting IV) is also relevant.

Targinact® is licensed for severe pain. Evidence to support promotional claims of improved pain control, better GI tolerability, and improved quality of life is based mainly on an uncontrolled, observational study.[40,41]

RCTs have been undertaken in relatively young (mid-50s) non-cancer patients with either moderate or severe pain, and with normal hepatic and renal function. Those unable to tolerate a 'restricted laxative regimen' were excluded, i.e. the most severely constipated. Although Targinact® improved bowel function and reduced the number of patients requiring laxatives, laxatives were taken only p.r.n.[42,43]

Targinact® is 40% more expensive than the equivalent dose of m/r oxycodone alone, and 2–3 times more expensive than an equivalent dose of morphine + regular laxatives. Because the benefit for patients taking laxatives *regularly* is uncertain, the Scottish Medicines Consortium, the Drugs and Therapeutics Bulletin and *PCF* do *not* recommend the use of Targinact®.[44]

If clinicians choose to prescribe Targinact®, its use should be restricted to occasions when the upward titration of regularly administered laxatives is ineffective (see p.42). Because constipation is generally multifactorial in origin,[45] Targinact® is likely to augment rather than replace laxatives.[42,43]

The m/r formulation of naloxone avoids a 'bolus dose', and >97% is removed by first-pass metabolism in the liver. Thus, the main effect of naloxone is on the GI tract, with insufficient amounts reaching the systemic circulation to adversely affect analgesia.[46,47] However, plasma concentrations of naloxone can increase significantly in:

- *hepatic impairment:* use of Targinact® requires caution in mild impairment and is contra-indicated in moderate–severe impairment
- *renal impairment:* use Targinact® with caution.

Dose recommendations:

- in opioid-naïve patients, generally start with oxycodone/naloxone 10mg/5mg b.d.
- in elderly/frail patients, 5mg/2.5mg b.d. may be more appropriate
- in those already taking strong opioids, switch to the equivalent dose of oxycodone
- maximum dose 40mg/20mg b.d.

When higher analgesic doses are required, the manufacturer recommends supplemental oxycodone m/r tablets, taken at the same time as the m/r combination tablets. However, this reduces the impact of the naloxone, and oxycodone:naloxone ratios >4:1 have no significant effect on bowel function.[42,48]

Common undesirable effects include nausea, vomiting, abdominal pain and diarrhoea. The manufacturer warns that patients on long-term opioids may develop opioid withdrawal symptoms when switched to Targinact®.

When converting from PO oxycodone to SC/IV oxycodone:

- the manufacturer recommends giving half the PO dose by injection; however, because mean oral bio-availability is 75% (range 60–87%), some centres use a conversion ratio of 1.5:1, e.g. oxycodone 30mg/24h PO → oxycodone 20mg/24h SC/IV
- if necessary, titrate the dose upwards, guided by p.r.n. use.

For patients transferring from **morphine** injections, use a 1:1 dose ratio (e.g. replace SC **morphine** 10mg by SC oxycodone 10mg), and titrate to optimize analgesia.

Two strengths of injection are available, 10mg/mL and high-strength 50mg/mL. The latter may be useful in situations where high doses cause volume difficulties for CSCI. However, there is an increased risk of serious mistakes being made when more than one strength is readily available.[50,51] There are also differences in compatibility with other drugs (see below) and, on a mg for mg basis, the high-strength injection costs about twice as much.

CSCI with oxycodone 10mg/mL

There are 2-drug compatibility data for mixtures in WFI with **clonazepam, dexamethasone, glycopyrronium, haloperidol, hyoscine *butylbromide*, hyoscine *hydrobromide*, levomepromazine, metoclopramide, midazolam,** and **octreotide**.

Concentration-dependent incompatibility may occur when oxycodone (hydrochloride) is mixed with **cyclizine** (lactate); for more details see Appendix 3, Chart A3.1, p776.

CSCI with oxycodone 50mg/mL

Differences in compatibility for the 10mg/mL and 50mg/mL formulations of oxycodone have been reported.[52,53] This may be due to the different ratios of excipients in each formulation (see p.669). It is important *not* to extrapolate compatibility information from one formulation to the other.

More details

For 2-drug and 3-drug compatibility data for oxycodone 10mg/mL in WFI, and for currently available data for oxycodone 50mg/mL, see Appendix 3, Charts A3.1 (p.776), A3.6 (p.786) and Table A3.1 (p.790).

Information on compatibility in 0.9% saline can be found on www.palliativedrugs.com Syringe Driver Survey Database.

Supply

Unless indicated otherwise, all preparations are **CD**.

Oxycodone (generic)
Injection 10mg/mL, 1mL amp = £1.50, 2mL amp = £3.

OxyNorm® (Napp)
Capsules 5mg, 10mg, 20mg, 5mg dose = £0.50.
Oral solution (sugar-free) 5mg/5mL, 5mg dose = £0.50.
Concentrated oral solution (sugar-free) 10mg/mL, 5mg dose = £0.50.
Injection 10mg/mL, 1mL amp = £1.50, 2mL amp = £3.
Injection 50mg/mL, 1mL amp = £14.

Modified-release
OxyContin® (Napp)
Tablets m/r 5mg, 10mg, 15mg, 20mg, 30mg, 40mg, 60mg, 80mg, 120mg 28 days @ 10mg, 15mg, 20mg, 30mg, 80mg and 120mg b.d. = £25, £37, £50, £75, £200 and £299 respectively.

Oxycodone/naloxone combined
Targinact® (Napp)
Tablets m/r containing oxycodone/naloxone in a fixed ratio of 2:1, 5mg/2.5mg, 10mg/5mg, 20mg/10mg, 40mg/20mg, 28 days @10mg/5mg b.d. = £35.

1 Kalso E (2005) Oxycodone. *Journal of Pain and Symptom Management*. **29 (suppl 5)**: s47–s56.
2 Davis MP *et al.* (2003) Normal-release and controlled-release oxycodone: pharmacokinetics, pharmacodynamics, and controversy. *Supportive Care in Cancer.* **11**: 84–92.
3 Shah S and Hardy J (2001) Oxycodone: a review of the literature. *European Journal of Palliative Care*. **8**: 93–96.
4 Poyhia R *et al.* (1993) Oxycodone: an alternative to morphine for cancer pain. A review. *Journal of Pain and Symptom Management.* **8**: 63–67.
5 Glare PA and Walsh TD (1993) Dose-ranging study of oxycodone for chronic pain in advanced cancer. *Journal of Clinical Oncology*. **11**: 973–978.
6 Poyhia R *et al.* (1993) A review of oxycodone's clinical pharmacokinetics and pharmacodynamics. *Journal of Pain and Symptom Management.* **8**: 63–67.
7 Poyhia R and Kalso EA (1992) Antinociceptive effects and central nervous system depression caused by oxycodone and morphine in rats. *Pharmacology and Toxicology.* **70**: 125–130.
8 Smith M *et al.* (2001) Oxycodone has a distinctly different pharmacology from morphine. *European Journal of Pain*. **15 (suppl A)**: 135–136.
9 Ross F and Smith M (1997) The intrinsic antinociceptive effects of oxycodone appear to be kappa-opioid receptor mediated. *Pain*. **73**: 151–157.
10 Yoburn B *et al.* (1995) Supersensitivity to opioid analgesics following chronic opioid antagonist treatment: relationship to receptor selectivity. *Pharmacology, Biochemistry and Behavior.* **51**: 535–539.
11 Chen Z *et al.* (1991) Mu receptor binding of some commonly used opioids and their metabolites. *Life Sciences*. **48**: 2165–2171.
12 Kalso E *et al.* (1990) Morphine and oxycodone in the management of cancer pain: plasma levels determined by chemical and radioreceptor assays. *Pharmacology and Toxicology*. **67**: 322–328.
13 Ross FB *et al.* (2000) Co-administration of sub-antinociceptive doses of oxycodone and morphine produces marked antinociceptive synergy with reduced CNS side-effects in rats. *Pain*. **84**: 421–428.
14 Grach M *et al.* (2004) Can coadministration of oxycodone and morphine produce analgesic synergy in humans? An experimental cold pain study. *British Journal of Clinical Pharmacology.* **58**: 235–242.
15 Lalovic B *et al.* (2006) Pharmacokinetics and pharmacodynamics of oral oxycodone in healthy human subjects: role of circulating active metabolites. *Clinical Pharmacology and Therapeutics*. **79**: 461–479.
16 Heiskanen T *et al.* (1998) Effects of blocking CYP2D6 on oxycodone. *Clinical Pharmacology and Therapeutics*. **64**: 603–611.
17 Beaver WT *et al.* (1978) Analgesic studies of codeine and oxycodone in patients with cancer. II. Comparisons of intramuscular oxycodone with intramuscular morphine and codeine. *Journal Pharmacology and Experiemental Therapeutics*. **207**: 101–108.
18 Zwisler ST *et al.* (2010) Impact of the CYP2D6 genotype on post-operative intravenous oxycodone analgesia. *Acta Anaesthesiologica Scandinavica*. **54**: 232–240.
19 de Leon J *et al.* (2003) Adverse drug reactions to oxycodone and hydrocodone in CYP2D6 ultrarapid metabolizers. *Journal of Clinical Psychopharmacology.* **23**: 420–421.
20 Lauretti GR *et al.* (2003) Comparison of sustained-release morphine with sustained-release oxycodone in advanced cancer patients. *British Journal of Cancer.* **89**: 2027–2030.
21 Curtis GB *et al.* (1999) Relative potency of controlled-release oxycodone and controlled-release morphine in a postoperative pain model. *European Journal of Clinical Pharmacology.* **55**: 425–429.
22 Mucci-LoRusso P *et al.* (1998) Controlled-release oxycodone compared with controlled-release morphine in the treatment of cancer pain: a randomized, double-blind, parallel-group study. *European Journal of Pain*. **2**: 239–249.
23 Bruera E *et al.* (1998) Randomized, double-blind, cross-over trial comparing safety and efficacy of oral controlled-release oxycodone with controlled-release morphine in patients with cancer pain. *Journal of Clinical Oncology.* **16**: 3222–3229.
24 Heiskanen T and Kalso E (1997) Controlled-release oxycodone and morphine in cancer related pain. *Pain*. **73**: 37–45.
25 Kalso E and Vainio A (1990) Morphine and oxycodone in the management of cancer pain. *Clinical Pharmacology and Therapeutics*. **47**: 639–646.
26 Kalso E *et al.* (1991) Intravenous morphine and oxycodone for pain after abdominal surgery. *Acta Anaesthesiologica Scandinavica*. **35**: 642–646.
27 Silvasti M *et al.* (1998) Comparison of analgesic efficacy of oxycodone and morphine in postoperative intravenous patient-controlled analgesia. *Acta Anaesthesiologica Scandinavica*. **42**: 576–580.
28 Glare P and Davis MP (2009) Oxycodone. In: MP Davis *et al.* (eds) *Opioids in Cancer Pain* (2e). Oxford University Press, Oxford, pp. 155–173.
29 Liukas A *et al.* (2011) Elimination of intravenous oxycodone in the elderly: a pharmacokinetic study in postoperative orthopaedic patients of different age groups. *Drugs Aging*. **28**: 41–50.
30 Leow K *et al.* (1992) Single-dose and steady-state pharmacokinetics and pharmacodynamics of oxycodone in patients with cancer. *Clinical Pharmacology and Therapeutics*. **52**: 487–495.
31 Poyhia R *et al.* (1992) The pharmacokinetics and metabolism of oxycodone after intramuscular and oral administration to healthy subjects. *British Journal of Clinical Pharmacology.* **33**: 617–621.
32 Hagelberg NM *et al.* (2011) Interaction of oxycodone and voriconazole-a case series of patients with cancer pain supports the findings of randomised controlled studies with healthy subjects. *European Journal of Clinical Pharmacology.* **67**: 863–864.
33 Baxter K (2011) Stockley's Drug Interactions (online edition). Pharmaceutical Press, London. Available from: www.medicinescomplete.com
34 Nieminen TH *et al.* (2010) Oxycodone concentrations are greatly increased by the concomitant use of ritonavir or lopinavir/ritonavir. *European Journal of Clinical Pharmacology.* **66**: 977–985.
35 Hagelberg NM *et al.* (2009) Voriconazole drastically increases exposure to oral oxycodone. *European Journal of Clinical Pharmacology.* **65**: 263–271.
36 Kleine-Bruggeney (2010) Pharmacogenetics in palliative care. *Forensic Science International*. epub doi:10.1016/j.forsciint.2010.1007.1003.
37 Nieminen TH *et al.* (2009) Rifampin greatly reduces the plasma concentrations of intravenous and oral oxycodone. *Anesthesiology.* **110**: 1371–1378.
38 Leppert W (2010) Role of oxycodone and oxycodone/naloxone in cancer pain management. *Pharmacological Reports*. **62**: 578–591.
39 Reid CM *et al.* (2006) Oxycodone for cancer-related pain: meta-analysis of randomized controlled trials. *Archives of Internal Medicine*. **166**: 837–843.
40 Schutter U *et al.* (2010) Innovative pain therapy with a fixed combination of prolonged-release oxycodone/naloxone: a large observational study under conditions of daily practice. *Current Medical Research Opinion*. **26**: 1377–1387.

41 Clemens KE *et al.* (2011) Bowel function during pain therapy with oxycodone/naloxone prolonged-release tablets in patients with advanced cancer. *International Journal of Clinical Practice.* **65**: 472–478.
42 Lowenstein O *et al.* (2009) Combined prolonged-release oxycodone and naloxone improves bowel function in patients receiving opioids for moderate–to–severe non-malignant chronic pain: a randomised controlled trial. *Expert Opinion in Pharmacotherapy.* **10**: 531–543.
43 Simpson K *et al.* (2008) Fixed-ratio combination oxycodone/naloxone compared with oxycodone alone for the relief of opioid-induced constipation in moderate-to-severe noncancer pain. *Current Medical Research Opinion.* **24**: 3503–3512.
44 Anonymous (2010) Targinact–opioid relief without constipation? *Drugs and Therapeutics Bulletin.* **48**: 138–141.
45 Larkin PJ *et al.* (2008) The management of constipation in palliative care: clinical practice recommendations. *Palliative Medicine.* **22**: 796–807.
46 Vondrackova D *et al.* (2008) Analgesic efficacy and safety of oxycodone in combination with naloxone as prolonged release tablets in patients with moderate to severe chronic pain. *Journal of Pain.* **9**: 1144–1154.
47 Sandner-Kiesling A *et al.* (2010) Long-term efficacy and safety of combined prolonged-release oxycodone and naloxone in the management of non-cancer chronic pain. *International Journal of Clinical Practice.* **64**: 763–774.
48 Meissner W *et al.* (2009) A randomised controlled trial with prolonged-release oral oxycodone and naloxone to prevent and reverse opioid-induced constipation. *European Journal of Pain.* **13**: 56–64.
49 Lugo RA and Kern SE (2004) The pharmacokinetics of oxycodone. *Journal of Pain and Palliative Care Pharmacotherapy.* **18 (4)**: 17–30.
50 NPSA (National Patient Safety Agency) (2008) Reducing risk of overdose with midazolam injection in adults. Rapid response report **11**. Available from: www.nrls.npsa.nhs.uk/resources
51 NPSA (National Patient Safety Agency) (2006) Ensuring safer practice with high dose ampoules of diamorphine and morphine *Safer Practice Notice.* **295**. Available from www.npsa.nhs.uk/resources
52 Gardiner P (2003) Compatibility of an injectable oxycodone formulation with typical diluents, syringes, tubings, infusion bags and drugs for potential co-administration. *Hospital Pharmacist* **10**: 354–361.
53 Hines S and Pleasance S (2009) Compatibility of an injectable high strength oxycodone formulation with typical diluents, syrings, tubings and infusion bags and drugs for potential co-administration. *European Journal of Hospital Pharmacy Practice.* **15**: 32–38.

OPIOID ANTAGONISTS — BNF 4.10 & 15.1.7

Pharmacology

Naloxone, **naltrexone**, **nalmefene** (not UK) and **methylnaltrexone** are generally classed as pure antagonists. They possess a high affinity for opioid receptors at which they have no intrinsic activity. They block access to the opioid receptors by opioid agonists/opioid analgesics; and, if administered after a strong opioid, they displace the latter because of their higher receptor affinity.[1]

However, the discovery that ultra-low doses of **naloxone** and **nalmefene** given postoperatively either potentiate the analgesic effect of **morphine** (and presumably of other agonist opioids) or reduce undesirable effects (nausea and vomiting, and pruritus), or both, means that the situation is more complex.[2–5] In fact, it is over 30 years since it was shown in post-dental extraction pain that **naloxone** could produce either analgesia (low-dose) or hyperalgesia (high-dose).[6] Further, in the same circumstances, **naloxone** 400microgram neutralizes the analgesic effect of **morphine** 8mg IV (as expected) but more than doubles the analgesic effect of **pentazocine** 60mg IV.[7] (**Pentazocine** is a partial μ and κ agonist and δ antagonist.)[8]

These phenomena are probably explained by **naloxone** having other effects beyond classical opioid receptor antagonism. A ligand binding to an opioid receptor can trigger either an inhibitory or excitatory response, dependent on the type of G protein coupled to the receptor, either G_I/G_O (inhibitory) or G_s (excitatory). The latter increases in various circumstances, e.g. chronic opioid use, nerve damage.[9] Thus, an inhibitory response contributes to typical opioid analgesic and other effects, whereas an excitatory response may contribute to tolerance and, when predominant, to opioid-induced hyperalgesia.[10]

Ultra-low levels of **naloxone** have been shown to inhibit excitatory signalling of opioid receptors by interfering with the scaffolding protein (filamin A) which couples Gs to the opioid receptor.[11] Another non-opioid receptor binding site of **naloxone** is the toll-like receptor 4 on glial cells; this interaction inhibits glial cell activation which appears important in CNS sensitization.[12,13] Thus, ultra-low dose **naloxone**, through effects at non-opioid receptor binding sites, can improve analgesia; an effect which is lost with higher doses because of classical opioid receptor antagonism. **Naltrexone** appears to demonstrate similar effects.[14–16] Nonetheless, the inherent risk of reversal of analgesia limits the widespread clinical application of this approach. Drugs which target only these non-opioid receptor binding sites are being developed.

Opioid antagonists have a role to play in the management of pruritus associated with chronic disease, notably in cholestasis.[17–19] Pruritus in cholestasis is caused by increased opioidergic tone secondary to an increase in plasma enkephalin concentration. Opioid antagonists are effective in counterbalancing the increased tone, and thus relieve the pruritus.[20] Unfortunately, an opioid-like withdrawal syndrome may be precipitated.[19] This can be avoided by using small incremental doses of the opioid antagonist (see p.437 and p.439).

As a general rule, patients with cholestatic jaundice and both pruritus and severe pain should *not* be treated with an opioid antagonist.[21] Instead, an alternative treatment for pruritus, e.g. **sertraline**, **rifampicin** should be used (Table 5.29 and Table 5.30), and the pain treated appropriately with both non-opioid and opioid analgesics.

An alternative, but less established approach, would be to use **buprenorphine** (see p.381). In case reports or small series, patients with cholestatic pruritus have responded to treatment with **buprenorphine** alone or in combination with ultra-low doses of **naloxone**.[22–25] Sometimes the use of ultra-low doses of **naloxone** or **naltrexone** have helped to improve both the pruritus and the pain.[26] However, there are insufficient data at present to recommend this approach outside of a specialist service.

In uraemic pruritus, the situation is more complex because there are several causal mechanisms, both peripheral (cutaneous) and central (neural).[27] The opioid system is involved, but in uraemia there is no increase in opioidergic tone (and thus no danger of a withdrawal syndrome if an opioid antagonist is given). Instead, the ratio between μ-opioid receptors (pruritus-inducible; relative increase in number) and κ-opioid receptors (pruritus-suppressive; relative decrease in number) alters in favour of the former.[28,29] This predisposes to the development of pruritus. It also suggests that both κ *agonists* and μ *antagonists* could bring relief. Thus, in an RCT lasting 2–4 weeks of **nalfurafine** (not UK), a novel κ agonist, 36% of subjects responded (at least 50% reduction in worst itching) compared with 15% in the placebo group.[30] **Naltrexone** has also been tried in this setting.[31]

However, RCTs have given conflicting results, e.g. benefit was seen in uraemic patients with very severe pruritus[32] but not in those with moderately severe pruritus.[33] One explanation is that, in uraemia, an opioid mechanism is important only in severe pruritus. The fact that **naltrexone** is non-selective and antagonizes both μ- and κ-opioid receptors may also be relevant.

Methylnaltrexone and **alvimopan** (not UK) are quaternary compounds which do not readily cross the blood-brain barrier and thus act as peripheral opioid antagonists. **Methylnaltrexone**, administered as an SC injection, is licensed for the treatment of opioid-induced constipation in advanced illness (see Box 5.W) and **alvimopan**, administered PO, for postoperative ileus.[34,35] They have not been formally studied in pruritus.

Uses

Naloxone is used principally to reverse life-threatening respiratory depression (see p.436). **Naloxone** and **naltrexone** are both used to:

- prevent relapse in opioid ex-addicts
- relieve pruritus associated with cholestasis.[19]

However, pruritus associated with chronic disease generally requires alternative specific measures (Table 5.29 and Table 5.30).

Although **naloxone** and **naltrexone** have been used in the past to correct opioid-induced GI disorders (i.e. delayed gastric emptying and constipation),[34] **methylnaltrexone** is now preferable (Box 5.W).

Table 5.29 Management of pruritus in non-skin diseases and weight of evidence[a] (also see p.579 and p.586)

Condition	*Treatment*	*Comment*
	Non-drug treatment	
Malignant extra-hepatic cholestasis	Stenting of common bile duct	
Uraemia	Modify dialysis regimen UVB phototherapy **A**[36]	
Hodgkin's lymphoma	Curative radiotherapy and/or chemotherapy	
	Specific drug treatment	
Cholestasis	Colestyramine 4g once daily–b.d. **A**[19]	Based on 2 methodologically poor RCTs; may cause nausea, vomiting and diarrhoea. Not of value in complete large duct biliary obstruction
	Rifampicin 300–600mg once daily **A**[19]	RCTs were only for 1–2 weeks; for chronic use, smaller starting doses are advised, i.e. 150mg once daily; rare reports of severe hepatotoxicity
	Naltrexone 50mg once daily **A**[19]	Transient opioid withdrawal effects common
	Sertraline 50–100mg each morning **A**[37]	
	17α-alkyl androgen, e.g.:[38,39]	
	methyltestosterone 25mg once daily *sublingual* (not UK)[39]	
	danazol 200mg once daily–t.d.s.	
Hodgkin's lymphoma	Corticosteroids ± palliative chemotherapy Cimetidine 800mg/24h **B**[40] Thalidomide 200mg at bedtime[41]	Cost of thalidomide is prohibitive and may cause severe neuropathy if used long-term (see p.519)
Paraneoplasia	Paroxetine 5–20mg once daily **A**[42] Thalidomide 100mg at bedtime[43]	Cost of thalidomide is prohibitive and may cause severe neuropathy if used long-term (see p.519)
Uraemia	Capsaicin cream 0.025–0.075% once daily–q.d.s. **A**[44,45]	Patients may find the burning sensation intolerable
	Gabapentin 100–300mg PO following dialysis **A**[46,47]	
	Nalfurafine 5microgram IV following dialysis **A** (not UK)[30]	
	Naltrexone 50mg once daily[31]	RCTs give diametrically opposite results (much benefit vs. no benefit).
	Thalidomide 100mg at bedtime **A**[48]	Cost of thalidomide is prohibitive and may cause severe neuropathy if used long-term (see p.519)
Spinal opioids	See Spinal analgesia, Box 21.C (p.688)	
Consider when specific treatments fail	Paroxetine 5–60mg once daily (or other SSRI)[49] Mirtazapine 7.5–15mg at bedtime	

a. strength of recommendations: grade **A** is based on evidence from ≥1 RCTs, and grade **B** on well-designed non-randomized studies;[50] where no grade is given, recommendation based on case reports and/or expert opinion.

Table 5.30 Management strategy for pruritus in non-skin diseases used in some centres[a,b]

Condition	*Step 1*	*Step 2*	*Step 3*
Cholestasis[c]	Naltrexone 12.5–250mg once daily **A**[19,51]	Sertraline[d] 50–100mg once daily **A**[37] *or* Rifampicin 150–300mg once daily **A**[19,52]	Methyltestosterone 25mg SL once daily (not UK)[38,39] *or* alternative, e.g. danazol 200mg once daily–t.d.s.[e]
Hodgkin's lymphoma[f]	Prednisolone 10–20mg t.d.s.	Cimetidine 800mg/24h **A**[40]	SSRI[d] *or* mirtazapine 15–30mg at bedtime *or* carbamazepine 200mg b.d.
Paraneoplastic pruritus[f]	Paroxetine[d] 5–20mg once daily **A**[42]	Mirtazapine 15–30mg at bedtime	Thalidomide 100mg at bedtime[g] *or* carbamazepine 200mg b.d.
Uraemia[h]	UVB phototherapy **A**[36] *or* (if localized) capsaicin cream 0.025–0.075% once daily–q.d.s. **A**[44,45]	Nalfurafine **A** (not UK)[30] Naltrexone 50mg once daily **A**[i, 31]	Gabapentin 100–300mg given three times a week after haemodialysis **A**[46,47]
Systemic opioid-induced pruritus[j]	Stat dose of H_1 antihistamine, e.g. chlorphenamine 4–12mg, if after 2–3h there is definite benefit, prescribe 4mg t.d.s.; if not, proceed to Step 2	Switch opioid[k], e.g. morphine → oxycodone[53]	Ondansetron 8mg PO b.d.
Other causes *or* origin unknown	Paroxetine[d] 5–20mg once daily	Mirtazapine 15–30mg at bedtime	Thalidomide 100mg at bedtime[g]

a. strength of recommendations: grade **A** is based on evidence from ⩾1 RCTs, and grade **B** on well-designed non-randomized studies;[50] where no grade is given, recommendation based on case reports and/or expert opinion
b. given PO unless stated otherwise
c. in total bile obstruction, where bile duct stenting is impossible or unwanted
d. fluvoxamine, paroxetine and sertraline all have an antipruritic effect[42,49] and any of these could probably be used; anecdotally, fluoxetine and citalopram are not effective
e. androgens may be hepatotoxic and may increase cholestasis while reducing pruritus
f. assuming that cytoreductive/anticancer treatment is impossible or unwanted
g. thalidomide is prohibitively expensive and may cause severe neuropathy if used long-term (see p.519)
h. after the haemodialysis regimen has been optimized
i. controlled trials give contradictory results (much benefit vs. no benefit)
j. pruritus after systemic opioids is uncommon, and poorly documented. Although some cases may be caused by cutaneous histamine release[54] and may be self-limiting, the most distressing cases are chronic and antihistamine-resistant[53]
k. methylnaltrexone has been used but the large doses required make it impractical and prohibitively expensive[55].

Box 5.W Methylnaltrexone

Methylnaltrexone is a quaternary opioid antagonist which does not readily cross the blood-brain barrier. It is authorized as a SC injection for use in patients with 'advanced illness' and opioid-induced constipation despite treatment with laxatives. A PO formulation is being developed.

Methylnaltexone is relatively expensive (£21 per 12mg vial) and should be considered only when the optimum use of laxatives is ineffective. Because constipation in advanced disease is generally multifactorial in origin,[56] methylnaltrexone is likely to augment rather than replace laxatives:

- about 1/3–1/2 of patients given methylnaltrexone have a bowel movement within 30min–4h, without loss of analgesia or the development of opioid withdrawal symptoms[57–61]
- dose recommendations:
  - ▷ for patients weighing 38–61kg, start with 8mg on alternate days
  - ▷ for patients weighing 62–114kg, start with 12mg on alternate days
  - ▷ outside this range, give 150microgram/kg on alternate days
  - ▷ the interval between administrations can be varied, either extended or reduced, but not more than once daily
- in severe renal impairment (creatinine clearance <30mL/min) reduce the dose:
  - ▷ for patients weighing 62–114kg, reduce to 8mg
  - ▷ outside this range, reduce to *75microgram/kg*, rounding up the dose volume to the nearest 0.1mL
- methylnaltrexone is contra-indicated in cases of known or suspected bowel obstruction; it should be used with caution in patients with conditions which may predispose to perforation (e.g. GI cancer, peptic ulcer, colonic pseudo-obstruction)
- common undesirable effects include abdominal pain/colic, diarrhoea, flatulence, nausea (these generally resolve after a bowel movement) and dizziness (postural hypotension can occur)
- serious adverse events are rare but include syncope, severe diarrhoea and cardiovascular collapse, and GI perforation (stomach, small and large bowel).[62]

A recent survey in one USA institution found that about one quarter of prescriptions of methylnaltrexone (mainly by generalists) were inappropriate with regard to indication or dose.[63]

1 Choi YS and Billings JA (2002) Opioid antagonists: a review of their role in palliative care, focusing on use in opioid-related constipation. *Journal of Pain and Symptom Management*. **24**: 71–90.

2 Gan T *et al.* (1997) Opioid-sparing effects of a low-dose infusion of naloxone in patient-administered morphine sulfate. *Anesthesiology*. **87**: 1075–1081.

3 Joshi G *et al.* (1999) Effects of prophylactic nalmefene on the incidence of morphine-related side effects in patients receiving intravenous patient controlled analgesia. *Anesthesiology*. **90**: 1007–1011.

4 Cepeda MS *et al.* (2004) Addition of ultralow dose naloxone to postoperative morphine PCA: unchanged analgesia and opioid requirement but decreased incidence of opioid side effects. *Pain*. **107**: 41–46.

5 Maxwell LG *et al.* (2005) The effects of a small-dose naloxone infusion on opioid-induced side effects and analgesia in children and adolescents treated with intravenous patient-controlled analgesia: a double-blind, prospective, randomized, controlled study. *Anesthesia and Analgesia*. **100**: 953–958.

6 Levine JD *et al.* (1979) Naloxone dose dependently produces analgesia and hyperalgesia in postoperative pain. *Nature*. **278**: 740–741.

7 Levine J and Gordon N (1988) Synergism between the analgesic actions of morphine and pentazocine. *Pain*. **33**: 369–372.

8 Hill RG (1992) Multiple opioid receptors and their ligands. *Frontiers of Pain*. **4**: 1–4.

9 Crain S and Shen K (2000) Antagonists of excitatory opioid receptor functions enhance morphine's analgesic potency and attenuate opioid tolerance/dependence liability. *Pain*. **84**: 121–131.

10 Sjogren P *et al.* (1994) Disappearance of morphine-induced hyperalgesia after discontinuing or substituting morphine with other opioid antagonists. *Pain*. **59**: 313–316.

11 Wang HY and Burns LH (2009) Naloxone's pentapeptide binding site on filamin A blocks Mu opioid receptor-Gs coupling and CREB activation of acute morphine. *PLoS One*. **4**: e4282.

12 Milligan ED and Watkins LR (2009) Pathological and protective roles of glia in chronic pain. *Nature Reviews Neurosciene*. **10**: 23–36.

13 Ren K and Dubner R (2008) Neuron-glia crosstalk gets serious: role in pain hypersensitivity. *Current Opinion in Anaesthesiology*. **21**: 570–579.

14 Chindalore VL *et al.* (2005) Adding ultralow-dose naltrexone to oxycodone enhances and prolongs analgesia: a randomized, controlled trial of Oxytrex. *Journal of Pain.* **6**: 392–399.

15 Largent-Milnes TM *et al.* (2008) Oxycodone plus ultra-low-dose naltrexone attenuates neuropathic pain and associated mu-opioid receptor-Gs coupling. *Journal of Pain.* **9**: 700–713.

16 Hay JL *et al.* (2011) Potentiation of buprenorphine antinociception with ultra-low dose naltrexone in healthy subjects. *European Journal of Pain.* **15**: 293–298.

17 Metze D *et al.* (1999) Efficacy and safety of naltrexone, an oral opiate receptor antagonist, in the treatment of pruritus in internal and dermatological diseases. *Journal of the American Academy of Dermatology.* **41**: 533–539.

18 Jones E *et al.* (2002) Opiate antagonist therapy for the pruritus of cholestasis: the avoidance of opioid withdrawal-like reactions. *Quarterly Journal of Medicine.* **95**: 547–552.

19 Tandon P *et al.* (2007) The efficacy and safety of bile Acid binding agents, opioid antagonists, or rifampin in the treatment of cholestasis-associated pruritus. *American Journal of Gastroenterology.* **102**: 1528–1536.

20 Davis M (2007) Cholestasis and endogenous opioids: liver disease and exogenous opioid pharmacokinetics. *Clinical Pharmacokinetics.* **46**: 825–850.

21 Lonsdale-Eccles AA and Carmichael AJ (2009) Opioid antagonist for pruritus of cholestasis unmasking bony metastases. *Acta Dermato Venereologica.* **89**: 90.

22 Juby L *et al.* (1994) Buprenorphine and hepatic pruritus. *British Journal of Clinical Practice.* **48**: 331.

23 Reddy L *et al.* (2007) Transdermal buprenorphine may be effective in the treatment of pruritus in primary biliary cirrhosis. *Journal of Pain and Symptom Management.* **34**: 455–456.

24 Marinangeli F *et al.* (2009) Intravenous naloxone plus transdermal buprenorphine in cancer pain associated with intractable cholestatic pruritus. *Journal of Pain and Symptom Management.* **38**: e5–8.

25 Zylicz Z *et al.* (2005) Severe pruritus of cholestasis in disseminated cancer: developing a rational treatment strategy. A case report. *Journal of Pain and Symptom Management.* **29**: 100–103.

26 Jones EA and Zylicz Z (2005) Treatment of pruritus caused by cholestasis with opioid antagonists. *Journal of Palliative Medicine.* **8**: 1290–1294.

27 Manenti L *et al.* (2009) Uraemic pruritus: clinical characteristics, pathophysiology and treatment. *Drugs.* **69**: 251–263.

28 Kumagai H et al. (2000) Endogenous opioid system in uraemic patients. *In: Joint Meeting of the Seventh World Conference on Clinical Pharmacology and IUPHAR — Division of Clinical Pharmacology and the Fourth Congress of the European Association for Clinical Pharmacology and Therapeutics.*

29 Odou P *et al.* (2001) A hypothesis for endogenous opioid peptides in uraemic pruritus: role of enkephalin. *Nephrology, Dialysis, Transplantation.* **16**: 1953–1954.

30 Wikstrom B *et al.* (2005) Kappa-opioid system in uremic pruritus: multicenter, randomized, double-blind, placebo-controlled clinical studies. *Journal of the American Society of Nephrology.* **16**: 3742–3747.

31 Quan Phan N (2010) Antipruritic treatment with systemic u-opioid receptor antagonists; a review. *Journal of the American Academy of Dermatology.* **63**: 680–688.

32 Peer G *et al.* (1996) Randomised crossover trial of naltrexone in uraemic pruritus. *Lancet.* **348**: 1552–1554.

33 Pauli-Magnus C *et al.* (2000) Naltrexone does not relieve uremic pruritus. *Journal of the American Society of Nephrology.* **11**: 514–519.

34 McNicol ED (2008) Mu-opioid antagonists for opioid-induced bowel dysfunction. *Cochrane Database of Systematic Reviews.* **2 (April 16)**: CD006332.

35 Becker G and Blum HE (2009) Novel opioid antagonists for opioid-induced bowel dysfunction and postoperative ileus. *Lancet.* **373**: 1198–1206.

36 Gilchrest B *et al.* (1997) Relief of uremic pruritus with ultraviolet phototherapy. *New England Journal of Medicine.* **297**: 136–138.

37 Mayo MJ *et al.* (2007) Sertraline as a first-line treatment for cholestatic pruritus. *Hepatology.* **45**: 666–674.

38 Ahrens E *et al.* (1950) Primary biliary cirrhosis. *Medicine.* **29**: 299–364.

39 Lloyd-Thomas H and Sherlock S (1952) Testosterone therapy for the pruritus of obstructive jaundice. *British Medical Journal.* **ii**: 1289–1291.

40 Aymard J *et al.* (1980) Cimetidine for pruritus in Hodgkin's disease. *British Medical Journal.* **280**: 151–152.

41 Goncalves F (2010) Thalidomide for the control of severe paraneoplastic pruritus associated with hodgkin's disease. Epub ahead of print. *American Journal of Hospice and Palliative Care.* **27**: 486–487.

42 Zylicz Z *et al.* (2003) Paroxetine in the treatment of severe non-dermatological pruritus: a randomized, controlled trial. *Journal of Pain and Symptom Management.* **26**: 1105–1112.

43 Smith J *et al.* (2002) Use of thalidomide in the treatment of intractable itch. Poster abstract 21. In: *Palliative Care Congress*; Sheffield, UK.

44 Breneman D *et al.* (1992) Topical capsaicin for treatment of hemodialysis-related pruritus. *Journal of the American Academy of Dermatology.* **26**: 91–94.

45 Makhlough A (2010) Topical capsaicin therapy for uremic pruritus in patients on hemodialysis. *Iranian Journal of Kidney Disease.* **4**: 137–140.

46 Gunal AI *et al.* (2004) Gabapentin therapy for pruritus in haemodialysis patients: a randomized, placebo-controlled, double-blind trial. *Nephrology, Dialysis, Transplantation.* **19**: 3137–3139.

47 Razeghi E *et al.* (2009) Gabapentin and uremic pruritus in hemodialysis patients. *Renal Failure.* **31**: 85–90.

48 Silva S *et al.* (1994) Thalidomide for the treatment of uremic pruritus: a crossover randomized double-blind trial. *Nephron.* **67**: 270–273.

49 Stander S *et al.* (2007) Clinical classification of itch: a position paper of the International Forum for the Study of Itch. *Acta Dermato Venereologica.* **87**: 291–294.

50 BMJ Publishing Group (2009) Resources for authors. Checklists and forms: clinical management guidelines. Available from: www.resources.bmj.com/bmj/authors/checklists-forms/clinical-management-guidelines

51 Wolfhagen F *et al.* (1997) Oral naltrexone treatment for cholestatic pruritus: A double-blind, placebo-controlled study. *Gastroenterology.* **113**: 1264–1269.

52 Ghent C and Carruthers S (1988) Treatment of pruritus in primary biliary cirrhosis with rifampin. Results of a double-blind crossover randomized trial. *Gastroenterology.* **94**: 488–493.

53 Tarcatu D *et al.* (2007) Are we still scratching the surface? A case of intractable pruritus following systemic opioid analgesia. *Journal of Opioid Management.* **3**: 167–170.

54 Krajnik M (2004) Opioid-induced pruritus. In: Z Zylicz *et al.* (eds) *Pruritus in advanced disease.* Oxford University Press, London, pp. 84–96.

55 Yuan CS *et al.* (1998) Efficacy of orally administered methylnaltrexone in decreasing subjective effects after intravenous morphine. *Drug Alcohol Dependence.* **52**: 161–165.
56 Larkin PJ *et al.* (2008) The management of constipation in palliative care: clinical practice recommendations. *Palliative Medicine.* **22**: 796–807.
57 Portenoy RK *et al.* (2008) Subcutaneous methylnaltrexone for the treatment of opioid-induced constipation in patients with advanced illness: a double-blind, randomized, parallel group, dose-ranging study. *Journal of Pain and Symptom Management.* **35**: 458–468.
58 Thomas J *et al.* (2008) Methylnaltrexone for opioid-induced constipation in advanced illness. *New England Journal of Medicine.* **358**: 2332–2343.
59 Slatkin N *et al.* (2009) Methylnaltrexone for treatment of opioid-induced constipation in advanced illness patients. *Journal of Supportive Oncology.* **7**: 39–46.
60 Michna E *et al.* (2011) Subcutaneous Methylnaltrexone for Treatment of Opioid-Induced Constipation in Patients With Chronic, Nonmalignant Pain: A Randomized Controlled Study. *Journal of Pain.*
61 Candy B *et al.* (2011) Laxatives or methylnaltrexone for the management of constipation in palliative care patients. *Cochrane Database of Systematic Reviews.* **19**: CD003448.
62 Mackey AC *et al.* (2010) Methylnaltrexone and gastrointestinal perforation. *Journal of Pain and Symptom Management.* **40**: e1–3.
63 Watkins JL *et al.* (2011) Utilization of methylnaltrexone (relistor) for opioid-induced constipation in an oncology hospital. *Pharmacy and Therapeutics.* **36**: 33–36.

NALOXONE — BNF 15.1.7

Class: Opioid antagonist.

Indications: Reversal of opioid-induced respiratory depression; acute opioid overdose; prevention of relapse in opioid ex-addicts (in combination products with **buprenorphine** (Suboxone®)); †pruritus due to cholestasis or spinal opioids.

Pharmacology

Naloxone is a potent opioid antagonist. It has a high affinity for opioid receptors and reverses the effect of opioid analgesics by displacement in a dose-related manner. Partial antagonism may be obtained by using small doses. Activity after oral administration is low; it is only one fifteenth as potent by mouth as by injection. Naloxone is rapidly metabolized by the liver, primarily to naloxone glucuronide which is excreted by the kidneys.

The most important clinical property of naloxone is reversal of opioid-induced respiratory depression (and other opioid effects) caused by either an overdose of an opioid (including **codeine** and **dextropropoxyphene**) or an exaggerated response to conventional doses. Antagonism of **buprenorphine** requires higher than usual doses of naloxone because of the former's high receptor affinity (see p.381).

Naloxone has been reported to be only partially effective in reversing the effects of **tramadol.**[1,2] However, in a series of 11 patients with a **tramadol** overdose, seven had a good response to naloxone, and only one had no response.[3] *Naloxone is not effective against respiratory depression caused by non-opioids, e.g. barbiturates.*

Both naloxone and **naltrexone** have been used to correct opioid-induced GI disorders (i.e. delayed gastric emptying and constipation) but their use risks antagonizing the analgesic effect of the opioid.[4]

Combined naloxone and **buprenorphine** SL tablets are available for the treatment of opioid dependency. A combination product containing m/r formulations of **oxycodone** and naloxone (Targinact®) is also available. Although primarily added to deter misuse (e.g. by crushing and injecting IV), the naloxone appears to reduce the impact of the opioid on the GI tract (see p.424). However, **methylnaltrexone**, a quaternary opioid antagonist free of central effects, is preferable for acute relief of severe opioid-related constipation (see Box 5.W, p.433).

Naloxone is also of benefit in patients with septic shock,[5] **morphine**-induced peripheral vasodilation,[6] ischaemic central neurological deficits[7,8] and post-stroke central pain.[9]

Postoperative pain studies indicate that *ultra-low* doses of naloxone can either potentiate the analgesic effect of **morphine** (and presumably of other agonist opioids) or reduce undesirable effects (e.g. nausea, vomiting, pruritus).[10–13] These phenomena are probably explained by **naloxone** having other effects beyond classical opioid receptor antagonism (see p.429). Thus, ultra-low dose **naloxone**, through effects at non-opioid receptor binding sites, can improve analgesia; an effect which is lost with higher doses because of classical opioid receptor antagonism. Potentially, ultra-low dose naloxone could have a place in the treatment of opioid-induced hyperalgesia. However, the inherent risk of reversal of analgesia limits the widespread clinical application of this approach, and it should only be undertaken by specialists in pain or palliative medicine. Reducing the dose of the offending opioid is the first and most important step.[14]

Naloxone by CIVI decreases scratching activity by patients with cholestatic pruritus (see p.437).[15,16] Thus, naloxone has a potential place in the emergency treatment of acute exacerbations of cholestatic pruritus. **Naltrexone** (see p.439) [17,18] and **nalmefene** (not UK),[19,20] which are both bio-available by mouth, can then be used long-term.

However, opioid antagonists can precipitate an opioid withdrawal-like reaction in patients with cholestasis, including hallucinations and dysphoria.[21,22] To avoid or minimize such a reaction, treatment must be started with a cautious low-dose infusion of naloxone (see p.437), low-dose **naltrexone** (see p.439) or PO **nalmefene** (not UK). Ultra-low dose naloxone is also used to relieve pruritus caused by spinal opioids, when other treatments have failed (see Box 21.C, p.688).

Bio-availability 6% PO.

Onset of action 1–2min IV; 2–5min SC/IM.

Plasma halflife about 1h.

Duration of action IV 15–90min.

Cautions

In patients receiving opioids for pain relief, naloxone should *not* be used for drowsiness and/or delirium which is not life-threatening because of the danger of reversing the opioid analgesia, and precipitating a major physical withdrawal syndrome.

Undesirable effects

Nausea and vomiting. Occasionally severe hypertension, pulmonary oedema, tachycardia, arrhythmias, cardiac arrest;[23] doses as small as 100–400microgram of naloxone have been implicated.[24] The mechanism of these sporadic events may be related to the centrally-mediated catecholamine responses to opioid reversal.[25]

Dose and use

Naloxone is best given IV but, if not practical, may be given IM or SC.

Opioid overdose

- give 400microgram–2mg IV every 2–3min p.r.n., up to a total of 10mg
- if the overdose is associated with a long-acting opioid (particularly **methadone** or **dextropropoxyphene**) or an m/r formulation, the duration of action of the opioid will exceed that of naloxone. Even if there is an initial response to naloxone, further IV doses are likely to be required, and it may be necessary to continue treatment with a closely monitored IV infusion of naloxone for up to 24h, and sometimes longer.

Reversal of respiratory depression caused by the medicinal use of opioids

- give 100–200microgram IV stat
- give further doses of 100microgram every 2min until respiratory function is satisfactory.

Further IV doses should be given after 1–2h if there is concern that further absorption of the opioid will result in delayed respiratory depression. Even lower doses have been recommended (Box 5.X). It is important to titrate dose against respiratory function and *not* the level of consciousness because total antagonism will cause a return of severe pain with hyperalgesia and, if physically dependent, severe physical withdrawal symptoms and marked agitation.[26]

Consider and address the possible cause(s) of the opioid overdose, e.g. excessive use in an opioid poorly-responsive pain, accumulation because of a long halflife (**methadone**) or reduced elimination because of renal impairment (**morphine**, **hydromorphone**). Wait until there has been a sustained improvement in consciousness before restarting a lower dose of opioid. It may be preferable to switch the type of opioid; seek specialist advice.

Box 5.X Naloxone for iatrogenic opioid overdose (based on the recommendations of the American Pain Society)[27]

If respiratory rate ≥8 breaths/min, and the patient easily rousable and not cyanosed, adopt a policy of 'wait and see'; consider reducing or omitting the next regular dose of morphine.

If respiratory rate <8 breaths/min, and the patient comatose/unconscious and/or cyanosed:
- dilute a standard ampoule containing naloxone 400microgram to 10mL with 0.9% saline for injection
- administer 0.5mL (20microgram) IV every 2min until the patient's respiratory status is satisfactory
- further boluses may be necessary because naloxone is shorter-acting than morphine (and other opioids)
- wait until there has been a sustained improvement in consciousness before restarting a lower dose of opioid (see text).

Cholestatic pruritus
- to avoid or minimize an opioid withdrawal-like syndrome, start with a sub-optimal dose of naloxone by CIVI, e.g. 0.002microgram/kg/min (about 160–200microgram/24h)[22]
- provided no withdrawal-like symptoms occur, the rate can be doubled every 3–4h; if symptoms occur, continue with the current dose until resolved
- after 18–24h, when a rate known to be associated with opioid antagonistic effects is reached (0.2microgram/kg/min), the infusion is stopped and **naltrexone** 12.5mg b.d.–25mg t.d.s. is started)[21,22]
- the dose is escalated over a few days until a satisfactory clinical response is obtained; at this stage the effective dose should be consolidated into a single daily maintenance dose
- the effective dose range for **naltrexone** is 25–250mg once daily;[22] for **nalmefene** (not UK), 25–120mg once daily.[19]

Supply
Naloxone hydrochloride (generic)
Injection 400microgram/mL, 1mL amp = £4; 1mg/mL, 2mL prefilled syringe = £8.

Minijet® Naloxone (UCB Pharma)
Injection 400microgram/mL, 1mL prefilled disposable syringe = £20, 2mL prefilled disposable syringe = £13, 5mL prefilled disposable syringe = £13.

1 Raffa RB *et al.* (1992) Opioid and nonopioid components independently contribute to the mechanism of action of tramadol, an 'atypical' opioid analgesic. *Journal of Pharmacology and Therapeutics*. **260**: 275–285.
2 Shipton EA (2000) Tramadol — present and future. *Anaesthesia and Intensive Care*. **28**: 363–374.
3 Marquardt KA *et al.* (2005) Tramadol exposures reported to statewide poison control system. *Annals of Pharmacotherapy*. **39**: 1039–1044.
4 McNicol ED (2008) Mu-opioid antagonists for opioid-induced bowel dysfunction. *Cochrane Database of Systematic Reviews*. **2 (April 16)**: CD006332.
5 Peters WP *et al.* (1981) Pressor effect of naloxone in septic shock. *Lancet*. **i**: 529–532.
6 Cohen RA and Coffman JD (1980) Naloxone reversal of morphine-induced peripheral vasodilatation. *Clinical Pharmacology and Therapeutics*. **28**: 541–544.
7 Baskin DS and Hosobuchi Y (1981) Naloxone reversal of ischaemic neurological deficits in man. *Lancet*. **ii**: 272–275.
8 Bousigue J-Y *et al.* (1982) Naloxone reversal of neurological deficit. *Lancet*. **ii**: 618–619.
9 Ray D and Tai Y (1988) Infusions of naloxone in thalamic pain. *British Medical Journal*. **296**: 969–970.
10 Gan T *et al.* (1997) Opioid-sparing effects of a low-dose infusion of naloxone in patient-administered morphine sulfate. *Anesthesiology*. **87**: 1075–1081.
11 Joshi G *et al.* (1999) Effects of prophylactic nalmefene on the incidence of morphine-related side effects in patients receiving intravenous patient-controlled analgesia. *Anesthesiology*. **90**: 1007–1011.
12 Cepeda MS *et al.* (2004) Addition of ultralow dose naloxone to postoperative morphine PCA: unchanged analgesia and opioid requirement but decreased incidence of opioid side effects. *Pain*. **107**: 41–46.
13 Maxwell LG *et al.* (2005) The effects of a small-dose naloxone infusion on opioid-induced side effects and analgesia in children and adolescents treated with intravenous patient-controlled analgesia: a double-blind, prospective, randomized, controlled study. *Anesthesia and Analgesia*. **100**: 953–958.
14 Twycross R *et al.* (2009) *Symptom Management in Advanced Cancer* (4e). palliativedrugs.com Ltd, Nottingham, pp. 43–45.

15 Bergasa N *et al.* (1992) A controlled trial of naloxone infusions for the pruritus of chronic cholestasis. *Gastroenterology.* **102**: 544–549.
16 Bergasa N *et al.* (1995) Effects of naloxone infusions in patients with the pruritus of cholestasis. *Annals of internal medicine.* **123**: 161–167.
17 Carson K *et al.* (1996) Pilot study of the use of naltrexone to treat the severe pruritus of cholestatic liver disease. *American Journal of Gastroenterology.* **91**: 1022–1023.
18 Wolfhagen F *et al.* (1997) Oral naltrexone treatment for cholestatic pruritus: A double-blind, placebo-controlled study. *Gastroenterology.* **113**: 1264–1269.
19 Bergasa N *et al.* (1998) Open-label trial of oral nalmefene therapy for the pruritus of cholestasis. *Hepatology.* **27**: 679–684.
20 Bergasa N *et al.* (1999) Oral nalmefene therapy reduces scratching activity due to the pruritus of cholestasis: a controlled study. *Journal of the American Academy of Dermatology.* **41**: 431–434.
21 Jones E and Dekker L (2000) Florid opioid withdrawal-like reaction precipitated by naltrexone in a patient with chronic cholestasis. *Gastroenterology.* **118**: 431–432.
22 Jones E *et al.* (2002) Opiate antagonist therapy for the pruritus of cholestasis: the avoidance of opioid withdrawal-like reactions. *Quarterly Journal of Medicine.* **95**: 547–552.
23 Partridge BL and Ward CF (1986) Pulmonary oedema following low-dose naloxone administration. *Anesthesiology.* **65**: 709–710.
24 Pallasch TJ and Gill CJ (1981) Naloxone associated morbidity and mortality. *Oral Surgery.* **52**: 602–603.
25 Smith G and Pinnock C (1985) Editorial: naloxone–paradox or panacea? *British Journal of Anaesthesia.* **57**: 547–549.
26 Cleary J (2000) Incidence and characteristics of naloxone administration in medical oncology patients with cancer pain. *Journal of Pharmaceutical Care in Pain and Symptom Control.* **8**: 65–73.
27 Miaskowski C et al. (2008) *Principles of analgesic use in the treatment of acute pain and cancer pain* (6e). American Pain Society, Skokie, Illinois, p.31.

NALTREXONE — BNF 4.10

Class: Opioid antagonist.

Indications: Prevention of relapse in opioid and †alcohol ex-addicts, †pruritus associated with cholestasis[1,2] and, possibly, chronic renal failure.[3,4]

Contra-indications: Patients currently dependent on opioids; acute hepatitis or hepatic failure; severe renal impairment (creatinine clearance <10mL/min).

Pharmacology

Naltrexone is a specific opioid antagonist with actions similar to those of **naloxone**.[5] Thus, it reversibly blocks the pharmacological effects of opioids at μ, κ and δ-opioid receptors. Compared with **naloxone**, naltrexone has a higher PO bio-availability, and a longer duration of action. Naltrexone is well absorbed from the GI tract but undergoes extensive first-pass metabolism.[6,7] It is extensively metabolized in the liver and the major metabolite, 6-β-naltrexol, may also possess weak antagonist activity. Naltrexone and its metabolites are excreted mainly in the urine. Less than 1% of an oral dose of naltrexone is excreted unchanged.[8]

In former drug addicts, naltrexone 100mg blocks the effect of a challenge of IV **diamorphine** 25mg:
- 96% at 24h
- 86% at 48h
- 46% at 72h.[9]

Thus, naltrexone is primarily used to prevent relapse in opioid ex-addicts by blocking the opioid 'high'. It is given PO once daily or three times a week. It is also available as a long-acting depot IM injection (duration of action of >1 month; licensed for use only in alcoholics) and a SC pellet implant (duration of action of weeks to months; unlicensed and only available through private addiction clinics in the UK).[10,11]

Naltrexone is also used to treat cholestatic pruritus (see p.439).[1,2] However, orally administered opioid antagonists can precipitate a transient opioid withdrawal-like reaction in patients with cholestasis, including hallucinations and dysphoria.[12,13] To avoid or minimize such a reaction, treatment must be started cautiously with a sub-optimal low dose. In an open study of patients with various skin and systemic disorders associated with pruritus, good relief was obtained with naltrexone in 70% of patients.[14] However, in the absence of controlled data, the results should be interpreted with caution. The use of naltrexone to relieve cholestatic jaundice may sometimes unmask or exacerbate underlying pain, necessitating discontinuation of naltrexone.[15]

The use of naltrexone will severely impede opioid analgesia.[16] The long-term use of naltrexone also increases the concentration of opioid receptors in the CNS and results in a temporary enhanced response to the subsequent administration of opioid analgesics.[17] The management of acute pain or postoperative pain in patients receiving long-term naltrexone requires careful consideration and detailed planning (Box 5.Y).[16]

Conversely, *ultra-low* dose naltrexone has been found to potentiate the analgesic effect of **methadone** and intrathecal **morphine**.[18,19] This phenomenon is probably explained by naltrexone having other effects beyond classical opioid receptor antagonism (see p.429). Thus, through effects at non-opioid receptor binding sites, ultra-low dose naltrexone can improve analgesia; an effect which is lost with higher doses because of classical opioid receptor antagonism. However, the inherent risk of reversal of analgesia limits the widespread clinical application of this approach.

Naltrexone has been used to correct opioid-induced GI disorders (i.e. delayed gastric emptying and constipation) but its use risks antagonizing the analgesic effect of the opioid.[20] However, **methylnaltrexone**, a quaternary opioid antagonist free of central effects, is preferable for acute relief of severe opioid-related constipation (see Box 5.W, p.433).

A combination product containing **morphine** and sequestered naltrexone is in development, primarily to deter misuse (e.g. by crushing and injecting IV).[21]

Bio-availability 5–40% PO.

Onset of action may precipitate withdrawal symptoms in <5min in opioid-dependent patients.

Time to peak plasma concentration 1–2h PO.

Plasma halflife 4h; 13h for 6-β-naltrexol.[22]

Duration of action 1–3 days.

Cautions

Opioid withdrawal-like syndrome in patients with cholestatic pruritus. Hepatic and renal impairment. Occasional hepatotoxicity;[23] the manufacturer advises checking LFTs before and at intervals during treatment.

Undesirable effects

Very common (>10% in detoxifying opioid addicts): insomnia, anxiety, nervousness, intestinal colic, nausea and vomiting, low energy, joint and muscle pain, headaches.

Dose and use

Cholestatic pruritus

If administered after initial naloxone infusion, see p.437.

If *de novo*:

- start with 12.5mg b.d. (some centres start with 1mg once daily)
- increase after 3 days to 25mg b.d./50mg once daily
- escalate slowly over several weeks
- the effective dose range is 25–250mg once daily.[13]

Uraemic pruritus

- start with 50mg once daily.[3,4]
- if ineffective after 1 week, consider increasing dose to 100mg once daily.

Supply

Nalorex® (Bristol-Myers Squibb)

Tablets 50mg scored, 28 days @ 50mg once daily = £22.

Opizone® (Genus)

Tablets 50mg scored, 28 days @ 50mg once daily = £23.

Box 5.Y Management of acute pain in patients receiving naltrexone

Elective surgery
The use of naltrexone must be identified well before the operation.

Ensure effective liaison between the substance misuse and acute pain teams.

Consider switching patients on depot injections to PO naltrexone before surgery.

Remove SC pellet implants when major surgery/severe postoperative pain anticipated. For minor surgery, leave the implant in-situ, *provided non-opioids are considered sufficient to manage the postoperative pain.*

Discontinue PO naltrexone 72h before the operation.

When possible use non-opioid analgesics, e.g. IV paracetamol, NSAID.

Anticipate that greater than usual doses of opioid may be required; conversely be aware of the potential for an increased response.

Unexpected severe acute pain, e.g. trauma, emergency surgery
When possible use non-opioid analgesics, e.g.:
- IV paracetamol and/or NSAID
- clonidine 1microgram/kg IV every 5min until satisfactory analgesia obtained, up to a total dose of 4microgram/kg; may be repeated after 4h
- ketamine 100microgram/kg IV every 5min until satisfactory analgesia obtained, plus a single dose of midazolam 20–40microgram/kg IV to minimize dysphoria; may be repeated after 30min; give further midazolam only if dysphoria present.

Note: there is a risk of marked sedation when ketamine and midazolam are combined in this way; to be used only by those competent in airway management.

In patients with no veins, clonidine and ketamine can be given SC; use the same doses as for IV but allow 15min between doses.

The above are generally used to achieve rapid pain relief until other measures can be instituted, e.g.:
- local anaesthetic blocks
- epidural analgesia (local anaesthetic ± clonidine).

1 Carson K *et al.* (1996) Pilot study of the use of naltrexone to treat the severe pruritus of cholestatic liver disease. *American Journal of Gastroenterology.* **91**: 1022–1023.
2 Wolfhagen F *et al.* (1997) Oral naltrexone treatment for cholestatic pruritus: A double-blind, placebo-controlled study. *Gastroenterology.* **113**: 1264–1269.
3 Peer G *et al.* (1996) Randomised crossover trial of naltrexone in uraemic pruritus. *Lancet.* **348**: 1552–1554.
4 Pauli-Magnus C *et al.* (2000) Naltrexone does not relieve uremic pruritus. *Journal of the American Society of Nephrology.* **11**: 514–519.
5 Verebey K *et al.* (1976) Naltrexone: disposition, metabolism and effects after acute and chronic dosing. *Clinical Pharmacology and Therapeutics.* **20**: 315–328.
6 Gonzalez J and Brogden R (1988) Naltrexone: a review of its pharmacodynamic and pharmacokinetic properties and therapeutic efficacy in the management of opioid dependence. *Drugs.* **35**: 192–213.
7 Crabtree B (1984) Review of naltrexone: a long-acting opiate antagonist. *Clinical Pharmacy.* **3**: 273–280.
8 Wall M *et al.* (1981) Metabolism and disposition of naltrexone in man after oral and intravenous administration. *Drug Metabolism and Disposition.* **9**: 369–375.
9 Verebey K (1981) The clinical pharmacology of naltrexone: pharmacology and pharmacodynamics. *NIDA Research Monograph.* **28**: 147–158.
10 Volpicelli JR *et al.* (1992) Naltrexone in the treatment of alcohol dependence. *Archives of General Psychiatry.* **49**: 876–880.
11 Swift RM *et al.* (1994) Naltrexone-induced alterations in human ethanol intoxication. *American Journal of Psychiatry.* **151**: 1463–1467.
12 Jones E and Dekker L (2000) Florid opioid withdrawal-like reaction precipitated by naltrexone in a patient with chronic cholestasis. *Gastroenterology.* **118**: 431–432.
13 Jones E *et al.* (2002) Opiate antagonist therapy for the pruritus of cholestasis: the avoidance of opioid withdrawal-like reactions. *Quarterly Journal of Medicine.* **95**: 547–552.
14 Metze D *et al.* (1999) Efficacy and safety of naltrexone, an oral opiate receptor antagonist, in the treatment of pruritus in internal and dermatological diseases. *Journal of the American Academy of Dermatology.* **41**: 533–539.

15 McRae CA *et al.* (2003) Pain as a complication of use of opiate antagonists for symptom control in cholestasis. *Gastroenterology.* **125**: 591–596.

16 Vickers AP and Jolly A (2006) Naltrexone and problems in pain management. *British Medical Journal.* **332**: 132–133.

17 Yoburn BC *et al.* (1988) Upregulation of opioid receptor subtypes correlates with potency changes of morphine and DADLE. *Life Sciences.* **43**: 1319–1324.

18 Cruciani RA *et al.* (2003) Ultra-low dose oral naltrexone decreases side effects and potentiates the effect of methadone. *Journal of Pain and Symptom Management.* **25**: 491–494.

19 Hamann S and Sloan P (2007) Oral naltrexone to enhance analgesia in patients receiving continuous intrathecal morphine for chronic pain: a randomized, double-blind, prospective pilot study. *Journal of Opioid Management.* **3**: 137–144.

20 McNicol ED (2008) Mu-opioid antagonists for opioid-induced bowel dysfunction. *Cochrane Database of Systematic Reviews.* **2 (April 16)**: CD006332.

21 Webster LR *et al.* (2010) Long-term safety and efficacy of morphine sulfate and naltrexone hydrochloride extended release capsules, a novel formulation containing morphine and sequestered naltrexone, in patients with chronic, moderate to severe pain. *Journal of Pain and Symptom Management.* **40**: 734–746.

22 Gutstein H and Akil H (2001) Opioid analgesics. In: J Hardman *et al.* (eds) *Goodman & Gilman's The Pharmacological Basis of Therapeutics* (10e). McGraw-Hill, New York; London.

23 Mitchell J (1986) Naltrexone and hepatotoxicity. *Lancet.* **1**: 1215.

6: INFECTIONS

ANTIBACTERIALS IN PALLIATIVE CARE

BNF Section 5 contains a comprehensive account of antibacterial use,[1] and many hospitals have antibacterial policies which govern local infection control and treatment, e.g. the prevention of methicillin-resistant *Staphylococcus aureus* (MRSA) infection and the prevention of *Clostridium difficile* infection. Advice sometimes varies from region to region. Thus, any specific recommendations about antibacterials in *PCF* should be considered in conjunction with local policy. When in doubt, seek advice from a local medical microbiologist.

Remember: always ask about drug allergies before prescribing an antibacterial.
The dose and frequency of many antibacterials are reduced in renal impairment.

Antibacterial resistance

Recent national and international surveillance has identified an increase in ESBL (Extended Spectrum Beta-Lactamase) positive enterobacteria, most commonly *Escherichia coli* and *Klebsiella pneumoniae*. These Gram-negative bacilli produce an enzyme which mediates antibacterial resistance, with up to 10% resistant to **gentamicin** and 3rd generation cephalosporins, e.g. **cefuroxime**, **cefotaxime** and **ceftazidime**. This possibility should be considered particularly in patients with:

- previous isolation of ESBL positive multiresistant Gram-negative organisms
- recurrent urinary or biliary tract infection (>2 episodes in the last year)
- persistent infection despite current or recent treatment (within the last week) with broad-spectrum antibacterials.

Appropriate specimens (including blood cultures) should be taken and any previous microbiology reviewed. If a multiresistant isolate is identified, treatment must be discussed with a medical microbiologist, and strict infection control procedures followed.

Penicillin allergy

Allergic reactions to penicillins occur in 1–10% of exposed individuals, and anaphylaxis in <0.05%. Those with a history of urticaria, rash or anaphylaxis immediately after starting a course of a penicillin should not receive a penicillin, beta-lactam antibacterial or a cephalosporin.

Those with a history of a minor rash (e.g. non-confluent, non-pruritic rash restricted to a small area of the body) or a rash that occurs >72 hours after a penicillin is started are probably *not* allergic to penicillin, and a penicillin need not be withheld if indicated. However, the possibility of an allergic reaction should be kept in mind. Other beta-lactam antibacterials (including cephalosporins) can be used in these patients.[1]

General considerations

Stop and think! In a moribund patient with progressive incurable disease, are you justified in giving antibacterials for an intercurrent infection which may be the natural endpoint of the dying process?

No evidence-based guidelines are available on the appropriate use of antibacterial drugs in patients receiving palliative care.[2] The information given in this chapter is limited to several common situations in palliative care, or to occasional events which demand decisive immediate action, such as:

- local infection causing severe pain (see below)
- ascending cholangitis associated with a biliary stent (see below)
- cellulitis in patients with lymphoedema (see p.455).

Antibacterials in end-stage disease should have the primary purpose of ameliorating distressing symptoms (including fever and malaise), and not simply delaying inevitable death. It has been claimed that the use of antibacterials for *symptomatic* infection (which implies a conscious patient) does *not* prolong survival (and thus prolong the process and distress of dying).[3] Even so, it is important *to stop and think*. If there is an automatic 'reflex' to prescribe antibacterials when infection is diagnosed, it is possible that they will be overprescribed, and dying prolonged.[4]

In one survey, 25% of patients with advanced cancer and definite infection died within 1 week of starting antibacterials, and a further 25% died within a week of completing a course of antibacterials.[5] Other surveys give comparable short survival times.[6,7] Further, a recent report suggests antibacterials given in the last week of life have little impact on symptoms.[2]

Several surveys give similar prevalence rates for symptomatic infection in *conscious* palliative care/hospice patients, namely about 40%,[3] and show that the response to antibacterials varies according to the site of infection (Table 6.1). Provided a patient does not have an indwelling urinary catheter, UTIs should generally be treated routinely unless there is an overriding reason for not doing so (see p.452).[3,5] Cough caused by infection is also significantly reduced by antibacterials.[5] On the other hand, the use of antibacterials to treat bacteraemia in a patient with *end-stage* progressive disease would appear to be futile (Table 6.1).

Table 6.1 Response to antimicrobials[a] in >600 home care patients[3]

Type of infection	*Number*	*Response (%)*[b]
UTI	265	79
RTI	221	43
Oral cavity[a]	63	46
Skin or SC	59	41
Bacteraemia	25	0

a. includes the use of antibacterials for infections at all sites, and of antifungals for oropharyngeal candidosis
b. reduction of fever ± amelioration of site-specific symptoms within 3 days.

Antibacterials to relieve infection-related pain

Antibacterials are essential in some patients for the relief of severe pain associated with infection around a malignant tumour in, for example, the neck, the gluteal muscles underlying an ulcerated cancer, or the perineum.[8] Sometimes there is a history of a rapid increase in pain intensity over several days which is poorly responsive to escalating doses of a strong opioid. The pain is often associated with fever and malaise, and may be complicated by delirium. Commonly, there will be a mixture of more superficial aerobic infection with deeper anaerobic infection. Treatment is similar to that recommended for ascending cholangitis (see below).

Ascending cholangitis

Ascending cholangitis may occur in patients with a partially obstructed or stented common bile duct. It often causes severe systemic disturbance and should be treated promptly, e.g.:

- **co-amoxiclav** 1,200mg IV q8h
- if a minor rash with a penicillin in the past (see p.443), **cefuroxime** 1,500mg IV q8h plus **metronidazole** 500mg IV q8h
- if the patient is in septic shock, also give a single dose of **gentamicin** 5mg/kg (maximum dose 500mg) IV over 20–30min
- if a risk of multiresistant Gram-negative bacilli (see p.443), serious penicillin allergy or in any doubt, consult a medical microbiologist.

When IV administration is difficult, alternatives include:

- **ceftazidime** 1g IM q8h, reconstituted with 3mL of WFI or 0.5–1% **lidocaine hydrochloride** solution (total injection volume = 3.8mL)
- in countries where it is available (not UK) **cefepime** 1g SC q8h reconstituted with 2.4mL of either 0.9% saline, 5% glucose (dextrose), WFI or 0.5–1% **lidocaine hydrochloride** solution (total injection volume = 3.6mL).

The doses and/or frequency of **co-amoxiclav**, **cefuroxime**, **ceftazidime**, **cefepime**, and **gentamicin** should be reduced in renal impairment.

Infection associated with an airway stent

The presence of an airway stent, whether for cancer or other obstruction, increases the risk of serious respiratory tract infection. In a systematic review of 500 patients, mortality rate was almost 70%.[9] Commonest pathogens are *Staphylococcus aureus* and *Pseudomonas aeruginosa*. Treatment should be commenced promptly and guided by the advice of a medical microbiologist.

Respiratory tract infection in the imminently dying patient

Occasionally, death rattle (noisy respiratory secretions) is caused by profuse purulent sputum from a chest infection, and an antibacterial is prescribed in the hope that it will reduce the copious purulent malodorous discharge from the mouth.[10] In this circumstance, the IV route is generally the best. However, if not practical, the IM or SC routes can be used instead.[11]

Some centres use single doses of **ceftriaxone**; either 1–2g IV or 1g IM reconstituted with 3.5mL **lidocaine** 1% (total injection volume = 4mL).[10] **Ceftriaxone** is a broad-spectrum antibacterial and has a long duration of action. Patients who responded did so within hours (marked reduction in purulent sputum and resolution of associated halitosis). Non-responders appeared not to benefit from a second dose after 24h.

Other centres give **ceftriaxone** by SC injection[12,13] and administer multiple doses if a patient survives > 1 day, e.g. **ceftriaxone** 1g vial reconstituted with 2.2mL **lidocaine** 1% (total injection volume = 2.8mL) 250mg–1g SC once daily. If a larger volume of **lidocaine** is added, e.g. 3.3mL (total injection volume = 3.9mL), the mixture can be administered as a divided dose, given at the same time but using two or more separate SC/IM sites[14] (see manufacturer's SPC for additional information and guidance).

The results of a survey suggest that the above are reasonably well tolerated, and have been used for up to 10 days when patients have not been imminently dying.[11]

The bio-availability (in volunteers) of **cefepime** SC is comparable with IM.[15] Further, when 1g is infused over 30min, pain at the injection site is absent or minimal. Thus, **cefepime** (not UK) could be a better option. Concern about the safety of **cefepime**[16] has been shown to be groundless.[17]

Supply

Co-amoxiclav (generic)
Injection (powder for reconstitution) co-amoxiclav 500/100 (amoxicillin 500mg as sodium salt, clavulanic acid 100mg as potassium salt), co-amoxiclav 1,000/200 (amoxicillin 1g as sodium salt, clavulanic acid 200mg as potassium salt), 2 days @ 1,200mg t.d.s = £15.

Cefuroxime
Zinacef® (GSK)
Injection (powder for reconstitution) 250mg, 750mg, 1.5g (IV only), 2 days @ 1,500mg t.d.s. = £28.

Ceftazidime (generic)
Injection (powder for reconstitution) 1g, 2g, 2 days @ 1g t.d.s. = £51.

Ceftriaxone (generic)
Injection (powder for reconstitution) 1g vial = £10, 2g vial = £20.

Gentamicin sulphate (generic)
Injection 40mg/mL, 1mL amp, 2mL amp, 2mL vial, all products = £1.50.

Also see **metronidazole**, p.451.

1 BNF (2010) British National Formulary (No. 60). British Medical Association and the Royal Pharmaceutical Society of Great Britain, London. Available from: www.bnf.org.
2 Nakagawa S *et al.* (2010) Can anti-infective drugs improve the infection-related symptoms of patients with cancer during the terminal stages of their lives? *Journal of Palliative Medicine*. **13**: 535–540.
3 Reinbolt RE *et al.* (2005) Symptomatic treatment of infections in patients with advanced cancer receiving hospice care. *Journal of Pain and Symptom Management*. **30**: 175–182.
4 Lam PT *et al.* (2005) Retrospective analysis of antibiotic use and survival in advanced cancer patients with infections. *Journal of Pain and Symptom Management*. **30**: 536–543.
5 Mirhosseini M *et al.* (2006) The role of antibiotics in the management of infection-related symptoms in advanced cancer patients. *Journal of Palliative Care*. **22**: 69–74.
6 Clayton J *et al.* (2003) Parenteral antibiotics in a palliative care unit: prospective analysis of current practice. *Palliative Medicine*. **17**: 44–48.
7 Brabin E and Allsopp L (2008) How effective are parenteral antibiotics in hospice patients? *European Journal of Palliative Care*. **15**: 115–117.
8 Bruera E and MacDonald N (1986) Intractable pain in patients with advanced head and neck tumors: a possible role of local infection. *Cancer Treatment Reports*. **70**: 691–692.
9 Agrafiotis M *et al.* (2009) Infections related to airway stenting: a systematic review. *Respiration*. **78**: 69–74.
10 Spruyt O and Kausae A (1998) Antibiotic use for infective terminal respiratory secretions. *Journal of Pain and Symptom Management*. **15**: 263–264.
11 palliativedrugs.com. (2010) Survey: SC/IM antibiotics — Do you use this route? Available from: www.palliativedrugs.com
12 Borner K *et al.* (1985) Comparative pharmacokinetics of ceftriaxone after subcutaneous and intravenous administration. *Chemotherapy*. **31**: 237–245.
13 Bricaire F *et al.* (1988) [Pharmacokinetics and tolerance of ceftriaxone after subcutaneous administration]. *Pathologie Biologie (Paris)*. **36**: 702–705.
14 Tahmasebi M (2005) Is there any possibility for injecting antibiotics subcutaneously? In: *Bulletin board*. Palliativedrugs.com Ltd. Available from: www.palliativedrugs.org/forum/read.php?f=1&i=8124&t=8016
15 Walker P *et al.* (2005) Subcutaneous administration of cefepime. *Journal of Pain and Symptom Management*. **30**: 170–174.
16 Yahav D *et al.* (2007) Efficacy and safety of cefepime: a systematic review and meta-analysis. *The Lancet Infectious Diseases*. **7**: 338–348.
17 FDA (2009) Cefepime (marketed as Maxipime) update of ongoing safety review. Available from: www.fda.gov/Safety/MedWatch/SafetyInformation/SafetyAlertsforHumanMedicalProducts/ucm167427.htm

OROPHARYNGEAL CANDIDOSIS BNF 5.2 & 12.3.2

Oral yeast carriage is present in about 1/3 of the general population. The prevalence in patients with advanced cancer is significantly higher (about 50–90%).[1] Thus, it is not surprising that oropharyngeal candidosis is a common fungal infection in the palliative care population of patients (13–30%).[2,3]

Many patients with oropharyngeal candidosis have concurrent oesophageal infection,[4] and some patients develop systemic fungal infections. Oral candidosis is associated with:

- poor performance status
- dry mouth
- dentures
- topical antibacterials and/or corticosteroids
- in AIDS with CD4 cell count $<$200cells/mm^3.[1–3]

Oral candidosis is *not* associated with the use of oral/parenteral antibacterials, and most data suggest that it is not associated with the use of oral/parenteral corticosteroids.[5]

Non-*Candida albicans* species are increasing being isolated from patients with oral candidosis.[2,3] The reason for this is thought to be related to increased use of antifungal drugs; the consequence of this change is an increased incidence of azole drug resistance (many non-*Candida albicans* species exhibit inherent azole drug resistance).[6]

Management strategy

Correct the correctable

Underlying causal factors must be considered and corrected if possible, particularly dry mouth and poor denture hygiene.

Dentures must be thoroughly cleaned at least once daily, brushing the denture with a nailbrush or denture brush, and using soap and water or an appropriate commercial product.[7] Dentures should also be soaked overnight in an appropriate antiseptic, e.g. **chlorhexidine** or dilute **sodium hypochlorite**. The latter should not be used for dentures with metal parts. Failure to sterilize the denture will lead to failure of antifungal treatment. The dentures should be thoroughly rinsed before re-insertion to prevent drug inactivation (see Dose and use).

Drug treatment

Oral candidosis generally responds to topical treatment, e.g. **nystatin**, **amphotericin** (not UK). A systematic review concluded that there is no difference in efficacy between topical and systemic treatments.[8] When efficacy, lack of resistance (see below), and cost are all taken into account, **nystatin** is probably the antifungal drug of choice for oral candidosis in non-immunocompromised patients.

On the other hand, because they are more convenient, many patients are treated systemically with a once daily azole antifungal, e.g. **fluconazole**. However, organisms resistant to one or more azole do occur. Recent data on the prevalence of resistant organisms in palliative care patients are:

- **itraconazole** 21%
- **fluconazole** 22%
- **ketoconazole** 8%
- **voriconazole** 3%.[9]

In practice, patients who have *not* received multiple courses of azoles will probably be sensitive to this group of drugs *unless* the causal yeast is a non-*Candida albicans* species. However, cross-resistance and cross-infection do occur and, if there is a high prevalence of azole resistance within the local patient population, then even azole-naïve patients may be infected with azole-resistant organisms. Local treatment protocols must take such factors into account.

Azole antifungals have an inhibitory effect on human cytochrome P450 enzymes (see p.735). This results in inhibition of adrenal steroid synthesis (cortisol, testosterone, oestrogens and progesterone) and of the metabolism of many drugs. Drug interactions are most likely with **ketoconazole** and **itraconazole**. They are generally less likely and less pronounced with **fluconazole** (a weaker CYP inhibitor), although several clinically important interactions have been reported with all of these.[10]

Potential topical treatments in resistant cases (or other special circumstances) include **chlorhexidine**,[1] gentian violet (e.g. 0.5–1%, 1.5mL applied twice daily),[11] and tea tree oil.[12]

Cautions

Because of a potential teratogenic risk, the manufacturers of **fluconazole** and **itraconazole** advise that women of child-bearing potential should use contraceptive precautions until the next menstrual period after completing treatment. Because of similar toxicological findings in animal studies with other azoles, it would be wise to extend this precaution to **ketoconazole** and **miconazole**.

The systemic absorption of **ketoconazole** is markedly reduced in hypochlorhydric states. Thus, absorption is impaired in patients taking antacids, **sucralfate** (has a weak antacid effect), H_2-receptor antagonists or a PPI. In hypochlorhydria, absorption from **itraconazole** capsules is variable, but from the oral solution absorption is reliable and bio-availability is higher. The absorption of **fluconazole** is not affected by antacids, **sucralfate**, H_2-receptor antagonists, PPIs or food.

Itraconazole may cause or worsen left ventricular dysfunction or CHF.

Renal impairment: reduce dose of **fluconazole** by 50% if creatinine clearance is <50mL/min; do not use **itraconazole** if creatinine clearance is <30mL/min (although the bio-availability of oral **itraconazole** may be reduced in renal impairment).

Hepatic impairment: serious or fatal hepatotoxicity may occur with **fluconazole**, **itraconazole**, and particularly **ketoconazole**. Indeed, for this reason, the MHRA (UK) has concluded that ketoconazole is 'not suitable as a first-line treatment or for superficial infections'.[13] Further, the MHRA advises monitoring liver function before starting treatment, 2 and 4 weeks after starting treatment, and monthly thereafter. The manufacturers of **fluconazole** and **itraconazole** advise monitoring liver function in patients receiving large doses and/or prolonged courses, and in patients with pre-existing liver dysfunction or liver disease. With all 3 drugs, treatment should be discontinued if symptoms suggestive of hepatotoxicity develop, e.g. jaundice, dark urine.

Drug interactions

Through inhibition of various cytochrome P450 enzymes, particularly CYP3A4, azoles produce clinically important increases in the plasma concentration of many drugs (see Cytochrome P450, p.735). Avoid concurrent administration of **itraconazole, ketoconazole** or **miconazole** with **astemizole**, **pimozide** or **quinidine** because of a risk of fatal cardiac arrhythmias.

Fluconazole, **itraconazole**, **miconazole** and **ketoconazole** increase the plasma concentration of **alfentanil**, **carbamazepine**, **dexamethasone**, **digoxin**, **glipizide**, **glyburide**, **methylprednisolone**, **midazolam**, **nifedipine**, **phenytoin**, **theophylline**, TCAs, most statins, and **warfarin**, and thus increase their toxicity and/or undesirable effects.

Strong CYP3A4 inducers, e.g. **carbamazepine**, **phenytoin**, **phenobarbital**, **rifampicin**, **rifabutin** and possibly *Hypericum perforatum* (St. John's wort), reduce **fluconazole**, **itraconazole**, and **ketoconazole** plasma concentrations, which may result in antifungal treatment failure.

Undesirable effects

Common (<10%, >1%): headache (azole antifungals), dizziness (**fluconazole** and **itraconazole**), GI symptoms, i.e. dyspepsia, nausea and vomiting, abdominal pain, diarrhoea (**fluconazole** and **itraconazole**), rashes, pruritus, hypokalaemia (**fluconazole** and **itraconazole**).
Uncommon, rare or very rare (<1%): anaphylaxis, hepatitis, cholestasis, hepatic failure, adrenal suppression (**itraconazole**), reduced libido, gynaecomastia, impotence, menstrual disturbances.

Dose and use

See Table 6.2. For patients being treated with topical **nystatin** suspension, **miconazole** oral gel or **amphotericin** lozenges (not UK), dentures should be removed temporarily before each dose is given. With all topical preparations food and drink should be avoided for 1h after each dose, and with **itraconazole** oral solution. Note:

- because **chlorhexidine** binds to **nystatin** and leads to inactivation of both drugs, **chlorhexidine** mouthwash should *not* be used at the same time as **nystatin** oral suspension.[14] The problem can be avoided if **chlorhexidine** is used ≥30min before **nystatin**
- the absorption of **ketoconazole** and **itraconazole** capsules is improved if taken with an acidic drink, e.g. cola.

Systemic drugs are more convenient than **nystatin**, and more suitable when candidosis involves the oesophagus. They also obviate the need for denture removal at each administration (although denture cleaning remains important; see Correct the correctable above).

Supply

Nystatin

Nystan® (Squibb)
Oral suspension 100,000 units/mL, 7 days @ 5mL q.d.s. = £10.

Miconazole

Daktarin® (Janssen-Cilag)
Oral gel 24mg/mL, 7 days @ 120mg q.d.s = £12.

Loramyc® (SpePharm)
Buccal tablet (muco-adhesive) 50mg, 7 days @ 50mg once daily = £23.

Fluconazole (generic)
Capsules 50mg, 150mg, 200mg, 7 days @ 50mg once daily = £1.

Diflucan® (Pfizer)
Capsules 50mg, 150mg, 200mg, 7 days @ 50mg once daily = £17.
Oral solution (powder for reconstitution) 50mg/5mL, 200mg/5mL, 7 days @ 50mg once daily = £17.

Itraconazole (generic)
Capsules (containing coated beads) 100mg, 14 days @100mg = £10.

Table 6.2 Antifungal treatment[15]

Class	*Drug*	*Recommended regimen*	*Comments*
Polyene group	Nystatin	Oral suspension 100,000 units/mL; 5mL q.d.s for 7 days (continue for 48h after lesions disappear); hold against lesions for at least 1min, and then swallow.	Smaller volumes make it more difficult to hold against lesions. The suspension has a high sugar content.
	Amphotericin (not UK)	Lozenges 10mg; 1 lozenge q.d.s for 10–14 days (continue for 48h after lesions disappear); place in the mouth and allow to dissolve.	Up to 2 lozenges q.d.s. in severe infections.
Azole group (imidazoles)	Miconazole	Oral gel 24mg/mL; 5–10mL oral gel q.d.s for 5–7 days (continue for 48h after lesions disappear); hold against lesions for as long as possible, and then swallow. Buccal tablet 50mg; attach 1 tablet to the upper gum once daily for 7–14 days.	Useful in management of angular cheilitis (has anti-staphylococcal action). Remove and brush dentures at night with gel.
	Ketoconazole	Tablet 200mg; 200mg once daily until symptoms have resolved (see text).	*Not* recommended as first line treatment (see text).
Azole group (triazoles)	Fluconazole	Capsules 50mg, 150mg, 200mg. Oral suspension 50mg/5mL and 200mg/5mL; 50–100mg once daily for 7 days.	Higher doses/longer courses may be required in immunosuppressed patients, and patients with more severe infections or those with dentures. No evidence to support a single 150mg dose for oral candidosis.
	Itraconazole	Capsules 100mg; 100mg once daily for 2 weeks. Oral solution 10mg/mL; 10–20mL b.d. for 2 weeks, use as a mouthwash and swallow.	Generally *not* used as first-line treatment. Higher doses may be required in immunosuppressed patients, and patients with more severe infections.

Sporanox® (Janssen-Cilag)
Capsules (containing coated beads) 100mg, 14 days @ 100mg once daily = £14.
Oral solution 10mg/mL, 14 days @ 100mg b.d. = £93.

Ketoconazole
Nizoral® (Janssen-Cilag)
Tablets 200mg, 7 days @ 200mg once daily = £3.50.

1 Finlay I and Davies A (2005) Fungal Infections. In: A Davies and I Finlay (eds) *Oral Care in Advanced Disease*. Oxford University Press, Oxford, pp. 55–71.
2 Davies AN *et al.* (2008) Oral candidosis in community-based patients with advanced cancer. *Journal of Pain and Symptom Management*. **35**: 508–514.
3 Davies AN *et al.* (2006) Oral candidosis in patients with advanced cancer. *Oral Oncology*. **42**: 698–702.
4 Samonis G *et al.* (1998) Oropharyngeal candidiasis as a marker for esophageal candidiasis in patients with cancer. *Clinical Infectious Diseases*. **27**: 283–286.
5 Samaranayake L (1990) Host factors and oral candidosis. In: L Samaranayake and T MacFarlane (eds) *Oral Candidosis*. Wright, London, pp. 66–103.
6 Bagg J *et al.* (2003) High prevalence of non-albicans yeasts and detection of anti-fungal resistance in the oral flora of patients with advanced cancer. *Palliative Medicine*. **17**: 477–481.
7 Sweeney P and Davies A (2010) Oral hygiene. In: A Davies and J Epstein (eds) *Oral Complications of Cancer and its Management*. Oxford University Press, Oxford, pp. 43–51.
8 Worthington HV *et al.* (2007) Interventions for treating oral candidiasis for patients with cancer receiving treatment. *Cochrane Database Systematic Reviews*. **1**: CD001972.pub 001972.
9 Davies A *et al.* (2006) Antifungal drug resistance amongst yeasts isolated from patients with advanced cancer. *Supportive Care in Cancer*. **14**: 645.
10 Baxter K (2011) Stockley's Drug Interactions (online edition). Pharmaceutical Press, London. Available from: www.medicinescomplete.com
11 Nyst MJ *et al.* (1992) Gentian violet, ketoconazole and nystatin in oropharyngeal and esophageal candidiasis in Zairian AIDS patients. *Annales de la Societe Belge de Medecine Tropicale*. **72**: 45–52.
12 Vazquez J (1999) Options for the management of mucosal candidiasis in patients with AIDS and HIV infection. *Pharmacotherapy*. **19**: 76–87.
13 MHRA (2008). Available from: www.mhra.gov.uk/Publications/Safetyguidance/DrugSafetyUpdate/CON014099
14 Barkvoll P and Attramadal A (1989) Effect of nystatin and chlorhexidine digluconate on Candida albicans. *Oral Surgery Oral Medicine and Oral Pathology*. **67**: 279–281.
15 Samaranayake K and Sitheeque M (2010) Oral fungal infections. In: A Davies and J Epstein (eds) *Oral Complications of Cancer and its Management*. Oxford University Press, Oxford, pp. 171–183.

METRONIDAZOLE — BNF 5.1.11 & 13.10.1.2

Class: Antibacterial and antiprotozoal.

Indications: Anaerobic and protozoal infections, *Helicobacter pylori* gastritis (see p.464), malodour caused by anaerobic infection (topical gel), †pseudomembranous colitis (see *Clostridium difficile* infection, p.461) bacterial vaginosis (vaginal gel).

Pharmacology

Metronidazole is highly active against anaerobic bacteria and protozoa. Although it has no activity against aerobic organisms *in vitro*, in mixed infections *in vivo* both aerobes and anaerobes appear susceptible. Unlike most other antibacterials, resistance to metronidazole among anaerobes is uncommon. Metronidazole can be applied topically to malodorous fungating cancers and decubitus ulcers.[1,2] The malodour is caused by volatile fatty acids produced by anaerobic bacteria. **Tinidazole** is similar to metronidazole with a longer duration of action; it causes less GI disturbance but costs more.[3]

Metronidazole is hepatically metabolized, and accumulation may occur in severe hepatic impairment; the resulting high plasma concentrations may exacerbate hepatic encephalopathy.
Bio-availability 100% PO; 60–80% PR; 20% PV.
Onset of action 20–60min PO; 5–12h PR.
Time to peak plasma concentration 1–2h PO; 3h PR.
Plasma halflife 6–11h.
Duration of action 8–12h.

Cautions

Metronidazole precipitates a **disulfiram**-like reaction with alcohol in about 25% of patients.[4,5] Like **disulfiram**, metabolites of metronidazole inhibit alcohol dehydrogenase, xanthine oxidase and aldehyde dehydrogenase. Inhibition of alcohol dehydrogenase leads to activation of microsomal enzyme oxidative pathways, generating ketones and lactate which may cause acidosis.[6] Xanthine oxidase inhibition can lead to noradrenaline (norepinephrine) excess.[6] Accumulation of acetaldehyde is probably responsible for most of the symptoms, e.g. flushing of the face and neck, headaches, epigastric discomfort, nausea and vomiting, and a fall in blood pressure.

Patients should be warned that if they drink alcohol when taking metronidazole they may have an unpleasant reaction, although generally this is little more than mild anorexia. However, the occasional patient may vomit profusely. The possibility of a reaction with liquid medicines containing alcohol, e.g. Oramorph®, should also be considered. In one patient, nausea and vomiting occurred during concurrent treatment with PO metronidazole and an alcohol-containing mouthwash (Corsodyl® mouthwash 30mL b.d.), some of which the patient swallowed rather than spitting out.[7] The risk of a reaction with metronidazole PV is small because absorption is low.[8]

Undesirable effects

Nausea and vomiting, unpleasant taste, furred tongue, GI disturbance. May cause darkening of urine; encephalopathy (very rare <0.01%); anaphylaxis has been reported.

Dose and use

In patients with incipient or actual hepatic encephalopathy, administer systemic doses once daily (i.e. reduce the daily dose to 1/3 of standard recommendation).

Metronidazole can be given PR if PO not possible: 1g PR q8h is equivalent to 400mg PO q8h (with or after food). Because prolonged rectal use causes proctitis, try to limit PR administration to 2–3 days or reduce to 1g PR q12h if PO medication cannot be restarted.

Anaerobic infections

Metronidazole 400mg PO t.d.s. for 2 weeks; 400mg PO b.d. in elderly debilitated patients, 400mg PO once daily if significant hepatic impairment.

Re-treat for 2 weeks if malodour or other symptoms and signs of infection recur, then continue indefinitely with 200mg b.d.

Fungating tumours

Metronidazole 0.75% gel is commercially available and should be applied topically liberally.[1,2,9,10] Some centres use a crushed 200mg tablet in lubricating gel.[11] The dose from a crushed tablet is several times greater than that from commercial products. The higher dose may have an observable impact (reduced odour) within 1 day compared with several days for commercial products, and is significantly cheaper. However, the lower concentration has been shown to be effective.[12,13]

Clostridium difficile infection (see p.461).

Helicobacter pylori gastritis (see p.464).

Supply

Metronidazole (generic)

Tablets 200mg, 400mg, 14 days @ 400mg t.d.s. = £2.50.

Oral suspension 200mg/5mL, 14 days @ 400mg t.d.s. = £34.

IV infusion 5mg/mL, 100mL = £3.50 (note: based on BNF pricing, this is *more expensive* than proprietary Metrolyl® injection).

Flagyl® (Winthrop)

Tablets 200mg, 400mg, 14 days @ 400mg t.d.s. = £19.

Oral suspension (Flagyl S®?) 200mg/5mL, 14 days @ 400mg t.d.s. = £47.

Suppositories 500mg, 1g, 3 days @ 1g t.d.s. and 11 days @ 1g b.d. = £72.

Metrolyl® (Sandoz)
Suppositories 500mg, 1g, 3 days @ 1g t.d.s. and 11 days @ 1g b.d. = £57.
IV infusion 5mg/mL, 100mL = £1.50 (note: based on BNF pricing, this is *cheaper* than generic injection).

Topical products
Anabact® (CHS)
Gel 0.75%, 15g = £4.50, 30g = £8.

Other topical metronidazole gels are available but are licensed for exacerbation of rosacea and are generally more expensive.

Crushed tablets in lubricating gel cost about £0.70 per topical application compared with £4.50 for proprietary gel.

Zidoval® (Meda)
Vaginal gel 0.75%, 40g pack with 5 applicators = £4.50.

1 Newman V *et al.* (1989) The use of metronidazole gel to control the smell of malodorous lesions. *Palliative Medicine*. **3**: 303–305.
2 Editorial (1990) Management of smelly tumours. *Lancet*. **335**: 141–142.
3 Carmine AA *et al.* (1982) Tinidazole in anaerobic infections: a review of its antibacterial activity, pharmacological properties and therapeutic efficacy. *Drugs*. **24**: 85–117.
4 deMattos H (1968) Relations between alcoholism and the gastrointestinal system. Experience using metronidazole. [In Portuguese]. *Hospital (Rio J)*. **74**: 1669–1676.
5 Penick S *et al.* (1969) Metronidazole in the treatment of alcoholism. *American Journal of Psychiatry*. **125**: 1063–1066.
6 Harries D *et al.* (1990) Metronidazole and alcohol: potential problems. *Scottish Medical Journal*. **35**: 179–180.
7 Dickman A (2007) *Personal communication*.
8 Plosker G (1987) Possible interaction between ethanol and vaginally administered metronidazole. *Clinical Pharmacy*. **6**: 189–193.
9 Ashford R *et al.* (1984) Double-blind trial of metronidazole in malodorous ulcerating tumours. *Lancet*. **1**: 1232–1233.
10 Thomas S and Hay N (1991) The antimicrobial properties of two metronidazole medicated dressings used to treat malodorous wounds. *Pharmaceutical Journal*. **246**: 264–266.
11 Twycross R *et al.* (2009) *Symptom Management in Advanced Cancer* (4e). palliativedrugs.com, Nottingham, p. 344.
12 Bower M *et al.* (1992) A double-blind study of the efficacy of metronidazole gel in the treatment of malodorous fungating tumours. *European Journal of Cancer*. **28A**: 888–889.
13 Finlay IG *et al.* (1996) The effect of topical 0.75% metronidazole gel on malodorous cutaneous ulcers. *Journal of Pain and Symptom Management*. **11**: 158–162.

URINARY TRACT INFECTIONS BNF 5.1.2, 5.1.8 & 5.1.13

Infections with strains of *Escherichia coli* and other Gram-negative bacilli which are resistant to several antibacterials, i.e. ESBL (Extended Spectrum Beta-Lactamase) positive enterobacteria, are increasing. Some are resistant to **gentamicin**, quinolones and cephalosporins as well as other antibacterials.[1]

This possibility should be considered in patients with recurrent urinary infection. Appropriate specimens (including blood cultures) should be taken and any previous microbiology reviewed. If a multiresistant isolate has been identified previously, e.g. a **gentamicin**-resistant coliform in urine, treatment should be discussed with a medical microbiologist because the usual first-line treatment may not be appropriate.

Urinary tract infection (UTI) is a common site of infection in terminally ill patients and, as in general medicine, *E. coli* is the commonest causal organism.[2] UTIs are more common in women than in men. Sixty percent of women in community settings presenting with suggestive symptoms have a UTI confirmed by microscopy and culture (MC&S).[3]

Diagnosis

If a woman has typical or severe symptoms and signs of a UTI, prompt empirical antibacterial treatment is indicated; dipstick testing (see below) is irrelevant.[3]

In the community in non-catheterized women, three symptoms independently predict UTI: cloudy urine, dysuria and recent-onset nocturia:
- presence of all three symptoms has a positive predictive value of 82%
- absence of all three symptoms had a negative predictive value of 67%.[3,4]

Thus, using a symptom score alone will lead to a missed diagnosis in about 1/3 of UTIs.

With dipsticks, nitrites are most predictive, followed by leucocytes (leucocyte esterase+ or greater) and blood (haemolysed trace or greater). For dipstick tests in combination:
- nitrite+ and *either* blood+ *or* leucocyte esterase+; positive predictive value 92%
- nitrite+ or leucocyte esterase and blood *both*+; positive predictive value about 80%
- nitrite, leucocyte esterase and blood *all*−; negative predictive value 76% (Box 6.A).[3,4]

Thus, the use of a dipstick alone will lead to a missed diagnosis in about 1/4 of UTIs.

Box 6.A Urine dipsticks and the diagnosis of UTIs in non-catheterized women with few or mild symptoms

Use a urine dipstick which measures urinary pH and specific gravity, and the presence and amount of:
- glucose
- ketone
- blood
- protein
- nitrite, a bacterial metabolite
- leucocyte esterase (produced by inflammation/infection).

When to do the test
- if patient has few or mild symptoms of UTI
- if typical or severe symptoms of UTI, prescribe an antibacterial in accord with local policy without using a dipstick.

How to do the test
- clean external genitalia with sterile 0.9% sodium chloride
- take a mid-stream specimen of urine (or in-and-out catheter sample under aseptic conditions)
- dip the whole strip into the urine container and remove immediately
- drag the edge of the strip against the container rim to remove excess urine and start timing
- compare each test pad on the strip to the corresponding row of colour blocks on the bottle label
- read each test pad at the time shown on the bottle, starting with the shortest time first.

Late readings are of no value.

Significance of the results

Nitrite positive or leucocyte and blood positive or all three positive: make a working diagnosis of UTI; prescribe an antibacterial in accord with local policy. Urine specimen for MC&S *not* required unless risk factors present e.g. recent hospital admission, recurrent UTIs.

Nitrite, leucocyte and blood all negative: tentatively exclude UTI; do *not* send urine specimen for MC&S unless definite urinary tract symptoms.

If empirical treatment fails in a woman, urine should be sent for MC&S to confirm the diagnosis and guide antibacterial choice. A negative culture may suggest an alternative diagnosis, e.g. urethritis caused by sexually transmitted infections (STIs, e.g. *Chlamydia*, *Neisseria*, *Trichomonas*) or interstitial cystitis.

MC&S should also be done routinely in patients at risk of a complicated UTI. For example, those with:
- impaired immunity, e.g. from immunosuppressive treatment or poorly controlled diabetes mellitus
- moderate–severe renal impairment

- an abnormal urinary tract
- a recent hospital admission.

In men who have a suspected UTI, send urine for MC&S before starting antibacterials.

In frail, elderly and hospitalized patients, diagnosis of a UTI is harder. *Symptom scores and dipsticks are less reliable.* Thus, unless there are symptoms or signs of systemic infection, delay starting an antibacterial until the results of MC&S are available.[3,5,6]

Management

Remember: always ask about drug allergies before prescribing an antibacterial.
The dose and frequency of many antibacterials are reduced in renal impairment.

If symptoms are moderate–severe, or urine dipstick test is positive, start antibacterial treatment according to local guidelines. Alternatively, consider:

- **trimethoprim** 200mg PO b.d.[3,7]
- **nitrofurantoin** 50mg PO q.d.s. or 100mg m/r PO b.d. *or*
- **co-amoxiclav** 375mg PO t.d.s. and **amoxicillin** 250mg PO t.d.s. (or **co-amoxiclav** 625mg PO t.d.s. whichever is cheaper locally).

Recommendations vary in relation to duration of antibacterial treatment from 3 days for an uncomplicated UTI in a woman to 7–14 days for children, men, and women with fever and/or loin pain (i.e. possible pyelonephritis).

If the patient is systemically unwell, or has pyelonephritis, consider IV **co-amoxiclav** 1.2g t.d.s. (but if history of penicillin allergy, give **ciprofloxacin** PO or IV instead, according to local guidelines). A single dose of IV **gentamicin** 5mg/kg should be given if there is severe sepsis or septic shock. Second-line antibacterials vary from region to region; if necessary, consult a medical microbiologist.

In catheterized patients, bacterial colonization is normal and is not necessarily harmful; it should not be investigated unless symptomatic. If UTI is clinically suspected, do not perform a urine dipstick test because it is unreliable but send urine for MC&S and start empirical treatment with either **trimethoprim** or **nitrofurantoin** (as above) for 7 days.[8] Do not use **trimethoprim** empirically if the patient has a history of recurrent UTIs or has taken **trimethoprim** in the last year. Changing the catheter before starting antibacterials for UTI improves clinical and bacteriological cure rates.[3,9]

Prophylactic antibacterials for routine catheter changes are not recommended unless the patient has a history of UTI associated with catheter changes.[3] However, antibacterial treatment for 2 days before removal of a catheter significantly reduces the risk of a subsequent UTI.[10,11]

Trimethoprim 300mg as a single-dose treatment is useful in frail patients, resulting in a 74% and 71% cure rate when tested 1 and 6 weeks later.[12,13] In patients with symptoms of a UTI after catheter removal, the cure rate for a single dose of **trimethoprim** was 79%, compared with a 10-day treatment cure rate of 81%, i.e. statistically identical.[10]

Alternative approaches

In catheterized patients, consider a urinary antiseptic to help prevent recurrent UTIs (but *not* for treatment), e.g. **methenamine hippurate** (see p.529) or **cranberry juice** (see p.531).

Supply

Amoxicillin (generic)
Capsules 250mg, 500mg, 7 days @ 250mg t.d.s. = £1.
Oral suspension 125mg/5mL, 250mg/5mL, 7 days @ 250mg t.d.s. = £1.50.

Co-amoxiclav (generic)
Tablets 250/125 (amoxicillin 250mg, clavulanic acid 125mg), 7 days @ 375mg t.d.s. = £3.
Tablets 500/125 (amoxicillin 500mg, clavulanic acid 125mg), 7 days @ 625mg t.d.s. = £6.
Oral suspension 250/62 (amoxicillin 250mg as trihydrate, clavulanic acid 62.5mg as potassium salt)/5mL 7 days @ 5mL or 10mL t.d.s = £6 or £12 respectively.
Injection (powder for reconstitution) 1000/200 (amoxicillin 1,000mg as sodium salt, clavulanic acid 200mg as potassium salt) 1.2g = £2.50.

Ciprofloxacin (generic)
Tablets 100mg, 250mg, 500mg, 750mg, 7 days @ 500mg b.d. = £1.
Infusion 2mg/mL, 400mg (200mL) bottle = £22.

Nitrofurantoin (generic)
Tablets 50mg, 100mg, 7 days @ 50mg q.d.s. = £2.
Oral suspension 25mg/5mL, 7 days @ 50mg q.d.s. = £65.

Macrobid® (Goldshield)
Capsules m/r 100mg, 7 days @ 100mg b.d. = £5.

Trimethoprim (generic)
Tablets 100mg, 200mg, 7 days @ 200mg b.d. = £1.
Oral suspension 50mg/5mL, 7 days @ 200mg b.d. = £8.

Gentamicin sulphate (generic)
Injection 40mg/mL, 1mL amp, 2mL amp, 2mL vial all = £1.50.

1 D'Agata EM (2004) Rapidly rising prevalence of nosocomial multidrug-resistant, Gram-negative bacilli: a 9-year surveillance study. *Infection Control and Hospital Epidemiology.* **25**: 842–846.
2 Vitetta L *et al.* (2000) Bacterial infections in terminally ill hospice patients. *Journal of Pain and Symptom Management.* **20**: 326–334.
3 CKS (2009) UTI in women. Available from: www.cks.nhs.uk/urinary_tract_infection_lower_women# (accessed June 2010)
4 Little P *et al.* (2009) Dipsticks and diagnostic algorithms in urinary tract infection: development and validation, randomised trial, economic analysis, observational cohort and qualitative study. *Health Technology Assessment.* **13**: iii–iv, ix–xi, 1–73.
5 Singh S et al. (2007) Treatment of Urinary Tract Iinfections in the Older Person. Medicines Information Leaflet. Vol 4 No.10. Oxford Radcliffe Hospital, Oxford.
6 CKS (2010) UTI in men. Available from: www.cks.nhs.uk/urinary_tract_infection_lower_men# (accessed June 2010)
7 Oxford Hospitals Adult Inpatient Pocket Antimicrobial Guide (2009) *Urinary tract infection.*
8 Schwartz DS and Barone JE (2006) Correlation of urinalysis and dipstick results with catheter-associated urinary tract infections in surgical ICU patients. *Intensive Care Medicine.* **32**: 1797–1801.
9 Raz R *et al.* (2000) Chronic indwelling catheter replacement before antimicrobial therapy for symptomatic urinary tract infection. *Journal of Urology.* **164**: 1254–1258.
10 Harding GK *et al.* (1991) How long should catheter-acquired urinary tract infection in women be treated? A randomized controlled study. *Annals of Internal Medicine.* **114**: 713–719.
11 Hustinx W *et al.* (1991) Impact of concurrent antimicrobial therapy on catheter-associated urinary tract infection. *Journal of Hospital Infection.* **18**: 45–56.
12 Brumfitt W *et al.* (1982) Comparative trial of trimethoprim and co-trimoxazole in recurrent urinary infections. *Infection.* **10**: 280–284.
13 Bailey R and Abbott G (1978) Treatment of urinary tract infection with a single dose of trimethoprim-sulfamethoxazole. *Canadian Medical Association Journal.* **118**: 551–552.

CELLULITIS IN A LYMPHOEDEMATOUS LIMB

Cellulitis, also called an acute inflammatory episode (AIE), is common in lymphoedema:
- mild: pain, increased swelling, erythema (well-defined or blotchy)
- severe: extensive erythema with well-defined margins, increased swelling, blistering and weeping skin; often accompanied by fever, nausea and vomiting, pain and, when the leg is affected, difficulty in walking.[1]

Management strategy
Preventive measures
Patients should be educated about:
- why they are susceptible to cellulitis, i.e. skin crevices harbour bacteria, reduced immunity[2]
- the consequences of cellulitis, i.e. increased swelling, more fibrosis, decreased response to compression treatment
- the importance of daily skin care to improve and maintain skin integrity. Risk factors for cellulitis include cracked or macerated interdigital skin, dermatitis, limb wounds (including leg ulcers), and weeping lymphangiectasia (leaking lymph blisters on the skin surface)

- reducing risk by, for example, reducing the swelling, protecting hands when gardening, cleaning cuts, treating fungal infections (e.g. **clotrimazole** 1% or **terbinafine** 1% cream b.d. for 2 weeks) and ingrowing toenails[3]
- the importance of seeking prompt medical attention and treatment; in situations when accessing medical care may be difficult, e.g. holidays, provide a 2-week supply of amoxicillin 500mg q8h (erythromycin 500mg q6h for those allergic to penicillin) to patients who have had cellulitis in the past.

Non-drug treatment

- compression garments should not be worn until the limb is comfortable
- daily skin hygiene should be continued; washing and gentle drying
- emollients should not be used in the affected area if the skin is broken
- if severe, bed rest is essential with the affected limb elevated in a comfortable position and supported on pillows.[3,4]

Drug treatment

Remember: always ask about drug allergies before prescribing an antibacterial.
The dose and frequency of many antibacterials are reduced in renal impairment.

Cellulitis should be treated promptly with antibacterials to prevent increased morbidity from increased swelling and accelerated fibrosis (see Quick practice guide, p.459). It is often difficult to isolate the responsible pathogen. Although cellulitis in a non-lymphoedematous limb may commonly be caused by *Staphylococcus aureus*,[5] most cellulitis in a lymphoedematous limb is believed to be caused by Group A *Streptococci*.[1,6,7] The advice of the British Lymphology Society/ Lymphoedema Support Network (www.thebls.com, October 2010) is summarized in Table 6.3.

The advice of a medical microbiologist should be obtained in unusual circumstances, e.g. cellulitis developing shortly after an animal lick or bite, and when the inflammation fails to respond to the recommended antibacterials.

Remember: Cellulitis is painful: analgesics should be prescribed regularly and p.r.n. Because of a possible relationship between skin infections, NSAIDs and necrotizing fasciitis, paracetamol and opioids are the preferred analgesics.[8,9]

Supply

Amoxicillin (generic)
Capsules 250mg, 500mg, 14 days @ 500mg t.d.s. = £3.
Oral suspension 125mg/5mL, 250mg/5mL, 14 days @ 500mg t.d.s. = £8.
Injection (powder for reconstitution) containing **amoxicillin** (as sodium salt) 1g vial = £1.

Flucloxacillin sodium (generic)
Capsules 250mg, 500mg, 14 days @ 500mg q.d.s. = £5.
Oral solution 125mg/5mL, 250mg/5mL, 14 days @ 500mg q.d.s. = £160.
Injection (powder for reconstitution) 1g vial = £5.

Erythromycin (generic)
Capsules enclosing e/c granules **erythromycin** 250mg, 14 days @ 500mg q.d.s. or 250mg once daily = £24 and £3 respectively.
Tablets e/c 250mg, 14 days @ 500mg q.d.s. or 250mg once daily = £8 and £1 respectively.
Oral suspension **erythromycin** (as ethyl succinate) 125mg/5mL, 250mg/5mL, 500mg/5mL, 14 days @ 500mg q.d.s. or 250mg once daily = £12 and £2.50 respectively.

Clarithromycin (generic)
Tablets 250mg, 500mg, 14 days @ 500mg b.d. or 250mg once daily = £11 and £3 respectively.

Klaricid® (Abbott)
Tablets **clarithromycin** 250mg, 500mg, 14 days @ 500mg b.d. or 250mg once daily = £23 and £7 respectively.
Oral suspension **clarithromycin** 125mg/5mL, 250mg/5mL, 14 days @ 500mg b.d. or 250mg once daily = £43 and £11 respectively.

Table 6.3 Antibacterials for cellulitis[a]

Situation	*First-line antibacterials*	*If allergic to penicillin*	*Second-line antibacterials*	*Comments*
Acute cellulitis + septicaemia (inpatient admission)	Amoxicillin 2g IV q8h *or* flucloxacillin 2g IV q6h[b,c]	Clindamycin 600mg IV q6h[10]	Clindamycin 600mg IV q6h (if poor or no response by 48h)	Switch to amoxicillin 500mg PO q8h or flucloxacillin 500mg PO q6h or clindamycin 300mg PO q6h when: • temperature down for 48h • inflammation much resolved • falling CRP. Then continue as below.
Acute cellulitis (home care)	Amoxicillin 500mg q8h[c]	Erythromycin[e] 500mg q6h *or* clarithromycin[e] 500mg q12h	Clindamycin 300mg q6h. If fails to resolve, convert to first-line IV regimen above	Give for a minimum of 2 weeks. Continue antibacterials until the acute inflammation has completely resolved; in severe cases this may take 1–2 months. (Note: residual 'staining' may persist beyond this.)
Prophylaxis if 2+ episodes of cellulitis per year	Phenoxymethylpenicillin 500mg once daily (1g if weight >75kg)	Erythromycin[e] 250mg once daily *or* clarithromycin[e] 250mg once daily	Clindamycin 150mg once daily *or* cefalexin 250mg once daily *or* doxycycline 50mg once daily	Continue for 2 years, after 1 year, halve the dose of phenoxymethylpenicillin; if an AIE develops after dose reduction/ discontinuation, treat the acute episode and then commence *life-long* prophylaxis
Emergency supply of antibacterials (in case of need when away from home)	Amoxicillin 500mg q8h	Erythromycin[e] 500mg q6h *or* clarithromycin[e] 500mg q12h	If fails to resolve, or the patient becomes generally unwell, convert to first-line IV regimen above	

a. PO unless stated otherwise
b. many hospital guidelines recommend single agent flucloxacillin[6]
c. gentamicin 5mg/kg IV daily for 1 week should be added if the anogenital region is involved, adjust dose according to renal function and assay
d. if *Staphylococcus aureus* infection suspected (folliculitis, pus formation, crusted dermatitis), flucloxacillin 500mg q6h should be added or used as a single agent
e. for patients taking astemizole, tolterodine or statins, do *not* prescribe macrolide antibacterials (clarithromycin, erythromycin); use cefalexin (but not in patients with a history of serious penicillin allergy, i.e. anaphylaxis) or doxycycline; see p.460.

Clindamycin (generic)
Capsules **clindamycin** (as hydrochloride) 150mg, 14 days @ 300mg q.d.s. or 150mg once daily = £84 and £11 respectively (note: based on BNF pricing, this is *more expensive* than proprietary Dalacin C® capsules).

Dalacin C® (Pharmacia)
Capsules **clindamycin** (as hydrochloride) 75mg, 150mg, 14 days @ 300mg q.d.s. or 150mg once daily = £64 and £8 respectively (note: based on BNF pricing, this is *cheaper* than generic capsules).
Injection **clindamycin** (as phosphate) 150mg/mL, 4mL amp = £13.

Gentamicin sulphate (generic)
Injection 40mg/mL, 1mL amp, 2mL amp, 2mL vial all = £1.50.

Phenoxymethylpenicillin potassium (generic)
Tablets 250mg, 14 days @ 500mg once daily = £2.50.
Oral solution 125mg/5mL, 250mg/5mL, 14 days @ 500mg once daily = £5.

Cefalexin (generic)
Capsules 250mg, 500mg, 14 days @ 250mg once daily = £1.
Tablets 250mg, 500mg, 14 days @ 250mg once daily = £1.
Oral solution 125mg/5mL, 250mg/5mL, 14 days @ = 250mg once daily £2.50.

Doxycycline (generic)
Capsules (as hyclate) 50mg, 100mg, 14 days @ 50mg once daily = £1.

Also see **Trimethoprim** (p.455).

1 Mortimer P (2000) Acute inflammatory episodes. In: RG Twycross *et al.* (eds) *Lymphoedema*. Radcliffe Medical Press, Oxford, pp. 130–139.
2 Mallon E *et al.* (1997) Evidence for altered cell-mediated immunity in postmastectomy lymphoedema. *British Journal of Dermatology*. **137**: 928–933.
3 Twycross R *et al.* (2000) *Lymphoedema*. Radcliffe Medical Press, Oxford.
4 Twycross RG *et al.* (2007) *Symptom Management in Advanced Cancer* (4e). Palliativedrugs.com Ltd, Nottingham.
5 Chira S and Miller LG (2010) Staphylococcus aureus is the most common identified cause of cellulitis: a systematic review. *Epidemiology Infection*. **138**: 313–317.
6 Leman P and Mukherjee D (2005) Flucloxacillin alone or combined with benzylpenicillin to treat lower limb cellulitis: a randomised controlled trial. *Emergency Medical Journal*. **22**: 342–346.
7 Cox NH (2008) Streptococcal cellulitis/erysipelas of the lower leg. In: William H et al (ed) *Evidence-Based Dermatology 2nd edition*. Blackwell Publishing, Oxford, pp. 406–417.
8 Anonymous (2007) Necrotising fasciitis, dermal infections and NSAIDs: caution. *Prescrire International*. **16**: 17.
9 British Lymphology Society. Available from: www.thebls.com
10 Bisno AL and Stevens DL (1996) Streptococcal infections of skin and soft tissues. *New England Journal of Medicine*. **334**: 240–245.

Quick Practice Guide: Cellulitis in Lymphoedema

Cellulitis is often associated with septicaemia (e.g. fever, flu-like symptoms, hypotension, tachycardia, delirium, nausea and vomiting). It may be difficult to identify the infective agent, but *Streptococcus* is the mostly likely pathogen.

Evaluation

1 Clinical features
- mild: pain, increased swelling, erythema (well-defined or blotchy)
- severe: extensive erythema with well-defined margins, increased swelling, blistering and weeping skin; often accompanied by fever, nausea and vomiting, pain and, when the leg is affected, difficulty in walking.

2 Diagnosis is based on pattern recognition and clinical judgement. The following information should be solicited:
- present history: date of onset, precipitating factor (e.g. insect bite or trauma), treatment received to date
- past history: details of previous cellulitis, precipitating factors, antibacterials taken
- examination: include sites of lymphatic drainage to and from inflamed area.

3 Establish a baseline
- extent and severity of rash: if well demarcated outline with pen and date
- level of systemic upset: temperature, pulse, BP, CRP, white cell count
- swab cuts or breaks in skin for microbiology before starting antibacterials.

4 Arrange admission to hospital for patients with septicaemia or who deteriorate or fail to improve despite antibacterials.

Antibacterials

5 To prevent increased swelling and accelerated fibrosis, cellulitis should be treated promptly with antibacterials *for a minimum of 2 weeks*. Continue antibacterials until the acute inflammation has completely resolved; this may take 1–2 months.

6 The advice of a microbiologist should be obtained in unusual circumstances, e.g. cellulitis developing shortly after an animal bite, and when the inflammation fails to respond to the recommended antibacterials.

7 Standard treatment at home (PO)

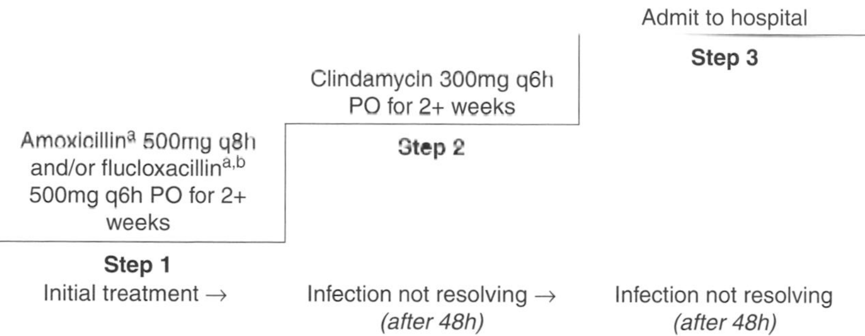

a. if a history of penicillin allergy, erythromycin 500mg q6h or clarithromycin 500mg q12h.

b. add or use as single agent if features suggest *Staphylococcus aureus* infection, e.g. folliculitis, pus, crusted dermatitis.

continued

8 Standard treatment in hospital (IV): choice of antibacterials may vary with local policy. The following are the recommendations of the British Lymphology Society and Lymphoedema Support Network. Switch to PO amoxicillin, flucloxacillin or clindamycin when no fever for 48h, inflammation settling and CRP falling (see 7 above).

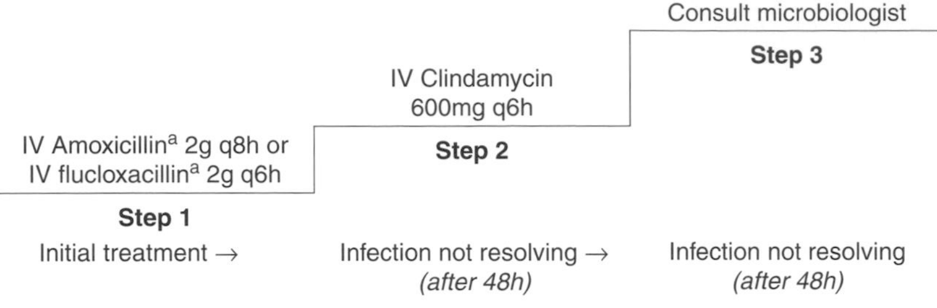

a. if a history of penicillin allergy, start on Step 2.

9 For anogenital cellulitis, first line treatment is amoxicillin 2g IV q8h plus gentamicin 5mg/kg IV once daily; the dose of the latter to be adjusted according to renal function and assay.

10 If ≥2 episodes of cellulitis/year, review skin condition and skin care regimen, and consider further steps to reduce limb swelling. Start antibacterial prophylaxis with:
- phenoxymethylpenicillin 500mg (1g in those >75kg) once daily for two years; halve the dose after one year if no recurrence
- if allergic to penicillin, erythromycin or clarithromycin 250mg once daily (but see 11 below)
- if cellulitis develops despite antibacterials, consider other once daily prophylactic antibacterials e.g. clindamycin 150mg, cefalexin 250mg or doxycycline 50mg; advice from a medical microbiologist and local specialist lymphoedema service is advised
- if cellulitis develops after discontinuation of antibacterials after 2 years, treat the acute episode, and then commence life-long prophylaxis
- if the patient has recurrent ano-genital cellulitis, give trimethoprim 100mg at bedtime.

11 Check for important drug interactions with macrolide antibacterials (clarithromycin, erythromycin) and, particularly, statins, astemizole or tolterodine (avoid concurrent use); alternative antibacterials are cefalexin 500mg q8h (but not in patients with a history of severe penicillin allergy) or doxycycline 200mg once daily stat, then 100mg once daily. For prophylaxis, prescribe cefalexin 250mg or doxycycline 50mg once daily.

General

12 Remember:
- if severe, bed rest and elevation of the affected limb on pillows is essential
- cellulitis is painful; analgesics should be prescribed regularly and p.r.n. It is recommended that NSAIDs are avoided as there may be an increased risk of necrotizing fasciitis.
- compression garments should not be worn until limb is comfortable
- daily skin hygiene should be continued; washing and gentle drying
- emollients should not be used in the affected area if the skin is broken.

13 Patients should be educated about cellulitis:
- why they are susceptible, i.e. skin crevices harbour bacteria, reduced immunity
- consequences, i.e. increased swelling, more fibrosis, decreased response to compression
- importance of daily skin care to improve and maintain skin integrity
- reducing risk, e.g. by protecting hands when gardening, cleaning cuts, treating fungal infections (terbinafine cream once daily for two weeks) and ingrowing toenails
- obtaining prompt medical attention if cellulitis occurs and, if a history of cellulitis, taking a 2-week supply of amoxicillin 500mg q8h (erythromycin 500mg q6h or clarithromycin 500mg q12h if allergic to penicillin) for emergency use when away from home.

CLOSTRIDIUM DIFFICILE INFECTION BNF 1.5, 5.1.7 & 5.1.11

Clostridium difficile infection is a complication of antibacterial treatment, particularly broad-spectrum antibacterials. A pseudomembranous colitis develops in severe cases (Box 6.B), with sloughing of the inflamed colonic epithelium. This manifests as foul-smelling diarrhoea mingled with mucus and blood. *C. difficile* infection has a mortality of up to 25% in elderly frail patients.[1] In England, NHS Trusts are obliged to report all cases of *C. difficile* infection in anyone over 2 years old, and regular updates on infection rates and outcomes are published by the Health Protection Agency (available from: www.hpa.org.uk/Topics/InfectiousDiseases/InfectionsAZ/ClostridiumDifficile/).

Box 6.B *Clostridium difficile* infection

Causal antibacterials[2]

Highest risk
Cephalosporins (second/third generation)
Clindamycin
Fluoroquinolones

Medium risk
Amoxicillin/ampicillin
Co-amoxiclav
Macrolides

Low risk
Aminoglycosides
Benzylpenicillin
Piptazobactam
Tetracyclines
Trimethoprim
Vancomycin

Clinical features
Watery diarrhoea + mucus ± blood
Abdominal pain and tenderness + tenesmus
Fever and malaise
± Nausea, vomiting, and anorexia
± Dehydration and delirium
± Leukocytosis

Symptoms generally begin within 1 week of starting antibacterial treatment or shortly after stopping, but may occur up to 2 months later.[3] It is caused by colonization of the GI tract by *C. difficile* and the production of toxins A and B which cause the mucosal damage. A failure to mount an immune response is associated with colonization and toxin production.

Although associated with hospital admission (Box 6.C), community-acquired cases are becoming more common.[4]

C. difficile is spread indirectly by the faecal–oral route by spores left on surfaces:

- asymptomatic colonization in the general population is about 5%
- asymptomatic colonization in hospital and nursing home populations may be ≤30%[3]
- in about 33% of those colonized, *C. difficile* produces diarrhoea-producing toxins.[6]

Diagnosis

- a high level of suspicion in high-risk patients who develop diarrhoea, e.g. >300mL of liquid faeces in 1 day or 2–6 loose stools in 36h, but the use of opioids, including **diphenoxlate** and **loperamide**, may modify the clinical picture, particularly in mild–moderate cases
- *C. difficile* is strongly anaerobic and difficult to culture; most laboratories no longer attempt to culture it routinely for diagnostic purposes, although molecular genetic methods may be used for typing and surveillance of particularly virulent strains[4,7]
- diagnosis is confirmed by the detection in the faeces of toxins produced by *C. difficile*[4,7]

- if in doubt, endoscopy, a CT scan or rectal biopsy may be of value, but endoscopy identifies pseudomembranous colitis in only about 50% of cases confirmed by laboratory criteria (a positive culture for *C difficile* and a positive faecal cytotoxin test)[4,8]
- a trial of therapy may be the most practical way of confirming the diagnosis.

Box 6.C Risk factors for *Clostridium difficile* infection

Patient-related factors
Age > 65 years
Previous infection with *C. difficile*

Treatment-related factors
Prolonged hospital admission: 1% incidence if < 1 week but 50% if > 4 weeks[5]
GI procedures (non-surgical or surgical)
Nasogastric tubes
PPIs
Radiotherapy

Antibacterial use
Prolonged antibacterial treatment
Use of high and medium risk antibacterials (see Box 6.B)

Underlying disease states
Cancer
COPD
Renal failure
Immunosuppression

Management strategy

Preventive measures

Spread of *C. difficile* is by the ingestion of spores from the environment around symptomatic patients. Environmental controls ('universal precautions') will generally prevent the spread of outbreaks:

- patients should be isolated while they have diarrhoea, and have their own commode
- carers should use gloves, gowns and disposable aprons when caring for infected patients and handling body fluids
- carers should thoroughly wash their hands before and after patient contact using antibacterial soap and water; *alcohol-based hand rubs are ineffective against C. difficile spores*[4]
  - ▷ the WHO produces a downloadable chart illustrating correct hand-washing technique (available from: www.who.int/gpsc/tools/Pocket-Leaflet.pdf)
- areas where there are patients with *C. difficile* should be thoroughly cleaned using chlorine disinfectants.[7,9]

Antibacterial prescribing policies should aim to minimize the use of broad-spectrum antibacterials, and to regulate treatment duration.[2,4,7,9]

Drug treatment

Metronidazole PO is the treatment of choice; it is as effective as **vancomycin** for mild–moderate infections, and much cheaper.[4,7,10] IV **metronidazole** has been used in patients unable to take oral formulations but treatment failures have occurred.[3]

Vancomycin must be given PO or PR, because it is not secreted into the GI tract after IV administration.[11] It is generally reserved for:

- patients with an ileus
- patients with severe infection, i.e. with any of the following: WBC > 15 × 10^9/L, acutely rising plasma creatinine (> 50% above baseline), temperature > 38.5°C, clinical or radiographic evidence of severe colitis[7]
- patients unable to tolerate **metronidazole** or being treated with alcohol-containing solutions (see p.451)
- non-responders to **metronidazole**.

UK guidelines recommend IV **metronidazole** with high-dose PO or intracolonic **vancomycin** in severe cases which have not responded to low-dose **vancomycin** or with life-threatening infection.[7]

Most patients show some symptom improvement in <2 days, e.g. reduction of fever. However, resolution of diarrhoea may take ≥6 days.[4] Other antibacterials are sometimes used.[7,11]

Dose and use

- **metronidazole:**
  - ▹ 400–500mg PO t.d.s. for 10–14 days for initial treatment of mild–moderate cases[7,12,13]
  - ▹ 500mg IV t.d.s. may be given in addition to high-dose PO or intracolonic **vancomycin** in severe cases which have not responded to low-dose **vancomycin** or in life-threatening infection[7]
- **vancomycin:**
  - ▹ 125mg PO q.d.s. for 10–14 days [7]
  - ▹ increase to 500mg PO q.d.s. if infection is severe, life-threatening, or fails to respond to low-dose treatment[7] *or*
  - ▹ if life-threatening, 500mg q.d.s. may be administered by the intracolonic (rectal) route.[7]

Relapse

About 20% of patients relapse, most in ≤3 weeks.[7,12] This may be caused by germination of residual spores within the colon, re-infection with *C. difficile* (50% of recurrences are caused by infection with a new strain)[13] or further antibacterial treatment:

- although mild relapses often resolve spontaneously, repeat treatment with **metronidazole** for 10–14 days is recommended[7,12]
- for a second or third relapse, or if the first relapse is severe, treat with **vancomycin** 125mg PO q.d.s. for 10–14 days
- for repeated relapses, consider prolonged treatment with a slowly decreasing dose of **vancomycin**, e.g. over 6 weeks:[7,13]
  - ▹ week 1, 125mg q.d.s.
  - ▹ week 2, 125mg b.d.
  - ▹ week 3, 125mg once daily
  - ▹ week 4, 125mg every other day
  - ▹ week 5 and 6, 125mg every 3 days
- this latter intermittent therapy allows spores to germinate on 'no antibacterial' days with subsequent destruction on 'antibacterial' days
- some centres add **rifampicin** 300mg PO b.d. for 10–14 days.[7,14]

Relapse because of resistance of *C. difficile* to antibacterial treatment is rare.[15]

Probiotics may reduce the incidence of relapse,[16–18] but are not used routinely, and are not recommended by UK guidelines.[7] Monoclonal antibodies against *C. difficile* toxins A and B are being investigated for the prevention of recurrence of *C. difficile* infection in patients already being treated with **metronidazole** or **vancomycin**.[19,20]

Supply

See **metronidazole**, p.450.

Vancomycin (generic)
Capsules 125mg, 250mg, 10 days @ 125mg q.d.s. = £189.
Injection (powder for reconstitution) 500mg, 1g vial = £7 and £15 respectively.

Vancocin® (Flynn)
Matrigel capsules 125mg, 10 days @ 125mg q.d.s. = £125.
Injection (powder for reconstitution) 500mg, 1g vial = £8 and £16 respectively.

Vancomycin *injection can be used to prepare an oral solution; add 10mL WFI to a 500mg vial of powder and give 2.5mL (125mg) q.d.s. diluted with water or fruit juice (other than grapefruit), 10-day course = £70.*

1 Pepin J *et al.* (2004) Clostridium difficile-associated diarrhea in a region of Quebec from 1991 to 2003: a changing pattern of disease severity. *Canadian Medical Association Journal.* **171**: 466–472.
2 Monaghan T *et al.* (2008) Recent advances in Clostridium difficile-associated disease. *Gut.* **57**: 850–860.

3 Fekety R (1997) Guidelines for the diagnosis and management of Clostridium difficile-associated diarrhea and colitis. American College of Gastroenterology, Practice Parameters Committee. *American Journal of Gastroenterology*. **92**: 739–750.
4 Shannon-Lowe J *et al.* (2010) Prevention and medical management of Clostridium difficile infection. *British Medical Journal*. **340**: c1296.
5 Johnson S *et al.* (1990) Nosocomial Clostridium difficile colonisation and disease. *Lancet*. **336**: 97–100.
6 Starr J (2005) Clostridium difficile associated diarrhoea: diagnosis and treatment. *British Medical Journal*. **331**: 498–501.
7 Department of Health (2009) Clostridium difficile infection: how to deal with the problem. Available from: www.dh.gov.uk/en/Publicationsandstatistics/Publications/PublicationsPolicyAndGuidance/DH_093220
8 Gerding DN *et al.* (1995) Clostridium difficile associated diarrhoea and colitis. Clinical Practice Guidelines by the Society for Healthcare Epidemiology (SHEA) and the Infectious Diseases Society of America (ISDA). Infection control and hospital epidemiology. 16.459–477. Available from: www.shea-online.org/Assets/files/position_papers/Cldiff95.PDF
9 Donaldson L and Beasley C (2005) Infection caused by Clostridium difficile. Letter from the Chief Medical Officer and Chief Nursing Officer. Department of Health. Available from: www.dh.gov.uk/en/Publicationsandstatistics/Lettersandcirculars/Professionalletters/Chiefmedicalofficerletters/DH_4125069
10 BNF (2011) Section 1.5. In: *British National Formulary (No 61)*. British Medical Association and Royal Pharmaceutical Society of Great Britain, London. Current BNF available from www.bnf.org.
11 Durai R (2007) Epidemiology, pathogenesis, and management of Clostridium difficile infection. *Digestive Diseases and Sciences*. **52**: 2958–2962.
12 Gilbert DN *et al.* (eds) (2008) *The Sanford guide to antimicrobial therapy 2008. Antimicrobial Therapy Inc, Sperryville.*
13 Malnick SD and Zimhony O (2002) Treatment of Clostridium difficile-associated diarrhea. *Annals of Pharmacotherapy*. **36**: 1767–1775.
14 Blondel-Hill E and Fryters S (eds) (2006) Bugs & Drugs (online edition) Capital Health. Edmonton. Available from: www.bugsanddrugs.ca/bugs_drugs_website/web-content/COMBINED_BandD2006_certified.pdf
15 Bricker E *et al.* (2005) Antibiotic treatment for Clostridium difficile-associated diarrhea in adults. *Cochrane Database of Systematic Reviews*. CD004610.
16 Surawicz CM *et al.* (2000) The search for a better treatment for recurrent Clostridium difficile disease: use of high-dose vancomycin combined with Saccharomyces boulardii. *Clinical Infectious Diseases*. **31**: 1012–1017.
17 Dendukuri N *et al.* (2005) Probiotic therapy for the prevention and treatment of Clostridium difficile-associated diarrhea: a systematic review. *Canadian Medical Association Journal*. **173**: 167–170.
18 Venuto C *et al.* (2010) Alternative therapies for Clostridium difficile infections. *Pharmacotherapy*. **30**: 1266–1278.
19 Lowy I *et al.* (2010) Treatment with monoclonal antibodies against Clostridium difficile toxins. *New England Journal of Medicine*. **362**: 197–205.
20 Kyne L (2010) Clostridium difficile–beyond antibiotics. *New England Journal of Medicine*. **362**: 264–265.

HELICOBACTER PYLORI GASTRITIS — BNF 1.3

Helicobacter pylori infection of the stomach is ubiquitous, with a global prevalence of about 50% of the adult population. However, infection rates are uneven; it is more prevalent among low socio-economic groups and in developing countries. Infection is generally acquired in childhood, and long-term infection predisposes to chronic gastritis, GI ulceration and subsequent gastric cancer.[1,2] Eradication of *H. pylori* with antibacterials and gastric acid suppressants (PPIs or H_2-receptor antagonists) is more cost-effective than acid suppression alone in relation to:

- relieving non-ulcer dyspepsia[3]
- healing peptic ulcers[3,4]
- preventing recurrent ulceration and bleeding.[4,5]

Evidence that *H. pylori* eradication lowers the risk of gastric cancer is accumulating.[6–12] Current European guidelines recommend eradication after gastric cancer resection, and in first-degree relatives of gastric cancer patients.[3] Further, eradication produces remission in a high proportion of patients with early-stage mucosa-associated lymphoid tissue (MALT) lymphoma, and is also recommended for this indication by European guidelines.[3]

H. pylori-associated type B chronic atrophic gastritis facilitates the development of gastropathy during treatment with NSAIDs (see p.299), and eradication probably improves the GI safety of NSAIDs.[7,13] Thus testing for and eradicating *H. pylori* is important in patients starting regular NSAID treatment, particularly if they have dyspepsia, a history of ulceration or a high risk of ulceration (see Box 5.C, p.299).[3,13–15]

The benefit of eradication is debatable in patients with established ulcers who need to continue taking an NSAID or low-dose aspirin.[3,15,16] In relation to ulcer healing, when given after discontinuing an NSAID in patients with NSAID-related bleeding, eradication is no more effective than **omeprazole** alone.[16]

Eradication alone is also less effective than PPI maintenance treatment in preventing recurrence of ulcers or upper GI bleeding in chronic NSAID users.[3] However, current European guidelines advise that eradication is of value in chronic NSAID users, although it is not in itself sufficient to prevent NSAID-induced ulcers.

The European guidelines also recommend a 'test-and-treat' approach to patients on long-term PPIs for preventing the recurrence of NSAID-induced ulcers, because eradication in *H. pylori*-positive patients reduces a PPI-*H. pylori* interaction which predisposes to atrophic gastritis.[3]

Management strategy

If possible, stop the NSAID

Patients on an NSAID who develop symptoms suggesting a GI ulcer should ideally stop taking the NSAID (or minimize the dose if this is not possible), start on a gastric acid suppressant, and be tested for *H. pylori*.[15,17]

Test for H. pylori

For patients starting on regular NSAID treatment or those with symptoms suggestive of an *uncomplicated* ulcer (e.g. gnawing or burning epigastric pain, worse at night or when the stomach is empty, and relieved by food or antacids), non-invasive tests are appropriate:
- faecal (stool) antigen tests detect *H. pylori*-associated antigens in faeces using specific antibodies. These tests have a specificity and sensitivity of >90% when performed accurately[13,18]
- urea breath tests involve ingesting ^{13}C-labelled urea, which is broken down by *H. pylori* to produce ammonia and labelled CO_2. This is then detected in expired air. These tests have excellent specificity, sensitivity and reliability.[13,19] The kits are more expensive than faecal antigen tests (£21 vs. £9) but, unlike faecal antigen tests, there are no further laboratory analysis costs. However, to avoid false-positive results, PPIs or H_2-receptor antagonists must be stopped 1–2 weeks before the test, and patients must fast for 6h immediately before.[19]

Both types of test are better markers of *active* infection than a serological antibody test, which does not distinguish between present and past infection with *H. pylori*. ^{13}C-labelled urea breath tests are preferred in the UK, based on patient acceptability, convenience and overall cost.[13]

An endoscopic examination and biopsy is recommended for patients with symptoms suggesting a *complicated* ulcer or gastric cancer (i.e. otherwise unexplained GI bleeding, iron-deficiency anaemia, GI obstruction or mass, dysphagia, persistent vomiting, anorexia or weight loss, severe abdominal pain suggesting perforation, or suspicious barium meal). Endoscopy is also recommended for patients >55 years old who have unexplained persistent dyspepsia alone.[17]

Eradication

Many *H. pylori* eradication regimens exist. In the UK, 1-week triple therapy regimens (two antibacterials and a gastroprotective drug) are recommended (Box 6.D). Eradication is achieved in about 85% of patients with fewer undesirable effects and greater adherence than 2-week regimens.[15]

Box 6.D First-line eradication regimens for *Helicobacter pylori* in the UK[15]

Standard regimens

Three drugs are taken b.d. for 1 week:
- a standard-dose PPI, e.g. lansoprazole 30mg, omeprazole 20mg or pantoprazole 40mg
- two of the following antibacterials:
  - amoxicillin 1g
  - clarithromycin 500mg *or*
  - metronidazole 400mg.

Resistance to amoxicillin is rare, whereas resistance to clarithromycin and metronidazole is common and can arise during treatment. Thus, if the patient has recently been treated with metronidazole for a different infection, choose clarithromycin for *H. pylori* eradication, and *vice versa*.

Other regimens exist, but are more expensive or involve taking doses t.d.s. (see BNF for more information).

Regimen suitable for patients allergic to penicillins

Three drugs are taken b.d. for 1 week:
- a standard-dose PPI, as above
- clarithromycin 250mg
- metronidazole 400mg.

Treatment failure generally indicates poor adherence or antibacterial resistance. Dual therapy regimens (one antibacterial and a PPI) are not recommended because they are less effective.[15]

Older **bismuth**-based regimens involve taking 4 different types of tablets/capsules up to q.d.s. for 2 weeks. Consequently, adherence is low and eradication failure relatively common. This type of regimen is now used in the UK only if the first-line eradication regimen fails; see BNF for details.[15] Alternatively, the patient can be referred for specialist treatment based on culture and sensitivity testing.

Newer regimens using different antibacterials or a sequential treatment approach are being investigated in an attempt to overcome the growing problem of resistance, but are not yet recommended for general use in the UK.[20–22]

Confirm eradication

Patients with, or at high risk of, ulcer complications (e.g. perforation or bleeding) should be retested to confirm eradication. A faecal antigen test is best because the accuracy of urea breath tests is affected by antibacterials and PPIs. It is necessary to delay urea breath retesting for 4 weeks after finishing antibacterial-containing eradication regimens and 2 weeks after completing a course of PPIs.[15] Serological testing does not help because antibodies persist long after *H. pylori* has been eradicated.[13]

Supply

For **lansoprazole** and **omeprazole**, see Proton pump inhibitors, p.30.

For **amoxicillin** and **clarithromycin**, see Cellulitis in a lymphoedematous limb, p.456.

For **metronidazole**, see p.451.

^{13}C-labelled urea breath tests

diabact UBT® (MDE)

Tablets 50mg, 1 kit (including 1 tablet, 4 breath-sample containers, straws) = £21 (analysis included).

Pylobactell® (Torbet)

Tablets soluble 100mg, 1 kit (including 6 breath-sample containers, 30mL mixing and administration vial, straws) = £21 (analysis included).

1 Czinn SJ (2005) Helicobacter pylori infection: detection, investigation, and management. *Journal of Pediatrics*. **146 (suppl)**: s21–26.

2 Guarner J (2004) The spectrum of gastric disease associated with Helicobacter pylori and other infectious gastritides. *Current Gastroenterology Reports*. **6**: 441–446.

3 Malfertheiner P *et al.* (2007) Current concepts in the management of Helicobacter pylori infection: the Maastricht III Consensus Report. *Gut*. **56**: 772–781.

4 Ford A *et al.* (2009) Eradication therapy for peptic ulcer disease in Helicobacter pylori positive patients. *Cochrane Database of Systematic Reviews*. **4**: CD003840.

5 Gisbert JP *et al.* (2010) Helicobacter pylori eradication therapy vs. antisecretory non-eradication therapy (with or without long-term maintenance antisecretory therapy) for the prevention of recurrent bleeding from peptic ulcer. *Cochrane Database of Systematic Reviews*. **2**: CD004062.

6 McCormack K (1989) Mathematical model for assessing risk of gastrointestinal reactions to NSAIDs. In: K Rainsford (ed) *Azapropazone — over two decades of clinical use*. Kluwer Academic Publishers, Boston, pp. 81–93.

7 Becker JC *et al.* (2004) Current approaches to prevent NSAID-induced gastropathy–COX selectivity and beyond. *British Journal of Clinical Pharmacology*. **58**: 587–600.

8 Sung JJ (2004) Should we eradicate Helicobacter pylori in non-steroidal anti-inflammatory drug users? *Alimentary Pharmacology and Therapeutics*. **20 (suppl 2)**: 65–70.

9 Di Leo V *et al.* (2005) Effect of Helicobacter pylori and eradication therapy on gastrointestinal permeability. Implications for patients with seronegative spondyloarthritis. *Journal of Rheumatology*. **32**: 295–300.

10 De Vries AC and Kuipers EJ (2007) Review article: Helicobacter pylori eradication for the prevention of gastric cancer. *Alimentary Pharmacology and Therapeutics*. **26 (suppl 2)**: 25–35.

11 Fuccio L *et al.* (2009) Meta-analysis: can Helicobacter pylori eradication treatment reduce the risk for gastric cancer? *Annals of internal medicine*. **151**: 121–128.

12 Hartgrink HH *et al.* (2009) Gastric cancer. *Lancet*. **374**: 477–490.

13 DTB (2005) H. pylori eradication in NSAID-associated ulcers. *Drug and Therapeutics Bulletin*. **43**: 37–40.

14 Hunt RH and Bazzoli F (2004) Review article: should NSAID/low-dose aspirin takers be tested routinely for H. pylori infection and treated if positive? Implications for primary risk of ulcer and ulcer relapse after initial healing. *Alimentary Pharmacology and Therapeutics*. **19 (suppl 1)**: 9–16.

15 BNF (2011) Section 1.3. In: *British National Formulary* (No. 61). British Medical Association and Royal Pharmaceutical Society of Great Britain, London. Current BNF available from: www.bnf.org/bnf/bnf/current/.

16 Chan FK *et al.* (1998) Does eradication of Helicobacter pylori impair healing of nonsteroidal anti-inflammatory drug associated bleeding peptic ulcers? A prospective randomized study. *Alimentary Pharmacology and Therapeutics*. **12**: 1201–1205.

17 NICE (2004) Dyspepsia. Management of dyspepsia in adults in primary care. In: *Clinical Guideline 17*. National Institute for Clinical Excellence. Available from: www.nice.org.uk/page.aspx?o = CG017
18 Schenk BE *et al.* (2000) Effect of Helicobacter pylori eradication on chronic gastritis during omeprazole therapy. *Gut*. **46**: 615–621.
19 Fallone CA *et al.* (2000) The urea breath test for Helicobacter pylori infection: taking the wind out of the sails of endoscopy. *Canadian Medical Association Journal*. **162**: 371–372.
20 Suzuki H *et al.* (2010) Helicobacter pylori eradication therapy. *Future Microbiology*. **5**: 639–648.
21 Marshall B (2008) Sequential therapy for Helicobacter pylori: a worthwhile effort for your patients. *Annals of Internal Medicine*. **148**: 962–963.
22 Jafri NS *et al.* (2008) Meta-analysis: sequential therapy appears superior to standard therapy for Helicobacter pylori infection in patients naive to treatment. *Annals of Internal Medicine*. **148**: 923–931.

7: ENDOCRINE SYSTEM AND IMMUNOMODULATION

BISPHOSPHONATES BNF 6.6.2 & 9.5.1.2

Indications: Licensed indications vary between products; consult the manufacturers' SPCs for details; they include tumour-induced hypercalcaemia, prophylactic use to reduce skeletal events associated with osteolytic lesions (multiple myeloma, metastatic cancer), metastatic bone pain (only **disodium pamidronate** is licensed for use in breast cancer and multiple myeloma); prevention/treatment of osteoporosis; Paget's disease.

Pharmacology

The bisphosphonates are stable analogues of pyrophosphate, a naturally occurring regulator of bone metabolism. They have a high affinity for calcium ions, and bind rapidly to hydroxyapatite crystals in mineralized bone. Bisphosphonates are subsequently released and taken up by osteoclasts, interfering with their function and/or inducing their apoptosis (programmed cell death). Nitrogen-containing bisphosphonates (e.g. **alendronate**, **ibandronic acid**, **disodium pamidronate**, **zoledronic acid**) inhibit the mevalonate pathway vital for normal cellular function (e.g. vesicular trafficking, cell signalling, cytoskeleton function) and non-nitrogen-containing bisphosphonates (**sodium clodronate**, **disodium etidronate**) form cytotoxic adenosine triphosphate (ATP) analogues.[1,2] These cellular effects also extend to macrophages, reducing the production of cytokines, and this anti-inflammatory effect may contribute to the analgesic effect of bisphosphonates.[3,4] Bisphosphonates interfere with the cancer-related increase in the number and activity of osteoclasts which cause bone pain by:

- producing an increasingly acidic environment (stimulating acid-sensing receptors on sensory nerves)
- destroying sensory nerves (producing neuropathic pain)
- causing mechanical instability as a result of the loss of bone mineral (stimulating mechanoreceptors on sensory nerves in the periosteum).[5]

In vitro and in animals, bisphosphonates also have a direct anticancer effect via inhibition of matrix metalloproteinase, altered cell adhesion, anti-angiogenic activity, reduction in release of local growth factors from bone and induction of apoptosis.[6,7] However, a cancer-promoting effect has been seen in some animal studies.[8] Bisphosphonates have no impact on the effect of parathyroid-related protein (PTHrP) or on renal tubular resorption of calcium.

Bisphosphonates are poorly absorbed PO and this is reduced further by food. They are rapidly taken up by the skeleton, particularly at sites of bone resorption and where the mineral is more exposed, and they remain there for weeks to months.[9] Most of the remainder is bound to plasma proteins. Bisphosphonates are not metabolized and are excreted unchanged via the kidneys. The plasma proportion of the drug is eliminated generally within 24h. Thereafter, elimination is much slower as the remainder gradually seeps out of bone.[10] Comparison of the halflives of different bisphosphonates is complicated by this multiphasic elimination. Other pharmacokinetic details are shown in Table 7.1.

Table 7.1 Bisphosphonates and the initial treatment of hypercalcaemia[11–13]

	Zoledronic acid	*Ibandronic acid*	*Disodium pamidronate*
IV dose	4mg	2–6mg	30–90mg
Onset of effect	<4 days	<4 days	<3 days
Maximum effect	4–7 days	7 days	5–7 days
Duration of effect	4 weeks	2.5 weeks (4mg) 4 weeks (6mg)	2.5 weeks
Restores normocalcaemia	90%	75%	70–75%

Tumour-induced hypercalcaemia

Bisphosphonates given IV are the treatment of choice for hypercalcaemia of malignancy.[14] The initial response is higher with **zoledronic acid** (~90%), with **ibandronic acid** equal to **disodium pamidronate** (~75%). A longer duration of response can be obtained with **zoledronic acid** and **ibandronic acid** compared with **disodium pamidronate**.[12,13] The SPC for **disodium pamidronate** recommends a scale of doses depending on the initial *corrected* calcium concentration (see p.473), with higher doses for higher initial calcium concentrations. However, one systematic review suggests that 90mg (the maximum recommended dose) should always be given to increase the likelihood of a response, and prolong its duration.[14]

Prophylactic use in patients with myeloma or bone metastases

Disodium pamidronate IV, **zoledronic acid** IV and **ibandronic acid** PO/IV given long-term decrease the incidence of new skeletal events in patients with bone metastases. Benefit is most evident for patients with breast cancer or myeloma but is less clear for other types of cancers.[15–20] Only studies ⩾6 months in duration have shown a reduction in vertebral and non-vertebral fractures, hypercalcaemia, and the need for radiotherapy. Studies ⩾2 years in duration have also shown a reduced need for orthopaedic surgery. The incidence and severity of pain is reduced with an NNT of 11 at 1 month and 7 at 3 months. There is no impact on survival or the occurrence of spinal cord compression.

Various national guidelines recommend, with provisos, the routine use of bisphosphonates for the treatment and prevention of skeletal complications in patients with:

- breast cancer with symptomatic bone metastases[21,22]
- myeloma whether or not bone lesions are evident[23,24]
- hormone-resistant prostate cancer with bone metastases (± symptoms); also for the relief of bone pain.[25,26]

The optimal duration of treatment is unclear, but bisphosphonates are generally continued for as long as they are tolerated, or there is a substantial decline in the patient's performance status. There is no consensus on the use of bisphosphonates in other cancers, although it has been suggested that, in any patient with a prognosis of ⩾4–6 months and multiple bone metastases, it is reasonable to consider their use.[27]

The ability of bisphosphonates to prevent the development of bone metastases is being investigated.[28]

Alternatives to bisphosphonates are being developed. For example, **denosumab** is a human monoclonal antibody which binds to receptor activator of nuclear factor kappa B ligand (RANKL). This prevents the ligand binding to the RANK receptor on osteoclasts, which is required for their activation.

In the USA, **denosumab** is approved for the prevention of skeletal-related events in patients with bone metastases from solid cancers, administered as a monthly SC injection. In RCTs, **denosumab** is more effective than **zoledronic acid** in delaying complications of bone metastases in both breast and prostate cancer, and is as effective in other cancer types.[29–31] Survival does not differ between the two treatments, except for patients with myeloma, where it was more favourable with **zoledronic acid**; thus myeloma is excluded from the indications for **denosumab**. As with bisphosphonates, undesirable effects include hypocalcaemia and osteonecrosis of the jaw (about 1% of patients with either); unlike bisphosphonates, **denosumab** does not impair renal function. However, at twice the price of **zoledronic acid**, some question if the modest gains provided by **denosumab** justify the increased cost.[32]

In the UK, **denosumab** is currently recommended only for the secondary prevention of osteoporotic fractures in postmenopausal women when bisphosphonates are contra-indicated or poorly tolerated.[33]

Bisphosphonates as adjuvant analgesics
Bisphosphonates have been used for metastatic bone pain and several regimens have been recommended for use when more conventional methods have been exhausted.[3,34–37] An effect is generally seen within 2 weeks. The evidence suggests that benefit is more likely in patients with breast cancer or myeloma, and with an IV bisphosphonate.[37] For moderate–severe bone pain, a more intensive, 'loading dose' regimen of **ibandronic acid** 6mg IV given on 3 consecutive days is being explored (see p.479).

Prophylactic use in patients treated for breast or prostate cancer
Oestrogen deficiency is induced in women treated for breast cancer by chemotherapy ± aromatase inhibitors. This increases the rate of bone loss and risk of fracture.[38] Oral bisphosphonates, e.g. **risedronate** 35mg once a week, can prevent the loss following chemotherapy and ongoing studies are examining their use with aromatase inhibitors.[38,39]

The increased bone loss associated with androgen deprivation treatment in men with prostate cancer is also prevented by bisphosphonates, e.g. **zoledronic acid** 4mg every 3 months.[40]

Cautions

Serious drug interactions: prolonged hypocalcaemia ± hypomagnesaemia may occur with the concurrent use of an aminoglycoside and a bisphosphonate, including PO **sodium clodronate**.[41] Risk of renal impairment increased by concurrent use with other nephrotoxic drugs.

Renal impairment (correct hypovolaemia before treatment and monitor renal function). Vitamin D deficiency (increased risk of hypocalcaemia);[42] unless being treated for tumour-related hypercalcaemia, daily oral supplements of elemental **calcium** 500mg and **vitamin D** 400 units are recommended, e.g. Calcichew® D3 Forte. Invasive dental procedures (risk of osteonecrosis of the jaw).

Undesirable effects
Very common (>10%): transient pyrexia and flu-like symptoms (more common with IV nitrogen-containing bisphosphonates; see below), fatigue, headache, anxiety, hypertension, anaemia, thrombocytopenia, cough, arthralgia, myalgia, bone pain, *asymptomatic hypocalcaemia, hypomagnesaemia, hypophosphataemia.*

Oral products in particular may cause anorexia, dyspepsia, nausea, vomiting, abdominal pain, diarrhoea or constipation.

Common (<10%, >1%): sleep disturbance, psychosis, tachycardia, atrial fibrillation or flutter, syncope, breathlessness, leucopenia, infusion site reactions, deterioration in renal function (see below), hypokalaemia, jaw osteonecrosis (see below).

Rare (<0.1%, >0.01%): ocular inflammation (see below), angioedema, collapsing focal segmental glomerulosclerosis (**disodium pamidronate**), nephrotic syndrome (**disodium pamidronate**), symptomatic hypocalcaemia (e.g. tetany).

Very rare (<0.01%): anaphylaxis, bronchospasm.

Systemic reactions after IV bisphosphonates
Acute systemic inflammatory reactions causing symptoms such as fever, myalgia, arthralgia, nausea and vomiting, occur in 25–50% of patients after IV bisphosphonates. They are possibly related to the release of cytokines from inflammatory cells. Generally, the onset is within 2 days of the infusion; the fever is mild, although rigors occasionally occur. There may be bone pain, generally < 12h of the infusion. These effects can be treated with **paracetamol** or NSAIDs, and resolve completely within 1–2 days. They generally lessen with repeat doses or with prophylactic **paracetamol** or NSAID.[43]

Renal toxicity

Bisphosphonates can affect renal function. High-dose (200–1,500mg/day for 2–5 days) short-duration (<2h) IVI of **sodium clodronate** (not UK) and **disodium etidronate** (not UK) can cause oliguria, tubulo-interstitial damage and acute renal failure, possibly via the formation of an insoluble calcium-bisphosphonate complex in the blood.[44,45] **Disodium pamidronate** also rarely causes collapsing focal segmental glomerulosclerosis, particularly in high doses, e.g. 180mg every 2–4 weeks. The probable mechanism is a direct toxic effect on glomerular capillary podocytes and renal tubules.[46]

The more potent third-generation bisphosphonates are given in much smaller doses and reach lower concentrations in the renal tubules. Nevertheless, renal impairment has occurred with **zoledronic acid** (see p.476) and **ibandronic acid** (see p.479).[47–51] The risk of renal toxicity is reduced by adhering to the recommended dose and infusion rate, ensuring adequate hydration, monitoring renal function and adjusting the dose of bisphosphonate as appropriate or discontinuing treatment if there is deterioration, and avoiding the concurrent use of other nephrotoxic drugs.

Jaw osteonecrosis

All bisphosphonates (and **denosumab**) have been implicated as a risk factor for jaw osteonecrosis.[32,52–54] Most reports involve the long-term use of **zoledronic acid** or **disodium pamidronate** for metastatic bone disease.[55] Although osteonecrosis has been reported after as little as 4 months of bisphosphonate use, generally, patients have been receiving bisphosphonates for years (mean and median duration of use vary around 1 and 2–3 years respectively). The true incidence of osteonecrosis is difficult to identify, but some studies put it as high as 10% of patients receiving long-term **zoledronic acid** and 4% of those receiving **disodium pamidronate**.[55] Other risk factors for jaw osteonecrosis include dental procedures (reported in about 60% of patients), poor dental health, blood clotting disorders, anaemia, and possibly chemotherapy and corticosteroids.

The jaw bones may be particularly susceptible to osteonecrosis because of the combination of repeated low-level local trauma (e.g. from chewing, dentures) and ease of infection from microbes. Trauma and infection increase the demand for bone repair which the bisphosphonate-inhibited bone cannot meet, resulting in localized bone necrosis; the anti-angiogenic effect of bisphosphonates may also contribute.[55]

Osteonecrosis can present as an asymptomatic bony exposure in one or more sites in the mandible or maxilla, or with orofacial pain, trismus, offensive discharge from a cutaneous fistula, chronic sinusitis because of an oro-antral fistula and numbness in the mandible or maxilla.[43] If probed, the necrotic bone is usually non-tender and may not bleed. There may be osteomyelitis with oral-cavity flora or *Actinomyces* species. Osteonecrosis may show as mottled bone on a plain radiograph and be confused with bone metastases on a bone scan. Pathological fracture can occur.

Management is based on clinical experience. Long-term outcomes are generally poor with relatively few patients experiencing improvement or resolution. Thus, prevention is an important part of the recommended approach:[43]

- *preventive dental treatment* before commencing long-term bisphosphonates, e.g. treat infection, teeth extractions
- *encourage good dental hygiene* including regular dental cleaning by a dentist or dental hygienist
- *avoid invasive dental procedures during treatment*
- *minimize trauma*, e.g. patients with dentures should wear soft liners.

If osteonecrosis occurs:

- *discontinue the bisphosphonate* but new lesions may continue to appear
- *treat infection*, e.g. antimicrobials, **chlorhexidine** mouthwash, periodic minor debridement and wound irrigation (major debridement is avoided as it may worsen the situation)
- *avoid major surgery* unless there is no alternative, e.g. due to sequestered bone, pathological fracture, or oro-antral fistula.

If urgent treatment precludes a prior dental examination, a dental referral and any treatment should be undertaken within 1–2 months for patients expected to receive long-term bisphosphonates.[55]

Ocular toxicity

A rare undesirable effect is ocular inflammation, causing eye pain, redness, swelling, abnormal vision or impaired eye movement (due to rectus muscle oedema).[56,57] Typically, the onset is within 2 days of the first or second infusion and affects both eyes. There may be other symptoms of an acute systemic inflammatory reaction (see above). An urgent ophthalmology assessment is required, followed by appropriate treatment. Patients with mild reactions, e.g. those which settle quickly without treatment, can generally continue to receive the same bisphosphonate. Those with more severe reactions, e.g. uveitis or scleritis, should not receive the same bisphosphonate again; some tolerate a switch to a non-nitrogen-containing bisphosphonate, but specialist advice should be sought from the ophthalmologist ± endocrinologist.[43]

Other emerging toxicities

Severe (sometimes incapacitating) musculoskeletal pain has been reported after days, months or years of bisphosphonate treatment. It has generally occurred with PO bisphosphonates used for osteoporosis and Paget's disease, but the FDA is also investigating a possible link with IV bisphosphonates. The pain is distinct from the arthralgia/myalgia associated with an acute systemic inflammatory reaction (see above), and may respond to temporary or permanent discontinuation of the bisphosphonate.[58]

Dose and use

On the grounds of cost, **disodium pamidronate** is still widely used as the bisphosphonate of first choice, and **zoledronic acid** tends to be reserved for patients who fail to respond to **disodium pamidronate**. The guidance below relates to **disodium pamidronate**; for **zoledronic acid** and **ibandronic acid**, see p.476 and p.479 respectively.

Tumour-induced hypercalcaemia

Stop and think! Are you justified in correcting a potentially fatal complication in a moribund patient?

The SPC for **disodium pamidronate** recommends a dose dependent on the initial albumin-corrected plasma calcium concentration (Box 7.A and Table 7.2). However, it has been suggested that the higher dose should be given irrespective of the initial calcium level to increase the probability of a response and prolong its duration.[14] Patients should be well hydrated, using 0.9% saline if necessary:

- standard and maximum recommended dose is 90mg IVI/treatment
- dilute the dose in 0.9% saline or 5% glucose; the concentration should not exceed 60mg/250mL
- the infusion rate should not exceed 1mg/min in patients with normal renal function; patients with mild–moderate renal impairment (creatinine clearance 30–90mL/min) do not require dose reduction but the infusion rate should not exceed 90mg/4h (about 20–22mg/h)
- for patients with severe renal impairment (creatinine clearance <30mL/min) see below
- repeat after 1 week if initial response inadequate
- repeat every 3–4 weeks according to plasma calcium concentration
- measure plasma creatinine before each dose, no dose adjustment is required in mild–moderate renal impairment.

In palliative care, treatment with a bisphosphonate is unlikely to be started in patients with hypercalcaemia and severe renal impairment (creatinine clearance <30mL/min). However, if considered appropriate, see below in the prophylactic use of **disodium pamidronate** in patients with multiple myeloma or breast cancer with bone metastases.

If the IV route is inaccessible, bisphosphonates can be administered by CSCI, together with SC hydration:[59,60]

- **disodium pamidronate** 90mg in 1L 0.9% saline over 12–24h
- **sodium clodronate** (not UK) 1,500mg in 50–250mL 0.9% saline or 5% glucose over 2–3h.

Box 7.A Correcting plasma calcium concentrations[a]

If the mean normal albumin for the local laboratory is 40g/L

Corrected calcium (mmol/L) = measured calcium + (0.022 × (40 − albumin g/L))

e.g. measured calcium = 2.45; albumin = 32

corrected calcium = 2.45 + (0.022 × 8) = 2.63mmol/L

(normal range = 2.12–2.65mmol/L)

a. most UK pathology laboratories will now automatically report an albumin-corrected plasma calcium concentration based on locally validated data.

Table 7.2 IV disodium pamidronate for hypercalcaemia[a]

Corrected plasma calcium concentration (mmol/L)	*Dose (mg)*
<3	15 or 30
3–3.5	30 or 60
3.5–4	60 or 90
>4	90

a. manufacturer's recommendations.

Prophylactic use to reduce the incidence of skeletal-related events in patients with multiple myeloma or breast cancer with bone metastases

For **disodium pamidronate**:

- patients should be well hydrated, using 0.9% saline if necessary
- dilute 90mg in a minimum of 375mL of 0.9% saline or 5% glucose; the concentration should not exceed 60mg/250mL
- in *breast cancer with bone metastases* give 90mg IVI over 1.5h every 3–4 weeks
- in *multiple myeloma* a slower infusion rate is recommended because of the greater risk of renal impairment/renal toxicity; give 90mg IVI over 4h every 4 weeks
- plasma creatinine should be measured before each dose. Treatment should be withheld if creatinine increases by:
  - ▹ ≥44micromol/L in patients with a normal baseline creatinine concentration (i.e. <124micromol/L), *or*
  - ▹ ≥88micromol/L in patients with a raised baseline creatinine concentration (i.e. >124micromol/L)
- treatment may be resumed at the same dose as before when plasma creatinine returns to within 10% of the baseline value
- discontinue treatment permanently if plasma creatinine fails to improve after 4–8 weeks.

Metastatic bone pain

Several regimens have been recommended for when more conventional methods have been exhausted:

- **disodium pamidronate** 90mg IVI (50% of patients respond, generally within 1–2 weeks); if helpful repeat 60–90mg every 3–4 weeks for as long as benefit is maintained[3]
- **disodium pamidronate** 120mg IVI, repeated p.r.n. every 2–4 months[36]
- **disodium pamidronate** 90–120mg IVI or **sodium clodronate** 600–1,500mg IVI (not UK), repeated p.r.n. In patients not responding to a first treatment, a second can be tried but, if still no response, discontinue.[37]

Supply

For **zoledronic acid** and **ibandronic acid**, see p.479 and p.482 respectively.

Disodium pamidronate (generic)
Injection 3mg/mL, 5mL and 10mL vial = £28 and £55 respectively; 6mg/mL, 10mL vial = £95; 9mg/mL, 10mL vial = £165; 15mg/mL, 1mL, 2mL, 4mL and 6mL vial = £30, £60, £119 and £170 respectively.

Aredia Dry Powder® (Novartis)
Injection (powder for reconstitution) 15mg vial = £30; 30mg vial = £60; 90mg vial = £170; supplied with diluent for reconstitution.

1 Fleisch H (1998) Bisphosphonates: mechanisms of action. *Endocrine Reviews*. **19**: 80–100.
2 Russell R *et al.* (1999) Bisphosphonates: pharmacology, mechanisms of action and clinical uses. *Osteoporosis International*. **9 (suppl 2)**: s66-s80.
3 Crosby V *et al.* (1998) A randomized controlled trial of intravenous clodronate. *Journal of Pain and Symptom Management*. **15**: 266–268.
4 Harada H *et al.* (2004) Effects of bisphosphonates on joint damage and bone loss in rat adjuvant-induced arthritis. *Inflammation Research*. **53**: 45–52.

5 Mantyh PW (2006) Cancer pain and its impact on diagnosis, survival and quality of life. *Nature Reviews Neuroscience*. **7**: 797–809.
6 Neville-Webbe H *et al.* (2002) The anti-tumour activity of bisphosphonates. *Cancer Treatment Reviews*. **28**: 305–319.
7 Green JR (2004) Bisphosphonates: preclinical review. *Oncologist*. **9 (suppl 4)**: 3–13.
8 Sevcik MA *et al.* (2004) Bone cancer pain: the effects of the bisphosphonate alendronate on pain, skeletal remodeling, tumor growth and tumor necrosis. *Pain*. **111**: 169–180.
9 Rogers MJ *et al.* (2000) Cellular and molecular mechanisms of action of bisphosphonates. *Cancer.* **88 (suppl 12)**: 2961–2978.
10 Barrett J *et al.* (2004) Ibandronate: a clinical pharmacological and pharmacokinetic update. *Journal of Clinical Pharmacology*. **44**: 951–965.
11 Purohit O *et al.* (1995) A randomised, double-blind comparison of intravenous pamidronate and clodronate in hypercalcaemia of malignancy. *British Journal of Cancer.* **72**: 1289–1293.
12 Major P *et al.* (2001) Zoledronic acid is superior to pamidronate in the treatment of hypercalcaemia of malignancy: a pooled analysis of two randomized, controlled clinical trials. *Journal of Clinical Oncology*. **19**: 558–567.
13 Ralston SH *et al.* (1997) Dose-response study of ibandronate in the treatment of cancer-associated hypercalcaemia. *British Journal of Cancer.* **75**: 295–300.
14 Saunders Y *et al.* (2004) Systematic review of bisphosphonates for hypercalcaemia of malignancy. *Palliative Medicine*. **18**: 418–431.
15 Wong R and Wiffen PJ (2002) Bisphosphonates for the relief of pain secondary to bone metastases. *Cochrane Database Systematic Reviews*. **2**: CD002068.
16 Ross JR *et al.* (2003) Systematic review of role of bisphosphonates on skeletal morbidity in metastatic cancer. *British Medical Journal*. **327**: 469.
17 Body JJ *et al.* (2004) Oral ibandronate improves bone pain and preserves quality of life in patients with skeletal metastases due to breast cancer. *Pain*. **111**: 306–312.
18 Body JJ *et al.* (2004) Oral ibandronate reduces the risk of skeletal complications in breast cancer patients with metastatic bone disease: results from two randomised, placebo-controlled phase III studies. *British Journal of Cancer.* **90**: 1133–1137.
19 Pavlakis N *et al.* (2005) Bisphosphonates for breast cancer. *Cochrane Database Systematic Reviews*. CD003474.
20 Yuen KK *et al.* (2006) Bisphosphonates for advanced prostate cancer. *Cochrane Database Systematic Reviews*. CD006250.
21 Warr D *et al.* (2004) Use of biphosphonates in women with breast cancer. Practice guideline report #1 11. In: *Cancer Care Ontario program in evidence-based care*. Available from: www.cancercare.on.ca/common/pages/UserFile.aspx?fileId = 34182
22 SIGN (Scottish Intercollegiate Guidelines Network) (2005) *Management of breast cancer in women. A national clinical guideline*. (No. 84). SIGN publication, Edinburgh (Scotland).
23 Smith A et *al.* (2006) Guidelines on the diagnosis and management of multiple myeloma 2005. *British Journal of Haematology*. **132**: 410–451.
24 Imrie K *et al.* (2007) The role of biphosphonates in the management of skeletal complications for patients with multiple myeloma: a clinical practice guideline. In: *Cancer Care Ontario program in evidence-based care*. Available from: www.cancercare.on.ca/common/pages/UserFile.aspx?fileId = 14146
25 British Association of Urological Surgeons (2005) Systemic management of metastatic bone disease. In: *Guidelines on the management and treatment of metastatic prostate cancer*, UK.
26 Berry S *et al.* (2005) The use of biphosphonates in men with hormone-refractory prostate cancer. Practice guideline report #3–14. In: *Cancer Care Ontario program in evidence-based care*. Available from: www.cancercare.on.ca/common/pages/userFile.aspx?fileId = 14032
27 Body JJ (2006) Bisphosphonates for malignancy-related bone disease: current status, future developments. *Supportive Care in Cancer.* **14**: 408–418.
28 Clemons M and Verma S (2005) Should oral bisphosphonates be standard of care in women with early breast cancer? *Breast Cancer Research and Treatment*. **90**: 315–318.
29 Stopeck AT *et al.* (2010) Denosumab compared with zoledronic acid for the treatment of bone metastases in patients with advanced breast cancer: a randomized, double-blind study. *Journal of Clinical Oncology*. **28**: 5132–5139.
30 Fizazi K *et al.* (2011) Denosumab versus zoledronic acid for treatment of bone metastases in men with castration-resistant prostate cancer: a randomised, double-blind study. *Lancet*. **377**: 813–822.
31 Henry DH *et al.* (2011) Randomized, double-blind study of denosumab versus zoledronic acid in the treatment of bone metastases in patients with advanced cancer (excluding breast and prostate cancer) or multiple myeloma. *Journal of Clinical Oncology*. **29**: 1125–1132.
32 West H (2011) Denosumab for prevention of skeletal-related events in patients with bone metastases from solid tumors: incremental benefit, debatable value. *Journal of Clinical Oncology*. **29**: 1095–1098.
33 NICE (2010) Technology appraisal guidance 204. Denosumab for the prevention of osteoporotic fractures in postmenopausal women. London UK. Available from: www.nice.org.uk/nicemedia/live/13251/51293/51293.pdf
34 Vorreuther R (1993) Biphosphonates as an adjunct to palliative therapy of bone metastases from prostatic carcinoma. A pilot study on clodronate. *British Journal of Urology*. **72**: 792–795.
35 O'Rourke N *et al.* (1995) Double-blind, placebo-controlled, dose response trial of oral clodronate in patients with bone metastases. *Journal of Clinical Oncology*. **13**: 929–934.
36 Vinholes J *et al.* (1996) Metabolic effects of pamidronate in patients with metastatic bone disease. *British Journal of Cancer.* **73**: 1089–1095.
37 Mannix K *et al.* (2000) Using bisphosphonates to control the pain of bone metastases: evidence-based guidelines for palliative care. *Palliative Medicine*. **14**: 455–461.
38 Eastell R (2007) Breast cancer and the risk of osteoporotic fracture: a paradox. *Journal of Clinical Endocrinology and Metaboloism*. **92**: 42–43.
39 Greenspan SL *et al.* (2007) Prevention of bone loss in survivors of breast cancer: a randomized, double-blind, placebo-controlled clinical trial. *Journal of Clinical Endocrinology and Metabolism*. **92**: 131–136.
40 Smith MR (2003) Bisphosphonates to prevent osteoporosis in men receiving androgen deprivation therapy for prostate cancer. *Drugs Aging*. **20**: 175–183.
41 Johnson M and Fallon M (1998) Symptomatic hypocalcaemia with oral clodronate. *Journal of Pain and Symptom Management*. **15**: 140–142.
42 Broadbent A *et al.* (2005) Bisphosphonate-induced hypocalcemia associated with vitamin D deficiency in a patient with advanced cancer. *American Journal of Hospice and Palliative Care*. **22**: 382–384.

43 Tanvetyanon T and Stiff PJ (2006) Management of the adverse effects associated with intravenous bisphosphonates. *Annals of Oncology.* **17**: 897–907.
44 Bounameaux HM *et al.* (1983) Renal failure associated with intravenous diphosphonates. *Lancet.* **1**: 471.
45 Kanis JA *et al.* (1983) Effects of intravenous diphosphonates on renal function. *Lancet.* **1**: 1328.
46 Markowitz GS *et al.* (2001) Collapsing focal segmental glomerulosclerosis following treatment with high-dose pamidronate. *Journal of the American Society of Nephrology.* **12**: 1164–1172.
47 Rosen LS *et al.* (2001) Zoledronic acid versus pamidronate in the treatment of skeletal metastases in patients with breast cancer or osteolytic lesions of multiple myeloma: a phase III, double-blind, comparative trial. *Cancer Journal.* **7**: 377–387.
48 Rosen LS *et al.* (2004) Zoledronic acid is superior to pamidronate for the treatment of bone metastases in breast carcinoma patients with at least one osteolytic lesion. *Cancer.* **100**: 36–43.
49 Markowitz GS *et al.* (2003) Toxic acute tubular necrosis following treatment with zoledronate (Zometa). *Kidney International.* **64**: 281–289.
50 Chang JT *et al.* (2003) Renal failure with the use of zoledronic acid. *New England Journal of Medicine.* **349**: 1676–1679.
51 Diel I *et al.* (2003) Renal safety of oral and intravenous ibandronate in metastatic bone disease: phase III clinical trial results. In: *15th Annual MASCC Meeting*; Berlin, 18–21 June.
52 FDA (2004) Drug Safety Revisions: Food and Drugs Administration Update. *P&T.* **29**: 733.
53 Ruggiero SL *et al.* (2004) Osteonecrosis of the jaws associated with the use of bisphosphonates: a review of 63 cases. *Journal of Oral and Maxillofacial Surgery.* **62**: 527–534.
54 CHM (2006) Osteonecrosis of the jaw with bisphosphonates. In: Current Problems in Pharmacovigilance. Commission on Human Medicines. Available from: www.mhra.gov.uk/Publications/Safetyguidance/CurrentProblemsinPharmacovigilance/CON2023859
55 Woo SB *et al.* (2006) Narrative review: bisphosphonates and osteonecrosis of the jaws. *Annals of internal medicine.* **144**: 753–761.
56 Fraunfelder FW and Fraunfelder FT (2003) Bisphosphonates and ocular inflammation. *New England Journal of Medicine.* **348**: 1187–1188.
57 Australian Adverse Drug Reactions Bulletin (2004) Bisphosphonates and ocular inflammation. Available from: www.tga.gov.au/hp/aadrb_0404.htm
58 FDA (2008) Information for healthcare professionals. Bisphosphonates (marketed as Actonel, Actonel+Ca, Aredia, Boniva, Didronel, Fosamax, Fosamax+D, Reclast, Skelid, and Zometa). Food and Drugs Administration. Available from: www.fda.gov/Drugs/DrugSafety/PostmarketDrugSafetyInformationforPatientsandProviders/ucm101551.htm
59 Roemer-Becuwe C *et al.* (2003) Safety of subcutaneous clodronate and efficacy in hypercalcemia of malignancy: a novel route of administration. *Journal of Pain and Symptom Management.* **26**: 843–848.
60 Duncan AR (2003) The use of subcutaneous pamidronate. *Journal of Pain and Symptom Management.* **26**: 592–593.

ZOLEDRONIC ACID BNF 6.6.2 & 9.5.1.2

Class: Bisphosphonate.

Indications: Tumour-induced hypercalcaemia; prophylactic use to reduce the incidence of skeletal-related events in patients with advanced cancer involving bone; †bone pain. Aclasta®: Paget's disease, osteoporosis in women (postmenopausal) or men.

Pharmacology

Zoledronic acid is a third-generation bisphosphonate and the most potent currently available.[1,2] In patients with hypercalcaemia, zoledronic acid 4mg is more effective than **disodium pamidronate** 90mg in achieving normocalcaemia (90% vs. 70%) and provides a longer median time to relapse, about 4 weeks vs. 2.5 weeks (see Table 7.1, p.470).[3] Zoledronic acid 8mg has been given to patients who do not respond to 4mg or to **disodium pamidronate**, and those who relapse within a few days of treatment. Normocalcaemia is achieved in 50% but the median duration of response is only 2 weeks.[3] However, because the incidence of renal impairment doubles with the 8mg dose, its use was abandoned in clinical trials and it is unlicensed.[4]

In patients with breast cancer, compared with placebo, zoledronic acid 4mg IV given monthly for 1 year reduces the risk of a bone metastatic event (fractures, hypercalcaemia, need for radiotherapy) by about 40%.[5] Treatment every 2 weeks provides no greater benefit.[6] Zoledronic acid is at least as effective as **disodium pamidronate** in reducing skeletal complications and pain scores in patients with multiple myeloma or breast cancer.[7–9] In one RCT, patients receiving zoledronic acid required less radiotherapy and less surgery than those receiving **disodium pamidronate**; NNTs were 4 and 20 respectively.[4] Zoledronic acid has reduced pain and markers of bone turnover in patients with breast cancer who have developed a skeletal-related event or progressive bone disease despite receiving **disodium pamidronate** or **disodium clodronate**.[9]

In patients with prostate cancer, compared with placebo, zoledronic acid 4mg IV given every 3 weeks for up to 2 years reduces the risk of skeletal complications by about 36%.[4,10] Baseline bone pain levels were low (mean composite Brief Pain Inventory score of 2/10) and over the course of the study, pain increased slightly in both groups; this was to a lesser degree with zoledronic acid which was significant at some but not all time points. However, about one third of patients had what is considered a clinically relevant improvement in bone pain (⩾2 point change in their pain score).[11]

Although licensed for all solid cancers, the evidence of benefit is generally weaker for other types of cancer.[12] The combination of zoledronic acid with radionucleotides, e.g. Strontium-89 and Samarium-153, is being explored to reduce skeletal complications. In addition to its effect on bone, there is emerging evidence that zoledronic acid may also have a direct anticancer effect.[13]

Zoledronic acid and **disodium pamidronate** are tolerated equally well.[7,8,10,12,14] Because of its slow release from bone back into the systemic circulation, zoledronic acid has a long terminal elimination halflife; it is excreted unchanged by the kidney. Dose reduction is required in patients with mild–moderate renal impairment (see Table 7.3).

In direct comparisons, the incidence of decreased renal function with zoledronic acid 4mg (about 10%) is similar to **disodium pamidronate** 90mg over 2h.[4,12] Decreased renal function was defined in terms of increases in plasma creatinine concentration:

- ⩾44micromol/L for patients with a normal baseline value
- ⩾88micromol/L for patients with an abnormal baseline value
- a doubling or more of the baseline value.

With zoledronic acid 4mg, increases in plasma creatinine lead to treatment delay or discontinuation in about 1% and 3% of patients respectively. Increases in creatinine levels >3 times the upper limit of normal were seen in 0.4% of patients.[7,15] There have been reports of life-threatening renal failure caused by toxic acute tubular necrosis in patients treated with zoledronic acid, e.g. 72 cases among >430,000 patients (i.e. <0.02%).[16–18] Other risk factors were often present, including dehydration, pre-existing renal impairment, and concurrent use of other nephrotoxic drugs.

Onset of decreased renal function varies, but often manifests within 2 months of starting treatment. Mild impairment tends to recover a few days–several months after discontinuing zoledronic acid. In those with renal failure, the damage is generally permanent.[19] The risk of renal toxicity is reduced by adhering to the recommended dose and infusion rate, ensuring adequate hydration, avoiding the concurrent use of other nephrotoxic drugs and monitoring renal function. The dose of zoledronic acid should be adjusted or discontinued if there is deterioration in renal function (see Dose and use).

Onset of action normocalcaemia achieved after a median of 4 days (ranging up to 10); pain relief up to 14 days.

Plasma halflife 1.75h; terminal elimination halflife 1 week.

Duration of action 4 weeks.

Cautions

Serious drug interactions: concurrent use with other nephrotoxic drugs, aminoglycosides (risk of prolonged hypocalcaemia and hypomagnesaemia), loop diuretics (risk of hypocalcaemia and dehydration), or **thalidomide** (increased risk of renal impairment in multiple myeloma patients).

Not recommended in severe renal impairment, i.e. creatinine clearance <30mL/min (see p.478); correct hypovolaemia before treatment and monitor renal function in patients with any degree of renal impairment.

To minimize the risk of osteonecrosis of the jaw, patients should undergo a dental examination before starting long-term zoledronic acid and avoid invasive dental procedures during treatment (see p.472).

Undesirable effects

Very common (>10%): fever, flu-like syndrome (fatigue, rigors, malaise, and flushing), headache, insomnia, dizziness, anxiety, depression, confusion, agitation, fatigue, weakness, paraesthesia, anaemia, neutropenia, cough, breathlessness, weight loss, abdominal pain, nausea, vomiting, constipation or diarrhoea, bone pain, myalgia, hypophosphataemia, hypomagnesaemia, hypokalaemia.

Common (<10%, >1%): asthenia, drowsiness, chest pain, leg oedema, hypotension, granulocytopenia, thrombocytopenia, pancytopenia, pleural effusion, stomatitis, mucositis, anorexia, renal impairment, jaw osteonecrosis, arthralgia, hypocalcaemia.
Rare (<0.1%): uveitis, episcleritis.

There are reports of severe (sometimes incapacitating) musculoskeletal pain arising days–years after starting treatment with a bisphosphonate (generally with PO use for osteoporosis and Paget's disease). This may respond to temporary or permanent discontinuation. The FDA is investigating a possible link with all bisphosphonates, including zoledronic acid.[20]

Dose and use

Tumour-induced hypercalcaemia (corrected plasma calcium >3mmol/L)

Stop and think! Are you justified in correcting a potentially fatal complication in a moribund patient?

- patients should be well hydrated
- give 4mg IVI in 100mL 0.9% saline or 5% glucose over 15min
- if plasma calcium does not normalize, repeat after 1 week[14]
- 8mg has been used in refractory hypercalcaemia[3] but is unlicensed because of concerns relating to renal impairment (see Pharmacology)
- measure plasma creatinine before each dose; no dose adjustment is needed in mild–moderate renal impairment for patients being treated for hypercalcaemia.

In palliative care, treatment with bisphosphonates will probably not be initiated in patients with hypercalcaemia and severe renal impairment. If it is considered appropriate, seek specialist renal/endocrinology advice.

Prophylactic use to reduce the incidence of skeletal-related events in patients with cancer involving the bones and for metastatic bone pain when more conventional methods have been exhausted

- patients should be well hydrated
- give 4mg IVI in 100mL 0.9% saline or 5% glucose over 15min every 3–4 weeks; with appropriate support, these can be given in the home setting[21,22]
- for dose in patients with renal impairment, see Table 7.3
- daily supplements of elemental **calcium** 500mg and **vitamin D** 400 units are recommended, e.g. Calcichew® D3 Forte[23]
- measure plasma creatinine before each dose; withhold treatment if creatinine increases by:
  - ⩾44micromol/L in patients with a normal baseline creatinine concentration (i.e. <124micromol/L) *or*
  - ⩾88micromol/L in patients with a raised baseline creatinine concentration (i.e. >124micromol/L)
- treatment may be resumed at the same dose as before if plasma creatinine returns to within 10% of the baseline value
- discontinue treatment permanently if plasma creatinine fails to improve after 4–8 weeks.

Table 7.3 Dose reduction for zoledronic acid in patients with cancer involving the bones and mild–moderate renal impairment[a,b,c]

Baseline creatinine clearance (mL/min)	*Recommended dose (mg)*	*Amount of concentrate (mL)*
>60	4.0 (i.e. no reduction)	5
50–60	3.5	4.4
40–49	3.3	4.1
30–39	3.0	3.8

a. manufacturer's recommendations for patients with multiple myeloma or bone metastases
b. no data exist for severe renal impairment (creatinine clearance <30mL/min) because these patients were excluded from the studies
c. reduced doses are diluted in 100mL 0.9% saline or 5% glucose and given IVI over 15min.

Supply

Zometa® (Novartis)

Injection (concentrate for dilution and use as an infusion) 4mg/5mL, 5mL vial = £183.

Note: zoledronic acid 50microgram/mL, 100mL (Aclasta®) given IVI over 15min is licensed for the treatment of Paget's disease and as an annual dose for osteoporosis in women (postmenopausal) or men.

1 Green J *et al.* (1994) Preclinical pharmacology of CGP 42'446 a new, potent, heterocyclic bisphosphonate compound. *Journal of Bone and Mineral Research*. **9**: 745–751.

2 Neville-Webbe H and Coleman RE (2003) The use of zoledronic acid in the management of metastatic bone disease and hypercalcaemia. *Palliative Medicine*. **17**: 539–553.

3 Major P *et al.* (2001) Zoledronic acid is superior to pamidronate in the treatment of hypercalcaemia of malignancy: a pooled analysis of two randomized, controlled clinical trials. *Journal of Clinical Oncology*. **19**: 558–567.

4 Rosen LS *et al.* (2001) Zoledronic acid versus pamidronate in the treatment of skeletal metastases in patients with breast cancer or osteolytic lesions of multiple myeloma: a phase III, double-blind, comparative trial. *Cancer Journal*. **7**: 377–387.

5 Kohno N *et al.* (2005) Zoledronic acid significantly reduces skeletal complications compared with placebo in Japanese women with bone metastases from breast cancer: a randomized, placebo-controlled trial. *Journal of Clinical Oncology*. **23**: 3314–3321.

6 Mystakidou K *et al.* (2006) A prospective randomized controlled clinical trial of zoledronic acid for bone metastases. *American Journal of Hospice and Palliative Medicine*. **23**: 41–50.

7 Rosen LS *et al.* (2003) Long-term efficacy and safety of zoledronic acid compared with pamidronate disodium in the treatment of skeletal complications in patients with advanced multiple myeloma or breast carcinoma: a randomized, double-blind, multicenter, comparative trial. *Cancer*. **98**: 1735–1744.

8 Rosen LS *et al.* (2004) Long-term efficacy and safety of zoledronic acid in the treatment of skeletal metastases in patients with nonsmall cell lung carcinoma and other solid tumors: a randomized, Phase III, double-blind, placebo-controlled trial. *Cancer*. **100**: 2613–2621.

9 Clemons MJ *et al.* (2006) Phase II trial evaluating the palliative benefit of second-line zoledronic acid in breast cancer patients with either a skeletal-related event or progressive bone metastases despite first-line bisphosphonate therapy. *Journal of Clinical Oncology*. **24**: 4895–4900.

10 Saad F *et al.* (2004) Long-term efficacy of zoledronic acid for the prevention of skeletal complications in patients with metastatic hormone-refractory prostate cancer. *Journal of the National Cancer Institute*. **96**: 879–882.

11 Weinfurt KP *et al.* (2006) Effect of zoledronic acid on pain associated with bone metastasis in patients with prostate cancer. *Annals of Oncology*. **17**: 986–989.

12 Rosen LS *et al.* (2004) Zoledronic acid is superior to pamidronate for the treatment of bone metastases in breast carcinoma patients with at least one osteolytic lesion. *Cancer*. **100**: 36–43.

13 Costa L *et al.* (2011) Anticancer evidence for zoledronic acid across the cancer continuum. *Critical Reviews in Oncology Hematology*. **77 (suppl 1)**: S31–37.

14 Perry CM and Figgitt DP (2004) Zoledronic acid: a review of its use in patients with advanced cancer. *Drugs*. **64**: 1197–1211.

15 Vogel CL *et al.* (2004) Safety and pain palliation of zoledronic acid in patients with breast cancer, prostate cancer, or multiple myeloma who previously received bisphosphonate therapy. *Oncologist*. **9**: 687–695.

16 Chang JT *et al.* (2003) Renal failure with the use of zoledronic acid. *New England Journal of Medicine*. **349**: 1676–1679.

17 Markowitz GS *et al.* (2003) Toxic acute tubular necrosis following treatment with zoledronate (Zometa). *Kidney International*. **64**: 281–289.

18 Munier A *et al.* (2005) Zoledronic acid and renal toxicity: data from French adverse effect reporting database. *Annals of Pharmacotherapy*. **39**: 1194–1197.

19 Tanvetyanon T and Stiff PJ (2006) Management of the adverse effects associated with intravenous bisphosphonates. *Annals of Oncology*. **17**: 897–907.

20 FDA (2008) Information for healthcare professionals. Bisphosphonates (marketed as Actonel, Actonel+Ca, Aredia, Boniva, Didronel, Fosamax, Fosamax+D, Reclast, Skelid, and Zometa). Food and Drugs Administration. Available from: www.fda.gov/Drugs/DrugSafety/PostmarketDrugSafetyInformationforPatientsandProviders/ucm101551.htm

21 Italiano A *et al.* (2006) Home infusions of biphosphonate in cancer patients: a prospective study. *Journal of Chemotherapy*. **18**: 217–220.

22 Wardley A *et al.* (2005) Zoledronic acid significantly improves pain scores and quality of life in breast cancer patients with bone metastases: a randomised, crossover study of community vs hospital bisphosphonate administration. *British Journal of Cancer*. **92**: 1869–1876.

23 Dhillon S *et al.* (2008) Zoledronic acid: a review of its use in the management of bone metastases of malignancy. *Drugs*. **68**: 507–534.

IBANDRONIC ACID — BNF 6.6.2 & 9.5.1.2

Class: Bisphosphonate.

Indications: Tumour-induced hypercalcaemia, prevention of skeletal events in patients with breast cancer and bone metastases; †metastatic bone pain. Bonviva®: Postmenopausal osteoporosis.

Pharmacology

Ibandronic acid is a third-generation bisphosphonate. Normocalcaemia is achieved in up to two thirds of hypercalcaemic patients after a single IV dose of 2mg, and in three quarters after 4mg. Increasing the dose to 6mg does not increase the response rate above this. Median times to relapse range from 2–4 weeks, depending on the dose (see Table 7.1, p.470).[1,2] In an open RCT, ibandronic acid 4mg IV was as effective as **disodium pamidronate** 60mg IV, with three quarters of patients achieving normocalcaemia after the first dose.[3] Ibandronic acid has not been compared with **zoledronic acid**, which is more effective than **disodium pamidronate** in hypercalcaemia.[4]

In patients with breast cancer, compared with placebo, ibandronic acid 50mg PO once daily or 6mg IV every 3–4 weeks reduces the risk of a bone metastatic event (fractures, need for radiotherapy or surgery) by about 30–40%.[5,6] Preliminary results also suggest that ibandronic acid 50mg PO once daily is as effective as **zoledronic acid** 4mg IV every 4 weeks in suppressing breast cancer-induced bone resorption.[7] The ability of ibandronic acid to prevent the development of bone metastases in women with breast cancer is being explored.[8] In two RCTs, ibandronic acid 50mg PO once daily and 6mg IV every 3–4 weeks improved bone pain and slowed the decline in quality of life in patients with breast cancer. The mean reduction in pain was respectively 0.1 and 0.3 on a 5-point pain scale, compared with an increase of 0.2 with placebo.[9] Although small, the baseline pain scores (median 1.3 and 1.0 respectively) and analgesic requirements were also low.

Open studies indicate benefit in patients with painful bone metastases from other types of cancer. In patients with prostate cancer given ibandronic acid 6mg IV for 3 consecutive days followed by 6mg IV every 4 weeks, one third became pain-free and two thirds had partial improvement after a mean of 3 days (range 1–5 days). Relief was maintained for a mean of 24 weeks (range 16–43 weeks).[10] In patients with various cancers (mostly breast cancer), ibandronic acid 4mg IV once daily for 4 consecutive days reduced bone pain within 1 week. Analgesia was maintained for $>$6 weeks. Quality of life and functional status were also improved. There was no overall reduction in opioid requirements.[11]

The bio-availability of ibandronic acid is low ($<$1%). It is reduced further (by up to 90%) by milk, food, antacids and medicines containing iron or calcium; and these should be avoided for 30–60min after administration. Despite poor bio-availability, ibandronic acid 50mg PO once daily achieves a similar mean plasma concentration (expressed as area under the concentration/time curve) to ibandronic acid 6mg IV once a month.[12] However, the actions of bisphosphonates are related to their concentrations in bone, not plasma,[13] and so clinical equivalence cannot be assumed. Around half of the dose is rapidly adsorbed onto bone and most of the remainder is bound to plasma proteins. Ibandronic acid is excreted unchanged via the kidneys. The plasma proportion of the drug is rapidly eliminated, mostly within 24h. Thereafter, elimination is much slower as the remainder gradually seeps out of bone.

Ibandronic acid and **disodium pamidronate** are equally well tolerated, and the incidence of undesirable effects with ibandronic acid is low during follow-up for up to 4 years.[3,14,15] Because of concerns about the renal effects of bisphosphonates (see p.472), the renal safety of ibandronic acid has been specifically examined. Undesirable renal effects are generally uncommon and occur at a similar or lower rate to placebo, e.g. an increase in plasma creatinine was observed in 6% of patients receiving ibandronic acid 6mg IV over 1–2h every 3–4 weeks for 2 years vs. 12% on placebo. Further, no deterioration in renal function has been seen with a 'loading dose' of ibandronic acid, i.e. 6mg IV over 1h on three consecutive days (even in patients with pre-existing renal impairment),[16,17] or when given over a shorter infusion time of 15min every 3–4 weeks for $\geqslant$1 year.[18] In a direct comparison, there were no renal effects among 37 patients receiving ibandronic acid, whereas one of 34 **disodium pamidronate**-treated patients developed renal failure.[3] Despite concerns of greater renal toxicity with **zoledronic acid** (see p.477), one small RCT (published as a meeting abstract), failed to find any clinically significant renal toxicity with either ibandronic acid 6mg IV or **zoledronic acid** 4mg IV given over 6 months to patients with breast cancer. Identical minimal changes in renal function were temporarily seen following either drug.[19]

Bio-availability <1% PO.
Time to peak plasma concentration <1h.
Onset of action normocalcaemia achieved after a median of <4 days;[1,2] bone pain relieved after a median of 3 days (range 1–5 days) with loading dose regimen.[10]
Plasma halflife 3h; terminal elimination halflife 10–60h.[13]
Duration of action hypercalcaemia 2.5 weeks (4mg IV), 4 weeks (6mg IV);[2] bone pain >6 weeks (4mg IV once daily for 4 days);[11] other IV regimens and PO no data.

Cautions

Pre-existing or bisphosphonate-induced hypocalcaemia (correct before starting treatment; calcium and vitamin D supplements should be given if dietary intake is inadequate). Hypovolaemia (correct before treatment and monitor renal function; avoid overhydration in patients at risk of heart failure). Moderate or severe renal impairment (dose reduction required if creatinine clearance <50mL/min). Concurrent use with aminoglycosides (both can lower plasma calcium and magnesium concentrations for prolonged periods).

Osteonecrosis of the jaw has been reported with ibandronic acid. To minimize the risk, carry out a dental examination before starting treatment and avoid invasive dental procedures while receiving treatment.

PO administration: oesophagitis and oropharyngeal, oesophageal and gastric ulceration (discontinue if dysphagia, pain on swallowing, retrosternal pain or heartburn occur). Concurrent use with NSAIDs (both can cause GI irritation and ulceration).

Undesirable effects

Very common (>10%): pyrexia.
Common (<10%, >1%): asthenia, flu-like symptoms, headache, hypocalcaemia, bone pain, myalgia. Oral products may cause nausea, dyspepsia, or oesophagitis.

Dose and use

When taken PO, to maximize absorption and to minimize undesirable gastro-oesophageal effects, ibandronic acid tablets are best taken after an overnight fast, with no food for at least another 30min. The tablets should be swallowed whole with a glass of *plain tap water* (not mineral water because this may contain considerable amounts of calcium) in an upright position. Patients should not lie down for 1h afterwards.

Patients treated with IVI ibandronic acid should be well hydrated. If necessary, rehydrate with an IVI of 0.9% saline. Renal function should be monitored (see below).

Tumour-induced hypercalcaemia

Stop and think! Are you justified in correcting a potentially fatal complication in a moribund patient?

- if the corrected plasma calcium is >3mmol/L give 4mg
- if the corrected plasma calcium is <3mmol/L give 2mg
- for both, the dose is given IVI in 500mL 0.9% saline *or* 5% glucose over 2h.

Prevention of skeletal events in patients with bone metastases from breast cancer

- 50mg PO once daily *or*
- 6mg IVI in 100mL 0.9% saline *or* 5% glucose over 15min every 3–4 weeks.

The 15min infusion regimen is recommended only for patients with normal renal function or mild renal impairment, i.e. creatinine clearance >50mL/min. See below for patients with more severe renal impairment.

Metastatic bone pain

- 50mg PO once daily *or*
- 6mg IVI in 500mL 0.9% saline or 5% glucose over 1h every 3–4 weeks.

For patients with moderate–severe bone pain, consider an initial 'loading dose' regimen, e.g. 6mg IVI daily for 3 days.[10]

In renal impairment

The SPC recommends a dose reduction in patients with moderate or severe renal impairment (creatinine clearance <50–30mL/min and <30mL/min respectively) being treated to prevent skeletal events in metastatic breast cancer:

- *PO treatment:*
  - ▹ in moderate renal impairment, give 50mg PO *alternate days*
  - ▹ in severe renal impairment, give 50mg PO *once a week*
- *IV treatment:* in moderate–severe renal impairment, adjust the dose according to creatinine clearance (Table 7.4).

Table 7.4 Prophylactic IV ibandronic acid in patients with metastatic breast cancer and renal impairment

Renal impairment	*Creatinine clearance (mL/min)*	*Dose and infusion time*[a]	*Infusion volume*[b]
Moderate	<50–30	4mg over 1h	500mL
Severe	<30	2mg over 1h	500mL

a. given every 3–4 weeks
b. use 0.9% saline or 5% glucose as diluent.

The SPC gives no recommended dose reductions for patients with moderate–severe renal impairment receiving ibandronic acid for bone pain or hypercalcaemia. However, prolonging the infusion time of a standard dose would provide an added safeguard (e.g. give over 2h instead of 1h).

Ibandronic acid is removed by haemodialysis. Following a single dose of 1mg IVI, the plasma concentration was successively reduced by approximately 50% at each of 3 sessions. Ibandronic acid was undetectable after the third session.[20]

Supply

Bondronat® (Roche)

Tablets 50mg, 28 days @ 50mg once daily = £184.

Injection (concentrate for dilution and use as an infusion) 1mg/mL, 2mL amp = £89; 6mL vial = £184.

Note: ibandronic acid 150mg tablets and 1mg/mL, 3mL pre-filled syringe (Bonviva®) *given once a month and every 3 months respectively are licensed for the treatment of postmenopausal osteoporosis.*

1 Pecherstorfer M *et al.* (1996) Randomized phase II trial comparing different doses of the bisphosphonate ibandronate in the treatment of hypercalcemia of malignancy. *Journal of Clinical Oncology.* **14**: 268–276.

2 Ralston SH *et al.* (1997) Dose-response study of ibandronate in the treatment of cancer-associated hypercalcaemia. *British Journal of Cancer.* **75**: 295–300.

3 Pecherstorfer M *et al.* (2003) Efficacy and safety of ibandronate in the treatment of hypercalcemia of malignancy: a randomized multicentric comparison to pamidronate. *Supportive Care in Cancer.* **11**: 539–547.

4 Major P *et al.* (2001) Zoledronic acid is superior to pamidronate in the treatment of hypercalcaemia of malignancy: a pooled analysis of two randomized, controlled clinical trials. *Journal of Clinical Oncology.* **19**: 558–567.

5 Body JJ *et al.* (2003) Intravenous ibandronate reduces the incidence of skeletal complications in patients with breast cancer and bone metastases. *Annals of Oncology.* **14**: 1399–1405.

6 Body JJ *et al.* (2004) Oral ibandronate reduces the risk of skeletal complications in breast cancer patients with metastatic bone disease: results from two randomised, placebo-controlled phase III studies. *British Journal of Cancer.* **90**: 1133–1137.

7 Body JJ (2005) Effect of oral ibandronate versus intravenous (i.v.) zoledronic acid on markers of bone resorption in patients with breast cancer and bone metastases: results from a comparative phase III trial. (Poster). In: *ASCO Annual Meeting* 13–17 May; Orlando, Florida.

8 Clemons M and Verma S (2005) Should oral bisphosphonates be standard of care in women with early breast cancer? *Breast Cancer Research and Treatment.* **90**: 315–318.

9 Body JJ *et al.* (2004) Oral ibandronate improves bone pain and preserves quality of life in patients with skeletal metastases due to breast cancer. *Pain.* **111**: 306–312.

10 Heidenreich A *et al.* (2002) Ibandronate in the treatment of prostate cancer associated painful osseous metastases. *Prostate Cancer and Prostatic Disease.* **5**: 231–235.

11 Mancini I *et al.* (2004) Efficacy and safety of ibandronate in the treatment of opioid-resistant bone pain associated with metastatic bone disease: a pilot study. *Journal of Clinical Oncology.* **22**: 3587–3592.

12 Leyland-Jones B (2004) Pharmacokinetic and clinical equivalence of oral and intravenous ibandronate for metastatic bone disease. *European Journal of Cancer Supplements*. **2 (suppl 5)**: 9–12.
13 Barrett J *et al.* (2004) Ibandronate: a clinical pharmacological and pharmacokinetic update. *Journal of Clinical Pharmacology*. **44**: 951–965.
14 McLachlan SA *et al.* (2003) Long-term safety of oral ibandronate for up to 4 years in patients with skeletal metastases from breast cancer. (Poster). In: *the IVth International Conference on Cancer-induced Bone Diseases* 7–9 December; San Antonio, Texas.
15 Rivkin S *et al.* (2003) Long-term safety of intravenous (i.v.) ibandronate by bolus injection or infusion for up to 4 years in metastatic bone disease: results of an open-label study. (Poster). In: *the IVth International Conference on Cancer-induced Bone Diseases* 7–9 December; San Antonio, Texas.
16 Bergner R *et al.* (2005) Renal safety of ibandronate in multiple myeloma patients with renal deterioration. *Cancer Treatment Reviews*. **31 (suppl 1)**: s45.
17 Heidenreich A *et al.* (2005) Renal safety of loading dose ibandronate in urologic patients with compensated renal insufficiency. *Cancer Treatment Reviews*. **31(suppl 1)**: s50.
18 von Moos R *et al.* (2010) Long-term renal safety profile of ibandronate 6 mg infused over 15 minutes. *Onkologie*. **33**: 447–450.
19 Luedders DW (2010) Lack of differences in nephrotoxicity of intravenous bisphosphonates in metastatic breast cancer. *Journal of Clinical Oncology*. **28 (Suppl May 20)**: 1122.
20 Bergner R *et al.* (2002) Elimination of intravenously administered ibandronate in patients on haemodialysis: a monocentre open study. *Nephrology Dialysis Transplantation*. **17**: 1281–1285.

SYSTEMIC CORTICOSTEROIDS — BNF 6.3.2

Indications: Suppression of inflammatory and allergic disorders, cerebral oedema, nausea and vomiting with chemotherapy; †see Box 7.B.

Box 7.B Off-label indications for systemic corticosteroids in advanced cancer[1,2]

This list of off-label uses does not claim to be totally comprehensive. Further, inclusion does not mean that a systemic corticosteroid is necessarily the treatment of choice. Further, the evidence-base for some indications is only 'expert opinion'.

Specific
Spinal cord compression[3]
Nerve compression
Breathlessness
 pneumonitis (after radiotherapy)
 lymphangitic carcinomatosis
 tracheal compression/stridor
Superior vena caval obstruction[4]
Obstruction of hollow viscus
 bronchus[5]
 ureter
 GI[6,7]
Radiation-induced inflammation
Discharge from rectal tumour (can give either PO or PR)
Paraneoplastic fever
Nausea and vomiting in cancer resistant to standard measures (see p.486)
Hypercalcaemia associated with cancer (an adjunct to SC calcitonin)[8,9]

Pain relief
Pain caused by a tumour in a confined organ or body cavity, e.g. raised intracranial pressure, bone pain

Anticancer hormone therapy
Breast cancer[10]
Prostate cancer[11]
Haematological malignancies
Lymphoproliferative disorders

General ('tonic')
To improve appetite
To enhance sense of wellbeing

Contra-indications: Systemic infection, unless considered to be life-saving and specific anti-infective therapy is employed.

Pharmacology

The adrenal cortex secretes **hydrocortisone** (cortisol) which has glucocorticoid activity and weak mineralocorticoid activity.[12] It also secretes aldosterone which has mineralocorticoid activity. Thus, in deficiency states, physiological replacement is best achieved with a combination of **hydrocortisone** and **fludrocortisone**, a mineralocorticoid.

In many disease states, corticosteroids are used primarily as potent anti-inflammatory agents. The anti-inflammatory action is mediated via several interacting mechanisms,[12] in contrast to the more specific impact of NSAIDs on prostaglandin synthesis (see p.294). Thus, as anti-inflammatory agents, corticosteroids are potentially more effective than NSAIDs. However, certainly when used long-term, corticosteroids are likely to cause more numerous and more serious undesirable effects (see below).

When comparing the relative anti-inflammatory (glucocorticoid) potencies of corticosteroids, their water-retaining properties (mineralocorticoid effect) should also be borne in mind (Table 7.5). Thus, **hydrocortisone** is not used for long-term disease suppression because large doses would be required which would cause troublesome fluid retention. On the other hand, its moderate anti-inflammatory effect makes it a useful corticosteroid for topical use in inflammatory skin conditions; both topical and systemic undesirable effects are minimal.

Prednisolone is the most frequently used corticosteroid for disease suppression. **Dexamethasone**, with high glucocorticoid activity but insignificant mineralocorticoid effect, is particularly suitable for high-dose anti-inflammatory therapy. It is 6–12 times more potent than **prednisolone**, i.e. 2mg of **dexamethasone** is approximately equivalent to 15–25mg of **prednisolone** (Box 7.C) and it has a long duration of action (Table 7.5). Some corticosteroid esters, e.g. of **betamethasone** and of **beclometasone**, exert a marked topical effect; use is made of this property with skin applications and bronchial inhalations (see p.582 and p.114).

Box 7.C Approximate equivalent anti-inflammatory doses of corticosteroids[a]

Cortisone acetate	25mg
Hydrocortisone	20mg
Prednisone	5mg
Prednisolone	5mg
Methylprednisolone	4mg
Triamcinolone	4mg
Betamethasone	750microgram
Dexamethasone	750microgram

a. this list takes no account of mineralocorticoid effects or variations in duration of action.

General 'tonic' use

The non-specific 'tonic' use of corticosteroids is based on the known general effects of this group of drugs. In patients with advanced cancer, treatment with corticosteroids may result in increased appetite, reduced nausea and improved well-being. In a recent qualitative study, patients initially reported distressing symptoms, physical deterioration, decreased autonomy, and a feeling of apprehension and foreboding. After treatment for one week with **betamethasone** 4mg once daily, most patients had improved symptom relief, and reported enhanced physical abilities, increased autonomy, and renewed hope.[13]

RCTs of corticosteroids specifically as appetite stimulants have used daily doses of **prednisolone** 15–40mg (or equivalent).[14–16] All showed benefit compared with placebo. In one, benefit was comparable for daily doses of **dexamethasone** of either 3mg or 6mg (equivalent to **prednisolone** 20mg or 40mg). Overall, over 50% of the patients reported benefit, which was still apparent after 4 weeks.[14,15,17]

Table 7.5 Selected pharmacokinetic details of commonly used corticosteroids[25,26]

Drug	*Anti-inflammatory potency*	*Approximate equivalent dose (mg)*	*Sodium-retaining potency*	*Oral bio-availability (%)*	*Onset of action*	*Peak plasma concentration*	*Plasma halflife (h)*	*Duration of action (h)*	*Relative affinity for lung tissue*	*Daily dose (mg) above which adrenal suppression possible*	
										Male	*Female*
Hydrocortisone	1	20	1	96	No data	1h PO	1.5	8–12	1	20–30	15–25
Prednisone[a] / Prednisolone	4	5	0.25	75–85	No data	1h PO	3.5	12–36	1.6	7.5–10	7.5
Dexamethasone	25–50[b]	0.5–1	<0.01	78	8–24h IM[c]	1–2h PO	4.5	36–54	1	1–1.15	1
Betamethasone				98	No data	10–36min IV	6.5	24–48			

a. biologically inert prednisone is converted by the liver to prednisolone
b. thymic involution assay
c. acute allergic reactions.

However, both corticosteroids and progestogens (see p.513) should *not* be regarded as 'anticachexia' agents. Any weight gain relates to fluid retention ± increased fat, rather than to increased skeletal muscle mass. This could make mobilizing more difficult in an already debilitated patient. In addition, the catabolic effect of corticosteroids on skeletal muscle, exacerbated by reduced levels of physical activity, may well further weaken the patient, rendering corticosteroids suitable for short-term use only.

Nausea and vomiting

Dexamethasone is an integral part of standard management of severe chemotherapeutic vomiting.[18] The anti-emetic effect is possibly mediated by a corticosteroid-induced reduction in the permeability of the chemoreceptor trigger zone and of the blood–brain barrier to emetogenic substances, and a reduction in the neuronal content of gamma-aminobutyric acid (GABA) in the brain stem.

In palliative care, **dexamethasone** is often used when all else fails as an 'add-on' anti-emetic (see p.226). However, there is some evidence that **dexamethasone** does not add to the anti-emetic efficacy of **metoclopramide** or phenothiazines in patients with advanced cancer.[19–21]

Obstructive syndromes

In obstructive syndromes (Box 7.B), corticosteroids may help by reducing inflammation at the site of the obstruction, thereby increasing the lumen of the obstructed hollow viscus. Corticosteroids (**dexamethasone** equivalent 6–16mg/24h) may improve bowel obstruction but do not affect survival. The incidence of undesirable events is low.[6] High-dose corticosteroids (**dexamethasone** equivalent 20–40mg/24h) relieved stridor within 12h in 3 patients with upper airway obstruction from infiltrating tumour.[5]

Brain metastases

Dexamethasone is recommended for treatment of adults with symptomatic brain metastases; no benefit is seen in patients with asymptomatic brain metastases. **Dexamethasone** 4–8mg/24h provides temporary symptomatic relief for patients with mild symptoms related to raised intracranial pressure from cerebral oedema. If patients have severe symptoms or are at risk of herniation, doses of ≥16mg/24h are recommended. Symptom relief from **dexamethasone** reduces over time and undesirable effects increase. Thus, ideally, the dose of **dexamethasone** should be reduced after one week and discontinued after 2–4 weeks.[22] However, unless patients receive additional treatment (e.g. palliative radiotherapy), they will experience a recurrence of their symptoms at some point as the dose of **dexamethasone** is decreased. Thus, it may be necessary to taper more slowly or continue 'maintenance' **dexamethasone** indefinitely in some patients.

Whole brain radiotherapy may cause nausea, vomiting, headache, fever and a transient worsening of neurological symptoms. **Dexamethasone** should be continued for one week after treatment and then tapered over 2–4 weeks.[23,24]

For pharmacokinetic details, see Table 7.5.

Cautions

Diabetes mellitus, psychotic illness. Although there is only a small increased risk of peptic ulceration with corticosteroids alone,[27] when given concurrently with NSAIDs, the risk is increased up to *15 times*.[28,29]

Prolonged courses of corticosteroids increase susceptibility to infections and their severity. Clinical presentation may be atypical; the signs of infection (including peritonitis) may be masked. Serious infections (e.g. septicaemia and tuberculosis) may reach an advanced stage before diagnosis. Live vaccines should not be given; the antibody response to other vaccines may be diminished.

In patients who have taken > 10mg **prednisolone** (or equivalent) daily for 3 weeks, the occurrence of any significant intercurrent illness, trauma or surgical procedure necessitates a temporary increase in corticosteroid dose (or, if stopped within the past 3 months, a temporary re-introduction) to compensate for a reduced adrenocortical response caused by the corticosteroid treatment.[30]

Drug interactions

Corticosteroids antagonize oral hypoglycaemics and **insulin** (glucocorticoid effect), antihypertensives and diuretics (mineralocorticoid effect). Increased risk of hypokalaemia if high doses of corticosteroids are prescribed with β_2 agonists (e.g. **salbutamol**, **terbutaline**).

The metabolism of corticosteroids is accelerated by anti-epileptics (**carbamazepine**, **phenobarbital**, **phenytoin**, **primidone**), and rifamycins (**rifabutin**, **rifampicin**). This is more pronounced with long-acting glucocorticoids; thus **phenytoin** may reduce the bioavailability of **dexamethasone** to 25–50%, and larger doses (double or more) will be needed when prescribed concurrently.[31] **Dexamethasone** itself can affect plasma **phenytoin** concentrations (may either rise or fall).

Concurrent prescription of a corticosteroid increases the INR in patients already taking **warfarin**, necessitating a dose reduction in about 50% of patients.[32] Thus, the INR should be checked weekly for 2–3 weeks when a corticosteroid is started or dose altered.

Undesirable effects

See Box 7.D–Box 7.G.

Box 7.D Undesirable effects of corticosteroids[28]

Glucocorticoid effects
Avascular bone necrosis
Cataract (prednisolone 15mg/24h or equivalent for several years = 75% risk; also seen with long-term inhaled steroids)[33]
Diabetes mellitus or deterioration of glycaemic control in known diabetics (see p.503)
Infection (increased susceptibility):
- candidosis (debatable, see p.446)
- septicaemia (may delay recognition)
- tuberculosis (may delay recognition)
- chickenpox[a]
- measles (increased severity)

Mental disturbances (Box 7.E)
Muscle wasting and weakness (Box 7.F)
Osteoporosis
Peptic ulceration (if given with an NSAID)[34]
Suppression of growth (in child)

Mineralocorticoid effects
Sodium and water retention → oedema
Potassium loss
Hypertension

Cushingoid features
Lipodystrophy after ≥8 weeks of treatment in 30–70% of patients (reversible on stopping treatment):
- moon face
- buffalo hump
- increased abdominal fat
- reduced subcutaneous fat in limbs

Acne
Bruising
Hirsuitism
Striae

a. if exposed to infection, non-immune patients should be given varicella-zoster immunoglobulin (see BNF section 6.3.2).

Box 7.E Corticosteroid-induced psychiatric disturbances[35–38]

Incidence
Reports range from 13–62% of those prescribed a corticosteroid.
Prevalence is higher in women, and more likely with higher doses.

Clinical manifestations
Symptoms generally occur 4–6 days after starting a corticosteroid, but this is highly variable and can occur even after cessation of treatment.
Manifestations are mostly mild or moderate, but can be severe, and include:
- depression (40%)
- mania (25%)

continued

Box 7.E Continued

- paranoid ('steroid') psychosis (15%)
- delirium (10%)
- bipolar disorder (5%).[36]

Educating patients about the possible risk of undesirable psychiatric effects may improve the reporting of symptoms.

Management

Reduce or discontinue the causal corticosteroid if possible.[35]

Environmental conditions should be optimized to minimize agitation.[39]

Symptoms may take 1–2 weeks to resolve.[37]

If the corticosteroid cannot be stopped, or symptoms are intolerable, atypical antipsychotics should be prescribed for patients with psychosis, aggression or agitation.

Although antidepressants may exacerbate agitation and psychosis, they are generally helpful in depressed patients who require long-term corticosteroids.

All patients with corticosteroid-induced psychiatric disturbance should be evaluated for suicidal ideation.

Prognosis

A history of:

- psychiatric disease does not make a corticosteroid-induced psychiatric disturbance more likely
- previous corticosteroid-induced disturbance does not necessarily mean that a second disturbance will occur if corticosteroids are represcribed.[38]

Box 7.F Systemic corticosteroid myopathy[40,41]

Glucocorticoids cause atrophy of limb and respiratory muscles. It is a dose-related effect which generally manifests only after $\geq$2 months of treatment with dexamethasone >4mg/24h or prednisolone >40mg/24h. Can occur earlier and with lower doses.

If the chronological sequence fits with corticosteroid myopathy, a presumptive diagnosis should be made and the following steps taken:

- explanation to patient and family
- discuss need to compromise between maximizing therapeutic benefit and minimizing undesirable effects
- halve corticosteroid dose (generally possible as a single step)
- consider changing from dexamethasone to prednisolone (non-fluorinated corticosteroids cause less myopathy)
- attempt further reductions in dose at intervals of 1–2 weeks
- arrange for physiotherapy (disuse exacerbates myopathy)
- emphasize that weakness should improve after 3–4 weeks (provided cancer-induced weakness does not supervene).

Box 7.G Pseudorheumatism

Patients receiving corticosteroids for rheumatoid arthritis occasionally develop myalgia, arthralgia, malaise, rhinitis, conjunctivitis, painful itchy skin nodules, weight loss and pyrexia; so-called steroid pseudorheumatism.[42]

It is sometimes also seen in cancer patients receiving large doses of corticosteroids or when a very high dose is reduced rapidly to a lower dose. Most likely to be affected are those:

- receiving 100mg of prednisolone/24h for several days in association with chemotherapy

continued

Box 7.G Continued

- with spinal cord compression given dexamethasone 96mg IV/24h for 3 days[43] (followed by a rapidly reducing oral dose)[a]
- on high doses of dexamethasone to reduce raised intracranial pressure associated with brain metastases
- reducing to an ordinary maintenance dose after a prolonged course.

a. such a high dose is unnecessary; 10mg IV is as effective as 96mg.[44,45]

Dose and use

Given the many and significant undesirable effects of corticosteroids, and the potentially deleterious effect of rapid withdrawal, corticosteroids should be prescribed cautiously:

- for defined symptoms potentially responsive to corticosteroid therapy
- always bearing in mind potential benefit vs. risk
- at a low–moderate dose, titrated to clinical effect
- for a time-limited trial
- discontinued if no clinical/symptomatic benefit seen *or*
- weaned to the lowest effective dose.[46]

If expected to take corticosteroids for ≥3 weeks, patients should be given a *Steroid Treatment* card (Box 7.H).

Box 7.H Example of a *Steroid Treatment* card

I am a patient on STEROID treatment which must not be stopped suddenly.

- If you have been taking this medicine for more than 3 weeks, the dose should be reduced gradually when you stop taking steroids unless your doctor says otherwise.
- Read the patient information leaflet given with the medicine.
- Always carry this card with you and show it to anyone who treats you (for example a doctor, nurse, pharmacist, or dentist).
- For 1 year after you stop the treatment, you must mention that you have taken steroids.
- If you become ill, or if you come into contact with anyone who has an infectious disease, consult your doctor promptly.
- If you have never had chickenpox, you should avoid close contact with people who have chickenpox or shingles. If you do come into contact with chickenpox, see your doctor urgently.
- Make sure that the information on the card about your current dose is kept up to date.

Except for **hydrocortisone**, corticosteroids can be given in a single daily dose each morning; this eases compliance and reduces the likelihood of corticosteroid-induced insomnia. Even so, **temazepam** or **diazepam** at bedtime is sometimes needed to counter insomnia or agitation. The initial dose varies according to indication and fashion.

All the doses below are PO unless otherwise stated. **Dexamethasone** has a PO bio-availability of about 80%; and, when necessary, many centres convert to SC/IV dexamethasone on a 1:1 basis (i.e. use the same dose for either route).

Replacement therapy: **hydrocortisone** 20mg each morning, 10mg each evening with **fludrocortisone** 100–300microgram each morning.
Anti-emetic: e.g. **dexamethasone** 8–20mg each morning (see Pharmacology section above; also p.226).[47–49]
Anorexia: **dexamethasone** 2–6mg or **prednisolone** 15–40mg each morning.[14–17]
Raised intracranial pressure: **dexamethasone** 8–16mg each morning.[50,51]
Obstruction of hollow viscus: **dexamethasone** 6–16mg each morning.[6]
Spinal cord compression: **dexamethasone** 16mg each morning.[45]

Discharge from rectal tumour or acute post-radiation proctitis: retention enema of **hydrocortisone acetate** 125mg PR or **prednisolone** 20mg PR every 1–2 days. If local application is impractical, PO corticosteroids can be used instead.

For inhaled corticosteroids, see p.114.
For depot corticosteroid injections, see p.555.
For topical corticosteroids, see p.582.
For CSCI, see p.666.

Stopping corticosteroids

If after 7–10 days the corticosteroid fails to achieve the desired effect, it should be stopped. It is often possible to stop corticosteroids abruptly (Box 7.I).[52] However, if there is uncertainty about disease or symptom resolution, withdrawal should be guided by monitoring disease activity or the symptom.

Particularly if it has been taken for >3 weeks, rapid withdrawal of a corticosteroid may result in a corticosteroid withdrawal syndrome. This may cause an array of symptoms and signs similar to those of pseudorheumatism (Box 7.G) together with adrenal insufficiency. The syndrome is treated by restarting the corticosteroid or increasing the dose to that given before the onset of withdrawal symptoms.[53]

In patients who are moribund and no longer able to swallow tablets, it is generally acceptable to discontinue corticosteroids abruptly,[46] although sometimes a maintenance dose may be indicated to prevent distress from symptomatic hypo-adrenalism.

Occasionally, a patient with a brain tumour or multiple brain metastases requests that **dexamethasone** is stopped because, despite its continued use, there is progressive physical deterioration and/or cognitive impairment. In this circumstance, it is often best to reduce the **dexamethasone** step by step on a daily basis. This gives the patient time to reconsider. Extra analgesics should be prescribed in case headache develops as the intracranial pressure increases:

- if already taking **paracetamol**, prescribe a weak opioid or a weak opioid-**paracetamol** combination p.r.n.
- if already taking a weak opioid, prescribe **morphine** 10–20mg PO or **morphine** 5–10mg SC p.r.n.
- if >2 p.r.n. doses have been given in the last 24h, increase the regular analgesic dose
- if the patient becomes drowsy or swallowing becomes difficult, switch PO anti-epileptics to a non-oral route, e.g. SC **midazolam** or IM/IV **phenobarbital** (see p.272) and possibly give both **morphine** and the anti-epileptic by CSCI.

If the patient becomes semicomatose and cannot communicate clearly, the presence of headache may manifest as grimacing or general restlessness. However, as in all moribund patients, it is important to exclude other common reasons for agitation, e.g. a full bladder or rectum, and discomfort and stiffness secondary to immobility.

Box 7.I Recommendations for withdrawing systemic corticosteroids[52]

Abrupt withdrawal

Systemic corticosteroids may be stopped abruptly in those whose disease is unlikely to relapse *and* have received treatment for <3 weeks *and* are not in the groups below.

Gradual withdrawal

Gradual withdrawal of systemic corticosteroids is advisable in patients who:

- have received more than 3 weeks treatment
- have received prednisolone >40mg/24h or equivalent, e.g. dexamethasone 4–6mg
- have had a second dose in the evening
- have received repeated treatments
- are taking a short course within 1 year of stopping long-term treatment
- have other possible causes of adrenal suppression.

During corticosteroid withdrawal the dose may initially be reduced rapidly (e.g. halving the dose daily) to physiological doses (prednisolone 7.5mg/24h or equivalent) and then more slowly (e.g. 1–2mg per week) to allow the adrenals to recover and to prevent a hypo-adrenal crisis (malaise, profound weakness, hypotension, etc.). The patient should be monitored during withdrawal in case of deterioration.

Supply

Dexamethasone formulations in the UK[54]

PO tablets are formulated as dexamethasone *base,* the two parenteral preparations available are formulated as dexamethasone *sodium phosphate*, but are different strengths (Table 7.6). BNF, SPCs and product labels now all use dexamethasone *base* for labelling and dosing advice.

For simplicity Organon's 4mg/mL ampoule is preferable when prescribing with the option for either PO or parenteral administration.

Dexamethasone (generic)
Tablets 500microgram, 2mg, 28 days @ 2mg once daily = £4.50.
Oral solution (sugar-free) 2mg/5mL, 28 days @ 2mg once daily = £40.
Injection 4mg/mL, 1mL amp = £1.
Injection 3.3mg/mL, 1mL amp = £1, 2mL vial = £2.

Table 7.6 Dexamethasone base and salt content in UK parenteral formulations

Manufacturer	*Presentation*	*Dexamethasone base (as on the label)*[a]	*Dexamethasone sodium phosphate*
Organon	1mL amp	4mg	5.2mg
Hospira	1mL amp	3.3mg	4.3mg
Hospira	2mL vial	6.6mg	8.6mg

a. dexamethasone base 1mg = dexamethasone sodium phosphate 1.3mg approximately.

Hydrocortisone (generic)
Tablets (scored) 10mg, 20mg, 28days @ 20mg each morning and 10mg each evening = £100.

Fludrocortisone
Florinef® (Squibb)
Tablets (scored) 100microgram, 28 days @ 100microgram each morning = £1.50.

Prednisolone (generic)
Tablets 1mg, 5mg, 25mg, 28 days @ 15mg once daily = £4.
Tablets e/c 2.5mg, 5mg, 28 days @ 15mg once daily = £15.
Tablets soluble 5mg, 28 days @ 15mg once daily = £27.

Rectal products
Hydrocortisone
Colifoam® (Meda)
Retention foam enema **hydrocortisone *acetate*** 10% (100mg/mL), 1 metered application = 125mg **hydrocortisone *acetate***, 14-application cannister with applicator = £9.

Prednisolone
Predenema® (Chemidex)
Retention enema **prednisolone** (as ***sodium metasulphobenzoate***) 20mg in 100mL, single standard tube or long tube = £1 and £1.50 respectively.

Predfoam® (Forest)
Retention foam enema **prednisolone** (as ***sodium metasulphobenzoate***) 20mg/metered application, 14-application canister with applicators = £7.

Predsol® (UCB Pharma)
Retention enema **prednisolone** (as ***sodium phosphate***) 20mg in 100mL, single = £1.
Suppositories **prednisolone** (as ***sodium phosphate***) 5mg, 10 = £1.50.

Note: **budesonide** rectal products are also available, but are much more expensive.

1 Hanks GW *et al.* (1983) Corticosteroids in terminal cancer — a prospective analysis of current practice. *Postgraduate Medical Journal.* **59**: 702–706.
2 Hardy J *et al.* (2001) A prospective survey of the use of dexamethasone on a palliative care unit. *Palliative Medicine.* **15**: 3–8.
3 NICE (2008) Matastatic spinal cord compression: diagnosis and management of patients at risk of or with metastatic spinal cord compression. (Clinical guideline 75.). National Institute for Health and Clinical Excellence, London. Available from: www.nice.org.uk/CG75
4 Rowell NP and Gleeson FV (2001) Steroids, radiotherapy, chemotherapy and stents for superior vena caval obstruction in carcinoma of the bronchus. *Cochrane Database of Systematic Reviews.* CD001316.
5 Elsayem A and Bruera E (2007) High-dose corticosteroids for the management of dyspnea in patients with tumor obstruction of the upper airway. *Supportive Care in Cancer.* **15**: 1437–1439.
6 Feuer DJ and Broadley KE (2009) Corticosteroids for the resolution of malignant bowel obstruction in advanced gynaecological and gastrointestinal cancer 2000 (2). Update 2009. *Cochrane Database of Systematic Reviews.* CD001219.
7 Laval G *et al.* (2000) The use of steroids in the management of inoperable intestinal obstruction in terminal cancer patients: do they remove the obstruction? *Palliative Medicine.* **14**: 3–10.
8 Ralston S *et al.* (1985) Comparison of aminohydroxypropylidene diphosphonate, mithramycin, and corticosteroids/calcitonin in treatment of cancer-associated hypercalcaemia. *Lancet.* **ii**: 907–910.
9 Percival R *et al.* (1984) Role of glucocorticoids in management of malignant hypercalcaemia. *British Medical Journal.* **289**: 287.
10 Minton MJ *et al.* (1981) Corticosteroids for elderly patients with breast cancer. *Cancer.* **48**: 883–887.
11 Tannock IF *et al.* (1996) Chemotherapy with mitoxantrone plus prednisone or prednisone alone for symptomatic hormone-resistant prostate cancer: a Canadian randomized trial with palliative end points. *Journal of Clinical Oncology.* **14**: 1756–1764.
12 Rhen T and Cidlowski JA (2005) Antiinflammatory action of glucocorticoids–new mechanisms for old drugs. *New England Journal of Medicine.* **353**: 1711–1723.
13 Lundstrom S *et al.* (2009) The existential impact of starting corticosteroid treatment as symptom control in advanced metastatic cancer. *Palliative Medicine.* **23**: 165–170.
14 Bruera E *et al.* (1985) Action of oral methylprednisolone in terminal cancer patients: a prospective randomized double-blind study. *Cancer Treatment Reports.* **69**: 751–754.
15 Moertel C *et al.* (1974) Corticosteroid therapy for preterminal gastrointestinal cancer. *Cancer.* **33**: 1607–1609.
16 Twycross RG and Guppy D (1985) Prednisolone in terminal breast and bronchogenic cancer. *Practitioner.* **229**: 57–59.
17 Willox JC *et al.* (1984) Prednisolone as an appetite stimulant in patients with cancer. *British Medical Journal.* **288**: 27.
18 Ioannidis JP *et al.* (2000) Contribution of dexamethasone to control of chemotherapy-induced nausea and vomiting: a meta-analysis of randomized evidence. *Journal of Clinical Oncology.* **18**: 3409–3422.
19 Bruera E *et al.* (2004) Dexamethasone in addition to metoclopramide for chronic nausea in patients with advanced cancer: a randomized controlled trial. *Journal of Pain and Symptom Management.* **28**: 381–388.
20 Davis MP *et al.* (2010) A systematic review of the treatment of nausea and/or vomiting in cancer unrelated to chemotherapy or radiation. *Journal of Pain and Symptom Management.* **39**: 756–767.
21 Glare PA *et al.* (2008) Treatment of nausea and vomiting in terminally ill cancer patients. *Drugs.* **68**: 2575–2590.
22 Vecht C *et al.* (1994) Dose-effect relationship of dexamethasone on Karnofsky performance in metastatic brain tumors. A randomized study of doses of 4, 8 and 16 mg per day. *Neurology.* **44**: 675–680.
23 Ryken TC *et al.* (2010) The role of steroids in the management of brain metastases: a systematic review and evidence-based clinical practice guideline. *Journal of Neuro-oncology.* **96**: 103–114.
24 Soffetti *et al.* (2006) EFNS guidelines on diagnosis and treatment of brain metastases. *European Journal of Neurology.* **13**: 674–681.
25 Swartz S and Dluhy R (1978) Corticosteroids: clinical pharmacology and therapeutic use. *Drugs.* **16**: 238–255.
26 Demoly P and Chung K (1998) Pharmacology of corticosteroids. *Respiratory Medicine.* **92**: 385–394.
27 Ellershaw J and Kelly M (1994) Corticosteroids and peptic ulceration. *Palliative Medicine.* **8**: 313–319.
28 Fardet L *et al.* (2007) Corticosteroid-induced adverse events in adults: frequency, screening and prevention. *Drug Safety.* **30**: 861–881.
29 Naesdal J and Brown K (2006) NSAID-associated adverse effects and acid control aids to prevent them: a review of current treatment options. *Drug Safety.* **29**: 119–132.
30 BNF (2011) Section 6.3.2. In: *British National Formulary No 61*. British Medical Association and the Royal Pharmaceutical Society of Great Britain, London.
31 Chalk J *et al.* (1984) Phenytoin impairs the bioavailability of dexamethasone in neurological and neurosurgical patients. *Journal of Neurology, Neurosurgery, and Psychiatry.* **47**: 1087–1090.
32 Hazlewood KA *et al.* (2006) Effect of oral corticosteroids on chronic warfarin therapy. *Annals of Pharmacotherapy.* **40**: 2101–2106.
33 Jick S *et al.* (2001) The risk of cataract among users of inhaled steroids. *Epidemiology.* **12**: 229–234.
34 Piper JM *et al.* (1991) Corticosteroid use and peptic ulcer disease: role of nonsteroidal anti-inflammatory drugs. *Annals of internal medicine.* **114**: 735–740.
35 Warrington TP and Bostwick JM (2006) Psychiatric adverse effects of corticosteroids. *Mayo Clinic Proceedings.* **81**: 1361–1367.
36 Hall R Psychiatric adverse drug reactions: steroid psychosis. Available from: www.drrichardhall.com/steroid.htm
37 Brown ES and Suppes T (1998) Mood symptoms during corticosteroid therapy: a review. *Harvard Review of Psychiatry.* **5**: 239–246.
38 Stiefel FC *et al.* (1989) Corticosteroids in cancer: neuropsychiatric complications. *Cancer Investigation.* **7**: 479–491.
39 Twycross R *et al.* (2009) *Symptom Management in Advanced Cancer* (4e). palliativedrugs.com, Nottingham, pp. 209–210.
40 Eidelberg D (1991) Steroid myopathy. In: DA Rottenberg (ed) *Neurological Complications of Cancer Treatment.* Butterworth-Heineman, Boston, pp. 185–191.
41 Schakman O *et al.* (2008) Mechanisms of glucocorticoid-induced myopathy. *Journal of Endocrinology.* **197**: 1–10.
42 Rotstein J and Good R (1957) Steroid pseudorheumatism. *AMA Archives of Internal Medicine.* **99**: 545–555.
43 Greenberg H *et al.* (1979) Epidural spinal cord compression from metastatic tumour: results with a new treatment protocol. *Annals of Neurology.* **8**: 361–366.
44 Delattre J-Y *et al.* (1988) High dose versus low dose dexamethasone in experimental epidural spinal cord compression. *Neurosurgery.* **22**: 1005–1007.
45 Vecht C *et al.* (1989) Initial bolus of conventional versus high-dose dexamethasone in metastatic spinal cord compression. *Neurology.* **39**: 1255–1257.

46 Rousseau P (2004) Sudden withdrawal of corticosteroids: a commentary. *American Journal of Hospice and Palliative Care.* **21**: 169–171.
47 Editorial (1991) Ondansetron versus dexamethasone for chemotherapy-induced emesis. *Lancet.* **338**: 478.
48 Sridhar K *et al.* (1992) Five-drug antiemetic combination for cisplatin chemotherapy. *Cancer Investigation.* **10**: 191–199.
49 Gralla R *et al.* (1999) Recommendations for the use of antiemetics: evidence-based, clinical practice guidelines. *Journal of Clinical Oncology.* **17**: 2971–2994.
50 Galicich JH and French LA (1961) The use of dexamethasone in the treatment of cerebral oedema resulting from brain tumours and brain surgery. *American Practitioner.* **12**: 169.
51 Kirkham S (1988) The palliation of cerebral tumours with high-dose dexamethasone: a review. *Palliative Medicine.* **2**: 27–33.
52 CSM (Committee on Safety of Medicines and Medicines Control Agency) (1998) Withdrawal of systemic corticosteroids. *Current Problems in Pharmacovigilance.* **24 (May)**: 5–7.
53 Margolin L *et al.* (2007) The steroid withdrawal syndrome: a review of the implications, etiology, and treatments. *Journal of Pain and Symptom Management.* **33**: 224–228.
54 Palliativedrugs.com (2010) Clarifying label changes to parenteral formulations of dexamethasone. Available from: www.palliativedrugs.com/news/december/clarifying-dexamethasone-prescribing.html

DEMECLOCYCLINE — BNF 5.1.3 & 6.5.2

Class: Tetracycline antibacterial and vasopressin receptor antagonist.

Indications: Symptomatic hyponatraemia caused by the syndrome of inappropriate antidiuretic hormone (ADH) secretion (SIADH).

Pharmacology

Demeclocycline is a tetracycline derivative. It induces nephrogenic diabetes insipidus, i.e. inhibits the action of ADH on renal tubules, probably by antagonism of arginine-vasopressin V_2-receptors, although its precise mechanism of action has not been fully elucidated.[1–3] There are at least three arginine-vasopressin receptor subtypes. V_2-receptors are concentrated in renal collecting tubules where antagonism leads to aquaresis, i.e. the excretion of water without significantly changing the total level of electrolyte excretion. V_2-receptors also occur in vascular endothelium where antagonism results in vasodilation.

The manufacturer's literature states that, in SIADH, demeclocycline should be used only if fluid restriction is ineffective. However, in palliative care, fluid restriction to 700–1,000mL/24h (or a daily urine output of <500mL) is burdensome and treatment with demeclocycline is generally preferable. The effect of demeclocycline is apparent after 3–5 days, and persists for several days after stopping treatment. There is no need to restrict fluid during treatment.

Tolvaptan is a recently introduced alternative arginine-vasopressin V_2 antagonist available for PO use (Box 7.J).

SIADH may be caused by many different medical conditions.[10] It also occurs with various drugs, notably TCAs, SSRIs, **carbamazepine**, phenothiazines, **lorazepam**, barbiturates. SIADH should be considered in all patients who develop hyponatraemia, drowsiness, confusion or convulsions while taking a TCA or SSRI. Risk factors for the development of SIADH with SSRIs include older age, female gender, low body weight and concurrent use of diuretics.[11]

Clinical features of SIADH depend on both the level and the rate of decline of the plasma sodium concentration (Box 7.K). Asymptomatic hyponatraemia indicates chronic rather than acute SIADH. Treatment is necessary only if the hyponatraemia is symptomatic.

If suspected, paired urine and serum samples should be obtained from the patient. The diagnosis of SIADH is based on the following criteria:

- hyponatraemia (<130mmol/L)
- low plasma osmolality (<270mosmol/L)
- urine osmolality >300mosmol/L (i.e. higher than plasma osmolality)
- urine sodium concentration always >20mmol/L, and generally >40mmol/L
- normal or moderately expanded plasma volume.[12]

Urine osmolality >100mosm/L but <300mosm/L may be consistent with a diagnosis of SIADH if there is co-existent renal tubular dysfunction, diuretic use or reset osmostat syndrome. In such cases, a raised urine sodium concentration (>30mmol/L) is more diagnostically reliable.[13,14]

Box 7.J Vasopressin receptor antagonists (VRAs, vaptans)

Conivaptan, a mixed V_1/V_2 antagonist, was approved by the US FDA in 2005 for IV use in euvolaemic and hypervolaemic hyponatraemia. Conivaptan results in a mean improvement in plasma sodium concentration of 6mmol/L with a daily dose of 40mg; and 9mmol/L with 80mg.[4,5]

Tolvaptan was approved by the US FDA in 2009 for PO use in euvolaemic and hypervolaemic hyponatraemia associated with heart failure, cirrhosis and SIADH (plasma sodium <125mmol/L or less marked but symptomatic hyponatraemia resistant to fluid restriction). It is approved in the EU for treatment of SIADH.[6,7] In patients who are not fluid-restricted, the plasma sodium concentration increases by 2–3mmol/L in the first 24h of treatment, with a mean increase of 7mmol/L after 1 month. Generally, plasma sodium increases more in patients with marked baseline hyponatraemia (<125mmol/L).[8]

Conivaptan (but not tolvaptan) is a potent inhibitor pf CYP3A4. The most common undesirable effects of conivaptan are infusion site reactions (24%), phlebitis (16%) and pain (8%). With tolvaptan, undesirable effects include dry mouth and thirst (20%), weakness (10%), nausea (9%), constipation (8%), urinary frequency (7%), dizziness (7%) and hyperglycaemia (5%). Hypernatremia developed in up to 10% of patients in some studies, and 3% experienced a rapid increase in serum sodium (>12mmol/L in 24h). Patients on concurrent fluid restriction were at greater risk of this.

No cases of osmotic demyelination leading to myelinosis have been reported. This may be because this tends to occur with rapid plasma sodium correction from a low baseline, e.g. 115mmol/L. Trials have excluded patients with hyponatraemia of this severity.[5]

VRAs are contra-indicated in patients with hypovolaemic hyponatraemia, e.g. caused by severe diarrhoea, vomiting, or adrenal insufficiency.[5,9]

The place of VRAs in the treatment of SIADH is unclear. Most trials include patients with any cause of hyponatremia and do not provide sub-group analysis, so specific regimens for SIADH are not clear. Efficacy of VRAs has not been compared to fluid restriction or demeclocyline. The impact of VRAs on medium and long-term morbidity or mortality in SIADH is not known. However, the cost of tolvaptan will restrict its use in palliative care (about £75/day).

Box 7.K Clinical features of SIADH

Plasma sodium 110–120mmol/L	**Plasma sodium <110mmol/L**
Anorexia	Multifocal myoclonus
Nausea and vomiting	Drowsiness
Lassitude	Seizures
Confusion	Coma

In practice, a plasma sodium concentration of ≤120mmol/L is sufficient to make a clinical diagnosis of SIADH in the absence of:

- severe vomiting
- diuretic therapy
- hypo-adrenalism
- hypothyroidism
- severe renal impairment.

Bio-availability 60–80%.
Onset of action 3–5 days.
Time to peak plasma concentration 3–4h.
Plasma halflife 12h.
Duration of action several days.

Cautions

Renal and hepatic impairment; lower doses advised to avoid excessive systemic accumulation. The absorption of demeclocycline is reduced by the concurrent administration of **iron**, **calcium**, **magnesium**, **aluminium** and **zinc**.

Demeclocycline depresses plasma prothrombin activity and, if used concurrently, the dose of **warfarin** may need to be reduced. Risk of oral contraceptive failure (as with all antibacterials). Avoid concurrent **penicillin** use (tetracyclines possibly antagonize the effect of penicillins). Risk of photosensitivity; warn patients not to expose skin to direct sunlight or sunlamps.

Undesirable effects

Nausea, vomiting, diarrhoea, renal impairment (more likely with daily dose of 1,200mg),[15] photosensitivity, discolouration of teeth during tooth development. Higher doses may lead to uraemia.

Dose and use

Treat the patient and not the biochemical results.

If symptomatic:

- start with 300mg b.d. on an empty stomach, e.g. 1h a.c., avoiding milk, antacids, **iron** and **zinc** preparations at the same time of day
- if necessary, increase to 300mg q.d.s. after 1 week.

In patients unable to take drugs PO, demeclocycline can be given PR dispersed in 5mL of a methylcellulose carrier.[16] However, the powder may cause local irritation and inflammation.

Supply

Ledermycin® (Goldshield)
Capsules 150mg, 28 days @ 300mg b.d. = £64.

Tolvaptan

Samsca® (Otsuka)
Tablets 15mg, 30mg, 28 days @ 15mg or 30mg daily = £2,091.

1 deTroyer A (1977) Demeclocycline. Treatment for syndrome of inappropriate antidiuretic hormone secretion. *Journal of the American Medical Association*. **237**: 2723–2726.

2 Forrest J *et al.* (1978) Superiority of demeclocycline over lithium in the treatment of chronic syndrome of inappropriate secretion of antidiuretic hormone. *New England Journal of Medicine*. **298**: 173–177.

3 Miyagawa C (1986) The pharmacologic management of the syndrome of inapprorpiate secretion of antidiuretic hormone. *Drug Intelligence and Clinical Pharmacy*. **20**: 527–531.

4 Ghali JK *et al.* (2006) Efficacy and safety of oral conivaptan: a V1A/V2 vasopressin receptor antagonist, assessed in a randomized, placebo-controlled trial in patients with euvolemic or hypervolemic hyponatremia. *Journal of Clinical Endocrinology and Metabolism*. **91**: 2145–2152.

5 Decaux G *et al.* (2008) Non-peptide arginine-vasopressin antagonists: the vaptans. *Lancet*. **371**: 1624–1632.

6 Amin A and Meeran K (2011) New drugs for hyponatraemia. *British Medical Journal*. **342**: 559–560.

7 Plosker GL (2010) Tolvaptan: Adis drug profile. *Drugs*. **70**: 443–454.

8 Schrier RW *et al.* (2006) Tolvaptan, a selective oral vasopressin V2-receptor antagonist, for hyponatremia. *New England Journal of Medicine*. **355**: 2099–2112.

9 Ali F *et al.* (2007) Therapeutic potential of vasopressin receptor antagonists. *Drugs*. **67**: 847–858.

10 Twycross R *et al.* (2009) *Symptom Management in Advanced Cancer* (4e). palliativedrugs.com, Nottingham, p. 236.

11 Jacob S and Spinler SA (2006) Hyponatremia associated with selective serotonin-reuptake inhibitors in older adults. *Annals of Pharmacotherapy*. **40**: 1618–1622.

12 Burtis CA *et al.* (eds) (2008) *Pituitary disorders.* (6e). WB Saunders, Philadelphia, pp. 746–747.
13 Smellie WS and Heald A (2007) Hyponatraemia and hypernatraemia: pitfalls in testing. *British Medical Journal.* **334**: 473–476.
14 Ellison DH and Berl T (2007) Clinical practice. The syndrome of inappropriate antidiuresis. *New England Journal of Medicine.* **356**: 2064–2072.
15 Trump D (1981) Serious hyponatremia in patients with cancer: management with demeclocycline. *Cancer.* **47**: 2908–2912.
16 Hussain I *et al.* (1998) Rectal administration of demeclocycline in a patient with syndrome of inappropriate ADH secretion. *International Journal of Clinical Practice.* **52**: 59.

DESMOPRESSIN BNF 6.5.2

Class: Vasopressin analogue.

Indications: Licensed indications vary between products and formulations (Table 7.7); see SPCs for details. Pituitary diabetes insipidus, nocturnal enuresis and nocturia, mild–moderate haemophilia and von Willebrand's disease, headache from a lumbar puncture, testing renal concentration capacity, testing fibrinolytic response, †treatment of severe surface bleeding or bleeding associated with severe renal or hepatic impairment.[1–3]

Contra-indications: See SPCs for details. Patients aged >65 years, current or previous hyponatraemia, coronary insufficiency, unstable angina, hypertension, concurrent use with diuretics, psychogenic and alcohol abuse-related polydipsia, moderate-severe renal impairment (creatinine clearance <50mL/min), type IIB or platelet-type (pseudo) von Willebrand's disease.

Pharmacology

Desmopressin is an analogue of the pituitary antidiuretic hormone, **vasopressin**. It stimulates arginine-vasopressin V_2-receptors in the medullary collecting tubules, increasing water resorption by the renal tubules, thereby reducing urine volume. The antidiuretic effect of desmopressin is 3–10 times greater than that of **vasopressin**, and it has a longer duration of action. Unlike **vasopressin**, it has no vasoconstrictor effect. Desmopressin is ineffective in nephrogenic diabetes insipidus.[4]

Desmopressin also stimulates V_2-receptors on endothelial cells, leading to the release of stored von Willebrand factor and factor VIII. This augments platelet function and enhances haemostasis; hence its use in certain bleeding states, including those associated with severe renal or hepatic impairment.[2,3,5]

Bio-availability 3–4% intranasal; 0.1–5% PO.
Onset of action 1h intranasal; 2h PO.
Plasma halflife 0.4–4h intranasal; 1.5–2.5h PO.
Duration of action 5–24h intranasal; 6–8h PO.

Cautions

Serious drug interactions: the concurrent use of drugs which increase the endogenous secretion of vasopressin increases the risk of symptomatic hyponatraemia, notably TCAs, SSRIs, **chlorpromazine**, opioids, NSAIDs, **lamotrigine** and **carbamazepine**.

Loperamide triples the desmopressin plasma concentration after PO administration.[6]

CHF, raised intracranial pressure, cystic fibrosis. Take care to avoid fluid overload because with excessive water intake there is an increased risk of hyponatraemia. The effect of desmopressin may be potentiated by drugs which cause fluid retention, e.g. NSAIDs and corticosteroids. In CKD, the antidiuretic effect is less. Food may reduce the absorption of tablets.

Undesirable effects

Common (<10%, >1%): tablets and high doses of nasal spray (≥40microgram/24h): headache, abdominal pain, nausea. Nasal spray: nosebleeds, nasal congestion or rhinitis, sore throat.
Rare or very rare (<0.1%): water retention and hyponatraemia; in extreme cases this may result in hyponatraemic seizures.

Dose and use

Global post-marketing data indicate a higher incidence of hyponatraemia in patients being treated with intranasal formulations compared with oral formulations.[5]

Keep to the recommended starting doses to minimize the risk of hyponatraemic seizures, and take precautions to avoid fluid overload particularly if at risk of developing raised intracranial pressure. Advise patients with nocturia or nocturnal enuresis to limit fluid intake to a minimum from 1h before until 8h after the dose.[7] If desmopressin is taken for nocturia, monitor the patient's blood pressure and weight. Patients should stop taking desmopressin if persistent nausea and vomiting, or diarrhoea develop, and seek medical advice.

Pituitary diabetes insipidus

Tablets should be used first line. The nasal spray should be used only where PO or SL are not suitable.

- start with 100microgram PO t.d.s., 60microgram SL t.d.s. (or 10–20microgram intranasally at bedtime)
- if ineffective, increase dose progressively every few days
- effective dose is generally 100–400microgram PO t.d.s., 120–240microgram SL t.d.s. (or 10 20microgram intranasally at bedtime–b.d.).

Refractory nocturia

Treat only with PO or SL tablets (Desmotabs® or Desmomelt® are the UK brands licensed for this indication):

- start with 200microgram PO or 120microgram SL at bedtime
- after 1–2 weeks, if ineffective, increase dose to 400microgram PO or 240microgram SL at bedtime.[4]

Nocturia associated with multiple sclerosis

Give only when other treatments have failed in adults under 65 years:

- 10–20microgram intranasally at bedtime
- dose not to be repeated within 24h.[4,8]

Severe surface bleeding and bleeding in renal impairment

Monitor blood pressure closely when using for haemostasis. If there is a progressive increase in body weight, plasma sodium concentration <130mmol/L or plasma osmolality <270mosmol/kg, the fluid intake must be reduced drastically and the injections stopped:

- give a single dose of desmopressin 0.3–0.4microgram/kg IVI in 50mL 0.9% saline over 20min or by SC injection (using the Octim® formulation to minimize injection volume)[2]
- if necessary, give repeat injections once daily up to a total of 4 days[9]
- if inadequate, consider giving cryoprecipitate, e.g. 2 pooled packs.

Because of the mechanism of action of desmopressin (releasing stored von Willebrand factor and factor VIII from the vascular endothelium) the second and subsequent injections provide only about two thirds of the benefit of the first injection.[9]

Severe bleeding in hepatic impairment

If **phytomenadione** injection (Konakion® MM) 10mg IV is insufficient (see p.542 = Vit K), administer desmopressin as for bleeding in renal impairment.[1,9]

Supply

Table 7.7 Main licensed indications for UK desmopressin formulations[a]

	Diabetes Insipidus[b]	*Nocturnal Enuresis*	*Nocturia associated with MS*
PO formulations			
DDAVP® tablets	Yes		
DDAVP® Melt SL tablets	Yes		
Desmotabs®		Yes	
Desmomelt®		Yes	
Nasal formulations			
Desmopressin generic	Yes		Yes
DDAVP® intranasal solution	Yes		Yes
Desmospray®	Yes		Yes

a. for full licensed indications see manufacturer's SPC
b. tablets should be used first-line following post-marketing data recommendations.

Desmopressin (generic)
Nasal spray 10microgram/metered spray, 60 dose bottle = £24.

DDAVP® (Ferring)
Tablets 100microgram, 200microgram, 28 days @ 200microgram t.d.s. = £82.
Tablets SL (DDAVP® Melt) 60microgram, 120microgram, 240microgram, 28 days @ 120microgram t.d.s. = £85.
Intranasal solution 100microgram/mL, 2.5mL dropper bottle and catheter = £10; *store in refrigerator at 2–8° C and protect from light.*
Injection 4microgram/mL, 1mL amp = £1.

Desmotabs® (Ferring)
Tablets 200microgram, 28 days @ 200microgram t.d.s. = £82.

Desmomelt® (Ferring)
Tablets SL 120microgram, 240microgram, 28 days @ 120microgram t.d.s. = £85.

Desmospray® (Ferring)
Nasal spray 10microgram/metered spray, 60 dose bottle = £25;
store at room temperature and protect from light.

Octim® (Ferring)
Nasal spray 150microgram/metered spray, 25 dose bottle = £577.
Injection 15microgram/mL, 1mL amp = £19;
store at room temperature and protect from light.

1 Blonski W *et al.* (2007) Coagulopathy in liver disease. *Current Treatment Options in Gastroenterology.* **10**: 464–473.
2 Hedges SJ *et al.* (2006) Evidence-based treatment recommendations for uremic bleeding. *Nature Clinical Practice Oncology.* **3**: 138–153.
3 Mannucci P (1997) Desmopressin (DDAVP) in the treatment of bleeding disorders: the first 20 years. *Blood.* **90**: 2515–2521.
4 Cvetkovic RS and Plosker GL (2005) Desmopressin: in adults with nocturia. *Drugs.* **65**: 99–107; discussion 108–109.
5 Van de Walle *et al.* (2007) Desmopressin 30 years in clinical use: A safety review. *Current Drug Safety.* **2**: 232–238.
6 Callreus T *et al.* (1999) Changes in gastrointestinal motility influence the absorption of desmopressin. *European Journal of Clinical Pharmacology.* **55**: 305–309.
7 BNF (2011) In: *British National Formulary* (No. 61). British Medical Association and the Royal Pharmaceutical Society of Great Britain, London.
8 Zahariou A *et al.* (2008) Maximal bladder capacity is a positive predictor of response to desmopressin treatment in patients with MS and nocturia. *International Urology and Nephrology.* **40**: 65–69.
9 Manucci (1992) Patterns of development of tachyphylaxis in patient with haemophilia and von Willebrand disease after repeated doses of desmopression (DDAVP). *British Journal of Haematology.* **82**: 87–93.

DRUGS FOR DIABETES MELLITUS BNF 6.1

Indications: Diabetes mellitus not controlled by diet.

Contra-indications: Oral hypoglycaemics should not be used during severe infection, after major trauma, or peri-operatively.

Glibenclamide and **chlorpropamide** (not UK) should not be used in the elderly and those with severe renal (creatinine clearance <20mL/min) or hepatic impairment because of their long plasma halflives.

Metformin should not be used in patients with severe renal impairment (creatinine clearance <30mL/min), and should be withheld during and for 48h after testing with IV iodinated contrast agents or until renal function is normal. Because of the risk of developing lactic acidosis, it should be withheld in patients with acute conditions which may cause tissue hypoxia or sudden deterioration in renal function, e.g. dehydration, severe infection, sepsis, shock, acute heart failure, respiratory failure, hepatic impairment, excessive alcohol intake.[1]

Thiazolidinediones, e.g. **pioglitazone**, should not be used in patients with CHF, severe hepatic impairment, at higher risk of fracture.

Background

Diabetes mellitus comprises a group of metabolic diseases characterized by hyperglycaemia resulting from defects in insulin secretion, insulin action or both.[2] There are two main types of diabetes mellitus (Box 7.L). Some patients can exhibit features of both type 1 and type 2 diabetes, making a definite classification difficult.

Box 7.L Classification of diabetes mellitus

Type 1 (the minority, <10%)
Typically develops in children, young people, and adults <30 years old. There is a lack of insulin because of immune-mediated destruction of the β-cells in the pancreas. Symptoms develop rapidly and the diagnosis is based on the presence of characteristic symptoms plus a high blood glucose concentration.

Type 2 (the majority)
Typically develops in adults >40 years old, although it is increasingly manifesting in younger people because of obesity. The pancreas does not produce sufficient insulin for the body's needs and generally there is also marked insulin resistance, i.e. cells are not able to respond to the insulin that is produced. Symptoms tend to develop gradually, with a long delay (possibly years) before diagnosis. Treatment is based on modification of diet and weight loss, together with various glucose-lowering drugs. *Some Type 2 diabetics need insulin.*

In the UK, 4% of the general population have diabetes mellitus,[3,4] and nearly 40% of cancer patients have impaired glucose tolerance demonstrated by an oral or IV glucose tolerance test.[5,6] In cancer, corticosteroids are the most common cause of drug-induced hyperglycaemia[7] (see p.503), but thiazides, **levothyroxine**, **furosemide**, **octreotide** and atypical antipsychotics (e.g. **risperidone**, **olanzapine**) are also potential precipitants.[8]

In patients with symptoms suggestive of diabetes mellitus (e.g. thirst, polydipsia and/or polyuria), a diagnosis can be made on the basis of the following criteria:

- fasting plasma glucose concentrations of ≥7.0mmol/L (normal <5.6mmol/L) or
- random plasma glucose concentrations of ≥11.1mmol/L or
- 2h post-load plasma glucose ≥11.1mmol/L (normal = <7.8mmol/L) during oral glucose tolerance test.[2,9]

The main goal of diabetic management in palliative care is to preserve quality of life. Thus, the aim of treatment is the prevention of symptoms from hyper- or hypoglycaemia, keto-acidosis and hyperosmolar non-ketotic states. Concern about long-term complications is no longer relevant.[10,11] Measuring glycated haemoglobin (HbA_{1c}) to determine the overall level of glycaemic control over 6–8 weeks is also irrelevant in most palliative care patients. Further:

- it is unnecessary to maintain theoretically ideal blood glucose levels to avoid long-term complications[10,12]
- rigid dietary control is not indicated when life expectancy is short
- when stable, monitoring is generally adequate with a fasting blood glucose fingerstick test twice a week
- although not always accurate, urine tests for glucose may well suffice.

In advanced cancer, insulin requirement often decreases because of weight loss, anorexia, nausea and vomiting, renal and/or hepatic impairment. Insulin doses in patients with type 1 diabetes will need to be reduced. Insulin-treated type 2 diabetics may be able to stop insulin, and tablet-treated type 2 diabetics may be able to stop tablets. If symptoms of hyperglycaemia develop, a blood glucose fingerstick test should be performed and hyperglycaemia treated accordingly (see below).[13]

Pharmacology

This section provides advice about management in the last few weeks and days of life. Because regimens are individually tailored, there is no standard approach and guidance from a diabetologist is invaluable. For corticosteroid-induced diabetes mellitus see Box 7.M, p.503.

Drug treatment in type 1 diabetes mellitus

Injections of **insulin** are an essential life-long treatment, including the last days of life. However, in most patients, the **insulin** requirement will diminish as death approaches. Generally, short-acting **insulins** (given to cover mealtimes) which produce a more rapid peak and have a greater risk of hypoglycaemia, are reduced or discontinued first. Intermediate- or long-acting **insulins** (given once daily or b.d. to provide background control) may subsequently need to be reduced as well.

Likewise, patients receiving mixed **insulins** may need to reduce or discontinue the short-acting **insulin** component. However, if a patient has months or weeks to live, it would be prudent to liaise with a diabetologist before making major changes to an established insulin regimen.

A decision to stop **insulin** completely should generally be taken only after discussion with the patient (if still has capacity) and the family. It is generally appropriate to stop **insulin** injections completely when the patient has become irreversibly unconscious as part of the dying process, and not because of hypoglycaemia or diabetic keto-acidosis, and when all other life-prolonging treatments have been stopped.[7]

If it is felt strongly that the **insulin** should be continued, a simple regimen can be used, e.g. once daily long-acting, or b.d. intermediate-acting **insulin**, with the minimum of routine monitoring, e.g. once daily.[14]

Drug treatment in type 2 diabetes mellitus

There are several different classes of oral antidiabetic drugs, with differing modes of action (Table 7.8). The risk of hypoglycaemia is greatest with insulin and the sulphonylureas. **Metformin** is recommended as first-line therapy for overweight or obese diabetics in particular.[2,15] However, it is unlikely to be appropriate in patients with advanced cancer because it promotes weight loss, and initially may cause nausea and diarrhoea, or other undesirable effects, in ≤20% of patients. It is contra-indicated in patients with CHF or with renal impairment because of the increased risk of lactic acidosis. **Metformin** is also best not used in elderly debilitated patients, particularly those with hepatic impairment or COPD. Although **metformin** has been associated with lactic acidosis in patients with deteriorating renal function or tissue hypoxia, recent evidence has cast doubt on this.[3,16] Hypoglycaemia is rare with **metformin**.

Generally, in debilitated or elderly patients, a sulphonylurea may be a more appropriate choice. However, because of their long plasma halflives, **glibenclamide** and **chlorpropamide** (not UK) are best avoided in palliative care patients. A relatively short-acting sulphonylurea such as **gliclazide** or **tolbutamide** should be prescribed with a realistic, safe target, e.g. a fasting or pre-meal glucose of 8–15mmol/L. Because different patients will have different thresholds for symptomatic hyperglycaemia, the upper limit may need to be reduced to avoid symptoms.[10]

Table 7.8 Oral antidiabetic drugs

Class	*Examples*	*Mechanism of action*	*Risk of hypoglycaemia*	*Comment*
Biguanides	Metformin	Decrease hepatic gluconeogenesis, and increase uptake of glucose by muscle	–	Tend to cause weight loss; may cause nausea and diarrhoea; low risk of lactic acidosis
Sulphonylureas	Gliclazide, tolbutamide, glibenclamide, chlorpropamide (not UK)	Increase insulin secretion	++ with longer-acting drugs, glibenclamide, chlorpropamide	Original class of oral antidiabetic drugs; relatively inexpensive
Meglitinides	Repaglinide	Increase insulin secretion	±	Relatively fast onset and short duration of action; permits a more flexible regimen
Thiazolidinediones	Pioglitazone, rosiglitazone (not UK)	Enhance the effect of insulin	±	2nd or 3rd line drugs; cause fluid retention, exacerbate CHF, and increase the risk of myocardial infarction;[17] also of fracture.[15] Rosiglitazone withdrawn in the EU and restricted in the USA.[18,19]
DPP-4 (dipeptidyl peptidase-4) inhibitors	Saxagliptin, sitagliptin, vildagliptin	Increase insulin secretion and lower glucagon secretion	±	Newly introduced; 2nd or 3rd line drugs, for use particularly if patient at high risk of hypoglycaemia[15]
GLP-1 (glucagon-like peptide-1) receptor agonist	Exenatide, liraglutide	Increase insulin secretion and lower glucagon secretion; slows gastric emptying and increase satiety	±	Newly introduced; 2nd or 3rd line drugs, for use particularly if a patient has a BMI $\geqslant$35kg/m^2.[15]

Meglitinides, e.g. **repaglinide,** are a new class of insulin secretagogue. They provide similar glucose control to sulphonylureas but act more rapidly and for a shorter time. This permits flexible 'pulse dosing' before meals, which may be useful in patients with a variable appetite and oral intake. For pharmacokinetic details, see Table 7.9. Meglitinides are significantly more expensive than sulphonylureas.

Table 7.9 Pharmacokinetics of selected oral hypoglycaemic drugs

	Repaglinide	*Tolbutamide*	*Gliclazide*
Bio-availability	56%	>95%	78%
Onset of action	15–60min	1–3h	3–4h
Time to peak plasma concentration	1h	3–5h	2–4h
Plasma halflife	1h	4.5–6.5h	10–12h
Duration of action	4–6h	≤12h	12–24h

Thiazolidinediones are used as second or third line therapy with **metformin** and/or a sulphonylurea. Thiazolidinediones are contra-indicated in patients with a higher risk of fracture (because they increase the risk of distal fracture, particularly in women)[20,21] or with CHF (because they cause fluid retention). All patients taking a thiazolidinedione should be monitored for symptoms and signs of CHF, e.g. excessive/rapid weight gain, cough, increasing breathlessness, and/or oedema.[15,22] Both **pioglitazone** and **rosiglitazone** are associated with CHF, but the risk of heart failure and death (but not acute myocardial infarction) is significantly greater with **rosiglitazone** which has resulted in its withdrawal in the EU and restricted use in the USA.[18,19,23]

Isolated spikes of hyperglycaemia should *not* be treated with stat doses of short/rapid-acting **insulin**. Instead, monitor with regular fingerstick tests (capillary blood glucose measurement) and adjust hypoglycaemic regimen if a particular pattern emerges.[24]

Insulin is sometimes needed in patients with type 2 diabetes. If the patient is already taking **metformin** or a sulphonylurea, usual practice is to start **insulin** in addition.[15] When adding **insulin** to oral hypoglycaemics to improve blood glucose control, 6–12 units of **isophane insulin** or long-acting **insulin** once daily may suffice.

In patients with advanced cancer and newly diagnosed type 2 diabetes mellitus, the relative advantages and disadvantages of **insulin** or oral hypoglycaemic drugs need to be considered alongside factors such as the patient's prognosis, oral nutritional intake and presence of other co-morbidities. **Insulin** provides rapid, effective and more predictable control, is easier to titrate, and has less risk of prolonged hypoglycaemia compared with some oral hypoglycaemics. It is a better choice in patients with:

- a short prognosis (≤3 months)
- co-morbidity contributing to hyperglycaemia, e.g. infection
- poor or erratic oral nutritional intake
- contra-indications to the use of oral hypoglycaemics
- severe symptoms from hyperglycaemia.

With oral hypoglycaemics, control may take several weeks, and be less effective, less predictable and harder to titrate than **insulin.**[8]

When deciding the starting dose of **insulin**, the patient's build, oral intake and the blood glucose levels must be taken into account. The dose is monitored to achieve a fasting blood glucose of 8–15mmol/L. Doses of 0.5 units/kg/day of a *long-acting* **insulin analogue**, e.g. **insulin glargine**, **insulin detemir** (both given once daily) or **isophane insulin** (given b.d., or just at bedtime) will provide only a basal insulin supply, and thus it does not matter if a patient on this amount is not eating.

However, in patients who are still eating and require larger doses than this, **insulin glargine** or **insulin detemir** are a better choice than **isophane insulin** because there is less likelihood of interprandial hypoglycaemia, they still generally need be given only once daily, and need not be given at the same time each day, thus easing the burden of injections on the patient/carer.[3,15,25] Given these advantages, it may be beneficial for patients on oral hypoglycaemics troubled by hypoglycaemic episodes or a burdensome tablet load to be switched to once daily injections of **insulin glargine** or **insulin detemir**. Blood glucose should be monitored before each dose until the **insulin** dose is stable. The frequency can then be reduced and the time of testing varied to monitor control during different parts of the day.

A sliding scale of a *rapid-acting* **insulin analogue** (e.g. **insulin aspart**, **insulin lispro**, available as pen devices) is occasionally necessary. An IV sliding scale of rapid-acting regular **soluble insulin** is generally reserved for patients with diabetic keto-acidosis or peri-operatively.

Corticosteroid-induced diabetes mellitus

Diabetes mellitus occurs in 2% of patients treated with corticosteroids.[26] It can occur with any corticosteroid or any formulation (including inhaled and topical),[27] and is dose-related.[28,29] The greatest rise in blood glucose is likely to occur 2–3h after taking a corticosteroid, returning to normal ≤12h later.[13] Thus, treatment with a longer acting product, whether a sulphonylurea (see Table 7.9) or **insulin**, may cause nocturnal hypoglycaemia. This should be taken into account when planning treatment.

Some recommend that **insulin** should be first-line treatment for all patients with corticosteroid-induced diabetes, particularly if they have high blood sugars at diagnosis (Box 7.M).[13,28]

Box 7.M Drug treatment for corticosteroid-induced diabetes mellitus

Do not consider starting drug treatment unless a prolonged course of corticosteroid treatment is planned (> 1 month) and the patient has symptomatic hyperglycaemia.

If glycaemic control in a patient with pre-existing diabetes mellitus deteriorates when corticosteroids are started, existing treatment should be adjusted accordingly.

No previous diabetic history

In patients with a prognosis of ≥2–3 months, a sulphonylurea should be started, e.g. gliclazide, tolbutamide (see Dose and use below).

However, in patients with a small food intake there is a risk of night-time or early morning hypoglycaemia, and repaglinide is a better choice because it has a shorter duration of action (Table 7.9).

In patients with a prognosis of ≤2–3 months, a once daily dose of 10 units of insulin glargine, insulin detemir or isophane insulin given at the same time as the once daily dose of corticosteroid may be sufficient to prevent symptomatic hyperglycaemia.[13]

Pre-existing non-insulin dependent diabetes mellitus

If hyperglycaemia remains despite maximal doses of an appropriate oral hypoglycaemic drug, insulin should be given *in addition*.

If high blood glucose levels are seen only after a once daily dose of a corticosteroid, a once daily dose of 10 units of insulin glargine, insulin detemir or isophane insulin given at the same time as the corticosteroid may be sufficient to prevent symptomatic hyperglycaemia.[13]

Sometimes, a much higher total daily dose of insulin is necessary, occasionally as much as 100 units.[10]

If tight glycaemic control is required, an ultra-short-acting insulin, e.g. aspart or lispro, can be given immediately before a meal to prevent post-prandial hyperglycaemia.[28] Advice should be sought from a diabetologist.

Reducing the corticosteroid dose

Insulin requirements decline in parallel. To help identify patients at high risk of nocturnal hypoglycaemia, blood glucose is best monitored before breakfast; if <8mmol/L the dose of insulin should be reduced.[28]

Cautions

Patients starting treatment with **insulin** must inform the Driver and Vehicle Licensing Agency (DVLA) if they intend to drive. Patients with impaired awareness of the onset of hypoglycaemia or frequent hypoglycaemic episodes are not allowed to drive. This includes some patients who are taking only oral hypoglycaemic drugs. Detailed guidance on eligibility to drive is available from the DVLA, www.dvla.gov.uk/medical.aspx.

The dose of **metformin** should be reduced in patients with creatinine clearance 30–45mL/min. After discontinuation, **glibenclamide** and **chlorpropamide** (not UK) can produce hypoglycaemia for 2–3 days, and up to 4 days if there is renal or hepatic impairment.

Hypoglycaemia

Hypoglycaemia is a lower than physiologically normal blood glucose level. It can be described as 'mild' if self-treated and 'severe' if assistance by another person is needed.[30] Any blood glucose less than 4mmol/L should be treated (Box 7.N). For patients at risk, it is helpful to have a 'hypo box' containing everything necessary for treating hypoglycaemia, and keep it in a prominent place.[24,30]

Box 7.N Treatment of hypoglycaemia[24]

1. If conscious, give quick-acting carbohydrate 15–20g PO of the patient's choice e.g:
   - 150–200mL of pure fruit juice
   - 90–120mL of Lucozade® (*not* diet version); this is preferable in renal patients
   - 120–150mL of Coca-Cola® (*not* diet version)
   - 5–7 Dextrosol® glucose tablets (or 4–5 Glucotabs®)
   - 3–4 heaped teaspoons or 4–5 lumps of sugar dissolved in water.
2. If the patient is not able to take tablets or drink but can still swallow, give 1.5–2 tubes of GlucoGel® or Dextrogel® squeezed into the mouth between the teeth and gums.
3. Repeat fingerstick test after 10–15min; if blood glucose <4mmol/L, repeat step 1 up to 3 times.
4. If blood glucose remains <4mmol/L after 45min or 3 cycles, give glucagon 1mg IM (can be given SC, but will act more slowly) *or* glucose 10% 100mL IV (if patient malnourished or cachectic).
5. When the blood glucose is >4mmol/L and the patient has recovered, give a long-acting carbohydrate of the patient's choice e.g.
   - two biscuits
   - one slice of bread/toast
   - 200–300mL glass of milk (not soya)
   - normal meal if due (must contain carbohydrate).

Note: patients given glucagon require a larger portion of long-acting carbohydrate to replenish glycogen stores.

6. Do *not* omit insulin injection if due, but consider reducing the dose.

In patients with long-standing diabetes, autonomic neuropathy may remove both the warning symptoms (sweating, tremor, pounding heart beat) and the counter-regulatory mechanism of an adrenaline (epinephrine)-induced increase in blood glucose. Such patients tend to present with pallor, mental detachment ± drowsiness ± clumsiness. Some become irritable and aggressive, and others slip rapidly into hypoglycaemic coma. Malnourished patients with reduced hepatic glycogen stores also have a reduced capacity to counteract hypoglycaemia. **Glucagon** treatment in these patients is likely to be less effective.[31]

If the patient is unconscious or having seizures or is very aggressive, check the airway and give high-flow oxygen via a mask, check breathing and circulation and obtain IV access. If the patient has an **insulin** infusion in situ, stop immediately. Give **glucagon** 1mg IM. This will be less appropriate in malnourished patients, so instead give 20% glucose 75mL IV (over 10–15min) *or* 10% glucose 150mL IV (over 10–15min). Repeat fingerstick test 10min later and repeat if blood glucose <4mmol/L.

If the patient is 'nil by mouth', give glucose IV as above until blood sugar >4mmol/L. Consider 10% glucose 100mL/h IV until the hypoglycaemic agent has been metabolized and blood glucose levels are stable.

If the patient is receiving enteral nutrition (PEG/NG feeding) and develops hypoglycaemia, give 15–20g quick-acting carbohydrate of the patient's choice, e.g. 25mL undiluted Ribena® (*not* diet version), 50–70mL of Ensure® Plus Juice or Fortijuice®, 3–4 heaped teaspoons of sugar dissolved in water. If necessary, proceed as above with IV glucose (**glucagon** is not recommended). When blood glucose is >4mmol/L and the patient has recovered, give a long acting carbohydrate, e.g. restart feed; if bolus feeding, give additional bolus feed (read nutritional information and calculate amount required to give 20g of carbohydrate).

Do *not* omit next **insulin** injection or start variable rate IV **insulin** infusion to 'stabilize' blood glucose. Instead, reduce the dose of hypoglycaemic to prevent further episodes of hypoglycaemia. If unsure of subsequent treatment, discuss with the diabetes team.

Drug interactions

The plasma concentration of sulphonylureas may be increased (effect enhanced) by **fluconazole** and **miconazole**, and decreased (effect reduced) by **rifampicin** and **rifabutin**.

Gemfibrozil increases plasma concentrations of **pioglitazone** and **repaglinide**, and this can result in severe hypoglycaemia; avoid concurrent use.

Undesirable effects

GI symptoms, e.g. nausea and diarrhoea, are common with **metformin**, particularly initially.

Dose and use

To maximize safety, all regular and single **insulin** (bolus) doses must be measured and administered using an **insulin** syringe or commercial **insulin** pen device. IV syringes must never be used because they are calibrated in mL and not in **insulin** units. *'Units' must always be written in full.* Abbreviations, e.g. 'U' or 'IU', should not be used; e.g. 10U could be mistakenly read as 100.[32]

Gliclazide

- start with 40–80mg each morning with breakfast
- if necessary, increase every 3 days to a maximum of 160mg b.d.

Tolbutamide

- start with 500mg b.d. with meals
- if necessary, increase every 3 days to a maximum of 1g b.d.

Metformin

- start with 500mg each morning with breakfast
- if necessary, increase by 500mg at weekly intervals
- maximum dose = 1g t.d.s.

Repaglinide

- start with 500microgram within 30min of main meals (or 1mg in patients previously treated with an alternative oral hypoglycaemic agent)
- if necessary, increase the dose at 1–2 week intervals to a maximum of 4mg q.d.s.

Insulin

- if the patient is already taking the maximum dose of an oral hypoglycaemic, and the fasting blood glucose is >12mmol/L, prescribe **insulin glargine** 6–12 units once daily at bedtime (best choice) or **isophane insulin** 6–12 units once daily at bedtime
- adjust the dose according to the response
- a preprandial sliding scale of short-acting **soluble insulin** is occasionally necessary (Table 7.10).

Table 7.10 Preprandial sliding scale of soluble insulin[a]

Preprandial blood glucose (mmol/L)	*Insulin dose (units)*
10–15	6
15–18	8
18–22	10
>22[b]	12

a. responses to insulin vary widely and sliding scales need to be individualized
b. patients with marked hyperglycaemia should have monitoring 2h after meals as well until the blood glucose is better controlled.

Supply

This is not a complete list; see BNF for additional details.

Gliclazide (generic)
Tablets 80mg (scored), 28 days @ 80mg each morning = £1.50.

Tolbutamide (generic)
Tablets 500mg, 28 days @ 500mg b.d. = £4.

Metformin (generic)
Tablets 500mg, 850mg, 28 days @ 500mg each morning = £1.
Oral solution (sugar-free) 500mg/5mL, 28 days @ 500mg each morning = £95.

Repaglinide
Prandin® (Daiichi Sankyo)
Tablets 500microgram, 1mg, 28 days @ 500microgram t.d.s. = £11.

Insulin
Most insulin products are also available as cartridges for use with dedicated re-usable injection pen devices or as prefilled disposable pen devices.

Short-acting insulin
Soluble insulin
Actrapid® (Novo Nordisk)
Injection 100 units/mL, 10mL multidose vial = £7.50.

Rapid-acting insulin analogues (e.g. aspart, glulisine, lispro)
Insulin aspart
Novorapid® (Novo Nordisk)
Injection 100 units/mL, 10mL multidose vial = £16.

Intermediate-acting insulin
Isophane insulin
Insulatard® (Novo Nordisk)
Injection 100 units/mL, 10mL multidose vial = £7.50.

Mixed preparations of short-acting with intermediate-acting insulins are available (biphasic isophane insulin, biphasic insulin aspart, biphasic insulin lispro).

Long-acting insulin (e.g. detemir, glargine, zinc suspension)
Insulin glargine (once daily, recombinant human insulin analogue)
Lantus® (Sanofi-Aventis)
Injection 100 units/mL, 10mL multidose vial = £26.

1 BNF (2011) In: *British National Formulary* (No. 61). British Medical Association and the Royal Pharmaceutical Society of Great Britain, London.
2 ADA (American Diabetes Association) (2008) Diagnosis and classification of diabetes mellitus. *Diabetes Care*. **31 (suppl 1)**: S55–60.
3 National Collaborating Centre for Chronic Conditions (2008) *Type 2 diabetes: national clinical guideline for management in primary and secondary care (update)*. London: Royal College of Physicians and NICE 2009.
4 YHPHO PBS Diabetes Prevalence Model Phase 3. Yorkshire and Humber Public Health Observatory. Available from: www.yhpho.org.uk

5 McCoubrie R *et al.* (2005) Managing diabetes mellitus in patients with advanced cancer: a case note audit and guidelines. *European Journal of Cancer Care (Engl).* **14**: 244–248.
6 Glicksman A and Rawson R (1956) Diabetes and altered carbohydrate metabolism in patients with cancer. *Cancer.* **9**: 1127–1134.
7 Poulson J (1997) The management of diabetes in patients with advanced cancer. *Journal of Pain and Symptom Management.* **13**: 339–346.
8 Twycross R *et al.* (2009) *Symptom Management in Advanced Cancer* (4e). palliativedrugs.com Nottingham, pp. 221–225.
9 Report of a WHO/IDF Consultation Definition and diagnosis of diabetes mellitus and intermediate hyperglycemia; 2006.
10 Usborne C and Wilding J (2003) Treating diabetes mellitus in palliative care patients. *European Journal of Palliative Care.* **10**: 186–188.
11 Angelo M *et al.* (2011) An approach to diabetes mellitus in hospice and palliative medicine. *Journal of Palliative Medicine.* **14**: 83–87.
12 Vandenhaute V (2010) Palliative Care and Type II Diabetes: A Need for New Guidelines? *American Journal of Hospice and Palliative Care.* Epub ahead of print.
13 Kilvert A *et al.* (2010) ABCD Position Statement: Diabetes and end of life care. Association of British Clinical Diabetologists. Available from: www.diabetologists-abcd.org.uk/
14 McCann M-A *et al.* (2006) Practical management of diabetes mellitus. *European Journal of Palliative Care.* **13**: 226–229.
15 NICE (2010) The management of type 2 diabetes. Clinical guideline 87. Issued May 2009 updated September 2010. Available from: http://guidance.nice.org.uk/CG87/NICEGuidance/pdf/English
16 Salpeter S *et al.* (2003) Risk of fatal and nonfatal lactic acidosis with metformin use in type 2 diabetes mellitus. *Cochrane Database of Systematic Reviews.* CD002967.
17 Loke YK *et al.* (2011) Comparative cardiovascular effects of thiazolidinediones: systematic review and meta-analysis of observational studies. *British Medical Journal.* **342**: d1309.
18 MHRA (2010) Rosiglitazone recommended withdrawal from clinical use. Drug Safety Update 4(3). Available from: www.mhra.gov.uk
19 FDA (2010) Decision on the continued marketing of rosiglitazone. Centre for Drug Evaluation and Research. Available from: www.fda.gov/Drugs/DrugsSafety/PostmarketDrugSafetyInformationforPatientsandProviders/ucm143349.htm
20 Loke YK *et al.* (2009) Long-term use of thiazolidinediones and fractures in type 2 diabetes: a meta-analysis. *Canadian Medical Association Journal.* **180**: 32–39.
21 Habib ZA *et al.* (2010) Thiazolidinedione use and the longitudinal risk of fractures in patients with type 2 diabetes mellitus. *Journal of Clinical Endocrinology and Metabolism.* **95**: 592–600.
22 Yki-Jarvinen H *et al.* (1992) Comparison of insulin regimens in patients with non-insulin-dependent diabetes mellitus. *New England Journal of Medicine.* **327**: 1426–1433.
23 Juurlink DN *et al.* (2009) Adverse cardiovascular events during treatment with pioglitazone and rosiglitazone: population based cohort study. *British Medical Journal.* **339**: b2942.
24 NHS (2010) Diabetes. The hospital management of hypoglycaemia in adults with diabetes mellitus. Available from: www.diabetes.nhs.uk/publications_and_resources/reports_and_guidance
25 Ciardullo AV *et al.* (2006) Effectiveness and safety of insulin glargine in the therapy of complicated or secondary diabetes: clinical audit. *Acta Diabetol.* **43**: 57–60.
26 Hardy J *et al.* (2001) A prospective survey of the use of dexamethasone on a palliative care unit. *Palliative Medicine.* **15**: 3–8.
27 van der Linden MW *et al.* (2009) Topical corticosteroids and the risk of diabetes mellitus: a nested case-control study in the Netherlands. *Drug Safety.* **32**: 527–537.
28 Oyer DS *et al.* (2006) How to manage steroid diabetes in the patient with cancer. *Journal of Supportive Oncology.* **4**: 479–483.
29 Asudani D and Calles-Escandon J (2007) Steroid Hyperglycaemia (letter reply). *Journal of Hospital Medicine.* **2(4)**: 285–286.
30 DCCT (1993) The effect of intensive treatment of diabetes on the development and progression of long-term complications in insulin-dependent diabetes mellitus. The Diabetes Control and Complications Trial Research Group. *New England Journal of Medicine.* **329**: 977–986.
31 Holroyde C *et al.* (1975) Altered glucose metabolism in metastatic carcinoma. *Cancer Research.* **35**: 3710–3714.
32 National Patient Safety Agency (NPSA) (2010) Safer administration of insulin. NPSA/2010/RRR13. Available from: www.npsa.nhs.uk

*OCTREOTIDE BNF 8.3.4.3

Class: Synthetic hormone.

Indications: Symptoms associated with unresectable hormone-secreting tumours, e.g. carcinoid, VIPomas, glucagonomas and acromegaly; prevention of complications after elective pancreatic surgery;[1] †bleeding oesophageal varices;[2] †salivary, pancreatic and enterocutaneous fistulas;[3,4] †intractable diarrhoea related to high output ileostomies,[5,6] AIDS, radiotherapy, chemotherapy or bone marrow transplant;[3,7–10] †inoperable bowel obstruction in patients with cancer;[11,12] †hypertrophic pulmonary osteo-arthopathy;[13] †ascites in cirrhosis and cancer;[14–16] †buccal fistula;[17] †death rattle (noisy respiratory secretions); †bronchorrhoea;[18] †reduction of tumour-related secretions.[14]

Pharmacology

Octreotide is a synthetic analogue of somatostatin with a longer duration of action.[19] Somatostatin is an inhibitory hormone found throughout the body. In the hypothalamus it inhibits the release of growth hormone, TSH, prolactin and ACTH. It inhibits the secretion of insulin, glucagon, gastrin and other peptides of the gastro-enteropancreatic system (i.e. peptide YY, neurotensin, VIP and substance P), reducing splanchnic blood flow, portal blood flow, GI motility, gastric, pancreatic and small bowel secretion, and increasing water and electrolyte absorption.[20] Somatostatin acts as an inhibitory neurotransmitter in the CNS and also inhibits cell proliferation.[21] In Type 1 diabetes mellitus, octreotide decreases insulin requirements. However, in Type 2 diabetes, octreotide suppresses both insulin and glucagon release, leaving plasma glucose concentrations either unchanged or slightly elevated.[22,23] Octreotide has a direct anticancer effect on solid tumours of the GI tract and prolongs survival.[24–27]

The inhibitory, antisecretory and absorptive effects of octreotide are utilized in a wide range of clinical settings:

Hormone-secreting tumours: octreotide improves symptoms by inhibiting hormone secretion, e.g.:
- 5HT in carcinoid (improving flushing and diarrhoea)
- VIP in VIPomas (improving diarrhoea)
- glucagon in glucagonomas (improving rash and diarrhoea).

Inoperable bowel obstruction in patients with cancer: octreotide can provide rapid relief of nausea and vomiting. The optimal dose has not been formally identified, but reports suggest <50% of patients respond to the typical starting dose of 300microgram/24h,[28] and 75–90% respond to 600–800microgram/24h.[12,29] Although doses of up to 1,500microgram/24h have been used,[30] a dose of 600–800microgram/24h is generally sufficient to identify those likely to respond.[29,31] In comparisons with **hyoscine *butylbromide*** (60–80mg/24h; p.14), octreotide (300–800microgram/24h) provides more effective and rapid relief of nausea and vomiting and reduction in NG tube output. However, in those patients responding to either drug, after about 4–6 days, overall symptom relief is similar, and NG tube removal possible with both.[29] (Although no head-to-head comparison has been published to date, it is likely that the same is true for **glycopyrronium**, p.11).

Ascites: octreotide 300microgram SC b.d. can suppress diuretic-induced activation of the renin-aldosterone-angiotensin system and its addition has improved renal function and Na^+ and water excretion in patients with cirrhosis and ascites receiving **furosemide** and **spironolactone** (p.60).[15] Octreotide is also reported to reduce the rate of formation of malignant ascites.[14,16] It may interfere with ascitic fluid formation through a reduction in splanchnic blood flow or as a result of a direct tumour antisecretory effect. Octreotide may also help improve the efficacy of diuretics as in cirrhosis.[32] Octreotide could be considered in patients with rapidly accumulating ascites requiring frequent paracentesis despite diuretic therapy (see **spironolactone** p.59). Octreotide may also help resolve chylous ascites and/or pleural effusion secondary to yellow nail syndrome,[33] ruptured thoracic duct,[34] cirrhosis,[35–37] peritoneal dialysis,[38] or cancer.[39]

Other antisecretory effects: octreotide reduces salivary production and may be of use in salivary or buccal fistulas (see **hyoscine *butylbromide*** p.14, **hyoscine *hydrobromide*** p.16, and **glycopyrronium** p.11).[4,17] Experience of its use in death rattle is limited and recommended only in the context of a clinical trial.[40] The use of octreotide led to rapid and complete control of bronchorrhoea (>1L/24h) in a patient with diffuse adenocarcinoma of the lung.[18] A systematic review supports the prophylactic use of octreotide with pancreatic surgery *for cancer*, to reduce the risk of complications, e.g. leak, fistula, but not with pancreatic surgery for other reasons.[1] Octreotide is recommended first-line for chemotherapy or radiotherapy-induced diarrhoea when severe (i.e. increase ≥7 stools/day over baseline, hospital admission and IV fluids >24h required) and second-line for less severe diarrhoea which does not respond to **loperamide** 16–24mg/24h (p.32).[9,10] For those who have experienced severe chemotherapy-induced diarrhoea, prophylactic depot octreotide is recommended for subsequent cycles. Octreotide has also been used for the treatment of enterovesical fistula,[41] and to improve mucous discharge from rectal cancers.[14]

Pain: octreotide is reported to have an analgesic effect in patients with cancer, e.g. in bone pain from metastatic carcinoid, in hypertrophic pulmonary osteo-arthopathy, pain arising from GI cancer, or when given IT.[13,42–44] However, a small RCT found octreotide to be no better than placebo.[45] Octreotide is also reported to be of value in chronic non-malignant pancreatic pain caused by hypertension in the scarred pancreatic ducts.[46,47] Benefit could be secondary to its antisecretory action;[48] suppressing exocrine function by administering **pancreatin** supplements (p.53) also reduces pain in 50–75% of patients with chronic pancreatitis.[49]

Miscellaneous: at doses far below those necessary for an antisecretory effect (e.g. 1microgram SC t.d.s.), octreotide protects the stomach from NSAID-related injury, probably via its ability to reduce NSAID-induced neutrophil adhesion to the microvasculature.[50] Somatostatin receptors have been identified on leukocytes and, in rats, octreotide has been shown to suppress inflammation.[51] A recent systematic review casts doubt on the value of octreotide in the management of bleeding oesophageal varices.[2]

Octreotide is generally given as a SC bolus or by CSCI[52] but can be given IV when a rapid effect is required. Octreotide has also been administered IT (as an analgesic).[44] A long-acting depot formulation is also available but evaluation has been generally limited to hormone-secreting tumours.[53] Benefit from depot octreotide has been reported in a RCT for the prevention of chemotherapy-related diarrhoea[7] and in cancer patients with bowel obstruction.[54,55] **Lanreotide** is an alternative sandostatin analogue available in depot formulations.

Onset of action 30min.

Time to peak plasma concentration 30min SC.

Plasma halflife 1.5h SC.

Duration of action 8h.

Cautions

Insulinoma (may potentiate hypoglycaemia). In Type 1 diabetes mellitus, **insulin** requirements may be reduced by up to 50%; monitor plasma glucose concentrations to guide any dose reduction needed with **insulin** or oral hypoglycaemic agents. Octreotide increases the bio-availability of **bromocriptine** by about 40% (consider when using the combination in acromegaly).[56]

Cirrhosis, renal failure requiring dialysis (both lead to reduced elimination which may necessitate a dose reduction). May cause gallstones (although the manufacturer advises ultrasound examination of the gallbladder before treatment and every 6–12 months thereafter, this is generally not necessary in palliative care). Avoid abrupt withdrawal of short-acting octreotide after long-term treatment (may precipitate biliary colic caused by gallstones/biliary sludge).

May cause bradycardia, conduction defects or arrhythmias; use with caution in at-risk patients. Monitor thyroid function during long-term treatment (may cause hypothyroidism).

Drug interactions

Octreotide markedly reduces plasma **ciclosporin** concentrations and inadequate immunosuppression may result. Increase the **ciclosporin** dose by 50% before starting octreotide, and monitor the plasma concentration daily to guide further adjustments.[56]

Undesirable effects

Bolus SC injection is painful (but less if the vial is warmed to room temperature). Dry mouth, flatulence (lowers oesophageal sphincter tone), nausea, abdominal pain, diarrhoea, steatorrhoea (GI undesirable effects may be reduced by administering octreotide between meals or at bedtime), impaired glucose tolerance, hypoglycaemia (shortly after starting treatment), persistent hyperglycaemia (during long-term treatment), gallstones (10–20% of patients on long-term treatment), pancreatitis (associated with gallstones).

Dose and use

The dose varies according to the indication (Table 7.11). To maximise the benefit (convenience and cost) of the multidose vials, the starting doses have been given in convenient fractions of 1mg (e.g. 250–500microgram rather than 300–600microgram). If necessary, the dose should be titrated upwards to achieve the desired response. When this has been achieved, it may subsequently be possible to reduce the dose to a lower maintenance level.

Table 7.11 Dose recommendations for SC octreotide

Indication	*Starting dose*[a]	*Maximum dose*[b]
Hormone-secreting tumours		
Acromegaly	100–200microgram t.d.s.	600microgram/24h[20]
Carcinoid, VIPomas, glucagonomas	50microgram once daily or b.d.	1,500microgram/24h; rarely 6,000microgram/24h[57]
Intractable diarrhoea (including that caused by chemotherapy and radiotherapy)	250–500microgram/24h	1,500microgram/24h,[9,10,58] occasionally higher
Intestinal obstruction	250–500microgram/24h	750microgram/24h, occasionally higher
Tumour-antisecretory effect	50–100microgram b.d.	600microgram/24h[14]
Ascites	250–500microgram/24h	600microgram/24h[16]
Bronchorrhoea	250–500microgram/24h[18]	
Hypertrophic pulmonary osteo-arthopathy	100microgram b.d.[13]	

a. doses 'rounded' to maximize benefit from multidose vials.
b. 'unrounded' doses derived from the literature.

Octreotide can be painful if given as a SC bolus injection. This can be reduced if the ampoule is warmed in the hand to body temperature before injection. To reduce the likelihood of inflammatory reactions at the skin injection site with CSCI, dilute to the largest volume possible and consider the use of 0.9% saline (see p.667).

CSCI compatibility with other drugs: There are 2-drug compatibility data for octreotide in 0.9% saline with **diamorphine, haloperidol, hyoscine *butylbromide*, hyoscine *hydrobromide*, midazolam, morphine sulphate, ondansetron**, and **oxycodone**.

Incompatibility may occur with **dexamethasone** or **levomepromazine**. More details and 3-drug compatibility data can be found on *www.palliativedrugs.com* Syringe Driver Survey Database.

For compatibility charts for mixing drugs in WFI see Appendix 3 (p.773).

Depot formulation

A depot formulation of octreotide 10–30mg, given every 4 weeks is available (Sandotatin LAR®). This has a relative bio-availability of about 60% compared to SC octreotide. Generally, the depot formulation is used only when symptoms have first been controlled with SC octreotide. Patients who have not previously received SC octreotide should have a test dose of 50–100microgram SC and, provided there are no unacceptable undesirable effects, then switch to the depot injection. The starting dose for those patients with acromegaly or gastroenteropancreatic tumours who have received a test dose or who are adequately controlled is 20mg every 4 weeks. The depot formulation requires deep IM injection into the gluteal muscle; to minimise irritation use alternate sides for subsequent injections.

In acromegaly, stop the SC dose of octreotide when the first depot injection is given; for other neuro-endocrine tumours continue the SC dose for a further 2 weeks.

In a recent survey, 40% of clinicians reported the use of depot formulations in the management of cancer-related bowel obstruction.[59] There is limited published experience of their use in this setting, although benefit in a small number of patients with ovarian cancer for up to 15 months has been reported.[55] A reduction in NG tube output and symptomatic benefit is evident within 24h.[54]

Lanreotide

Patients can be started directly on either of the long acting formulations. However for palliative care, use of the Somatuline Autogel® may be preferable as it is given by deep SC injection into the superior, external quadrant of the buttock:

- start with 60mg every 4 weeks for the first 3 months
- if necessary, increase to 120mg every 4 weeks.

Supply

For full details of storage and reconstitution details, see manufacturer's SPC.

For prolonged storage, keep all *unopened* ampoules, vials and pre-filled syringes in a refrigerator. Once opened, a multidose vial can be kept for up to 2 weeks at room temperature for day-to-day use.

Octreotide (generic)
Injection (as acetate) 50microgram/mL, 1mL amp = £4; 100microgram/mL, 1mL amp = £7; 500microgram/mL, 1mL amp = £34 (note: based on BNF pricing this is more expensive than proprietary Sandostatin® ampoules).
Injection (as acetate) 200microgram/mL multidose vial, 1mg in 5mL = £70.

Sandostatin® (Novartis)
Injection (as acetate) 50microgram/mL, 1mL amp = £3; 100microgram/mL, 1mL amp = £6; 500microgram/mL, 1mL amp = £27 (note: based on BNF pricing this is cheaper than generic ampoules).
Injection (as acetate) 200microgram/mL multidose vial, 1mg in 5mL = £70.

Sandostatin LAR® (Novartis)
Depot injection (microsphere powder for aqueous suspension), octreotide (as acetate) 10mg vial = £638; 20mg vial = £850; 30mg vial = £1,063 (all supplied with diluent filled syringe) for deep IM injection every 28 days.

Lanreotide
Somatuline LA® (Ipsen)
Long acting injection (copolymer microparticles for aqueous suspension), lanreotide (as acetate) 30mg vial (with vehicle) = £323 for IM injection every 14days.

Somatuline Autogel® (Ipsen)
Depot injection (prefilled syringe), lanreotide (as acetate) 60mg = £551; 90mg = £736; 120mg = £937 for deep SC injection into the superior, external quadrant of the buttock every 28 days.

1 Gurusamy KS *et al.* (2010) Somatostatin analogues for pancreatic surgery. *Cochrane Database of Systematic Reviews.* **2**: CD008370.
2 Gotzsche PC and Hrobjartsson A (2008) Somatostatin analogues for acute bleeding oesophageal varices. *Cochrane Database of Systematic Reviews.* **3**: CD000193.
3 Harris A (1992) Octreotide in the treatment of disorders of the gastrointestinal tract. *Drug Investigation.* **4**: 1–54.
4 Spinelli C *et al.* (1995) Postoperative salivary fistula: therapeutic action of octreotide. *Surgery.* **117**: 117–118.
5 Dorta G (1999) Role of octreotide and somatostatin in the treatment of intestinal fistulae. *Digestion.* **60 (suppl 2)**: 53–56.
6 Farthing MJ (1994) Octreotide in the treatment of refractory diarrhoea and intestinal fistulae. *Gut.* **35 (suppl 3)**: s5–10.
7 Rosenoff SH *et al.* (2006) A multicenter, randomized trial of long-acting octreotide for the optimum prevention of chemotherapy-induced diarrhea: results of the STOP trial. *Journal of Supportive Oncology.* **4**: 289–294.
8 Crouch M *et al.* (1996) Octreotide acetate in refractory bone marrow transplant-associated diarrhea. *Annals of Pharmacotherapy.* **30**: 331–336.
9 Benson AB *et al.* (2004) Recommended Guidelines for the Treatment of Cancer Treatment-Induced Diarrhea. *Journal of Clinical Oncology.* **22**: 2918–2926.
10 Maroun JA *et al.* (2007) Prevention and management of chemotherapy-induced diarrhea in patients with colorectal cancer: a consensus statement by the Canadian Working Group on Chemotherapy-Induced Diarrhea. *Current Oncology.* **14**: 13–20.
11 Mercadante S *et al.* (2007) Medical treatment for inoperable malignant bowel obstruction: a qualitative systematic review. *Journal of Pain and Symptom Management.* **33**: 217–223.
12 Ripamonti C and Mercadante S (2004) How to use octreotide for malignant bowel obstruction. *Journal of Supportive Oncology.* **2**: 357–364.
13 Johnson S *et al.* (1997) Treatment of resistant pain in hypertrophic pulmonary arthropathy with subcutaneous octreotide. *Thorax.* **52**: 298–299.
14 Harvey M and Dunlop R (1996) Octreotide and the secretory effects of advanced cancer. *Palliative Medicine.* **10**: 346–347.
15 Kalambokis G *et al.* (2005) Renal effects of treatment with diuretics, octreotide or both, in non-azotemic cirrhotic patients with ascites. *Nephrology, Dialysis, Transplantation.* **20**: 1623–1629.

16 Caims W and Malone R (1999) Octreotide as an agent for the relief of malignant ascites in palliative care patients. *Palliative Medicine*. **13**: 429–430.
17 Lam C and Wong S (1996) Use of somatostatin analog in the management of traumatic parotid fistula. *Surgery*. **119**: 481–482.
18 Hudson E *et al.* (2006) Successful treatment of bronchorrhea with octreotide in a patient with adenocarcinoma of the lung. *Journal of Pain and Symptom Management*. **32**: 200–202.
19 Lamberts SWJ *et al.* (1996) Octreotide. *New England Journal of Medicine*. **334**: 246–254.
20 Gyr K and Meier R (1993) Pharmacodynamic effects of sandostatin in the gastrointestinal tract. *Digestion*. **54**: 14–19.
21 Patel YC (1999) Somatostatin and its receptor family. *Frontiers in Neuroendocrinology*. **20**: 157–198.
22 Davies R *et al.* (1989) Somatostatin analogues in diabetes mellitus. *Diabetic Medicine*. **6**: 103–111.
23 Lunetta M *et al.* (1997) Effects of octreotide on glycaemic control, glucose disposal, hepatic glucose production and counterregulatory hormone secretion in type 1 and type 2 insulin treated diabetic patients. *Diabetes Research and Clinical Practice*. **38**: 81–89.
24 Deming DA *et al.* (2005) A dramatic response to long-acting octreotide in metastatic hepatocellular carcinoma. *Clinical Advances in Hematology and Oncology*. **3**: 468–472; discussion 472–464.
25 Kouroumalis E *et al.* (1998) Treatment of hepatocellular carcinoma with octreotide: a randomised controlled study. *Gut*. **42**: 442–447.
26 Pandha H and Waxman J (1996) Octreotide in malignant intestinal obstruction. *Anti-cancer Drugs*. **7**: 5–10.
27 Cascinu S *et al.* (1995) A randomised trial of octreotide vs best supportive care only in advanced gastrointestinal cancer patients refractory to chemotherapy. *British Journal of Cancer*. **71**: 97–101.
28 Shima Y *et al.* (2008) Clinical efficacy and safety of octreotide (SMS201-995) in terminally ill Japanese cancer patients with malignant bowel obstruction. *Japanese Journal of Clinical Oncology*. **38**: 354–359.
29 Mystakidou K *et al.* (2002) Comparison of octreotide administration vs conservative treatment in the management of inoperable bowel obstruction in patients with far advanced cancer: a randomized, double-blind, controlled clinical trial. *Anticancer Research*. **22**: 1187–1192.
30 Weber C and Zulian GB (2009) Malignant irreversible intestinal obstruction: the powerful association of octreotide to corticosteroids, antiemetics, and analgesics. *American Journal of Hospice and Palliative Care*. **26**: 84–88.
31 Riley J and Fallon M (1994) Octreotide in terminal malignant obstruction of the gastrointestinal tract. *European Journal of Palliative Care*. **1**: 23–25.
32 Kalambokis G *et al.* (2006) The effects of treatment with octreotide, diuretics, or both on portal hemodynamics in nonazotemic cirrhotic patients with ascites. *Journal of Clinical Gastroenterology*. **40**: 342–346.
33 Widjaja A *et al.* (1999) Octreotide for therapy of chylous ascites in yellow nail syndrome. *Gastroenterology*. **116**: 1017–1018.
34 Ferrandiere M *et al.* (2000) Chylous ascites following radical nephrectomy: efficacy of octreotide as treatment of ruptured thoracic duct. *Intensive Care and Medicine*. **26**: 484–485.
35 Zhou DX *et al.* (2009) The effectiveness of the treatment of octreotide on chylous ascites after liver cirrhosis. *Digestive Diseases and Sciences*. **54**: 1783–1788.
36 Pfammatter R *et al.* (2001) Treatment of hepatic hydrothorax and reduction of chest tube output with octreotide. *European Journal of Gastroenterology and Hepatology*. **13**: 977–980.
37 Dumortier J *et al.* (2000) Successful treatment of hepatic hydrothorax with octreotide. *European Journal of Gastroenterology and Hepatology*. **12**: 817–820.
38 Lee PH *et al.* (2005) Octreotide therapy for chylous ascites in a chronic dialysis patient. *Nephrology (Carlton)*. **10**: 344–347.
39 Mincher L *et al.* (2005) The successful treatment of chylous effusions in malignant disease with octreotide. *Clinical Oncology*. **17**: 118–121.
40 Clark K *et al.* (2008) A pilot phase II randomized, cross-over, double-blinded, controlled efficacy study of octreotide versus hyoscine hydrobromide for control of noisy breathing at the end-of-life. *Journal of Pain and Palliative Care Pharmacotherapy*. **22**: 131–138.
41 Shinjo T *et al.* (2009) Treatment of malignant enterovesical fistula with octreotide. *Journal of Palliative Medicine*. **12**: 965–967.
42 Katai M *et al.* (2005) Octreotide as a rapid and effective painkiller for metastatic carcinoid tumor. *Endocrine Journal*. **52**: 277–280.
43 Befon S *et al.* (2000) Continuous subcutaneous octreotide in gastrointestinal cancer patients: pain control and beta-endorphin levels. *Anticancer Research*. **20**: 4039–4046.
44 Penn RD *et al.* (1992) Octreotide: A potent new nonopiate analgesic for intrathecal infusion. *Pain*. **49**: 13–19.
45 De-Conno F *et al.* (1994) Subcutaneous octreotide in the treatment of pain in advanced cancer patients. *Journal of Pain and Symptom Management*. **9**: 34–38.
46 Donnelly PK *et al.* (1991) Somatostatin for chronic pancreatic pain. *Journal of Pain and Symptom Management*. **6**: 349–350.
47 Okazaki K *et al.* (1988) Pressure of papillary zone and pancreatic main duct in patients with chronic pancreatitis in the early state. *Scandinavian Journal of Gastroenterology*. **23**: 501–506.
48 Lembcke B *et al.* (1987) Effect of the somatostatin analogue sandostatin on gastrointestinal, pancreatic and biliary function and hormone release in man. *Digestion*. **36**: 108–124.
49 Mossner J *et al.* (1989) Influence of treatment with pancreatic extracts on pancreatic enzyme secretion. *Gut*. **3**: 1143–1149.
50 Scheiman J *et al.* (1997) Reduction of NSAID induced gastric injury and leucocyte endothelial adhesion by octreotide. *Gut*. **40**: 720–725.
51 Karalis K *et al.* (1994) Somatostatin analogues suppress the inflammatory reaction in vivo. *Journal of Clinical Investigations*. **93**: 2000–2006.
52 Mercadante S (1995) Tolerability of continuous subcutaneous octreotide used in combination with other drugs. *Journal of Palliative Care*. **11 (4)**: 14–16.
53 Scherubl H *et al.* (1994) Treatment of the carcinoid syndrome with a depot formulation of the somatostatin analogue lanreotide. *European Journal of Cancer*. **30A**: 1590–1591.
54 Massacesi C and Galeazzi G (2006) Sustained release octreotide may have a role in the treatment of malignant bowel obstruction. *Journal of Palliative Medicine*. **20**: 715–716.
55 Matulonis UA *et al.* (2005) Long-acting octreotide for the treatment and symptomatic relief of bowel obstruction in advanced ovarian cancer. *Journal of Pain and Symptom Management*. **30**: 563–569.
56 Baxter K (ed) (2008) *Stockley's Drug Interactions* (8e). Pharmaceutical Press, London.
57 Harris A and Redfern J (1995) Octreotide treatment of carcinoid syndrome: analysis of published dose-titration data. *Alimentary Pharmacology and Therapeutics*. **9**: 387–394.

58 Cello J *et al.* (1991) Effect of octreotide on refractory AIDS-associated diarrhea. A prospective, multicenter clinical trial. *Annals of internal medicine*. **115**: 705–710.
59 Palliativedrugs.com (2010) Octreotide — What is your experience? Available from: www.palliativedrugs.com/download/100401_octreotide.pdf

PROGESTOGENS BNF 6.4.1.2 & 8.3.2

Class: Sex hormones.

Indications: Licensed indications vary between products; consult SPCs for details. Hormone therapy in endometrial cancer (use in breast, prostate and renal cancer has diminished);[1] anovulatory uterine bleeding; secondary amenorrhoea; mild–moderate endometriosis; †anorexia and cachexia in cancer, AIDS, other end-stage chronic diseases and the frail elderly; †post-castration hot flushes in both women and men.

Contra-indications: Medroxyprogesterone acetate (MPA) oestrogen-progestogen-dependent cancer, hepatic impairment, history of (or high risk of developing) thrombo-embolism, active thrombophlebitis, undiagnosed abnormal vaginal bleeding, pregnancy (known or suspected).

Pharmacology

In addition to natural **progesterone**, there are several classes of synthetic progestogens, e.g. derivatives of retroprogesterone, progesterone, and 17α-hydroxyprogesterone (**cyproterone, MPA, megestrol acetate**).[2] Whereas all derivatives have a progestogenic effect on the uterus, there are differences in other biological effects (Table 7.12).

Table 7.12 Comparison of the biological effects of natural progesterone and selected synthetic progestogens[2]

Progestogen	*Effect*[a]		
	Androgenic	*Anti-androgenic*	*Anti-mineralocorticoid*
Progesterone	−	+	+
Cyproterone acetate	−	++	−
Megestrol acetate	+	+	−
MPA	+	−	−

Key: ++ = effect present; + = weak effect; − = no effect.
a. all the above possess similar progestogenic, anti-gonadotrophic, anti-oestrogenic and glucocorticoid effects.

In palliative care, progestogens are used mainly in selected patients with cachexia-anorexia, although their efficacy in cachexia is debatable (see next section). Progestogens may improve appetite by increasing levels of orexigenic neurotransmitters in the hypothalamus (e.g. neuropeptide Y), counteracting the anorexic effects of cytokines on the hypothalamus, or by interfering with the production of cytokines via their glucocorticoid anti-inflammatory effect.[3,4] *In vitro*, cytokine release from peripheral blood mononucleocytes are inhibited by both **MPA** and **megestrol acetate** in concentrations that would be achieved by daily doses of 1,500–2,000mg and 320–960mg respectively.[3] The release of serotonin was also inhibited and was considered one possible mechanism by which progestogens have an anti-emetic effect.[3]

Bio-availability of **MPA** and **megestrol acetate** is low (Table 7.13). Both **MPA** and **megestrol acetate** are highly protein-bound, mainly to albumin. **MPA** is metabolized extensively in the liver, and excreted mainly as glucuronides, whereas **megestrol acetate** is excreted mainly unchanged in the urine.

Table 7.13 Selected pharmacokinetic data[5,6]

	Medroxyprogesterone acetate	*Megestrol acetate*
Bio-availability	1–10%	No absolute data; reduced by 25% in fasting state
Time to peak plasma concentration	2–7h	3–5h
Plasma halflife	38–46h	24–42h

Cachexia and anorexia

Cachexia is common in cancer and other chronic diseases, impairing quality of life and increasing morbidity and mortality.[7] Cachexia is characterized by the loss of skeletal muscle ± body fat that cannot be fully reversed by conventional nutritional support. Loss of skeletal muscle is associated with impaired physical function and quality of life, whereas loss of fat (the body's main energy store) is associated with reduced survival. Recommended diagnostic criteria for cancer cachexia are:

- involuntary weight loss >5% in the past 6 months, *or*
- weight loss >2% in patients with either a BMI of <20kg/m^2 or skeletal muscle sarcopenia (absolute muscularity <5th centile of sex-specific norm).[8]

In cancer, a negative protein and energy balance is driven by the combination of reduced food intake (anorexia) and abnormal host metabolism resulting from factors produced by the cancer, e.g. proteolysis-inducing factor, or by the host in response to the cancer, e.g. cytokines.[9] One outcome of this is a chronic inflammatory state, as evidenced by a raised serum CRP, the level of which relates to the degree and rate of weight loss.[10] Cytokines such as interleukin-1 and tumour necrosis factor-α act on the hypothalamus and skeletal muscle leading to anorexia, inefficient energy expenditure, wasting of skeletal muscle and loss of body fat. The management of cachexia requires both of these main mechanisms to be addressed, and explains why increasing nutritional intake alone is generally ineffective.[9,11–13]

Recent recommendations emphasize the importance of early identification and intervention, and recognize that once cachexia is advanced (patient has severe muscle wasting, ongoing catabolism, WHO performance status 3–4, metastatic disease refractory to therapy and a prognosis of <3 months) a response to treatment is unlikely, and that the focus in these circumstances should be on symptom relief and psychosocial support.[8]

Megestrol acetate is used to stimulate appetite and weight gain in patients with cancer or AIDS. Several systematic reviews of the literature (about 30 trials, >4,000 patients) have concluded that appetite (NNT 3) and weight (NNT 8) is improved in patients with cancer, but have been unable to comment for other groups, because of insufficient numbers. For appetite stimulation, 160mg/day is as effective as a higher dose. For weight gain there appears to be more of a dose-response, although one review found no difference in outcomes between ≤800mg and >800mg daily.[14–16] However, the studies in the reviews used body weight as a primary outcome measure, and none accurately evaluated changes in body composition.

In those studies that have evaluated body composition, both **megestrol acetate** and **MPA** appear to increase fat mass, but not fat-free mass, the part which includes skeletal muscle.[4,17–19] Thus it is likely that the gain in weight with progestogens (and corticosteroids), rather than representing the ideal increase in skeletal muscle *and* fat, is a less helpful retention of fluid or increase in fat only. This could make mobilizing more difficult in an already debilitated patient. In addition, the catabolic effect of progestogens on skeletal muscle could further weaken the patient. Catabolism may result from the glucocorticoid effect of progestogens but they also suppress the amount and function of testosterone, which is anabolic.

Others have noted that progestogens lead to a substantial improvement in appetite in <30% of patients, or have questioned the clinical relevance of the magnitude of weight gain seen (≈1kg), or have highlighted the occurrence of undesirable effects of deep vein thrombosis (5%) and male impotence (10–25%).[4,18–24] Further, in the USA, where **megestrol acetate** is increasingly used in frail, elderly nursing home residents with weight loss from any cause, a recent study suggests its use is associated with a significant increase in all-cause mortality but not weight. The reasons for this are unclear but venous thrombo-embolism may play a role as the incidence of DVT was 6-fold higher with **megestrol acetate**.[25]

Progestogens are much more expensive than **dexamethasone** or **prednisolone**. **Megestrol acetate** 800mg/day and **dexamethasone** 3mg/day are comparable with regard to appetite stimulation and non-fluid weight gain, although the latter was not accurately evaluated.[26] In this study, a high proportion of patients discontinued **dexamethasone** (36%) or **megestrol acetate** (25%) because of undesirable effects. **Dexamethasone** was more likely to cause cushingoid changes, myopathy, heartburn and peptic ulcers; **megestrol acetate** was associated with increased thrombo-embolism.[26] **Dexamethasone** is a fluorinated corticosteroid, a class which is more prone to cause muscle catabolism.[27] Thus, ideally, **dexamethasone** should be limited to short-term use only.

If long-term use of a corticosteroid is contemplated, a switch to the non-fluorinated **prednisolone** 10–20mg/day should be considered.[4] However, for patients expected to live months rather than weeks, progestogens may be more appropriate. Caution is still required as long-term progestogens can also cause cushingoid changes (25% of patients after 3 months in one study),[28] muscle catabolism and suppression of the hypothalamic-pituitary-adrenal axis. The latter may present with non-specific symptoms and a high level of clinical suspicion is required.[29] Additional corticosteroid replacement therapy would be a reasonable precaution in patients with serious infections or undergoing surgery.[4,30,31] Adrenal suppression is secondary to a central glucocorticoid effect on the hypothalamus and is dose-related; maximal suppression is seen with daily doses of **megestrol acetate** 200mg and **MPA** 1,000mg.[28]

The combination of a progestogen and an NSAID has been investigated.[32,33] **Megestrol acetate** 160mg t.d.s. together with **ibuprofen** 400mg t.d.s. resulted in improved quality of life and weight gain. However, this was probably caused by fluid retention, because total body water increased *even though there was no clinical oedema*.[32] The combination of **MPA** 500mg b.d. and **celecoxib** 200mg b.d. also stabilized weight and improved systemic symptoms.[33] Because the NSAID probably provided benefit by reducing the chronic inflammatory response (CRP levels were reduced), others have used **indomethacin** alone.[34]

In conclusion, progestogens and systemic corticosteroids (see p.483) are useful *appetite stimulants* which can increase calorie intake and as such may be indicated in selected patients for anorexia. Progestogens may be better for long-term use than corticosteroids, but significant undesirable effects can occur. Starting doses should be low and titrated to the lowest effective dose. Both progestogens and corticosteroids are best *not* regarded as *'anticachexia' agents*; any weight gain is likely to be because of an increase in fat and fluid retention, and the catabolism of skeletal muscle *increased*, particularly in inactive people.

Cautions

May suppress the hypothalamic-pituitary-adrenal axis.[35] Possibility of glucocorticoid effects. May cause or worsen diabetes mellitus.

MPA: discontinue if any of the following develop: jaundice, hepatic impairment, significant increase in blood pressure, thrombo-embolic event (e.g. stroke, myocardial infarction, DVT, pulmonary embolism), new onset migraine, severe visual disturbances. May exacerbate hypercalcaemia, migraine, epilepsy, asthma, cardiac and renal impairment.

Megestrol acetate: history of thrombophlebitis, severe hepatic impairment.

Undesirable effects

Thrombo-embolism (5%).

Frequency not stated: hyperglycaemia, depression, insomnia, fatigue, hypertension, oedema/fluid retention, nausea, vomiting, constipation, cushingoid changes, bone mineral density loss, reduced libido, impotence, altered menstruation, breast tenderness, urticaria, acne.

Rare (<0.1%): jaundice, alopecia, hirsutism.

Dose and use

Appetite stimulation

- start with **megestrol acetate** 80–160mg PO each morning
- if initial response poor, consider doubling the dose after 2 weeks[36,37]
- maximum dose generally 800mg PO daily.

MPA 400mg PO each morning–b.d. is an alternative in countries where higher strength tablets are available (e.g. 100mg, 200mg and 400mg).

Hot flushes after surgical or chemical castration

- **MPA** 5–20mg b.d.–q.d.s. *or*
- **megestrol acetate** 80mg each morning; 40mg is used in countries where the oral suspension is readily available. The effect manifests after 2–4 weeks.[38]

Supply

Megestrol acetate

Megace® (Bristol-Myers Squibb)
Tablets (scored) 160mg, 28 days @ 160mg each morning = £18.
Oral suspension 40mg/mL, 28 days @ 160mg each morning = £127. Unlicensed in UK, can import via IDIS, 240mL bottle = £270 (see Obtaining unlicensed products, p.769).

Medroxyprogesterone acetate

Provera® (Pharmacia)
Tablets 2.5mg, 5mg, 10mg, 100mg, 200mg, 400mg, 28 days @ 5mg b.d. = £7; @ 400mg each morning = £55.

Climanor® (Resource Medical)
Tablets 5mg, 28 days @ 5mg b.d. = £7.

1 Decruze SB and Green JA (2007) Hormone therapy in advanced and recurrent endometrial cancer: a systematic review. *International Journal of Gynecology Cancer.* **17**: 964–978.
2 Schindler AE *et al.* (2003) Classification and pharmacology of progestins. *Maturitas.* **46 (suppl 1)**: s7–s16.
3 Mantovani G *et al.* (1998) Cytokine involvement in cancer anorexia/cachexia: role of megestrol acetate and medroxyprogesterone acetate on cytokine downregulation and improvement of clinical symptoms. *Critical Reviews in Oncogenesis.* **9**: 99–106.
4 MacDonald N (2005) Anorexia-cachexia syndrome. *European Journal of Palliative Care.* **12 (suppl)**: 8s–14s.
5 Par Pharmaceuticals *Data on file.*
6 Deschamps B *et al.* (2009) Food effect on the bioavailability of two distinct formulations of megestrol acetate oral suspension. *International Journal of Nanomedicine.* **4**: 185–192.
7 Laviano A *et al.* (2003) Cancer anorexia: clinical implications, pathogenesis, and therapeutic strategies. *Lancet Oncology.* **4**: 686–694.
8 Fearon K *et al.* (2010) Definition and classification of cancer cachexia: an international consensus framework. *Lancet Oncology* **12**: 489–495.
9 Gordon JN *et al.* (2005) Cancer cachexia. *Qjm.* **98**: 779–788.
10 Scott HR *et al.* (2002) The systemic inflammatory response, weight loss, performance status and survival in patients with inoperable non-small cell lung cancer. *British Journal of Cancer.* **87**: 264–267.
11 Davis MP *et al.* (2004) Appetite and cancer-associated anorexia: a review. *Journal of Clinical Oncology.* **22**: 1510–1517.
12 Ramos EJ *et al.* (2004) Cancer anorexia-cachexia syndrome: cytokines and neuropeptides. *Current Opinion in Clinical Nutrition and Metabolic care.* **7**: 427–434.
13 Laviano A *et al.* (2005) Therapy insight: Cancer anorexia-cachexia syndrome–when all you can eat is yourself. *Nature Clinical Practice Oncology.* **2**: 158–165.
14 Pascual Lopez A *et al.* (2004) Systematic review of megestrol acetate in the treatment of anorexia-cachexia syndrome. *Journal of Pain and Symptom Management.* **27**: 360–369.
15 Berenstein EG and Ortiz Z (2005) Megestrol acetate for the treatment of anorexia-cachexia syndrome. *Cochrane Database of Systematic Reviews.* **2**: CD004310.
16 Lesniak W *et al.* (2008) Effects of megestrol acetate in patients with cancer anorexia-cachexia syndrome–a systematic review and meta-analysis. *Polskie Archiwum Medycyny Wewnetrznej.* **118**: 636–644.
17 Loprinzi C *et al.* (1993) Body-composition changes in patients who gain weight while receiving megestrol acetate. *Journal of Clinical Oncology.* **11**: 152–154.
18 Loprinzi CL *et al.* (1993) Phase III evaluation of four doses of megestrol acetate as therapy for patients with cancer anorexia and/or cachexia. *Journal of Clinical Oncology.* **11**: 762–767.
19 Simons JP *et al.* (1998) Effects of medroxyprogesterone acetate on food intake, body composition, and resting energy expenditure in patients with advanced, nonhormone-sensitive cancer: a randomized, placebo-controlled trial. *Cancer.* **82**: 553–560.
20 Jatoi A *et al.* (2002) Dronabinol versus megestrol acetate versus combination therapy for cancer-associated anorexia: a North Central Cancer Treatment Group study. *Journal of Clinical Oncology.* **20**: 567–573.
21 Jatoi A *et al.* (2003) On appetite and its loss. *Journal of Clinical Oncology.* **21 (suppl 9)**: 79–81.
22 Jatoi A *et al.* (2004) An eicosapentaenoic acid supplement versus megestrol acetate versus both for patients with cancer-associated wasting: a North Central Cancer Treatment Group and National Cancer Institute of Canada collaborative effort. *Journal of Clinical Oncology.* **22**: 2469–2476.
23 Kropsky B *et al.* (2003) Incidence of deep-venous thrombosis in nursing home residents using megestrol acetate. *Journal of the American Medical Directors Association.* **4**: 255–256.
24 Garcia VR and Juan O (2005) Megestrol acetate-probably less effective than has been reported! *Journal of Pain and Symptom Management.* **30**: 4; author reply 5–6.
25 Bodenner D *et al.* (2007) A retrospective study of the association between megestrol acetate administration and mortality among nursing home residents with clinically significant weight loss. *American Journal Geriatric Pharmacotherapy.* **5**: 137–146.

26 Loprinzi CL *et al.* (1999) Randomized comparison of megestrol acetate versus dexamethasone versus fluoxymesterone for the treatment of cancer anorexia/cachexia. *Journal of Clinical Oncology.* **17**: 3299–3306.
27 Faludi G *et al.* (1966) Factors influencing the development of steroid-induced myopathies. *Annals of the New York Academy of Sciences.* **138**: 62–72.
28 Willemse PH *et al.* (1990) A randomized comparison of megestrol acetate (MA) and medroxyprogesterone acetate (MPA) in patients with advanced breast cancer. *European Journal of Cancer.* **26**: 337–343.
29 Dev R *et al.* (2007) Association between megestrol acetate treatment and symptomatic adrenal insufficiency with hypogonadism in male patients with cancer. *Cancer.* **110**: 1173–1177.
30 Naing KK *et al.* (1999) Megestrol acetate therapy and secondary adrenal suppression. *Cancer.* **86**: 1044–1049.
31 Lambert C *et al.* (2002) Effects of testosterone replacement and/or resistance exercise on the composition of megestrol acetate stimulated weight gain in elderly men: a randomized controlled trial. *Journal of Clinical Endocrinology and Metabolism.* **87**: 2100–2106.
32 McMillan DC *et al.* (1999) A prospective randomized study of megestrol acetate and ibuprofen in gastrointestinal cancer patients with weight loss. *British Journal of Cancer.* **79**: 495–500.
33 Cerchietti LC *et al.* (2004) Effects of celecoxib, medroxyprogesterone, and dietary intervention on systemic syndromes in patients with advanced lung adenocarcinoma: a pilot study. *Journal of Pain and Symptom Management.* **27**: 85–95.
34 Bosaeus I *et al.* (2002) Dietary intake, resting energy expenditure, weight loss and survival in cancer patients. *Journal of Nutrirtion.* **132 (suppl)**: 3465s-3466s.
35 Villarroel *et al.* (2008) Megestrol acetate-induced adrenal insufficiency. *Clinical Translational Oncology.* **10**: 235–237.
36 Donnelly S and Walsh TD (1995) Low-dose megestrol acetate for appetite stimulation in advanced cancer. *Journal of Pain and Symptom Management.* **10**: 182–183.
37 Vadell C *et al.* (1998) Anticachectic efficacy of megestrol acetate at different doses and versus placebo in patients with neoplastic cachexia. *American Journal of Clinical Oncology.* **21**: 347–351.
38 Loprinzi CL *et al.* (1996) Megestrol acetate for the prevention of hot flashes. *New England Journal of Medicine.* **331**: 347–352.

DANAZOL — BNF 6.7.2

Class: Anabolic steroid, 17α-alkyl androgen.

Indications: Endometriosis, benign fibrocystic breast disease, †hereditary angioedema,[1,2] †pruritus associated with obstructive jaundice, †idiopathic immune thrombocytopenia, †gynaecomastia.

Contra-Indications: Thrombo-embolic disorders; severe cardiac, hepatic or renal impairment (*except when indicated for cholestatic pruritus,* see Table 5.29, p.431); androgen-dependent tumour; undiagnosed genital bleeding; porphyria; pregnancy; breast-feeding.

Pharmacology

Danazol is a chemically modified testosterone. It suppresses the pituitary-ovarian axis by inhibiting the pituitary output of gonadotrophins. The beneficial effect of 17α-alkyl androgens in hepatic (cholestatic) pruritus was discovered serendipitously some 60 years ago when the co-incidental use of **methyltestosterone** in a patient with primary biliary cirrhosis resulted in relief from the associated pruritus.[3] Hepatic pruritus is central in origin and is associated with enhanced opioidergic tone, secondary to the increased production of endogenous opioids.[4–6] In intrahepatic cholestasis, an opioid antagonist such as **naloxone** (see p.435) or **naltrexone** (see p.438) is the treatment of choice.[7]

It is possible that, when opioids are needed for concurrent cancer pain, a 17α-alkyl androgen is one alternative.[8] The mechanism of action is uncertain, but 17α-alkyl androgens are directly toxic to hepatocytes.[9–11] Thus, it is possible that danazol causes focal cell damage which limits the ability of the cholestatic liver to produce enkephalins. Androgens themselves can cause cholestatic jaundice,[12,13] and have occasionally caused severe hepatic impairment.[14,15] By mouth, 17α-alkyl androgens (e.g. **methyltestosterone**) are more bio-available than other androgens (e.g. **testosterone**) because of the reduction in first-pass hepatic metabolism in androgens with a 17α-alkyl radical.[16] Danazol also has additional effects on the liver which are not shared by **testosterone**.[17] The antipruritic effect is maintained even if the cholestasis is exacerbated by the androgen itself.[16] Androgens and oestrogens sometimes relieve non-specific pruritus in the elderly.[18]

A recent meta-analysis suggests that anabolic steroids may increase body weight and lean body mass in HIV-infected individuals, though the change is small and may not be clinically significant.[19]

Bio-availability 11% (fasting), 44% (after lipid-rich meal);[20] doubling the dose increases the plasma concentration by only 35–40%.

Onset of action 5–10 days in hepatic pruritus.
Time to peak plasma concentration <2h.
Plasma halflife 4.5h (single dose); >24h (multiple doses).
Duration of action >24h.

Cautions

Hepatic or renal disease, fluid retention, cardiovascular disease, hypertension, epilepsy, diabetes mellitus, lipoprotein disorder, polycythaemia, migraine. Discontinue if female virilization occurs (may become irreversible if treatment continued), or if symptoms of raised intracranial pressure or thrombo-embolism arise.

Danazol inhibits CYP3A4 and may enhance the activity of several drugs, including **carbamazepine**, **ciclosporin**, **warfarin**, and possibly **tacrolimus**. It can cause insulin resistance.

The concurrent use of danazol and a statin has been associated with acute renal impairment, pancreatitis and rhabdomyolysis.[21,22]

Monitor liver function and blood count every 6 months during long-term treatment. May cause false results with thyroid function tests.

Undesirable effects

Related to inhibition of the pituitary-ovarian axis: amenorrhoea, hot flushes, sweating, reduction in breast size, reduced libido, vaginitis, emotional lability.
Related to androgenic activity: acne, oily skin or hair, mild hirsutism, deepening of the voice, androgenic alopecia, and rarely clitoral hypertrophy. Paradoxically, testicular atrophy may occur.
Other effects: include cramps, nausea, photosensitivity, severe hepatotoxicity (occasional), benign intracranial hypertension (rare).

Dose and use

Pruritus

Moisturizing the skin with an emollient is always the first step. In patients with an extrahepatic obstruction (e.g. because of pancreatic cancer, lymphadenopathy), the treatment of choice is generally stenting of the bile duct.

When this is not feasible or when associated with intrahepatic cholestasis, one of several drugs can be used, and the choice depends on both individual circumstances and local fashion:

- **naltrexone** 12.5–250mg once daily[5–7]
- **rifampicin** 150–300mg once daily[23]
- **paroxetine** 5–20mg once daily[24]
- danazol 200mg once daily–t.d.s.[25]

Benefit from danazol is generally seen after about 5–10 days.[26,27] Androgenic changes may be ameliorated by reducing the dose from once daily to 3 times weekly or even less.[16]

Alternative 17α-alkyl androgens in some countries (not UK) include:

- **norethandrolone** 10mg b.d.–t.d.s.
- **methyltestosterone** 25mg once daily SL.

Supply

Danazol (generic)
Capsules 100mg, 200mg, 28 days @ 200mg once daily = £33 (note: based on BNF pricing, this is *more expensive* than proprietary danazol capsules).

Danol® (Sanofi-Aventis)
Capsules 100mg, 200mg, 28 days @ 200mg once daily = £15 (note: based on BNF pricing, this is *cheaper* than generic danazol capsules).

Paroxetine (generic)
Tablets 20mg, 30mg, 28 days @ 20mg once daily = £2.50.

Seroxat® (GSK)
Tablets (scored) 10mg, 20mg, 30mg, 28 days @ 10mg once daily = £12.
Oral suspension 10mg/5mL, 28 days @ 10mg once daily = £9.

Rifampicin (generic)
Capsules 150mg, 300mg, 28 days@ 150mg once daily = £6.

Rifadin® (Sanofi-Aventis)
Capsules 150mg, 300mg, 28 days@ 150mg once daily = £5.
Oral syrup 100mg/5mL, 28 days @ 150mg once daily = £6.

Also see **naltrexone**, p.438.

1 Hosea SW and Frank MM (1980) Danazole in the treatment of hereditary angioedema. *Drugs.* **19**: 370–372.
2 MacFarlane JT and Davies D (1981) Management of hereditary angio-oedema with low-dose danazol. *Br Med J (Clin Res Ed).* **282**: 1275.
3 Ahrens E *et al.* (1950) Primary biliary cirrhosis. *Medicine.* **29**: 299–364.
4 Jones E and Bergasa N (1990) The pruritus of cholestasis. From bile acids to opiate agonists. *Hepatology.* **11**: 884–887.
5 Jones E and Dekker L (2000) Florid opioid withdrawal-like reaction precipitated by naltrexone in a patient with chronic cholestasis. *Gastroenterology.* **118**: 431–432.
6 Jones EA and Bergasa N (2004) The pruritus of cholestasis and the opioid neurotransmitter system. In: Z Zylicz *et al.* (eds) *Pruritus in advanced desease.* Oxford University Press, Oxford, pp. 56–60.
7 Jones E and Bergasa N (1999) The pruritus of cholestasis. *Hepatology.* **29**: 1003–1006.
8 Twycross RG *et al.* (2003) Itch: scratching more than the surface. *Quarterly Journal of Medicine.* **96**: 7–26.
9 Welder A *et al.* (1995) Toxic effects of anabolic-androgen steroids in primary rat hepatic cell cultures. *Journal of Pharmacological and Toxicological Methods.* **33**: 187–195.
10 Ohsawa T and Iwashita S (1986) Hepatitis associated with danazol. *Drug Intell Clin Pharm.* **20**: 889.
11 Fermand JP *et al.* (1990) Danazol-induced hepatocellular adenoma. *American Journal of Medicine.* **88**: 529–530.
12 Boue F *et al.* (1986) Danazol and cholestatic hepatitis. *Annals of Internal Medicine.* **105**: 139–140.
13 Silva MO *et al.* (1989) Danazol-induced cholestasis. *American Journal of Gastroenterology.* **84**: 426–428.
14 Gurakar A *et al.* (1994) Androgenic/anabolic steroid-induced intrahepatic cholestasis: a review with four additional case reports. *Journal of Oklahoma State Medical Association.* **87**: 399–404.
15 Piekarska A and Wojcik K (2009) Modern anabolics and anticatabolics: The scope of the hepatologist's knowledge. *Experimental and Clinical Hepatology.* **5**: 7–11.
16 Lloyd-Thomas H and Sherlock S (1952) Testosterone therapy for the pruritus of obstructive jaundice. *British Medical Journal.* **ii**: 1289–1291.
17 Fernandez L *et al.* (1994) Stanozolol and danazol, unlike natural androgens, interact with the low affinity glucocorticoid-binding sites from male rat liver microsomes. *Endocrinology.* **134**: 1401–1408.
18 Feldman S *et al.* (1942) Treatment of senile pruritus with androgens and estrogens. *Archives of Dermatology and Syphilology Chicago.* **46**: 112–127.
19 Johns KKJ *et al.* (2005) Anabolic steroids for the treatment of weight loss in HIV-infected individuals. *Cochrane Database of Systematic Reviews.* **4**: CD005483.
20 Sunesen VH *et al.* (2005) Effect of liquid volume and food intake on the absolute bioavailability of danazol, a poorly soluble drug. *Eur J Pharm Sci.* **24**: 297–303.
21 Hsieh CY and Chen CH (2008) Rhabdomyolysis and pancreatitis associated with coadministration of danazol 600 mg/d and lovastatin 40 mg/d. *Clinical Therapeutics.* **30**: 1330–1335.
22 Andreou ER and Ledger S (2003) Potential drug interaction between simvastatin and danazol causing rhabdomyolysis. *Canadian Journal of Clinical Pharmacology.* **10**: 172–174.
23 Ghent C and Carruthers S (1988) Treatment of pruritus in primary biliary cirrhosis with rifampin. Results of a double-blind crossover randomized trial. *Gastroenterology.* **94**: 488–493.
24 Zylicz Z *et al.* (2003) Paroxetine in the treatment of severe non-dermatological pruritus: a randomized, controlled trial. *Journal of Pain and Symptom Management.* **26**: 1105–1112.
25 Twycross RG and Zylicz Z (2004) Systemic therapy: making rational choices. In: Z Zylicz *et al.* (eds) *Pruritus in advanced disease.* Oxford University Press, London, pp. 161–178.
26 Sherlock S (1981) *Diseases of the Liver and Biliary System* (6e). Blackwell Scientific, Oxford.
27 Sherlock S and Dooley J (1993) *Diseases of the Liver and Biliary System* (9e). Blackwell Scientific, Oxford.

*THALIDOMIDE — BNF 8.2.4

Class: Biologic response modifier.

Indications: Multiple myeloma (with concurrent **melphalan** and **prednisone** as first-line treatment in patients ⩾65 years or ineligible for high dose chemotherapy), †cutaneous manifestations of lepromatous leprosy (erythema nodosum leprosum), †graft versus host disease

(GVHD), †recurrent aphthous stomatitis in HIV infection and connective tissue disease (Behcet's syndrome), †paraneoplastic sweating, †paraneoplastic and uraemic pruritus, †cachexia in HIV and cancer, †intractable GI bleeding, †intractable irinotecan-induced diarrhoea, †discoid lupus erythematosus, †rheumatoid arthritis, †prevention of graft rejection.[1,2]

Contra-indications: Because it causes severe congenital abnormalities (absent or shortened limbs), thalidomide is contra-indicated in pregnant women and in women with childbearing potential unless strict contraception is implemented (see Dose and use).[3]

Pharmacology

Thalidomide is an immunomodulator with anticytokine, anti-integrin, and anti-angiogenic properties.[4,5] It was withdrawn from use as a non-barbiturate hypnotic with anti-emetic properties in the early 1960s after it became apparent that it was teratogenic.[6] Subsequently, it has been found to have immunomodulatory properties with potential for the treatment of various conditions.[7] However, its use is closely monitored and it is prohibitively expensive (see Supply).

Thalidomide inhibits the synthesis of the pro-inflammatory cytokine tumour necrosis factor α (TNF-α) by monocytes,[8] and stimulates interleukin-2 and interferon-γ production (thereby stimulating human T lymphocytes).[9] It also inhibits chemotaxis of neutrophils and monocytes. Thalidomide also has an antiproliferative and pro-apoptotic activity in tumour cells.[10]

Thalidomide antagonizes PGE_2, PGF_2, histamine, serotonin, and acetylcholine.[11] It also affects several other mechanisms associated with inflammation and immunomodulation.[12] These properties probably account for the prevention of **irinotecan**-induced diarrhoea,[13] and for the amelioration of paraneoplastic sweating[14] and paraneoplastic pruritus.[15]

Thalidomide also inhibits angiogenesis, a property which is the basis for investigational studies in oncology.[16,17] Thalidomide suppresses vascular endothelial growth factor (VEGF), a potent angiogenic factor secreted by cancer cells in response to hypoxia. This property also provides the rationale underlying the use of thalidomide in refractory GI bleeding.[18–21]

Analogues of thalidomide with similar anti-angiogenic, immunomodulatory and anti-inflammatory properties have been developed.[22] For example, **lenalidomide** is licensed in the USA and Europe for certain myelodysplastic syndromes which cause transfusion-dependent anaemia[23–25] and, with concurrent **dexamethasone**, as a second-line treatment in multiple myeloma.[26] However, **lenalidomide** is also presumed to carry serious teratogenic risk, is restricted in its availability, and is very expensive. Further, there is a dearth of experience with **lenalidomide** in symptom management and palliative care, and no obvious advantage over thalidomide.

The metabolism of thalidomide is by non-enzymatic hydrolysis in the plasma. Hepatic metabolism is minor.[27] Studies in patients with hepatic and renal impairment have not been performed.

Bio-availability 67–93% PO in animals, no data in humans.

Onset of action varies from 2 days for lepromatous leprosy and paraneoplastic sweating to 1–2 months for GVHD and 2–3 months for rheumatoid arthritis.

Time to peak plasma concentration 2–6h, delayed by food.

Plasma half-life 6h (200mg/24h)–18h (800mg/24h).[12]

Duration of action 24h.

Cautions

Treat as a 'cytotoxic' when handling. Thalidomide potentiates the sedative properties of barbiturates and alcohol, and increases the likelihood of extrapyramidal effects with **chlorpromazine** and **reserpine**.[11] Thalidomide should be used cautiously with other drugs which cause drowsiness, neuropathy or reduce the effectiveness of oral contraception (e.g. HIV protease inhibitors, **rifampicin**, **rifabutin**, **phenytoin**, **carbamazepine**).[11,28]

Undesirable effects

Low grade peripheral neuropathy occurs in $>$80% of patients receiving thalidomide, and severe neuropathy in 3–5%, generally after treatment lasting $>$6 months.[29,30] The incidence is higher in elderly patients, women, and in patients with pre-existing neuropathy or who are treated with neurotoxic chemotherapy, e.g. **vincristine, cisplatin, paclitaxel.**[30] Generally, the peripheral neuropathy presents as distal paraesthesia or dysaesthesia with or without sensory loss. Physical examination may be normal or show mildly decreased sensation in the distal limbs. Strength is usually preserved, but reflexes, particularly ankle jerks, may be depressed or absent. These symptoms, which are progressive, typically begin in the distal lower limbs and extend proximally and into the upper limbs.[31]

Although some studies have found a relationship between the cumulative dose and the occurrence of neuropathy,[32] others have not.[33] Nerve conduction studies typically show results consistent with a sensory axonal neuropathy. If a patient develops neuropathy, dose reduction or cessation may be required to decrease the likelihood of chronic painful neuropathy (see Dose and use).[34,35]

Some 80% of patients experience a mild decrease in bowel motility; this may reflect autonomic dysfunction, and can exacerbate constipation.[36] Somnolence or sedation may also occur and is the reason for taking the daily thalidomide dose at bedtime.[37]

Thalidomide and **lenalidomide** increase the risk of VTE in patients with multiple myeloma, particularly when used in combination with high-dose corticosteroids and/or chemotherapy, and thromboprophylaxis is recommended.[37,38] Both thalidomide and **lenalidomide** increase the risk of arterial thrombosis, e.g. myocardial infarction, stroke.[39] The MHRA recommends thromboprophylaxis for patients at increased thrombotic risk for the first five months of treatment.[39]

Thalidomide is associated with arrhythmia, hypotension, and oedema. Sinus bradycardia, generally mild, has been reported in ≤25% of patients.[40] Severe sinus bradycardia occurs in only 1–3% of patients.[16] Mild peripheral oedema has been reported in 15%.[8] Orthostatic hypotension and dizziness also have been reported with thalidomide.[41] A dose-dependent decrease in supine systolic and diastolic pressures is seen up to 2h after dosing.[42] However, symptom control doses should not affect blood pressure.

A pruritic and maculopapular rash may occur 10–14 days after starting treatment, starting on the trunk and extending to the back and proximal limbs. This is generally mild and resolves with the use of an emollient and dose reduction.[43] Severe skin reactions, such as Stevens-Johnson syndrome and toxic epidermal necrolysis, may also occur.[44] Skin complications seem more likely when thalidomide is combined with corticosteroids.

Tumour flare (a temporary increase in size of a cancerous lesion) may occur. When thalidomide is used to treat chronic lymphocytic leukaemia, some patients have experienced increased lymphadenopathy, enlargement of the spleen, and an increased lymphocyte count.[45]

Other undesirable effects include seizures,[41] altered temperature sensitivity, irregular menstrual cycles, and hypothyroidism. Thalidomide can increase HIV viral load.[46] Myelosuppression is rare.

Dose and use

Thalidomide is prohibitively expensive and cost alone will severely limit its use. In palliative care, thalidomide should *never* be considered as a first-line treatment. Its use should be considered only when more conventional treatments have failed and a full review of the potential benefits and harms has been undertaken with specialist colleagues.

There are several potential uses for thalidomide in palliative care (Table 7.14).[47] Female patients prescribed thalidomide must be counselled about the need for contraception, and male patients must use a condom. Written consent should be obtained.[48] Contraception should be used for ≥4 weeks before starting, during, and for 4 weeks after stopping treatment. Regular pregnancy testing is advised throughout treatment. Because thalidomide is present in the semen of men treated with the drug, even after vasectomy a latex condom must be used during sexual intercourse with women of childbearing potential.[49]

Table 7.14 Potential uses of thalidomide in palliative care[a]

Indication	*Dose*
Aphthous ulcers in HIV+ disease	100–200mg at bedtime for 10 days[50]
Paraneoplastic sweating	100–200mg at bedtime[51,52]
Paraneoplastic and uraemic pruritus	100–200mg at bedtime[15,53,54]
Cachexia in HIV+ disease and cancer	100–200mg at bedtime[55–57]
GI bleeding associated with angiodysplasia/ radiation proctitis	100–300mg at bedtime[21]
Intractable irinotecan-induced diarrhoea	400mg at bedtime[13,58]

a. Thalidomide is *not* the first-line treatment for any of these indications.

For dose modifications if peripheral neuropathy occurs (i.e. paraesthesia, weakness and/or loss of reflexes), see Table 7.15.[3]

Table 7.15 Dose changes in thalidomide-related neuropathy[a]

Grade	*Impact of neuropathy*	*Dose modification*[b]
1	No loss of function	Consider reducing dose if symptoms worsen
2	Interfering with function but not with activities of daily living	Reduce dose or interrupt treatment. If no improvement or further deterioration, stop treatment. If improves to grade 1 or better, restart treatment (if the benefit/risk ratio remains favourable)
3	Interfering with activities of daily living	Stop treatment
4	Disabling	Stop treatment

a. based on first-line use in multiple myeloma
b. monitor the patient regularly during treatment, e.g. monthly in women of child-bearing potential, otherwise every 3 months.

Supply

In the UK, thalidomide is available through a strictly monitored Thalidomide Celgene pregnancy prevention programme (www.celgene.co.uk/hcp_thalidomide_hcpip.aspx). Both prescribers and pharmacies must be registered with the programme to prescribe, order and supply thalidomide.

Lenalidomide is similarly monitored through the Revlimid pregnancy prevention programme (www.celgene.co.uk/hcp_revlimid.aspx).

Thalidomide Celgene® (Celgene)
Capsules 50mg, 28 days @ 200mg at bedtime = £1,194.

Lenalidomide
Revlimid® (Celgene)
Capsules 5mg, 10mg, 15mg, 25mg, 28 days @ 10mg once daily = £5,040.

1 Calabrese L and Fleischer A (2000) Thalidomide: current and potential clinical applications. *American Journal of Medicine*. **108**: 487–495.
2 Chen M *et al.* (2010) Innovative uses of thalidomide. *Dermatologic Clinics*. **28**: 577–586.
3 SPC (2010) Thalidomide Celgene accessed 12/2010. Available from: www.medicines.org.uk
4 Jacobson J (2000) Thalidomide: a remarkable comeback. *Expert Opinion in Pharmacotherapy*. **1**: 849–863.
5 De Sanctis JB *et al.* (2010) Pharmacological properties of thalidomide and its analogues. *Recent Patents on Inflammation and Allergy Drug Discovery*. **4**: 144–148.
6 Marriott J *et al.* (1999) Thalidomide as an emerging immunotherapeutic agent. *Trends in Immunology Today*. **20**: 538–540.
7 Peuckmann V *et al.* (2000) Potential novel uses of thalidomide: focus on palliative care. *Drugs*. **60**: 273–292.

8 Sampaio E *et al.* (1991) Thalidomide selectively inhibits tumour necrosis factor alpha production by stimulated human monocytes. *Journal of Experimental Medicine*. **173**: 699–703.
9 Corral LG and Kaplan G (1999) Immunomodulation by thalidomide and thalidomide analogues. *Annals of the Rheumatic Diseases*. **58 (suppl 1)**: 1107–113.
10 Hideshima T *et al.* (2000) Thalidomide and its analogs overcome drug resistance of human multiple myeloma cells to conventional therapy. *Blood*. **96**: 2943–2950.
11 Radomsky C and Levine N (2001) Thalidomide. *Dermatologic Clinics*. **19**: 87–103.
12 Bousvaros A and Mueller B (2001) Thalidomide in gastrointestinal disorders. *Drugs*. **61**: 777–787.
13 Govindarajan R *et al.* (2000) Effect of thalidomide on gastrointestinal toxic effects of irinotecan. *Lancet*. **356**: 566–567.
14 Deaner P (2000) The use of thalidomide in the management of severe sweating in patients with advanced malignancy: trial report. *Palliative Medicine*. **14**: 429–431.
15 Smith J *et al.* (2002) Use of thalidomide in the treatment of intractable itch. In: International Journal of Palliative Nursing (ed) *Palliative Care Congress*; Sheffield. Mark Allen.
16 Eisen T (2000) Thalidomide in solid tumors: the London experience. *Oncology (Williston Park)*. **14 (12) (suppl 13)**: 17–20.
17 Eleutherakis-Papaiakovou V *et al.* (2004) Thalidomide in cancer medicine. *Annals of Oncology*. **15**: 1151–1160.
18 Bauditz J *et al.* (2004) Thalidomide for treatment of severe intestinal bleeding. *Gut*. **53**: 609–612.
19 Craanen ME *et al.* (2006) Thalidomide in refractory haemorrhagic radiation induced proctitis. *Gut*. **55**: 1371–1372.
20 Karajeh MA *et al.* (2006) Refractory bleeding from portal hypertensive gastropathy: a further novel role for thalidomide therapy? *European Journal of Gastroenterology and Hepatology*. **18**: 545–548.
21 Lambert K and Ward J (2009) The use of thalidomide in the management of bleeding from a gastric cancer. *Palliative Medicine*. **23**: 473–475.
22 Li S *et al.* (2010) Recent advances of IMiDs in cancer therapy. *Current Opinion in Oncology*. **22**: 579–585.
23 List A *et al.* (2005) Efficacy of lenalidomide in myelodysplastic syndromes. *New England Journal of Medicine*. **352**: 549–557.
24 Giagounidis AA *et al.* (2006) Biological and prognostic significance of chromosome 5q deletions in myeloid malignancies. *Clinical Cancer Research*. **12**: 5–10.
25 Naing A *et al.* (2006) Developmental therapeutics for myelodysplastic syndromes. *Journal of the National Comprehensive Cancer Network*. **4**: 78–82.
26 Richardson P *et al.* (2010) Lenalidomide in multiple myeloma: an evidence-based review of its role in therapy. *Core Evidence*. **4**: 215–245.
27 Prescribing Information (2008) Thalomid(R) thalidomide, 2001a. Ref Type: Generic.
28 Thomas D and Kantarjian H (2000) Current role of thalidomide in cancer treatment. *Current Opinion in Oncology*. **12**: 564–573.
29 Dimopoulos MA and Eleutherakis-Papaiakovou V (2004) Adverse effects of thalidomide administration in patients with neoplastic diseases. *American Journal of Medicine*. **117**: 508–515.
30 Mileshkin L *et al.* (2006) Development of neuropathy in patients with myeloma treated with thalidomide: patterns of occurrence and the role of electrophysiologic monitoring. *Journal of Clinical Oncology*. **24**: 4507–4514.
31 Wulff CH *et al.* (1985) Development of polyneuropathy during thalidomide therapy. *British Journal of Dermatology*. **112**: 475–480.
32 Fullerton P and O'Sullivan D (1968) Thalidomide neuropathy: a clinical, electrophysiological, and histological follow up study. *Journal of Neurology, Neurosurgery and Psychiatry*. **31**: 543–551.
33 Chapon F *et al.* (1985) [Neuropathies caused by thalidomide]. *Rev Neurol (Paris)*. **141**: 719–728.
34 Gardner-Medwin J *et al.* (1994) Clinical experience with thalidomide in the management of severe oral and genital ulceration in conditions such as Behcet's disease. *Annals of Rheumatic Diseases*. **128**: 443–450.
35 Ochonisky S *et al.* (1994) Thalidomide neuropathy incidence and clinico-electrophysiologic findings in 42 patients. *Archives of Dermatology*. **130**: 66–69.
36 Grover JK *et al.* (2002) The adverse effects of thalidomide in relapsed and refractory patients of multiple myeloma. *Annals of Oncology*. **13**: 1636–1640.
37 Palumbo A *et al.* (2008) Prevention of thalidomide- and lenalidomide-associated thrombosis in myeloma. *Leukemia*. **22**: 414–423.
38 Uaprasert N *et al.* (2010) Venous thromboembolism in multiple myeloma: current perspectives in pathogenesis. *European Journal of Cancer*. **46**: 1790–1799.
39 MHRA (2011) Drug safety update. **4**, issues 7 and 12. Available from: www.mhra.gov.uk/Safetyinformation/DrugSafetyUpdate
40 Kaur A *et al.* (2003) Thalidomide-induced sinus bradycardia. *Annals of Pharmacotherapy*. **37**: 1040–1043.
41 Clark T *et al.* (2001) Thalidomid (Thalidomide) capsules: A review of the first 18 months of spontaneous postmarketing adverse event surveillance, including off-label prescribing. *Drug Safety*. **24**: 87–117.
42 Noormohamed F *et al.* (1999) Pharmacokinetics and hemodynamic effects of single oral doses of thalidomide in asymptomatic human immunodeficiency virus-infected subjects. *AIDS Research and Human Retroviruses*. **15**: 1047–1052.
43 Ng SS *et al.* (2002) Thalidomide, an antiangiogenic agent with clinical activity in cancer. *Biomed Pharmaco*. **56**: 194–199.
44 Rajkumar SV *et al.* (2000) Life-threatening toxic epidermal necrolysis with thalidomide therapy for myeloma. *New England Journal of Medicine*. **343**: 972–973.
45 Chanan-Khan A *et al.* (2005) Results of a phase I clinical trial of thalidomide in combination with fludarabine as initial therapy for patients with treatment-requiring chronic lymphocytic leukemia (CLL). *Blood*. **106**: 3348–3352.
46 Marriott J *et al.* (1997) A double-blind placebo-controlled phase II trial of thalidomide in asymptomatic HIV-positive patients: clinical tolerance and effect on activation markers and cytokines. *AIDS Research and Human Retroviruses*. **13**: 1625–1631.
47 Davis M and Dickerson E (2001) Thalidomide: dual benefits in palliative medicine and oncology. *American Journal of Hospice and Palliative Care*. **18**: 347–351.
48 Powell R and Gardner-Medwin J (1994) Guideline for the clinical use and dispensing of thalidomide. *Postgraduate Medical Journal*. **70**: 901–904.
49 Teo SK *et al.* (2001) Thalidomide is distributed into human semen after oral dosing. *Drug Metabolism and Disposition*. **29**: 1355–1357.
50 Jacobson J *et al.* (1997) Thalidomide for the treatment of oral aphthous ulcers in patients with human immunodeficiency virus infection. *New England Journal of Medicine*. **336**: 1487–1493.
51 Deaner P (1998) Thalidomide for distressing night sweats in advanced malignant disease. *Palliative Medicine*. **12**: 208–209.
52 Calder K and Bruera E (2000) Thalidomide for night sweats in patients with advanced cancer. *Palliative Medicine*. **14**: 77–78.
53 Goncalves F (2010) Thalidomide for the control of severe paraneoplastic pruritus associated with Hodgkin's disease. *American Journal of Hospice and Palliative Care*. **27**: 486–487

54 Silva S *et al.* (1994) Thalidomide for the treatment of uremic pruritus: a crossover randomized double-blind trial. *Nephron.* **67**: 270–273.

55 Boasberg P *et al.* (2000) Thalidomide induced cessation of weight loss and improved sleep in advanced cancer patients with cachexia. *ASCO Online*. **Abstract 2396**.

56 Mantovani G *et al.* (2001) Managing cancer-related anorexia/cachexia. *Drugs.* **61**: 499–514.

57 Gordon JN *et al.* (2005) Thalidomide in the treatment of cancer cachexia: a randomised placebo controlled trial. *Gut.* **54**: 540–545.

58 Govindarajan R (2000) Irinotecan and thalidomide in metastatic colorectal cancer. *Oncology (Williston Park)*. **14 (12) (suppl 13)**: 29–32.

8: URINARY TRACT DISORDERS

TAMSULOSIN — BNF 7.4.1

Class: Uroselective α_1-adrenergic receptor antagonist (α_1 antagonist).[1]

Indications: Symptoms associated with benign prostatic hypertrophy (e.g. hesitancy of micturition, straining and poor urinary stream), †radiation-induced urethritis, †medical management of urinary stones,[2] †management of acute urinary retention before removing urinary catheter.[3]

Contra-indications: Symptomatic postural hypotension.

Pharmacology

Tamsulosin is a selective and competitive antagonist at post-synaptic α_1-adrenergic receptors, particularly subtype α_{1A}, in the prostate. It relaxes the smooth muscle of the prostate gland and bladder neck.[4–7] Smooth muscle hyperplasia is estimated to be responsible for nearly half of the obstructive component in benign prostatic hyperplasia. Consequently, tamsulosin reduces functional prostatic obstruction and increases maximum urinary flow rate. Thus, it should be prescribed for men with troublesome moderate–severe lower urinary tract symptoms (LUTS) and a moderately enlarged prostate gland (<30g). RCT data indicate that tamsulosin improves LUTS by 20–50%, compared to 20–30% for placebo.[8]

For men with troublesome moderate–severe LUTS and a greater degree of prostatic enlargement (>30g) at risk of progressive obstruction, a combination of tamsulosin and a 5α-reductase inhibitor, e.g. **dutasteride** or **finasteride**, should be considered. Whereas tamsulosin generally improves symptoms within several days with a full response by 6 weeks, 5α-reductase inhibitors improve symptoms only after 3–6 months.[3,9]

Tamsulosin may also antagonize α_{1A}- and α_{1D}-adrenergic receptors in the bladder, inhibiting detrusor contractions and improving detrusor instability and urinary storage symptoms such as frequency, urgency and incontinence. Inhibition of α-adrenergic receptors in the sympathetic nervous system and spinal cord may also contribute to its effects.[7] Tamsulosin is metabolized in the liver, primarily by CYP2D6 and CYP3A4; <10% is excreted unchanged in the urine.

Tamsulosin 400–800microgram/24h reduces external beam radiotherapy-induced LUTS in patients with prostate cancer. When started at least 5 days before prostate radiation brachytherapy, tamsulosin also reduces short-term LUTS.[10]

Other less specific α_1 antagonists are available, e.g. **prazosin**. Symptomatic and urodynamic efficacy is similar but, unlike **prazosin**, tamsulosin generally does *not* cause postural hypotension either when given alone or with commonly used antihypertensive drugs, e.g. **atenolol**, **enalapril** and **nifedipine**.[11–13] **Prazosin** also needs to be taken b.d. rather than once daily; lower cost is its only advantage.

An alternative approach to the management of urinary hesitancy, when urinary obstruction has been excluded, is to use either a muscarinic drug, e.g. **bethanechol** 10–25mg t.d.s., or an anticholinesterase, e.g. **distigmine bromide** 5mg each morning (30min before breakfast). Because of their different mechanism of action, they can be used concurrently with tamsulosin and they improve symptoms more rapidly than 5α-reductase inhibitors.

Bio-availability m/r ~100% PO fasting, reduced by 30% p.c.;[7] Flomaxtra® XL 55–59%, not affected by food.

Onset of action m/r 4–8h; maximum benefit 4–8 weeks.
Time to peak plasma concentration 1h; m/r 4h fasting, 6h p.c.;[7] Flomaxtra® XL 4–6h, not affected by food.
Plasma halflife 5–7h; m/r 9–13h (healthy volunteers), 14–15h (elderly);[7] Flomaxtra® XL 19h (single dose), 15h (steady-state).
Duration of action <24h.

Cautions

Severe hepatic or renal impairment. Concurrent use with epidural **morphine**, **sildenafil** or other α_1 antagonists increases the risk of postural hypotension. Tamsulosin may increase the anticoagulant effect of **warfarin**. *In vitro* studies suggest that **diclofenac** and **warfarin** may increase the elimination of tamsulosin. **Cimetidine** decreases the elimination of tamsulosin.[7]

Undesirable effects

For more information, see National Clinical Guidelines Centre information.[3]
Very common (>10%): dizziness, orthostatic hypotension.
Common (<10%, >1%): headache, asthenia, drowsiness or insomnia, amblyopia, chest pain, rhinitis, sinusitis, pharyngitis, cough, bitter taste, nausea, abdominal discomfort, diarrhoea, back pain, reduced libido, ejaculatory impairment, impotence or erectile dysfunction.
Uncommon (<1%, >0.1%): syncope, palpitations, vomiting, constipation, rash, pruritus, gynaecomastia.
Very rare (<0.01%, >0.001%): priapism.

Dose and use

Hesitancy of micturition

- tamsulosin 400microgram m/r once daily (take at the same time each day, preferably 30min p.c.)
- if necessary, increase to 800microgram m/r once daily after 2–4 weeks[7]
- to avoid damaging the m/r properties, do not open, crush or chew the capsules.

Supply

Tamsulosin (generic)
Capsules m/r 400microgram, 28 days @ 400microgram once daily = £4.50.

Flomaxtra® XL (Astellas)
Capsules m/r 400microgram, 28 days @ 400microgram once daily = £10.

1 Hieble JP *et al.* (1995) International Union of Pharmacology. X. Recommendation for nomenclature of alpha 1-adrenoceptors: consensus update. *Pharmacological Reviews.* **47**: 267–270.
2 Nargund VH and Grey AD (2008) Tamsulosin MR and OCAS (modified release and oral controlled absorption system): current therapeutic uses. *Expert Opinion in Pharmacotherapy.* **9**: 813–824.
3 National Clinical Guidelines Centre (2009) *The management of lower urinary tract systems in men.* National Clinical Guidelines Centre for Acute Care at The Royal College of Physicians, London.
4 Hieble J and Ruffolo R (1996) The use of alpha-adrenoceptor antagonists in the pharmacological management of benign prostatic hypertrophy: an overview. *Pharmacological Research.* **33**: 145–160.
5 Kenny B *et al.* (1996) Evaluation of the pharmacological selectivity profile of alpha 1 adrenoceptor antagonists at prostatic alpha 1 adrenoceptors: binding, functional and in vivo studies. *British Journal of Pharmacology.* **118**: 871–878.
6 Pupo A *et al.* (1999) Effects of indoramin in rat vas deferens and aorta: concomitant alpha 1-adrenoceptor and neuronal uptake blockade. *British Journal of Pharmacology.* **127**: 1832–1836.
7 Lyseng-Williamson KA *et al.* (2002) Tamsulosin: an update of its role in the management of lower urinary tract symptoms. *Drugs.* **62**: 135–167.
8 Wilt TJ *et al.* (2003) Tamsulosin for benign prostatic hyperplasia. *Cochrane Database of Systematic Reviews.* **1**: CD002081.
9 NHS (2009) NHS clinical knowledge summaries. Prostate-benign hyperplasia-management. Available from: www.cks.nhs.uk/prostate_benign_hyperplasia/management
10 Crawford ED and Kavanagh BD (2006) The role of alpha-blockers in the management of lower urinary tract symptoms in prostate cancer patients treated with radiotherapy. *American Journal of Clinical Oncology.* **29**: 517–523.
11 Lowe FC (1997) Coadministration of tamsulosin and three antihypertensive agents in patients with benign prostatic hyperplasia: pharmacodynamic effect. *Clinical Therapeutics.* **19**: 730–742.
12 Michel MC *et al.* (1998) Tamsulosin: real life clinical experience in 19,365 patients. *European Urology.* **34 (suppl 2)**: 37–45.
13 Clifford G and Farmer R (2000) Medical therapy for benign prostatic hyperplasia: a review of the literature. *European Urology.* **38**: 2–19.

OXYBUTYNIN BNF 7.4.2

Class: Antimuscarinic (anticholinergic).

Indications: Symptoms of an overactive bladder, including urge incontinence, urinary frequency, urgency, caused by either idiopathic detrusor instability or a neurogenic bladder (detrusor hyperreflexia); nocturnal enuresis associated with an overactive bladder.

Contra-indications: Bladder outflow obstruction, GI obstruction including paralytic ileus, predisposition to narrow-angle glaucoma, myasthenia gravis.

Pharmacology

Bladder muscle (detrusor) contains all subtypes of muscarinic receptor. M_2 and M_3 predominate, with M_2 outnumbering M_3 by 3:1. M_3 receptors are particularly important in relation to detrusor contraction; the function of M_2 receptors is less clear.

Oxybutynin hydrochloride has an antimuscarinic effect on bladder innervation. It is relatively selective for M_1 and M_3 receptor subtypes (see p.4). It also has a direct papaverine-like antispasmodic effect on the detrusor.[1] It inhibits bladder contraction, relieves spasm induced by various stimuli, increases bladder capacity, and delays the desire to void in patients with a neurogenic bladder. Oxybutynin also has a topical anaesthetic effect on the bladder mucosa.[2] Oxybutynin has an active metabolite, N-desethyloxybutynin. It is not clear what proportion of its total effects are due to the metabolite. The plasma halflife of oxybutynin increases in the elderly, generally allowing smaller doses to be given.

Newer antimuscarinics, e.g. **darifenacin**, have higher M3 receptor selectivity than older ones, e.g. oxybutynin and **tolterodine**.[3,4] There is no consistent evidence that any one urinary antimuscarinic has greater efficacy than the others, but there is a trend in favour of m/r formulations and higher doses of some newer drugs, e.g. **fesoterodine** and **solifenacin**.[5] However, because of the low cost of generic oxybutynin, it is still first-line treatment for overactive bladder.[5]

Urinary antimuscarinics reduce frequency by 15–20% (vs. 10% with placebo); leakage episodes 45–75% (vs. 20–45%); urgency 40% (vs. 35%), and have subjective improvement rates of 40–70% (vs. 20–50%).[6,7]

Antimuscarinics differ in their ability to cross the blood-brain barrier, and thus in their propensity to cause CNS effects, e.g. cognitive impairment, delirium. Oxybutynin (a tertiary amine) enters the CNS relatively easily, whereas **trospium** (a quaternary ammonium compound) does not. Surprisingly, there is no hard clinical evidence that any one urinary antimuscarinic causes fewer CNS effects. This may be because most RCTs have not evaluated such effects.[3,7,8]

On the other hand, m/r and TD formulations of oxybutynin (and all the other urinary antimuscarinics) are better tolerated than normal-release oxybutynin;[7] and m/r **tolterodine** 4mg once daily definitely causes fewer undesirable effects than oxybutynin.[7] It is as effective as oxybutynin 5mg t.d.s. Thus, if oxybutynin is not tolerated, m/r **tolterodine** would be a good alternative. Alternatively, consider one of the newer more selective antimuscarinics, e.g. **fesoterodine** and **solifenacin**.[6,9] For further options, see Box 8.A.

Box 8.A Alternative drugs for urinary frequency and bladder spasms

Other drugs with antimuscarinic properties, e.g. amitriptyline or imipramine 25–50mg at bedtime.

Musculotropic drugs, flavoxate 200–400mg t.d.s.; less effective but fewer undesirable effects.

NSAIDs, e.g. naproxen 250–500mg b.d. may reduce nocturia.[12]

For isolated or persistent nocturia, consider a loop diuretic, e.g. furosemide 40mg once daily in the late afternoon (e.g. 1700–1800h). If unhelpful, vasopressin analogues, e.g. desmopressin, are of value; hyponatraemia is a possible complication.[12]

Short-term topical intravaginal oestrogens may improve incontinence and frequency in postmenopausal women with vaginal atrophy.[9]

Bio-availability 2–11% PO (normal-release); increased by 50% with m/r tablets (with a corresponding reduction in the amount of N-desethyloxybutynin).[10]
Onset of action 30–60min PO (normal-release).
Time to peak plasma concentration 30–60min PO (normal-release); 4–6h (m/r, after first dose);[10,11] 24–48h TD.
Plasma halflife 2–3h PO (normal-release); 4–5h in the elderly (normal-release); 12–14h (m/r).[10,11]
Duration of action 6–10h PO (normal-release); >24h (m/r); >4 days TD.

Cautions

See Antimuscarinics, p.4.

Undesirable effects

Undesirable effects are common with all antimuscarinic drugs, including dry mouth, cognitive impairment and delirium (particularly in the frail and elderly), nausea and abdominal discomfort (see p.5).[13] Skin reactions are common with TD oxybutynin.

Dose and use

Normal-release

- start with 5mg b.d., but 2.5mg b.d. in the over 60s and the very frail
- if necessary, increase to 5mg q.d.s.[9]

Modified-release

- start with 5mg once daily
- if necessary, increase in 5mg/day steps at weekly intervals
- maximum recommended dose 30mg once daily.

TD patches

- apply 1 patch (3.9mg/24h) twice weekly to clean, dry skin on abdomen, hip or buttock; avoid application to same site within 1 week.

Supply

Oxybutynin (generic)
Tablets 2.5mg, 3mg, 5mg, 28 days @ 5mg b.d. = £6.

Cystrin® (Sanofi-Aventis)
Tablets 3mg, 5mg, 28 days @ 5mg b.d. = £15.

Ditropan® (Sanofi-Aventis)
Tablets 2.5mg, 5mg, 28 days @ 5mg b.d. = £9.
Oral solution 2.5mg/5mL, 28 days @ 5mg b.d. = £26.

Modified-release
Lyrinel® XL (Janssen-Cilag)
Tablets m/r 5mg, 10mg, 28 days @ 10mg once daily = £21.

Transdermal
Kentera® (Recordati)
TD patches 36mg (releasing 3.9mg/24h), 28 days @ 1 patch twice weekly = £27.

Tolterodine
Detrusitol® (Pharmacia)
Tablets 1mg, 2mg, 28 days @ 2mg b.d. = £31.

Modified-release
Detrusitol® XL (Pharmacia)
Capsules m/r 4mg, 28 days @ 4mg once daily = £26.

1 Andersson K (1988) Current concepts in the treatment of disorders of micturition. *Drugs*. **35**: 477–494.
2 Robinson T and Castleden C (1994) Drugs in focus: 11. Oxybutynin hydrochloride. *Prescribers' Journal*. **34**: 27–30.
3 Abrams P *et al.* (2006) Muscarinic receptors: their distribution and function in body systems, and the implications for treating overactive bladder. *British Journal of Pharmacology*. **148**: 565–578.
4 Andersson KE (2002) Potential benefits of muscarinic M3 receptor selectivity. *European Urology Supplements*. **1**: 23–28.
5 NICE (2006) Urinary incontinence: the management of urinary incontinence in women. In: Clinical guidelines. National Institute for Health and Clinical Excellence. Available from: http://guidance.nice.org.uk/CG40
6 Novara G *et al.* (2008) A systematic review and meta-analysis of randomized controlled trials with antimuscarinic drugs for overactive bladder. *European Urology*. **54**: 740–763.
7 Chapple CR *et al.* (2008) The effects of antimuscarinic treatments in overactive bladder: an update of a systematic review and meta-analysis. *European Urology*. **54**: 543–562.
8 Wagg A (2008) Recent advances in the treatment of urinary incontinence in older women. *Current Opinion in Urology*. **18**: 383–388.
9 NHS (2009) NHS clinical knowledge summaries. Incontinence - urinary, in women. Available from: www.cks.nhs.uk/incontinence_urinary_in_women
10 Gupta SK and Sathyan G (1999) Pharmacokinetics of an oral once-a-day controlled-release oxybutynin formulation compared with immediate-release oxybutynin. *Journal of Clinical Pharmacology*. **39**: 289–296.
11 Janssen-Cilag (2009) SPC for Lyrinel XL. Available from: www.medicines.org.uk/EMC/medicine/12229/SPC/LyrinelXLprolongedreleasetablet/
12 NICE (2010) The management of lower urinary tract symptoms in men. Clinical guideline CG97. Available from: http://guidance.nice.org.uk/CG97
13 Donnellan C *et al.* (1997) Oxybutynin and cognitive dysfunction. *British Medical Journal*. **315**: 1363–1364.

METHENAMINE HIPPURATE — BNF 5.1.13

The use of methenamine hippurate as a specific *lower* urinary tract antibacterial is now relatively uncommon. However, methenamine may reduce the frequency of catheter blockage in people with a long-term indwelling urinary catheter.

Class: Urinary antiseptic (antibacterial).

Indications: Prophylaxis against blockage of indwelling urinary catheters.

Contra-indications: Methenamine hippurate should not be used in severe renal impairment (creatinine clearance <10mL/min; eGFR <10mL/min/1.73m^2), infection of the *upper* urinary tract (pyelonephritis), metabolic acidosis, hepatic impairment, severe dehydration, or gout.

Pharmacology

Unlike most antibacterials, methenamine does *not* act by impairing bacterial protein synthesis. In an acid environment (pH <5.5), methenamine hippurate dissociates into methenamine and hippuric acid. Methenamine is then converted to formaldehyde which is responsible for the bactericidal effect.[1,2] Urea-splitting bacteria, e.g. *Pseudomonas aeruginosa*, by producing ammonia increase the alkalinity of urine and tend to inhibit the formation of formaldehyde, thereby neutralizing the effect of methenamine. However, hippuric acid maintains an acidic environment, and thus facilitates the formation of formaldehyde. Nearly all bacteria are sensitive to formaldehyde at concentrations of ≥20microgram/mL. It is because of this distinct mode of action that methenamine can be classified separately as a urinary antiseptic.

In patients with a normal renal tract, methenamine hippurate has limited effectiveness in preventing symptomatic UTIs. Prophylactic oral antibacterials, and possibly **cranberry juice**, are more effective than methenamine hippurate.[3–5]

An intrinsic limitation of using urinary antiseptics to treat or prevent catheter encrustation is that some urine-colonizing bacteria produce secretions which eventually thicken enough to form a protective biofilm attached to the catheter surface. This can embed both the bacteria and phosphate crystals in a matrix which is impervious to urinary antiseptics or acidifying catheter patency solutions.[6]

In catheterized patients, formaldehyde remains in the bladder only for a short time. Thus, intermittent clamping may increase the effectiveness of methenamine hippurate. In patients with spinal cord compression above spinal cord level T7, catheter clamping should be avoided because of the risk of autonomic dysreflexia.[7]

A recent RCT in people after spinal cord injury (some with indwelling urethral or suprapubic catheters, others using intermittent self-catheterization, some reflex voiding) compared methenamine hippurate with **cranberry juice** and placebo, and found that the incidence of symptomatic UTIs was the same in all three groups.[8] Indeed, international guidelines state that the benefit from prophylactic antibiotics and urinary antiseptics for catheter-associated UTIs has never been established in an RCT.[5] However, in an RCT in people with an indwelling urinary catheter after a stroke, methenamine hippurate significantly decreased the need for antibacterial treatment for symptomatic UTIs[9] and in a second RCT reduced catheter blockage, doubling the interval between catheter changes from 1 to 2 weeks.[10]
Bio-availability readily absorbed.
Onset of action >2h.
Plasma halflife 4h.
Duration of action no data.

Cautions

With chronic use, the formaldehyde produced from methenamine may irritate and inflame the bladder mucosa, and lead to painful and frequent voiding, haematuria and proteinuria.

Methenamine hippurate should not be administered concurrently with sulphonamides because of the possibility of crystalluria. Methenamine hippurate should *not* be given concurrently with alkalinizing agents, e.g. **potassium citrate**, because of the need for an acid urinary environment.

Undesirable effects

May occasionally cause dyspepsia, nausea and vomiting, rash, pruritus.

Dose and use

The optimum dose for a urinary antiseptic in patients with an indwelling catheter is unknown. The following reflects practice at some centres:
- methenamine hippurate 1g b.d.–q8h[2,11]

The tablets may be crushed and taken with milk or fruit juice.

Nitrofurantoin 50–100mg once daily is used for the same purpose at other centres.[4,9]

Supply

Hiprex® (Meda)
Tablets 1g, 28 days @ 1g b.d. or 1g t.d.s. = £6 and £9 respectively.

1 Strom JJ and Jun H (1993) Effect of urine pH and ascorbic acid on the rate of conversion of methenamine to formaldehyde. *Biopharmaceutics and Drug Disposition*. **14**: 61–69.
2 Sweetman SC (ed) (2007) *Martindale: The complete drug reference* (35e). Pharmaceutical Press, London, pp. 266–267.
3 Lee BSB *et al.* (2007) Methenamine hippurate for preventing urinary tract infections. *Cochrane Database of Systematic Reviews*. **4**: CD003265. DOI: 003210.001002/14651858.CD14003265.pub14651852.
4 Brumfitt W *et al.* (1981) Prevention of recurrent urinary infections in women: a comparative trial between nitrofurantoin and methenamine hippurate. *Journal of Urology*. **126**: 71–74.
5 European Association of Urology (2009) Guidelines on urological infections. Available from: www.library.nhs.uk/GUIDELINESFINDER/ViewResource.aspx?resID=283008
6 Getliffe K (2002) Managing recurrent urinary catheter encrustation. *British Journal of Community Nursing*. **7**: 574, 576, 578–580.
7 Saint S and Lipsky BA (1999) Preventing catheter-related bacteriuria: should we? Can we? How? *Archives of Internal Medicine*. **159**: 800–808.
8 Lee BB *et al.* (2007) Spinal-injured neuropathic bladder antisepsis (SINBA) trial. *Spinal Cord*. **45**: 542–550.
9 Nyren P *et al.* (1981) Prophylactic methenamine hippurate or nitrofurantoin in patients with an indwelling urinary catheter. *Annals of Clinical Research*. **13**: 16–21.
10 Norberg A *et al.* (1980) Randomized double-blind study of prophylactic methenamine hippurate treatment of patients with indwelling catheters. *European Journal of Clinical Pharmacology*. **18**: 497–500.
11 Cronberg S *et al.* (1987) Prevention of recurrent acute cystitis by methenamine hippurate: double blind controlled crossover longterm study. *British Medical Journal*. **294**: 1507–1508.

CRANBERRY JUICE

Class: Herbal remedy.

Indications: †Prophylaxis against urinary tract infections (UTIs).

Pharmacology

Cranberry juice inhibits bacterial adherence to the urinary tract mucosa by disrupting the binding of bacterial macromolecules to receptors on mucosal epithelial cells.[1,2] This effect, which has been demonstrated *in vitro* in *Escherichia coli*, is produced by the pro-anthrocyanidins (tannins) and fructose present in cranberries.[3,4] Cranberry juice has also shown *in vitro* activity against *Staphylococcus aureus, Klebsiella pneumoniae, Pseudomonas aeruginosa* and *Proteus mirabilis*.[5] Blueberry juice also contains pro-anthrocyanidins, and may possess anti-adhesive activity, but clinical trials are lacking.[3] These natural juices could be a useful alternative to antibacterials for preventing UTIs, and could thus reduce the development of resistant organisms.[3]

The benefit of cranberry juice is limited to the prevention of UTIs; it does not cure established infection.[5,6] It reduces the frequency of symptomatic UTIs caused by *Escherichia coli*,[7] and the frequency of infections over 1 year in women with recurrent UTIs.[4] The addition of **ascorbic acid** (vitamin C) is not necessary. Evidence for effectiveness in the elderly (both men and women) is less clear, and there is no evidence of effectiveness in people with an indwelling urinary catheter.[3,4,8]

The optimum dose form is not clear, but most research has been done with fruit juice.[4] Juices with a fruit content of 25–33% have been used in most studies.[2,3] Volumes larger than 300mL/24h do not increase efficacy, and are associated with more undesirable effects.[5,7] Further, the relatively high drop-out rate in the clinical studies suggests that long-term consumption of cranberry juice is unacceptable to some patients.[4]

The NHS Clinical Knowledge Summary suggests that high-strength cranberry capsules (cranberry extract ≥200mg/capsule) may be more effective than the juice because they contain higher concentrations of the active substances; each 200mg of cranberry extract is equivalent to about 5g of fresh cranberries. Capsules may also be preferred by patients because they avoid the high fluid volume, bitter taste and high sugar content of the juice.[9] However, there is little research regarding the efficacy of cranberry capsules.[5]

Pharmacokinetic data not available.

Cautions

Like many other fruits and berries, cranberry juice contains significant amounts of salicylic acid (7mg/L). Theoretically, large amounts of cranberry juice could trigger an allergic reaction in people with **aspirin** allergy or asthma.[5]

In very large doses, e.g. 3–4L/24h of juice, cranberry can cause GI upset and diarrhoea. Consuming more than 1L/24h over a prolonged period may increase the risk of uric acid kidney stone formation (300mL of cranberry juice contains approximately 19mg of oxalate).[5]

Cranberry juice contains various anti-oxidants, including flavonoids, which are known to inhibit cytochrome P450 activity.[10] This was originally thought to explain several case reports, including one fatality,[11–14] in which the regular use of cranberry juice was linked to an increase in, or fluctuation of, INR values in patients taking **warfarin** (predominantly metabolized by CYP2C9, see p.735).[15] These cases led the CSM to recommend avoiding the concurrent use of cranberry products and **warfarin**, unless the benefit (prevention of UTI) outweighed the risks,[12] and this is still the official UK position.[16]

However, health authorities in other countries, e.g. Canada and the USA, do not consider the risk sufficiently high to issue a regulatory warning.[17,18] Patients on stable **warfarin** doses who drank cranberry juice 250mL once daily for 1 week showed no significant increase in anticoagulant activity.[19] Further, in volunteers, drinking cranberry juice 200mL t.d.s. did not significantly affect the pharmacokinetic profiles of **warfarin**, **tizanidine** or **midazolam**, which are probes for CYP2C9, CYP1A2 and CYP3A4 respectively.[20] On the other hand, the quantities of flavonoids in different commercial brands of cranberry juice may differ and it is unclear whether other mechanisms are also involved. Thus, an interaction with **warfarin** cannot be entirely ruled out, particularly if large volumes of cranberry juice are drunk regularly or when cranberry products other than juice are taken.[21–23] Accordingly, if a patient taking **warfarin** consumes large amounts of cranberry juice or takes other cranberry supplements, the INR should be monitored more closely.[23]

Dose and use

Drink as fruit juice, 150mL b.d. or 300mL once daily, or take as high-strength capsules containing cranberry extract 200–1,000mg once daily (200mg of extract is equivalent to about 5g of fresh cranberries). Benefit is seen only after 4 weeks or more.

Supply

Available OTC. ~~NHS~~

1 Liu Y (2006) Role of cranberry juice on molecular-scale surface characteristics and adhesion behaviour of Escherichia coli. *Biotechnology and Bioengineering*. **93**: 297–305.
2 Liu Y *et al.* (2008) Cranberry changes the physiochemical surface properties of E.coli and adhesion with uroepithelial cells. *Colloids and Surfaces B: Biointerfaces*. **65**: 35–42.
3 Jepson R (2007) A systematic review of the evidence for cranberries and blueberries in UTI prevention. *Molecular Nutrition and Food Research*. **51**: 738–745.
4 Jepson RG and Craig JC (2008) Cranberries for preventing urinary tract infections. In: *Cochrane Database of Systematic Reviews* 1: CD001321. Available from: www.mrw.interscience.wiley.com/cochrane/clsysrev/articles/CD001321/ frame.html.
5 Natural Medicines Comprehensive Database (2008) Cranberry. In: *Natural Medicines Comprehensive Database*. Available from: www.naturaldatabase.com
6 Tong H *et al.* (2006) Effect of ingesting cranberry juice on bacterial growth in urine. *American Journal of Health-System Pharmacy*. **63**: 1417–1419.
7 Avorn J *et al.* (1994) Reduction of bacteriuria and pyuria after ingestion of cranberry juice. *Journal of the American Medical Association*. **271**: 751–754.
8 McMurdo ME *et al.* (2005) Does ingestion of cranberry juice reduce symptomatic urinary tract infections in older people in hospital? A double-blind, placebo-controlled trial. *Age and Ageing*. **34**: 256–261.
9 NHS (2009) NHS clinical knowledge summaries. Urinary tract infection (lower)–women–management. Available from: www.cks.nhs.uk/urinary_tract_infection_lower_women/view_whole_topic#384750002
10 Hodek P *et al.* (2002) Flavonoids-potent and versatile biologically active compounds interacting with cytochromes P450. *Chemico-Biological Interactions*. **139**: 1–21.
11 Suvarna R *et al.* (2003) Possible interaction between warfarin and cranberry juice. *British Medical Journal*. **327**: 1454.
12 CSM (Committee on Safety of Medicines) (2004) Interaction between warfarin and cranberry juice: new advice. *Current Problems in Pharmacovigilance*. **30 (October)**: 10.
13 MHRA (2003) Possible interaction between warfarin and cranberry juice. *Current Problems in Pharmacovigilance*. **29 (Sept)**: 8.
14 Grant P (2004) Warfarin and cranberry juice: an interaction? *Journal of Heart Valve Disease*. **13**: 25–26.
15 Rettie AE *et al.* (1992) Hydroxylation of warfarin by human cDNA-expressed cytochrome P-450: a role for P-4502C9 in the etiology of (S)-warfarin-drug interactions. *Chemical Research in Toxicology*. **5**: 54–59.
16 MHRA (2009) Public assessment report. Warfarin: changes to product safety information December 2009. Available from: www.mhra.gov.uk/home/groups/pl-p/documents/websiteresources/con065506.pdf
17 Health Canada (2004) Suspected warfarin-cranberry juice interaction. *Canadian Adverse Reaction Newsletter*. **14 (July): 2.**
18 Health Canada (2007) Cranberry. Available from: www.hc-sc.gc.ca/dhp-mps/prodnatur/applications/licen-prod/monograph/mono_cranberry-canneberge-eng.php
19 Li Z *et al.* (2006) Cranberry does not affect prothrombin time in male subjects on warfarin. *Journal of the American Dietetic Society*. **106**: 2057–2061.
20 Lilja JJ *et al.* (2007) Effects of daily ingestion of cranberry juice on the pharmacokinetics of warfarin, tizanidine, and midazolam–probes of CYP2C9, CYP1A2, and CYP3A4. *Clinical Pharmacology and Therapeutics*. **81**: 833–839.
21 Aston JL *et al.* (2006) Interaction between warfarin and cranberry juice. *Pharmacotherapy*. **26**: 1314–1319.
22 Welch J and Forster K (2007) Probable elevation in international normalized ratio from cranberry juice. *Journal of Pharmacy Technology*. **23**: 104–107.
23 O'Mara N (2007) Does a cranberry juice-warfarin interaction really exist? Detail document. *Pharmacist's Letter/Prescriber's Letter*. **23**: 1–3.

CATHETER PATENCY SOLUTIONS — BNF 7.4.4

Indications: Catheter blockage.

General considerations

Catheters can block because of blood clots, bladder mucosal debris, small calculi and/or phosphate encrustations on the surface of an indwelling catheter. Encrustations are associated with colonization of the urine by urease-producing bacteria, e.g. *Proteus mirabilis*, *Pseudomonas aeruginosa* and *Klebsiella*. Urease breaks down urea to form ammonia, increasing the alkalinity of the urine and leading to the deposition of mainly phosphate crystals on the surface of the catheter.

Some bacteria produce secretions which eventually thicken enough to form a protective biofilm attached to the catheter surface. This can embed both bacteria and phosphate crystals in a matrix which is impervious to acidifying solutions or urinary antiseptics. Thus, repeated blockage with encrustation generally means that the catheter needs to be changed.[1,2]

The main purpose of a catheter patency solution is to reduce the frequency of catheter blockage. Although a Cochrane review found insufficient evidence to make firm recommendations,[3] the BNF states that **sodium chloride** 0.9% is generally adequate as a mechanical flush for removing mucosal debris or small blood clots, and that **solution G** (containing **citric acid** 3%) may be helpful in dissolving retained blood clots.[4]

Irrigation does *not* cure infection.[5,6] Although the BNF states that **chlorhexidine** 0.02% irrigation can be used in the management of common bladder infections, it is ineffective against most *Pseudomonas* species, and may irritate the bladder mucosa, and cause a burning sensation or haematuria.[4]

In a palliativedrugs.com survey, **sodium chloride** 0.9% was most commonly used for both flushing out cell debris or blood clots (75% of respondents) and treating or preventing encrustation (>50%). **Solution G** was next most popular for these indications (<10% and 20–25% respectively). Few respondents used other solutions.[7]

Use of irrigations to prevent catheter-related infections is *not* recommended by NICE.[8] Consideration should be given to the long-term use of a PO urinary antiseptic to acidify the urine and to reduce the frequency of infection (see **Methenamine hippurate**, p.529). Cranberry juice was also commonly prescribed by respondents in the palliativedrugs.com survey, although most did not use urine-acidifying or antiseptic agents.[7]

Dose and use

To reduce the likelihood of encrustations causing a blockage, latex catheters should be changed:
- uncoated every 2 weeks
- teflon-coated every 4 weeks
- silicone-coated every 6 weeks.[4,9]

If the catheter is to be left for longer periods, a silicone catheter should be used with a catheter patency solution.[4] These catheters are designed to remain in place for up to 3 months.[9]

However, some patients are more prone to recurrent encrustation than others. If encrustations regularly cause blockage, keep a diary over ⩾3 re-catheterizations, calculate the average time for which a catheter remains patent, then schedule a catheter change before a blockage is likely.[2]

For flushing out blockages caused by mucosal debris or small blood clots:
- start with **sodium chloride** 0.9% p.r.n.
- if necessary, use routinely every few days or even every day[7]
- if this is inadequate for dissolving retained clots, change to **solution G**.

For prevention of phosphate encrustations or calculi:[1,7]
- start with **sodium chloride** 0.9% p.r.n. or **solution G** once or twice a week
- if necessary, increase frequency.

Commercially available sachets are preferable to using a bladder syringe, because they are less likely to force encrusted material (which contains bacteria) higher up the urinary tract.

Supply

Sodium chloride 0.9%

OptiFlo S® (Bard)
Sachet 50mL, 100mL = £3.50 for both sizes.

Uriflex S® (Coloplast)
Sachet 100mL = £2.50.

Uro-Tainer sodium chloride® (B. Braun Medical)
Sachet 50mL, 100mL = £3.50 for both sizes.

Solution G containing **citric acid** 3.23% with magnesium oxide, sodium bicarbonate and disodium edetate.
OptiFlo G® (Bard)
Sachet 50mL, 100mL = £3.50 for both sizes.

Uriflex G® (Coloplast)
Sachet 100mL = £2.50.

Uro-Tainer Twin Suby G® (B. Braun Medical)
Dual-chamber sachet (each chamber contains 30mL) = £4.50.

Other irrigating solutions are available but are not featured here.

1 Williams C and Tonkin S (2003) Blocked urinary catheters: solutions are not the only solution. *British Journal of Community Nursing*. **8**: 321–326.
2 Getliffe K (2002) Managing recurrent urinary catheter encrustation. *British Journal of Community Nursing*. **7**: 574, 576, 578–580.
3 Hagen S (2010) Washout policies in long-term indwelling urinary catheterisation in adults. *Cochrane Database of Systematic Reviews*. **3**: CD004012.
4 BNF (2010) Section 7.4.4. In: *British National Formulary (No 60)*. British Medical Association and Royal Pharmaceutical Society of Great Britain, London. Current BNF available from: www.bnf.org.
5 Getliffe K (1996) Bladder instillations and bladder washouts in the management of catheterized patients. *Journal of Advanced Nursing*. **23**: 548–554.
6 Pomfret I *et al.* (2004) Using bladder instillations to manage indwelling catheters. *British journal of Nursing*. **13**: 261–267.
7 Palliativedrugs.com (2010) Survey: urinary catheter patency solutions — do you use them? Available from: www.palliativedrugs.com/latest/december/urinary-catheter-patency-solutions-do-you-use-them.html
8 NICE (2003) Infection control. Prevention of healthcare-associated infections in primary and community care. Clinical guideline CG2. Available from: http://guidance.nice.org.uk/CG2
9 Kelly A (2004) Nursing practice guidelines. Urinary catheterisation. *City Hospital, University Hospital and Rushcliffe PCT, Nottingham*.

DISCOLOURED URINE

Patients need to be warned about drugs and other substances which can discolour urine (Box 8.B). If the urine is red, it may be assumed to be blood, and cause alarm.

The colour-banding in Box 8.B is approximate, i.e. a drug listed under 'brown/orange/yellow' will most likely cause discolouration at some point in that range. Sometimes the colour is pH dependent. Further information on causes of discoloured urine is available from: www.wrongdiagnosis.com/symptoms/urine_color_changes/causes.htm.

Note: urine colour will vary according to the concentration or dilution of the urine. Colouring agents in processed food can also affect urine colour.

Box 8.B Selected causes of discoloured urine[a]

Black/dark brown
Iron (ferrous salts)
Methocarbamol

Brown/orange/yellow
Aloe
Carrots
Cascara
Chloroquine
Chlorzoxazone (not UK)
Dantrolene
Fluorescein
Heparin
Nitrofurantoin

continued

Box 8.B Continued

Paprika
Phenazopyridine (not UK)
Primaquine
Quinine
Retinol (vitamin A)
Riboflavin (vitamin B_2)
Rifampicin
Senna (pH dependent)
Sulfasalazine
Sulphonamides
Warfarin

Brown/red/pink
Beetroot (alkaline urine)
Blackberries (acid urine)
Dantron
Daunorubicin
Doxorubicin
Entacapone
Ibuprofen
Levodopa
Metronidazole (acid urine)
Napthalene-based dyes in foods and medicines, e.g. Ponceau 4R
Phenolphthalein (alkaline urine)
Phenothiazines
Phenytoin
Rhubarb (in several proprietary laxatives; pH dependent)
Senna (alkaline urine)

Purple
Degradation of tryptophan by urinary bacteria (see text)

Blue/green
Amitriptyline[1]
Chlorophyll breath mints
FD & C Dye No. 1 (used in foods and medicines)
Hydroquinone
Indometacin
Magnesium salicylate
Phenols
Promethazine (injection)
Propofol[2]
Pseudomonas aeruginosa (pyocyanin; alkaline urine)
Resorcinol
Thymol
Triamterene

Milky Colour
Diffuse glomerular nephritis
Lipids
Neutrophils
Phosphates
Radiographic dyes
Urates

a. discolouration which occurs only when urine is left 'on standing' has not been included.

Purple urine bag syndrome is caused by the breakdown of dietary tryptophan metabolites by bacteria in urine, ultimately producing indigo (blue) and indirubin (red) in alkaline urine.[3–5] Chronic urinary tract infection, long-term catheterization, constipation and immobility are the main risk factors. Although harmless, purple urine bag syndrome causes the urine to develop a strong, unpleasant odour, which becomes more noticeable over time and in warm conditions. This distresses patients more than the discolouration. Changing the drainage bag more frequently, e.g. every 3 days rather than every 5–7 days, helps to avoid the build-up of the odour. Indwelling long-term catheters may also need changing more often than normal.[5]

1 Beeley L (1986) What drugs turn urine green? *British Medical Journal.* **293**: 750.
2 Leclercq P *et al.* (2009) Green urine. *Lancet.* **373**: 1462.
3 Al-Jubouri MA and Vardhan MS (2001) A case of purple urine bag syndrome associated with Providencia rettgeri. *Journal of Clinical Pathology.* **54**: 412.
4 Ribeiro JP *et al.* (2004) Case report: purple urine bag syndrome. *Critical Care (London, England).* **8**: R137.
5 Robinson J (2003) Purple urinary bag syndrome: a harmless but alarming problem. *British Journal of Community Nursing.* **8**: 263–266.

9: NUTRITION AND BLOOD

ANAEMIA

Anaemia is common in cancer and other forms of chronic disease. The main causes are:

- anaemia of chronic disease
- iron deficiency
- folate deficiency
- malignant infiltration of the marrow
- haemolytic anaemia
- renal failure.

The commonest form in cancer is anaemia of chronic disease (ACD). This is a paraneoplastic phenomenon and relates partly to cytokine-mediated suppression of endogenous erythropoietin production and disturbance of iron homeostasis.[1] It is important to distinguish between the various types of anaemia because treatment differs. Diagnostic features of ACD are:

- normochromic-normocytic anaemia (vs. hypochromic-microcytic in iron deficiency)
- low/low–normal plasma transferrin concentration (effectively the same measurement as TIBC; vs. high/high–normal in iron deficiency)
- low transferrin saturation (vs. low–very low in iron deficiency)
- low plasma iron
- high/high–normal plasma ferritin concentration, although the ferritin rises during acute phase response, e.g. to trauma, infection and some cancers (vs. low in iron deficiency)
- low reticulocyte count (also low in iron deficiency)
- bone marrow appearance generally unremarkable; may show abnormal iron distribution
- increased marrow iron stores
- reduced iron within maturing erythroblasts.

There are two potential treatment options:

- intermittent blood transfusions[2]
- SC **erythropoietin**.[3]

About 75% of patients with ACD respond to **erythropoietin** treatment. In patients already transfusion-dependent, about half will become transfusion-independent.[4,5] However, because of increased tumour progression and reduced survival time in cancer patients treated with **erythropoietin**,[6,7] NICE now recommends that it (with IV **iron**) should be used only for:

- **platinum**-induced anaemia in women with ovarian cancer who are symptomatic with an Hb ≤8 g/dL
- patients with profound cancer-treatment related anaemia which is likely to have an impact on survival but who cannot be given blood transfusions.[8]

1 Weiss G and Goodnough LT (2005) Anemia of chronic disease. *New England Journal of Medicine*. **352**: 1011–1023.
2 MHRA (2008) Drug safety update. 2 (1, August): 3–4. Available from: www.mhra.gov.uk/Publications/Safetyguidance/index.htm
3 Ludwig H (2002) Anemia of hematologic malignancies: what are the treatment options? *Seminars in Oncology*. **29 (3 suppl 8)**: 45–54.
4 Seidenfeld J *et al.* (2001) Epoetin treatment of anemia associated with cancer therapy: a systematic review and meta-analysis of controlled clinical trials. *Journal of the National Cancer Institute*. **93**: 1204–1214.
5 Turner R *et al.* (2001) Epoetin alfa in cancer patients: evidence-based guidelines. *Journal of Pain and Symptom Management*. **22**: 954–965.
6 Steensma DP (2007) Erythropoiesis stimulating agents. *British Medical Journal*. **334**: 648–649.

7 Bohlius J (2009) Recombinant human erythropoiesis-stimulating agents and mortality in patients with cancer: a met-analysis of randomized trails. *Lancet.* **373**: 1532–1542.

8 NICE (2008) Epoetin alfa, epoetin beta and darbepoetin alfa for cancer treatment-induced anaemia. *Technology appraisal guidance TA142*. National Institute for Clinical Excellence. Available from: http:/guidance.nice.org.uk//TA142

FERROUS SULPHATE BNF 9.1.1.1

Class: Elemental salt.

Indications: Prevention and treatment of iron deficiency anaemia.

Contra-indications: Anaemia not caused by iron deficiency; haemosiderosis, haemochromatosis.

Pharmacology

Ferrous salts are better absorbed than ferric salts. Because there are only marginal differences in terms of efficiency of iron absorption, the choice of ferrous salt is based mainly on the incidence of undesirable effects and cost. Some undesirable effects relate directly to the amount of elemental iron, and improved tolerance after switching to another salt may be because the elemental iron content is less (Table 9.1). M/r formulations are designed to reduce undesirable effects by releasing iron gradually as the tablet or capsule passes down the GI tract. However, these products are likely to carry most of the iron past the first part of the duodenum into parts of the intestine where iron absorption is poor. Such products have no therapeutic advantage and should not be used.[1]

Dietary accessible (non-haem) iron absorption may be increased by a high intake of red meat, poultry, fish or **ascorbic acid** (e.g. from fruits) but reduced by a high intake of phytates (e.g. in whole-grain cereals), polyphenols (e.g. in tea and coffee), and **calcium** (e.g. in dairy products).[2]

Table 9.1 Elemental ferrous iron content of different iron salts

Iron salt	*Amount (mg)*	*Ferrous content (mg)*
Ferrous fumarate	200	65
Ferrous sulphate, dried (anhydrous)	200	65
Ferrous sulphate	300	60
Ferrous gluconate	300	35

Some oral formulations contain **ascorbic acid** or chelated iron. These modifications have been shown experimentally to produce a modest increase in the absorption of iron. However, the therapeutic advantage is minimal, and the cost may be increased.[1] Further, **ascorbic acid** may increase GI irritation. There is no clinical justification for the inclusion of other therapeutically active ingredients such as the B group of vitamins (except **folic acid** for pregnant women).

In the treatment of iron deficiency, Hb should rise by about 1g/dL/week. After the Hb has risen to normal, treatment should be continued for a further 3 months to replenish the iron stores. Epithelial tissue changes such as atrophic glossitis and koilonychia also improve but generally more slowly.

Drug interactions

Because of decreased absorption of iron, the other drug or both, ferrous sulphate should not be administered concurrently with antacids, bisphosphonates, **calcium** salts, **colestyramine**, **demeclocycline**, **levodopa**, **levothyroxine**, **penicillamine**, quinolone antibacterials, tetracyclines, and **zinc**.

Undesirable effects

Dyspepsia, nausea, epigastric pain, constipation and diarrhoea. Nausea and epigastric pain are dose-related but the relationship between dose and altered bowel habit is not so clear.[1]

Elderly patients are more likely to develop constipation, occasionally leading to faecal impaction; m/r products are more likely to cause diarrhoea.
Note: liquid formulations may stain teeth. Urine and stools are discoloured (black), and this may result in a false positive faecal occult blood test.

Dose and use

The diagnosis of iron deficiency should be confirmed before iron supplements are prescribed (see Anaemia, p.537). The PO dose of **elemental iron** for iron-deficiency anaemia is 100–200mg/24h. This can be provided, for example, as dried (anhydrous) ferrous sulphate 200mg b.d.–t.d.s (= elemental iron 130–195mg/24h).

Doses >600mg/24h of dried (anhydrous) ferrous sulphate exceed the maximal absorption capacity and increase undesirable effects. If undesirable GI effects occur:

- reduce the dose
- take with food (but may reduce absorption by up to 50%)
- switch to an alternative iron salt with a lower elemental iron content
- switch to a liquid formulation (may be less damaging to GI mucosa)[3]
- dilute liquid formulations and swallow through a straw to prevent discolouration of the teeth.

Consider prophylaxis in patients at high risk of iron deficiency, e.g. those with a poor diet, malabsorption, and after total or sub-total gastrectomy; for example, prescribe dried (anhydrous) ferrous sulphate 200mg once daily (elemental iron 65mg).

Supply

Ferrous sulphate, dried (generic)
Tablets 200mg (65mg iron), 28 days @ 200mg t.d.s. (195mg elemental iron/24h) = £3.50.

Ferrous *fumarate*
Fersaday® (Goldshield)
Tablets 322mg (100mg iron), 28 days @ 322mg b.d. (200mg elemental iron/24h) = £2.

Fersamal® (Goldshield)
Tablets 210mg (68mg iron), 28 days @ 210mg t.d.s. (204mg elemental iron/24h) = £1.50.
Oral suspension 140mg (45mg iron)/5mL, 28 days @ 280mg (10mL) b.d. (180mg elemental iron/24h) = £10.

Galfer® (Thornton & Ross)
Capsules 305mg (100mg iron), 28 days @ 305mg b.d. (200mg elemental iron/24h) = £1.50.
Oral syrup 140mg (45mg iron)/5mL, 28 days @ 280mg (10mL) b.d. (180mg elemental iron/24h) = £11.

Ferrous *gluconate* (generic)
Tablets 300mg (35mg iron), 28 days @ 600mg t.d.s. (210mg elemental iron/24h) = £18.
This is not a complete list; see BNF for more information.

1 BNF (2011) Oral Iron, Section 9.1.1.1 (No. 61). In: *British National Formulary*. British Medical Association and the Royal Pharmaceutical Society of Great Britain.
2 Heath AL and Fairweather-Tait SJ (2002) Clinical implications of changes in the modern diet: iron intake, absorption and status. *Best Practice and Research Clinical Haematology*. **15**: 225–241.
3 Ji H and Yardley JH (2004) Iron medication-associated gastric mucosal injury. *Archives of Pathology and Laboratory Medicine*. **128**: 821–822.

ASCORBIC ACID (VITAMIN C) BNF 9.6.3

Class: Vitamin.

Indications: Scurvy, †decubitus ulcers, †furred tongue (topical), †urinary infection.

Pharmacology

Ascorbic acid (vitamin C) is a powerful reducing agent. It is obtained from dietary sources of fresh fruit and vegetables, e.g. blackcurrants, kiwifruit, broccoli, red pepper and oranges. It cannot be synthesized by the body. It is involved in the hydroxylation of proline to hydroxyproline, which is necessary for the formation of collagen. The failure of this accounts for most of the clinical effects found in deficiency (scurvy), e.g. keratosis of hair follicles with 'corkscrew hair', perifollicular haemorrhages, swollen spongy infected and bleeding gums, loose teeth, spontaneous bruising and haemorrhage, anaemia and failure of wound healing. Repeated infections are also common. In healthy adults, a dietary intake of about 30–60mg/24h is necessary; in scurvy, a rapid clinical response is seen with ≥250mg/24h in divided doses.

Absorption occurs mainly from the proximal small intestine by a saturable process. In health, body stores of ascorbic acid are about 1.5g, although larger stores may occur with intakes higher than 200mg/24h. It is excreted mainly as oxalic acid and unchanged ascorbic acid. Ascorbic acid is used to acidify urine in patients with alkaline urine and recurrent urinary infections.

A beneficial effect of megadose ascorbic acid therapy has been claimed for many conditions,[1] including colds, asthma, atherosclerosis, cancer, psychiatric disorders, increased susceptibility to infections, infertility and osteogenesis imperfecta. Ascorbic acid has also been tried in the treatment of wound healing, pain in Paget's disease and opioid withdrawal. There is little evidence to substantiate these claims. A systematic review of vitamin C for the prevention and treatment of cancer found no evidence of benefit.[2] However, vitamin C deficiency is common in cancer patients, and low plasma concentrations are associated with shorter survival.[3]

Vitamin C alone or with β-carotene and vitamin E does not prevent the development of colorectal adenoma.[4] However, ascorbic acid does reduce the severity of a cold but not its incidence.[5] On the other hand, enthusiasm for high-dose ascorbic acid for HIV+ people waned after many died from disease progression.[6] Although it has been postulated that ascorbic acid might help prevent ischaemic heart disease, in contrast to other anti-oxidant vitamins, little benefit is seen in RCTs.[7,8] Of more concern are data which indicate that a total daily dose as small as 500mg has a pro-oxidant effect which could result in genetic mutation.[9]

Undesirable effects

GI symptoms may occur at doses of >1g/24h.[10] Doses of >3g/24h may result in acidosis, diarrhoea, glycosuria, oxaluria and renal stones. Tolerance may occur with prolonged use of large doses, resulting in symptoms of deficiency when intake is returned to normal. If allowed to dissolve in the mouth, the acidity of effervescent tablets can break down tooth enamel and may cause localized oesophagitis if patients lie down immediately after taking them.

Dose and use

Furred tongue

- place one quarter of a 1g effervescent tablet on the tongue and allow it to dissolve; repeat up to q.d.s. for ≤1 week
- do not use if the patient has a sore mouth.

Acidification of urine

- 100–200mg b.d.; test urine with litmus paper until constant acid result is obtained (note: may alter the excretion of some drugs).

Enhancement of healing

- 100mg b.d. for 4 weeks.

Vitamin C deficiency

- for florid scurvy, give 100mg t.d.s. for 4 weeks
- otherwise, give 100mg once daily; continue indefinitely in undernourished patients.

Supply
Ascorbic acid (generic)
Tablets 50mg, 100mg, 200mg, 500mg, 28 days @ 100mg t.d.s. = £4.
Tablets effervescent 1g, available OTC.
Injection 100mg/mL, 5mL amp = £4.50.

1 Ovesen L (1984) Vitamin therapy in the absence of obvious deficiency. What is the evidence? *Drugs*. **27**: 148–170.
2 Coulter ID *et al.* (2006) Antioxidants vitamin C and vitamin e for the prevention and treatment of cancer. *Journal of General Internal Medicine*. **21**: 735–744.
3 Mayland CR *et al.* (2005) Vitamin C deficiency in cancer patients. *Palliative Medicine*. **19**: 17–20.
4 Greenberg E *et al.* (1994) A clinical trial of antioxidant vitamins to prevent colorectal adenoma. Polyp Prevention Study Group. *New England Journal of Medicine*. **331**: 141–147.
5 Hemila H (1994) Does vitamin C alleviate the symptoms of the common cold? a review of current evidence. *Scandinavian Journal of Infectious Diseases*. **26**: 1–6.
6 Abrams D (1990) Alternative therapies in HIV infection. *AIDS*. **4**: 1179–1187.
7 Rimm E (1993) Vitamin E consumption and the risk of coronary heart disease in men. *New England Journal of Medicine*. **328**: 1450–1456.
8 Stampfer M (1993) Vitamin E consumption and the risk of coronary disease in women. *New England Journal of Medicine*. **328**: 1444–1449.
9 Podmore I *et al.* (1998) Vitamin C exhibits pro-oxidant properties. *Nature*. **392**: 559.
10 Beveridge C (2002) Basic Nutrition. In: C Repchinsky and C LeBlanc (eds) *Patient Self Care* (1e). Canadian Pharmacists Association, Ottawa, pp. 339–358.

PHYTOMENADIONE (VITAMIN K_1) — BNF 9.6.6

Class: Vitamin.

Indications: Vitamin K deficiency, reversal of anticoagulant effects of **warfarin**, †bleeding tendency in patients with hepatic impairment, †hypoprothrombinaemia induced by salicylates, sulfonamides, **quinidine**, **quinine** and antibacterials.

Pharmacology
Phytomenadione (vitamin K_1) is the active form of vitamin K, a fat-soluble vitamin. It is necessary for the synthesis of several coagulation factors (II, VII, IX, X), and of proteins involved in bone calcification. Oral coumarin anticoagulants (e.g. **warfarin**) act by interfering with vitamin K metabolism in the liver; their effect is antagonized by exogenous vitamin K. Phytomenadione is present in green vegetables and is synthesized by bacteria in the GI tract.

Hepatic stores of vitamin K are depleted in <3 days of dietary restriction. In patients with advanced cancer, $>20\%$ are vitamin K deficient.[1] Patients who are malnourished, have fat malabsorption (e.g. in biliary obstruction or liver disease), or are having prolonged courses of antibacterials which sterilize the GI tract are at risk of deficiency and a rapid rise in prothrombin time and activated partial thromboplastin time (APTT).

Menadiol sodium phosphate is a water-soluble synthetic vitamin K derivative which can be given PO to prevent vitamin K deficiency in patients with fat malabsorption, or to correct dietary deficiency.

Phytomenadione is *not* indicated routinely in hepatic failure, nor even in moribund patients with manifestations of a bleeding diathesis (e.g. petechiae, purpura, multiple bruising, nose and gum bleeds), and it should not be used merely to prevent an imminent inevitable death. Its use is limited to conscious patients with a reasonable performance status for whom other supportive measures are deemed appropriate (e.g. blood transfusion). Failure to respond to phytomenadione may indicate that a coagulation defect exists, e.g. clotting factor deficiency caused by impaired hepatic synthesis.
Plasma halflife 1.5–3h.

Cautions
Oral absorption of **menadiol sodium phosphate** is reduced by concurrent administration with **colestyramine** or **liquid paraffin (mineral oil)**.

Undesirable effects

Hypersensitivity/anaphylaxis after IV use.

Dose and use

Konakion® MM can be administered by slow IV injection over 3–5minutes or by IVI diluted in 50mL of 5% glucose over 20–30minutes; *it must not be given IM.*

Reversal of warfarin anticoagulation

Use the British Society for Haematology guidelines.[2,3]

Prevention of vitamin K deficiency in malabsorption

- give **menadiol phosphate** 10mg PO once daily
- check prothrombin time after 3 days and, if still raised, increase dose progressively up to 40mg once daily (rarely necessary)
- if serious bleeding:
  - ▹ phytomenadione injection (Konakion® MM) 10mg IV (see above)
  - ▹ if IV access difficult, consider Konakion® *MM Paediatric* 10mg IM
  - ▹ 4 units of fresh frozen plasma, or factor concentrates, or prothrombin complex concentrates may also be necessary.[4]

Correction of a bleeding tendency in hepatic failure

- give **menadiol phosphate** 10mg PO once daily
- check prothrombin time after 3 days and, if still raised, increase the dose progressively up to 40mg once daily (rarely necessary)
- if **menadiol phosphate** unavailable, consider giving phytomenadione injection (Konakion® MM) 2.5–10mg *by mouth*
- if serious bleeding, give phytomenadione injection (Konakion® MM) 10mg IV (see above) then proceed as for malabsorption above.

In patients with hepatic impairment, the risk of venous thrombosis is often paradoxically increased. Thus, in this situation, prothrombin complex concentrates should be used only in emergency situations after specialist advice.

Note: **desmopressin** may improve haemostasis in patients with hepatic platelet dysfunction (see p.496).

Supply

Menadiol phosphate (generic)

Tablets menadiol sodium phosphate equivalent to 10mg of menadiol phosphate, 7days @ 10mg once daily = £4.

Phytomenadione

Konakion® MM (*Roche*)

Injection (colloidal) phytomenadione 10mg/mL in a mixed micelles vehicle, 1mL amp = £0.50. For IV use only, do not use IM. Can be used PO off-label.

Konakion® MM Paediatric (*Roche*)

Injection (colloidal) phytomenadione 10mg/mL in a mixed micelles vehicle, 0.2mL (2mg) amp = £1. *Konakion® MM Paediatric may be administered PO, IM, IV.*

1 Harrington DJ *et al.* (2008) A study of the prevalence of vitamin K deficiency in patients with cancer referred to a hospital palliative care team and its association with abnormal haemostasis. *Journal of Clinical Pathology.* **61**: 537–540.

2 BNF (2011) Section 2.8.2. Oral anticoagulants. In: *British National Formulary.* British Medical Association and the Royal Pharmaceutical Society of Great Britain, London.

3 Baglin TP *et al.* (2006) Guidelines on oral anticoagulation (warfarin): third edition–2005 update. *British Journal of Haematology.* **132**: 277–285.

4 Blonski W *et al.* (2007) Coagulopathy in liver disease. *Current Treatment Options in Gastroenterology.* **10**: 464–473.

POTASSIUM BNF 9.2.1.1

Class: Elemental salt.

Indications: Hypokalaemia (<3.5mmol/L).

Pharmacology

In palliative care, hypokalaemia is most common in patients receiving non-potassium-sparing diuretics, particularly if also taking a corticosteroid. Hypokalaemia is also associated with chronic diarrhoea and persistent vomiting. Correction of hypokalaemia is important in patients taking **digoxin** or other anti-arrhythmic drugs because of the risk of an arrhythmia. Potassium supplements are seldom required with small doses of diuretics given to treat hypertension.

When larger doses of thiazide or loop diuretics are given to eliminate oedema, potassium-sparing diuretics (e.g. **amiloride**, **spironolactone**) rather than potassium supplements are preferable. Dietary supplements also help to maintain plasma potassium; 10mmol of potassium is contained in a large banana and in 250mL of orange juice.

When treating hypokalaemia, potassium chloride is generally the salt of choice because of associated hypochloraemia. However, occasionally, hypokalaemia is associated with a hyperchloraemic metabolic acidosis, and an alkalinizing salt will be preferable, e.g. potassium *bicarbonate* or potassium *citrate* (not UK). Co-existing hypomagnesaemia should always be corrected (see p.545).

Drugs are a common cause of hyperkalaemia in hospitalized patients (see Cautions), particularly in association with pre-existing or new renal impairment. When *mild–moderate* (i.e. 5.5–6.9mmol/L, with no ECG changes or symptoms), dose reduction or stopping the causal drug may be all that needs to be done. However, other causes may need to be considered, e.g. hypo-aldosteronism, tumour lysis syndrome, **digoxin** toxicity. Spurious results can also occur, e.g. as a result of haemolysis, marked leukocytosis or thrombocytosis. Repeating the sample and/or obtaining advice from the clinical chemistry laboratory may be necessary. For the treatment of *severe* hyperkalaemia, see below.

Cautions

Hyperkalaemia may result if used concurrently with drugs which increase the plasma potassium concentration, e.g. ACE inhibitors, potassium-sparing diuretics, **ciclosporin**. Use smaller doses of potassium if there is renal impairment (common in the elderly).

Undesirable effects

Oesophageal or GI ulceration, nausea and vomiting. Liquid or effervescent formulations are distasteful.

Dose and use

The normal adult daily requirement and the typical dietary intake of potassium is 40–80mmol. Whenever possible, orange juice and bananas should be used as a palatable source of potassium (see Pharmacology above). To minimize nausea and vomiting, potassium supplements are best taken during or after a meal.

Slow-K® tablets must be swallowed whole to preserve the m/r mechanism. Because this is difficult for some patients, liquid or effervescent products are generally preferable.

Prevention of hypokalaemia

- potassium *chloride*, e.g. Sando-K® 1–2 tablets b.d. (24–48mmol/24h K^+) *or*
- prescribe a potassium-sparing diuretic, e.g. **amiloride** 5–10mg once daily (maximum 20mg once daily) or **spironolactone** 25–200mg/24h.

Treatment of hypokalaemia

- potassium *chloride*, e.g. Sando-K® 2 tablets t.d.s. (72mmol/24h K^+)
- if the patient is hyperchloraemic, prescribe potassium *bicarbonate* effervescent tablets BPC 1968 instead
- if hypokalaemia persists, investigate for possible magnesium deficiency (see p.545).

Emergency treatment of hyperkalaemia

Stop and think! Are you justified in correcting a potentially fatal complication in a moribund patient?

Urgent treatment is required when hyperkalaemia is severe (≥7mmol/L) or with any level ≥5.5mmol/L accompanied by ECG changes (e.g. reduced or absent P waves, PR prolongation, QRS widening) and/or symptoms (e.g. muscle weakness, paraesthesia, palpitation). An approach is summarized in Box 9.A. However, this is only part of the management of hyperkalaemia and specialist advice should be obtained as necessary.

Box 9.A Emergency treatment of severe hyperkalaemia[1–3]

Stop potentially contributory or antagonistic drugs

These include ACE inhibitors, potassium-sparing diuretics, NSAIDS and potassium-containing laxatives (e.g. Movicol®).

β-blockers and digoxin should also be stopped as they antagonize the effect of insulin and β_2 agonists (see below).

Reduce the risk of cardiac arrhythmia

This is always the first step.

Give calcium gluconate 10mL of 10% solution IV over 2min; any improvement in ECG abnormalities will be seen in <3min; *stop if bradycardia develops*

If necessary, repeat the same dose every 10min until improvement is obtained; some patients require up to 50mL

Duration of action is 30–60min, and further doses may be required.

Note. Calcium gluconate can precipitate digoxin toxicity; give in 100mL of 5% dextrose IV over 20min in patients using digoxin (seek specialist advice).

Shift potassium into cells

When hyperkalaemia is severe (≥7mmol/L), insulin is generally given.

β_2 agonists (e.g. salbutamol) can be as effective.

Both reduce the plasma potassium concentration by about 0.5–1mmol/L.

Some guidelines do not recommended β_2 agonists as a sole treatment because some patients, e.g. those who are dialysis dependent or using β-blockers or digoxin, are less likely to respond.

The combination of insulin with nebulized salbutamol is more effective than either alone, with the latter helping to reduce the hypoglycaemic effect of the insulin.

These interventions do not remove potassium from the body, but buy time for more definitive treatment to be carried out.

Insulin

- add 10 units soluble insulin (e.g. Actrapid®) to 50mL dextrose 50% and give IV over 5min
- onset of effect 15min, duration of action at least 1h and commonly 4–6h
- if it becomes necessary to repeat the dose of insulin, additional glucose is not required if plasma glucose is ≥15mmol/L.

β_2 agonist

- give salbutamol 10–20mg nebulized over 10–30min (10mg in patients with ischaemic heart disease)
- when a nebulizer is not available, use salbutamol 1,200microgram (12 puffs) inhaled over 2min via a spacer device
- onset of effect 5–30min, duration of action 2h or more.

Monitoring treatment

- recheck urea and electrolytes after 30min; if there is a good response, check again 1–2h after the last intervention
- when insulin used, check blood glucose after 30min and then q1h for 6h, as delayed hypoglycaemia can occur.

continued

Box 9.A Continued

Other measures
If the combined approach above fails to work, emergency dialysis may be necessary to remove potassium from the body (if appropriate to the patient's overall circumstances).

Calcium polystyrene sulphonate resin (Calcium Resonium®) 15g PO q.d.s. is also used together with regular lactulose to increase potassium loss from the GI tract. However, it is *not* an emergency treatment because it has a slow onset of action (4–24h); it can also be poorly tolerated.

Supply

Potassium *chloride*
Sando-K® (HK Pharma)
Tablets effervescent potassium bicarbonate and chloride equivalent to potassium 470mg (12mmol K^+) and chloride 285mg (8mmol Cl^-), 28 days @ 2 t.d.s. (72mmol/24h K^+ and 48mmol/24h Cl^-) = £13.

Modified-release
Slow-K® (Alliance)
Tablets m/r potassium chloride 600mg (8mmol K^+ and 8mmol Cl^-), 28 days @ 2 t.d.s. (48mmol/24h K^+ and Cl^-) = £3.50.

Potassium *bicarbonate*
Effervescent potassium tablets BPC 1968 (generic)
Tablets effervescent potassium bicarbonate 500mg, potassium acid tartrate 300mg (6.5mmol K^+), 28 days @ 2 q.d.s. (52mmol/24h K^+) = £134; dose depends on acid-base balance as well as plasma potassium concentration.

1 GAIN (Guidelines and Audit Implementation Network) (2008) Guidelines for the treatment of hyperkalaemia in adults. Available from: www.gain-ni.org/Library/Guidelines/hyperkalaemia_guidelines.pdf
2 Mahoney BA (2009) Emergency interventions for hyperkalaemia. *Cochrane Database of Systematic Reviews.* **3**: CD003235.
3 Mandelberg A *et al.* (1999) Salbutamol metered-dose inhaler with spacer for hyperkalemia: how fast? How safe? *Chest.* **115**: 617–622.

MAGNESIUM BNF 9.5.1.3

Class: Metal element.

Indications: Hypomagnesaemia, constipation (see p.49), †arrhythmia, †eclampsia, †asthma, †myocardial infarction.

Pharmacology

Magnesium is the second most abundant intracellular ion after potassium. It is involved in numerous enzymatic reactions and is a co-factor for many biological processes, most of which use ATP. It is important for bone mineralization, muscular relaxation and neurotransmission.[1,2]

The recommended total daily intake is about 6–12mmol/24h. Magnesium competes with calcium for absorption in the small intestine, probably by active transport. Magnesium salts are generally poorly absorbed PO and have a laxative effect. The normal serum magnesium is 0.7–1.1mmol/L. Intracellular magnesium is mostly bound to ribosomes, phospholipids and nucleotides.[1] Magnesium is excreted by the kidneys, 3–12mmol/24h. Magnesium and calcium share the same transport system in the renal tubules and there is a reciprocal relationship between the amounts excreted.

Magnesium deficiency can result from:
- an inadequate dietary intake
- alcoholism

- reduced absorption, e.g. small bowel resection, cholestasis, pancreatic insufficiency
- excessive loss from the GI tract, e.g. diarrhoea, stoma, fistula
- excessive loss from the kidney, e.g. interstitial nephritis, diuretic phase of acute tubular necrosis, drug-induced (loop diuretic, aminoglycosides, **amphotericin**, **ciclosporin**, **cisplatin**)
- endocrine disorders, e.g. hyperparathyroidism, hyperthyroidism, SIADH.

The risk of hypomagnesaemia with **cisplatin** is dose-dependent and increases with cumulative doses (40% cycle 1 → 100% cycle 6).[3] It can persist for 4–5 months, and sometimes years, after completing treatment.[4,5] Although generally mild and asymptomatic, it can be severe and symptomatic.

When magnesium deficiency develops acutely, the symptoms may be obvious and severe, particularly muscle cramps, which aids diagnosis (Box 9.B). In chronic deficiency, symptoms may be insidious in onset, less severe and non-specific.

In animal studies, magnesium deficiency results in an increased release of substance P and other mediators from nerve endings. These activate immune cells to release histamine and cytokines, producing a pro-inflammatory state and increased levels of oxygen-derived free radicals and nitric oxide. Manifestations include:[6,7]

- cutaneous vasodilatation → erythema and oedema
- leucocytosis
- inflammatory lesions in cardiac muscle
- atherogenesis
- increased levels of oxidative stress
- hyperalgesia.

In humans, the incidence of magnesium deficiency increases with aging (due to poor diet, reduced intestinal absorption, increased urinary loss etc.), and both magnesium deficiency and aging are associated with low-grade inflammation and excessive production of oxygen-derived free radicals. This has led some to postulate that magnesium deficiency is a contributing factor in age-related diseases such as diabetes, cardiac failure, and hypertension.[7,8]

Serum magnesium is associated with muscle performance, e.g. in the elderly[9] and in patients with coronary artery disease.[10] In the latter, the use of magnesium supplements improved exercise capacity. However, evidence that the use of magnesium supplements or the correction of mild magnesium deficiency, e.g. in patients with diabetes, is of consistent benefit is currently lacking.[2]

Box 9.B Symptoms and signs of magnesium deficiency and excess

Magnesium deficiency	**Magnesium excess**
Muscle	Muscle
weakness	weakness
tremor	hypotonia
twitching	loss of reflexes
cramps	Sensation of warmth (IV)
tetany (positive Chvostek's sign)	Flushing (IV)
Paraesthesia	Drowsiness
Apathy	Slurred speech
Depression	Double vision
Delirium	Delirium
Choreiform movements	Hypotension
Nystagmus	Cardiac arrhythmia
Seizures	Respiratory depression
Prolonged QT interval	Nausea and vomiting
Cardiac arrhythmia, including *torsade de pointes*	Thirst
Increased pain (?)	Hypermagnesaemia
Hypomagnesaemia (not always)	
Hypokalaemia	
Hypocalcaemia	
Hypophosphataemia	

Hypermagnesaemia is rare and is seen most often in patients with renal impairment who take OTC medicines containing magnesium. Serum concentrations >4mmol/L produce drowsiness, vasodilation, slowing of atrioventricular conduction and hypotension. Over 6mmol/L there is profound CNS depression and muscle weakness (Box 9.B). **Calcium gluconate** IV is used to help reverse the effects of hypermagnesaemia.

When drugs such as **cisplatin** cause severe renal wasting of magnesium, hypomagnesaemia is generally present and aids diagnosis. If necessary, this can be confirmed by the high urinary excretion of magnesium. In deficiency states which develop more insidiously the serum magnesium is an insensitive guide to total body stores and hypomagnesaemia is not always present.[11 12] In this situation, the finding of a low urinary excretion of magnesium may help the diagnosis. Currently, the best method for detecting magnesium deficiency is the magnesium loading test (Box 9.C).

If it is not possible to perform a magnesium loading test, hypokalaemia (± hypocalcaemia) not responding to potassium supplementation should raise the possibility of magnesium deficiency, and a trial of magnesium replacement therapy should be considered.[2]

Box 9.C The magnesium loading test[13]

Collect pre-infusion urine sample for urinary magnesium (Mg)/creatinine (Cr) ratio. Measure Mg and Cr in mmol/L; divide the Mg value by the Cr value to calculate the Mg/Cr ratio.

By IVI over 4h, give 0.1mmol/kg of elemental magnesium, using magnesium sulphate 50% (contains elemental magnesium 2mmol/mL; see Supply), diluted to 50mL with 5% glucose.

Simultaneously, start a 24h urine collection for magnesium and creatinine. Measure the total amounts of magnesium and creatinine excreted in mmol (*not* the concentrations in mmol/L).

Calculate % magnesium retention:

$$1-\left[\frac{\text{24h urinary Mg (mmol)} - (\text{pre-infusion urinary Mg/Cr ratio (mmol/L)} \times \text{24h urinary Cr (mmol)})}{\text{dose of elemental magnesium infused (mmol)}}\right]\times 100$$

>50% retention implies definite deficiency.

Magnesium is also an NMDA-receptor-channel blocker (see p.593) and this probably accounts for its analgesic effect (Box 9.D).[15–18] However, despite the overall positive outcome from numerous RCTs, the role of IV or spinal magnesium as an analgesic in palliative care is yet to be determined and ideally such use should be in the setting of a clinical trial.

Box 9.D Magnesium as an analgesic

A number of studies have explored the effects of magnesium, mainly as an adjuvant analgesic for postoperative pain, with mixed results.

A systematic review of 14 studies concluded that there is no convincing evidence of reduced postoperative pain intensity or decreased analgesic requirements when magnesium was used as an adjuvant.[19]

However, of the nine RCTs undertaken since this systematic review, all but two have reported reduced postoperative pain and analgesic requirements.[20–28,29,30]

Further, five RCTs of spinal magnesium have all reported lower pain scores and decreased analgesic requirements.[31–35]

Cautions

Generally, parenteral magnesium should not be given to patients with heart block or severe renal impairment. Risk of hypermagnesaemia in patients with renal impairment.

Undesirable effects

Flushing, sweating and sensation of warmth IV; diarrhoea PO. Also see features of magnesium excess in Box 9.B.

Dose and use

Severe (plasma magnesium <0.5mmol/L) and symptomatic hypomagnesaemia generally involves the need to replace >1mmol/kg of magnesium; the route of choice is IVI, given in divided doses over 3–5 days.[2,36] Mild or asymptomatic hypomagnesaemia may be treated PO.

If the cause of the magnesium deficiency persists, PO maintenance therapy will be needed.

Prevention of deficiency

- magnesium-rich foods, e.g. meat, seafood, green leafy vegetables, cereals and nuts
- potassium-sparing diuretics also preserve magnesium, e.g. **amiloride**.

IV correction of chronic deficiency

Because the degree of deficiency is difficult to determine from the plasma magnesium, replacement is empirical, guided by symptoms, plasma magnesium and renal function:

- on the first day give 25–50mmol, then 25mmol each day until the deficiency is corrected
- use magnesium sulphate injection 50% (contains elemental magnesium 2mmol/mL; see Supply) 12.5–25mL, add to 250mL 0.9% saline or 5% glucose
- infuse over 1.5h (restricting the infusion rate to ≤0.6mmol/min avoids exceeding the maximum renal tubular resorption capacity for magnesium)
- if undesirable effects occur, e.g. hypotension, increase infusion time up to 4h.

In mild–moderate renal impairment reduce doses by 50% and monitor plasma magnesium daily. In severe renal impairment, avoid IV replacement if possible.

IVI is the parenteral route of choice. If PO and IV routes are not feasible, options include (in order of preference):

- IM magnesium sulphate: in severe deficiency, give ≤1mmol/kg/24h in divided doses, e.g. multiple injections spread over 4h of magnesium sulphate 50% (elemental magnesium 2mmol/mL, see Supply); can be painful
- CSCI magnesium sulphate: data are limited, but use of an isotonic solution is recommended, i.e. 25mmol of magnesium sulphate in 100mL WFI.[37,38]

Patients receiving cisplatin chemotherapy

Routine monitoring of magnesium levels and the provision of magnesium supplementation in the IV hydration fluid is recommended (Table 9.2).[3]

Table 9.2 Magnesium supplementation in patients receiving cisplatin

Cisplatin dose (mg/m^2)	*Magnesium/cycle (mmol)*
≤60	40
61–100	60
>100	80

PO maintenance

To prevent recurrence of the deficit, prescribe magnesium 24mmol/24h in divided doses. PO is used unless poorly tolerated or ineffective, e.g. malabsorption. The main limiting factor is diarrhoea, but this is uncommon with doses <40mmol/24h. It may be reduced by taking magnesium with or after food.

None of the PO products are licensed for magnesium deficiency. The BNF suggests magnesium glycerophosphate; alternatives include preparations normally used as antacids or laxatives (see Supply).

Supply

Magnesium *glycerophosphate*

All products are unlicensed; available as a named patient supply from IDIS, Special Products Limited or Mitovie Pharma (see Obtaining unlicensed products, p.769).

Tablets elemental magnesium 4mmol, 100 = £40; *some brands may be chewable.*

Tablets chewable elemental magnesium 4mmol, 50 = £20.

Oral liquid elemental magnesium 1mmol/mL, 200mL = £35 (from Special Products Limited).

Magnesium *hydroxide*

Oral suspension (magnesium hydroxide mixture BP 415mg/5mL) elemental magnesium 7mmol/5mL, available OTC as Milk of Magnesia®; *do not store in a cold place.*

Magnesium *sulphate*

Oral powder elemental magnesium 4mmol/1g, available OTC as Epsom Salts; dissolve in water.

Injection 20% (200mg/mL), elemental magnesium 0.8mmol/mL, 20mL amp = £3.

Injection 50% (500mg/mL), elemental magnesium 2mmol/mL, 2mL, 5mL and 10mL amp = £2.50, £3 and £1 respectively.

Injection (prefilled syringe) 50% (500mg/mL) elemental magnesium 2mmol/mL, 4mL, 10mL syringe = £8 and £5 respectively.

1 Romani A (2007) Regulation of magnesium homeostasis and transport in mammalian cells. *Archives of Biochemistry and Biophysics.* **458**: 90–102.

2 Martin KJ *et al.* (2009) Clinical consequences and management of hypomagnesemia. *Journal of the American Society of Nephrology.* **20**: 2291–2295.

3 Hodgkinson E *et al.* (2006) Magnesium depletion in patients receiving cisplatin-based chemotherapy. *Clinical Oncology.* **18**: 710–718.

4 Schilsky RL *et al.* (1982) Persistent hypomagnesemia following cisplatin chemotherapy for testicular cancer. *Cancer Treatment Reports.* **66**: 1767–1769.

5 Buckley JE *et al.* (1984) Hypomagnesemia after cisplatin combination chemotherapy. *Archives of Internal Medicine.* **144**: 2347–2348.

6 Mazur A *et al.* (2007) Magnesium and the inflammatory response: Potential physiopathological implications. *Archives of Biochemistry and Biophysics.* **458**: 48–56.

7 Tejero-Taldo MI *et al.* (2006) The nerve-heart connection in the pro-oxidant response to Mg-deficiency. *Heart Failure Reviews.* **11**: 35–44.

8 Barbagallo M *et al.* (2009) Magnesium homeostasis and aging. *Magnesium Research.* **22**: 235–246.

9 Dominguez LJ *et al.* (2006) Magnesium and muscle performance in older persons: the InCHIANTI study. *American Journal of Clinical Nutrition.* **84**: 419–426.

10 Pokan R *et al.* (2006) Oral magnesium therapy, exercise heart rate, exercise tolerance, and myocardial function in coronary artery disease patients. *British Journal of Sports Medicine.* **40**: 773–778.

11 Dyckner T and Wester P (1982) Magnesium deficiency — guidelines for diagnosis and substitution therapy. *Acta Medica Scandinavica.* **661**: 37–41.

12 Ismail Y and Ismail AA (2010) The underestimated problem of using serum magnesium measurements to exclude magnesium deficiency in adults; a health warning is needed for "normal" results. *Clinical Chemistry and Laboratory Medicine.* **48**: 323–327.

13 Ryzen E *et al.* (1985) Parenteral magnesium testing in the evaluation of magnesium deficiency. *Magnesium.* **4**: 137–147.

14 Crosby V *et al.* (2000) The importance of low magnesium in palliative care. *Palliative Medicine.* **14**: 544.

15 Mauskop A *et al.* (1995) Intravenous magnesium sulphate relieves migraine attacks in patients with low serum ionised magnesium levels: a pilot study. *Clinical Science.* **89**: 633–636.

16 Tramer M *et al.* (1996) Role of magnesium sulphate in postoperative analgesia. *Anesthesiology.* **84**: 340–347.

17 Crosby V *et al.* (2000) The safety and efficacy of a single dose (500mg or 1g) of intravenous magnesium sulfate in neuropathic pain poorly responsive to strong opioid analgesics in patients with cancer. *Journal of Pain and Symptom Management.* **19**: 35–39.

18 Bondok RS and Abd El-Hady AM (2006) Intra-articular magnesium is effective for postoperative analgesia in arthroscopic knee surgery. *British Journal of Anaesthesia.* **97**: 389–392.

19 Lysakowski C *et al.* (2007) Magnesium as an adjuvant to postoperative analgesia: a systematic review of randomized trials. *Anesthesia and Analgesia.* **104**: 1532–1539.

20 Tauzin-Fin P *et al.* (2006) Intravenous magnesium sulphate decreases postoperative tramadol requirement after radical prostatectomy. *European Journal of Anaesthesiology.* **23**: 1055–1059.

21 Ozcan PE *et al.* (2007) Role of magnesium sulfate in postoperative pain management for patients undergoing thoracotomy. *Journal of Cardiothoracic and Vascular Anesthesia.* **21**: 827–831.

22 Mentes O *et al.* (2008) Effect of intraoperative magnesium sulphate infusion on pain relief after laparoscopic cholecystectomy. *Acta Anaesthesiologica Scandinavica.* **52**: 1353–1359.

23 Ryu JH *et al.* (2008) Effects of magnesium sulphate on intraoperative anaesthetic requirements and postoperative analgesia in gynaecology patients receiving total intravenous anaesthesia. *British Journal of Anaesthesia.* **100**: 397–403.

24 Dabbagh A *et al.* (2009) Intravenous magnesium sulfate for post-operative pain in patients undergoing lower limb orthopedic surgery. *Acta Anaesthesiologica Scandinavica.* **53**: 1088–1091.
25 Kogler J (2009) The analgesic effect of magnesium sulfate in patients undergoing thoracotomy. *Acta Clinica Croatica.* **48**: 19–26.
26 Turhanoglu S *et al.* (2009) Magnesium sulfate reduces postoperative morphine requirement after remifentanil-based anesthesia. *Medical Science Monitor.* **15**: 15–19.
27 Hwang JY *et al.* (2010) I.V. infusion of magnesium sulphate during spinal anaesthesia improves postoperative analgesia. *British Journal of Anaesthesia.* **104**: 89–93.
28 Saadawy IM *et al.* (2010) Lidocaine vs. magnesium: effect on analgesia after a laparoscopic cholecystectomy. *Acta Anaesthesiologica Scandinavica.* **54**: 549–556.
29 Paech MJ *et al.* (2006) Does magnesium sulfate reduce the short- and long-term requirements for pain relief after caesarean delivery? A double-blind placebo-controlled trial. *American Journal of Obstetrics and Gynecology.* **194**: 1596–1602; discussion 1602–1593.
30 Tramer MR and Glynn CJ (2007) An evaluation of a single dose of magnesium to supplement analgesia after ambulatory surgery: randomized controlled trial. *Anesthesia and Analgesia.* **104**: 1349–1374.
31 Bilir A *et al.* (2007) Epidural magnesium reduces postoperative analgesic requirement. *British Journal of Anaesthesia.* **98**: 519–523.
32 Arcioni R *et al.* (2007) Combined intrathecal and epidural magnesium sulfate supplementation of spinal anesthesia to reduce post-operative analgesic requirements: a prospective, randomized, double-blind, controlled trial in patients undergoing major orthopedic surgery. *Acta Anaesthesiologica Scandinavica.* **51**: 482–489.
33 Farouk S (2008) Pre-incisional epidural magnesium provides pre-emptive and preventive analgesia in patients undergoing abdominal hysterectomy. *British Journal of Anaesthesia.* **101**: 694–699.
34 Ghatak T *et al.* (2010) Evaluation of the effect of magnesium sulphate vs. clonidine as adjunct to epidural bupivacaine. *Indian Journal of Anaesthesia.* **54**: 308–313.
35 Yousef AA and Amr YM (2010) The effect of adding magnesium sulphate to epidural bupivacaine and fentanyl in elective caesarean section using combined spinal-epidural anaesthesia: a prospective double blind randomised study. *International Journal of Obstetrics and Anesthesia.* **19**: 401–404.
36 Miller S (1995) Drug-induced hypomagnesaemia. *Hospital Pharmacy.* **30**: 248–250.
37 Anonymous (2010) How is acute hypomagnesaemia treated in adults. UK Medicines Information. Medicines Q&A 350.2.
38 Anonymous (2009) Can magnesium sulphate be given subcutaneously? UK Medicines Information. Medicines Q&A 14.3.

ZINC — BNF 9.5.4 & 9.8.1

Class: Metal element.

Indications: Zinc deficiency, Wilson's disease (Wilzin®), †anorexia due to taste changes, †wound healing.

Pharmacology

Zinc is an essential trace element with multiple functions. It is present in >300 enzymes, and has catalytic, structural and regulatory functions (Box 9.E).[1–3] It occurs in all tissues, particularly muscle and bone, and to a lesser extent in skin and liver. Most is intracellular, and much is intranuclear. Plasma contains only 0.1% of the body's zinc, mostly bound to albumin.[4]

Homeostasis is achieved primarily through regulation of the intestinal absorption. When dietary zinc is high, intestinal metal-binding proteins increase, and these slow absorption.[1] With a very high intake, secondary homeostatic mechanisms operate, e.g. increased renal excretion and redistribution of tissue zinc.[4]

There are no significant stores of zinc in the body and a constant dietary intake is essential. The UK reference nutrient intake (RNI) for daily dietary (elemental) zinc is 5.5–9.5mg in men and 4–7mg for women.[2,5] In contrast, the EU recommended daily allowance is 15mg.[2,6] Sources include meat, sea food, dairy products, wholegrain cereals, legumes and nuts. Bio-availability of dietary zinc is about 20–30%, and is lower from plant sources because of phytate-binding.[2]

Excessive intake is generally safe. However, acute and chronic poisoning has been reported.[1,7] Prolonged ingestion of high doses (50–300mg/24h elemental zinc) is associated with impaired immune function with leucopenia and neutropenia, sideroblastic anaemia and reduced ferritin levels. It can lead to secondary copper deficiency with increased LDL:HDL cholesterol ratio and HbA_{1c}.[1,7] The safe upper levels for elemental zinc intake recommended in the UK are 25mg/day from supplements and 42mg/day in total (i.e. from supplements and diet combined).[6,7]

In the brain, the main effect of zinc is to reduce neuronal excitability.[8] However, as a consequence of various insults (e.g. trauma, ischaema, hypoglycaemia) zinc may accumulate to toxic levels and cause neural damage and apoptosis. Zinc also appears to have a role in the pathogenesis of neurodegerative disease. Thus, zinc-dependent proteins have been implicated in MND/AML, and zinc induces amyloid deposition in Alzheimer's disease.[8] It is concentrated in and

Box 9.E Physiological functions of zinc

Gene expression and cellular stability
Zinc-dependent RNA and DNA polymerases and reverse transcriptase
Cell proliferation and differentiation
Regulation of apoptosis (cell-specific; either increases or decreases)
Zinc-fingers transcription factors
Structural maintenance of biomembranes

Homeostasis and metabolism
Cellular signal and transmission
Hormone storage, synthesis and action, e.g. sex and thyroid hormones
Metabolism of proteins, carbohydrates and lipids
Tissue growth and repair
Neurosensory (cognition, behavioural response, taste, smell, appetite)

Anti-oxidant
Protects from free radical reactions
Component of super oxide dismutase (SOD)
Induces metal-binding protein production
Membrane stabilization

Anti-inflammatory
Inhibits expression of pro-inflammatory cytokines (IL-4, IL-6, and TNF-α)

Immune response
Thymulin activity
T-cell maturation and differentiation
Regulates cytokine production
Natural killer cell activity
T-lymphocyte activation
Direct effect on DNA for immune cell proliferation

around plaques, but no clinical benefit is seen with **clioquinol**, a metal protein-attenuating compound, which interacts with zinc and promotes solubilization of amyloid.[9]

Zinc concentrations can be measured in the cellular components of blood (RBC, mononuclear cells and platelets), plasma, urine, faeces, skin, hair and saliva. Cellular zinc is sensitive but measurement is complex.[10] Consequently, plasma concentration is widely used instead, with zinc deficiency defined as < 15micromol/L.[11] However, plasma zinc may not reflect total body zinc, and is influenced by various factors, e.g. plasma protein, drugs (see Cautions), infection, and inflammation.[2,7,10,12] Thus, when zinc deficiency is clinically suspected, even if the plasma zinc concentration is within the normal range, a therapeutic trial of replacement therapy should be considered.

Zinc deficiency can occur relatively rapidly as a result of inadequate dietary intake, poor intestinal absorption or increased loss due to conditions such as cancer, malabsorption, alcoholism, renal disease, sickle cell anaemia and AIDS. Metal-binding proteins, in addition to binding zinc and other heavy metals such as copper, have a protective role scavenging toxic metals and free radicals, and improving immunity. However, in stressful states, e.g. inflammation and with increasing age, levels increase and bind more intracellular zinc. Consequently, the persistent sequestration of zinc leads to reduced bio-availability and a relative deficiency state.[1,13] The effects of zinc deficiency are numerous and reflect its multifunctional role and importance in gene expression, protein synthesis and enzyme function (Box 9.F).[1,2,13]

There are conflicting reports regarding the relationship between zinc and cancer. Some studies show no effect, others a protective effect and some an increased risk. A possible explanation is the proliferative and apoptotic actions of zinc are cell-specific. For example, in prostate, ovarian, oesophageal, and hepatocellular cancers, malignant cells are unable to accumulate zinc, resulting in a loss of zinc-induced apoptosis. Zinc deficiency leads to an increased risk and, conversely, supplementation has an anti-cancer effect. Oxidative stress and chronic inflammation have been

Box 9.F Consequences of zinc deficiency

Immunological
Increased risk of infections due to impaired cellular immunity
Reduced neutrophils, monocytes, natural killer cells
Reduced T-helper$_1$ cytokines (IL-2 and IFN-γ)
Reduced thymulin activity
Increased inflammation secondary to increased pro-inflammatory cytokines, NO, COX-2 and NF-κB

Other cellular effects
Increased apoptosis
Increased oxidative stress with lipid peroxidation of mitochondrial membranes

Haematological
Defective platelet aggregation
Iron-deficiency anaemia

Neuropsychological
Impaired smell, taste and vision
Impaired cognition
Behavioural disturbance
Depression

Gastro-intestinal
Anorexia
Diarrhoea
Gastric acid and pepsin secretion causing mucosal damage

Hormonal
Thyroid hormone function
Hypogonadism and infertility

Dermatological
Dermatitis
Alopecia
Nail dystrophy
Delayed wound healing

implicated as possible causal mechanisms.[14] In contrast, breast and pancreatic cancers have a high zinc concentration which enhances cell proliferation.[15]

Zinc supplements are of benefit in the common cold. A recent Cochrane review concluded that, in otherwise healthy people, zinc lozenges and syrup reduce the severity and duration of symptoms if started within 24h of the onset of symptoms. Lozenges were less well tolerated but, because the studies used different doses (30–190mg/24h) for different lengths of time, general recommendations could not be made.[16] Patients with impaired immunity have not been investigated.

In zinc-deficient patients, supplements promote wound healing.[2] However, a Cochrane review (based on poor quality studies) found no strong evidence of benefit on leg ulcer healing.[17] There is inconclusive or insufficient evidence regarding zinc's effectiveness as a treatment for male infertility and age-related macular degeneration.[2,18]

Supplementation improves zinc deficiency, disturbances of taste and smell, and dry mouth (xerostomia).[19,20] It can help idiopathic taste disorders[21] but not if drug-induced.[11] Supplements can also prevent or reduce radiotherapy-induced taste changes.[22] The beneficial effect on zinc-related anorexia is linked to an increase in leptin levels and by influencing the hypothalamic neuropeptides which regulate appetite.[23] The effect on leptin possibly involves increased cytokine production.[24] Zinc is also used to prevent the absorption of copper in Wilson's disease.

Bio-availability of zinc supplements is salt-dependent, e.g. gluconate $>$ sulphate $>$ oxide.[25]

Cautions

Acute renal impairment (may accumulate). If taken for prolonged periods, monitor zinc and copper plasma concentrations, FBC and plasma cholesterol to detect incipient zinc toxicity and copper deficiency.

Drug interactions

PO zinc decreases GI absorption of chelating agents (**penicillamine**, **trientine**), fluoroquinolone antibacterials, **iron**, and tetracyclines. Absorption of PO zinc is decreased by **calcium** and **iron** supplements, chelating agents (**penicillamine**, **trientine**), phosphorus-containing products, and tetracyclines. Separating administration times by 2–3h avoids these interactions.

Thiazides and loop diuretics increase the urinary excretion of zinc which, if used long-term, may lead to deficiency.

Undesirable effects

More common: gastric irritation, gastritis, dyspepsia, abdominal pain, nausea, vomiting, diarrhoea; these can be reduced by giving PO zinc with or after food.
Less common: headache, lethargy and irritability.

Dose and use

Zinc deficiency

- elemental zinc up to 50mg PO t.d.s., e.g. Solvazinc® 1 tablet (elemental zinc 45mg) dissolved in water once daily–t.d.s. p.c. *or*
- add zinc sulphate 2mL once daily to an IVI; this provides elemental zinc 6.5mg.

Wilson's disease

Zinc *acetate* is available for use ± chelating agents (**penicillinamine**, **trientine**) under specialist supervision to decrease copper absorption from the GI tract in Wilson's disease.[2] See BNF section 9.8.1.

Supply

Zinc sulphate (generic)
Injection 14.6mg/mL (elemental zinc 3.3mg/mL), 10mL vial = £2.50.

Solvazinc® (Galen)
Tablets effervescent zinc sulphate monohydrate 125mg (elemental zinc 45mg), 28 days @ 1 tablet t.d.s. = £12.

Many zinc products are available OTC (citrate, gluconate, glycinate, oxide and sulphate salts) as dietary supplements and as symptomatic treatment for the common cold.

1 Stefanidou M *et al.* (2006) Zinc: a multipurpose trace element. *Archives of Toxicology*. **80**: 1–9.
2 Mason P (2006) Physiological and medicinal zinc. *Pharmaceutical Journal*. **276**: 271–274.
3 Frassinetti S *et al.* (2006) The role of zinc in life: a review. *Journal of Environmental Pathology, Toxicology and Oncology*. **25**: 597–610.
4 King JC *et al.* (2000) Zinc homeostasis in humans. *Journal of Nutritrion*. **130**: 1360S–1366S.
5 COMA (1991) Committee on Medical Aspects of Food and Nutrition Policy. Dietary reference values for food energy and nutrients for the United Kingdom. Report of the panel on dietary reference values. HMSO, London.
6 Mason P (2003) Upper safety limits for vitamins–why have different authorities set different guidance? *Pharmaceutical Journal*. **271**: 55–57.
7 EVM (2003) Expert Group on Vitamins and Minerals. Risk assessment: zinc: In: Safe upper levels for vitamins and minerals. pp253–262. Food Standards Agency, London. Available from: www.food.gov.uk
8 Frederickson CJ *et al.* (2005) The neurobiology of zinc in health and disease. *Nature Reviews Neuroscience*. **6**: 449–462.
9 Sampson E *et al.* (2008) Metal protein attenuating compounds for the treatment of Alzheimers Disease. *Cochrane Database of Systematic Reviews*. **1**: CD005880.
10 Hambridge M (2003) Biomarkers of trace mineral intake and status. *Journal of Nutritrion*. **133**: 948S–955S.
11 Heyneman CA (1996) Zinc deficiency and taste disorders. *Annals of Pharmacotherapy*. **30**: 186–187.
12 Alpers DH (1994) Zinc and deficiencies of taste and smell. *Journal of the American Medical Association*. **272**: 1233–1234.
13 Vasto S *et al.* (2007) Zinc and inflammatory/immune response in aging. *Annals of the New York Academy of Sciences*. **1100**: 111–122.
14 Prasad AS *et al.* (2009) Zinc in cancer prevention. *Nutrition and Cancer*. **61**: 879–887.

15 Franklin RB and Costello LC (2009) The important role of the apoptotic effects of zinc in the development of cancers. *Journal of Cellular Biochemistry.* **106**: 750–757.
16 Singh M and Das RR (2011) Zinc for the common cold. *Cochrane Database of Systematic Reviews.* **2**: CD001364.
17 Wilkinson E *et al.* (1998) Oral zinc for arterial and venous ulcers. *Cochrane Database of Systematic Reviews.* **4**: CD001273.
18 Anonymous (2003) Antioxidant vitamins and zinc for macular degeneration. *Medical Letter on Drugs and Therapeutics.* **45**: 45–46.
19 Tanaka M (2002) Secretory function of the salivary gland in patients with taste disorders or xerostomia: correlation with zinc deficiency. *Acta Otolaryngol Suppl.* 134–141.
20 Henkin RI *et al.* (1999) Efficacy of exogenous oral zinc in treatment of patients with carbonic anhydrase VI deficiency. *American Journal of Medical Sciences.* **318**: 392–405.
21 Heckmann SM *et al.* (2005) Zinc gluconate in the treatment of dysgeusia–a randomized clinical trial. *Journal of Dental Research.* **84**: 35–38.
22 Ripamonti C *et al.* (1998) A randomized, controlled clinical trial to evaluate the effects of zinc sulfate on cancer patients with taste alterations caused by head and neck irradiation. *Cancer.* **82**: 1938–1945.
23 Shay NF and Mangian HF (2000) Neurobiology of zinc-influenced eating behavior. *Journal of Nutritrion.* **130**: 1493S–1499S.
24 Mantzoros CS *et al.* (1998) Zinc may regulate serum leptin concentrations in humans. *Journal of American College of Nutrition.* **17**: 270–275.
25 Mittmann (2001) Bioverfügbarkeit von Zink-Präparaten. *J Pharmakol Ther.* **10**: 143–153.

10: MUSCULOSKELETAL AND JOINT DISEASES

DEPOT CORTICOSTEROID INJECTIONS BNF 10.1.2.2

Indications: Inflammation of joints and soft tissues, †pain in superficial bones (e.g. rib, scapula, iliac crest), †intractable pain caused by spinal metastases, †malignant (peritoneal) ascites.

Contra-indications: Untreated local or systemic infection. Must not be given IV or IT.

Pharmacology

Corticosteroids have an anti-inflammatory effect; they reduce the concentration of algesic substances present in inflammation which sensitize nerve endings.[1] Further, in animal studies, when injected locally around an injured nerve, corticosteroids have been shown to have a direct inhibitory effect on the spontaneous activity associated with nerve injury.[2]

For many years depot injections of corticosteroids have been given epidurally in selected patients with non-malignant radicular (nerve root) compression pain associated with spinal pathology, e.g. lumbar disc herniation, sciatica.[3] However, a systematic review found only weak RCT evidence for their efficacy.[4] Even so, in patients with spinal metastases and intractable radicular pain, clinical experience indicates that ED depot corticosteroids can be helpful.

Cautions

Current or history of severe affective disorders (e.g. depression, bipolar disorder) or steroid-induced psychosis, epilepsy, glaucoma, myasthenia gravis, hypertension, CHF, predisposition to thrombophlebitis, peptic ulceration, diverticulitis, ulcerative colitis, severe hepatic impairment, renal impairment, hypothyroidism, osteoporosis.

Depot formulations may result in symptomatic hyperglycaemia for several days in patients with diabetes mellitus and suppression of the hypothalamic-pituitary-adrenal axis for up to 4 weeks. Injection under a rib may be complicated by a pneumothorax.

Corticosteroids may mask or alter the presentation of infection in immunocompromised patients; such patients should not receive live vaccines and, if exposed to chickenpox, should receive *Varicella zoster* immunoglobulin.

Undesirable effects

Undesirable effects associated with systemic corticosteroids can also occur with depot injections (see p.487). These include antagonism of antihypertensive, antidiabetic and diuretic drugs, and increased risk of hypokalaemia if used concurrently with β_2 agonists (e.g. **salbutamol, terbutaline**) or other potassium-wasting drugs.

Occasionally, a patient develops lipodystrophy (local fat necrosis) which results in an indentation of the overlying skin.

ED injection of **methylprednisolone *acetate*** (unlicensed route) has been associated with wound dehiscence and with loss of sphincter control.

Dose and use

Injection into and/or over a painful bone secondary[5]

- infiltrate the skin and SC tissues overlying the point of maximal bone tenderness with local anaesthetic
- with the tip of the needle pressing against the tender bone, inject depot **methylprednisolone *acetate*** 80mg in 2mL
- if there are 2 painful bones, inject 40mg at each spot; generally limit the total amount given at any one time to 80mg.

Also, for rib lesions, reposition the needle under the rib and inject 5mL of **bupivacaine** 0.5% to anaesthetize the intercostal nerve. Complete or good relief occurs in about 70% of patients. If of benefit, injections can be repeated if the pain returns but not more than every 2 weeks.

Epidural injection[3]

Depot **methylprednisolone *acetate*** 80mg in 2mL (unlicensed route). A single ED injection is given, followed if necessary by a further 1–2 injections at 3–4 week intervals. The effect of ED corticosteroids is unpredictable and may not peak until 1 week after an injection. Depot corticosteroids cannot be injected through an epidural bacterial filter. In some countries, depot **triamcinolone** or a *non-depot* formulation of **dexamethasone sodium phosphate** is used for ED injection.

Malignant (peritoneal) ascites

After a preliminary paracentesis, inject intra-abdominally:

- **triamcinolone *acetonide*** 8mg/kg, up to a maximum of 520mg (13 vials) *or*
- **triamcinolone *hexacetonide*** (not UK) 10mg/kg, up to a maximum of 640mg *or*
- **methylprednisolone *acetate*** 10mg/kg, up to a maximum of 640mg (8 × 2mL vials).

In an open study, the mean interval between paracentesis increased from 9 to 18 days.[6]

Supply

Methylprednisolone *acetate*

Depo-Medrone® (Pharmacia)

Depot injection (aqueous suspension) 40mg/mL, 1mL vial = £3, 2mL vial = £5, 3mL vial = £7.

Triamcinolone *acetonide*

Kenalog® Intra-articular/Intramuscular (Squibb)

Depot injection (aqueous suspension) 40mg/mL, 1mL vial = £1.50.

1 Pybus P (1984) Osteoarthritis: a new neurological method of pain control. *Medical Hypothesis*. **14**: 413–422.

2 Devor M *et al.* (1985) Corticosteroids reduce neuroma hyperexcitability. In: HL Fields *et al.* (eds) *Advances in Pain Research and Therapy* Vol 9. Raven Press, New York, pp. 451–455.

3 McLain RF *et al.* (2004) Epidural steroids for back and leg pain: mechanism of action and efficacy. *Cleveland Clinic Journal of Medicine*. **71**: 961–970.

4 Armon C *et al.* (2007) Assessment: use of epidural steroid injections to treat radicular lumbosacral pain: report of the Therapeutics and Technology Assessment Subcommittee of the American Academy of Neurology. *Neurology*. **68**: 723–729.

5 Rowell NP (1988) Intralesional methylprednisolone for rib metastases: an alternative to radiotherapy? *Palliative Medicine*. **2**: 153–155.

6 Mackey J *et al.* (2000) A phase II trial of triamcinolone hexacetanide for symptomatic recurrent malignant ascites. *Journal of Pain and Symptom Management*. **19**: 193–199.

RUBEFACIENTS AND OTHER TOPICAL PRODUCTS — BNF 10.3.2

Indications: Soft tissue pains (rubefacients, topical NSAIDs), pain relief in osteo-arthritis (**capsaicin** cream 0.025%, topical NSAIDs),[1] post-herpetic and diabetic neuralgia (**capsaicin** cream 0.075%),[2] peripheral neuropathic pain in non-diabetic patients (**capsaicin** TD patch 8%), †notalgia paraesthetica, †severe skin reaction to an indwelling SC cannula and/or phlebitis (**kaolin** poultice).

Contra-indications: Inflamed or broken skin.
Capsaicin TD patch 8%: do not apply to the face or head.
Topical NSAIDs: if nasal polyps or history of asthma, angioedema, urticaria or acute rhinitis precipitated by aspirin or another NSAID.

Pharmacology

Rubefacients act by counter-stimulation of the skin, closing the pain 'gate' in the dorsal horn of the spinal cord.[3,4] Further benefit is obtained by the inclusion of **menthol**. This cools the skin for several hours by acting on heat-sensitive transient receptor potential (TRP) channels expressed on sensory nerve endings.[5,6] **Menthol**-containing rubefacients have been used as 'home remedies' for tension headache, muscle spasm, and joint pain. (**Menthol** is also an ingredient in several topical antipruritic products, see p.586.) Warm **kaolin** poultices also act by counter-stimulation, substituting the pleasure of warmth for the stinging/burning of the inflamed skin.

Capsaicin

Capsaicin is a naturally occurring alkaloid found in the fruits of various species of *Solanaceae* (the nightshade family) and in pepper plants of the genus *Capsicum* (chilli peppers).[7] It acts by depleting substance P (SP) at sensory nerve endings. In animals, **capsaicin** has also been shown to be neurotoxic, particularly for nociceptive C fibres.[8]

Application of **capsaicin** causes an initial release of SP from C fibres which manifests as a burning or stinging sensation (see Undesirable effects below) with subsequent depletion on continued use. Axonal transport of SP to synaptic terminals is reduced and synthesis inhibited.[9] **Capsaicin** may also elevate the thresholds for the release of SP and other neurotransmitters. Reduced availability of SP diminishes pain transmission. After stopping topical **capsaicin**, SP stores revert to pretreatment levels and neuronal sensitivity returns to normal.[10–12]

A Cochrane review found weak supporting evidence for the analgesic use of **capsaicin** (both cream and TD formulations), and concluded that **capsaicin** could provide useful pain relief for patients who did not respond to, or could not tolerate, standard treatments.[13] In an open study of topical **capsaicin** cream 0.025% in post-axillary dissection pain, 12/18 women reported benefit after 1 month, eight of whom had good or excellent responses; and, after 6 months, most still had good relief.[14] A placebo-controlled RCT of **capsaicin** cream 0.075% for 6 weeks gave comparable results; 8/13 patients had ≥50% improvement, 5 of whom had a good or excellent result.[15] Benefit was seen mainly in relation to stabbing pain.

A TD patch containing **capsaicin** 8% has recently been marketed for non-diabetic painful neuropathy, e.g. post-herpetic or HIV. Two studies have reported moderate (20–30%) improvement in pain scores over 3 months.[16,17] However, to date, no RCTs have been published comparing TD **capsaicin** patches with standard systemic adjuvant analgesics (see p.281). Cost alone is likely to restrict its use to specialist pain clinics.

Capsaicin cream is of benefit in histamine-related pruritus, aquagenic pruritus, and pruritus associated with uraemia, nodular prurigo, psoriasis and post-axillary dissection syndrome (see p.586).[6] Benefit is also seen with pruritus caused by notalgia paraesthetica (nerve injury, often caused by entrapment, of the dorsal ramus of the T2–T6 thoracic nerves which causes pruritus and/or altered sensation in the areas of skin between or below the shoulder blade on either side of the back).[18,19]

Topical NSAIDs

Topical NSAIDs are of value for the relief of pain associated with soft tissue trauma, e.g. strains and sprains,[20–22] inflammation of superficial joints,[23] early osteo-arthritis.[1]

Topically applied salicylates and some other NSAIDs can achieve local high SC concentrations and therapeutically effective concentrations within synovial fluid and peri-articular tissues similar to those seen after PO administration.[24–27]

A Cochrane review compared topical NSAIDs with placebo in *acute* musculoskeletal pain over 1–2 weeks and found that topical NSAIDs had an NNT of 4.5 when a 50% reduction in pain was used as the measure of clinical success. Topical **diclofenac**, **ibuprofen**, **ketoprofen** and **piroxicam** were effective, whereas **indometacin** and **benzydamine** were no better than placebo.[20] A second Cochrane review concluded that, in *chronic* musculoskeletal pain, rubefacients containing salicylates were less effective than topical NSAIDs; and, in *acute* musculoskeletal pain, they were little better than placebo.[28] However, different formulations of the same drug can result in major differences in effectiveness.[29]

Pharmacokinetic details for **capsaicin** products and topical NSAIDs are shown in Table 10.1.

Table 10.1 Pharmacokinetic details for capsaicin products and topical NSAIDs

	Capsaicin cream 0.025% and 0.075%	*Capsaicin TD patch 8%*	*Topical NSAIDs*
Onset of action	Counter-stimulation generally immediate. 1 week in osteo-arthritis but full effect may not be seen for ≤2 months. 2–4 weeks in neuralgia	1–14 days in peripheral neuropathy	Product- and drug-dependent
Duration of action	No data; manufacturers advise applying q4–6h	No data; manufacturers advise a 3-month gap between applications	Product and drug dependent; manufacturers advise applying b.d.–q.d.s.

Cautions

General

Avoid contact with eyes, mucous membranes, and inflamed or broken skin; discontinue if rash develops. Do not cover with occlusive dressings or tight bandages.

Capsaicin cream 0.025% and 0.075%

Avoid hot baths or showers immediately before application because this can enhance the burning sensation. Avoid inhaling the vapour from the cream. Wash hands immediately after application.

*Capsaicin TD patch 8%

Unstable or poorly controlled blood pressure, heart disease (see Undesirable effects). The painful burning sensation may necessitate local cooling (e.g. with a cold compress) or systemic analgesia. Avoid inhaling the vapour from the patch. Special precautions are required for handling (see Dose and use).

Topical NSAIDs

History of peptic ulcer, renal disease or asthma. May cause photosensitivity, particularly **ketoprofen**. Avoid exposing the treated area to sunlight when using topical **ketoprofen** and for 2 weeks afterwards.

Provided very large amounts are not applied, undesirable effects and drug interactions are much less likely with topical NSAIDs than with systemic NSAIDs because plasma concentrations are much lower.

Undesirable effects

The commonest undesirable effect of **capsaicin** cream is tingling, stinging or burning at the site of application. This effect is thought to be related to the initial release of SP from C fibres. The stinging and burning generally decreases with continued applications, often clearing in a few days but sometimes persisting for >4 weeks. Some patients discontinue treatment because of this. Runny eyes and respiratory tract irritation, causing coughing and sneezing, may result from rubbing the eyes and/or inhaling **capsaicin** vapour when applying the cream. Breathlessness and exacerbation of asthma have occurred occasionally.

Almost all patients experience local erythema and a burning sensation with **capsaicin** TD patches. Other common local effects (1–10% of patients) are itching, blistering, swelling and dryness. Uncommon symptoms (1–10 per 1,000 patients) include raised blood pressure, arrhythmia, palpitations, loss of taste sensation, muscle spasm, reduced sensation in limbs, local wheals, prickling sensation and bruising.

Large quantities of topical NSAIDs have been associated with systemic effects (e.g. hypersensitivity, rash, asthma, renal impairment[30]) and potentiation of **warfarin**, occasionally leading to bleeding.[31] Local reactions include drying, reddening, burning sensations, and contact dermatitis. A Cochrane review found that, in short-term studies, topical NSAIDs and placebo produced a similar incidence of local reactions and systemic undesirable effects (about 6% and 3% respectively).[20]

Dose and use

Capsaicin cream 0.025–0.075%

- apply a pea-sized amount t.d.s.–q.d.s.

The initial burning sensation felt after the application of **capsaicin** cream is intensified and/or prolonged when larger quantities are applied (particularly with the higher-strength cream), or if applied less frequently than t.d.s. If the burning is severe, topical **lidocaine** or another local anaesthetic can be applied before **capsaicin** in the first few weeks of treatment.

Because heat and humidity influence dysaesthesia, patients should avoid excessive sweating and not take a hot bath immediately before application. Occlusion and tight bandaging should also be avoided.

Patients should apply the cream using gentle massage, avoiding contact with eyes, mucous membranes and broken/inflamed skin. *Patients must wash their hands after applying the cream to avoid subsequent unintentional contact with the eyes.*

Capsaicin TD patch 8%

Health professionals should wear nitrile gloves when handling the patches and cleansing solution; latex gloves do *not* provide adequate protection:

- mark out the most painful areas with ink
- depending on the size of the painful areas, up to 4 patches may be applied simultaneously, or a patch may be cut to fit
- wash the skin in the treatment area with soap and water and dry thoroughly; any hair may be clipped but not shaved
- because most patients experience a burning sensation when the patches are applied, pre-treat the area with topical **lidocaine** or another local anaesthetic 1h before applying the patches
- leave patches in place for:
  - ▹ 30min if applied to the feet
  - ▹ 1h if applied elsewhere
  - ▹ if necessary, disposable socks or an open-weave bandage can be used to keep the patch in place
- when removing patches, roll them inwards to enclose the remaining **capsaicin**
- use the cleansing gel supplied to remove any traces of **capsaicin** from the patient's skin, both after any accidental contact and after removing the patches; leave the gel on the skin for 1min, then wipe off
- wash the skin with soap and water after using the cleansing gel
- treatment can be repeated after 3 months if necessary.

Used patches, gloves, wipes, socks and bandages should be placed in a plastic bag and disposed of safely.

Topical NSAIDs

- generally apply b.d.–q.d.s.

Kaolin poultice

- generally apply b.d.

Supply

For **menthol** products, see p.588.

Kaolin (generic)
Poultice 200g = £3.

Kaolin Poultice K/L Pack® (K/L)
Poultice 4 × 100g pouches = £6.

Capsaicin
Zacin® (Cephalon)

Cream 0.025%, 45g = £18.
Axsain® (Cephalon)
Cream 0.075%, 45g = £14.

Qutenza® (Astellas)
TD patch 8% (contains 179mg **capsaicin**), 1 patch (with cleansing gel) = £210.

Topical NSAIDs
Diclofenac
Mobigel® (Goldshield)
Spray containing **diclofenac *sodium*** 4%, 25g = £5 (smaller packs available OTC).

Voltarol Emulgel® (Novartis)
Gel containing **diclofenac *diethylammonium*** 1.16% (equivalent to **diclofenac *sodium*** 1%), 20g (hospital only) = £1.50; 100g = £7 (also available OTC).
Also see **diclofenac**, p.315.

Felbinac
Traxam® (Goldshield)
Foam 3.17%, 100g = £7.
Gel 3%, 100g = £7.

Ibuprofen (generic)
Gel 5%, 30g = £2, 50g = £2.50, 100g = £6.

Fenbid® Forte (Goldshield)
Forte gel 10%, 100g = £7 (smaller packs available OTC).

Ibugel Forte® (Dermal)
Forte gel 10%, 100g = £6.
Also see **ibuprofen** p.320.

This is not a complete list; see BNF for more details.

---

1 NHS (2008) Clinical knowledge summaries. Osteoarthritis. Available from: www.cks.nhs.uk/osteoarthritis#-324225
2 NHS (2008) Clinical knowledge summaries. Post-herpetic neuralgia-management. Available from: www.cks.nhs.uk/post_herpetic_neuralgia
3 Melzack R and Wall P (1965) Pain mechanisms: a new theory. *Science*. **150**: 971–979.
4 Melzack R (1991) The gate control theory 25 years later: new perspectives on phantom limb pain. In: M Bond *et al.* (eds) *Proceedings of the VIth World Congress on Pain*. Elsevier Science, Amsterdam, pp. 9–21.
5 Peier AM *et al.* (2002) A TRP channel that senses cold stimuli and menthol. *Cell*. **108**: 705–715.
6 Patel T *et al.* (2007) Menthol: a refreshing look at this ancient compound. *Journal of the American Academy of Dermatology*. **57**: 873–878.
7 Towlerton GR and Rice AS (2003) Topical analgesics for chronic pain. In: AS Rice *et al.* (eds) *Clinical Pain Management: Chronic Pain*. Arnold, London, pp. 213–226.
8 Chung JM *et al.* (1993) Chronic effects of topical application of capsaicin to the sciatic nerve on responses of primate spinothalamic neurons. *Pain*. **53**: 311–321.
9 Gamse R *et al.* (1982) Capsaicin applied to peripheral nerve inhibits axoplasmic transport of substance P and somatostatin. *Brain Research*. **239**: 447–462.
10 Gamse R *et al.* (1981) Differential effects of capsaicin on the content of somatostatin, substance P, and neurotensin in the nervous system of the rat. *Naunyn Schmiedebergs Archives of Pharmacology*. **317**: 140–148.
11 Fitzgerald M (1983) Capsaicin and sensory neurones: a review. *Pain*. **15**: 109–130.
12 LaMotte RH *et al.* (1988) Hypothesis for novel classes of chemoreceptors mediating chemogenic pain and itch. In: R Dubner *et al.* (eds) *Proceedings of the Vth World Congress on Pain*. Elsevier, New York, pp. 529–535.
13 Derry S *et al.* (2009) Topical capsaicin for chronic neuropathic pain in adults. *Cochrane Database of Systematic Reviews*. **4**: CD007393.
14 Watson C *et al.* (1989) The postmastectomy pain syndrome and the effect of topical capsaicin. *Pain*. **38**: 177–186.
15 Watson CPN and Evans RJ (1992) Post-mastectomy pain syndrome and topical capsaicin: a randomized trial. *Pain*. **51**: 375–379.
16 Backonja M *et al.* (2008) NGX-4010, a high-concentration capsaicin patch, for the treatment of postherpetic neuralgia: a randomised, double-blind study. *Lancet Neurology*. **7**: 1106–1112.
17 Simpson DM *et al.* (2008) Controlled trial of high-concentration capsaicin patch for treatment of painful HIV neuropathy. *Neurology*. **70**: 2305–2313.
18 Bernstein JE (1988) Capsaicin in dermatologic disease. *Seminars in Dermatology*. **7**: 304–309.
19 Breneman D *et al.* (1992) Topical capsaicin for treatment of hemodialysis-related pruritus. *Journal of the American Academy of Dermatology*. **26**: 91–94.
20 Massey T *et al.* (2010) Topical NSAIDS for acute pain in adults. *Cochrane Database of Systematic Reviews*. **6**: CD007402.
21 Mason L *et al.* (2004) Topical NSAIDs for chronic musculoskeletal pain: systematic review and meta-analysis. *BMC Musculoskeletal Disorders*. **5**: 28.

22 Moore R *et al.* (1998) Quantitative systematic review of topically applied non-steroidal anti-inflammatory drugs. *British Medical Journal*. **316**: 333–338.
23 Underwood M *et al.* (2008) Advice to use topical or oral ibuprofen for chronic knee pain in older people: randomised controlled trial and patient preference study. *British Medical Journal*. **336**: 138–142.
24 Mondino A *et al.* (1983) Kinetic studies of ibuprofen on humans. Comparative study for the determination of blood concentrations and metabolites following local and oral administration. *Medizinische Welt*. **34**: 1052–1054.
25 Chlud K and Wagener H (1987) Percutaneous nonsteroidal anti-inflammatory drug (NSAID) therapy with particular reference to pharmacokinetic factors. *EULAR Bulletin*. **2**: 40–43.
26 Peters H *et al.* (1987) Percutaneous kinetics of ibuprofen (German). *Aktuelle Rheumatologie*. **12**: 208–211.
27 Dominkus M *et al.* (1996) Comparison of tissue and plasma levels of ibuprofen after oral and topical administration. *Arzneimittelforschung*. **46**: 1138–1143.
28 Matthews P *et al.* (2010) Topical rubefacients for acute and chronic pain in adults. *Cochrane Database of Systematic Reviews*. **11**: CD007403.
29 Haroutiunian S *et al.* (2010) Topical NSAID therapy for musculoskeletal pain. *Pain Medicine*. **11**: 535–549.
30 O'Callaghan C *et al.* (1994) Renal disease and use of topical NSAIDs. *British Medical Journal*. **308**: 110–111.
31 Makris UE *et al.* (2010) Adverse effects of topical nonsteroidal antiinflammatory drugs in older adults with osteoarthritis: a systematic literature review. *Journal of Rheumatology*. **37**: 1236–1243.

SKELETAL MUSCLE RELAXANTS — BNF 10.2.2

Skeletal muscle relaxants are used to relieve painful chronic muscle spasm and spasticity associated with neural injury, e.g. paraplegia, post-stroke, multiple sclerosis, and sometimes motor neurone disease/amyotrophic lateral sclerosis (MND/AML).[1] †**Baclofen** is also used to relieve hiccup.

Baclofen, **diazepam** and **tizanidine** act principally on spinal and supraspinal sites within the CNS; **dantrolene** (and **quinine**) acts on muscle (Table 10.2). There is no clear evidence that any one drug is superior to any other.[2,3] The use of **diazepam** as a muscle relaxant is discussed on p.137 and p.140.

All skeletal muscle relaxants may reduce voluntary muscle power. This may be a disadvantage in people with hemiplegia or paraplegia if increased spastic muscle tone is what enables them to walk or function more independently. Thus, dose escalation to the maximum recommended dose should be spread out over 4–8 weeks to balance the benefits of reduced spasticity with possible loss of functional performance and independence. On the other hand, in patients unable to use their limbs because of severe spasticity or paralysis or motor weakness, the dose can be escalated more rapidly. For these patients, sedation is likely to be the dose-limiting factor.[4]

Drug treatment of lower limb muscle cramp is similar to that of spasticity.[5] **Quinine** has traditionally been used to relieve nocturnal cramp, but this is now discouraged (Box 10.A). **Baclofen**, **diazepam**, **dantrolene** and **tizanidine** are all currently approved for use in patients with spasticity. If there are no concurrent indications for a benzodiazepine, **baclofen** should generally be prescribed as the first-line drug, particularly if long-term treatment is likely. **Gabapentin** in doses of up to 900mg t.d.s. is also an effective treatment, although it has only been studied in the short-term.[11,12]

More invasive treatments include IT **phenol**. This is neurotoxic and can cause urinary and faecal incontinence. The use of indwelling devices to deliver IT **baclofen** has largely replaced the use of **phenol**.[5,12]

Botulinum toxin (BTX) injections are largely reserved for treatment of contractures. The BTX-type A light chain acts as a zinc endopeptidase and interferes with acetylcholine release.[13] The toxin is injected into each spastic muscle separately and reduces spasticity in a dose-dependent manner.[14] Its use is rarely relevant in palliative care. It has been used for the management of drooling in people with neurodegenerative disorders, e.g. MND/ALS.

Box 10.A Quinine and cramp

A recent Cochrane review found moderate evidence that quinine is more effective than placebo in reducing the frequency and intensity of cramp at doses of 200–500mg/24h.[6]

Withdrawal rates because of undesirable effects were similar to placebo (1.5% vs. 1.4%). Less than 1/1,000 patients had a serious undesirable event (leucopenia, thrombocytopenia, severe rash, myalgia, severe nausea), all of which resolved on discontinuation.

Minor undesirable effects (quinine 13% vs. placebo 10%) were most commonly GI symptoms or headache.[6]

However, various regulatory agencies consider that, because alternatives are available, the risks associated with using quinine for cramp are generally unacceptably high:

- rare but serious undesirable effects:
  - ▹ thrombocytopenia, possibly leading to severe bleeding
  - ▹ haemolytic-uraemic syndrome, possibly leading to permanent renal damage
- toxicity in overdose resulting in permanent blindness or death
- serious drug interactions with, e.g. digoxin, warfarin.[7,8]

Consequently, the MHRA advises that quinine should not be used for nocturnal cramps unless the following criteria are all met:

- treatable causes have been ruled out
- non-pharmacological measures have failed[9]
- they regularly cause loss of sleep
- they are very painful or frequent.

If quinine is considered necessary, suitable doses are:

- quinine *sulphate* 200mg at bedtime, increased if necessary to 300mg at bedtime
- quinine *bisulphate* 300mg at bedtime.

During the early stages of treatment, patients should be monitored for signs of thrombocytopenia, e.g. unexplained petechiae, bruising or bleeding.

Treatment should be discontinued after 4 weeks if there is no benefit, and interrupted approximately every 3 months to re-evaluate benefit.[7,10]

Table 10.2 Oral drugs used to treat spasticity

Drug	*Starting dose*	*Maximum dose*	*Undesirable effects*	*Monitoring*	*Precautions*
Diazepam	5mg at bedtime	60mg/24h	Weakness, sedation, cognitive impairment, depression	Accumulation; prolonged halflife with cimetidine	Abrupt cessation may result in rebound anxiety and insomnia
Baclofen	5mg once daily–t.d.s.	20mg q.d.s.	Weakness, sedation, fatigue, dizziness, nausea, hepatotoxicity	LFTs	Abrupt cessation may result in agitation, psychosis and seizures
Tizanidine	2–4mg at bedtime	12mg t.d.s.	Drowsiness, dry mouth, dizziness, hepatotoxicity	LFTs	Do not use with antihypertensives or clonidine
Dantrolene	25mg once daily	100mg q.d.s.	Weakness, sedation, diarrhoea, hepatotoxicity	LFTs	

1 Zafonte R *et al.* (2004) Acute care management of post-TBI spasticity. *Journal of Head Trauma Rehabilitation.* **19**: 89–100.
2 Shakespeare DT *et al.* (2003) Anti-spasticity agents for multiple sclerosis. *Cochrane Database of Systematic Reviews.* **4**: CD001332.
3 Chou R *et al.* (2004) Comparative efficacy and safety of skeletal muscle relaxants for spasticity and musculoskeletal conditions: a systematic review. *Journal of Pain and Symptom Management.* **28**: 140–175.
4 Noth J and Fink GR (2004) Spasticity. In: R Voltz *et al.* (eds) *Palliative care in neurology* (No. 69). Oxford University Press, Oxford, p. 154.
5 Kita M and Goodkin D (2000) Drugs used to treat spasticity. *Drugs.* **59**: 487–495.
6 El Tawil S *et al.* (2010) Quinine for muscle cramps. *Cochrane Database of Systematic Reviews.* **12**: CD005044.
7 MHRA (2010) Quinine: not to be used routinely for nocturnal leg cramps. Drug Safety Update. **3 (June)**: 3–4. Available from: www.mhra.gov.uk/home/idcplg?IdcService=GET_FILE&dDocName=CON084657&RevisionSelectionMethod=LatestReleased
8 FDA (2010) Qualaquin (quinine sulfate): New Risk Evaluation and Mitigation Strategy — Risk of serious hematological reactions. Available from: www.fda.gov/Safety/MedWatch/SafetyInformation/SafetyAlertsforHumanMedicalProducts/ucm218424.htm
9 Twycross R *et al.* (2009) *Symptom Management in Advanced Cancer* (4e). palliativedrugs.com, Nottingham, pp. 273–276.
10 NHS (2010) Clinical Knowledge Summary. Leg cramps–unknown cause–management. Available from: www.cks.nhs.uk/leg_cramps/drugs_in_this_topic#-338896
11 Paisley S *et al.* (2002) Clinical effectiveness of oral treatments for spasticity in multiple sclerosis: a systematic review. *Multiple Sclerosis.* **8**: 319–329.
12 Royal College of Physicians (2004) Multiple Sclerosis: National clinical guidelines for diagnosis and management in primary and secondary care. Available from: http://bookshop.rcplondon.ac.uk/details.aspx?e = 13
13 Brin M (1997) Dosing, administration and a treatment algorithm for use of botulinum toxin A for adult-onset of spasticity. *Muscle and Nerve.* **20 (Suppl 6)**: 208–220.
14 Royal College of Physicians of London (2009) Spasticity in adults: management using botulinum toxin. National guidelines. Available from: http://bookshop.rcplondon.ac.uk/details.aspx?e = 272

BACLOFEN — BNF 10.2.2

Class: Skeletal muscle relaxant.

Indications: Spasticity ± painful flexor muscle spasms of voluntary (skeletal) muscle resulting from spinal or CNS lesions, †hiccup.

Contra-indications: PO: Peptic ulcer (baclofen stimulates gastric acid secretion). **IT:** treatment-resistant epilepsy.

Pharmacology

Baclofen is a chemical congener of the naturally occurring neurotransmitter, GABA.[1] It acts upon the GABA-receptor, inhibiting the release of the excitatory amino acids glutamate and aspartate, principally at the spinal level and also at supraspinal sites, thereby decreasing spasm in skeletal muscle.[2,3] It is preferable to **diazepam** for long-term use (e.g. in patients with chronic neurological disease such as multiple sclerosis) because it avoids the problem of **diazepam** dependence. Further, its use is not associated with tolerance; it retains its antispasmodic effects even after many years of continued use.[4] Baclofen relieves hiccup, possibly by a direct effect on the diaphragm.

Bio-availability >90% PO.
Onset of action 3–4 days.
Time to peak plasma concentration 0.5–3h.
Plasma halflife 3.5h; 4.5h in the elderly.
Duration of action 6–8h.[5]

Cautions

Withdrawal: abrupt withdrawal of PO baclofen may precipitate serious psychiatric reactions, e.g. agitation, confusion, hallucinations, paranoia, delusions, psychosis. Thus, discontinue by gradual dose reduction over 1–2 weeks, or longer if withdrawal symptoms occur.[6] Sudden withdrawal of IT baclofen or failure of the IT pump may lead to a potentially fatal withdrawal syndrome (see Box 21.A, p.684).

Use with caution in patients with severe psychiatric disorders, epilepsy, Parkinson's disease, respiratory impairment, stroke, history of peptic ulceration, liver disease (monitor LFTs), diabetes mellitus, hesitancy of micturition (may precipitate urinary retention), patients who use spasticity to maintain posture or to aid function. Drowsiness may affect skilled tasks and driving; effects of alcohol enhanced.

Renal impairment

Some patients treated with baclofen for spasticity have a low muscle mass, resulting in plasma creatinine concentrations which overestimate renal function. Because baclofen toxicity has been seen in patients with renal impairment, those with a GFR of 30–60mL/min/1.73m^2 should start with very low doses at long intervals and titrate to effect, and people with a GFR of $<$30mL/min/1.73m^2 should be prescribed an alternative drug (e.g. **tizanidine**, **dantrolene**).[7] However, advice on suitable doses and dose intervals in renal impairment varies:

- the *Renal Drug Handbook (3e)* advises:
  - ▹ for patients with creatinine clearance (Cl_{cr}) 10–20mL/min, start with 5mg b.d. and then titrate to response
  - ▹ for patients with Cl_{cr} $<$10mL/min, start with 5mg once daily then titrate to response[8]
- the manufacturer's SPC states that signs of overdose have been seen in renal patients taking $>$5mg once daily, and thus advises:
  - ▹ 5mg once daily for patients with renal impairment (degree not stated) or undergoing regular haemodialysis
  - ▹ baclofen should be used in patients with end-stage renal disease (CKD stage 5; GFR $<$15mL/min) only if benefit outweighs risk, and with close monitoring for signs of overdose, e.g. drowsiness, lethargy.

Note: the starting dose intervals and titration steps given in Dose and use below are more conservative than those in the SPC.

Undesirable effects

Very common (>10%): sedation, drowsiness, nausea.
Common (<10%, >1%): dizziness, fatigue, muscle hypotonia, pain or weakness, ataxia, tremor, insomnia, headache, visual disturbances, nystagmus, psychiatric disturbances, hypotension, respiratory depression, dry mouth, vomiting, constipation or diarrhoea, urinary frequency or incontinence, dysuria, hyperhidrosis, rash.
Uncommon, rare or very rare (<1%, >0.001%): paradoxical increase in spasticity, seizures (particularly in known epileptics), joint pain, hypothermia, paraesthesia, taste disturbance, abdominal pain, hepatic impairment, urinary retention, impotence.

Dose and use

PO starting doses are the same for muscle spasm, spasticity and hiccup:

- start with 5mg b.d.–t.d.s., preferably p.c.
- increase if necessary by 5mg b.d.–t.d.s. every 3 days but more slowly if troublesome undesirable effects, particularly in the elderly
- effective doses for hiccup are often relatively low, e.g. 5–10mg t.d.s., although it may be necessary to increase the dose to 20mg t.d.s.
- for spasticity, the effective dose is generally $\leqslant$20mg t.d.s. (maximum 100mg/24h)
- effective doses for muscle spasm fall somewhere in the middle.

With spasticity, if no improvement with maximum tolerated dose after 6 weeks, *withdraw gradually over 1–2 weeks.*

An undesirable degree of hypotonia may occur, but can generally be relieved by reducing the daytime dose and increasing the evening dose.

An IT injection is available for specialist use in patients with severe chronic spasticity in whom PO treatment is ineffective or poorly tolerated (see Spinal analgesia, p.681).

Supply

Baclofen (generic)
Tablets (scored) 10mg, 28 days @ 5mg t.d.s. = £1.
Oral solution 5mg/5mL, 28 days @ 5mg t.d.s. = £14.

Lioresal® (Novartis)
Tablets (scored) 10mg, 28 days @ 5mg t.d.s. = £4.50.
Oral solution (sugar-free) 5mg/5mL, 28 days @ 5mg t.d.s. = £10; *raspberry flavoured.*
****IT injection*** 50microgram/mL, 1mL amp (for test dose) = £2; 500microgram/mL, 20mL amp (for use in implantable pump) = £49; 2mg/mL, 5mL amp (for use with implantable pump) = £49.

1 Zafonte R *et al.* (2004) Acute care management of post-TBI spasticity. *Journal of Head Trauma Rehabilitation.* **19**: 89–100.
2 Guelaud C *et al.* (1995) Baclofen therapy for chronic hiccup. *European Respiratory Journal.* **8**: 235–237.
3 Ramirez FC and Graham DY (1992) Treatment of intractable hiccup with baclofen: results of a double-blind randomized, controlled, crossover study. *American Journal of Gastroenterology.* **87**: 1789–1791.
4 Gaillard JM (1977) Comparison of two muscle relaxant drugs on human sleep: diazepam and parachlorophenylgaba. *Acta Psychiatrica Belgica.* **77**: 410–425.
5 Kochak GM *et al.* (1985) The pharmacokinetics of baclofen derived from intestinal infusion. *Clinical Pharmacology and Therapeutics.* **38**: 251–257.
6 CSM (Committee on Safety of Medicines and Medicines Control Agency) (1997) Reminder! Severe withdrawal reactions with baclofen can be prevented by gradual dose reduction. *Current Problems in Pharmacovigilance.* **23**: 6.
7 Su W *et al.* (2009) Reduced level of consciousness from baclofen in people with low kidney function. *British Medical Journal.* **339**: b4559.
8 Ashley C and Currie A (2009) *The Renal Drug Handbook* (3e). Radcliffe Publishing Ltd, Oxford.

DANTROLENE SODIUM — BNF 10.2.2

Class: Skeletal muscle relaxant.

Indications: Chronic severe spasticity of skeletal muscle.

Contra-indications: Hepatic impairment, particularly active liver disease, e.g. hepatitis or cirrhosis (may cause severe liver damage); acute muscle spasm or where spasm is useful in maintaining posture, balance or walking.

Pharmacology

Unlike **baclofen** and **diazepam**, dantrolene acts directly on skeletal muscle by binding to ryanodine receptors, thereby reducing the amount of intracellular calcium available for contraction.[1] It produces fewer central undesirable effects than **baclofen** and **diazepam** and, if necessary, can be used concurrently with these drugs in an attempt to produce a better balance between muscle relaxation and undesirable effects, e.g. unacceptable drowsiness.[2]
Bio-availability 35% PO.
Onset of action up to 1 week.
Time to peak plasma concentration up to 3h.
Plasma halflife 5–9h.
Duration of action no data.

Cautions

Compromised pulmonary function, particularly COPD; predisposition to or actual cardiovascular impairment. Drowsiness may affect the performance of skilled tasks, e.g. driving; effects of alcohol enhanced.

Because of the risk of hepatotoxicity with long-term use, discontinue if no benefit is observed after 6 weeks of treatment. Perform LFTs before starting treatment and then at regular intervals, e.g. monthly, throughout treatment; if possible, avoid concurrent use of other hepatotoxic drugs.

Undesirable effects

Transient drowsiness, dizziness, muscle weakness, diarrhoea. Severe hepatotoxicity develops rarely, generally after 1–6 months, and is more likely in people over 30 years old, women (particularly those taking oral contraceptives), and with doses >400mg/24h. Fatalities have occurred only with doses >200mg/24h.[3,4]

Dose and use

The dose of dantrolene should be built up slowly:

- start with 25mg once daily
- initially increase by no more than 25mg/24h weekly
- above 100mg/24h, larger increments are permissible (see SPC)
- usual effective dose 75mg t.d.s.
- maximum recommended dose 100mg q.d.s.

Supply

Dantrium® (SpePharm)
Capsules 25mg, 100mg, 28 days @ 75mg t.d.s. = £43.

1 Zafonte R *et al.* (2004) Acute care management of post-TBI spasticity. *Journal of Head Trauma Rehabilitation.* **19**: 89–100.
2 Krause T *et al.* (2004) Dantrolene–a review of its pharmacology, therapeutic use and new developments. *Anaesthesia.* **59**: 364–373.
3 Utili R *et al.* (1977) Dantrolene-associated hepatic injury. Incidence and character. *Gastroenterology.* **72**: 610–616.
4 Wilkinson S *et al.* (1979) Hepatitis from dantrolene sodium. *Gut.* **20**: 33–36.

TIZANIDINE — BNF 10.2.2

Class: Skeletal muscle relaxant.

Indications: Spasticity in multiple sclerosis, spinal cord injury or disease.

Contra-indications: Severe hepatic impairment, patients for whom spasm is useful in maintaining posture, balance or walking, concurrent use with potent CYP1A2 inhibitors, e.g. **ciprofloxacin**, **fluvoxamine**.

Pharmacology

Tizanidine, like **clonidine**, is a central α_2 agonist within the CNS at supraspinal and spinal levels.[1] It inhibits spinal polysynaptic reflex activity. This reduces the sympathetic outflow which in turn reduces muscle tone. Tizanidine has no direct effect on skeletal muscle, neuromuscular junctions or monosynaptic spinal reflexes. Tizanidine reduces pathologically increased muscle tone, including resistance to passive movements, and alleviates painful spasms and clonus.[2] In spasticity, tizanidine is comparable in efficacy to **diazepam** and **baclofen**,[3] and has superior tolerability.[4]

Tizanidine is well absorbed but undergoes extensive first-pass metabolism in the liver to inactive metabolites which are mostly excreted by the kidneys. Wide interindividual variability in the effective plasma concentration means that the optimal dose must be titrated slowly over 2–4 weeks. Maximum effects occur within 2h of administration.[5]

Bio-availability 40% PO.
Onset of action 1–2h; peak response 8 weeks.
Time to peak plasma concentration 1.5h.
Plasma halflife 2.5h; up to 14h ± 10h in renal failure.[6]
Duration of action 'relatively short' (manufacturer's SPC).

Cautions

Renal impairment; elderly; concurrent administration with drugs which prolong the QT interval; concurrent administration with hypotensive drugs or **digoxin** which may potentiate hypotension or bradycardia.

LFTs should be monitored monthly for the first 4 months; discontinue if liver enzymes remain persistently > 3 times the upper limit of normal. Avoid abrupt withdrawal, particularly after long-term use or high doses (risk of rebound hypertension and tachycardia); monitor blood pressure during withdrawal. Drowsiness may affect performance of skilled tasks, e.g. driving; effects of alcohol enhanced.

Drug interactions

Tizanidine plasma concentrations are increased by CYP1A2 inhibitors, potentially leading to severe hypotension. Thus, avoid concurrent use with potent CYP1A2 inhibitors, e.g. **ciprofloxacin** (and possibly **enoxacin** (not UK)), **fluvoxamine**, and use with caution with moderately strong inhibitors, e.g. **norfloxacin, oestrogens, progestogens.**[7]

Undesirable effects

Drowsiness, weakness and dry mouth in more than two thirds of those taking it,[8] although drowsiness and weakness may be less than with **diazepam** and **baclofen**.[9] Hypotension and dizziness, nausea and other GI disturbances. Less frequently insomnia, bradycardia, hallucinations and hepatotoxicity.

Dose and use

- start with 2mg once daily
- if necessary, increase by 2mg every 3–4 days
- doses above 2mg/24h should be divided, and given b.d.–q.d.s.
- effective dose generally ≤24mg/24h, in 3–4 divided doses
- maximum recommended dose 36mg/24h.

A slow titration helps to reduce undesirable effects. Elderly patients and those with severe renal impairment (creatinine clearance <30mL/min) should undergo an even slower titration. Because of the prolonged plasma halflife, slow titration with a *single* daily dose is recommended by the manufacturer.

Supply

Tizanidine (generic)
Tablets 2mg, 4mg, 28 days @ 8mg t.d.s. = £21.

Zanaflex® (Cephalon)
Tablets 2mg, 4mg, 28 days @ 8mg t.d.s = £112.

1 Zafonte R *et al.* (2004) Acute care management of post-TBI spasticity. *Journal of Head Trauma Rehabilitation*. **19**: 89–100.
2 Wallace J (1994) Summary of combined clinical analysis of controlled clinical trials with tizanidine. *Neurology*. **44 (11 suppl 9)**: s60–s69.
3 Lataste X *et al.* (1994) Comparative profile of tizanidine in the management of spasticity. *Neurology*. **44 (11 suppl 9)**: s53–s59.
4 Kamen L *et al.* (2008) A practical overview of tizanidine use for spasticity secondary to multiple sclerosis, stroke, and spinal cord injury. *Current Medical Research and Opinion*. **24**: 425–439.
5 Wagstaff A and Bryson H (1997) Tizanidine. A review of its pharmacology, clinical efficacy and tolerability in the management of spasticity associated with cerebral and spinal disorders. *Drugs*. **53**: 435–452.
6 Keyser E and Ohnhaus E (1986) *Data on file*. Pharmacokinetic study with Sirdalud (tizanidine, DS 103–282) in patients with renal insufficiency.
7 Baxter K (ed) (2010) Stockley's Drug Interactions (online edition). The Pharmaceutical Press, London. Available from: www.medicinescomplete.com
8 Nance P *et al.* (1997) Relationship of the antispasticity effect of tizanidine to plasma concentration in patients with multiple sclerosis. *Archives of Neurology*. **54**: 731–736.
9 Smith H and Barton A (2000) Tizanidine in the management of spasticity and musculoskeletal complaints in the palliative care population. *American Journal of Hospice and Palliative Care*. **17**: 50–58.

11: EAR, NOSE AND OROPHARYNX

MOUTHWASHES — BNF 12.3.4

Mouthwashes can cleanse and freshen the mouth. Generally, a tepid saline solution or **compound sodium chloride mouthwash BP** is probably as beneficial as any other type of mouthwash. Mouth swabs containing **glycerol** (glycerine) should *not* be used because **glycerol** tends to have a drying effect.[1]

Chlorhexidine inhibits the formation of plaque on teeth, and is useful when toothbrushing is not possible. It does not remove established plaque, which should be removed by professional dental cleaning. **Chlorhexidine** is also used to prevent/treat various oral infections (e.g. periodontal disease, oral candidosis),[2,3] and to sterilize dentures and other prostheses.[4] Because it has a prolonged duration of action, it generally needs to be used only b.d. **Chlorhexidine** can stain the teeth (and tongue), and this can be exacerbated by drinking tea and coffee; this staining can be removed by professional dental cleaning. Most brands of **chlorhexidine** mouthwash contain alcohol which may cause discomfort. Diluting the mouthwash with an equal amount of water may help reduce the discomfort.[4] Curasept ADS 220® is alcohol-free; it is not currently available on NHS prescriptions, but can be bought from dentists or via internet shopping sites.

Because **chlorhexidine** binds to **nystatin** and leads to inactivation of both drugs, **chlorhexidine** mouthwash should *not* be used at the same time as **nystatin** oral suspension.[5] The problem can be overcome if **chlorhexidine** is used ≥30min before **nystatin**.

Hydrogen peroxide mouthwash is used as a non-specific cleansing agent; the 'frothing' action of the mouthwash encourages disintegration of oral debris. **Hydrogen peroxide** is also used in the treatment of certain types of periodontal disease (involving anaerobic organisms). **Ascorbic acid** (vitamin C) effervescent tablets can also be used for debriding the tongue (see p.540) but should not be used in patients with a sore mouth. Pineapple contains a proteolytic enzyme, ananase, and can also used to clean a coated mouth.[6,7] Any form of pineapple can be used except pineapple tinned in *syrup* because the syrup destroys the ananase. Pineapple is unsuitable for patients with an inflamed or ulcerated mouth because the juice is acidic.

Sodium bicarbonate mouthwash has been advocated as a symptomatic treatment for oral mucositis.[8]

Supply and use

For liquid mouthwashes, rinse the mouth with the recommended volume for about 30–60sec, and then spit out.

Saline solution

Add 1 heaped teaspoonful of table salt to a glass of tepid water and stir well to dissolve. Use p.r.n.

Sodium chloride mouthwash, compound BP

Mouthwash containing **sodium chloride** 1.5%, **sodium bicarbonate** 1% in peppermint-flavoured chloroform water; can be prepared locally. Dilute 15mL with an equal volume of warm water and use p.r.n.

Chlorhexidine gluconate (generic)

Mouthwash 0.2%, 300mL = £2. Use 10mL undiluted or diluted with an equal volume of water b.d.

Corsodyl® (GSK Consumer Healthcare)
Mouthwash 0.2%, 300mL = £2, 600mL = £4; *original or mint flavour.* Use 10mL undiluted or diluted with an equal volume of water b.d.
Oral spray 0.2%, 60mL = £4; *mint flavour.* Spray on to tooth and gum surfaces, using up to 12 actuations b.d.
Dental gel 1%, 50g = £1. Use as a toothpaste b.d.

Curasept ADS 220® (Curaprox)
Mouthwash 0.2%, 200mL, can be bought from dentists or internet shopping sites, recommended retail price = £4.50; *alcohol-free.*

Hydrogen peroxide
Peroxyl® (Colgate Palmolive)
Mouthwash 1.5%, 300mL = £3.50. Use 10mL undiluted after meals and at bedtime.

1 Poland JM *et al.* (1987) Comparing Moi-Stir to lemon-glycerin swabs. *American Journal of Nursing.* **87**: 422–424.
2 Chow A (2010) Oral bacterial infections. In: AN Davies and JB Epstein (eds) *Oral Complications of Cancer and its Management.* Oxford University Press, Oxford, pp. 185–193.
3 Finlay I and Davies A (2005) Fungal Infections. In: A Davies and I Finlay (eds) *Oral Care in Advanced Disease.* Oxford University Press, Oxford, pp. 55–71.
4 Sweeney P (2005) Oral hygiene. In: A Davies and I Finlay (eds) *Oral Care in Advanced Disease.* Oxford University Press, Oxford, pp. 21–35.
5 Barkvoll P and Attramadal A (1989) Effect of nystatin and chlorhexidine digluconate on Candida albicans. *Oral Surgery Oral Medicine and Oral Pathology.* **67**: 279–281.
6 Regnard C *et al.* (1997) Mouth care, skin care, and lymphoedema. *British Medical Journal.* **315**: 1002–1005.
7 Twycross RG *et al.* (2009) *Symptom Management in Advanced Cancer.* (4e). palliativedrugs.com Ltd., Nottingham, pp. 64–65.
8 National Cancer Institute (2010) Oral complications of chemotherapy and head/neck radiation (PDQ). Available from: www.cancer.gov/cancertopics/pdq/supportivecare/oralcomplications/

ARTIFICIAL SALIVA AND TOPICAL SALIVA STIMULANTS — BNF 12.3.5

Dry mouth (xerostomia) is managed by saliva stimulants or substitutes. Although 99% of saliva is water, the remaining 1% comprises a wide range of electrolytes and molecules which are important for saliva's many roles, e.g. lubricant, cleansing, antimicrobial, taste, digestion, buffering, and mineralization of teeth.[1] This may explain why sipping water, iced drinks or sucking ice chips gives only short-lived relief.

Artificial saliva is a poor substitute for natural saliva. Thus, *unless a main salivary duct is blocked*, a saliva stimulant is preferable. Chewing gum acts as a saliva stimulant and is as effective as, and preferred to, **mucin**-based artificial saliva.[2] The gum should be sugar-free and, in patients with dentures, low-tack, e.g. Orbit®.

If dry mouth remains a problem, an alternative topical saliva stimulant can be tried, e.g. Salivix® or SST® (acidic; use with caution, see below). However, in some patients, **pilocarpine** or **bethanechol** should be considered (see p.572). For patients who do not respond to or cannot tolerate saliva stimulants, artificial saliva is an option, e.g. AS Saliva Orthana®, Biotène Oralbalance® or BioXtra®.

The ideal artificial saliva should be easy to use, pleasant, effective and well tolerated.[3] Further, it should have a neutral pH (to prevent demineralization of the teeth), and contain fluoride (to enhance remineralization of the teeth).[4] Acidic products also predispose to certain oral infections (e.g. dental caries, oral candidosis). Some products contain **lactoperoxidase** which, in natural saliva, enhances the production of hypothiocyanite, an antibacterial ion. Thus, theoretically, **lactoperoxidase** could enhance the effect of artificial saliva. However, there is no evidence that this is the case.

Generally, RCTs indicate that **mucin**-based products are better tolerated and more effective than cellulose-based ones, e.g. **carboxymethylcellulose (carmellose)**,[5–7] with some patients finding cellulose-based products no better than frequent sips of fluid. The **mucin** comes from the stomach of pigs, and this may be an issue for some patients (e.g. Jews, Muslims, vegetarians). There is no good evidence that gels are more effective/last longer than sprays.

Undesirable effects

Unpleasant taste, irritation of the mouth, nausea and/or diarrhoea in ≥30% of patients.[2,8]

Dose and use

PCF regards sugar-free chewing gum as the saliva stimulant of choice for most patients. For patients with dentures, it should be low-tack, e.g. Orbit®.

Artificial salivas with a neutral pH are preferred for long-term use by *PCF*. Artificial salivas or topical saliva stimulants with an acidic pH should be avoided in dentate patients (demineralization of teeth) or in those with stomatitis/mucositis (increased pain). Acidic products also predispose to dental caries and oral candidosis.

The duration of effect of artificial salivas is relatively short, due to a combination of swallowing and evaporation. Thus, artificial salivas and topical saliva stimulants may need to be taken every 30–60min, and also before (and sometimes during) meals. Proprietary artificial salivas include:

- **mucin**-based sprays and lozenges (AS Saliva Orthana®); neutral pH
- **hydroxyethylcellulose**-based gels containing **lactoperoxidase** (Biotène Oralbalance®, BioXtra®); neutral pH.

Proprietary topical saliva stimulants include:

- pastilles containing **malic acid** and **acacia** gum (Salivix®); acidic pH
- orodispersible tablets containing **citric** and **malic acids**, with a calcium buffer to attempt to prevent demineralization of teeth (SST®); avoid if salivary duct blocked; acidic pH.

AS Saliva Orthana®, Salivix® pastilles and **lactoperoxidase** gels are classified in the UK as borderline substances and have ACBS approval for dry mouth associated with radiotherapy or sicca syndrome. The prescriber must endorse an NHS FP10 prescription for one of these products with 'ACBS', otherwise the Prescription Pricing Authority will investigate whether it has been issued for an approved indication. SST® is licensed for patients with salivary gland impairment but patent salivary ducts.

Supply

Topical saliva stimulants

Salivix® (Galen)

Pastilles (sugar-free) containing **malic acid** and **acacia** gum, 50 = £3.50.

SST® (Medac)

Tablets orodispersible (sugar-free) containing **citric acid** and **malic acid** in a sorbitol base, 100 = £5.

Artificial saliva products

AS Saliva Orthana® (AS Pharma)

Oral spray containing gastric **mucin** (porcine) 3.5%, xylitol 2%, sodium fluoride 4.2mg/L, 50mL bottle = £5; 450mL refill = £34.

Lozenges containing gastric **mucin** (porcine) 65mg, xylitol 59mg in a sorbitol base, 30 = £3.50.

Biotène Oralbalance® (GSK)

Saliva replacement gel containing **lactoperoxidase**, lactoferrin, lysozyme, glucose oxidase, 50g = £4, 24 x 12.4mL tubes (for hospital use) = £30.

Mouth moisturizing liquid containing **lactoperoxidase**, lactoferrin, lysozyme, glucose oxidase, calcium, 45mL spray bottle = £7.

BioXtra® (RIS Products)

Saliva replacement gel containing **lactoperoxidase**, lactoferrin, lysozyme, 40mL tube = £4, 50mL spray = £4.

Chewing gum containing **lactoperoxidase**, lactoferrin, lysozyme, 20-piece pack = £4.

1 Davies A (2005) Salivary gland dysfunction. In: A Davies and I Finlay (eds) *Oral Care in Advanced Disease*. Oxford University Press, Oxford, pp. 97–114.

2 Davies AN (2000) A comparison of artificial saliva and chewing gum in the management of xerostomia in patients with advanced cancer. *Palliative Medicine*. **14**: 197–203.

3 Epstein JB and Stevenson-Moore P (1992) A clinical comparative trial of saliva substitutes in radiation-induced salivary gland hypofunction. *Special Care Dentistry.* **12**: 21–23.
4 Davies A (2010) Salivary gland dysfunction. In: AN Davies and JB Epstein (eds) *Oral Complications of Cancer and its Management.* Oxford University Press, Oxford, pp. 203–223.
5 S'Gravenmade E *et al.* (1974) The effect of mucin-containing artificial saliva on severe xerostomia. *International Journal of Oral Surgery.* **3**: 435–439.
6 Vissink A *et al.* (1983) A clinical comparison between commercially available mucin- and CMC-containing saliva substitutes. *International Journal of Oral Surgery.* **12**: 232–238.
7 Visch L *et al.* (1986) A double-blind crossover trial of CMC- and mucin-containing saliva substitutes. *International Journal of Oral and Maxillofacial Surgery.* **15**: 395–400.
8 Davies A *et al.* (1998) A comparison of artificial saliva and pilocarpine in the management of xerostomia in patients with advanced cancer. *Palliative Medicine.* **12**: 105–111.

PILOCARPINE — BNF 11.6 & 12.3.5

Class: Parasympathomimetic.

Indications: Xerostomia (dry mouth) after radiotherapy for head and neck cancer, dry mouth (and dry eyes) in Sjögren's syndrome and †drug-induced dry mouth.

Contra-indications: Intestinal or urinary obstruction, or when increased intestinal or urinary tract motility could be harmful (e.g. after recent surgery); asthma; when miosis could be harmful (e.g. narrow-angle glaucoma, acute iritis).

Pharmacology

Pilocarpine is a parasympathomimetic (predominantly muscarinic) drug with mild β-adrenergic activity which stimulates secretion from exocrine glands, including salivary glands.[1] A systematic review suggests that 40–50% of patients with radiotherapy-induced dry mouth respond to pilocarpine, with a time to response of up to 12 weeks.[2] However, undesirable effects are common, and were the main reason for withdrawal from studies (6–15% of patients taking 5mg t.d.s.).

About 90% of patients with drug-induced dry mouth respond to pilocarpine with benefit seen within 24h.[3] In an RCT, half of the patients preferred pilocarpine because it was more effective, and half preferred the comparator **mucin**-based artificial saliva, mainly because it was a spray and not a tablet.[3] Undesirable effects were much more common in patients receiving pilocarpine (84% vs. 22%), which resulted in a quarter of the patients withdrawing from the study. Alternatives to pilocarpine are used at some centres, e.g. **bethanechol**.[4–6] However, generally topical measures should be tried before resorting to a parasympathomimetic (see p.570).

Bio-availability 96% PO.
Onset of action 20min (drug-induced dry mouth); up to 3 months (after radiation).
Time to peak plasma concentration 1h.
Plasma halflife 1h.
Duration of action 3–5h (single dose).

Cautions

Pilocarpine may antagonize the effects of antimuscarinic drugs, e.g. inhaled **ipratropium bromide**. Concurrent use with β antagonists (β-blockers) may cause cardiac conduction disturbances.

Cognitive or psychiatric disorder, epilepsy, parkinsonism. Miosis may affect vision and driving ability, particularly at night. Cardiovascular disease (changes in haemodynamics or heart rhythm), hyperthyroidism, COPD (increased bronchial smooth muscle tone, airway resistance and bronchial secretions). Peptic ulcer (increased acid secretion), gallstones or biliary tract disease (increased biliary smooth muscle contraction). Mild–moderate hepatic impairment (reduce dose); avoid in severe hepatic impairment (no human data on metabolism and excretion). Renal impairment (no reliable human data on metabolism and excretion), kidney stones (potential for renal colic). Increased sweating may exacerbate dehydration in patients unable to drink sufficient fluids.

Undesirable effects

Very common (>10%): headache, flu-like syndrome, nausea, urinary frequency, sweating.
Common (<10%, >1%): dizziness, asthenia, chills, blurred vision, eye pain, conjunctivitis, flushing, palpitations, hypertension (after initial hypotension), rhinitis, abdominal pain, dyspepsia, vomiting, diarrhoea or constipation, rash, pruritus.

Dose and use

Pilocarpine should generally be used only when topical measures are insufficient (see p.570). In drug-induced dry mouth, the effective dose is generally 5mg t.d.s. or less, whereas after radiotherapy the effective dose is generally 5–10mg t.d.s.:

- start with 5mg t.d.s. with meals or 4mg if using eyedrop formulation; this is 2 drops of a 4% solution (see comment about cost in Supply)
- the last dose of the day should be taken with the evening meal
- if necessary and if tolerated, increase the dose after 2 days if the dry mouth is drug-induced, and after 4 weeks if radiation-induced
- maximum dose 10mg t.d.s.
- if no improvement, stop after 4 days if the dry mouth is drug-induced, and after 12 weeks if radiation-induced.

In patients with mild–moderate hepatic impairment start on a lower dose, e.g. 5mg once daily, and work up to 5mg t.d.s. if well tolerated.

If **bethanechol** is used instead for drug-induced dry mouth:

- start with 25mg t.d.s. 30min a.c.
- reduce dose to 10mg t.d.s. if patients experience excessive salivation.

Undesirable effects are similar to pilocarpine but generally less severe, either because the equivalent dose is less or the muscarinic receptor binding pattern of **bethanechol** is different.

Supply

Note: **Bethanechol** tablets are cheaper than pilocarpine tablets. However, it is cheaper still to give pilocarpine *eyedrops* PO. The use of the eyedrops in this way is off label.

Pilocarpine (generic)
Eyedrops 4% (40mg/1mL), 10mL lasts 33 days @ 2 drops/4mg PO t.d.s. = £3.50.

Salagen® (Novartis)
Tablets 5mg, 28 days @ 5mg t.d.s. = £51.

Bethanechol
Myotonine® (Glenwood)
Tablets 10mg, 25mg, 28 days @ 25mg t.d.s. = £5.

1 Anonymous (1994) Oral pilocarpine for xerostomia. *Medical Letter on Drugs and Therapeutics*. **36**: 76.
2 Davies A and Shorthose K (2007) Parasympathomimetic drugs for the treatment of salivary gland dysfunction due to radiotherapy. *Cochrane Database of Systematic Reviews*. CD003782.
3 Davies A *et al.* (1998) A comparison of artificial saliva and pilocarpine in the management of xerostomia in patients with advanced cancer. *Palliative Medicine*. **12**: 105–111.
4 Everett H (1975) The use of bethanechol chloride with tricyclic antidepressants. *American Journal of Psychiatry*. **132**: 1202–1204.
5 Epstein J *et al.* (1994) A clinical trial of bethanechol in patients with xerostomia after radiotherapy. A pilot study. *Oral Surgery, Oral Medicine and Oral Pathology*. **77**: 610–614.
6 Davies A (2005) Salivary gland dysfunction. In: A Davies and I Finlay (eds) *Oral Care in Advanced Disease*. Oxford University Press, Oxford, pp. 97–114.

DRUGS FOR ORAL INFLAMMATION AND ULCERATION BNF 12.3.1

'Oral stomatitis' is a term applied to diffuse inflammatory, erosive and ulcerative conditions affecting the mucous membranes of the mouth, whereas 'oral mucositis' tends to be restricted to stomatitis caused by local radiotherapy, chemotherapy or other anti-cancer modalities.

The causes of oral ulceration include trauma (physical, chemical), recurrent aphthous ulceration, infection, cancer, skin conditions, nutritional deficiencies, GI conditions, haematopoietic disorders and drug treatment. It is important to determine the cause so that, if appropriate, specific treatment is given as well as symptomatic treatment. For example, ill-fitting dentures which cause traumatic ulceration (and/or mucosal hyperplasia) should be relined, or ideally replaced.[1]

Management strategy

The symptomatic management of oral inflammation and ulceration involves measures which:

- maintain oral hygiene
- relieve the pain
- protect ulcerated mucosa
- treat secondary infection
- reduce the inflammation.

Advice should be sought from an oral medicine specialist if unexplained ulceration persists for >3 weeks.

Maintain oral hygiene

Simple mouthwashes, e.g. water or 0.9% **saline**, can be soothing, help to maintain oral hygiene, and prevent secondary infection (see p.569). The temperature of the mouthwash appears to be important, with tepid ones being more soothing than cold or warm ones.

Pain relief

Topical and systemic analgesics are used.

Topical analgesics

Topical analgesics include local anaesthetics, NSAIDs (e.g. **benzydamine**, **choline salicylate**), opioids (e.g. **morphine**); and also **diphenhydramine**[2] and **doxepin**.[3]

The efficacy of topical local anaesthetics relates to the formulation, duration of application (at least 5min is required) and site of application. They are less effective in more keratinized areas of the mouth, e.g. the palate.[4] Some systemic absorption of the local anaesthetic occurs, which is increased by mucosal inflammation. However, plasma levels are generally low, and toxicity has been reported only in exceptional circumstances (see p.61).

With all topical local anaesthetics care must be taken not to produce anaesthesia of the pharynx before meals because this might lead to choking and aspiration:

- **lidocaine** ointment 5% (has a water miscible base), applied a.c. and p.r.n.
- **lidocaine** spray 10%, applied thinly to the ulcer using a cotton bud a.c. and p.r.n.
- various OTC products.

Benzydamine is an NSAID with local anaesthetic and antimicrobial effects. It is available as an oral rinse or spray, and can ease the discomfort associated with various causes of oral stomatitis, including local radiotherapy. **Choline salicylate** dental gel is a weak analgesic, and excessive usage or confinement under a denture can result in oral irritation and/or ulceration. Other related options include **diclofenac** dispersible tablets and **flurbiprofen** lozenges (can also result in oral ulceration):

- **benzydamine** 0.15% oral rinse (Difflam®), rinse or gargle 15mL for 20–30sec before spitting out, repeat q3h–q1.5h p.r.n. Dilute with an equal volume of water if the full-strength oral rinse causes stinging[5]
- **choline salicylate** 8.7% oral gel (e.g. Bonjela®), apply 1–2cm by gentle massage q3h p.r.n.; maximum recommended dose 6 applications/day.

Opioids have a topical analgesic effect on inflamed tissue and can be used as a mouthwash. Some recommend that the mouthwash is subsequently swallowed in order to combine a systemic analgesic effect with the topical one:

- locally prepared **morphine sulphate** 0.2% (2mg/mL) solution, take 10mg in 5mL q4h–q3h, hold in the mouth for 2min *and then spit out or swallow*; some patients need higher doses, occasionally 30mg q4h–q3h[6,7]

- locally prepared **morphine sulphate** 1–5mg/mL gel, initially 3mL q8h–q4h, hold in mouth for 10min *and then spit out or swallow* (see p.366).

Systemic analgesics

Systemic analgesics include non-opioids and opioids given as for other pains, balancing benefit against undesirable effects. For severe mucositis (patient unable to eat ± unable to drink) with inadequate pain relief from topical measures, a parenteral opioid should be administered either by patient-controlled analgesia, or continuous infusion with boluses as required. **Ketamine** is also of benefit in this situation.[8] Chemotherapy patients often have a permanent IV access, and ideally this should be used for administering parenteral analgesics.

Protect the ulcerated areas

Coating agents are of limited value. They can be difficult to apply, and they do not relieve persistent pain caused by oral inflammation. However, by adhering to and coating the denuded surface, they may help to reduce contact pain, e.g. from eating or drinking. Available agents include:

- **carmellose (carboxymethylcellulose) sodium** (Orabase® paste, Orahesive® powder) apply the paste to, or sprinkle the powder onto, the sore area p.c.
- **polyvinylpyrrolidine** and **sodium hyaluronate** oral gel (Gelclair®) t.d.s. p.r.n.; mix contents of 1 sachet with 40mL water, rinse around mouth for at least 1min, gargle and then spit out
- **sucralfate** is *not* of benefit in radiation-induced oral mucositis,[9] but may help in other types of oral stomatitis; it can be given in a suspension 1g/5mL q.d.s.

Treat secondary infection

Consider the use of **chlorhexidine** mouthwash; ideally, this should be alcohol-free, although the alcohol-free formulation is not currently available on NHS prescriptions (see p.570).

Reduce the inflammation

Topical corticosteroids are useful in the management of certain types of oral ulceration, e.g. recurrent aphthous ulceration (see Box 11.A). However, corticosteroids do *not* feature in the management of oral mucositis. Systemic corticosteroids are generally reserved for severe ulcerative conditions, e.g. pemphigus vulgaris.

Box 11.A Treatment of aphthous ulcers

Corticosteroids

Corticosteroids are useful for recurrent attacks. Use as soon as symptoms/ulcers appear; avoid in oral infections:

- hydrocortisone oromucosal tablets 2.5mg q.d.s. for up to 5 days; tablets are placed at the site of the ulcers and left to dissolve
- beclometasone aerosol inhaler 50 or 100microgram sprayed into the mouth b.d., when a more potent corticosteroid is needed for difficult-to-reach sites such as the soft palate and oropharynx (unlicensed indication)
- betamethasone soluble tablets 500microgram, dispersed in 20mL water and rinsed around the mouth q.d.s.; also suitable when a more potent corticosteroid is needed for difficult-to-reach sites (unlicensed indication).

Antiseptic and antibacterial mouthwashes

Useful when there are multiple ulcers and when not accessible to covering pastes, e.g.:

- chlorhexidine gluconate mouthwash 0.2%, ideally alcohol-free (see p.570)
- doxycycline suspension 100mg in 10mL q.d.s. for 3 days (prepared by mixing the contents of a capsule with a small quantity of water); rinse around the mouth for 2–3min and then spit out (unlicensed indication)
- in some countries, tetracycline suspension 250mg in 10mL[10] or minocycline suspension 10mg in 5mL[11] are used instead.

Supply
The following list is selective.

Topical analgesics
Lidocaine (generic)
Ointment 5% in a water-miscible base, 15g = £1.

Xylocaine® (AstraZeneca)
Spray 10%, 50mL = £3. Apply thinly to ulcer using cotton bud (unlicensed indication).

Benzydamine
Difflam® (3M)
Oral rinse (mouthwash) 0.15%, 200mL = £2.50, 300mL = £4.
Oromucosal spray 0.15%, 30mL = £3.

Choline salicylate dental gel BP
Bonjela® (Reckitt Benckiser)
Oral gel 8.7%, 15g = £2; also available OTC.

Diclofenac
Voltarol® (Novartis)
Tablets dispersible 50mg, 28 days @ 50mg t.d.s. = £25.

Flurbiprofen
Strefen® (Reckitt Benckiser)
Lozenges 8.75mg, 16 = £2.

Morphine
Mouthwash 0.2% (2mg/mL in water), locally prepared.
Oral gel 0.1–0.5% (1–5mg/mL), locally prepared.

Coating agents
Orabase® (ConvaTec)
Oral paste containing **carmellose sodium** 16.7%, **gelatin** 16.7% and **pectin** 16.7%, 30g = £2, 100g = £4.50.

Orahesive® (ConvaTec)
Powder containing **carmellose sodium**, **gelatin** and **pectin**, equal parts, 25g = £2.50.

Gelclair® (Cambridge Laboratories)
Oral gel containing **polyvinylpyrrolidine** and **sodium hyaluronate**, 28 days @ 1 sachet t.d.s. = £125.

Sucralfate
Antepsin® (Chugai)
Oral suspension 1g/5mL, 250mL = £6; *aniseed or caramel flavour.*

Antiseptic and antibacterial mouthwashes
For **chlorhexidine gluconate** mouthwashes, see p.570.

Doxycycline (generic)
Capsules 100mg (as hyclate), 3 days @ 100mg q.d.s. = £2.

Corticosteroids
Hydrocortisone
Corlan® Pellets (UCB)
Oromucosal tablets 2.5mg (as sodium succinate), 5 days @ 1 q.d.s. = £2.

Beclometasone (generic)
Aerosol inhalation 50microgram/metered spray, 200-dose inhaler = £3; 100microgram/metered spray, 200-dose inhaler = £6.

Betamethasone
Betnesol® (UCB)
Tablets soluble 500microgram, 28 days @ 500microgram q.d.s. = £6.

1 Walls A (2005) Domiciliary dental care. In: A Davies and I Finlay (eds) *Oral Care in Advanced Disease*. Oxford University Press, Oxford, pp. 37–45.
2 NIH Consensus Development Conference Statement (1989) Oral complications of cancer therapies, prevention and treatment. *NIH Consensus Statement*. **7**: 1–11.
3 Epstein JB *et al.* (2007) Management of pain in cancer patients with oral mucositis: follow-up of multiple doses of doxepin oral rinse. *Journal of Pain and Symptom Management*. **33**: 111–114.
4 Meecham J (2005) Oral pain. In: A Davies and I Finlay (eds) *Oral Care in Advanced Disease*. Oxford University Press, Oxford, pp. 134–143.
5 Kim J *et al.* (1985) A clinical study of benzydamine for the treatment of radiotherapy induced mucositis of the orpharynx. *International Journal of Tissue Reaction*. **7**: 215–218.
6 Cerchietti LC *et al.* (2002) Effect of topical morphine for mucositis-associated pain following concomitant chemoradiotherapy for head and neck carcinoma. *Cancer*. **95**: 2230–2236.
7 Cerchietti L and Cerchietti L (2007) Morphine mouthwashes for painful mucositis. *Supportive Care in Cancer*. **15**: 115–116; author reply 117.
8 Jackson K *et al.* (2001) 'Burst' ketamine for refractory cancer pain: an open-label audit of 39 patients. *Journal of Pain and Symptom Management*. **22**: 834–842.
9 Keefe DM *et al.* (2007) Updated clinical practice guidelines for the prevention and treatment of mucositis. *Cancer*. **109**: 820–831.
10 Barrons RW (2001) Treatment strategies for recurrent oral aphthous ulcers. *American Journal of Health-System Pharmacy*. **58**: 41–50; quiz 51–43.
11 Gorsky M *et al.* (2007) Topical minocycline and tetracycline rinses in treatment of recurrent aphthous stomatitis: a randomized cross-over study. *Dermatology Online Journal*. **13**: 1.

CERUMENOLYTICS BNF 12.1.3

Indications: Impacted earwax (cerumen).

Contra-indications: perforated ear drum, presence of myringotomy tubes (grommets), recent ear surgery.

Pharmacology

Cerumen impaction is defined as an accumulation of earwax which causes symptoms, prevents adequate examination of the ear, or both; it does not necessarily imply complete obstruction.[1,2] Symptoms associated with impacted earwax include deafness, tinnitus, fullness, itching, otalgia, discharge, and chronic cough. Asymptomatic earwax does *not* need to be removed.

Earwax is secreted to provide a protective film on the skin of the external ear canal. It is generally expelled naturally. The risk of impaction is increased in children, the elderly, people with learning disabilities, and when natural expulsion is obstructed, e.g. by anatomical abnormalities of the ear canal, hearing aids, or inappropriate use of 'cotton buds' to clean the ears.[1,3]

Cerumenolytics are classified as either water-based (e.g. water, 0.9% saline, 5% **sodium bicarbonate**), oil-based (e.g. **almond oil**, **olive oil**), or non-water/non-oil based (e.g. **urea-hydrogen peroxide**).[4] Water-based products are true cerumenolytics (i.e. break up keratin within earwax),[5] whereas oil-based products lubricate and soften the earwax. The mechanism of action of non-water/non-oil-based products is unclear.

Evidence is too limited to indicate if one type of cerumenolytic is more effective than any other.[1,6] An *in vitro* study lends strong support to the use of just water.[5]

Systematic reviews have concluded that cerumenolytics can clear earwax in about one third of cases in 4 days, thereby obviating the need for syringing.[4,6] For these patients, self-treatment with clean tap water will be the most cost-effective treatment.

Syringing without pre-treatment with a cerumenolytic is effective in about three quarters of patients, but may be more difficult than after pre-treatment.[3,4,6] After pre-treatment, success approaches 100%.[1] Pre-treatment with water 15–30min before syringing is as effective as applying drops b.d. for several days.[4,7] It works in 'nearly all cases', and is more convenient for patients than having to wait several days.[8]

Syringing can cause undesirable effects, including pain, minor damage to the external ear canal, and otitis externa; less commonly perforation of the tympanic membrane and vertigo (the latter generally if the water is too cold).[1]

In those few cases where syringing fails to remove the wax, commonsense dictates that drops should be continued for several more days before a further attempt.[3,8]

There is no evidence to support any type of manual removal of earwax.[1] However, many practitioners consider manual techniques to be standard practice.

Management strategy

PCF regards water (tap or sterile) or 0.9% saline as the cerumenolytics of choice.

- use drops alone for at least 4 days (e.g. 3–4 drops b.d.)
- if this fails, proceed to syringing
- if this fails, use drops for 3–4 more days and syringe again
- if syringing fails on the second occasion, proceed to manual removal using curette, probe, forceps, suction or hook.

To minimize the risk of damaging the ear canal and tympanic membrane, manual removal after failed syringing is best undertaken by those with specialist training.[1,3]

Supply

Although OTC products are available, their relative effectiveness is unproven and they appear to be no better than water or 0.9% saline. Thus, none is recommended. Some proprietary products contain potentially irritant constituents.[2]

0.9% Saline (generic)
Injection (use as ear drops) 5mL = £0.50.
Nose drops (use as ear drops), 10mL = £0.50; available OTC.

1 Browning G (2008) Ear Wax. In: *BMJ Clinical Evidence*. Available from: www.clinicalevidence.bmj.com/ceweb/conditions/ent/0504/0504-get.pdf
2 Roland PS *et al.* (2008) Clinical practice guideline: cerumen impaction. *Otolaryngology — Head and Neck Surgery*. **139 (3 suppl 2)**: S1–S21.
3 McCarter DF *et al.* (2007) Cerumen impaction. *American Family Physician*. **75**: 1523–1528.
4 Hand C and Harvey I (2004) The effectiveness of topical preparations for the treatment of earwax: a systematic review. *British Journal of General Practice*. **54**: 862–867.
5 Chalishazar U and Williams H (2007) Back to basics: finding an optimal cerumenolytic (earwax solvent). *British Journal of Nursing*. **16**: 806–808.
6 Burton MJ and Doree CJ (2009) Ear drops for the removal of ear wax. *Cochrane Database of Systematic Reviews*. **1**: CD004326.
7 Pavlidis C and Pickering JA (2005) Water as a fast acting wax softening agent before ear syringing. *Australian Family Physician*. **34**: 303–304.
8 Eekhof JA *et al.* (2001) A quasi-randomised controlled trial of water as a quick softening agent of persistent earwax in general practice. *British Journal of General Practice*. **51**: 635–637.

12: SKIN

EMOLLIENTS **BNF 13.2.1**

Indications: Dry or rough skin.

Introduction

Emollients soften and increase the hydration of the outermost layer of the epidermis (stratum corneum). This increases the integrity and resilience of the skin and so helps to protect the skin from irritants, allergens, and microbes.[1] Emollients also hydrate skin by preventing loss of water. Older patients are particularly likely to develop dry skin (asteotic dermatitis). Other common causes include:

- varicose (stasis) dermatitis
- drying environments
- excessive washing
- diuretics
- drug reactions
- radiotherapy.

Types of emollients

Emollients vary in greasiness depending on the amount of oil and water they contain (Table 12.1). Creams and ointments are most commonly used. However, other formulations may be used for specific indications. The choice of emollient depends on many factors.

Ointments are greasy because of their structure, even when their water content is high. Anhydrous ointments provide an occlusive film of oil over the surface of the skin. The water trapped under the ointment passes back into the stratum corneum which then swells up, improving skin barrier function.

Some creams contain **propylene glycol** which gives a smoother texture, and facilitates application. The properties of oily lotions are comparable to creams but, because they are more liquid, they can be applied more easily to large areas and are easier to apply to hairy skin. Both creams and oily lotions have a cooling effect on the skin (heat lost by evaporation of the water content).

Humectants are substances which attract moisture to, and retain it in, the stratum corneum, e.g. **urea**, **glycerol**, **lactic acid**, **alpha-hydroxy acids** and **propylene glycol**.[2] Adequate hydration is generally obtained with creams containing **urea** 5–10%[3,4] and, for patients with only mild–moderate dryness, this may be more cosmetically acceptable than using an ointment. **Urea** at higher concentrations of 20–30% is antipruritic, breaks down keratin, decreases the thickness of the stratum corneum, and is used in scaling conditions such as ichthyosis.[3] However, humectants may be irritating, particularly on inflamed skin, when humectant-free creams or ointments may be preferable.

Proprietary emollients often contain additives and fragrances (perfumes) which are potentially allergenic (Table 12.2). Concern about **lanolin** is largely misplaced; many emollients contain refined ('hypo-allergenic') **lanolin** which is rarely responsible for contact dermatitis.[5]

Table 12.1 Emollient formulations

	Ointments	*Creams*	*Lotions*	*Sprays*	*Soap Substitutes*	*Bath additives*
Description	Grease-based	Emulsions of water and oil; vary from more greasy products (water-in-oil, 'rich creams') to more aqueous ones (oil-in-water, 'light creams')	Solutions, suspensions or emulsions from which water evaporates leaving a thin coating of powder or oil	Oil in volatile silicone	May be in the form of creams, lotions or ointments	Oil; often contain an antimicrobial or antipruritic
Features	Increased absorption	Cosmetically acceptable Suitable for face and flexures May be used for large areas	Suitable for wet rashes and hairy areas Spread well Useful for soaks or wet dressings	Spray on, so application is quick No touching the skin No contamination from the hands	Unlike soaps, do not have detergent properties	Widely used despite the absence of scientific evidence of benefit
Potential limitations	Messy Difficult to apply to hairy areas May occlude hair follicles Perspiration can be trapped under the ointment, causing discomfort from excessive body heat and moisture Avoid applying to large areas	May contain fragrances or preservatives	Only emulsions containing oil have an emollient effect; other lotions are drying Often contain alcohol which will sting broken skin	Make skin and surfaces slippery		Make skin and surfaces slippery; particular care needed when bathing Additives can cause contact dermatitis if used excessively

Table 12.2 Potential skin allergens in emollients

Allergen	*Comment*
Fragrances (perfumes)[a,3,6]	
Preservatives (particularly parabens and cresols)[a,3,6]	In many creams and lotions, and in some ointments
Emulsifying agents and ointment bases (particularly sodium lauryl sulphate and cetostearyl alcohols)[a,3,6]	In many creams, lotions and ointments
Wool fat derivatives (includes lanolin)[a,3,6]	In many creams and ointments
Topical local anaesthetics	
Neomycin	
Ethyl alcohol	In some products and skin wipes
Rubber additives (plasticizers, preservatives)	Undersheets, elastic stockings, etc.
Paraphenylenediamine, chromates	In leather
Tea tree oil[7]	

a. Section 13.1.3 of the BNF lists potential sensitizers which mainly fall into these categories.

Cautions

Official advice states that emollients containing **arachis** (peanut) **oil** should not be used by patients with peanut or soya allergy.[8] However, unlike *crude* **arachis oil**, the *refined* oil used in pharmaceutical products is not allergenic, and thus is highly unlikely to cause allergic reactions in people with (whole) peanut allergy.[9,10]

Clothing and dressings in contact with paraffin-based emollients, e.g. **emulsifying ointment BP** or **liquid paraffin and white soft paraffin ointment NPF**, are easily ignited by a naked flame. The risk is increased when the products are applied to large areas of the body, and clothing or dressings become soaked with them. Patients should keep away from fire or flames, and not smoke when using these products, particularly if applying large quantities.[11]

In hairy patients prone to folliculitis, to reduce the risk of further episodes, creams and ointments should be applied using downward strokes in the direction of hair growth, particularly on the legs.[12]

Dose and use

Choice of emollient involves consideration of:

- patient preference
- area to be treated, e.g. ointments are generally acceptable for the legs and trunk but not the face, and ointment may be necessary for the thicker skin of the palms and soles
- ingredients; does it contain known or potential allergens?
- degree of dryness; very dry skin often requires an ointment initially
- packaging, e.g. patients with weak hands find removing screw-tops or squeezing tubes difficult
- patient's lifestyle
- season; ointments are less well tolerated in the summer
- cost-effectiveness; **aqueous cream BP** is the cheapest product but does not suit everyone.

Note: in children with atopic dermatitis (eczema), **aqueous cream** has sometimes caused burning/stinging ± erythema when used as an emollient, rather than just as a soap substitute.[13] If this occurs, another emollient (e.g. Cetraben®, Diprobase®) can be substituted.

Emollients should be applied as frequently as needed to keep the skin well hydrated. This is generally twice daily. Very dry skin may require more frequent applications. Enough emollient should be applied to make the skin glisten.[12] However, if the emollient is applied too thickly, it may make the patient uncomfortable, hot or itchy, and may stain clothing.

The emollient should be applied immediately after a bath or shower when the skin is most hydrated. The patient should shake off excess water or lightly dab dry with a soft towel, and then apply the emollient to the damp skin. Emollients are essential for maintaining skin condition and should continue to be used at least once daily even when the dryness has improved/resolved.

It is helpful to demonstrate the use of the recommended emollient (or one of comparable consistency) to the patient and the family or carers. This is particularly useful in patients with unsightly skin who may feel ostracized, and for whom physical contact (touch) generally provides real psychological benefit.

In practice, *the best emollient is the one which a patient is happy to use*. This implies that it is both cosmetically acceptable and effective, and preferably should not be expensive. For example, many patients like the silky feel of **colloidal oatmeal** (e.g. Aveeno®), particularly on their hands and face. Average quantities required for b.d. application for 1 week are shown in Table 12.3.

Table 12.3 Quantities required for b.d. application for 1 week

	Creams and ointments (g)	*Lotions (mL)*
Face	15–30	100
Groins and genitalia	15–25	100
Both hands	25–50	200
Scalp	50–100	200
Both arms or both legs	100–200	200
Trunk	400	500

A light cream (e.g. **aqueous cream BP**, Cetraben®, Diprobase®) or emollient lotion b.d. generally suffices with mild–moderate degrees of dryness (Table 12.4). For severe dryness an ointment will be needed (e.g. Hydromol®, Epaderm®).

Soap should *not* be used because of its drying effect on the skin. It contributes to the breakdown of the skin barrier by raising the pH; this enhances protease activity, inhibts lipid synthesis, and promotes bacterial colonization. Use instead a soap substitute (e.g. **aqueous cream BP**, **emulsifying ointment BP**, Cetraben® cream, Dermol® cream or lotion) or a proprietary soap-free cleanser (e.g. E45® Emollient Wash Cream or Oilatum® Shower Emollient).

An emollient bath additive, such as Dermalo® or E45® Emollient Bath Oil, can also be used when bathing. It is advisable to use a bath mat to prevent slipping when using such products in the bath or shower.

When there is active skin disease causing inflammation and eroded or cracked skin, apply a moderately potent topical corticosteroid once daily–b.d. to the affected area for 3–7 days or until the inflammation settles, e.g. **clobetasone butyrate** 0.05% or **betamethasone valerate** 0.025% ointment. In practice, topical corticosteroids are prescribed mostly for dermatoses of the face and hands. Current best practice is to apply the corticosteroid 30–60min before or after the emollient has been applied.

If secondary infection is suspected, a topical antifungal and/or antibacterial should be prescribed ± a topical corticosteroid; various combination products are available. *To minimize the risk of developing resistance, products containing antimicrobials must not be used p.r.n. but as a full course for 7 days.*

If emollient-related contact dermatitis is suspected, patch testing with the standard set of potential allergens may identify an allergen. If allergy is confirmed, a product which does not contain the allergen (and, ideally, any other added preservatives or fragrances) should be prescribed. However, not all contact dermatitis is allergic; sometimes it is caused by direct chemical irritation.

Lymphoedema

Skin care is just one component of multimodal lymphoedema management.[14,15] The following advice must be applied within the broader management context.

The choice depends on the state of the skin but also on current fashion and local contracts:[16]

- if not obviously dry and flaky, a light cream, can be applied once daily–b.d. as a prophylactic measure, e.g. **aqueous cream BP** or an alternative (see Table 12.4)

- if the skin is dry ± cracked, apply **liquid and white soft paraffin ointment NPF (liquid paraffin in white soft paraffin** 50/50)
- if there is a build-up of scales wash the affected area with a light cream (see Table 12.4) using a circular motion in order to soften and lift off the scales; then apply **liquid and white soft paraffin ointment NPF**, and cover with a hydrocolloid dressing (e.g. Granuflex®) and bandage; repeat every 1–3 days until the skin condition is good
- if there are toe web fissures, take scrapings to look for fungus and, if present, treat appropriately, e.g. **clotrimazole** 1% or **terbinafine** 1% cream b.d. for 2 weeks.

Note:

- ointments are generally needed for only 1–2 weeks
- some people prefer coconut oil because it has a skin-cooling effect.

Table 12.4 Emollient and additive content of selected topical products[a]

	Wool fat derivatives e.g. lanolin	*Soft paraffin (petrolatum) or liquid paraffin (mineral oil)*	*Sensitizing preservative*	*Fragrance*
Ointments				
Emulsifying ointment BP	–	+	–	–
White soft paraffin BP	–	+	–	–
Liquid paraffin and white soft paraffin ointment NPF	–	+	–	–
Epaderm®	–	+	–	–
Hydromol®	–	+	–	–
Oils				
Coconut oil BP	–	–	–	–
Water-in-oil (rich) creams				
Hydrous ointment BP	+	+	–	–
Aquadrate®	–	+	–	–
Lipobase®	–	+	+	–
Unguentum M®	–	+	–	–
Oil in water (light) creams				
Aqueous cream BP	–	+	–	–
Aveeno®	–	+	+	–
Cetraben®	–	+	+	–
Dermol®	–	+	–	–
Diprobase®	–	+	+	–
E45®	+[b]	+	+	–
E45® Itch relief	–	+	+	–
Hydromol®	–	+	+	–
Ultrabase®	–	+	+	+
Zerobase®	–	+	+	–
Lotions				
Aveeno®	–	+	+	–
Dermol®	–	+	–	–
E45®	+[b]	+	+	–
Keri®	+	+	+	+

a. products which do not contain wool fat derivatives or liquid/soft paraffin generally contain plant-based oils or fatty acid derivatives

b. hypo-allergenic lanolin.

Antipruritic emollients

If pruritus is caused by dry skin, rehydration of the skin will correct it. Thus, all emollients are antipruritic in this sense. However, some products have a specific antipruritic agent added, and can provide extra benefit in some patients (see p.586).

Supply

This is not a complete list; see BNF for additional options.

Pharmaco-economics

Before prescribing a relatively expensive proprietary product, check to see whether, content for content, there is a cheaper essentially equivalent product.

Emollients

Aqueous cream BP (generic)
Cream (oil-in-water) containing **emulsifying ointment BP** 30%, phenoxyethanol 1% in water, 100g = £1, 500g = £2.

Cetraben® (Genus)
Cream containing **white soft paraffin** 13.2%, **light liquid paraffin** 10.5%, 50g pump-dispenser pack = £1, 150g pump-dispenser pack = £3, 500g pump-dispenser pack = £5, 1kg pump-dispenser pack = £11.

Colloidal oatmeal
Aveeno® (J&J)
Cream 100mL = £4.
Lotion 400mL = £6.
Bath oil 250mL = £4.50.
Colloidal bath additive 10 sachets = £7.
All classified in the UK as borderline substances; prescriptions must be endorsed ACBS.

Dermol® (Dermal)
Cream containing **benzalkonium chloride** 0.1%, **chlorhexidine hydrochloride** 0.1%, **liquid paraffin** 10%, **isopropyl myristate** 10%, 100g = £3, 500g pump-dispenser pack = £7.
Lotion Dermol® 500, containing **benzalkonium chloride** 0.1%, **chlorhexidine hydrochloride** 0.1%, **liquid paraffin** 2.5%, **isopropyl myristate** 2.5%, 500mL pump-dispenser pack = £6.

Diprobase® (Schering-Plough)
Cream (oil-in-water) containing **liquid paraffin** 6%, **white soft paraffin** 15%, **cetostearyl alcohol** 7.2%, cetomacrogol 2.25%, 50g = £1.50, 500g pump-dispenser pack = £7.

E45® (Crookes)
Cream (oil-in-water) containing **liquid paraffin** 12.6%, **white soft paraffin** 14.5%, **hypo-allergenic lanolin** 1%, 50g = £1.50, 500g pump-dispenser pack = £5.
Lotion containing **light liquid paraffin** 4%, **white soft paraffin** 10%, **hypo-allergenic lanolin** 1%, 200mL = £2.50, 500mL pump-dispenser pack = £4.50; *classified in the UK as a borderline substance; prescriptions must be endorsed ACBS.*

Epaderm® (Mölnlycke)
Cream containing **yellow soft paraffin** 15%, **liquid paraffin** 10%, **emulsifying wax** 5%, 50g pump-dispenser pack = £1.50, 500g pump-dispenser pack = £7.
Ointment containing **emulsifying wax** 30%, **yellow soft paraffin** 30%, **liquid paraffin** 40%, 125g = £3.50, 500g = £6, 1kg = £12.

Hydromol® (Alliance)
Cream containing **sodium pidolate** 2.5%, **liquid paraffin** 13.8%, 50g = £2, 100g = £4, 500g = £11.
Ointment containing **yellow soft paraffin** 30%, **emulsifying wax** 30%, **liquid paraffin** 40%, 125g = £3, 500g = £5, 1kg = £9.

Hydrous ointment BP (generic)
Cream (water-in-oil) containing dried **magnesium sulphate** 0.5%, **wool alcohols ointment** 50%, phenoxyethanol 1% in water, 500g = £2.

Liquid paraffin and white soft paraffin ointment NPF (generic)
Ointment containing **liquid paraffin** 50%, **white soft paraffin** 50%, 500g = £4.

Petroleum jelly (generic)
Ointment containing **white** or **yellow soft paraffin BP**, 100g = £0.50.

Unguentum M® (Almirall)
Cream (water-in-oil) containing **saturated neutral oil, liquid paraffin, white soft paraffin**, 100g = £3, 500g = £8.

With humectants
Aquadrate® (Alliance)
Cream (water-in-oil) containing **urea** 10%, 100g = £4.50.

E45 Itch Relief® (Crookes)
Cream (oil-in-water) containing **urea** 5%, **macrogol lauryl ether** 3%, 100g = £3.50, 500g pump-dispenser pack = £16.

Non-soap cleansers
Emulsifying ointment BP (generic)
Ointment containing **emulsifying wax** 30%, **white soft paraffin** 50%, **liquid paraffin** 20%, 500g = £2.

E45® Emollient Wash Cream (Crookes)
Wash cream containing **soap substitute, zinc oxide** 5% in emollient base, 250mL pump-dispenser pack = £3; *classified in the UK as a borderline substance; prescriptions must be endorsed ACBS.*

Oilatum® Shower Emollient (Stiefel)
Shower gel containing **light liquid paraffin** 70%, 150g = £5.

Bath oils
Dermalo® (Dermal)
Bath oil containing **liquid paraffin** 65%, **acetylated wool alcohols** 5%, 500mL = £3.50.

E45 Emollient Bath Oil® (Crookes)
Bath oil containing **liquid paraffin** 91%, **cetyl dimeticone** 5%, 500mL = £5; *classified in the UK as a borderline substance; prescriptions must be endorsed ACBS.*

Mild topical corticosteroid
Hydrocortisone (generic)
Cream 1%, 30g – £3.

Mildison® (Astellas)
Cream 1%, 30g – £2.50.

Moderately potent topical corticosteroids
Betamethasone valerate
Betnovate-RD® (GSK)
Cream 0.025%, 100g = £3.50; *this is 1/4 of the strength of Betnovate® cream.*
Ointment 0.025%, 100g = £3.50; *this is 1/4 of the strength of Betnovate® ointment.*

Clobetasone butyrate
Eumovate® (GSK)
Cream 0.05%, 30g = £2, 100g = £6.
Ointment 0.05%, 30g = £2, 100g = £6.

Antifungal creams
Clotrimazole (generic)
Cream 1%, 20g = £2.

Terbinafine (generic)
Cream 1%, 15g = £4.50; 30g = £3.50.

For more antifungal products, see Barrier products, p.591, and the *BNF.*

1 Cork MJ and Danby S (2009) Skin barrier breakdown: a renaissance in emollient therapy. *British Journal of Nursing*. **18**: 872, 874, 876–877.
2 Kraft JN and Lynde CW (2005) Moisturizers: what they are and a practical approach to product selection. *Skin Therapy Letter.* **10 (5)**: 1–8.
3 Sibbald D (2002) Dermatitis. In: C Repchinsky (ed) *Patient Self-care (2e)*. Canadian Pharmacists Association, Ottawa, pp. 479–505.
4 Fluhr JW *et al.* (2008) Emollients, moisturizers, and keratolytic agents in psoriasis. *Clinics in Dermatology.* **26**: 380–386.

5 Hoppe U (ed) (1999) *The Lanolin Book*. Beierdorf AG, Hamburg.
6 Voegeli D (2008) Care or harm: exploring essential components in skin care regimens. *British Journal of Nursing*. **17**: 24–30.
7 Rubel DM *et al.* (1998) Tea tree oil allergy: what is the offending agent? Report of three cases of tea tree oil allergy and review of the literature. *Australasian Journal of Dermatology*. **39**: 244–247.
8 MHRA (2003) Medicines containing peanut (arachis) oil. *Current Problems in Pharmacovigilance*. **29 (September)**: 5.
9 Hourihane JO *et al.* (1997) Randomised, double blind, crossover challenge study of allergenicity of peanut oils in subjects allergic to peanuts. *British Medical Journal*. **314**: 1084–1088.
10 Keating MU *et al.* (1990) Immunoassay of peanut allergens in food-processing materials and finished foods. *Journal of Allergy and Clinical Immunology*. **86**: 41–44.
11 BNF (2010) Section 13.2.1. In: *British National Formulary* (No. 60). British Medical Association and the Royal Pharmaceutical Society of Great Britain, London. Current BNF available from www.bnf.org.
12 Lawton S (2009) Practical issues for emollient therapy in dry and itchy skin. *British Journal of Nursing*. **18**: 978–984.
13 Cork MJ *et al.* (2003) An audit of adverse drug reactions to aqueous cream in children with atopic eczema. *The Pharmaceutical Journal*. **271**: 747–748.
14 Twycross R *et al.* (2009) *Symptom Management in Advanced Cancer* (4e). palliativedrugs.com, Nottingham, pp. 108–111.
15 Twycross R *et al.* (2000) *Lymphoedema*. Radcliffe Medical Press, Oxford.
16 Linnitt N (2000) Skin management in lymphoedema. In: RG Twycross *et al.* (eds) *Lymphoedema*. Radcliffe Medical Press, Oxford, pp. 118–129.

TOPICAL ANTIPRURITICS BNF 13.2.1 & 13.3

Indication: Pruritus which fails to respond to an emollient and/or specific treatment.

Background

Pruritus may be caused by systemic disease (e.g. drug hypersensitivity, obstructive jaundice, endocrine disease, malignant disease), skin disease (e.g. eczema, urticaria, psoriasis, scabies) or drugs (e.g. opioids).

Dryness of the skin (xerosis) is the commonest cause of pruritus without an accompanying rash, and an emollient is the first-line treatment (see p.579). Dryness is associated with normal ageing, inflammatory skin conditions (e.g. atopic dermatitis), systemic disease (e.g. hypothyroidism, renal failure), and cachexia and general debility in advanced cancer.

Whenever possible, the treatment of pruritus should be cause-specific.[1,2] For example, in skin disorders:

- scabies → treat patient and the whole family with **permethrin** or **malathion**
- atopic dermatitis → topical corticosteroid (+ emollient)[3]
- contact dermatitis → topical corticosteroid, identify causal substance and avoid further contact.

In systemic disorders or when caused by opioids, a range of options exist (see Table 5.29, p.431 and Table 5.30, p.432). A topical antipruritic should be considered only if a bland emollient and cause-specific treatment fail to relieve.

Although topical products are not convenient to apply regularly to the whole body, many patients with generalized pruritus have patches of more intense discomfort, and may benefit from more limited application.

Pharmacology

Traditional topical antipruritics include **phenol**, **menthol** and **camphor**. **Phenol** 0.5–3% acts by anaesthetizing cutaneous nerve endings. **Menthol** 0.5–2% and **camphor** 0.5–3% may relieve pruritus by cooling the skin by acting on heat-sensitive transient receptor potential (TRP) channels expressed on sensory nerve endings.[4,5] Cooling the skin is known to reduce the intensity of histamine-induced pruritus, and patients who suffer from chronic pruritic conditions such as atopic dermatitis, psoriasis and uraemic pruritus often find that cold showers reduce the pruritus. **Menthol** 1% can be added to an emollient,[6] and products containing these substances are available OTC.

Capsaicin is a naturally occurring alkaloid found in the fruits of various species of *Solanaceae* (the nightshade family) and in pepper plants of the genus *Capsicum* (chilli peppers).[7] It acts by depleting substance P at sensory nerve endings. **Capsaicin** products are useful in relieving neuropathic pain (see Rubefacients and other topical products, p.556). Benefit has also been reported in histamine-related pruritus, aquagenic pruritus, and pruritus associated with uraemia, nodular prurigo, psoriasis and post-axillary dissection syndrome.[4] **Capsaicin** has also been used successfully in the treatment of intractable pruritus ani.[8]

In practice, **capsaicin** will be applied to relatively limited areas of the skin. It often initially causes localized burning and stinging. This irritation subsides with repeated use but patients may have difficulty continuing treatment. Patients should use **capsaicin** q.d.s. to overcome the irritation, after which the frequency of applications can be reduced. The topical anaesthetic **EMLA (eutectic mixture of local anaesthetics, lidocaine** 2.5% and **prilocaine** 2.5%), used in conjunction with **capsaicin**, may reduce the initial irritation.[9] Excessive use of **EMLA** may result in acute transient systemic local anaesthetic neurotoxicity.[10]

Polidocanol (macrogol lauryl ether) is an anionic detergent with local anaesthetic properties.[11] Benefit has been reported in patients with pruritus associated with atopic dermatitis, non-atopic dermatitis and psoriasis, with the regular application of a cream containing 5% **urea** and 3% **polidocanol** (E45® Itch Relief Cream).[12,13] Benefit has also been reported in patients with pruritus associated with chronic renal failure who regularly used a **polidocanol**-containing bath oil (Balneum Plus®).[14]

Crotamiton 10% lotion (Eurax®) has a mild antiscabetic effect which is probably the reason for its reputation as an antipruritic. However, in an RCT in patients with chronic pruritic dermatoses, **crotamiton** lotion was no more effective than its vehicle.[15]

Topical H_1 antihistamines, e.g. **diphenhydramine**, are of benefit only when the pruritus is cutaneous in origin and related to histamine release.[1] Topical **diphenhydramine** can cause contact dermatitis and photosensitivity; if used, limit to a few days.

A **coal tar**-based shampoo, e.g. Polytar®, has a long tradition of use with scalp pruritus.

Doxepin

Doxepin is a TCA which is a potent H_1- and H_2-receptor antagonist. Its affinity for H_2-receptors is 6 times that of **cimetidine**.[16] It is also antimuscarinic, and may antagonize the pruritic effects of substance P at skin receptors. **Amitriptyline** is similar in potency to **doxepin** as an H_1 antihistamine, but other TCAs are much less so.[17] Patients with chronic urticaria who do not respond to conventional H_1 antihistamines may well benefit from **doxepin** 10–75mg PO at bedtime.[18]

Doxepin 5% cream is reported to be of benefit in some patients with atopic dermatitis[16,19,20] but long-term independent studies are lacking.[21] It is not generally suitable for children. It is possible that the benefit is systemic rather than topical. About 15% of patients complain initially of localized stinging or burning, and a similar proportion complain of drowsiness, secondary to systemic absorption.[19] The sedation may help the antipruritic effect.

Doxepin cream is less effective than systemic treatment[22] and, depending on the products prescribed, can be more expensive than **doxepin** capsules plus an emollient. Allergic contact dermatitis may occur.[19] Patients with contact allergy should not take the drug by mouth.[23]

Cautions

Because of:

- the risk of contact dermatitis, *discourage* the use of topical H_1 antihistamines and of local anaesthetics
- their drying effect, *discourage* the use of products containing **calamine** unless they contain oil (e.g. **calamine oily lotion BP**).

Calamine oily lotion BP contains *refined* **arachis** (peanut) **oil**, and official advice states that emollients containing **arachis** (peanut) **oil** should not be used by patients with peanut or soya allergy.[24,25] However, unlike *crude* **arachis oil**, the *refined* oil is not allergenic, and is highly unlikely to cause allergic reactions in people with (whole) peanut allergy.[26,27]

Polytar® products also contain traces of **arachis** (peanut) **oil** from the **coal tar** extraction process, and thus might cause allergic reactions in people with peanut or soya allergy.

Patients prescribed **doxepin**, either systemically or topically, should avoid the concurrent use of drugs which inhibit cytochrome P450, e.g. **cimetidine**, imidazole antifungals and macrolide antibacterials (see Cytochrome P450, p.735). As with other TCAs, MAOIs should be discontinued ⩾2 weeks before starting treatment with **doxepin**. Monitor carefully in patients with glaucoma, a tendency to urinary retention, severe liver disease or a history of mania.

Use

Because pruritus is commonly associated with dry skin, an emollient (moisturizer) should be tried first (see p.579). A light cream (oil-in-water), e.g. Cetraben®, often suffices with mild–moderate degrees of dryness. **Aqueous cream BP** is an option but at many centres is used only as a soap substitute. Products containing **colloidal oatmeal** (Aveeno®) are popular because of their silky feel (see p.584). Storing creams and lotions in a refrigerator may increase benefit.

Menthol 0.5%–2% (or **camphor** 0.5–3%) can be added to a bland emollient, and applied topically t.d.s.–q.d.s. Proprietary products include **menthol** 0.5–2% in **aqueous cream** (Dermacool®).

Calamine lotion BP contains **phenol** 0.5%, and can be strengthened by adding a further 0.5%. Although the vehicle is drying, it can be formulated as an oily lotion. **Phenolated calamine lotion USP** contains **phenol** 1%. However, because it is unsightly, **calamine** is unlikely to be acceptable except on a short-term basis, e.g. in acute contact dermatitis.

Supply

Several products available OTC contain **menthol** and **camphor** (with contents as high as 8–11%). These are marketed for rheumatic aches and pains, e.g. Tiger Balm®. Others are mainly intended for use on insect bites and the unit size is small.

Menthol

Dermacool® (Pern Consumer Products)
Cream 0.5%, 1%, 2% in **aqueous cream BP**, 100g tube (1% only), 50g pump spray (2% only), 500g pot (all strengths), available OTC.

Deep Freeze® (Mentholatum)
Gel 2% (Cold Gel®), 100g, available OTC.
Spray 2% (Cold Spray®), 150mL spray can, available OTC.
Deep Freeze® is marketed for minor sports injuries.

Phenol

Chymol Emollient Balm® (Almus)
Ointment containing **phenol** 2.4%, **eucalyptus oil** 1.2%, **methylsalicylate** 0.8% and **terpineol** 4%, 40g, available OTC.

Polidocanol (macrogol lauryl ether)

Balneum Plus® (Almirall)
Bath oil containing **soya oil** 83%, mixed **lauromacrogols** 15%, 500mL = £7.

E45 Itch Relief® (Crookes)
Cream (oil-in-water) containing **urea** 5%, **macrogol lauryl ether** 3%, 100g = £3.50.

Doxepin

Sinepin® (Marlborough)
Capsules 25mg, 50mg, 28 days @ 25mg, 50mg, 75mg at bedtime = £4, £6 and £9 respectively.

Xepin® (CHS)
Cream 5%, 30g = £12.

Other H_1 antihistamines include **hydroxyzine**, **chlorphenamine**, and **cetirizine**.

1 Zylicz Z *et al.* (eds) (2004) *Pruritus in Advanced Disease*. Oxford University Press, Oxford.
2 Twycross R *et al.* (2009) *Symptom Management in Advanced Cancer* (4e). palliativedrugs.com, Nottingham, pp. 321–329.
3 Cork MJ (1999) Taking the itch out of eczema: how careful use of emollients can break the itch-scratch cycle of atopic eczema. *Asthma Journal*. **4**: 16–20.
4 Patel T *et al.* (2007) Menthol: a refreshing look at this ancient compound. *Journal of the American Academy of Dermatology*. **57**: 873–878.
5 Peier AM *et al.* (2002) A TRP channel that senses cold stimuli and menthol. *Cell*. **108**: 705–715.
6 Anonymous (2005) Pharmacy information pointers. The preparation of menthol (1 per cent w/w) in aqueous cream BP. *Pharmaceutical Journal*. **274**: 469.
7 Towlerton GR and Rice AS (2003) Topical analgesics for chronic pain. In: AS Rice *et al.* (eds) *Clinical Pain Management: Chronic Pain*. Arnold, London, pp. 213–226.
8 Lysy J *et al.* (2003) Topical capsaicin–a novel and effective treatment for idiopathic intractable pruritus ani: a randomised, placebo controlled, crossover study. *Gut*. **52**: 1323–1326.
9 Yosipovitch G and Hundley JL (2004) Practical guidelines for relief of itch. *Dermatology Nursing*. **16**: 325–328; quiz 329.

10 Brosh-Nissimov T *et al.* (2004) Central nervous system toxicity following topical skin application of lidocaine. *European Journal of Clinical Pharmacology.* **60**: 683–684.
11 Vieluf D *et al.* (1992) Dry and itching skin—therapy with a new preparation, containing urea and polidocanol. *Zeitschrift fur Hautkrankheiten.* **67**: 816–821.
12 Hauss H *et al.* (1993) Comparative study of a formulation containing urea and polidocanol and a greasy cream containing linoleic acid in the treatment of dry, pruritic skin lesions [in German]. *Dermatosen in Beruf und Umwelt Occupational and Environmental Dermatoses.* **41**: 184–188.
13 Freitag G and Hoppner T (1997) Results of a postmarketing drug monitoring survey with a polidocanol-urea preparation for dry, itching skin. *Current Medical Research and Opinion.* **13**: 529–537.
14 Wasik F *et al.* (1996) Relief of uraemic pruritus after balneological therapy with a bath oil containing polidocanol (Balneum Hermal Plus). An open clinical study. *Journal of Dermatological Treatment.* **7**: 231–233.
15 Smith E *et al.* (1984) Crotamiton lotion in pruritus. *International Journal of Dermatology.* **23**: 684–685.
16 Drake L *et al.* (1994) Relief of pruritus in patients with atopic dermatitis after treatment with topical doxepin cream. The Doxepin Study Group. *Journal of the American Academy of Dermatology.* **31**: 613–616.
17 Figge J *et al.* (1979) Tricyclic antidepressants: potent blockade of histamine H_1 receptors of guinea pig ileum. *European Journal of Pharmacology.* **58**: 479–483.
18 Figueiredo A *et al.* (1990) Mechanism of action of doxepin in the treatment of chronic urticaria. *Fundamental and Clinical Pharmacology.* **4**: 147–158.
19 DTB (2000) Doxepin cream for eczema? *Drug and Therapeutics Bulletin.* **38**: 31.
20 Breneman D *et al.* (1997) Doxepin cream relieves eczema-associated pruritus within 15 minutes and is not accompanied by a risk of rebound upon discontinuation. *Journal of Dermatological Treatment.* **8**: 161–168.
21 Hoare C *et al.* (2000) Systematic review of treatments for atopic eczema. *Health Technology Assessment.* **4**: 1–191.
22 Smith P and Corelli R (1997) Doxepin in the management of pruritus associated with allergic cutaneous reactions. *Annals of Pharmacotherapy.* **31**: 633–635.
23 Bonnel RA *et al.* (2003) Allergic contact dermatitis from topical doxepin: Food and Drug Administration's postmarketing surveillance experience. *Journal of the American Academy of Dermatology.* **48**: 294–296.
24 MHRA (2003) Medicines containing peanut (arachis) oil. *Current Problems in Pharmacovigilance.* **29 (September)**: 5.
25 Anonymous (2003) Peanut allergy research is published. *Pharmaceutical Journal.* **270**: 391.
26 Keating MU *et al.* (1990) Immunoassay of peanut allergens in food-processing materials and finished foods. *Journal of Allergy and Clinical Immunology.* **86**: 41–44.
27 Hourihane JO *et al.* (1997) Randomised, double blind, crossover challenge study of allergenicity of peanut oils in subjects allergic to peanuts. *British Medical Journal.* **314**: 1084–1088.

BARRIER PRODUCTS — BNF 13.2.2

Indications: Skin protection, napkin rash.

Introduction

Barrier products contain water-repellent substances which help to protect the skin, and prevent maceration and infection. They can be used around stomas and in the perineal and peri-anal areas in patients with urinary or faecal incontinence. Most barrier creams and ointments are silicone-, titanium- or **zinc oxide**-based.[1]

Zinc cream BP, **zinc and castor oil ointment BP** and Siopel® contain *refined* **arachis** (peanut) **oil**. However, unlike *crude* **arachis oil**, the *refined* oil is not allergenic, and thus is highly unlikely to cause allergic reactions in people with (whole) peanut allergy.[2,3]

A cream is less greasy than an ointment and is easier to apply and wash off, e.g. Drapolene® (**benzalkonium chloride** 0.01% and **cetrimide** 0.2% in **white soft paraffin**, **cetyl alcohol** and **wool fat**) and Sudocrem® (**zinc oxide** 15%, hypo-allergenic **lanolin** 4%). Some products include **dimeticone**, e.g. Conotrane®, or other water-repellent silicone.

If a dressing is needed because of skin damage, a barrier product such as Cavilon No-Sting Barrier Film® will coat the skin with a film for ≤72h, and will prevent the dressing from adhering to the skin.

Cautions

If the damaged skin is infected, because they prevent topical antimicrobials from penetrating into the skin, the use of a barrier product should generally be delayed until the infection has been successfully treated.

Use

Ensure that infection is treated promptly with topical antifungals (more common) and/or antibacterials (less common).

Intertrigo

Intertrigo is an inflammatory dermatosis of skin folds primarily caused by skin on skin friction. Exacerbating factors, e.g. obesity, lack of air, heat and moisture, cause skin maceration and inflammation. Secondary fungal or bacterial infection is common. The wet component is the most easily modified, and drying the involved skin is essential. Initial treatment may comprise:

- cleanse with a soap substitute (e.g. **aqueous cream BP**, **emulsifying ointment BP**, Cetraben® cream, Dermol® cream or lotion) or a proprietary soap-free cleanser (e.g. E45® Emollient Wash Cream or Oilatum® Shower Emollient)
- dry well; blow-drying with a hand-held hair dryer is generally effective
- if infection is likely, because fungal infection is more common, a topical broad-spectrum antifungal should be prescribed, e.g. **clotrimazole**
- if inflammation is present, a mild topical corticosteroid for 3–7 days often accelerates improvement, e.g. **hydrocortisone** 1% cream or ointment (see p.585); combination products containing both an antifungal and **hydrocortisone** 1% are available
- an absorbent powder, e.g. ZeaSORB® (**aldioxa** and **chloroxylenol**) may be helpful
- when the wetness and infection has settled, then begin to use a barrier product.

Protection around a stoma

Many products designed to protect the skin around a stoma from liquid effluent are available; a stoma-care nurse can advise on product selection. Sprays or wipes which dry to form a protective film are commonly used.[4] An alcohol-free formulation is preferable because it is less likely to sting or irritate the skin.

Stoma therapists frequently use Comfeel® barrier cream prophylactically if the stoma effluent is liquid or if the stoma bag is being changed more than once daily. It is gently rubbed in and any excess wiped off. If the skin becomes red and sore, Cavilon No-Sting Barrier Film® is used instead.

Short-term use of a topical corticosteroid can be used to treat moderate–severe inflammation. Foam preparations are well tolerated, e.g. Bettamousse® (unlicensed use; this product is licensed as a scalp application).

Incontinence

After cleansing with a soap substitute and gently drying, apply a barrier product to the affected area whenever the dressing or padding is changed.[1]

Supply

The following is only a selection of the available products.

Ointments

Zinc ointment BP (generic)
Ointment containing **zinc oxide** 15% in a **white soft paraffin, hard paraffin, cetyl alcohol** and **wool fat** base, 25g = £0.50.

Zinc and castor oil ointment BP (generic)
Ointment containing **zinc oxide** 7.5% in a **castor oil, arachis** (peanut) **oil, white beeswax** and **cetostearyl alcohol** base, 100g = £1.

Creams

Conotrane® (Astellas)
Cream containing **dimeticone 350** 22% and **benzalkonium chloride** 0.1%, 100g = £1, 500g = £3.50.

Drapolene® (Chefaro)
Cream containing **benzalkonium chloride** 0.01% and **cetrimide** 0.2% in a **white soft paraffin**, **cetyl alcohol** and **wool fat** base, 100g = £1.50, 200g = £2.50, 350g = £4.

Sudocrem® (Forest)
Cream containing **zinc oxide** 15%, hypo-allergenic **lanolin** 4%, 125g = £2, 250g = £3, 400g = £4.50.

Stoma products

Comfeel® barrier cream (Coloplast)
Cream 60g = £4.50.

Cavilon No-Sting Barrier Film® (3M)
Foam applicator 5 × 1mL = £5; 5 × 3mL = £8.
Pump spray 28mL = £7.

Absorbent dusting powder
ZeaSORB® (Stiefel)
Dusting powder containing **aldioxia** 0.22%, **chloroxylenol** 0.5%, 50g = £2.50.

Antifungal products
Clotrimazole (generic)
Cream 1%, 20g = £2.

Canesten® (Bayer Consumer Care)
Cream 1%, 20g = £2, 50g = £3.50.
Solution 1%, 20mL = £2.50.
Spray 1%, 40mL = £5; *contains isopropyl alcohol.*

Miconazole (generic)
Cream 2%, 20g = £2, 45g = £2.

Daktarin® (Janssen-Cilag)
Cream 2%, 30g = £2.
Powder spray 0.16%, 100g = £2.50.

Topical corticosteroids
For **hydrocortisone** 1%, see p.585.

Bettamousse® (UCB)
Foam (scalp application) containing **betamethasone valerate** 0.12%, 100g = £9.

Combined antifungal and topical corticosteroid products
Canestan HC® (Bayer Consumer Care)
Cream containing **clotrimazole** 1% and **hydrocortisone** 1%, 30g = £2.50.

Daktacort® (Janssen-Cilag)
Cream containing **miconazole** 2% and **hydrocortisone** 1%, 30g = £2.

1 Nazarko L (2007) Managing a common dermatological problem: incontinence dermatitis. *British Journal of Community Nursing*. **12**: 358–363.
2 Keating MU *et al.* (1990) Immunoassay of peanut allergens in food-processing materials and finished foods. *Journal of Allergy and Clinical Immunology*. **86**: 41–44.
3 Hourihane JO *et al.* (1997) Randomised, double blind, crossover challenge study of allergenicity of peanut oils in subjects allergic to peanuts. *British Medical Journal*. **314**: 1084–1088.
4 Twycross R *et al.* (2009) *Symptom Management in Advanced Cancer* (4e). palliativedrugs.com, Nottingham, pp. 334–340.

13: ANAESTHESIA

*KETAMINE — BNF 15.1.1

Class: General anaesthetic.

Indications: Induction and maintenance of anaesthesia; †pain unresponsive to standard treatments (postoperative, neuropathic, inflammatory, ischaemic limb, myofascial and procedure-related).[1–3]

Contra-indications: Any situation in which an increase in blood pressure or intracranial pressure would constitute a hazard. Acute intermittent porphyria.

Pharmacology

The NMDA-receptor-channel complex is closely involved in the development of central sensitization of dorsal horn neurones which transmit pain signals (Figure 13.1).[4] At normal resting membrane potentials, the channel is blocked by magnesium and is inactive.[5] When the resting membrane potential is changed as a result of prolonged excitation, the channel unblocks and calcium moves into the cell. This results in neuronal hyperexcitability and consequently a reduction in opioid-responsiveness, hyperalgesia and allodynia. These effects are probably mediated by the intracellular formation of nitric oxide.[6]

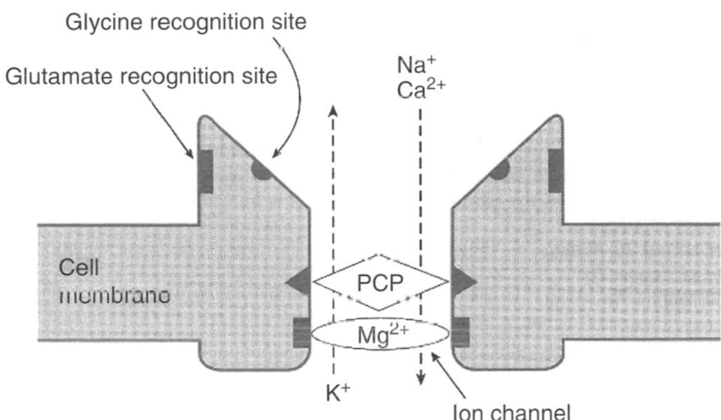

Figure 13.1 Diagram of NMDA (excitatory)-receptor-channel complex. The channel is blocked by Mg^{2+} when the membrane potential is at its resting level (voltage-dependent block) and by drugs which act at the phencyclidine (PCP) binding site in the glutamate-activated channel, e.g. dextromethorphan, ketamine, methadone (use-dependent block).[4]

Ketamine is a dissociative anaesthetic which has analgesic properties in sub-anaesthetic doses.[3,7] Ketamine is the most potent NMDA-receptor-channel blocker available for clinical use, binding to the phencyclidine site when the channels are in the open activated state.[8] It may also bind to a second membrane-associated site which decreases the frequency of channel opening.[9]

In some countries, both the racemic mixture and the *S*-enantiomer are commercially available for clinical use; in the UK only the racemic mixture is marketed, but the *S*-entantiomer can be imported (see Supply). Because of its greater affinity and selectivity for the NMDA-receptor, the *S*-enantiomer (parenterally) is about 4 times more potent an analgesic than the *R*-enantiomer, and twice as potent as the racemic mixture.[10–12] When equi-analgesic doses are compared, the *S*-enantiomer is also associated with lower levels of undesirable effects, e.g. anxiety, tiredness, cognitive impairment.[11,13] However, no significant differences in efficacy or tolerability were found between the PO racemic mixture (median dose 320mg/24h), the *S*-enantiomer or placebo in patients with cancer-related neuropathic pain.[14]

Ketamine has other actions, some of which may also contribute to its analgesic effect. These include interactions with other calcium and sodium channels, dopamine receptors, cholinergic transmission, noradrenergic and serotoninergic re-uptake (intact descending inhibitory pathways are necessary for analgesia), together with opioid-like and anti-inflammatory effects.[15,16] Ketamine also appears to have a rapid antidepressant effect in patients with major depression.[17]

The analgesic effects of ketamine have been utilized in a wide range of clinical settings using a variety of regimens and routes of administration.

Postoperative analgesia: Two systematic reviews of 37 RCTs of sub-anaesthetic doses of ketamine as an adjunct to opioid-based postoperative analgesia concluded that:

- IV and ED ketamine reduce opioid requirements and possibly chronic post-surgical pain
- CIVI (typically 120–600microgram/kg/h) is best for surgery associated with high opioid requirements, although a single IV dose (typically 150microgram–1mg/kg) may suffice for minor surgery
- adding ketamine to IV patient-controlled analgesia (PCA) is *not* effective.[18,19]

Chronic non-cancer pain: A review of sub-anaesthetic doses of ketamine for chronic non-cancer pain (mostly neuropathic but also ischaemic, fibromyalgia, post-whiplash, etc.) identified 29 RCTs and concluded that:

- ketamine provides relief
- undesirable effects can limit its use
- because of a lack of data, long-term use should be restricted to a controlled trial.[20]

There is RCT evidence of benefit in complex regional pain syndrome type 1.[21,22]

Cancer pain: A systematic review of ketamine as an adjunct to opioids in cancer pain found only two studies of sufficient quality[23,24] and concluded that there was insufficient robust evidence to reach a conclusion.[20] Thus, in patients with cancer, evidence of ketamine's efficacy as an analgesic is mainly from case reports, retrospective surveys or uncontrolled studies in patients with refractory neuropathic, bone and mucositis-related pain.[23–39] Generally, ketamine is used in addition to **morphine** or alternative strong opioid when further opioid increments have been ineffective or precluded by unacceptable undesirable effects. When used in this way, ketamine is generally administered PO or SC/CSCI.[27,33] It can also be administered IM, IV, SL, intranasally, PR and spinally (preservative-free formulation).[24,40–45] However, for spinal routes, concerns have been raised about the potential for neurotoxicity.[46] Ketamine has been given by CIVI in adults and children in combination with opioids (**fentanyl**, **morphine**) $\pm$ **midazolam** to control intractable pain and agitation.[47–49]

Miscellaneous: Ketamine can provide analgesia during painful procedures, e.g. change of burns dressings.[50] Topical ketamine has been applied to the skin in various non-cancer pains,[51,52] and used as an oral rinse in radiation-induced mucositits.[53]

'Burst' ketamine: There is some evidence that short-term 'burst' treatment with ketamine may have relatively long-term benefit in both cancer and non-cancer pain. For example, in patients taking regular strong opioids for ischaemic limb pain, a single 4h IV infusion of ketamine 600microgram/kg reduced opioid requirements during a week of observation.[54] Ketamine 100mg/24h by CIVI for 2 days in a cancer patient, repeated a month later, reduced opioid requirements by 70%.[55] In several case series of cancer patients with severe intractable pain from various causes, 'burst' ketamine 100–500mg/24h by CSCI for 3–5 days relieved pain in about 50% of patients.[35,37,56] Relief lasted from several days to 4 weeks, and occasionally for 2 months. In one study using this regimen, although there were no withdrawals, one quarter of patients experienced severe undesirable effects, such as sedation and confusion.[35]

There is increasing concern about the potential for urinary tract toxicity with ketamine (see Box 13.A). Thus, in patients with a prognosis of months–years, it is probably best to first try a 'burst' approach and limit the long-term regular use of ketamine to situations where this fails. Even then, after 2–3 weeks of satisfactory analgesia with regular ketamine, an attempt can be made to tail off the ketamine over several weeks. Although this may fail and the dose need to be increased again, for some patients benefit persists off ketamine for weeks-months, or with a smaller maintenance dose.[57]

PO ketamine undergoes extensive first-pass hepatic metabolism mainly to norketamine (via CYP3A4).[58] As an *anaesthetic*, norketamine is about one third as potent as parenteral ketamine. However, as an *analgesic* it is equipotent. The maximum blood concentration of norketamine is greater after PO administration than after an injection,[59] and in chronic use norketamine may be the main analgesic agent.

Ketamine causes tachycardia and intracranial hypertension. After anaesthetic use, most patients experience vivid dreams, misperceptions, hallucinations and alterations in body image and mood as emergent (psychotomimetic) phenomena, i.e. as the effects of a bolus dose wear off. These occur to a lesser extent with the sub-anaesthetic analgesic doses given PO or CSCI, and generally can be controlled by concurrent administration of a benzodiazepine (e.g. **diazepam**, **midazolam**) or **haloperidol**.[24,60,61] Sub-anaesthetic doses of ketamine are associated with impaired attention, memory and judgement, and it is used as a pharmacological model for acute schizophrenia.[3]

Less than 10% of ketamine is excreted unchanged, half in the faeces and half renally. Norketamine is excreted renally. Long-term use of ketamine leads to hepatic enzyme induction and enhanced ketamine metabolism.

Bio-availability 93% IM; 45% nasal; 30% SL; 30% PR; 20% PO.[62,63]
Onset of action 5min IM; 15–30min SC; 30min PO.
Time to peak plasma concentration no data SC; 30min PO; 1h norketamine.[64]
Plasma halflife 1–3h IM; 3h PO; 12h norketamine.[65]
Duration of action 30min–2h IM; 4–6h PO, sometimes longer.[66]

Cautions

Current or past history of psychiatric disorder; epilepsy, glaucoma, hypertension, heart failure, ischaemic heart disease and a history of cerebrovascular accidents.[67] Severe hepatic impairment (consider dose reduction).

Plasma concentration increased by **diazepam**. CYP3A4 inhibitors, e.g. **clarithromycin**, **ketoconazole**, increase plasma concentrations of ketamine and reduce those of norketamine, but the clinical relevance of this is unclear.[68]

Undesirable effects

Generally dose-related. Occur in about 40% of patients when given CSCI; less PO: psychotomimetic phenomena (euphoria, dysphasia, blunted affect, psychomotor retardation, vivid dreams, nightmares, impaired attention, memory and judgement, illusions, hallucinations, altered body image), delirium, dizziness, diplopia, blurred vision, nystagmus, altered hearing, hypertension, tachycardia, hypersalivation, nausea and vomiting, erythema and pain at injection site. Urinary tract toxicity (Box 13.A).

When used at higher doses in anaesthesia, tonic-clonic movements are very common (>10%); however, these have not been reported after PO use or with lower parenteral analgesic doses. Ketamine can be abused (or diverted) and careful monitoring is essential.

Dose and use

Because of concerns about urinary tract toxicity (see Box 13.A), consider using ketamine long-term only if a 'burst' approach has failed (see Pharmacology).

Dose recommendations vary considerably but ketamine is often started in a low dose PO (see below). An oral solution can be obtained as a special order or prepared by a local pharmacy (Box 13.B). Alternatively, patients can be supplied with vials of ketamine and 1mL graduated syringes. Two needles (one as an air vent) should be inserted in the stopper of the vial to facilitate withdrawing the ketamine; sterility is not necessary for PO administration.

Box 13.A Ketamine and urinary tract toxicity

The use of ketamine can cause urinary tract symptoms, e.g. frequency, urgency, urge incontinence, dysuria, and haematuria.[69,70] The causal agent has not been determined, but direct irritation by ketamine and/or its metabolites is a possibility.

Investigations have revealed interstitial cystitis, detrusor overactivity, decreased bladder capacity, vesico-ureteric reflux, hydronephrosis, papillary necrosis, and renal impairment. Irreversible damage leading to renal failure has occurred.

The largest case series involved 59 people who had used 'street' ketamine over a prolonged period (6 months–several years).[69]

A small series of three chronic pain patients developed urinary symptoms after receiving ketamine PO 650–800mg/24h for 5–18 months.[71] However, urinary symptoms developed after only 9 *days* in a 16 year-old receiving ketamine PO 8mg/kg/24h.[72]

Thus, when patients on ketamine experience urinary symptoms with no evidence of bacterial infection, practitioners should consider discontinuing the ketamine and seeking the advice of a urologist.

Symptoms generally settle several weeks after stopping ketamine; ideally this should be done gradually to avoid worsening pain (see Dose and use).[73]

Box 13.B Preparation of ketamine oral solution: pharmacy guidelines

Use ketamine 100mg/mL 10mL vials because this is the cheapest concentration. Raspberry Syrup BP can be used for dilution but this is too sweet for some patients. Alternatively, use purified water as the diluent and ask patients to add their own flavouring, e.g. fruit cordial, just before use to disguise the bitter taste.

To prepare 100mL of 50mg/5mL oral solution:
- 10mL vial of ketamine 100mg/mL for injection
- 90mL purified water.

Store in a refrigerator with an expiry date of 1 week from manufacture.

In some centres, an initial test dose is given to assess tolerability and efficacy. The prophylactic concurrent administration of a benzodiazepine or an antipsychotic is also routine in some but not all centres, where it is reserved for more select circumstances (see below). Long-term success, i.e. both pain relief and tolerable undesirable effects, varies from $<$20% to about 50%.[31,41,42,74]

By mouth[27,33,75–77]

Use direct from vial or dilute for convenience to 50mg/5mL (patient adds flavouring of choice, e.g. fruit cordial, to mask the bitter taste):
- start with 10–25mg t.d.s.–q.d.s and p.r.n.
- if necessary, increase dose in steps of 10–25mg up to 100mg q.d.s.
- maximum reported dose 200mg q.d.s.[75,77]
- give a smaller dose more frequently if psychotomimetic phenomena or drowsiness occur which do not respond to a reduction in opioid
- once analgesia has been obtained, some centres try withdrawing the ketamine over several weeks and benefit can persist off ketamine for weeks–months; the course of ketamine is repeated if the pain recurs.

Sublingual[45]

- start with 10–25mg
- place SL and ask patient not to swallow for 2min
- use a high concentration to minimize dose volume; retaining $>$2mL is difficult.

Subcutaneous[33]

- typically 10–25mg p.r.n., some use 2.5–5mg
- if necessary, increase dose in steps of 25–33%.

CSCI[25–27,29,60,78]

Because ketamine is irritant, dilute to the largest volume possible, and consider the use of 0.9% saline as the diluent (see p.667):

- start with 1–2.5mg/kg/24h
- if necessary, increase by 50–100mg/24h
- maximum reported dose 3.6g/24h.

Alternatively, give as short-term 'burst' therapy:[35,37,56]

- start with 100mg/24h
- if 100mg not effective, increase after 24h to 300mg/24h
- if 300mg not effective, increase after a further 24h to 500mg/24h
- stop 3 days after last dose increment.

Half of patients respond and the regimen can be repeated p.r.n.; the duration of benefit varies and undesirable effects are common. The use of prophylactic **diazepam**, **lorazepam**, **midazolam** or **haloperidol** is recommended (see text).

CSCI compatibility with other drugs: There are 2-drug compatibility data for ketamine in 0.9% saline with **alfentanil**, **clonazepam**, **dexamethasone** (low-dose), **diamorphine**, **haloperidol**, **levomepromazine**, **metoclopramide**, **midazolam**, **morphine sulphate** and **oxycodone**.

Ketamine is *incompatibile* with **phenobarbital**. More details, 2-drug and 3-drug compatibility charts can be found on *www.palliativedrugs.com* Syringe Driver Survey Database.

For compatibility charts for mixing drugs in WFI, see Appendix 3, p.773.

Intravenous[33,79]

For cancer pain:

- typically 2.5–5mg p.r.n.

To cover procedures which may cause severe pain:

- 500microgram–1mg/kg (typically 25–50mg; some start with 5–10mg), given over 1–2min preceded by, e.g. **lorazepam** 1mg or **midazolam** 100microgram/kg (typically 5–10mg; some start with 1–2mg) to reduce emergent phenomena.

The right dose should provide analgesia within 1–5min lasting for 10–20min. Note: there is a risk of marked sedation when ketamine and a benzodiazepine are combined in this way; use only if competent in airway management and when the patient can be adequately monitored. Procedures of longer duration may require ketamine CIVI; obtain advice from an anaesthetist.

CIVI[49,80]

- start with 50–200microgram/kg/h and titrate as necessary *or*
- give a single 'burst' of 600microgram/kg up to a maximum of 60mg over 4h (reduce dose by 1/3–1/2 in elderly/frail patients); monitor blood pressure at baseline and then hourly:
  - ▷ if necessary, repeat daily for up to 5 days
  - ▷ if *no* analgesic response to an infusion, increase the dose of the next one by 30%
  - ▷ further dose titrate according to response and/or undesirable effects
  - ▷ repeat the above if the pain subsequently recurs.[57]

In some centres, the background opioid dose is routinely reduced by 25–50% when starting parenteral ketamine. If the patient becomes drowsy, the dose of opioid should be reduced. If a patient experiences dysphoria or hallucinations, the dose of ketamine should be reduced and a benzodiazepine prescribed, e.g. **diazepam** 5mg PO stat & at bedtime, **lorazepam** 1mg PO stat & b.d., **midazolam** 5mg SC stat and 5–10mg CSCI, or **haloperidol**, e.g. 2–5mg PO stat & at bedtime, or 2–5mg SC stat and 2–5mg CSCI.[61] In patients at greatest risk of dysphoria, i.e. those with high anxiety levels, these measures may be more effective if given before starting ketamine.[8]

When switching from CSCI to PO after just a few days, a conversion ratio of 1:1 should be used.[32,81] However, after weeks–months of use, some have found that a *smaller* total daily dose (25–50% of the parenteral dose) can maintain a similar level of analgesia, e.g. CSCI 400mg/24h → PO 150mg/24h.[30] In both instances, the patient should be monitored closely and the dose titrated accordingly. When switching from PO to CSCI or CIVI, it is advisable to commence on a small dose and titrate as required.

Withdrawal phenomena do not generally occur on stopping ketamine. However, after long-term use it is preferable to discontinue ketamine gradually; whole body hyperalgesia and allodynia have been reported after the sudden cessation of ketamine after 3 weeks of use.[73]

Supply

Oral solution (sugar-free) made to order in strengths ranging from 5mg/5mL to 500mg/5mL and pack sizes ranging from 50mL to 500mL; *flavours include blackcurrant, lemon, peppermint, raspberry, and unflavoured.* Prices vary, contact Customer Services for details, e.g. 50mg/5mL, 28 days @ 50mg q.d.s. = £165, based on a 500mL pack of unflavoured solution. (Unlicensed, available as a special order from Martindale; see Obtaining unlicensed products, p.769).

Ketalar® (Pfizer)

Injection 10mg/mL, 20mL vial = £5; 50mg/mL, 10mL vial = £9; 100mg/mL, 10mL vial = £16. *Although use as an analgesic is unlicensed, ketamine injection can be prescribed both in hospitals and in the community. Community pharmacies can order ketamine injection through their Alliance Healthcare wholesale account. To initiate an account, contact head office (tel: 020 8391 2323).*

Ketanest S®

***Injection* ketamine (S-) hydrochloride** (esketamine hydrochloride) *equivalent to ketamine (S-) base* 5mg/mL, 20mL vial = £44. (Unlicensed, available as a named patient supply from IDIS; see Obtaining unlicensed products, p.769).

***Injection (preservative-free)* ketamine (S-) hydrochloride** (esketamine hydrochloride) *equivalent to ketamine (S-) base* 5mg/mL, 5mL amp = £8; 25mg/mL, 2mL amp = £18. (Unlicensed, available as a named patient supply from IDIS; see Obtaining unlicensed products, p.769).

1 Persson J *et al.* (1998) The analgesic effect of racemic ketamine in patients with chronic ischemic pain due to lower extremity arteriosclerosis obliterans. *Acta Anaesthesiologica Scandinavica.* **42**: 750–758.

2 Graven-Nielsen T *et al.* (2000) Ketamine reduces muscle pain, temporal summation, and referred pain in fibromyalgia patients. *Pain.* **85**: 483–491.

3 Visser E and Schug SA (2006) The role of ketamine in pain management. *Biomed Pharmacother.* **60**: 341–348.

4 Richens A (1991) The basis of the treatment of epilepsy: neuropharmacology. In: M Dam (ed) *A Practical Approach to Epilepsy.* Pergamon Press, Oxford, pp. 75–85.

5 Mayer M *et al.* (1984) Voltage-dependent block for Mg^{2+} of NMDA responses in spinal cord neurones. *Nature.* **309**: 261–263.

6 Elliott K *et al.* (1994) The NMDA receptor antagonists, LY274614 and MK-801, and the nitric oxide synthase inhibitor, NG-nitro-L-arginine, attenuate analgesic tolerance to the mu-opioid morphine but not to kappa opioids. *Pain.* **56**: 69–75.

7 Fallon MT and Welsh J (1996) The role of ketamine in pain control. *European Journal of Palliative Care.* **3**: 143–146.

8 Oye I (1998) Ketamine analgesia, NMDA receptors and the gates perception. *Acta Anaesthesiologica Scandinavica.* **42**: 747–749.

9 Orser B *et al.* (1997) Multiple mechanisms of ketamine blockade of N-methyl-D-aspartate receptors. *Anesthesiology.* **86**: 903–917.

10 Oye I *et al.* (1991) The chiral forms of ketamine as probes for NMDA receptor function in humans. In: T Kameyama (ed) *NMDA receptor Related Agents: biochemistry, pharmacology and behavior.* NPP, Ann Arbor, Michigan, pp. 381–389.

11 White PF *et al.* (1980) Pharmacology of ketamine isomers in surgical patients. *Anesthesiology.* **52**: 231–239.

12 Mathisen L *et al.* (1995) Effect of ketamine, an NMDA receptor inhibitor, in acute and chronic orofacial pain. *Pain.* **61**: 215–220.

13 Pfenninger EG *et al.* (2002) Cognitive impairment after small-dose ketamine isomers in comparison to equianalgesic racemic ketamine in human volunteers. *Anesthesiology.* **96**: 357–366.

14 Fallon MT *et al.* (2008) A randomised, double-blind, placebo-controlled, parallel group study, comparing oral racemic ketamine and S-ketamine in the treatment of cancer-related neuropathic pain (Meeting abstract). *Palliative Medicine.* **22**: 440.

15 Meller S (1996) Ketamine: relief from chronic pain through actions at the NMDA receptor? *Pain.* **68**: 435–436.

16 Kawasaki C *et al.* (2001) Ketamine isomers suppress superantigen-induced proinflammatory cytokine production in human whole blood. *Can J Anaesth.* **48**: 819–823.

17 Diazgranados N *et al.* (2010) A randomized add-on trial of an N-methyl-D-aspartate antagonist in treatment-resistant bipolar depression. *Archives of General Psychiatry.* **67**: 793–802.

18 Subramaniam K *et al.* (2004) Ketamine as adjuvant analgesic to opioids: a quantitative and qualitative systematic review. *Anesthesia and Analgesia.* **99**: 482–495.

19 Bell RF (2009) Perioperative ketamine for acute postoperative pain. *Cochrane Database of Systematic Reviews 2006.* **1 (Updated 2009)**

20 Bell RF (2009) Ketamine for chronic non-cancer pain. *Pain.* **141**: 210–214.

21 Sigtermans MJ *et al.* (2009) Ketamine produces effective and long-term pain relief in patients with Complex Regional Pain Syndrome Type 1. *Pain.* **145**: 304–311.

22 Schwartzman RJ *et al.* (2009) Outpatient intravenous ketamine for the treatment of complex regional pain syndrome: a double-blind placebo controlled study. *Pain.* **147**: 107–115.

23 Yang CY *et al.* (1996) Intrathecal ketamine reduces morphine requirements in patients with terminal cancer pain. *Canadian Journal of Anaesthesia.* **43**: 379–383.

24 Mercadante S *et al.* (2000) Analgesic effect of intravenous ketamine in cancer patients on morphine therapy: a randomized, controlled, double-blind, crossover, double-dose study. *Journal of Pain and Symptom Management.* **20**: 246–252.

25 Oshima E *et al.* (1990) Continuous subcutaneous injection of ketamine for cancer pain. *Canadian Journal of Anaesthetics*. **37**: 385–392.
26 Cherry DA *et al.* (1995) Ketamine as an adjunct to morphine in the treatment of pain. *Pain*. **62**: 119–121.
27 Luczak J *et al.* (1995) The role of ketamine, an NMDA receptor antagonist, in the management of pain. *Progress in Palliative Care*. **3**: 127–134.
28 Mercadante S (1996) Ketamine in cancer pain: an update. *Palliative Medicine*. **10**: 225–230.
29 Bell R (1999) Low-dose subcutaneous ketamine infusion and morphine tolerance. *Pain*. **83**: 101–103.
30 Fitzgibbon EJ *et al.* (2002) Low dose ketamine as an analgesic adjuvant in difficult pain syndromes: a strategy for conversion from parenteral to oral ketamine. *J Pain Symptom Manage*. **23**: 165–170.
31 Kannan TR *et al.* (2002) Oral ketamine as an adjuvant to oral morphine for neuropathic pain in cancer patients. *Journal of Pain and Symptom Management*. **23**: 60–65.
32 Benitez-Rosario M *et al.* (2003) A retrospective comparison of the dose ratio between subcutaneous and oral ketamine. *Journal of Pain and Symptom Management*. **25**: 400–402.
33 Kotlinska-Lemieszek A and Luczak J (2004) Subanesthetic ketamine: an essential adjuvant for intractable cancer pain. *Journal Pain Symptom Management*. **28**: 100–102.
34 Fitzgibbon EJ and Viola R (2005) Parenteral ketamine as an analgesic adjuvant for severe pain: development and retrospective audit of a protocol for a palliative care unit. *Journal of Palliative Medicine*. **8**: 49–57.
35 Jackson K and Howell D *Personal communication*.
36 Lauretti G *et al.* (1999) Oral ketamine and transdermal nitroglycerin as analgesic adjuvants to oral morphine therapy and amitriptyline for cancer pain management. *Anesthesiology*. **90**: 1528–1533.
37 Jackson K *et al.* (2001) 'Burst' ketamine for refractory cancer pain: an open-label audit of 39 patients. *Journal of Pain and Symptom Management*. **22**: 834–842.
38 Lossignol DA *et al.* (2005) Successful use of ketamine for intractable cancer pain. *Support Care Cancer*. **13**: 188–193.
39 James PJ *et al.* (2010) The addition of ketamine to a morphine nurse- or patient-controlled analgesia infusion (PCA/NCA) increases analgesic efficacy in children with mucositis pain. *Paediatric Anaesthesia*. **20**: 805–811.
40 Lin T *et al.* (1998) Long-term epidural ketamine, morphine and bupivacaine attenuate reflex sympathetic dystrophy neuralgia. *Canadian Journal of Anaesthesia*. **45**: 175–177.
41 Haines D and Gaines S (1999) N of 1 randomised controlled trials of oral ketamine in patients with chronic pain. *Pain*. **83**: 283–287.
42 Batchelor G (1999) Ketamine in neuropathic pain. *The Pain Society Newsletter*. **1**: 19.
43 Beltrutti D *et al.* (1999) The epidural and intrathecal administration of ketamine. *Current Review of Pain*. **3**: 458–472.
44 Carr DB *et al.* (2004) Safety and efficacy of intranasal ketamine for the treatment of breakthrough pain in patients with chronic pain: a randomized, double-blind, placebo-controlled, crossover study. *Pain*. **108**: 17–27.
45 Mercadante S *et al.* (2005) Alternative treatments of breakthrough pain in patients receiving spinal analgesics for cancer pain. *J Pain Symptom Manage*. **30**: 485–491.
46 Vranken JH *et al.* (2005) Neuropathological findings after continuous intrathecal administration of S(+)-ketamine for the management of neuropathic cancer pain. *Pain*. **117**: 231–235.
47 Berger J *et al.* (2000) Ketamine-fentanyl-midazolam infusion for the control of symptoms in terminal life care. *American Journal of Hospice and Palliative Care*. **17 (2)**: 127–132.
48 Enck R (2000) A ketamine, fentanyl, and midazolam infusion for uncontrolled terminal pain and agitation. *American Journal of Hospice and Palliative Care*. **17 (2)**: 76–77.
49 Conway M *et al.* (2009) Use of continuous intravenous ketamine for end-stage cancer pain in children. *Journal of Pediatric Oncology Nursing*. **26**: 100–106.
50 Richardson P and Mustard L (2009) The management of pain in the burns unit. *Burns*. **35**: 921–936.
51 Finch PM *et al.* (2009) Reduction of allodynia in patients with complex regional pain syndrome: A double-blind placebo-controlled trial of topical ketamine. *Pain*. **146**: 18–25.
52 Gammaitoni A *et al.* (2000) Topical ketamine gel: possible role in treating neuropathic pain. *Pain Medicine*. **1**: 97–100.
53 Slatkin NE and Rhiner M (2003) Topical ketamine in the treatment of mucositis pain. *Pain Medicine*. **4**: 298–303.
54 Mitchell AC and Fallon MT (2002) A single infusion of intravenous ketamine improves pain relief in patients with critical limb ischaemia: results of a double blind randomised controlled trial. *Pain*. **97**: 275–281.
55 Mercadante S *et al.* (2003) Burst ketamine to reverse opioid tolerance in cancer pain. *Journal of Pain and Symptom Management*. **25**: 302–305.
56 Wilcock A (2005) *Data on file*. Burst ketamine in cancer patients.
57 Fallon M (2010) Personal communication.
58 Hijazi Y *et al.* (2002) Contribution of CYP3A4, CYP2B6, and CYP2C9 isoforms to N-demethylation of ketamine in human liver microsomes. *Drug Metabolism & Disposition*. **30**. 853–858.
59 Clements JA *et al.* (1982) Bio-availability, pharmacokinetics and analgesic activity of ketamine in humans. *Journal of Pharmaceutical Sciences*. **71**: 539–542.
60 Hughes A et al. (1999) Ketamine. *CME Bulletin Palliative Medicine*. **1**: 53.
61 Giannini A *et al.* (2000) Acute ketamine intoxication treated by haloperidol: a preliminary study. *American Journal of Therapeutics*. **7**: 389–391.
62 Chong CC *et al.* (2006) Bioavailability of Ketamine After Oral or Sublingual Administration. *Pain Medicine*. **7**: 469–469.
63 Yanagihara Y *et al.* (2003) Plasma concentration profiles of ketamine and norketamine after administration of various ketamine preparations to healthy Japanese volunteers. *Biopharm Drug Dispos*. **24**: 37–43.
64 Grant IS *et al.* (1981) Pharmacokinetics and analgesic effects of IM and oral ketamine. *British Journal of Anaesthesia*. **53**: 805–810.
65 Domino E *et al.* (1984) Ketamine kinetics in unmedicated and diazepam premedicated subjects. *Clinical Pharmacology and Therapeutics*. **36**: 645–653.
66 Rabben T *et al.* (1999) Prolonged analgesic effect of ketamine, an N-methyl-D-aspartate receptor inhibitor, in patients with chronic pain. *Journal of Pharmacology and Experimental Therapeutics*. **289**: 1060–1066.
67 Ward J and Standage C (2003) Angina pain precipitated by a continuous subcutaneous infusion of ketamine. *J Pain Symptom Manage*. **25**: 6–7.
68 Hagelberg N *et al.* (2010) Clarythromycin, a potent inhibitor of CYP3A, greatly increases exposure to oral S-ketamine. *European Journal of Pain*. **14**: 625-629.
69 Chu PS *et al.* (2008) The destruction of the lower urinary tract by ketamine abuse: a new syndrome? *BJU Int*. **102**: 1616–1622.
70 Shahani R *et al.* (2007) Ketamine-associated ulcerative cystitis: a new clinical entity. *Urology*. **69**: 810–812.

71 Storr TM and Quibell R (2009) Can ketamine prescribed for pain cause damage to the urinary tract? *Palliative Medicine*. **23**: 670–672.
72 Gregoire MC *et al.* (2008) A pediatric case of ketamine-associated cystitis (Letter-to-the-Editor RE: Shahani R, Streutker C, Dickson B, et al: Ketamine-associated ulcerative cystitis: a new clinical entity. Urology 69: 810–812, 2007). *Urology*. **71**: 1232–1233.
73 Mitchell AC (1999) Generalized hyperalgesia and allodynia following abrupt cessation of subcutaneous ketamine infusion. *Palliat Med*. **13**: 427–428.
74 Enarson M *et al.* (1999) Clinical experience with oral ketamine. *Journal of Pain and Symptom Management*. **17**: 384–386.
75 Clark JL and Kalan GE (1995) Effective treatment of severe cancer pain of the head using low-dose ketamine in an opioid-tolerant patient. *Journal of Pain and Symptom Management*. **10**: 310–314.
76 Broadley K *et al.* (1996) Ketamine injection used orally. *Palliative Medicine*. **10**: 247–250.
77 Vielvoye-Kerkmeer A (2000) Clinical experience with ketamine. *Journal of Pain and Symptom Management*. **19**: 3.
78 Lloyd-Williams M (2000) Ketamine for cancer pain. *Journal of Pain and Symptom Management*. **19**: 79–80.
79 Mason KP *et al.* (2002) Evolution of a protocol for ketamine-induced sedation as an alternative to general anesthesia for interventional radiologic procedures in pediatric patients. *Radiology*. **225**: 457–465.
80 Hocking G *et al.* (2007) Ketamine: does life begin at 40? *Pain Clinical Updates IASP.* **XV. Issue 3**.
81 Benitez-Rosario MA *et al.* (2011) A strategy for conversion from subcutaneous to oral ketamine in cancer pain patients: efficacy of a 1:1 ratio. *Journal of Pain and Symptom Management.* **10**: 1098-1105.

*PROPOFOL — BNF 15.1.1

Class: General anaesthetic.

Indications: Induction and maintenance of general anaesthesia, continuous conscious sedation (surgical or diagnostic procedures, intubated and mechanically ventilated patients on intensive care units), †refractory agitated delirium or intolerable distress in the imminently dying, †intractable nausea and vomiting.[1]

Contra-indications: Continuous conscious sedation in children ≤16 years. When used for sedation in children in intensive care, the death rate increased 2–3 times.[2] However, propofol is used at some centres to enable radiotherapy in children.[3]

Allergy to eggs, soya or peanuts (the available products contain purified egg phosphatide as an emulsifying agent and soya bean oil).[4]

Pharmacology

Propofol is an ultrafast-acting IV anaesthetic agent. It is rapidly metabolized, mainly in the liver, to inactive compounds which are excreted in the urine. The incidence of untoward haemodynamic changes is low. Propofol reduces cerebral blood flow, cerebral metabolism and, less consistently, intracranial pressure.[5] The reduction in intracranial pressure is greater if the baseline pressure is raised. On discontinuation patients rapidly regain consciousness (10–30min) without residual drowsiness.

In palliative care, propofol is occasionally used, when other approaches have failed, to relieve agitated delirium or intolerable distress in the imminently dying.[6] Careful titration generally permits ‘conscious sedation’, i.e. patients open their eyes on verbal command, possess intact autonomic reflexes, and tolerate mild noxious stimuli.[1] Such use has also been described in children at the end of life.[7]

Propofol also has an anti-emetic effect resulting in less postoperative vomiting compared with other anaesthetic agents.[8–10] Specific postoperative anti-emetic regimens have been designed.[11–13] Chemotherapy-related nausea and vomiting is also helped by adjunctive propofol.[14] In patients receiving non-platinum regimens who were refractory to a combination of **dexamethasone** and a $5HT_3$ antagonist, propofol was of benefit in ≥80%.[15] In palliative care, propofol has also been used to relieve refractory nausea and vomiting in dying patients.[1] Most of the patients probably had bowel obstruction, and it was more effective in relieving nausea than vomiting.

Animal studies suggest that the mechanism of action of propofol as an anti-emetic is by inhibition of serotonin release by enhancing GABA activity, possibly by a direct GABA-mediated action on $5HT_3$-receptors in the area postrema/chemoreceptor trigger zone.[16]

Propofol also has antipruritic, anxiolytic, bronchodilatory, muscle relaxant and anti-epileptic properties. A possible role in refractory status epilepticus requires further clarification.[17,18] Transient excitatory phenomena are seen occasionally (e.g. myoclonus, opisthotonus, tonic-clonic

activity), during induction or recovery when blood levels are low, and presumably at a time when inhibitory centres but not excitatory centres have been depressed.[5,19,20]
Onset of action 30sec.
Time to peak effect 5min.
Plasma halflife 2–4min initial distribution phase; 30–60min slow distribution and initial elimination phase; 3–12h terminal elimination phase. The terminal elimination halflife may increase with prolonged use.
Duration of action 3–10min after single IV bolus.[21,22]

Cautions

Risk of cardiorespiratory depression. Involuntary movements and seizures have been reported, particularly in epileptics, during induction or recovery.[19,23] With prolonged use in acute intensive care, metabolic acidosis, hyperlipidaemia and hepatomegaly have been reported.[2] Although in this setting it is good practice to check plasma lipid levels in patients receiving propofol for ⩾3 days, it is unnecessary in patients whose expected prognosis is only days.

Diprivan® contains disodium edetate (EDTA), a chelating agent which can reduce circulating concentrations and increase urinary losses of trace metals, e.g. zinc. Supplements should be considered for patients who are not imminently dying and who are likely to receive prolonged propofol treatment, particularly those at high risk of deficiency, e.g. from fluid loss, catabolic states or infection.

Undesirable effects

Very common (>10%): local pain at the injection site.
Common (<10%, >1%): headache, hypotension, bradycardia, transient apnoea.
Uncommon (<1%, >0.1%): thrombosis, phlebitis.
Rare: misuse resulting in addiction and/or death. Concerns over a growing incidence among medical staff with access to propofol, e.g. anaesthetists, has prompted moves to designate propofol a controlled drug, particularly in the USA.[24,25]

Dose and use

Propofol is an emulsion of oil-in-water. This gives it a white appearance and makes it a potential growth medium. Diprivan® contains EDTA, a chelating agent which binds to divalent metal ions and reduces their availability for bacterial growth, replication and cell wall integrity. However, the concentration (0.005%) is sufficient only to *retard* microbial growth for up to 12h in the event of accidental contamination.[26] The generic products available in the UK contain no preservatives. Thus, with all propofol products, strict aseptic technique must be employed to prevent microbial contamination *and the container and IV line renewed every 6–12h, in accordance with the individual manufacturer's instructions*. The propofol products available in the UK should not be infused through a microbiological filter.

The use of propofol in palliative care should be restricted to units with access to the necessary expertise and equipment.
Undiluted propofol requires a computer-controlled volumetric infusion pump or IV syringe pump (see manufacturer's SPC for full details).

Undiluted propofol is given by CIVI as a 1% (10mg/mL) or 2% (20mg/mL) solution. Pain at the IV injection site is common but can be minimized by:
- using the antecubital vein (or a large vein in the fore-arm) instead of a hand vein[27,28]
- co-administration of the first dose with **lidocaine**: mix 20 parts propofol injection 1% with 1 part **lidocaine** injection 0.5% or 1% immediately before administration.

Note: *propofol 2% injection should not be mixed with **lidocaine** or any other drug.*
Diluted propofol injection 1% can be administered through a less sensitive infusion control device, e.g. an in-line burette or drop counter, after dilution with 5% glucose (Diprivan® and generic products) or 0.9% saline (generic products only; see SPCs for full details). Dilution is advised with less sensitive infusion control devices because the weaker concentration reduces the risk of severe overdose if the infusion runs fast. The concentration of propofol in the diluted

solution must not be less than 2mg/mL because this can disrupt the emulsion. Diluted propofol should be used within 6h. *Propofol injection 2% should not be diluted.*

Compatibility: Propofol injection 1% is compatible with **alfentanil** and **lidocaine**, and can be diluted with 5% glucose (dextrose) before use (see manufacturer's SPC for details). *Propofol injection 2% should not be diluted or mixed with any other drugs.* Both 1% and 2% propofol can be added through a Y-connector to a running infusion of 5% glucose, 0.9% saline or 4% glucose +0.18% saline; the Y-connector should be placed as close to the injection site as possible.

Refractory agitated delirium or intolerable distress in the imminently dying

Consider propofol only if standard treatments have failed, i.e. a sedative antipsychotic + a benzodiazepine (Figure 13.2).[1,29–31] However, generally, **phenobarbital** should be used in preference to propofol because it is less complicated for clinical staff to titrate and monitor (see p.270).

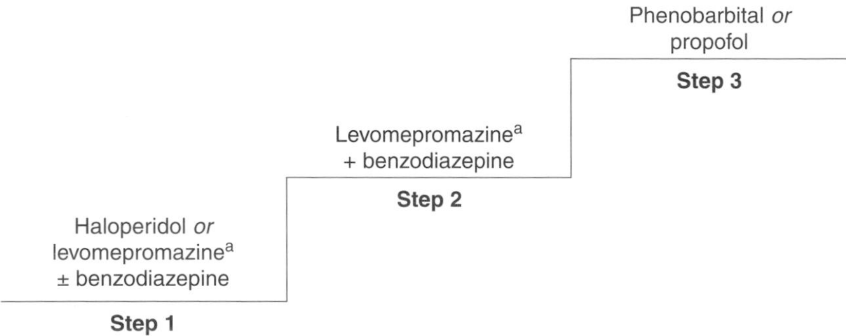

Figure 13.2 Drug treatment used at some centres for irreversible agitated delirium or intolerable distress in the imminently dying.

a. in countries where levomepromazine is not available, e.g. the USA, chlorpromazine is used instead.

Aim to titrate the dose until *conscious sedation* is achieved, i.e. patients open their eyes on verbal command but are not distressed by nursing interventions (e.g. mouth care, turning):

- remain with the patient throughout the initial titration process to ensure an effective and safe dose is found
- generally start with propofol 1mg/kg/h IV
- if necessary, increase by 0.5mg/kg/h every 5–10min until a satisfactory level of sedation is achieved; smaller dose steps can be used to fine-tune the treatment; most patients respond well to 1–2mg/kg/h
- to increase the level of sedation quickly, a bolus dose can be given by increasing the rate to 1mg/kg/*min* for 2–5min
- monitor the patient closely during the first hour of treatment with respect to symptom relief and/or level of sedation, and then after 2, 6, and 12h
- continue to monitor the effect of propofol and the level of sedation at least twice daily
- if the patient is too sedated (i.e. does not respond to a verbal command to open their eyes, shows no response to noxious stimuli) and/or there is evidence of drug-induced respiratory depression, the infusion should be turned off for 2–3min and restarted at a lower rate; occasionally this leads to a progressive reduction in dose because the patient has become unconscious as a result of their disease
- tolerance can develop, necessitating a dose increase, but generally not within 1 week
- long-term use of doses >4mg/kg/h is not recommended because of increasing risk of undesirable effects
- if the patient does not respond to propofol 4mg/kg/h alone, supplement with **midazolam** by CSCI

- it is important to replenish the infusion quickly when a container empties, because the effect of an infusion of propofol wears off after 10–30min
- *because propofol has no analgesic properties, analgesics should be continued.*

Intractable nausea and vomiting

The use of propofol as an anti-emetic should be considered only if all other treatments have failed (see Quick Practice Guide, p.225).[1] Dose titration is generally slower for intractable nausea and vomiting than for terminal agitation:

- remain with the patient for at least 10min following any dose change to ensure that excessive sedation does not occur
- generally start with propofol 0.5mg/kg/h
- if necessary, increase by 0.25–0.5mg/kg/h every 30–60min until a satisfactory response is obtained; smaller dose steps can be used to fine-tune the treatment
- most patients respond well to 0.5–1mg/kg/h; doses > 1mg/kg/h may result in sedation
- monitor the patient closely during the first hour of treatment with respect to symptom relief and/or level of sedation and then after 2, 6, and 12h
- continue to monitor the effect of propofol and level of sedation at least twice daily
- if the patient is too sedated, the infusion should be turned off for 2–3min and then restarted at a lower rate
- if the patient responds well, reduce the infusion rate on a trial basis after 18–24h
- tolerance can develop, necessitating a dose increase, but generally not within 1 week
- it is important to replenish the infusion quickly when a container empties, because the effect of an infusion of propofol wears off after 10–30min
- when used solely for its anti-emetic effect in the last days of life, some centres reduce the dose of, or even discontinue, propofol when the patient becomes unconscious.

Supply

Propofol (generic)

Injection (emulsion) 10mg/mL (1%), 20mL amp = £4, 50mL infusion bottle = £10, 100mL infusion bottle = £19.

Injection (emulsion) 20mg/mL (2%), 50mL vial = £21.

Diprivan® (AstraZeneca)

Injection (emulsion) 10mg/mL (1%), 20mL amp = £1, 50mL pre-filled syringe = £5.

Injection (emulsion) 20mg/mL (2%), 50mL pre-filled syringe = £5.

1 Lundstrom S *et al.* (2005) When nothing helps: propofol as sedative and antiemetic in palliative cancer care. *Journal of Pain and Symptom Management.* **30**: 570–577.
2 Anonymous (2001) Propofol (Diprivan) infusion: sedation in children aged 16 years or younger contraindicated. *Current Problems in Pharmacovigilance.* **27**: 10.
3 Harris EA (2010) Sedation and anesthesia options for pediatric patients in the radiation oncology suite. *International Journal of Pediatrics.* EPUB article ID 870921.
4 Hofer KN *et al.* (2003) Possible anaphylaxis after propofol in a child with food allergy. *Annals of Pharmacotherapy.* **37**: 398–401.
5 Mirenda J and Broyles G (1995) Propofol as used for sedation in the ICU. *Chest.* **108**: 539–548.
6 McWilliams K *et al.* (2010) Propofol for terminal sedation in palliative care: a systematic review. *Journal of Palliative Medicine.* **13**: 73–76.
7 Hooke MC *et al.* (2007) Propofol use in pediatric patients with severe cancer pain at the end of life. *Journal of Pediatric Oncology Nursing.* **24**: 29–34.
8 Tramer M *et al.* (1997) Meta-analytic comparison of prophylactic antiemetic efficacy for postoperative nausea and vomiting: propofol anaesthesia vs omitting nitrous oxide vs total i.v. anaesthesia with propofol. *British Journal of Anaesthesia.* **78**: 256–259.
9 Sneyd JR *et al.* (1998) A meta-analysis of nausea and vomiting following maintenance of anaesthesia with propofol or inhalational agents. *European Journal of Anaesthesiology.* **15**: 433–445.
10 DeBalli P (2003) The use of propofol as an antiemetic. *International Anesthesiology Clinics.* **41**: 67–77.
11 Fujii Y *et al.* (2001) Small doses of propofol, droperidol, and metoclopramide for the prevention of postoperative nausea and vomiting after thyroidectomy. *Otolaryngology–Head and Neck Surgery.* **124**: 266–269.
12 Gan TJ *et al.* (1997) Determination of plasma concentrations of propofol associated with 50% reduction in postoperative nausea. *Anesthesiology.* **87**: 779–784.
13 Gan TJ *et al.* (1999) Patient-controlled antiemesis: a randomized, double-blind comparison of two doses of propofol versus placebo. *Anesthesiology.* **90**: 1564–1570.
14 Scher C *et al.* (1992) Use of propofol for the prevention of chemotherapy-induced nausea and emesis in oncology patients. *Canadian Journal of Anaesthesia.* **39**: 170–172.
15 Borgeat A *et al.* (1994) Adjuvant propofol enables better control of nausea and emesis secondary to chemotherapy for breast cancer. *Canadian Journal of Anaesthesia.* **41**: 1117–1119.

16 Cechetto DF *et al.* (2001) The effects of propofol in the area postrema of rats. *Anesthesia and Analgesia*. **92**: 934–942.
17 Rossetti AO (2007) Which anesthetic should be used in the treatment of refractory status epilepticus? *Epilepsia*. **48 (suppl 8)**: 52–55.
18 Garcia Penas JJ *et al.* (2007) Status epilepticus: evidence and controversy. *Neurologist*. **13 (6 Suppl 1)**: S62–73.
19 Sneyd JR (1999) Propofol and epilepsy. *British Journal of Anaesthesia*. **82**: 168–169.
20 Meyer S *et al.* (2009) Propofol: pro- or anticonvulsant drug? *Anesthesia and Analgesia*. **108**: 1993–1994; author reply 1994.
21 Fechner J *et al.* (2004) Comparative pharmacokinetics and pharmacodynamics of the new propofol prodrug GPI 15715 and propofol emulsion. *Anesthesiology*. **101**: 626–639.
22 Jungheinrich C *et al.* (2002) Pharmacokinetics of the generic formulation Propofol 1 Fresenius in comparison with the original formulation (Disoprivan 1). *Clinical Drug Investigation*. **22**: 417–427.
23 AstraZeneca (2006) *Data on file*.
24 Charatan F (2009) Concerns mount over misuse of anaesthetic propofol among US health professionals. *British Medical Journal*. **339**: b3673.
25 Wilson C *et al.* (2010) The abuse potential of propofol. *Clinical Toxicology*. **48**: 165–170.
26 AstraZeneca (2010) *Personal communication*.
27 Wijeysundera DN and Kavanagh BP (2011) Prevention of pain from propofol injection. *British Medical Journal*. **342**: d1102.
28 Jalota L *et al.* (2011) Prevention of pain on injection of propofol: systematic review and meta-analysis. *British Medical Journal*. **342**: d1110.
29 Mercadante S *et al.* (1995) Propofol in terminal care. *Journal of Pain and Symptom Management*. **10**: 639–642.
30 Moyle J (1995) The use of propofol in palliative medicine. *Journal of Pain and Symptom Management*. **10**: 643–646.
31 Cheng C *et al.* (2002) When midazolam fails. *Journal of Pain and Symptom Management*. **23**: 256–265.

A USA version of this monograph has been published as: Lundström S *et al.* (2010) Propofol. *Journal of Pain and Symptom Management*. **40**: 466–470.

14: GUIDANCE ABOUT PRESCRIBING IN PALLIATIVE CARE

In recent years, both national drug regulatory authorities and the general public have become increasingly concerned about the possibility of dangerous/life-threatening adverse drug events. Official documents and drug manufacturers' information increasingly include a warning along the lines of:

> 'Use the lowest effective dose for the shortest possible time in order to reduce the risk of serious adverse events.'

This advice is, of course, one of the general foundational principles of therapeutic drug use; the advice is simply underlining 'good practice'. Official documents and drug manufacturers' information also highlight when caution is necessary in relation to, for example, hepatic and renal impairment.

In palliative care, many patients are elderly and debilitated, and many have impaired organ function. Accordingly, in *PCF*, it is assumed that prescribers will adopt an appropriately cautious approach in relation to both dose and duration of treatment (also see *Getting the most out of PCF*, p.xix).

This chapter, in addition to offering general advice about 'safe prescribing', emphasizes the special needs of children and the elderly, and examines the impact of hepatic and renal impairment.

GENERAL PRINCIPLES

Always remember: drugs are not the total answer for the relief of pain and other symptoms. For many symptoms, the concurrent use of non-drug measures is equally important, and sometimes more important. An holistic approach to patient care is outlined in various national service provision guidelines.[1–3]

The use of drugs should always be within the context of a systematic approach, which is encapsulated in the acronym ***EEMMA***:

- ***E****valuation* of the impact of the illness on the patient and family, and of the causes of the patient's symptoms (often multifactorial)
- ***E****xplanation* to the patient before starting treatment about what is going on, and what is the most appropriate course of action
- ***M****anagement:* correct the correctable, non-drug treatment, drug treatment
- ***M****onitoring:* frequent review of the impact of treatment; optimizing the doses of symptom relief drugs to maximize benefit and minimize undesirable effects
- ***A****ttention to detail:* do not make unwarranted assumptions; listen actively to the patient, respond to non-verbal and verbal cues.

In palliative care, the axiom *diagnosis before treatment* still holds true. Even when cancer is responsible, a symptom may be caused by different mechanisms. For example, in lung cancer, vomiting may be caused by hypercalcaemia or by raised intracranial pressure (to name just two possible causes). Treatment often varies with the cause.

Attention to detail

Attention to detail includes *precision in taking a drug history.* Thus, if a patient says, 'I take **morphine** every 4 hours', the doctor should ask, 'Tell me, when do you take your first dose?' 'And your second dose?', etc. When this is done, it often turns out that the patient is taking **morphine** q.d.s. rather than q4h, and possibly p.r.n. rather than prophylactically. One 90-year-old woman interpreted '**paracetamol** four times a day' as meaning 0800h, 1200h, 1600h, and 2000h. Although pain-free during the day, she regularly woke between 0200h and 0300h in excruciating pain - so much so that she dreaded going to bed at night. Retiming her medication, so that the doses were more equally spaced out around the clock (on waking, 1200h, 1800h, bedtime), resulted in a pain-free night.

Attention to detail also means giving *clear instructions for drug regimens.* 'Take as much as you like, as often as you like', is a recipe for anxiety and poor symptom relief. The drug regimen should be written out for the patient and their family to work from. Times to be taken, name of drugs, reason for use ('for pain', 'for bowels', etc.) and dose (x mL, y tablets) should all be stated (Figure 14.1 and Figure 14.2). This will need to be modified if both the patient and the immediate family cannot read. The patient should also be advised how to obtain further supplies, e.g. from the general practitioner.

When prescribing an additional drug, it is important to ask:
'What is the treatment goal?'
'How can it be monitored?'
'What is the risk of undesirable effects?'
'What is the risk of drug interactions?'
'Is it possible to stop any of the current medications?'

Safe prescribing

Safe prescribing is a skill, and is crucial to success in symptom management. It extends to considering size, shape and taste of tablets and solutions, and avoiding doses which force patients to take more tablets, and/or open more containers, than would be the case if doses were 'rounded up' to a more convenient tablet size. For example, m/r **morphine** 100mg (one tablet, one container) is easier for the patient than 90mg (two tablets and two containers: 60mg + 30mg).

Safe prescribing requires good communication with patients, carers, and other professionals. Poor communication contributes to one half of preventable drug errors.[4] A lack of information and involvement may leave patients dissatisfied.[5] Good communication includes clear documentation (e.g. allergies, co-morbidities, prescription writing).[6–8] The use of a patient's 'logbook' is to be encouraged; this would include important contact names and telephone numbers.

Safe prescribing practice is particularly important in palliative care where polypharmacy, debility, co-morbidities (e.g. renal impairment), involvement of multiple health professionals, and the use of higher risk medications are among the many factors which make such patients particularly vulnerable to problems with adherence (compliance), undesirable effects, medication errors, drug interactions and other potentially preventable burdens.

Monitoring medication

It is often difficult to predict the optimum dose of a symptom relief drug, particularly opioids, laxatives and psychotropics. Further, undesirable effects put drug adherence in jeopardy. Thus, arrangements must be made for monitoring the effects of medication. The responsibility for such monitoring must be clearly stated. Shared decision-making is a definite risk factor for medication errors.[5,9]

Compromise is sometimes necessary

It may be necessary to compromise on complete relief in order to avoid unacceptable undesirable effects. Antimuscarinic effects, e.g. dry mouth or visual disturbance, may limit dose escalation. Also, with inoperable bowel obstruction, it may be better to aim to reduce the incidence of vomiting to once or twice a day rather than to seek to abolish it altogether.

Hospice Home Care

Name *Linda Barton* **Age** *58* **Date** *15 December 2011*

Tablets/Medicines	2 am	On waking	10 am	2 pm	6 pm	Bed time	Purpose
MORPHINE (Oramorph 2 mg in 1 mL)		*10 mL*	*10 mL*	*10 mL*	*10 mL*	*20 mL*	*pain relief*
METOCLOPRAMIDE (10 mg tablet)		*1*	*1*	*1*	*1*	*1*	*anti-sickness*
IBUPROFEN (400 mg tablet)		*2*		*2*		*2*	*pain relief*
SENNA (tablet)			*2*			*2*	*for bowels*
TEMAZEPAM (20 mg tablet)						*1*	*for sleep*

If troublesome pain: take an extra 10 mL of MORPHINE between regular doses.
If bowels remain constipated: increase SENNA to 3 tablets twice a day.

- Keep this chart with you so you can show your doctor or nurse this list of what you are taking.
- Ask for a fresh supply of your medication 2–3 days before you need it.
- Sometimes your medication may be supplied in different strengths or presentations. If you have any concerns about this, check with your pharmacist.
- In an emergency, phone ______________________ and ask to speak to ______________

Figure 14.1 Example of a patient's home medication chart (q4h).

Hospice Home Care

Name *Nicolas Crowthorne* **Age** *65* **Date** *15 December 2011*

Tablets/Medicines	*Breakfast*	*Midday meal*	*Evening meal*	*Bedtime*	Purpose
ASILONE (suspension)	*10mL*	*10mL*	*10mL*	*10mL*	*for hiccups*
MORPHINE (MST 100 mg tablet)	*1*			*1*	*pain relief*
NAPROXEN (500 mg tablet)	*1*			*1*	*pain relief*
SENNA (tablet)	*2*	*2*	*2*	*2*	*for bowels*
HALOPERIDOL (1.5 mg tablet)				*1*	*anti-sickness*
DIAZEPAM (5 mg tablet)				*1*	*for sleeping and relaxation*

If troublesome pain: take MORPHINE SOLUTION (2mg in 1mL) 10 mL, up to every hour.
If troublesome hiccup: take extra 10 mL of ASILONE, up to every 2 hours.

- Keep this chart with you so you can show your doctor or nurse this list of what you are taking.
- Ask for a fresh supply of your medication 2–3 days before you need it.
- Sometimes your medication may be supplied in different strengths or presentations. If you have any concerns about this, check with your pharmacist.
- In an emergency, phone ______________________ and ask to speak to ______________

Figure 14.2 Example of a patient's home medication chart (q.d.s.).

Rescue ('as needed') medication

Patients need advice about what to do for episodic symptoms, particularly break-through (episodic) pain. Generally with drugs, it is good practice to err on the side of generosity in relation to the recommended frequency of p.r.n. medication. However, it does depend on the class and formulation of the drug in question, and whether the patient is an inpatient or at home.

In all circumstances, it is important that the permitted frequency is stated clearly on the patient's medication chart (see Figure 14.1 and Figure 14.2), and also verbally explained to the patient and the family.

Regular m/r strong opioid medication at home

The *corresponding* normal-release opioid analgesic formulation should also be prescribed q1h p.r.n. in an appropriate dose (see p.279).

Regular normal-release strong opioid medication at home

The *same* normal-release opioid analgesic formulation should also be prescribed routinely q1h p.r.n.

With regular normal-release strong opioid medication, if a patient needs an *occasional* rescue dose, say, 40min or less before the next regular dose is due, it may suffice to give the next regular dose early. However, opinion is divided. Some specialists say that a p.r.n. dose should be given, followed in due course by the regular dose.

Regular analgesic medication other than a strong opioid

Paracetamol and NSAIDs are often prescribed at the maximum recommended dose. In this case, a normal-release opioid analgesic should be prescribed *q1h p.r.n.*, either a weak opioid or a low dose of a strong opioid.

Recommendations for anti-emetics, laxatives, and psychotropics have been given in their respective sections.

Inpatients

Recommendations can be more generous because there are trained personnel to monitor the effect of any additional medication, and thus prevent serious toxicity. For example, prescribing a range of permitted doses allows nurses to increase the amount given on their own initiative.

Example: Patient taking m/r **morphine** 100mg b.d.
Expected p.r.n. dose = 1/10–1/6 of total 24h dose, i.e. 20–30mg
Chart **morphine** normal-release tablets/suspension 20–30mg q1h p.r.n.

In practice, nurses tend to start with the lower dose, but increase to the top of the range if necessary. If two consecutive top-of-the-range doses at the maximum permitted frequency are insufficient, medical advice should be obtained and alternative measures considered, e.g. rapid titration with IV **morphine** (see p.366 and Boxes 5.K and 5.L, p.367), with a subsequent upward adjustment of the regular PO dose.

SC DRUG ADMINISTRATION BY INFORMAL CARERS

Injections are regularly given by relatives and other informal carers to children or adults with, for example, diabetes mellitus or cystic fibrosis. In palliative care, there are occasions when it is helpful to train one or more relative or other informal carer to give SC injections (including Controlled Drugs):

- regular medication which cannot be taken by a less invasive route
- emergency medication for symptoms which may develop particularly during a patient's last days.

Clear procedures are necessary to ensure the safety of the patient, support for the carer, and to comply with Nursing and Midwifery Council standards for medicines management (Box 14.A).[10] Examples of procedures and documentation are available on www.palliativedrugs.com document library, filed under medication issues (subcutaneous administration).

Some emergency medication can be given SL rather than by injection. The same procedures and safeguards are needed when delegating the administration of any medicinal product to a relative or other informal carer.

Box 14.A Procedures and safeguards for informal carers giving SC injections[11,12]

Careful evaluation of the situation by the healthcare team.

Signed consent obtained from the patient (if feasible).

Informal carers, particularly if qualified nurses or doctors, must not be pressured to give injections, and should be able to discontinue at any time.

Carer's fears must be explored, including the possibility of the patient dying shortly after an injection.

Carers must:
- be trained and assessed as competent, and this must be documented and retained
- be provided with written information for each drug, including the name, dose, indication, likely undesirable effects, time before a repeat dose is permitted, maximum number of injections/24h
- keep a record of all injections given, including date, time, drug strength, formulation and dose, and name of person giving the injection
- be provided with contact telephone numbers for both in- and out-of-hours.

Regular support and review of the situation must be carried out by healthcare professionals.
Close liaison with the primary health care team, and all out-of-hours services.

PRESCRIBING FOR CHILDREN

The background for this section is given in Box 14.B.

Box 14.B Evaluation of symptoms in dying children

It is estimated that $>$7 million children worldwide could benefit from palliative care.[13] In England, the prevalence rate for the under 20s is estimated to be 16 per 10,000 population aged 0–19.[14]

Although cancer is the second most common condition (after trauma) causing death in children, most children needing palliative care have diagnoses other than cancer. The largest group have neurological or neuromuscular disorders, e.g. hypoxic brain injury or inherited progressive metabolic, muscle or degenerative disease.

The need for palliative care may extend over many years, sometimes from the time of diagnosis, and is commonly needed in parallel with ongoing treatment of the underlying condition and of any intercurrent illness.

Evaluation is inherently more difficult than in most adults. Further, in children with life-limiting conditions, it is often difficult to identify the end-stage, particularly with disorders other than cancer.

Common problems include cerebral irritability, intractable seizures, skeletal muscle spasm, pain, swallowing and feeding difficulties, gastro-oesophageal reflux, breathlessness and troublesome secretions.

Symptom evaluation is particularly difficult in children with cognitive impairment.[15,16] As far as possible, use self-reporting tools appropriate to the child's age and ability.[17–20]

A parent's report and staff observation are important.

Symptom scales and diaries aid continuity between different carers, and across different settings, e.g. home, school, hospital, hospice, and respite centre.

Ongoing care should be under the direction of a multiprofessional team, including specialist paediatric palliative care,[21] ideally with advice from a paediatric pharmacist.

There are several respected sources providing guidance about prescribing for children generally[22–25] and more specifically in palliative care.[13,26,27] A Master Formulary is available from the Association for Paediatric Palliative Medicine.[28]

There is still a dearth of paediatric data for pharmacokinetics, pharmacodynamics, and drug safety.[29] In order to increase the body of knowledge, significant undesirable effects in children should be reported:

- in UK:
  - ▹ through the Yellow Card Scheme, www.yellowcard.gov.uk
  - ▹ through the PaedPalCare list, www.act.org.uk
- other countries have similar national and specialist reporting schemes, e.g.:
  - ▹ FDA Medwatch, www.fda.gov/Safety/MedWatch/default.html (USA)
  - ▹ Medeffect, www.hc-sc.gc.ca/dhp-mps/medeff/index-eng.php (Canada)
  - ▹ Canadian Network of Palliative Care for Children, http://cnpcc.ca/
  - ▹ pediatric pain mailing list, http://pediatric-pain.ca/ppml/ppmlist.html (Canada)
- to www.palliativedrugs.com.

Extra care is required when prescribing for children:

- *avoid drugs as far as possible:* first consider non-drug options, and prescribe only if there is a clear indication
- *simplify regimens:* try to avoid the need to administer drugs during school time
- *limit the range of medications:* become familiar with the use of a limited range of drugs and their effects in children
- check dose calculations.

Children should be involved (at a level appropriate to their age and understanding) in decisions about taking drugs. Children are at increased risk of medication errors because of:

- lack of evidence-based data
- the diversity and rarity of their conditions
- the need to calculate and adjust the dose for the age and/or weight of the child
- the lack of suitable dose formulations
- variations in recommended doses and administration regimens
- inconsistent presentation of recommended dose information (e.g. microgram/kg per dose, microgram/kg/h, mg per dose, total 24h dose).

Particular care is required when prescribing in the neonatal period (prematurity and first 28 days of life) because of immature renal function and liver enzyme pathways, immature reticular activating systems, and differing volumes of distribution.

As far as possible, drugs should be prescribed within the terms of their licence.[24,30] However, as in adult palliative care, there are likely to be many occasions when it is necessary to prescribe drugs 'off-label', i.e. beyond their approved indications and/or routes of administration (see p.xxiii).

Deciding the dose

Paediatric dosing needs to be based on the physiological characteristics of the child, and the pharmacokinetics of the drug.[31] Dosing by age may be misleading, particularly in palliative care where, because of underlying disease, children are unlikely to be close to the mean weight for their age. Thus, generally, the dose is better determined by *body weight* than by age.

Using body surface area is more accurate because it tends to mirror physiological processes more closely, and this should be used particularly when calculating doses of cytotoxic drugs. Generally, doses in children should not exceed the maximum adult dose.

There is little evidence-based data for drug doses in children, and practice has often evolved from personal experience and case series. Flexible personalized schedules are acceptable for many drugs so as to make it as straightforward as possible for the child, and thus increase adherence to the regimen and minimize disruption to schooling and sleep. However, regular timing is important for some drugs, e.g. antibacterials.

Drug formulation and administration

A liquid may be easier to administer than tablets or capsules, particularly for young children who are very unwell and/or have dysphagia. Some children may prefer the taste of tablets to nauseating syrups. On the other hand, m/r tablets must not be crushed because this will accelerate drug delivery and absorption, sometimes dangerously (see p.693).

Although unpleasant taste may affect adherence, the taste of a medication can often be masked with small quantities of food or fruit juice. However, medication should not be added to a feeding bottle.

An oral syringe should be used for accurate measurement of liquid medicines. The use of alternative routes of administration (buccal, intranasal, PR, SC, IV) is relatively common in children. Some already have a central venous line which can be accessed by carers. If available, this route is generally the most appropriate for continuous infusions.

Many children with life-limiting illnesses or life-threatening conditions are fed by nasogastric tubes or gastrostomy (see p.693).[32] The presence of a feeding tube may mean that, during the last few hours or days, a CSCI/CIVI is not needed. However, vigilance is required because, close to death, GI absorption can become impaired. There is also the risk that medicines may continue to be administered via a feeding tube, even when no longer necessary or appropriate. Regular review is essential.

The IM route is particularly distressing for children, and should generally be avoided. The SC route may be appropriate and acceptable for children, and is the route of choice for continuous infusions if there is no permanent central venous access.

Pharmacological considerations

Polypharmacy

Children with life-limiting or life-threatening illnesses are often on complicated regimens with multiple medications. This increases the possibility of undesirable drug effects and interactions (particularly with anti-epileptic drugs). Further, large volumes of liquid may be needed when administering multiple medications. Regimens should be reviewed regularly and simplified whenever possible. In this, the help of a paediatric pharmacist is invaluable.

Pharmacokinetics and pharmacodynamics

Compared with adults, children under 12 years tend to absorb and metabolize drugs differently:

- *neonates (< 1 month)* have relatively low renal and hepatic clearances, and higher volumes of distribution, resulting in a prolonged halflife for many drugs; this may necessitate relatively lower doses at longer intervals (compared with infants and children, on a weight for weight basis). Drugs primarily metabolized by the liver should be administered with extreme care until the age of 2 months[31]
- *infants and children (1 month–12 years)* have relatively high drug clearances, and normal volumes of distribution, resulting in a shorter halflife for many drugs; this may necessitate relatively higher doses at shorter intervals (compared with adults)
- *hepatic impairment* may not necessitate dose reduction; children without liver disease have a large reserve of hepatic metabolic capacity. Liver volumes increase with age and are more closely correlated to surface area rather than to weight.[31]

Thus, special consideration is required with:

- *neonates (particularly if premature) and infants:* because liver enzyme systems may not be fully developed, metabolic pathways can differ from those in older children (e.g. **alfentanil**, **midazolam**, **morphine** all have longer elimination halflives in neonates and infants)[31]
- *hypoproteinaemia:* the effects of highly protein-bound drugs (e.g. benzodiazepines, **phenytoin**, **prednisolone**, **warfarin**) may be increased
- *coagulation impairment:* gives rise to an increased response to oral anticoagulants.

In addition, immaturity of renal function in children can result in lower renal drug clearance, particularly in neonates.

Monitoring drug concentrations

Monitoring serum drug concentrations is generally of limited value, and additional venepunctures are distressing for children. Monitor the serum concentration only when dose adjustment on a clinical basis is known to be inadequate, e.g. **gentamicin**, **phenobarbital**, **phenytoin**, **teicoplanin**.

Specific cautions when prescribing for children

Anti-epileptics

Many children with life-limiting or life-threatening conditions are on complicated anti-epileptic regimens. Interactions are common between anti-epileptics, and are mostly caused by liver enzyme induction or inhibition. They are variable and unpredictable and may increase toxicity without a corresponding increase in anti-epileptic effect. Anti-epileptics also have significant interactions with other drugs (see p.237). Specialist paediatric neurology advice is recommended when titrating or reducing anti-epileptics in children.

Generally, anti-epileptic medication should *not* be stopped in the terminal phase, although absorption and administration may prove unpredictable. An alternative route of administration, and the addition or substitution of SC **midazolam** or **phenobarbital** may be necessary. Some anti-epileptics (**carbamazepine**, **clonazepam**, **diazepam**, **lorazepam**, **phenobarbital** and **valproate**) can be given PR, but may require dose adjustment.[33] For example, the dose of **carbamazepine** should be increased by 25% when converting from PO to PR.[34]

Rectal administration may also be possible for **lamotrigine**[35] and **vigabatrin**, but strong evidence is lacking.

Corticosteroids

In paediatric palliative care, the commonest reason for prescribing a corticosteroid is headache and vomiting caused by raised intracranial pressure associated with progressive intracranial tumours. Compared with adults, children seem to experience a more rapid onset of relatively severe undesirable effects (particularly cushingoid facies, proximal myopathy, weight gain, and changes in mood and behaviour). Thus, corticosteroids should be used at the lowest effective dose and for the shortest possible time.

Some centres use short courses of corticosteroids (e.g. **dexamethasone** ≤500microgram/kg/day for 3–5 days) repeated as dictated by symptoms. However, good symptom management may necessitate daily administration, despite the increased undesirable effects and increased difficulty when attempting to wean a child off corticosteroids.[36,37] A gastroprotective drug may need to be prescribed concurrently.

Opioids

Opioids can generally be used safely in children, just as in adults, although this may require careful explanation to parents and carers to allay fears. The transmucosal route (buccal, SL) is often used for p.r.n. doses of **morphine** or **fentanyl** to relieve break-through (episodic) pain. As in adults, doses of transmucosal fentanyl products should be titrated against the child's pain. The needed dose may not correlate closely with background opioid requirements, although these should be taken into account.

The use of some drugs is limited in children by the lack of an appropriate formulation. However, **fentanyl** and **buprenorphine** patches are being increasingly used as a convenient long-acting opioid formulation for children. In view of the risk of fatal respiratory depression, TD medications should be used only in children already taking opioids regularly. Particular care should be exercised if a child becomes pyrexial because this is likely to accelerate the rate of diffusion from the patch.

Other than with inappropriately used TD products, there is little evidence of opioids causing serious respiratory depression in children when the dose is individually titrated against a child's pain, except in neonates. In this group, there is a documented incidence of late respiratory depression (>4h after administration of normal-release **morphine**).[38] Compared with doses in children aged 2–12 years, the recommended doses per kg are lower in those under 2 years, and much lower in neonates (<1 month).

Of the undesirable effects of opioids, pruritus and urinary retention are probably more common, and nausea probably less common than in adults (although this may be under-diagnosed).[39]

Phenothiazines

Although evidence is sparse, children may have an age-related increased risk of dystonic reactions with D_2 antagonists, e.g. phenothiazines and **metoclopramide** (also see Drug-induced movement disorders, p.745). Such drugs should be used with caution particularly in those <20 years old.[40,41]

PRESCRIBING FOR THE ELDERLY

Particular care is required when prescribing for the elderly.[42,43] The following should be kept in mind:

- *avoid drugs whenever possible:* always consider non-drug options first; prescribe drugs only when clearly indicated
- *simplify regimens:* avoid complicated or frequent dose regimens; whenever possible give medication once daily or b.d.
- *limit the range of drugs:* become familiar with the use of a limited range of drugs and their effects in the elderly
- *long-acting antidiabetic drugs:* **chlorpropamide** (not UK) and **glibenclamide** are best avoided
- *dose reduction:* doses should generally be lower than for younger patients, e.g. start with about 50% of the normal adult dose.

Form of medicine

Frail elderly patients may have difficulty swallowing tablets. They should be instructed to take tablets or capsules with fluid in an upright position to minimize the possibility of them remaining in the mouth or oesophagus, and causing ulceration (e.g. NSAIDs, **temazepam**). Alternative formulations (e.g. liquid) or routes of administration (e.g. SC) may be preferable.

Polypharmacy

Elderly patients are more likely to be receiving multiple drugs for existing diseases and the addition of more drugs for the relief of symptoms will increase the risk of drug interactions (see Cytochrome P450, p.735), undesirable effects, and may affect adherence (compliance). Thus, medicines should be reviewed regularly and any of doubtful benefit should be stopped. These include prophylactic drugs which become irrelevant for a patient with a poor prognosis, e.g. statins.

Pharmacokinetics

One of the most important changes to occur with increasing age, which influences the pharmacokinetics of many drugs, is the progressive decline in renal function. Drugs are excreted more slowly and a lower dose may suffice, particularly those with a narrow therapeutic ratio, e.g. **digoxin** (see Renal impairment, p.618). Acute illness, particularly accompanied by dehydration, can lead to a rapid further reduction in renal clearance.

Drug monitoring

With highly protein-bound drugs, if the serum drug concentration is used to monitor treatment, changes in serum protein concentrations can lead to difficulty in interpreting the results:

- *albumin* binds acidic drugs, e.g. **phenytoin**, and when reduced by malnutrition, cirrhosis, nephrotic syndrome, end-stage renal disease, etc., the proportion of unbound (active) drug is likely to increase, even though the total serum drug concentration may decrease or remain normal
- *α_1-acid glycoprotein* (an acute phase protein) binds basic drugs, e.g. **lidocaine**, and when increased by infection, inflammatory disease, cancer, etc., the total serum drug concentration will increase, but the proportion of unbound (active drug) may decrease or remain normal.

Thus, a patient with hypo-albuminaemia may have a low total **phenytoin** serum concentration but a therapeutic unbound concentration, and increasing the dose to achieve a 'therapeutic' total concentration may result in toxicity.

Conversely, a patient with an acute illness may have a high total **lidocaine** serum concentration but a therapeutic unbound concentration, and reducing the dose to achieve a 'therapeutic' total concentration may result in loss of effect.

Thus, measuring free (unbound) levels of highly protein-bound drugs is preferable. If this is not possible, formulas to 'correct' for low serum protein concentrations are available for some drugs. For example, the following formula can be used to correct the total **phenytoin** concentration in someone with hypo-albuminaemia:[44]

$$\text{Corrected total phenytoin concentration} = \frac{\text{observed concentration}}{(0.02 \times \text{albumin}) + 0.1}$$

Pharmacodynamics

The aging body shows increased sensitivity to drugs, e.g. centrally-acting drugs such as opioids, benzodiazepines and antipsychotics. This increases the risk of delirium, postural hypotension and falls (Box 14.C).

Box 14.C Specific cautions when prescribing for the elderly

Antihypertensives, antiparkinsonian drugs, digoxin, psychotropics
Undesirable effects are more common. Use smaller doses and monitor closely.

Co-trimoxazole, mianserin
Avoid if possible because of increased risk of drug-induced bone marrow depression.

Diuretics
Do not use long-term to treat simple gravitational or hypoproteinaemic oedema.

Night sedatives (hypnotics)
Use a short course of a drug with a short halflife. Benzodiazepines impair balance and their use may result in falls. There is no evidence that zopiclone or zolpidem are better tolerated.

NSAIDs
Serious or fatal bleeding is more common. A special hazard in patients with heart disease (fluid retention) or renal impairment (may exacerbate). Use non-drug methods and paracetamol before prescribing an NSAID in low dose, e.g. naproxen 250mg b.d. or ibuprofen 200–400mg t.d.s.

Warfarin
A lower maintenance dose is generally required, and the outcome of bleeding is often more serious.

HEPATIC IMPAIRMENT

Because the liver is the main site for the metabolism of most drugs, hepatic impairment, particularly when moderate–severe, may lead to changes in pharmacokinetics and pharmacodynamics.[45] These changes can include:

- increased bio-availability
- accumulation of drugs or metabolites
- prolonged halflife
- disruption of the blood-brain barrier resulting in higher CNS concentrations of some drugs.[46,47]

Such changes result from how the liver disease impacts on drug:

- absorption, e.g. reduced bile salts in cholestasis → reduced absorption of lipid soluble drugs
- distribution, e.g.:
  - ▹ ascites → increased volume of distribution of water-soluble drugs
  - ▹ hypo-albuminaemia → increased level of active unbound drug in those which are highly protein-bound (also see monitoring **phenytoin** levels, p.258)
- metabolism, e.g.:
  - ▹ decreased hepatic blood flow and drug extraction → increased bio-availability
  - ▹ decreased function of cytochrome P450 and other enzymes (see below) → increased bio-availability

- excretion, e.g.:
  - ▹ cholestasis → reduced elimination of drugs excreted in bile
  - ▹ hepatic and renal impairment can occur concurrently (hepatorenal syndrome, see below) → necessitates further consideration and caution
- pharmacodynamics; there may be altered sensitivity to the effects of drugs, e.g.:
  - ▹ antihypertensives → increased risk of hypotension
  - ▹ diuretics → reduced response
  - ▹ NSAIDs → increased risk of GI bleeding; fluid retention
  - ▹ opioids, benzodiazepines, psychotropics → increased sedation; may precipitate encephalopathy (see below)
  - ▹ oral anticoagulants → increased risk of bleeding
  - ▹ oral hypoglycaemics → increased risk of hypoglycaemia.

Hepatic metabolism involves:[48]

- *phase I:* cytochrome P450 enzymes in the endoplasmic reticulum (see Cytochrome P450, p.735)
- *phase II:* various enzymes, e.g. glucuronyl transferases, in the endoplasmic reticulum and cytosol
- *phase III:* active drug transport across cell membranes, e.g. P-glycoprotein.

The effect of liver disease on drug metabolism depends on:

- *drug:* generally the liver converts active lipophilic drugs into inactive hydrophilic metabolites for excretion by the kidneys; sometimes pro-drugs are metabolized into active forms, e.g. **codeine → morphine**
- *disease severity:* because of the large hepatic reserve, impaired hepatic elimination only occurs in severe disease
- *enzymes:* generally phase II enzymes are affected less than phase I enzymes, which are also affected to different degrees, e.g. CYP1A2, 2C19 > 2A6, 3A4 > 2C9, 2E1
- *disease process:* e.g. acute hepatitis impairs phase I > phase III, whereas the opposite occurs in cholestasis; drugs excreted unchanged in the bile, e.g. **rifampicin**, **fusidic acid**, may accumulate in cholestasis.

Severe and rapidly deteriorating liver disease impairs renal function (hepatorenal syndrome). However, even moderate hepatic impairment reduces renal clearance and will necessitate a reduction in dose of renally excreted drugs.[49] Serum creatinine is an insensitive guide to glomerular filtration rate (GFR) in patients with cirrhosis (reduced muscle mass; reduced conversion of creatine → creatinine). Ideally, creatinine clearance should be used, but it can overestimate GFR in cirrhosis.[48]

Many drugs can precipitate hepatic encephalopathy by causing sedation (e.g. opioids, benzodiazepines, psychotropics), hypokalaemia (e.g. diuretics, corticosteroids), or constipation (e.g. opioids).

Thus, in liver disease, the metabolism of different drugs is not uniformly affected, and it is not possible to predict from routine LFTs how the metabolism of a particular drug will be impaired. Despite this, for many drugs, there are few data on the effects of hepatic impairment on their metabolism; often this is limited to changes in halflife which occur in cirrhosis.

The Child-Pugh score

The Child-Pugh total score gives a general indication of the degree of hepatic impairment in cirrhosis, and is mainly used as a prognostic aid (Table 14.1). It stratifies into three classes: total score 5–6 = A; 7–9 = B; ≥10 = C.

Table 14.1 Child-Pugh Criteria of Liver Disease (see text for classification)

Factor	*Units*	*Score of 1*	*Score of 2*	*Score of 3*
Serum bilirubin	micromol/L	<34	34–51	>51
	mg/dL	<2.0	2.0–3.0	>3.0
Serum albumin	g/L	>35	30–35	<30
	g/dL	>3.5	3.0–3.5	<3.0
INR		<1.7	1.7–2.3	>2.3
Ascites		None	Easily controlled	Poorly controlled
Hepatic encephalopathy		None	Minimal	Advanced

Clinical recommendations

Hepatotoxic drugs should be avoided or used with extra care. Drugs causing dose-related toxicity do so at lower doses in patients with hepatic impairment, and drugs producing idiosyncratic reactions do so more frequently. Information on the halflives in cirrhosis or hepatic impairment of selected drugs is available elsewhere.[50]

Analgesics: Non-opioids

A single-dose study of **paracetamol** in patients with liver disease found that, in mild liver disease, plasma halflife was similar to that in healthy controls (predictable considering that **paracetamol** is eliminated principally by glucuronidation) but that, in severe liver failure, its halflife was nearly doubled.[51]

Aspirin and **ibuprofen** have similar pharmacokinetics in patients with moderate–severe liver disease.[52,53] On the other hand, **naproxen** has a greatly increased halflife in patients with hepatic disorders,[54] and it is recommended that the dose is halved.[46]

Analgesics: Opioids

Except for **morphine** and **buprenorphine**, the major metabolic pathway for most opioids is oxidation. This is reduced in patients with hepatic cirrhosis, resulting in:

- decreased drug clearance, particularly for **alfentanil**, **dextropropoxyphene**, **pentazocine**, **pethidine** (meperidine), and **tramadol** *and/or*
- increased oral bio-availability caused by a reduced first-pass metabolism, for **dextropropoxyphene**, **dihydrocodeine**, **pentazocine** and **pethidine.**[55]

Codeine, **dextropropoxyphene** and **pethidine** are generally best not used in moderate–severe hepatic impairment.[56] Care also needs to be taken to avoid constipation with opioids, as increased bowel transit time can result in increased ammonia absorption, and precipitate encephalopathy.[57]

To a large extent, **tramadol** and **codeine** are pro-drugs activated by metabolism in the liver. They are both best avoided in moderate–severe liver impairment.

There have been several studies on the plasma clearance and elimination halflife of **morphine** in patients with various degrees of hepatic failure or cirrhosis. More recent studies have found a decreased plasma clearance and prolonged elimination halflife in patients with cirrhosis, compared with patients without liver disease, thus necessitating a reduction in dose and a decreased frequency of administration.[58,56,59]

In end-stage cirrhosis, **oxycodone** has severely impaired elimination which returns to within normal limits after liver transplantation.[60] **Oxycodone** is best avoided in severe cirrhosis. In contrast, **fentanyl** pharmacokinetics are not altered.[61] This may be because of the large volume of distribution of **fentanyl**, with only a small fraction in the central compartment for hepatic uptake. In this case, its terminal halflife would better reflect its slow release from tissue depots rather than its hepatic elimination.[61] Thus, **fentanyl** may be the opioid of choice in patients with moderate–severe liver failure or cirrhosis.

Anti-arrthymics

The halflife of **lidocaine** and **mexiletine** is tripled in cirrhosis. Thus, if used, reduce the dose to 25% of the usual dose.[62]

Antibacterials

Most of the commonly used antibacterials seem to be safe when used for patients with liver disease. Although there is generally no need to alter the dose of **ampicillin** in cirrhosis, patients with co-existing renal impairment may need a reduced dose.[63] **Ceftriaxone** and **metronidazole** show no significant change in pharmacokinetics in patients with severe liver disease.[62]

Rifampicin is used to palliate the symptoms of cholestatic pruritus; its elimination halflife has been shown to be almost doubled in patients with severe hepatic impairment compared with controls.[64]

Antidepressants

The halflife of **amitriptyline** is unchanged, so the dose is unchanged.[62] In contrast, the dose of **fluoxetine** should be halved, and **paroxetine** should be started at a reduced dose.

Anti-emetics

There are few data on the halflife life changes for **cyclizine**, **haloperidol**, **metoclopramide** or **prochlorperazine**. However, **metoclopramide** is reported to be safe in liver failure.[65]

Clearance of **ondansetron** is progressively reduced with increasing hepatic impairment. Patients with severe hepatic impairment should have their dose of this drug limited to 8mg/24h.[66]

Anti-epileptics

In the presence of liver disease **carbamazepine** should be avoided.[67] The halflife of **valproate** is significantly prolonged in cirrhosis and in acute hepatitis, but generally it is not necessary to adjust the dose.[68] Thus it may be used with caution. There are no data for **gabapentin** or **pregabalin**.

Antipsychotics

There are limited data on the antipsychotics. It is known that **chlorpromazine** has an unchanged halflife, but there may be increased sensitivity to its effects.

Benzodiazepines

Sedatives have been implicated as common precipitants of coma in patients with hepatocellular disease,[69] even in usual doses.[70]

Midazolam is extensively metabolized in the liver via oxidation.[71] Elimination is significantly reduced in cirrhosis. However, the hypnotic effects were reported to be similar in both cirrhosis and healthy controls. Even so, it is best to start with a reduced dose of **midazolam** in advanced cirrhosis, and titrate as necessary.[71]

The halflife of **diazepam** in cirrhosis more than doubles.[72] Given its long halflife in healthy subjects (≤5 days, with an active metabolite with a halflife of ≤8 days), it should be used with great caution, preferably only p.r.n.

In contrast, **oxazepam** was found to have unaltered disposition and elimination in acute viral hepatitis and mild–moderate cirrhosis.[69] This may be partly because conjugation of the drug occurs in organs other than the liver. However, in patients with severe decompensated cirrhosis and encephalopathy, clearance is decreased.[73] Thus, although **oxazepam** can be used in normal doses in mild–moderate liver disease, great caution must be exercised in severe liver impairment.

No changes in the halflife of **lorazepam** and **temazepam** were shown in patients with cirrhosis.[70,74] This is not surprising because they are also eliminated through glucuronidation as opposed to oxidation. Hence there should be little change in dose.

Diuretics

Spironolactone and **furosemide** are commonly used to control ascites and oedema, and both have no major change in their pharmacokinetics in liver disease.[75,76] However, over-vigorous treatment of ascites in such patients may lead to dehydration and oliguria, which may impair drug elimination and cause problems.[76]

RENAL IMPAIRMENT

Renal impairment has important effects on both the pharmacokinetic and pharmacodynamic properties of many drugs. The most important is the effect on excretion of a drug or its metabolites (if active) leading to:

- accumulation of drug or metabolite
- a prolonged halflife
- a longer time to reach steady-state.

This is relevant in relation to, for example, **digoxin**, **gabapentin** and **pregabalin**, **insulin**, **lithium**, **LMWH**, morphine-6-glucuronide.

Other aspects of pharmacokinetics which may be affected include:

- hypo-albuminaemia can lead to an increase in the proportion of free drug in highly protein-bound drugs, resulting in a greater therapeutic effect and, if the serum drug concentration is used to monitor treatment, difficulty in interpreting the results, e.g. **phenytoin** (see p.258)
- reduced efficacy of some drugs acting on the kidneys, e.g. diuretics
- increased sensitivity to the therapeutic and undesirable effects of some drugs, even if elimination is unimpaired, possibly through increased permeability of the blood-brain barrier in the presence of uraemia, e.g. psycho-active drugs
- increased nephrotoxic effect of a drug, e.g. **allopurinol**, aminoglycosides, **ciclosporin**, **lithium**, NSAIDs; this may be particularly important for patients with mild–moderate renal impairment which is made worse by such drugs.

Some of these problems can be overcome by:
- avoiding drugs which are nephrotoxic
- using alternative drugs which are not renally excreted
- reducing the total daily maintenance dose of a renally excreted drug, either by reducing the size of the individual doses or by increasing the interval between doses
- taking special care with drugs with a narrow therapeutic index, where undesirable effects are likely with accumulation of the drug or its metabolites.

Advice about opioid choice in patients with renal impairment is given in the generic monograph on Strong opioids (p.345).

Principles of dose adjustment in renal impairment

The need for dose reduction in renal impairment depends on the extent to which the drug and any active metabolite are renally excreted and how serious any undesirable effects of the drug may be:
- for drugs with minimal undesirable effects, a simple scheme for dose reduction is sufficient, i.e. start low and monitor for efficacy and toxicity
- for drugs with a small safety margin, dose adjustments should be based on a measure of renal function, e.g. creatinine clearance, often estimated using the Cockcroft-Gault formula (see below)
- for drugs where both efficacy and/or toxicity are closely related to serum concentration, ongoing treatment must be adjusted according to clinical response and serum concentration, e.g. **gentamicin**.

Measuring renal function

The glomerular filtration rate (GFR) is the best overall measure of renal function, but the most accurate ways of measuring GFR are impractical for routine use. Serum creatinine concentration has traditionally been used as a proxy but is only a rough guide because a significant proportion of renal function may be lost before creatinine levels rise above the upper limit of normal, particularly in patients with a low body muscle mass or low protein intake. One approach is to use a formula-based *estimation* of GFR (eGFR), which takes into account some of the factors that complicate serum creatinine interpretation, e.g. Modification of Diet in Renal Disease (MDRD) study formula.[77]

Screening for, assessing and monitoring renal disease

The 4-variable (serum creatinine, age, sex, and ethnic origin) MDRD study formula is the nationally adopted standard in England.[43] It is more accurate than the Cockcroft-Gault formula with 90% of estimates $<$60mL/min/1.73m^2 within 30% of the true value. Changes in MDRD eGFR are more reliable than single estimates, with a decrease of $\gtrsim$15% likely to represent a true change in renal function.[77] Five stages of renal disease are categorized according to MDRD eGFR (Table 14.2).[78]

Table 14.2 Diagnostic stages of renal disease

Stage	*eGFR (mL/min/1.73m^2)*	*Description*[a]
1	$>$90	Normal renal function but renal disease based on urine findings, or presence of structural abnormalities or genetic trait
2	60–89	Mildly reduced renal function in the presence of renal disease (as above); in the absence of renal disease, an eGFR $\geq$60mL/min/1.73m^2 is considered normal
3	30–59	Moderately reduced renal function
4	15–29	Severely reduced renal function
5	$<$15	Very severe, established (end-stage) renal failure

a. evidence of damage or a reduced eGFR must be present for $>$3 months.

The MDRD eGFR is expressed as a normalized value, i.e. what that individual's GFR would be if they had a body surface area of $1.73m^2$. *Thus, the MDRD eGFR is not generally considered appropriate for considering drug clearance and dose adjustment because this should be based on an individual's absolute GFR.* For example, for individuals with a body surface area $<1.73m^2$, the MDRD eGFR could overestimate renal function and potentially lead to drug overdosing, with the converse being true for individuals with a body surface area $>1.73m^2$. The MDRD formula may also be misleading in situations where creatinine production, volume of distribution or excretion rate are altered, and in patients with a clearance of <50mL/min.[79] Further, it has not been validated for use in:

- children <18 years old
- pregnancy
- acute renal impairment
- oedematous states
- malnourished patients
- muscle wasting disease states
- amputees.

Thus, in palliative care patients who are elderly, malnourished, cachectic and/or oedematous, renal impairment may exist even when the serum creatinine or the MDRD eGFR are within normal limits, and it may be prudent to assume that there is at least mild renal impairment in such patients. Even when abnormal, the serum creatinine or the MDRD eGFR may both underestimate the actual degree of renal impairment.

Modifying drug dose based on renal function

In patients known to have chronic renal impairment or those at high risk of renal impairment, e.g. the elderly, and those with hypertension or diabetes, renal function should be checked before prescribing a drug which may need dose modification. A baseline serum creatinine and MDRD eGFR (bearing in mind the above limitations) can help to indicate the need for dose modification and serial measurements used to monitor the effect of the drug on renal function.

However, *when considering dose adjustment guidelines, creatinine clearance or an absolute MDRD eGFR should be calculated.* Because most dose adjustment guidelines are currently based on an estimated creatinine clearance using the Cockcroft-Gault formula, this should be used in preference. Alternatively, the MDRD eGFR can be converted to an absolute value:

Cockcroft-Gault formula

$$\text{Creatinine clearance} = \frac{F \times [140 - \text{age}] \times [\text{weight (kg)}]}{\text{serum creatinine (micromol/L)}}$$

F = 1.23 (male) or 1.04 (female)

Converting the MDRD eGFR to an absolute value:
Absolute eGFR (mL/min) = MDRD eGFR (mL/min/$1.73m^2$) × (body surface area/1.73) (m^2)

Body surface area (m^2) = $\sqrt{((\text{height (cm)} \times \text{weight (kg)})/3{,}600)}$

The Cockcroft-Gault formula, by taking weight rather than body surface area into account, tends to overestimate or underestimate creatinine clearance in obese and underweight patients respectively. As with the MDRD eGFR, it can be misleading in situations where creatinine production, volume of distribution or excretion rate are altered and similar precautions regarding the interpretation of results in palliative care patients will apply. It is not appropriate to use when renal function is changing rapidly.

Dose adjustment can then be made using the advice given in *PCF* or other resources such as the manufacturer's SPC, *The Renal Drug Handbook*,[80] *Drug Prescribing in Renal Failure*[81] and the *BNF*. It should be noted that the advice will vary.[82] For example, the *BNF* advice on dose adjustment is now generally expressed in terms of MDRD eGFR. Nonetheless, it points out that this:

- should not be used to adjust doses of nephrotoxic drugs or drugs with a narrow therapeutic index; use instead serum drug concentrations or creatinine clearance calculated using the Cockcroft-Gault formula

- should not be used to adjust drug doses in patients at both extremes of weight; use instead the absolute GFR or creatinine clearance calculated using the Cockcroft-Gault formula
- is not validated for use in children under 18 years.

PCF favours the dose adjustment guidance in *The Renal Drug Handbook* (generally based on creatinine clearance calculated using the Cockcroft-Gault formula) and reflects this unless stated otherwise. Nonetheless, given the limitations of the estimates of creatinine clearance, any guidance should be regarded only as useful approximations of a safe starting dose. Subsequent further adjustments are then based on response and undesirable effects, with monitoring of serum drug concentrations undertaken when appropriate.[83]

For *prescribing purposes*, renal impairment is generally arbitrarily divided into mild, moderate and severe, corresponding to creatinine clearances of 20–50mL/min, 10–20mL/min and <10mL/min respectively. However, the cut-off points vary slightly between sources.

When a drug dose modification has been necessary, or for drugs known to cause renal impairment, a clinical review and evaluation of renal function should be carried out within 2 weeks, or at anytime if drug-induced nephrotoxicity is suspected, e.g. symptoms such as rash, arthralgia, oedema.[77]

Patients requiring dialysis

For guidance on drug use in dialysis, generally consult specialist renal pharmacists and/or the literature. For example, because dialysis can remove **gabapentin**, a low dose is given after each dialysis session.

TRANSDERMAL PATCHES AND MRI

Broadly speaking, TD patches contain the drug either in a reservoir or embedded within a matrix. This is protected by a backing on the outside, and a removable liner covering the surface to be applied to the skin. Some TD patches contain metal in their backing (Box 14.D). This is potentially dangerous because, if such a patch is worn during MRI, the patient may develop a burn under the patch.[84,85]

Thus, TD patches with metal in the backing must be removed immediately before MRI, and replaced with a new patch immediately afterwards (Box 14.D). Although some patches have metal in the liner, this is irrelevant because the liner is removed before application. *If in doubt, double-check.*

(Box 14.D) is correct as of August 2010 for products distributed *in the UK*. For other countries, check the product literature, and/or contact the manufacturer directly.

Box 14.D TD patches (UK) and MRI, compiled from manufacturers' information: *correct as of August 2010*

Need to remove before MRI	**No need to remove before MRI**
Clonidine (Catapres TTS®; not UK but may be imported, US product contains metal)[86]	Buprenorphine (BuTrans®, Transtec®)
Glyceryl trinitrate (Transiderm Nitro®)	Estradiol HRT (Elleste MX®, Femtarix®)
Hyoscine (Scopoderm TTS®)	Estradiol ± progestogen for hormone replacement therapy (HRT) (Estraderm MX®, Estraderm TTS®, Estradot®, Evorel®, Evorel Conti®, Evorel Sequi®, FemSeven®, FemSeven Conti®, FemSeven Sequi®, Progynova TS®)
Some nicotine patches (Nicotinell®, NiQuitin®)	Ethinylestradiol + norelgestromin for contraception (Evra®)
Rotigotine (Neupro®)	
Some testosterone patches (Andropatch®)	

continued

Box 14.D *Continued*

Contain metal salts; manufacturers advise removal before MRI
Diclofenac (Voltarol gel patch®)
Lidocaine (Versatis®)
Nicotine (Nicorette Invisi®)
Salicylic acid (Scholl® callous removal pads, Scholl® corn pads/plasters)

No need to remove before MRI
Fentanyl (Durogesic DTrans® and all UK generics)
Glyceryl trinitrate (Deponit®, Minitran®, Nitro-Dur®)
Menthol (Deep Freeze®)
Some nicotine patches (NicAssist®, Nicorette®, NiQuitin Clear®)
Oxybutynin (Kentera®)
Rivastigmine (Exelon®)
Some testosterone patches (Intrinsa®)

1 Marie Curie Palliative Care Institute (2008) Liverpool Care Pathway for the Dying Patient (LPC), National LCP Renal Project Group Guidelines for LCP Drug Presribing in Advanced Chronic Kidney Disease. Available from: www.mcpcil.org.uk/about_the_institute/news/june_2008/06_june_2008
2 NICE (2004) Guidance on cancer services: improving supportive and palliative care for adults with cancer: the manual. National Institute for Clinical Excellence, London. Available from: www.nice.org.uk/page.aspx?o = csgspfullguideline
3 Thomas K (2003) The gold standards framework in community palliative care. *European Journal of Palliative Care.* **10**: 113–115.
4 Rothschild JM *et al.* (2002) Analysis of medication-related malpractice claims: causes, preventability, and costs. *Archives of Internal Medicine.* **162**: 2414–2420.
5 Spinewine A *et al.* (2005) Appropriateness of use of medicines in elderly inpatients: qualitative study. *British Medical Journal.* **331**: 935.
6 Kanjanarat P *et al.* (2003) Nature of preventable adverse drug events in hospitals: a literature review. *American Journal of Health System Pharmacy.* **60**: 1750–1759.
7 Jones TA and Como JA (2003) Assessment of medication errors that involved drug allergies at a university hospital. *Pharmacotherapy.* **23**: 855–860.
8 Neale G *et al.* (2001) Exploring the causes of adverse events in NHS hospital practice. *Journal of the Royal Society of Medicine.* **94**: 322–330.
9 Dean B *et al.* (2002) Causes of prescribing errors in hospital inpatients: a prospective study. *Lancet.* **359**: 1373–1378.
10 Nursing and Midwifery Council (2007) Standards for medicines management. Available from: www.nmc-uk.org/Documents/Standards/nmcStandardsForMedicinesManagementBooklet.pdf
11 Bradford and Airedale NHS Trust (2006) Subcutaneous drug administration by carers (adult palliative care). Available from: www.palliativedrugs.com document library
12 NHS National Prescribing Centre (2009) A guide to good practice in the management of controlled drugs in primary care (England) 3rd Edition.
13 International Children's Palliative Care Network (2008). Available from: www.icpcn.org.uk
14 Cochrane H *et al.* (2007) Palliative Care statistics for children and young adults. In: *Health and Care Partnerships Analysis.* Department of Health, London.
15 Regnard C *et al.* (2007) Understanding distress in people with severe communication difficulties: developing and assessing the Disability Distress Assessment Tool (DisDAT). *Journal of Intellectual Disability Research.* **51**: 277–292.
16 Regnard C *et al.* (2003) Difficulties in identifying distress and its causes in people with severe communication problems. *International Journal of Palliative Nursing.* **9**: 173–176.
17 Herr K *et al.* (2006) Pain assessment in the nonverbal patient: position statement with clinical practice recommendations. *Pain Management Nursing.* **7**: 44–52.
18 Gauvain-Piquard A *et al.* (1999) The development of the DEGR(R): A scale to assess pain in young children with cancer. *European Journal of Pain.* **3**: 165–176.
19 Hain RD (1997) Pain scales in children: a review. *Palliative Medicine.* **11**: 341–350.
20 Wong D and Baker C (1988) Pain in children: comparison of assessment scales. *Pediatric Nursing.* **14**: 9017.
21 Department of Health (2008) Better Care. Better Lives. Available from: www.dh.gov.uk/en/Publicationsandstatistics/Publications/PublicationsPolicyAndGuidance/DH_083106
22 Royal College of Paediatrics and Child Health (RCPCH) (2007) *Medicines for Children* (3e). RCPCH, London.
23 General Medical Council (GMC) (2007) 0-18. Guidance for all doctors. Available from: www.gmc-uk.org/static/documents/content/GMC_0-18_0911.pdf
24 BNFC (2007) *British National Formulary for Children.* BMJ Publishing Group Ltd, RPS Publishing, RCPCH Publications Ltd, London. Current BNFC available from: www.bnfc.org/bnfc/bnfc/current/.
25 Ballantine N and Fitzmaurice N (2006) Chapter 18. Using Medications. In: A Goldman *et al.* (eds) *Oxford Textbook of Palliative Care for Children.* Oxford University Press, Oxford.
26 Jassal S (2008) Basic symptom control in paediatric palliative care: the Rainbows Children's Hospice Guidelines. Available from: www.act.org.uk
27 Hain R and Jassal S (2010) *Paediatric Palliative Medicine. Oxford Specialist Handbooks in Paediatrics.* Oxford University Press, Oxford.
28 Jassal S and Hain RD (2011) Association for Paediatric Medicine Master Formulary. Available from: www.act.org.uk/APPM

29 Stephenson T (2005) How children's responses to drugs differ from adults. *British Journal of Clinical Pharmacology.* **59**: 670–673.
30 AAP (American Academy of Pediatrics) (2006) Uses of drugs not described in the package insert (off-label uses) Available from: www.aappolicy.aappublications.org/cgi/content/full/pediatrics;110/1/181
31 Bartelink IH *et al.* (2006) Guidelines on paediatric dosing on the basis of developmental physiology and pharmacokinetic considerations. *Clinical Pharmacokinetics.* **45**: 1077–1097.
32 White R and Bradnam V (2007) *Handbook of Drug Administration via Enteral Feeding Tubes.* Pharmaceutical Press, London.
33 Smith S *et al.* (2001) Guidelines for rectal administration of anticonvulsant medication in children. *Paediatric and Perinatal Drug Therapy.* **4**: 140–147.
34 Arvidsson J *et al.* (1995) Replacing carbamazepine slow-release tablets with carbamazepine suppositories: a pharmacokinetic and clinical study in children with epilepsy. *Journal of Child Neurology.* **10**: 114–117.
35 Birnbaum AK *et al.* (2000) Rectal absorption of lamotrigine compressed tablets. *Epilepsia.* **41**: 850–853.
36 Waterson G (2006) Corticosteroids in the palliative phase of brain tumours. *Archives of Disease in Childhood.* **86 (suppl 1)**: A76.
37 Glaser AW *et al.* (1997) Corticosteroids in the management of central nervous system tumours. Kids Neuro-Oncology Workshop (KNOWS). *Archives of Disease in Childhood.* **76**: 76–78.
38 Zernikow B *et al.* (2006) Paediatric cancer pain management using the WHO analgesic ladder-results of a prospective analysis from 2265 treatment days during a quality improvement study. *European Journal of Pain.* **10**: 587–595.
39 Hain RDW (2006) Pharmacodynamics of morphine and M6G in children with cancer: analgesia and adverse effects. *International Conference in Paediatric Palliative Care.*
40 Grosset KA and Grosset DG (2004) Prescribed drugs and neurological complications. *Journal of Neurology, Neurosurgery, and Psychiatry.* **75 Suppl 3**: iii2–8.
41 van Harten PN *et al.* (1999) Acute dystonia induced by drug treatment. *British Medical Journal.* **319**: 623–626.
42 Fick DM *et al.* (2003) Updating the Beers criteria for potentially inappropriate medication use in older adults: results of a US consensus panel of experts. *Archives of Internal Medicine.* **163**: 2716–2724.
43 DoH (2001) *National Service Framework for Older People.* HMSO, London.
44 Ashley C and Currie A (2004) *The Renal Drug Handbook* (2e). Radcliffe Medical Press Ltd, Oxford.
45 Bower M *et al.* (2010) Endocrine and metabolic complications of advanced cancer. In: Hanks G *et al.* (eds) *Oxford Textbook of Palliative Medicine* (4e). Oxford University Press, Oxford, pp. 1015–1033.
46 Williams RL *et al.* (1984) Naproxen disposition in patients with alcoholic cirrhosis. *European Journal of Clinical Pharmacology.* **27(3)**: 291–296.
47 Garg RK (2005) Anesthetic considerations in patients with hepatic failure. *International Anesthesiology Clinics.* **43**: 45–63.
48 Pirmohamed M (2006) Prescribing in liver disease. *Medicine.* **35**: 31–33.
49 Morgan TR *et al.* (1995) Protein consumption and hepatic encephalopathy in alcoholic hepatitis. VA Cooperative Study Group #275. *Journal of the American College of Nutrition.* **14**: 152–158.
50 Rhee C and Broadbent AM (2007) Palliation and liver failure: Palliative medications dosage guidelines. *Journal of Palliative Medicine.* **10**: 677–685.
51 Forrest JA *et al.* (1979) Paracetamol metabolism in chronic liver disease. *European Journal of Clinical Pharmacology.* **15**: 427–431.
52 Roberts MS *et al.* (1983) Pharmacokinetics of aspirin and salicylate in elderly subjects and in patients with alcoholic liver disease. *European Journal of Clinical Pharmacology.* **25**: 253–261.
53 Juhl RP *et al.* (1983) Ibuprofen and sulindac kinetics in alcoholic liver disease. *Clinical Pharmacology & Therapeutics.* **34**: 104–109.
54 Calvo MV *et al.* (1980) Naproxen disposition in hepatic and biliary disorders. *International Journal of Clinical Pharmacology, Therapy, & Toxicology.* **18**: 242–246.
55 Pond SM *et al.* (1980) Enhanced bioavailability of pethidine and pentazocine in patients with cirrhosis of the liver. *Aust NZ J Med.* **10**: 515–519.
56 Tegeder I *et al.* (1999) Pharmacokinetics of opioids in liver disease. *Clinical Pharmacokinetics.* **37**: 17–40.
57 Riordan SM and Williams R (1997) Treatment of hepatic encephalopathy.[see comment] *New England Journal of Medicine.* **337**: 473–479.
58 Crotty B *et al.* (1989) Hepatic extraction of morphine is impaired in cirrhosis. *European Journal of Clinical Pharmacology.* **36**: 501–506.
59 Hasselstrom J *et al.* (1990) The metabolism and bioavailability of morphine in patients with severe liver cirrhosis. *British Journal of Clinical Pharmacology.* **29**: 289–297.
60 Tallgren M *et al.* (1997) Pharmacokinetics and ventilatory effects of oxycodone before and after liver transplantation. *Clinical Pharmacology & Therapeutics.* **61**: 655–661.
61 Haberer JP *et al.* (1982) Fentanyl pharmacokinetics in anaesthetized patients with cirrhosis. *British Journal of Anaesthesia.* **54**: 1267–1270.
62 Bass NM and Williams RL (1988) Guide to drug dosage in hepatic disease. *Clinical Pharmacokinetics.* **15**: 396–420.
63 Lewis GP and Jusko WJ (1975) Pharmacokinetics of ampicillin in cirrhosis. *Clinical Pharmacology & Therapeutics.* **18**: 475–84.
64 Acocella G *et al.* (1972) Kinetics of rifampicin and isoniazid administered alone and in combination to normal subjects and patients with liver disease. *Gut.* **13**: 47–53.
65 Uribe M *et al.* (1985) Successful administration of metoclopramide for the treatment of nausea in patients with advanced liver disease. A double-blind controlled trial. *Gastroenterology.* **88**: 757–762.
66 Figg WD *et al.* (1996) Pharmacokinetics of ondansetron in patients with hepatic insufficiency. *Journal of Clinical Pharmacology.* **36**: 206–215.
67 Micromedex T (2005) Micromedex Health Series. Thomson Micromedex. Available from: www.micromedex.com
68 Klotz U *et al.* (1978) Disposition of valproic acid in patients with liver disease. *European Journal of Clinical Pharmacology.* **13**: 55–60.
69 Shull HJ *et al.* (1976) Normal disposition of oxazepam in acute viral hepatitis and cirrhosis. *Annals of Internal Medicine.* **84**: 420–425.
70 Kraus JW *et al.* (1978) Effects of aging and liver disease on disposition of lorazepam. *Clinical Pharmacology & Therapeutics.* **24**: 411–419.
71 Pentikainen PJ *et al.* (1989) Pharmacokinetics of midazolam following intravenous and oral administration in patients with chronic liver disease and in healthy subjects. *Journal of Clinical Pharmacology.* **29**: 272–277.
72 Klotz U *et al.* (1975) The effects of age and liver disease on the disposition and elimination of diazepam in adult man. *Journal of Clinical Investigation.* **55**: 347–359.

73 Sonne J *et al.* (1990) Glucuronidation of oxazepam is not spared in patients with hepatic encephalopathy. *Hepatology.* **11**: 951–956.
74 Ghabrial H *et al.* (1986) The effects of age and chronic liver disease on the elimination of temazepam. *European Journal of Clinical Pharmacology.* **30**: 93–97.
75 Verbeeck RK *et al.* (1982) Furosemide disposition in cirrhosis. *Clinical Pharmacology & Therapeutics.* **31**: 719–725.
76 Abshagen U *et al.* (1977) Disposition kinetics of spironolactone in hepatic failure after single doses and prolonged treatment. *European Journal of Clinical Pharmacology.* **11**: 169–176.
77 Anonymous (2006) The patient, the drug and the kidney. *Drug and Therapeutics Bulletin.* **44**: 89–95.
78 Royal College of Physicians of London and Renal Association (2006) Chronic Kidney disease in adults: UK guidelines for identification, management and referral. Available from: www.renal.org/CKDguide/full/CKDprintedfullguide.pdf
79 Holweger K *et al.* (2008) Novel algorithm for more accurate calculation of renal function in adults with cancer. *Annals of Pharmacotherapy.* **42**: 1749–1757.
80 Ashley C and Currie A (2009) *The Renal Drug Handbook* (3e). Radcliffe Publishing Ltd, Oxford.
81 Brier M and Aronoff G (2007) *Drug Prescribing in Renal Failure 5e.* ACP Press, Philadelphia.
82 Vidal L *et al.* (2005) Systematic comparison of four sources of drug information regarding adjustment of dose for renal function. *British Medical Journal.* **331**: 263.
83 Davison SN *et al.* (2010) Management of pain in renal failure. In: EJ Chambers *et al.* (eds) *Supportive Care for the Renal Patient* (2e). Oxford University Press, Oxford, pp. 139–188.
84 Institute for Safe Medication Practices (2004) Medication Safety Alert. Burns in MRI patients wearing transdermal patches. Available from: www.ismp.org/Newsletters/acutecare/articles/20040408.asp?ptr = y
85 MHRA (2007) *Device Bulletin. Safety guidelines for magnetic resonance imaging equipment in clinical use. DB2007(03).* MHRA and Department of Health, London, p. 46.
86 Hulisz DT (2008) Are topical patches safe during MRI or CT Scans? Medscape Pharmacists. Available from: www.medscape.com/viewarticle/572561

15: OPIOID DOSE CONVERSION RATIOS

General approach

It is crucial to appreciate that conversion ratios are *never* more than an approximate guide. Thus, careful monitoring during conversion is necessary to avoid both underdosing and excessive dosing. See also Opioid switching ('rotation'), p.354

This chapter provides a summary of selected opioid dose conversion ratios. These can be used to calculate equivalent doses of opioids when switching from a weak opioid to **morphine**, or from one strong opioid to another. Caution is always necessary. Conversion ratios are *never* more than an approximate guide because of:

- wide interindividual variation in opioid pharmacokinetics; influencing factors include age, ethnicity, renal or hepatic impairment
- other variables including dose and duration of opioid treatment, direction of switch in opioid, nutritional status and concurrent medications
- their method of derivation, e.g. single dose rather than chronic dose studies using a range of clinical doses.

Careful monitoring is particularly necessary when:

- switching at high doses
- there has been a recent rapid escalation of the first opioid
- switching to **methadone**.

Explicit guidance on switching opioids is difficult because both the reasons for switching and the patient's circumstances differ. One guideline, based on expert consensus, recommends routinely reducing the calculated equivalent dose of the new opioid by 25–50% (see p.354). Various patient factors are then taken into account to modify the rule, e.g. no reduction in a young patient in severe pain switching at low dose, or an even bigger reduction in an older delirious patient in moderate pain switching at high dose.

Certainly, a dose reduction of at least 50% would seem prudent when switching at high doses (e.g. **morphine** or equivalent doses of ≥1g/24h), in elderly or frail patients, because of intolerable undesirable effects (e.g. delirium), or when there has been a recent rapid escalation of the first opioid (possibly due to opioid-induced hyperalgesia). In such circumstances, p.r.n. doses can be relied on to make up any deficit while re-titrating to a satisfactory dose of the new opioid.

A separate strategy is necessary for **methadone** (see p.416).

Determining the dose of the second opioid

Select the appropriate Table based on the routes of administration:

Route	*Table*	*Page*
PO to PO	15.1	627
PO to TD	15.2	628
PO to SC/IV	15.3	631
SC/IV to SC/IV	15.4	632

The Tables relate mainly to switching to or from **morphine**. If switching from an opioid other than **morphine** to another opioid, it will be necessary to convert the dose of the first opioid to **morphine** equivalents, and then use that quantity to determine the dose of the second opioid. With any switch:

- round the calculated dose up or down to the nearest convenient dose of the formulation concerned, e.g. tablet, TD patch, ampoule
- decide on an appropriate p.r.n. dose.

The conversion ratios in this chapter are based on referenced sources given in the various individual opioid monographs. Where these differ significantly from the manufacturers' recommended ratios, the latter are included for comparison.

Table 15.1 PCF recommended dose conversion ratios: PO to PC

Conversion	*Ratio*	*Calculation*	*Example*	*Monograph*
Codeine to morphine	10:1	Divide 24h codeine dose by 10	Codeine 240mg/24h PO → morphine 24mg/24h PO	Codeine, p.332
Dihydrocodeine to morphine	10:1	Divide 24h dihydrocodeine dose by 10	Dihydrocodeine 240mg/24h PO → morphine 24mg/24h PO	Dihydrocodeine, p.335
Hydrocodone to morphine	1.5:1	Divide 24h hydrocodone dose by 1.5 (decrease dose by 1/3)	Hydrocodone 60mg/24h PO → morphine 40mg/24h PO	Not UK
Tramadol to morphine	10:1	Divide 24h tramadol dose by 10	Tramadol 400mg/24h PO → morphine 40mg/24h PO	Tramadol, p.340
Morphine to hydromorphone	5:1[a]	Divide 24h morphine dose by 5	Morphine 60mg/24h PO → hydromorphone 12mg/24h PO	Hydromorphone, p.414
	7.5:1[b]	*Divide 24h morphine dose by 7.5*	*Morphine 60mg/24h PO → hydromorphone 8mg/24h PO*	Hydromorphone, p.414
Morphine to methadone	Variable	See methadone, p.4 6		
Morphine to oxycodone	1.5:1	Divide 24h morphine dose by 1.5 (decrease dose by 1/3)	Morphine 30mg/24h PO → oxycodone 20mg/24h PO	Oxycodone, p.424
	2:1[b]	*Divide 24h morphine dose by 2*	*Morphine 30mg/24h PO → oxycodone 15mg/24h PO*	Oxycodone, p.424

a. for converse, some use 1:4, e.g. hydromorphone 8mg/24h PO → morphine 32mg/PO
b. italicized entries = manufacturers' recommendations.

Table 15.2 PCF recommended dose conversion ratios: PO to TD

Conversion	*Ratio*	*Calculation*	*Example*	*Monograph*
Morphine to buprenorphine	100:1	Multiply 24h morphine dose in mg by 10 to obtain 24h buprenorphine dose in microgram; divide answer by 24 to obtain microgram/h patch strength	Morphine 300mg/24h PO → buprenorphine 3000microgram/24h → 125microgram/h; *round up* to 70microgram/h × 2 or *round down* to 70+35microgram/h patches	Buprenorphine, p.381
	75–115:1[a]	*Use the manufacturer's guidelines in SPC, summarized in Box 15A, p.629*		Buprenorphine, p.381
Morphine to fentanyl	100:1	Multiply 24h morphine dose in mg by 10 to obtain 24h fentanyl dose in microgram; divide answer by 24 to obtain microgram/h patch strength	Morphine 300mg/24h PO → fentanyl 3,000microgram/24h → 125microgram/h; give as 100+25microgram/h patches	Fentanyl, p.390
	150:1[a]	*Use the manufacturer's guidelines in SPC, e.g. for DTrans® summarized in Box 15B, p.630*	*The doses will be smaller than those obtained with the PCF preferred dose conversion ratio*	Fentanyl, p.390

a. italicized entries = manufacturers' recommendations.

For determining the appropriate p.r.n. morphine dose for patients receiving TD buprenorphine or TD fentanyl, see p.388 and 398 respectively.

Box 15.A Edited extract from manufacturer's recommendations for starting TD buprenorphine (for full details, see SPC)

BuTrans® 5, 10 and 20microgram/h transdermal patch
Patients aged 18 years and over
The lowest BuTrans® dose (BuTrans® 5microgram/h TD patch) should be used as the initial dose. Consideration should be given to the previous opioid history of the patient as well as to the current general condition and medical status of the patient.

Conversion from opioids
BuTrans® can be used as an alternative to treatment with other opioids. Such patients should be started on the lowest available dose (BuTrans® 5microgram/h TD patch) and continue taking short-acting supplemental analgesics during titration, as required.

Transtec® 35, 52.5 and 70microgram transdermal patch
Patients over 18 years of age
The Transtec® dose should be adapted to the condition of the individual patient (pain intensity, suffering, individual reaction). The lowest possible dose providing adequate pain relief should be given.

Initial dose selection
Patients on no analgesics or on a WHO Step I (non-opioid) or a Step II (weak opioid) analgesic should begin with Transtec® 35microgram/h. The administration of a non-opioid analgesic can be continued, depending on the patient's overall medical condition.

When switching from a Step III (strong opioid) analgesic to Transtec®, the nature of the previous medication, administration and the mean daily dose should be taken into account in order to avoid the recurrence of pain. It is generally advisable to titrate the dose individually, starting with the lowest TD patch strength (Transtec® 35microgram/h). Clinical experience has shown that patients who were previously treated with higher doses of a strong opioid (approximately 120mg oral morphine per day) may start therapy with the next higher TD patch strength (i.e. 52.5microgram/h).

Sufficient supplementary immediate release analgesics should be made available during dose titration.

The necessary strength of Transtec® must be adapted to the requirements of the individual patient and checked at regular intervals.

After application of the first Transtec® TD patch the buprenorphine serum concentrations rise slowly and there is unlikely to be a rapid onset of effect. Consequently, a first evaluation of the analgesic effect should only be made after 24h.

The previous analgesic medication (with the exception of transdermal opioids) should be given in the same dose during the first 12h after switching to Transtec® and appropriate rescue medication given on demand in the following 12h.

Box 15.B Extract from manufacturer's recommendations for starting Durogesic DTrans® (for full details see SPC)[a]

Durogesic DTrans® 12/25/50/75/100microgram/h transdermal patch
Adults:
Initial dose selection
The initial Durogesic DTrans® dose should be based on the patient's opioid history, including the degree of opioid tolerance, if any, as well as on the current general condition and medical status of the patient.

In strong opioid-naive patients, Durogesic DTrans® dose 25microgram/h, should be used as the initial dose.

In opioid-tolerant patients, the initial dose of Durogesic DTrans® should be based on the previous 24h opioid analgesic requirement. A recommended conversion scheme from oral morphine to Durogesic DTrans® is given below:

Oral 24h morphine (mg/day)	Durogesic DTrans® (microgram/h)
<90	25
90–134	37
135–189	50
190–224	62
225–314	75
315–404	100
405–494	125
495–584	150
585–674	175
675–764	200
765–854	225
855–944	250
945–1034	275
1035–1124	300

Previous analgesic therapy should be phased out gradually from the time of the first patch application until analgesic efficacy with Durogesic DTrans® is attained. For both strong opioid-naive and opioid-tolerant patients, the initial evaluation of the analgesic effect of Durogesic DTrans® should not be made until the patch has been worn for 24h due to the gradual increase in serum fentanyl concentrations up to this time.

a. guidance varies between makes of TD fentanyl; see individual SPC.

Table 15.3 PCF recommended dose conversion ratios; PO to SC/IV

Conversion	*Ratio*	*Calculation*	*Example*	*Monograph*
Hydromorphone to hydromorphone	2:1	Divide 24h hydromorphone dose by 2	Hydromorphone 32mg/24h PO → hydromorphone 16mg/24h SC/IV	Hydromorphone, p.414
Methadone to methadone	2:1[a]	Divide 24h methadone dose by 2	Methadone 30mg/24h PO → methadone 15mg/24h SC/IV	Methadone, p.416
Morphine to alfentanil	30:1	Divide 24h morphine dose by 30	Morphine 30mg/24h PO → alfentanil 1mg/24h SC/IV	Alfentanil, p.374
Morphine to diamorphine	3:1	Divide 24h morphine dose by 3	Morphine 30mg/24h PO → diamorphine 10mg/24h SC/IV	Diamorphine, p.371
Morphine to hydromorphone	10–15:1	Divide 24h morphine dose by 10–15	Morphine 30mg/24h PO → hydromorphone 2mg/24h SC/IV	Hydromorphone, p.414
Morphine to methadone	Variable	See methadone, p.416		
Morphine to morphine	2:1	Divide 24h morphine dose by 2	Morphine 30mg/24h PO → morphine 15mg/24h SC/IV	Morphine, p.362
Morphine to oxycodone	2:1	Divide 24h morphine dose by 2	Morphine 60mg/24h PO → oxycodone 30mg/24h SC/IV	Oxycodone, p.424
Oxycodone to oxycodone	1.5:1[b]	Divide 24h oxycodone dose by 1.5 (decrease dose by 1/3)	Oxycodone 30mg/24h PO → oxycodone 20mg/24h SC/IV	Oxycodone, p.424
	2:1[c]	*Divide 24h oxycodone dose by 2*	*Oxycodone 30mg/24h PO → oxycodone 15mg/24h SC/IV*	Oxycodone, p.424

a. because mean oral bio-availability is 80% (range 40–100%), some centres use 1:1, e.g. methadone 30mg/24h PO → methadone 30mg/24h SC/IV, see p.416

b. because mean oral bio-availability is 75% (range 60–87%), some centres use a conversion ratio of 1.5:1 rather than 2:1

c. italicized entry = manufacturer's recommendation.

Table 15.4 PCF recommended dose conversion ratios; SC/IV to SC/IV

Conversion	*Ratio*	*Calculation*	*Example*	*Monograph*
Morphine to alfentanil	15:1	Divide 24h morphine dose by 15	Morphine 30mg/24h SC/IV → alfentanil 2mg/24h SC/IV	Alfentanil, p.374
Morphine to buprenorphine	30–40:1	Divide 24h morphine dose in mg by 30–40	Morphine 40mg/24h SC/IV → buprenorphine 1mg/24h SC/IV	Buprenorphine, p.381
Morphine to hydromorphone	5:1	Divide 24h morphine dose by 5	Morphine 30mg/24h SC/IV → hydromorphone 6mg/24h SC/IV	Hydromorphone, p.414
Morphine to methadone	Variable	See methadone, p.416		
Morphine to oxycodone	1:1	Use same dose as 24h morphine dose	Morphine 30mg/24h SC/IV → oxycodone 30mg/24h SC/IV	Oxycodone, p.424

16: DRUG TREATMENT IN THE IMMINENTLY DYING

In this chapter, in addition to the general discussion, advice is included about end-stage renal disease, heart failure and idiopathic Parkinson's disease (IPD). In essence, palliative care in all these situations is similar to palliative care in cancer, but with certain specific exceptions. These are detailed in the respective sections.

DIAGNOSING IMMINENT DEATH

In advanced cancer, if a patient is deteriorating without an obvious reversible cause:
- *month by month*, they probably have several months to live
- *week by week*, they probably have only weeks to live
- *day by day*, they probably have only days to live.

Estimating the prognosis in other end-stage diseases is generally less straightforward. However, in the absence of a reversible cause for deterioration, the following features collectively indicate that a patient probably has only days to live:
- physically wasted and profoundly weak → bedbound
- drowsy for much of the day → coma
- very limited attention span → disoriented (→ delirium)
- unable to take tablets or has great difficulty swallowing them
- little or no oral intake of food and fluid.[1–3]

Ideally, discussions about Advance Care Planning will already have taken place, and the carers will be aware of the patient's and family's wishes in relation to end-of-life care.[4,5] As death approaches, good communication becomes even more essential, both within the multiprofessional caring team and with the patient and family, particularly about uncertainties.

'GIVE DEATH A CHANCE'

In patients who are close to death it is often appropriate to 'give death a chance'. All patients must die eventually; ultimately nature will take its course. In this respect, the skill is to decide when the burdens of any life-sustaining treatment are likely to outweigh any benefits, and thus when to allow death to occur without further medical impediment. On the other hand, measures which provide comfort and symptom relief must be continued.

For example, an antibacterial is generally appropriate for the patient with advanced cancer who develops a chest infection when still relatively active and independent. However, in those who have become bedbound as a result of general progressive deterioration, and seem close to death, pneumonia should still be allowed to be 'the old person's friend'. In such circumstances it is generally appropriate *not* to prescribe an antibacterial (see p.443).

If it is difficult to make a decision, the '2-day rule' should be invoked, namely, if after 2–3 days of straightforward symptom management the patient is clearly holding his own, prescribe an antibacterial but, if the patient is clearly much worse, do not.[6]

On the other hand, not all end-stage patients who develop a chest infection die from it. A few recover spontaneously, and some progress to a 'grumbling pneumonia' but no further. A continuing wet cough may cause distress and, possibly, loss of sleep. In circumstances when the patient is neither better nor worse after 3–4 days, an antibacterial may be indicated for symptom relief.

REVIEWING GOALS AND MEDICATION

In England, the Liverpool Care Pathway (LCP) for the dying patient is a nationally recommended tool to facilitate high-quality terminal care.[7–9] Although originally used with patients dying from cancer in hospital, it is increasingly used in other settings, and for patients dying from other end-stage diseases.[10] Similar care pathways are used in other countries.[11–13]

At the most basic level, the LCP is a way of acknowledging that death is most probably imminent, and that it is now appropriate to focus primarily on comfort measures.[7,14,15] A standard protocol is used, which becomes part of the patient's clinical records. (Note: because of unexpected improvement, it is sometimes necessary to take a patient off the Pathway.)

Polypharmacy is a common burden for patients with any form of end-stage disease. It is thus important to try and simplify medication. The LCP includes a checklist which facilitates both stopping existing drugs and anticipatory prescribing of emergency drugs for common end-of-life problems:

- *simplifying medication:* particularly stopping long-term prophylactic medication, e.g. statins, antihypertensives, oral hypoglycaemics, **warfarin**, but also laxatives and antidepressants when the patient becomes moribund/comatose
- *anticipatory prescribing:* using the guidelines supplied to prescribe p.r.n. medication in case the patient develops pain, breathlessness, vomiting, delirium, etc., and ensuring that drugs are generally prescribed both PO and SC/IV (also see Chapter 17, Pre-emptive prescribing in the community, p.649)
- *IV hydration:* is it still appropriate? Should it be stopped?

In patients with insulin-dependent diabetes mellitus, the dose of **insulin** should be reduced as oral intake diminishes, and the regimen simplified (see p.500). However, a decision to stop **insulin** completely should normally be taken only after discussion with the patient (if they still have capacity) and the family.

Even so, it is generally appropriate to stop **insulin** injections completely when the patient has become irreversibly unconscious as part of the dying process, and not because of hypoglycaemia or diabetic keto-acidosis, and when all other life-sustaining treatments have been stopped.[16] However, if it is felt strongly that the **insulin** should be continued, a simple regimen of once daily long- or b.d. intermediate-acting **insulin** can be used, with the minimum of routine monitoring, e.g. once daily (see p.500).[17]

For advice about stopping **dexamethasone** in patients with intracranial malignancy, see p.486.

Finally, in the last days, some nursing procedures normally regarded as essential may be discontinued. For example, standard care of pressure areas may cause a moribund patient to become distressed. If so, such care should be reduced or stopped.

'AS NEEDED' MEDICATION

When a patient is likely to have difficulty with swallowing, non-oral as well as PO p.r.n. medication should be prescribed to cover common distressing situations. In some countries, SL, PR and TD products are preferred but, in the UK, SC injections are generally used, e.g.:

- analgesics: e.g. **morphine** SC *q1h* p.r.n. (dose depends on regular dose)
- anti-emetics: e.g. **metoclopramide** 10–20mg SC *q1h* or **levomepromazine** 6–25mg SC *q1h* p.r.n.
- sedative, anti-epileptic: e.g. **midazolam** 2.5–10mg SC *q1h* p.r.n.
- antisecretory drug: e.g. **hyoscine *butylbromide*** 20mg or **glycopyrronium** 200microgram SC *q1h* p.r.n.
- delirium: **haloperidol** 1–5mg SC *q1h* p.r.n.

Charting all these drugs for possible q1h administration facilitates rapid initial dose titration. In practice, after the first 2–3 doses, it would be uncommon for them to be given so frequently, particularly **levomepromazine** (also see Chapter 17, Pre-emptive prescribing in the community, p.649).

MAINTAINING COMFORT

Symptom relief in the last days of a patient's life is generally a continuation of what is already being done. However, previously well-managed symptoms can recur or new symptoms develop.[18–22] The same principles of management apply as before.[23] However, because time is short, there is a greater need for urgency; tomorrow may be too late.

In patients close to death, incontinence is generally best managed by an indwelling urinary catheter.[24] This provides maximum comfort with minimum ongoing disturbance.

Pain

Most patients dying from cancer need a strong opioid. Expressed in oral **morphine** equivalents, data from several specialist palliative care centres indicate that:

- the median dose in the last 24h of life is 30–150mg
- individual dose requirements vary widely, e.g. 7.5–2,000mg/24h.[25–27]

Generally, pain will not be troublesome at the very end if relief has previously been good. However, even when the patient is close to death, careful evaluation is still necessary. Dying patients may call out to check whether someone is with them, that they are not alone. These cries may be misinterpreted as pain, and be a source of concern to family and carers.

Some patients show signs of discomfort when being turned in bed, even when apparently deeply unconscious, and may moan or cry out. Although, for example, this may be pain caused by joint stiffness, it could equally be an 'alarm response' to an unexpected disturbance. Disturbance distress is likely to be reduced by warning a patient (even when unconscious) of any intended interventions by describing the procedure to be undertaken, and by gentle slow handling.

Even so, new pains are relatively common in the last days.[20] Causes include:

- painful bedsore (consider the local application of a local anaesthetic gel ± topical **morphine**; see p.366)
- distended bladder (relieve by catheterization).

Occasionally, patients who have been taking an NSAID for metastatic bone pain suffer renewed pain after 12–24h if the NSAID is stopped when swallowing tablets is no longer possible. In this circumstance, an NSAID can be given as a liquid, suppository or injection, (see p.308).

When a patient can no longer swallow medication PO, a strong opioid should be continued by an alternative route; abrupt discontinuation risks a renewed pain ± withdrawal symptoms, e.g. restlessness, diarrhoea.

Severe breathlessness

Patients often fear suffocating to death and a positive approach to the patient, their family and colleagues about the relief of terminal breathlessness is important:

- no patient should die with distressing breathlessness
- failure to relieve terminal breathlessness is a failure to utilize drug treatment correctly.

Because of the distress, inability to sleep and exhaustion, patients and their carers generally accept that drug-related drowsiness may need to be the price paid for greater comfort. However, unless there is overwhelming distress, deep sedation (reduced awareness/consciousness) is *not* the initial step. Some patients become mentally brighter when anxiety is reduced by light sedation (see p.638), and there is an associated improvement in their breathlessness. Even so, because increasing drowsiness also generally reflects a deteriorating clinical condition, it is important to stress the gravity of the situation and the aim of treatment to the relatives.

Drug treatment typically comprises:[28]

- parenteral administration of an opioid and a sedative-anxiolytic, e.g. **morphine** and **midazolam** or **lorazepam** by CSCI and p.r.n.
- **haloperidol** if the patient develops an agitated delirium (may be aggravated by a benzodiazepine; see p.638).

Death rattle (noisy respiratory secretions)

In most cases, an antimuscarinic is the drug of choice (see p.4 and Quick Practice Guide below). This needs to be given promptly because it does not affect existing pharyngeal secretions. Such drugs are probably most effective for rattle associated with the pooling of saliva in the pharynx and least effective for rattle caused by bronchial secretions (as a result of infection or oedema) or related to the reflux of gastric contents. Note:

- by injection, the efficacy of the different drugs is broadly similar,[29] and the rattle is reduced in 1/2–2/3 of patients[30]
- **hyoscine *hydrobromide*** crosses the blood-brain barrier and possesses anti-emetic and sedative properties,[31] but there is also a risk of developing or exacerbating delirium
- **atropine** also dries secretions and, like **hyoscine**, it crosses the blood-brain barrier but it tends to stimulate rather than sedate, and could increase the need for **midazolam** or **haloperidol**

Although in the UK, antimuscarinics are generally given SC for death rattle, in some countries, the SL route is preferred. For example, **glycopyrronium** 0.01% oral solution prepared locally from **glycopyrronium** powder, 1mL (100microgram) SL q6h p.r.n. (see p.12).

Quick Practice Guide: Management of death rattle (noisy respiratory secretions)

Death rattle is a term used to describe noisy rattling breathing which occurs in about 50% of patients near the end of life. It is caused by fluid pooling in the hypopharynx which arises from one or more sources:

- saliva (most common)
- respiratory tract infection
- pulmonary oedema
- gastric reflux.

Rattling breathing can also occur in patients with a tracheostomy and infection. Because the patient is generally semiconscious or unconscious, drug treatment for death rattle is mainly for the benefit of relatives, other patients and staff.

Non-drug treatment

- ease the family's distress by explaining that the semiconscious/unconscious patient is not distressed by the rattle
- position the patient semiprone to encourage postural drainage; but upright or semirecumbent if the cause is pulmonary oedema or gastric reflux
- oropharyngeal suction but, because it is distressing to many moribund patients, generally reserve for unconscious patients.

Drug treatment

Saliva

Because they do not affect existing secretions, an antisecretory drug should be given SC (see Table) or SL (see Box) as soon as the onset of the rattle begins. SL use is unlicensed and less well supported by the literature.

Antimuscarinic antisecretory drugs for death rattle: typical SC doses

Drug	*Stat and p.r.n. SC dose*	*CSCI dose/24h*
Atropine	400microgram	1,200–2,000microgram
Glycopyrronium	200microgram	600–1,200microgram
Hyoscine *butylbromide*	20mg	20–120mg
Hyoscine *hydrobromide*	400microgram	1,200–2,000microgram
Hyoscyamine (l-atropine; not UK)	200microgram	600–1,000microgram

Antimuscarinic antisecretory drugs for death rattle: typical SL doses

Atropine 1% ophthalmic solution, 4 drops SL q4h p.r.n. (Note: drop size varies with applicator and technique, dose per drop may vary from 200–500microgram, i.e. 800microgram–2mg/dose).

Glycopyrronium 0.01% oral solution, 1mL (100microgram) SL q6h p.r.n., can be prepared locally from glycopyrronium powder.

Hyoscyamine drops 125microgram/mL, 2mL (250microgram) SL q4h p.r.n. (not UK).

Note:

- by injection, the efficacy of the different drugs is broadly similar, and the rattle is reduced in 1/2–2/3 of patients
- hyoscine *hydrobromide* crosses the blood-brain barrier and possesses anti-emetic and sedative properties, but there is also a risk of developing or exacerbating delirium
- atropine and hyoscyamine also cross the blood-brain barrier but tend to stimulate rather than sedate; concurrent use with midazolam or haloperidol is more likely to be necessary.

Respiratory tract infection

Occasionally it is appropriate to prescribe an antibiotic in an imminently dying patient if death rattle is caused by profuse purulent sputum associated with an underlying chest infection:

- e.g. ceftriaxone, mix 1g ampoule with 2.1mL lidocaine 1% (total volume 2.6–2.8mL), and give 250–1,000mg SC/IM once daily
- some centres use larger volumes of lidocaine 1% (up to 4mL) and administer a divided dose at separate SC/IM sites once daily or give b.d.

Pulmonary oedema

Consider furosemide 20–40mg SC/IM/IV q2h p.r.n.
Note: beware precipitating urinary retention.

Gastric reflux

Consider metoclopramide 20mg SC/IV q3h p.r.n., but do not use concurrently with an antimuscarinic because the latter blocks the prokinetic effect of the former.

Rattling breathing causing distress to a patient

In a semiconscious patient, if rattling breathing is associated with breathlessness, supplement the above with an opioid (e.g. morphine) ± an anxiolytic sedative (e.g. midazolam).

Noisy tachypnoea in the moribund

Noisy tachypnoea in the moribund is distressing for the family and other patients, even though the patient is not aware. It represents a desperate last attempt by a patient's body to respond to irreversible terminal respiratory failure ± airway obstruction.

Consider alleviating the noise by reducing the depth and rate of respiration to 10–15/min with **diamorphine/morphine**, best initially titrated IV to identify an effective dose. This may be double, or even treble, the previously satisfactory analgesic dose. When there is associated heaving of the shoulders and chest, **midazolam** should be given as well, e.g. 5–10mg IV.

The **diamorphine/morphine** ± **midazolam** can be repeated IV/SC hourly as needed.

Severe acute stridor as a terminal event

This may be caused by haemorrhage into a tumour pressing on the trachea. Administer **diazepam/midazolam** IV until the patient is asleep (5–20mg). If IV administration is not possible, alternatives include **midazolam** 10mg IM or **diazepam** solution 10mg PR.

Myoclonus

Multifocal myoclonus is a central pre-epileptiform phenomenon. It is exacerbated by hypoglycaemia and, in the moribund, may be caused or exacerbated by dopamine antagonists (antipsychotics, **metoclopramide**) and opioids (particularly at higher doses) or as a result of drug withdrawal (benzodiazepines, barbiturates, anti-epileptics, alcohol).

It is seen in cancer patients dying with encephalopathy associated with organ failure, e.g. renal failure, hepatic failure. It occurs with cerebral oedema and hypoxia, and also with hyponatraemia. Treat with a benzodiazepine (see p.137).

Grand mal seizure

See p.237.

Agitation and delirium

Drugs are only part of the management of agitation in a patient who is imminently dying.[32]

Note:
- mild delirium is not always easy to detect
- an antipsychotic is essential if a patient manifests features suggestive of delirium
- the use of a benzodiazepine alone may precipitate or exacerbate delirium[33]
- if in doubt, treat an agitated imminently dying patient with both an antipsychotic and **midazolam**.

Delirium develops in most dying cancer patients at some point in the last week of life.[34,35] It is generally best treated with **haloperidol** ± **midazolam** given p.r.n. or by CSCI in an individually optimized dose. If delirium is not controlled on **haloperidol** 10–15mg/24h, a more sedating antipsychotic should be given instead, e.g. SC **levomepromazine** (see p.164).

Good practice dictates a step-by-step approach (Figure 16.1 and Box 16.A). Thus, sedation is not 'all or none' but a continuum from p.r.n. sedation to continuous deep sedation.

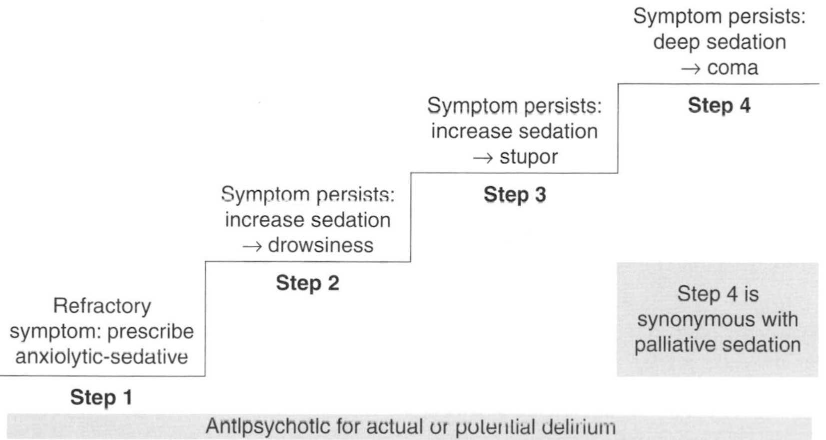

Figure 16.1 Progressive and proportionate treatment for an intolerable refractory symptom in the imminently dying.

Box 16.A Drugs for sedation in the imminently dying

For more information, see respective drug monographs.

First-line drugs

Midazolam
- start with 5–10mg stat and q1h p.r.n.
- if necessary, increase progressively to 20mg SC/IV stat
- maintain with CSCI/CIVI 10–60mg/24h.

Although some centres, if necessary, titrate the dose of midazolam up to 200mg/24h,[36] it is probably better to add in an antipsychotic if midazolam 30–40mg/24h is inadequate to settle the patient (see p.143).

Haloperidol
- start with 5–10mg q1h p.r.n. (2.5–5mg q4h in the elderly)
- if necessary, increase progressively to 10mg IV stat
- maintain with CIVI/CSCI 10–20mg/24h (see p.159).

continued

Box 16.A Continued

Second-line drugs
Levomepromazine
Generally given only if it is intended to reduce a patient's level of consciousness:
- start with 25mg SC stat and q1h p.r.n. (12.5mg in the elderly)
- if necessary, titrate dose according to response
- maintain with 50–300mg/24h CSCI.

Although high-dose levomepromazine (≥100mg/24h) is generally best given by CSCI, smaller doses can be conveniently given as an SC bolus at bedtime–b.d., and p.r.n. (see p.164).

If levomepromazine is not available, use chlorpromazine; doses generally need to be higher, e.g. double those of levomepromazine.

Third-line drugs
Phenobarbital
Because of the irritant nature of the injection (and the volume after dilution), stat doses are generally given IV, but can be followed by CSCI:
- dilute 200mg (in 1mL ampoule) to 10mL with WFI
- start with 100–200mg IV stat and q1h p.r.n.
- maintain with 600–1,200mg/24h CSCI

if necessary, increase the dose progressively to 2,400mg/24h, or even higher (see p.272).

Propofol
Some centres use propofol instead of phenobarbital. This is a specialist only treatment, and necessitates an IVI and appropriate variable-rate syringe driver (see p.600).[37]

Abrupt deep sedation is rarely necessary, e.g. sudden massive arterial haemorrhage. Particularly for existential distress, *respite* deep sedation for a few hours (up to 1–2 days in some centres) is an important step.[38]

In the imminently dying, it is uncommon to lighten the depth of the sedation once the patient is settled. However, at one centre, after the patient's distress has been relieved, medication is scaled down so that the patient is physically and mentally comfortable (albeit drowsy/sleeping for most/all of the time) but can be roused for short periods to permit meaningful communication:

> 'Our target in sedation is calming and comfort without lowering the level of consciousness deep enough to lose communication.'[36]

END-STAGE RENAL DISEASE

The two groups of patients for consideration in the last days of life are:
- those already on dialysis in whom a decision to stop dialysis has been made
- those who are chronic kidney disease (CKD) stage 5 (eGFR < 15mL/min), and are being treated with maximum conservative management (i.e. all renal care except dialysis; this includes, for example, **erythropoietin**).

For the patient who stops dialysis the mean survival is 8–10 days, whereas the duration of survival in the conservatively managed group is very variable, ranging from weeks to more than a year. Indicators that death may be approaching are similar to other non-malignant conditions:
- declining physical function
- increasing dependence
- increasing number of symptoms.[39]

Patients with advanced kidney disease experience more symptoms than patients with advanced cancer, with a mean of 20 symptoms in the last month of life.[40] Common symptoms in the last days include:

- breathlessness (may relate to fluid overload and acidosis)
- myoclonic jerks and seizures (relate to both increased drug toxicity and uraemia)
- delirium (also relates to both increased drug toxicity and uraemia).[41]

Other symptoms particularly associated with advanced kidney disease may continue to be a major problem, e.g. pruritus (see Table 5.30, p.432) and restless legs. **Clonazepam** in low doses (i.e. a starting dose of 500microgram PO/SC at bedtime, increased to a maximum dose of 2mg/24h) is often helpful in relieving restless legs; myoclonus, and also neuropathic pain.

Occasionally, with severe fluid overload, if the patient still has a dialysis line in place, it may be appropriate to have a few hours of ultra-filtration to correct the overload.

Anticipatory prescribing

Note the following:

- prescribe **fentanyl** (see p.390) or **alfentanil** (see p.374) instead of **morphine**
- halve the dose of **haloperidol**, **metoclopramide** and **midazolam** because of reduced clearance and the risk of accumulation, and an increased likelihood of dystonic reactions with **metoclopramide**
- do *not* give **cyclizine** by CSCI because it is not compatible with **alfentanil** and **hyoscine *butylbromide***; it also exacerbates dry mouth
- do *not* use **hyoscine *hydrobromide*** for retained secretions/death rattle because of an increased risk of sedation and delirium; instead use **hyoscine *butylbromide*** (dose unchanged) or **glycopyrronium** (halve dose).[42]

Prescribers should indicate clearly that **fentanyl/alfentanil** should be used for breathlessness (as well as pain), possibly in association with low-dose **midazolam**, i.e. 2.5mg p.r.n q1h.

Simplifying long-term medication

Patients with advanced kidney disease typically take numerous drugs to manage the various aspects of their kidney disease and co-morbidities. These drugs can be divided into categories according to function (see below). When to stop drugs as the end of life approaches will depend on:

- how close to death they are
- the purpose of the drug
- likely effects from stopping it
- the burden of taking tablets.

Drugs for mineral and bone disease

Calcium and vitamin D preparations should be continued while the patient is swallowing or until they stop dialysis because of the risk of hypocalcaemia. This is particularly important for the patient who has had a parathyroidectomy. However, for those who have not and are taking **cinacalcet**, a calcimimetic, this may generally be stopped earlier. Phosphate binders can be reduced or stopped as intake reduces because their effect is on the food which is eaten.

Drugs for anaemia

For as long as it is desirable to maintain the haemoglobin for optimal symptom relief, **iron** (given as an infusion at dialysis) can be continued, as can **erythropoietins** until the final weeks.

Diuretics for fluid control

Patients may be taking high doses of diuretics, these should be continued as long as their absence is likely to exacerbate symptoms.

Cardiovascular disease

Most end-stage kidney patients are prescribed statins for primary prevention of cardiovascular disease; and may also be taking **aspirin** and antihypertensives. These should generally be continued until dialysis is stopped.

Drugs to maintain dialysis access

Warfarin should be continued until dialysis stops.

END-STAGE HEART FAILURE

In some *cancer patients*, congestive heart failure (CHF) is a significant cause of breathlessness. It is important to recognize this, and treat appropriately.

General guidance about the care of patients with end-stage CHF is available from NICE[43] and elsewhere.[44–46] Additional resources include:

- *Supportive Care in Heart Failure*[47]
- *Heart Failure and Palliative Care: a team approach*[48]
- *Heart Improvement Programme* (website).[49]

This section provides guidance about which drugs can be stopped to ease a patient's 'tablet burden' without adversely affecting the level of comfort.[50] In end-stage CHF, it is important *not* to stop 'disease control' medication which also has an important contribution in symptom relief. Unlike cancer, where disease-specific treatment tends to become increasingly burdensome and futile (and possibly counterproductive), the continued disease-specific treatment of CHF generally continues to be essential for symptom management even when end-stage (Figure 16.2)[43] If in doubt, obtain advice from the patient's cardiologist or specialist heart failure nurse.

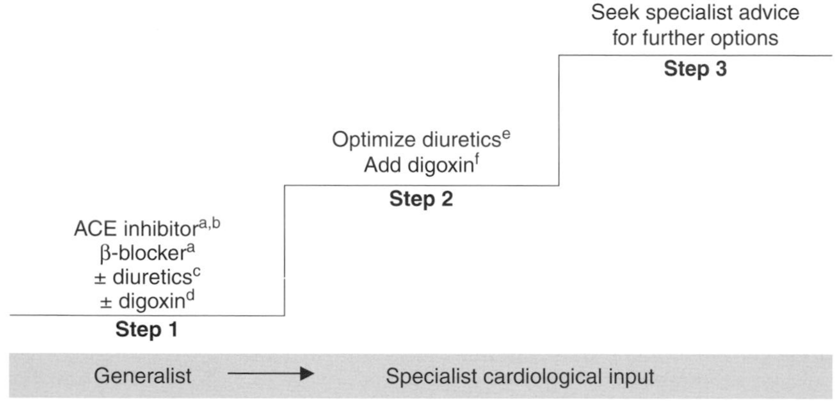

Figure 16.2 Synopsis of drug treatment for CHF caused by left ventricular systolic dysfunction.

a. in all patients who are stable, i.e. minimal or no signs of fluid overload or depletion, even if asymptomatic;
b. if an ACE inhibitor is not tolerated, substitute an angiotensin-II antagonist, e.g. losartan; if an angiotensin-II antagonist is not tolerated, substitute hydralazine and isosorbide dinitrate;
c. in patients with signs of fluid overload;
d. in patients with atrial fibrillation;
e. combine a loop diuretic with spironolactone (see p.59);
f. if not already taking it, i.e. patients in sinus rhythm.

Drugs that improve survival and symptoms

Angiotensin-converting enzyme (ACE) inhibitors; β-blockers; angiotensin receptor blockers

These should be continued because there is good evidence that they slow progression of CHF, prolong survival, and improve symptom control.[51–54] Indications for considering a dose reduction or discontinuation on either a temporary or permanent basis are:

- symptomatic hypotension
- deteriorating renal function
- excessive tablet burden.

The patient's clinical condition and renal function should be monitored closely, and further dose adjustments made (up or down) as necessary.

Aldosterone antagonist
Both **spironolactone** (see p.59) and **eplerenone** also benefit survival and symptom control.[55,56] They should be continued as long as hyperkalaemia is not unacceptably high (see p.60) and renal function is not deteriorating.

Drugs that primarily improve symptoms in advanced disease
Loop diuretics
Furosemide (see p.55) and **bumetanide** are widely used and provide the third intervention in 'triple therapy' for CHF.[57,58] Overall, they also increase survival. In very end-stage disease, the increasing dose required may exacerbate renal dysfunction. However, unless the patient becomes anuric or clinically hypovolaemic, a loop diuretic should be continued for symptom management. **Furosemide** by CSCI may reduce the need for hospital admission (see p.57).[59]

Anti-arrhythmic drugs
Anti-arrhythmic drugs can generally be considered for discontinuation at a relatively early stage. Most anti-arrhythmics lower blood pressure and can contribute to fatigue. However, if *symptomatic* tachycardias are present, or rate control is also helping angina symptoms, it may be best to continue. **Amiodarone** has a very long halflife (some 6 months) and thus can generally be stopped in end-stage CHF.

Anti-anginal agents
These can be discontinued if the patient has no angina. However, low-dose **isosorbide mononitrate**, with an 8h nitrate-free interval/24h, may help breathlessness.

Drugs for longer-term goals
Statins
Cholesterol-lowering drugs can generally be the first to be discontinued because they have no symptom-relieving properties (and have no proven prognostic benefit in CHF).[60]

Antihypertensive drugs
These are generally also inappropriate in end-stage disease.

Digoxin
In atrial fibrillation, **digoxin** may be important in rate control. Uncontrolled fast atrial fibrillation may be unpleasant for the patient and exacerbate symptoms. Care is needed because, if renal failure develops as the heart failure progresses, accumulation will necessitate dose reduction and possibly discontinuation. In sinus rhythm, unless there is clear history of benefit, **digoxin** could be stopped and the situation kept under review.

Antiplatelet agents
These have never been shown to improve prognosis in CHF. Indeed, **aspirin** is associated with an increase in hospital admissions in patients with CHF,[61] and possibly with increased mortality.[62] This probably relates to the fact that, in heart failure patients critically dependent on upregulation of vasodilator PGs, **aspirin** (and other NSAIDs) will attenuate the beneficial effect of ACE-inhibitors, and possibly of β-blockers.[63] Thus, **aspirin** in any dose should be stopped in end-stage heart failure.

Further, analgesic doses of all NSAIDs cause sodium and water retention, antagonizing the effect of diuretics. However, when no effective alternative exists (e.g. severe inflammatory joint pain), an occasional p.r.n. dose or a short course of an NSAID over 3–7 days may need to be given, with monitoring of daily weight. If fluid retention occurs, an increased dose of loop diuretic is given for the remainder of the course of the NSAID.

Warfarin
Warfarin is used to reduce the risk of stroke, particularly in patients with atrial fibrillation. When patients are close to death, the decision to withdraw **warfarin** is generally straightforward. The difficulty is when the patient is still ambulant but frail and at risk of falling, and with an INR remaining steady within the normal therapeutic range. Even so, at the same time, the risks are definitely beginning to increase and it now seems safer to stop the **warfarin**. In practice this requires time and counselling because many patients are anxious about stopping **warfarin**, fearing an immediate stroke.

Drugs for co-morbidities

Drugs for co-morbid conditions need to be reviewed as in any other end-stage disease, bearing in mind the likely impact of discontinuation, e.g. thyroid replacement therapy. For drugs which may be detrimental as far as the heart failure is concerned but beneficial for a co-morbid condition, there will be need to review the potential balance between benefit and harm, e.g. NSAIDs. As always, an individual value judgement will be necessary.

END-STAGE IDIOPATHIC PARKINSON'S DISEASE

Patients can die *with* concurrent idiopathic Parkinson's disease (IPD) or *from* IPD and, as such, patients can be at differing stages of disease as they approach death. One of the key challenges is trying to avoid centrally acting D_2 antagonists (e.g. antipsychotics, **metoclopramide**), because they exacerbate IPD, particularly rigidity and the consequential pain.

Although predicting prognosis in IPD is often difficult, a progressive decline in physical status, continuing weight loss, recurrent infections, cognitive impairment, swallowing problems, and episodes of aspiration pneumonia strongly suggest that the patient has reached the end-stage. Given the unreliability of prognostication, frequent review is necessary. When deterioration is rapid, this may need to be daily (see p.634). Each patient requires careful individual evaluation; and, when possible, there should be ongoing liaison with an IPD specialist.

A rapid decline from diagnosis (within 3–5 years) with a poor response to **levodopa** could indicate a 'PD plus syndrome' (e.g. progressive supranuclear palsy, multisystem atrophy). Most of these patients die some 6–9 years after diagnosis. The approach to palliative care in these conditions is the same as for IPD.

In the last few days of life the patient with IPD is likely to be rigid, wasted, unable to swallow, and confused (delirium).[64] An attempt to continue dopaminergic drugs should be made in patients dying with concurrent IPD (see below). On the other hand, in patients dying from IPD, withdrawal of dopaminergic drugs is sometimes appropriate because of loss of efficacy and/or increased undesirable effects, e.g. agitation, delirium, hallucinations.[65]

Rigidity

Rigidity is not always a major issue for patients with end-stage IPD, and many tolerate a reduction in their often complex IPD drug regimens. On the other hand, important causes of rigidity towards the end of life are:

- not getting dopaminergic drugs on time
- an inability to swallow medication
- worsening IPD which is less dopamine-responsive.

Thus, if the patient can still swallow, ensure that medication is given on time, and consider prescribing p.r.n. doses of dispersible Madopar®, e.g. 62.5mg (= **benserazide** 12.5mg + **levodopa** 50mg)

If the patient is not able swallow, consider giving previous dopaminergic medication via an existing PEG or an NG tube. Alternatively, discuss the use of one of the following parenteral dopamine agonists with a PD specialist:

- TD rotigotine:
  - ▹ start with a 2mg/24h patch; use a fresh site each day
  - ▹ if necessary, after 1 week, increase to 4mg/24h
  - ▹ maximum recommended dose = 8mg/24h
- SC **apomorphine**; also prescribe prophylactic **domperidone** to prevent almost inevitable nausea.[66]

Note: both **rotigotine** and **apomorphine** can cause delirium ± agitation; generally use only with guidance from a PD specialist.

Note: if dopaminergic medication is stopped, a CSCI of **midazolam** may help relieve rigidity. Optimal nursing care and gentle physiotherapy are also crucial.

Pain

Careful evaluation is needed to determine if pain is related to rigidity or to some other cause. Different pains often require different approaches to management:

- if related to rigidity, see above
- If not, consider:
  - ▷ non-drug treatment (e.g. positioning, nursing care, physiotherapy, TENS, massage, heat) *and*
  - ▷ drug treatment (see p.277).

Nausea and vomiting

Many drugs used for nausea and vomiting are D_2 antagonists, e.g. **metoclopramide**, **haloperidol**, **prochlorperazine** (see p.219), and ideally should be avoided in IPD because they will exacerbate rigidity and bradykinesia. Anecdotal reports suggest that **cyclizine** may also exacerbate IPD.

Anti-emetics least likely to exacerbate IPD are:

- **domperidone** (available as a suppository; see p.229)
- **ondansetron** (see p.234)
- **hyoscine *hydrobromide*** (see p.16), but may exacerbate delirium.

Despite being D_2 antagonists, it may be necessary to prescribe small doses of **levomepromazine** (e.g. 2.5–5mg at bedtime, see p.164) or **olanzapine** (e.g. 1.25–2.5mg at bedtime, see p.166) if all else fails.

Delirium and agitation

Remember: both **rotigotine** and **apomorphine** can cause delirium ± agitation.

There may well be need for a 'trade-off' between increased rigidity (and the consequential pain) and the relief of an agitated delirium. However, there are many potential causes for delirium and agitation in end-stage IPD and, as always, a systematic approach is necessary (see p.639):

- if feasible, treat any obvious underlying cause, e.g. constipation and/or urinary retention
- review dopaminergic drugs; discuss with the PD team the best order for stopping these
- this generally results in **levodopa** monotherapy, and perhaps reducing the dose of this as well
- if the patient can swallow, consider **quetiapine** (e.g. 25mg once daily–b.d.), an atypical antipsychotic available only as an oral product but the one least likely to cause extrapyramidal movement disorders
- if the patient cannot swallow, consider a benzodiazepine (see p.132), e.g.:
  - ▷ **midazolam** 2.5mg SC p.r.n.
  - ▷ **lorazepam** 0.5–1mg SC p.r.n.

  but be aware that this may sometimes exacerbate delirium
- if the situation remains unmanageable, prescribe an injectable antipsychotic, e.g. **levomepromazine** 6.25–12.5mg SC p.r.n. (see p.164).

The use of **levomepromazine** will generally result in a reduction in the patient's level of consciousness, but will exacerbate PD less than **haloperidol**.

Some patients with PD also have dementia, commonly Alzheimer's or dementia with Lewy bodies (DLB).[67,68] Extra care needs to be taken in DLB. About 50% of such patients are over-sensitive to antipsychotics and, if used, they will experience a marked exacerbation of the PD, reduced level of consciousness, increased delirium, and possibly neuroleptic (antipsychotic) malignant syndrome (see p.155).

AS DEATH APPROACHES

Even when there is nothing new to offer, it is important for the doctor to:

- continue to visit
- quietly indicate:
  'The important thing now is to keep you as comfortable as possible'
- continue to inform the family of the changing situation:
  'He is very weak now, but may still live for several days'
  'Although he seems better today, he's remains very weak. . . He could quickly deteriorate and die in just a few days'
- control agitation even if it results in sedation (see p.639)
- listen to the nurses.

1 Ellershaw JE *et al.* (1995) Dehydration and the dying patient. *Journal of Pain and Symptom Management.* **10**: 192–197.
2 Higgs R (1999) The diagnosis of dying. *Journal of the Royal College of Physicians of London.* **33**: 110–112.
3 Twycross R *et al.* (2009) *Symptom Management in Advanced Cancer* (4e). palliativedrugs.com, Nottingham, pp. 423–424.
4 Thomas K and Lobo B (eds) (2010) *Advance Care Planning in End of Life Care.* Oxford University Press, Oxford.
5 Twycross R *et al.* (2009) *Symptom Management in Advanced Cancer* (4e). palliativedrugs.com, Nottingham, pp. 407–421.
6 Twycross R *et al.* (2009) *Symptom Management in Advanced Cancer* (4e). palliativedrugs.com, Nottingham, pp. 407–438.
7 Ellershaw J and Wilkinson S (2010) *Care of the Dying. A Pathway to Excellence* (2e). Oxford University Press, Oxford.
8 NICE (2004) Improving supportive and palliative care for adults with cancer. National Institute for Health and Clinical Excellence, London, UK. Available from: http://guidance.nice.org.uk/CSGSP
9 Anonymous (2010) *The route to success in end of life care – achieving quality in acute hospitals.* National End of Life Care Programme, London.
10 Liverpool Care Pathway and Marie Curie Cancer Care (2010) The Liverpool care pathway for the dying patient. Version 12. Available from: http://www.mcpcil.org.uk/liverpool-care-pathway
11 Luhrs CA *et al.* (2005) Pilot of a pathway to improve the care of imminently dying oncology inpatients in a Veterans Affairs Medical Center. *Journal of Pain and Symptom Management.* **29**: 544–551.
12 Bookbinder M *et al.* (2005) Improving end-of-life care: development and pilot-test of a clinical pathway. *Journal of Pain and Symptom Management.* **29**: 529–543.
13 Ellershaw J (2002) Clinical pathways for care of the dying: an innovation to disseminate clinical excellence. *Journal of Palliative Medicine.* **5**: 617–621.
14 Swart S *et al.* (2006) Dutch experiences with the Liverpool Care Pathway. *European Journal of Palliative Care.* **13(4)**: 156–159.
15 Jack BA *et al.* (2003) Nurses' perceptions of the Liverpool Care Pathway for the dying patient in the acute hospital setting. *International Journal of Palliative Nursing.* **9**: 375–381.
16 Poulson J (1997) The management of diabetes in patients with advanced cancer. *Journal of Pain and Symptom Management.* **13**: 339–346.
17 McCann M-A *et al.* (2006) Practical management of diabetes mellitus. *European Journal of Palliative Care.* **13**: 226–229.
18 Fainsinger R *et al.* (1991) Symptom control during the last week of life on a palliative care unit. *Journal of Palliative Care.* **7 (1)**: 5–11.
19 Ventafridda V *et al.* (1990) Symptom prevalence and control during cancer patients' last days of life. *Journal of Palliative Care.* **6 (3)**: 7–11.
20 Lichter I and Hunt E (1990) The last 48 hours of life. *Journal of Palliative Care.* **6 (4)**: 7–15.
21 Wilkes E (1984) Dying now. *Lancet.* **1**: 950–952.
22 Exton-Smith AN (1961) Terminal illness in the aged. *Lancet.* **2**: 305–308.
23 Twycross R *et al.* (2009) *Symptom Management in Advanced Cancer* (4e). palliativedrugs.com, Nottingham.
24 Fainsinger RL *et al.* (1992) The use of urinary catheters in terminally ill cancer patients. *Journal of Pain and Symptom Management.* **7**: 333–338.
25 Wilcock A and Chauhan A (2007) Benchmarking the use of opioids in the last days of life. *Journal of Pain and Symptom Management.* **34**: 1–3.
26 Good PD *et al.* (2005) Effects of opioids and sedatives on survival in an Australian inpatient palliative care population. *Internal Medicine Journal.* **35**: 512–517.
27 Thorns A and Sykes N (2000) Opioid use in last week of life and implications for end-of-life decision-making. *Lancet.* **356**: 398–399.
28 Navigante AH *et al.* (2006) Midazolam as adjunct therapy to morphine in the alleviation of severe dyspnea perception in patients with advanced cancer. *Journal of Pain and Symptom Management.* **31**: 38–47.
29 Wildiers H *et al.* (2009) Atropine, hyoscine butylbromide, or scopolamine are equally effective for the treatment of death rattle in terminal care. *Journal of Pain and Symptom Management.* **38**: 124–133.
30 Hughes A *et al.* (2000) Audit of three antimuscarinic drugs for managing retained secretions. *Palliative Medicine.* **14**: 221–222.
31 Back I *et al.* (2001) A study comparing hyoscine hydrobromide and glycopyrrolate in the treatment of death rattle. *Palliative Medicine.* **15**: 329–336.
32 Twycross R *et al.* (2009) *Symptom Management in Advanced Cancer* (4e). palliativedrugs.com, Nottingham, pp. 430–432.
33 Breitbart W *et al.* (1996) A double-blind trial of haloperidol, chlorpromazine, and lorazepam in the treatment of delirium in hospitalized AIDS patients. *American Journal of Psychiatry.* **153**: 231–237.
34 Massie MJ *et al.* (1983) Delirium in terminally ill cancer patients. *Amercian Journal of Psychiatry.* **140**: 1048–1050.
35 Bruera E *et al.* (1987) Delirium and severe sedation in patients with terminal cancer. *Cancer Treatment Reports.* **71**: 787–788.
36 Muller-Busch HC *et al.* (2003) Sedation in palliative care – a critical analysis of 7 years experience. *BMC Palliative Care.* **2**: 2.
37 Lundstrom S *et al.* (2005) When nothing helps: propofol as sedative and antiemetic in palliative cancer care. *Journal of Pain and Symptom Management.* **30**: 570–577.
38 Twycross R *et al.* (2009) *Symptom Management in Advanced Cancer* (4e). palliativedrugs.com, Nottingham, pp. 432–435.

39 Murtagh F and Sheerin N (2010) Conservative management of end-stage renal disease. In: Chambers EJ *et al.* (eds) *Supportive Care for the Renal Patient* (2e). Oxford University Press, Oxford.
40 Murtagh FE *et al.* (2010) Symptoms in the month before death for stage 5 chronic kidney disease patients managed without dialysis. *Journal of Pain and Symptom Management.* **40**: 342–352.
41 Twycross R *et al.* (2009) *Symptom Management in Advanced Cancer* (4e). palliativedrugs.com, Nottingham.
42 Liverpool Care Pathway and Marie Curie Cancer Care Guidelines for LCP drug prescribing in advanced chronic kidney disease.
43 NICE (2010) Clinical Guideline 108. Chronic heart failure: management of chronic heart failure in adults in primary and secondary care.
44 Arnold JM *et al.* (2006) Canadian Cardiovascular Society consensus conference recommendations on heart failure 2006: diagnosis and management.[erratum appears in Canadian Journal of Cardiology. 2006 Mar 1;22(3):271]. *Canadian Journal of Cardiology.* **22**: 23–45.
45 Swedberg K *et al.* (2005) Guidelines for the diagnosis and treatment of chronic heart failure: full text (update 2005). European Heart Journal. Available from: 10.1093/eurheartj/ehi205
46 Hunt SA *et al.* (2005) Guideline Update for the Diagnosis and Management of Chronic Heart Failure in the Adult. ACC/AHA. Available from: http://circ.ahajournals.org/cgi/content/full/112/12/e154f
47 Beattie J and Goodlin S (eds) (2008) *Supportive Care in Heart Failure.* Oxford University Press, Oxford.
48 Johnson MJ and Lehman R (eds) (2006) *Heart Failure and Palliative Care: a team approach.* Radcliffe Publishing Ltd., Oxford.
49 NHS (2007) Supportive and Palliative Care in Heart Failure. In: *Heart Improvement Programme.* Available from: http://www.heart.nhs.uk/endoflifecare/hip.htm
50 Cleland JG *et al.* (2000) Polypharmacy (or polytherapy) in the treatment of heart failure. *Heart Failure Monitor.* **1**: 8–13.
51 Jong P *et al.* (2002) Angiotensin receptor blockers in heart failure: meta-analysis of randomized controlled trials. *Journal of the American College of Cardiology.* **39**: 463–470.
52 Shibata MC *et al.* (2001) Systematic review of the impact of beta blockers on mortality and hospital admissions in heart failure. *European Journal of Heart Failure.* **3**: 351–357.
53 The SOLVD Investigators (1991) Effect of enalapril on survival in patients with reduced left ventricular ejection fractions and congestive heart failure. The SOLVD Investigators. *New England Journal of Medicine.* **325**: 293–302.
54 Consensus Trial Study Group (1987) Effects of enalapril on mortality in severe congestive heart failure. Results of the Cooperative North Scandinavian Enalapril Survival Study (CONSENSUS). *New England Journal of Medicine.* **316**: 1429–1435.
55 Pitt B *et al.* (1999) The effect of spironolactone on morbidity and mortality in patients with severe heart failure. Randomized Aldactone Evaluation Study Investigators. *New England Journal of Medicine.* **341**: 709–717.
56 Pitt B *et al.* (2003) Eplerenone, a selective aldosterone blocker, in patients with left ventricular dysfunction after myocardial infarction. *New England Journal of Medicine.* **348**: 1309–1321.
57 McMurray JJ and Pfeffer MA (2005) Heart failure. *Lancet.* **365**: 1877–1889.
58 Faris R *et al.* (2006) Diuretics for heart failure. *Cochrane Database of Systematic Reviews.* CD003838.
59 Zacharias H *et al.* (2011) Is there a role for subcutaneous furosemide in the community and hospice management of end-stage heart failure? *Palliative Medicine.* Epub ahead of print.
60 McGowan MP and Treating to New Target Study G (2004) There is no evidence for an increase in acute coronary syndromes after short-term abrupt discontinuation of statins in stable cardiac patients. *Circulation.* **110**: 2333–2335.
61 Massie BM *et al.* (2009) Randomized trial of warfarin, aspirin, and clopidogrel in patients with chronic heart failure: the Warfarin and Antiplatelet Therapy in Chronic Heart Failure (WATCH) trial. *Circulation.* **119**: 1616–1624.
62 Cleland JG (2002) Is aspirin 'the weakest link' in cardiovascular prophylaxis? The surprising lack of evidence supporting the use of aspirin for cardiovascular disease. *Progress in Cardiovascular Diseases.* **44**: 275–292.
63 Davie AP *et al.* (2000) Even low-dose aspirin inhibits arachidonic acid-induced vasodilation in heart failure. *Clinical Pharmacology and Therapeutics.* **67**: 530–537.
64 Goy ER *et al.* (2008) Neurologic disease at the end of life: caregiver descriptions of Parkinson disease and amyotrophic lateral sclerosis. *Journal of Palliative Medicine.* **11**: 548–554.
65 National Council of Palliative Care (NCPC) Neurological Conditions Group (2011) Consensus statement for the management of symptoms in idiopathic Parkinsons's Disease (PD) and related conditions in the last few days of life.
66 Dewhurst F *et al.* (2009) The pragmatic use of apomorphine at the end of life. *Palliative Medicine.* **23**: 777–779.
67 McKeith IG *et al.* (2005) Diagnosis and management of dementia with Lewy bodies: third report of the DLB Consortium. *Neurology.* **65**: 1863–1872.
68 McKeith I (2002) Dementia with Lewy bodies. *British Journal of Psychiatry.* **180**: 144–147.

17: PRE-EMPTIVE PRESCRIBING IN THE COMMUNITY

Rapid access to drugs in the community is important to avoid crises at home and to reduce unwanted or unnecessary admissions in the last days of life.[1–3] Both enteral and parenteral formulations of drugs to relieve pain, nausea and vomiting, breathlessness, noisy respiratory secretions ('death rattle'), restlessness/agitation, delirium and seizures, need to be available.[4,5] The Department of Health (London) recommends that generally patients should be able to receive needed medication at the same time and in the same place as the out-of-hours (OOH) consultation.[6] Ways of enabling this include:

- *Anticipatory prescribing:* encouraging prescribers to think ahead and prescribe extra medication to manage sudden changes in the patient's condition, or pro-actively prescribe injectable drugs commonly used at the end of life which are then available in the home on an 'if needed' basis.[1,7]
- *Just in case* boxes are standard boxes containing drugs specifically prescribed for the patient, and left in the home.[8,9] Examples of the use of *Just in case* boxes are readily available.[6,10] The boxes generally contain a small selection of injectable drugs in a tamper-proof box, the choice based on local guidelines for care in the last days of life. Additional emergency supplies may be indicated for selected patients, e.g. for someone with MND/ALS (see below)[11] or a *Crisis haemorrhage* pack for those at risk of a major haemorrhage.
- *Breathing Space* boxes (now known as *Just in Case* kits) are designed for patients with end-stage MND at risk of severe breathlessness, panic or choking. On request, the MND Association provides the box free of charge to the GP; it contains information for both the patient and the GP. The GP is asked to prescribe appropriate drugs, e.g. **midazolam**, **glycopyrronium**, **diamorphine**, and keep them in the box in the patient's home.[11]
- *Palliative care emergency* kits contain various drugs and equipment which can be carried in an OOH service provider's car; they generally include a wider range of drugs than in a *Just in case* box and also a syringe driver. To carry CDs they must able to demonstrate compliance with current Home Office regulations.[12]
- *Extended pharmacy schemes* are nominated community palliative care pharmacies which offer extended opening hours, and agree to carry an extended palliative care stock.

Examples of local practice are available in the document library on www.palliativedrugs.com, filed under medication issues (out of hours issues).

Just in case boxes

The Gold Standards Framework (GSF) recommends the following for a *Just in case* box:

- SC formulations for pain, nausea and vomiting, agitation/restlessness and death rattle (2mL syringes and needles)
- ± rectal diazepam
- local prescribing algorithms
- signed permissions for medication administration
- patient information.[3,9]

Typical injectable drugs include:

- **diamorphine, morphine** or **oxycodone** for pain
- **cyclizine, haloperidol** or **levomepromazine** for nausea and vomiting
- **midazolam** for agitation/restlessness
- **glycopyrronium, hyoscine** ***hydrobromide*** or **hyoscine** ***butylbromide*** for respiratory secretions.

Some boxes also include rectal **diazepam** or **lorazepam** tablets (for SL use).

A syringe driver may be left with the box.[6] WFI and a small sharps disposal container are also recommended.[10]

The cost of a *Just in case* box will depend on its contents, and how many amps of each drug are prescribed. Typically, a box will contain 2–5 amps of each injectable drug (Table 17.1).[8]

Table 17.1 Cost of *Just in case* drugs[13]

Drug	*Strength and form*	*Cost/amp*[a]
Diamorphine hydrochloride	5mg amp, powder for reconstitution	£3
	10mg amp, powder for reconstitution	£3.50
Morphine sulphate	10, 15, 20 and 30mg/mL; 1mL and 2mL amps	£1–1.50
Cyclizine	50mg/mL, 1mL amp	£1
Midazolam	2mg/mL, 5mL amp	£1
	5mg/mL, 2mL amp	£1
Hyoscine *hydrobromide*	400microgram/mL, 1mL amp	£3
	600microgram/mL, 1mL amp	£3
Glycopyrronium	200microgram/mL, 1mL amp	£1
	200microgram/mL, 3mL amp	£1
Diazepam rectal solution	5mg and 10mg rectal tube	£2

a. cost rounded up to nearest 50p.

If the patient is at risk of a crisis such as catastrophic haemorrhage, it is important to ensure that sufficient ampoules are provided to deal with this (should it occur), but not forgetting that non-drug measures are generally equally or more important.[14,15] If crisis medication is supplied (Table 17.2), it should be:

- readily available in the patient's home
- rapid in onset (2–5 min)
- already drawn up and kept in a fridge because there is rarely time to prepare an injection or calmly measure a SL dose
- if possible, given by the nearest carer, whether professional or informal (see p.609).

Table 17.2 Crisis drugs prepared in advance for a major haemorrhage in order of speed of onset

Drug	*Route*	*Dose*	*Speed of onset*
Midazolam	IV	10mg	2–3min (see p.141)
	IM	10mg	5–15min
Lorazepam	SL[a]	4mg (1mL)	5min (see p.146)
Midazolam	Buccal/SL[b]	10mg (1mL)[c]	15min (see p.141)

a. use the contents of an ampoule for injection

b. unlicensed buccal liquid 10mg/mL; available as a special order from Special Products Ltd; see Obtaining unlicensed products, p.769. Needs to be ordered in advance for an individual patient

c. if buccal liquid unavailable, midazolam injection can be used instead. However, this will increase the volume (10mg = 2mL of 5mg/mL injection), and this may be more than some patients can retain easily in their mouth.

The 'nearest carer' will generally be a family member or other informal carer. Thus, it is necessary to train such carers to give medication SL or by injection, whichever is the case (see p.609).

In catastrophic haemorrhage, the SC route is inappropriate because of likely peripheral shutdown and unpredictable absorption. IV is ideal but, failing that, it should be given IM (deltoid may be quicker than gluteal).[16,17]

Boxes should generally be stored in a cool, dry, low-access area. **Lorazepam** injection needs refrigeration.

Procedures need to be in place to ensure the security of the box during the acquisition process, while stored in the patient's home, and during return to the pharmacy after use. In order to confirm that medication has not been unlawfully diverted, there must be an 'audit trail' documenting the ordering, dispensing and delivery of the drugs to the patient, and return of unused medication to the pharmacy.

A medication log included in the box can act as both an administration record and a stock balance sheet. The medication should be in a suitably robust container, fastened with a combination lock or a tamper-evident security tag. Unless specifically directed otherwise, it should be opened only by the community nurse who will be preparing the drugs for use by the patient/carer, or by a physician.

If the box is ordered before the last few days of life, there needs to be a robust procedure for reviewing the contents regularly, expiry dates, drug administration directions and medication doses as the patient's clinical condition changes. A prompt should be included in the box to ensure early medical review if any of the drugs are administered.[18] It is also essential that the patient and carer are told about:

- the contents of the emergency box
- the proper use of the medication, including training in the administration of SL/SC drugs when necessary (see p.609)
- who to contact in the event of an emergency.

The administration of emergency medication in a patient's home at the end of life carries a high risk for error. In order to avoid confusion at the time of use, concise, well-written and illustrated *patient and carer information material* should be included in the box.

Palliative care emergency kits for out-of-hours (OOH) services

The provision of and contents of palliative care emergency kits are dependent on the OOH service provider. The ideal is to 'keep it simple', i.e. to restrict the number of products to no more than 6–7. Some drugs will overlap OOH emergency medication needed in other clinical situations. Kits can be kept in the OOH provider's car, and also in OOH provider bases. Standardization across a geographical area is recommended, and helps staff to be familiar with what is available. A starting point is the National out-of-hours formulary palliative care core drug list:[19]

- **diamorphine** (injection)
- **cyclizine** (injection)
- **dexamethasone** (tablet)
- **hyoscine *butylbromide*** (injection)
- **ketorolac** or **diclofenac** (injection)
- **levomepromazine** (injection)
- **midazolam** (injection).

It is expected that these drugs will be part of a special locally available tamper-proof palliative care container. Local discussions will be necessary to determine optimum access. The quantities supplied should be enough to allow optimum symptom relief until formal review by the palliative care team or GP.

Other drugs useful in palliative care appear in other sections of the National out-of-hours Formulary:

- **haloperidol** and **diazepam** (oral and injectable) are under 'Psychiatric emergencies'
- antacids, **domperidone** (oral), **glycerol** suppositories, anti-spasmodic agents, **loperamide**, **metoclopramide** (injectable), **phosphate** enema and **prochlorperazine** (buccal) are under 'Gastro-intestinal'
- **codeine** (oral), **diamorphine** (injectable), a locally negotiated NSAID (oral and injectable) and **paracetamol** (oral) are under 'Analgesics'
- **naloxone** is in its own section for opioid overdose.

Local guidelines for the use of these drugs for palliative care, contact numbers for specialist advice, equipment to allow administration (including syringe drivers), and guidance on any local arrangements for rapid access to higher strengths of **diamorphine** or other injectable strong opioids should be included with the kit or be easily accessible, remembering the wide range of care settings an OOH service provider may cover.

Extended pharmacy schemes

These are generally PCT-commissioned, and involve networks of community pharmacies able to offer extended opening hours, and carrying a locally agreed palliative care stock list (Table 17.3) Some also agree to provide palliative care information, advice and an emergency contacts list for patients, carers and clinicians.[6]

Table 17.3 Lothian Community Pharmacy Palliative Care Networks Pan-Lothian Stock List October 2010[20]

Drug	*Form*	*Strength*	*Quantity stocked*
Alfentanil	Injection	1mg/2mL	1×10
Cyclizine	Injection	50mg/mL	2×5
Dexamethasone	Tablets	2mg	1×50
Dexamethasone (Organon)[a]	Injection	4mg/mL	1×10
Diamorphine hydrochloride	Injection	10mg	2×5
	Injection	30mg	2×5
	Injection	100mg	1×5
Diazepam	Rectal tubes	10mg/2.5mL	1×5
Fentanyl	TD patches	12microgram/h	1×5
	TD patches	25microgram/h	1×5
Glycopyrronium	Injection	200microgram/mL	1×10
Haloperidol	Injection	5mg/mL	2×5
Hyoscine *butylbromide* (Buscopan®)	Injection	20mg/mL	2×10
Hyoscine *hydrobromide*	Injection	400microgram/mL	1×10
Levomepromazine	Injection	25mg/mL	1×10
	Tablets[b]	6mg	1×28
Metoclopramide	Injection	10mg/2mL	2×12
Midazolam	Injection[c]	10mg/2mL	2×10
Morphine sulphate	Oral liquid	10mg/5mL	1×100mL
	Oral liquid	100mg/5mL	1×30mL
	Injection	10mg/mL	2×10
	Injection	30mg/mL	2×10
Morphine sulphate m/r (MST continus®)	Granules for oral suspension	30mg sachet	1×30
Oxycodone hydrochloride	Oral liquid	5mg/5mL	1×250mL
	Injection	20mg/2mL	1×5
Phenobarbital	Injection	200mg/mL	1×5
Sodium Chloride	Infusion	0.9%	20×500mL
WFI (10mL amps)	Injection	–	2×10

a. dexamethasone 4mg/mL refers specifically to the Organon product. The comparable Hospira product contains dexamethasone 3.3mg/mL

b. levomepromazine 6mg tablets are a named-patient product

c. the strength of midazolam stocked is 10mg/2mL; other strengths should not be used as they are too dilute for preparation of syringes for syringe drivers.

Achieving success

The success of any scheme will depend on generating and maintaining high levels of awareness across normal hours and OOH service providers. OOH service providers may employ large numbers of part-time staff working sporadic or infrequent shifts, covering the whole of emergency medicine, of which palliative care will be one small part. Straightforward up-to-date information about any local schemes for accessing drugs OOH needs to be integrated into induction and training sessions, any service handbooks, and be easily available at the point of need in service cars and at service bases.

1 Allanson H (2004) Delivering the out-of-hours review: securing proper access to medicines in the out-of-hours period. Department of Health. Available from: http://www.out-of-hours.info/documents.php
2 NICE (2004) Improving supportive and palliative care for adults with cancer. National Institute for Health and Clinical Excellence, London, UK. Available from: http://guidance.nice.org.uk/CSGSP
3 Gold Standards Framework (2010) Out of hours. Available from: www.goldstandardsframework.org.uk/GSFInPrimary+Care/OOHs
4 Wowchuk SM *et al.* (2009) The palliative medication kit: an effective way of extending care in the home for patients nearing death. *Journal of Palliative Medicine.* **12**: 797–803.
5 Dawkins L (2007) 'Just-in-case' medication boxes for palliative care patients. *End of Life Care.* **1**: 65–69.
6 Allanson H (2008) Medicines in unplanned care toolkit. NHS Medicines Management Network Northwest and Department of Health. Available from: www.palliativedrugs.com/download/110111_Master_Medicines_in_unplanned_Medicines_Toolkit_26_11_2008.pdf
7 Palmer E and Howarth J (2005) Palliative Care for the Primary Care Team (also available on gp-palliativecare.co.uk). In. Quay Books, London.
8 Amass C and Allen M (2005) How a "just in case" approach can improve out-of-hours palliative care. *The Pharmaceutical Journal.* **275**: 22–23.
9 Gold Standards Framework (2006) Check list of contents for "Just in Case Boxes". Available from: www.goldstandards-framework.nhs.uk/Resources/Gold%20Standards%20Framework/Test%20Content/SuggestedContentsForAJustInCaseBox.pdf
10 Gold Standards Framework (2006) Examples of Good Practice Resource Guide — Just in case boxes. Available from: www.goldstandardsframework.nhs.uk/Resources/Gold%20Standards%20Framework/Test%20Content/ExamplesOfGoodPracticeResourceGuideJustInCaseBoxes.pdf
11 Motor Neurone Disease Association (2010) Breathing space (Just in Case) kit. Available from: www.mndassociation.org/for_professionals/association_resources/jic_kit.html
12 National Prescribing Centre (2009) A guide to good practice in the management of controlled drugs in primary care (England) 3rd edition. Available from: http://www.npci.org.uk/cd/public/docs/controlled_drugs_third_edition.pdf
13 BNF (2010) British National Formulary (No. 60). British Medical Association and the Royal Pharmaceutical Society of Great Britain, London. Available from: www.bnf.org
14 North Cumbria Palliative Care Service Crisis Management Group (2006) Guidance for healthcare staff for managing catastrophic haemorrhage. Available from: www.palliativedrugs.com Document library.
15 Yorkshire Palliative Medicine Clinical Guidelines Group (2008) Guidelines on the management of bleeding for palliative care patients with cancer. Available from: www.palliativedrugs.com Document library
16 Lazebnik N *et al.* (1989) Intravenous, deltoid, or gluteus administration of meperidine during labor? *American Journal of Obstetrics and Gynecology.* **160**: 1184–1189.
17 British Association of Head and Neck Oncology Nurses (1999) Guidelines for carotid haemorrhage. Available from: http://www.bahnon.org.uk/Public/KnowledgeCentre/tabid/81/Default.aspx (subscription required).
18 Gold Standards Framework (2006) Check list for developing Just in Case boxes. Available from: www.goldstandardsframework.nhs.uk/Resources/Gold%20Standards%20Framework/Test%20Content/HowToDevelopJustInCaseBoxesInALocalArea.pdf
19 NHS (2010) Electronic drug tariff. Part XVIIC — National out-of-hours formulary. Available from: www.ppa.org.uk/edt/March_2010/mindex.htm
20 Lothian Community Pharmacy Palliative Care Networks (2010) Pan-Lothian stock list October 2010. Available from: www.nhslothian.scot.nhs.uk/Services/A-Z/PalliativeCare/PharmacyServices/Documents/NetworkCommunityPharmacyMedicineList.pdf

18: MANAGEMENT OF POSTOPERATIVE PAIN IN OPIOID-DEPENDENT PATIENTS

Opioid-dependent patients include those using long-term opioids for:

- pain relief (mainly cancer but increasingly non-cancer pain)
- long-term opioid maintenance for opioid dependence
- current substance misuse.

All such patients will require *additional* opioids to relieve any superadded pain. It is thus crucially important that pre-operative, peri-operative and postoperative doses take this into account, and that *extra amounts* of a strong opioid are prescribed. Almost certainly, these will be larger than the typical doses used by non-opioid-dependent patients in these circumstances.[1] For example, if only typical postoperative doses are prescribed (e.g. **morphine** 2.5–10mg IV/SC q1h p.r.n.), patients who are tolerant to higher doses may experience little or no pain relief.

Because tolerance to undesirable effects, e.g. respiratory depression, develops more rapidly than to analgesia (often within days or 1–2 weeks at most), opioids can be safely titrated to the higher doses required in opioid-dependent patients.

Further, a sudden significant reduction in overall opioid dose may well precipitate an opioid withdrawal syndrome, possibly accompanied by *hyperalgesia*. This will magnify the postoperative pain and any other underlying pain. Thus, under-prescribing could lead to devastating overwhelming pain.

As far as possible, a multidisciplinary approach should be adopted, e.g. pre-operative consultation with the patient's substance misuse team, the anaesthetist and the acute pain team, to develop a pain management plan which should include intra-operative and postoperative monitoring, with dose adjustments made by an experienced anaesthetist. There are no uniform recommendations, but Box 18.A outlines the general approach.[2–12] Addicts receiving maintenance therapy with **methadone** or high-dose SL **buprenorphine**, or **naltrexone** require additional considerations (see below).

Addicts receiving methadone maintenance therapy

Generally, **methadone** maintenance therapy is administered once daily, which is adequate to prevent opioid withdrawal symptoms for 24h, but not to relieve pain. In acute pain, generally the maintenance dose is continued at the same dose, but can be used to contribute towards analgesia *by halving the dose and administering it b.d.* When the PO route can not be used, SC or CSCI are alternative routes of administration (see p.416).

Addicts receiving high-dose SL buprenorphine maintenance therapy

Buprenorphine acts as a partial agonist at the μ-opioid receptor, to which it binds with a higher affinity than other μ-opioid receptor agonists. Thus, when **buprenorphine** is present in sufficient amounts, it will antagonize the analgesic effects of other μ-opioid receptor agonists. This is likely only with the higher doses used SL for opioid maintenance, i.e. ≥16mg/day (see p.381). This has led some to advocate discontinuing high-dose SL **buprenorphine** 5–7 days before elective surgery to avoid compromising postoperative pain relief, and to manage withdrawal symptoms with **methadone** instead.[14] On the other hand, various μ-opioid receptor agonists have been successfully used for postoperative pain in patients on SL **buprenorphine** 2–32mg/day, although higher doses than usual may be required.[15,16]

Box 18.A Management of postoperative pain in opioid-dependent patients

1 Consider local anaesthetic or multimodal approaches to analgesia, e.g. regional blocks, paracetamol, NSAIDs, ketamine, clonidine, etc.

2 Identify the baseline opioid dose; in patients misusing opioids this may mean a 'best guess' estimate.

3 Generally, the baseline opioid dose should be continued as a regular prescription.

4 Reduce the baseline dose if:
- the surgery will improve the pre-operative pain
- the baseline opioid needs to be replaced by an alternative opioid; because of possible incomplete cross-tolerance, reduce the dose calculated from equipotency tables by at least 1/3, particularly when dealing with large doses, e.g. ⩾ morphine 1g PO/24h or equivalent (see p.354).

5 If PO is not possible immediately postoperatively, an alternative route, e.g. CSCI or CIVI should be used to deliver the baseline dose. This can also be done via IV patient-controlled analgesia (PCA) (see point 11).

6 Before restarting PO m/r opioids, ensure that GI function has returned to normal. Gastric stasis can lead to delayed dissolution and drug absorption, followed by 'dose-dumping' when motility improves, with consequential overdose. Conversely, surgery which increases GI transit time (e.g. small bowel resection), may render the use of m/r products inappropriate.

7 It is sometimes recommended that fentanyl TD patches are removed before surgery. However, if the surgery is unlikely to lead to major changes in skin perfusion and the ongoing opioid requirements are unlikely to change, it is best to leave TD patches in place, and give additional p.r.n. opioid.

8 If TD patches are removed, pain relief will persist for several hours because fentanyl is sequestrated widely throughout the body, particularly in adipose tissue (see p.390). Note: in postoperative patients, after a patch has been removed, the mean time for the plasma fentanyl concentration to drop below the minimum effective level is 16h, with a range of 2–23h.[13]

9 Continue long-term ED or IT pumps unchanged unless the surgery is expected to reduce the pain for which these are being used.

10 Prescribe an appropriate dose of a strong opioid for p.r.n. use; typically equivalent to 1/10–1/6 of the total daily dose.

11 With IV PCA, a larger bolus dose is generally necessary compared with the typical bolus dose of morphine 1mg. PCA can also be used to continuously deliver part or all of the baseline opioid dose.

Example
Patient on long-term morphine 300mg/day PO = 100mg/day IV = 4mg/h IV.
PCA background infusion = 2–3mg/h IV.
PCA bolus dose = 2mg IV with a 5min lockout period between doses.

With addicts, if there is considerable uncertainty about their opioid intake, it may be safer to underestimate both the background infusion dose and bolus dose required.

12 Close monitoring is required to:
- identify inadequate dosing (unrelieved pain, withdrawal phenomena)
- ensure rapid dose titration
- prevent excessive dosing (sedation, respiratory depression)
- ensure that bolus doses are not being misused.

For someone on high-dose SL **buprenorphine** who experiences acute pain unexpectedly, options include:

- regional anaesthesia
- optimizing the use of non-opioid analgesics (see Box 18.A)
- prescribing a μ-opioid receptor agonist, e.g. IV **morphine**, **fentanyl**; higher doses than usual may be required
- progressively increasing the SL **buprenorphine** dose up to 24–32mg/day, and give in divided doses t.d.s.–q.d.s.[14,16]

Addicts receiving long-term naltrexone therapy

The opioid antagonist **naltrexone** is used to prevent relapse in opioid ex-addicts (by blocking the opioid 'high'), and in the treatment of alcohol dependence. It blocks all types of opioid receptor, and is long-acting. It thus prevents/blocks opioid analgesia. Analgesia for these patients is even more challenging (see Box 5.Y, p.440).[17]

1 Rapp SE *et al.* (1995) Acute pain management in patients with prior opioid consumption: a case-controlled retrospective review. *Pain.* **61**: 195–201.
2 Macintyre PE (2001) Safety and efficacy of patient-controlled analgesia. *British Journal of Anaesthesia.* **87**: 36–46.
3 Mitra S and Sinatra RS (2004) Perioperative management of acute pain in the opioid-dependent patient. *Anesthesiology.* **101**: 212–227.
4 Lewis NL and Williams JE (2005) Acute pain management in patients receiving opioids for chronic and cancer pain. *Continuing Education in Anaesthesia; critical care and pain.* **5**: 127–129.
5 Roberts DM and Meyer-Witting M (2005) High-dose buprenorphine: perioperative precautions and management strategies. *Anaesthesia and Intensive Care.* **33**: 17–25.
6 Alford DP *et al.* (2006) Acute pain management for patients receiving maintenance methadone or buprenorphine therapy. *Annals of Internal Medicine.* **144**: 127–134.
7 British Pain Society (2006) Pain and substance misuse: improving the patient experience. A consensus document for consultation. British Pain Society, London. Available from: www.britishpainsociety.org
8 James C and Williams JE (2006) How should postoperative pain in patients on long-term opioids be managed? *British Journal of Hospital Medicine (London).* **67**: 500.
9 Mackenzie JW (2006) Acute pain management for opioid dependent patients. *Anaesthesia.* **61**: 907–908.
10 Macintyre PE and Ready LB (2006) *Acute Pain Management — A Practical Guide* (2e). Saunders Ltd., p. 272.
11 Mehta V and Langford RM (2006) Acute pain management for opioid dependent patients. *Anaesthesia.* **61**: 269–276.
12 Macintyre P *et al.* (2010) APM:SE Working Group of the Australian and New Zealand College of Anaesthetists and Faculty of Pain Medicine. In: *Acute Pain Medicine Management Scientific Evidence* (3e). ANZCA & FPM, Melbourne.
13 Grond S *et al.* (2000) Clinical pharmacokinetics of transdermal opioids: focus on transdermal fentanyl. *Clinical Pharmacokinetics.* **38**: 59–89.
14 Savage SR *et al.* (2008) Challenges in using opioids to treat pain in persons with substance use disorders. *Addiction Science and Clinical Practice.* **4**: 4–25.
15 Kornfield H and Manfredi L (2010) Effectiveness of full agonist opioids in patients stablized on buprenorphine undergoing major surgery: A case series. *American Journal of Therapeutics.* **17**: 523–528.
16 Heit HA and Gourlay DL (2008) Buprenorphine: new tricks with an old molecule for pain management. *Clinical Journal of Pain.* **24**: 93–97.
17 Vickers AP and Jolly A (2006) Naltrexone and problems in pain management. *British Medical Journal.* **332**: 132–133.

19: ANALGESIC DRUGS AND FITNESS TO DRIVE

Several classes of centrally-acting analgesics have the potential to influence driving performance. Doctors have a duty of care to inform patients of this risk and advise them appropriately. As a minimum, patients should be reminded that it is their legal responsibility to ensure that they only drive if they feel 100% safe to do so. However, the impact of ceasing to drive can be considerable and impairment from stable doses of centrally-acting analgesics is not inevitable.

This chapter summarizes the evidence regarding the effect of opioids, anti-epileptics, antidepressants, benzodiazepines and cannabinoids on driving performance and the risk of a motor vehicle accident. Although the evidence is sometimes conflicting, the information provided here will assist health professionals when advising patients. Such advice will need to be tailored to individual circumstances, including the influence of the disease itself (e.g. risk of seizures), frailty, visual disturbances, the presence of pain, and the use of other sedative drugs (e.g. antimuscarinics).

Driving performance and drugs

Evaluating the impact of drugs on driving can be difficult. Driving performance is affected by multiple mechanisms from altered attention and reaction time to impaired judgment and risk taking. Studying actual or simulated driving, or surrogate laboratory markers of such skills, may not capture all influences on driving performance.[1] Although studying analgesic use among people involved in road traffic accidents avoids this problem, confounding factors include multiple drug use and impairment caused by pain and the illness itself.[2] Further, driving performance is impaired in some patients with chronic non-cancer pain not receiving centrally-acting medication.[3] Indeed, cognitive performance may improve with effective long-term opioid analgesia.[4,5] In a comparison of cancer patients (± **morphine** analgesia) with healthy volunteers, cognitive impairment was associated with cancer rather than **morphine**.[6]

Guidance for patients receiving a potentially sedating analgesic

In the UK, no distinction is made between illicit and prescribed drugs in terms of liability to prosecution for attempting to drive while intoxicated.[7]

The evidence, summarized in Table 19.1, suggests that patients should be warned not to drive after starting and when titrating potentially sedating medication, or after taking a dose for breakthrough (episodic) pain. They should be warned that sedation will be increased by the concurrent use of alcohol (even within normal alcohol driving limits) or other sedating medication, whether obtained by prescription, over-the-counter, or for illicit use.

More specifically, patients receiving opioids, anti-epileptics and antidepressants can consider driving once a stable dose is achieved if they are not affected by drowsiness, nor impaired by the disease itself. If possible, use a less sedating drug, e.g. consider the use of an SSRI rather than a TCA when treating depression. For benzodiazepines, particularly if taken in the daytime and/or those with a long halflife, the risk is more persistent, and consideration should be given to using a less sedating alternative, e.g. an SSRI for anxiety, or not driving. The risk with stable doses of prescribed cannabinoids is unclear.

Providing the patient with written information also helps (Box 19.A). Other examples of information leaflets are available at www.palliativedrugs.com; select *Document library* and search under prescribing issues, driving on medication.

Table 19.1 Drugs and driving: a summary of the evidence

Class of drug	*Impact on risk of a motor vehicle accident*	*Comments*
Opioids	No increased risk with chronic stable dose carefully titrated to avoid drowsiness and cognitive impairment[1,2,8–14]	Cognition and driving performance impaired for about 1 week after start of treatment or after dose increment.[15,16] The risk is shared by weak opioids.[17] Additional transient impairment with doses for break-through (episodic) pain
Anti-epileptics	No increased risk with chronic stable dose carefully titrated to avoid drowsiness and cognitive impairment[18]	Cognition impaired by multiple, high-dose anti-epileptics; marginally less with newer drugs (e.g. gabapentin) compared with older drugs (e.g. carbamazepine)[19,20]
Antidepressants	Sedative antidepressants double the risk in the elderly (>65 years) but not other age groups[18,21–24]	Sedative antidepressants impair performance for about 1 week after start of treatment (mianserin ⩾2 weeks). SSRIs appear to cause less impairment[7,25]
Benzodiazepines	60–80% increase in risk[26]	Risk partially decreases with time; related to dose, halflife and concurrent alcohol. Risk from nocturnal use of shorter halflife benzodiazepines is unclear[26,27]
Cannabinoids	Risk likely to be increased initially. Degree of tolerance to chronic stable dose is uncertain	Most studies deal with illicit use, frequently confounded by alcohol consumption and risk-taking behaviours[28,29]

Risk from specific analgesic drug classes

Opioids

Driving performance does not appear to be affected by stable doses of appropriately titrated strong opioids:[1,8–14]

- cognition returns to normal after about 1 week after the start of treatment or after dose increments[16]
- long-term opioid analgesia for cancer pain[14] and non-cancer pain[11,13] has little or no impact on surrogate laboratory measures of driving performance compared with:
  - ▷ healthy volunteers[11]
  - ▷ cancer patients not taking opioids[14]
  - ▷ patients with various causes of cerebral impairment who had passed a standardized fitness-to-drive test[13]
- patients with non-cancer pain taking opioids at stable doses for ⩾1 week do not differ from those not taking opioids or from healthy volunteers in tests of actual driving performance.[15]

The results of epidemiological studies are mixed.[26,31] However, an increased risk of road traffic accidents among drivers using opioid analgesics appears unlikely if confounding variables are taken into account:

- new vs. long-term use
- opioids vs. other psychotropics taken concurrently
- prescription vs. illicit use
- opioids vs. the pain itself.[2]

The optimal interval between dose initiation or increase and returning to driving is unclear and may vary between individuals and formulation used, e.g. steady-state plasma concentrations of TD **fentanyl** are generally achieved after 36–48h but, according to the manufacturers, this is sometimes achieved only after 6–12 days (see p.390).

Box 19.A Example of a patient information leaflet: Strong painkillers and driving[10,30]

The medicines you are taking do not automatically disqualify you from driving in the United Kingdom. However, some painkillers can affect the speed of your reactions or general alertness. Both the label and the Patient Information Leaflet will warn you that drowsiness can occur. If receiving such medication, or other sedative drugs, it is important that you take the following precautions:

Do not drive

- unless you feel 100% safe to do so
- if you feel sleepy
- after taking other sedative drugs, whether or not recommended by your doctor, or after drinking alcohol
- after taking extra 'rescue' doses of a sedative painkiller, e.g. for at least 3 hours after an extra dose of morphine
- after starting or increasing the dose of a sedative painkiller; wait until any sleepiness wears off, generally about 5 days, but sometimes longer.

Restarting driving

You may try driving when you feel 100% safe to do so and you no longer feel sleepy. Begin by making a short trip:

- on roads that are quiet and familiar
- at a quiet time of day when the light is good
- with a companion who may take over driving if required.

If you and your companion are happy with your attentiveness, reactions and general ability, then you may start to drive. Do not exhaust yourself by driving long distances. If you are in any doubt, discuss with your doctor or other health professional.

Who to inform if you are planning to drive

- *your doctor*, who can warn you about medication which might affect the speed of your reactions or general alertness
- *your insurance company*, to be sure that you are covered (note: it may help if you send the company a copy of this leaflet).

Although you do not necessarily need to inform the DVLA that you are taking regular painkillers, in practice insurance companies generally advise this. However, in relation to cancer, the DVLA will need to be informed if you have a brain tumour, a secondary tumour in your brain or if you have had a fit or problems with eyesight. *If in doubt, discuss with your doctor or the DVLA medical advisory helpline* (0870 600 0301; and have your driving licence number ready).

Anti-epileptics

Several studies have examined the cognitive effects of anti-epileptics in patients with epilepsy or healthy volunteers. Marked cognitive impairment is associated with the use of multiple or high-dose anti-epileptics, particularly **phenobarbital**. Newer drugs, e.g. **gabapentin**, may cause marginally less impairment than older drugs, e.g. **carbamazepine**, **valproate**.[19,20] In a case-control study, anti-epileptics did not increase the risk of a motor vehicle accident.[18]

Antidepressants

Using a standard on-the-road test, sedating antidepressants (e.g. **amitriptyline**, **doxepin**, **imipramine**, **mirtazapine**, **mianserin**) were found initially to impair driving performance. Performance returned to baseline within 1 week, except for **mianserin** which still caused impairment when the study ended after 2 weeks.[25] Less sedating drugs, e.g. SSRIs, appear to cause less impairment, but studies of airline pilots suggest that this can still be to a degree which necessitates caution.[7,25]

Even though lower doses of antidepressants are generally used for analgesia, performance in driving tests was impaired in patients with neuropathic pain after the first dose of **amitriptyline** 25mg but had returned to baseline when evaluated 2 weeks later.[3] The possibility of pharmacokinetic interactions and additive sedation with other analgesics should also be remembered.

In three case-control studies across all age groups, antidepressants did not increase the risk of a motor vehicle accident.[18,21,22] However, when older people were considered separately, the risk was doubled.[23,24]

Benzodiazepines

Benzodiazepines increase the risk of motor vehicle accidents by 60–80%. The risk is highest in those taking higher doses, drugs with a longer halflife, or concurrent alcohol.[26] The risk only partially decreases with time.[27]

Simulated driving tests show impaired reaction times, tracking and co-ordination with the acute use of benzodiazepines. In multiple-dose studies the degree of attenuation of impairment over time was variable.[32]

The risk from a bedtime dose of a hypnotic benzodiazepine with a short halflife is unclear; studies of airline pilots suggest that shorter-acting benzodiazepines do not cause a detectable sedating effect the following morning.[7] However, the results of case-control studies examining the risk of motor vehicle accidents are conflicting. **Zopiclone** is *not* a safer alternative.[26]

Cannabinoids

Most studies consider the risk from the illicit use of the whole cannabis plant. Interpretation is hampered by associated alcohol consumption, risk-taking behaviour (potentially a cause and/or effect of cannabis use), and methodological limitations. However, when taken together, these studies suggest that cannabis causes dose-dependent impairment of driving ability.[7,28,29] The risk of motor vehicle accidents is approximately doubled, and is further increased by concurrent alcohol consumption.[28] Some studies suggest a degree of insight into the impairment, and an ability to compensate partially for it (e.g. by driving more cautiously).

These studies are unlikely to reflect the risk associated with stable doses of prescribed cannabinoids (see p.213). Those which controlled for alcohol use or risk-taking behaviour generally found a reduced or even absent risk.[28] Further, stable doses may allow tolerance to impairment to develop, as with many psychotropics. For example, 6 patients with multiple sclerosis and painful spasticity showed no impairment of laboratory markers of driving ability after receiving **nabilone** 2mg/day for 4 weeks.[33] However, caution is necessary, particularly in physically debilitated patients, and they should be advised not to drive during initial dose titration. Once on a stable dose, and having evaluated the degree of psychomotor impairment caused of cannabinoids, restarting driving can be discussed.

1 Fishbain D *et al.* (2003) Are opioid-dependent/tolerant patients impaired in driving-related skills? A structured evidence-based review. *Journal of Pain and Symptom Management.* **25**: 559–577.
2 Fishbain D *et al.* (2002) Can patients taking opioids drive safely? A structured evidence-based review? *Journal of Pain and Palliative Care Pharmacotherapy.* **16 (1)**: 9–28.
3 Veldhuijzen DS *et al.* (2006) Effect of chronic nonmalignant pain on highway driving performance. *Pain.* **122**: 28–35.
4 Tassain V *et al.* (2003) Long term effects of oral sustained release morphine on neuropsychological performance in patients with chronic non-cancer pain. *Pain.* **104**: 389–400.
5 Jamison RN *et al.* (2003) Neuropsychological effects of long-term opioid use in chronic pain patients. *Journal of Pain and Symptom Management.* **26**: 913–921.
6 Clemons M *et al.* (1996) Alertness, cognition and morphine in patients with advanced cancer. *Cancer Treat Reviews.* **22**: 451–468.
7 Carter T (2006) *Fitness to Drive: A Guide for Health Professionals.* Royal Society of Medicine Press, London.
8 Kress HG and Kraft B (2005) Opioid medication and driving ability. *European Journal of Pain.* **9**: 141–144.
9 Brandman JF (2005) Cancer patients, opioids, and driving. *Journal of Supportive Oncology.* **3**: 317–320.
10 Pease N *et al.* (2004) Driving advice for palliative care patients taking strong opioid medication. *Palliative Medicine.* **18**: 663–665.
11 Sabatowski R *et al.* (2003) Driving ability under long-term treatment with transdermal fentanyl. *Journal of Pain and Symptom Management.* **25**: 38–47.
12 Chapman S (2001) The effects of opioids on driving ability in patients with chronic pain. *American Pain Society Bulletin.* **1**: 1.
13 Galski T *et al.* (2000) Effects of opioids on driving ability. *Journal of Pain and Symptom Management.* **19**: 200–208.
14 Vainio A *et al.* (1995) Driving ability in cancer patients receiving longterm morphine analgesia. *Lancet.* **346**: 667–670.
15 Byas-Smith MG *et al.* (2005) The effect of opioids on driving and psychomotor performance in patients with chronic pain. *Clinical Journal of Pain.* **21**: 345–352.
16 Bruera E *et al.* (1989) The cognitive effects of the administration of narcotic analgesics in patients with cancer pain. *Pain.* **39**: 13–16.
17 Bachs LC *et al.* (2009) The risk of motor vehicle accidents involving drivers with prescriptions for codeine or tramadol. *Clinical Pharmacology and Therapeutics.* **85**: 596–599.

18 Neutel I (1998) Benzodiazepine-related traffic accidents in young and elderly drivers. *Human Psychopharmacology.* **13 (suppl)**: s115–s123.
19 Aldenkamp AP *et al.* (2003) Newer antiepileptic drugs and cognitive issues. *Epilepsia.* **44 (suppl 4)**: 21–29.
20 Brunbech L and Sabers A (2002) Effect of antiepileptic drugs on cognitive function in individuals with epilepsy: a comparative review of newer versus older agents. *Drugs.* **62**: 593–604.
21 McGwin G, Jr. *et al.* (2000) Relations among chronic medical conditions, medications, and automobile crashes in the elderly: a population-based case-control study. *American Journal of Epidemiology.* **152**: 424–431.
22 Barbone F *et al.* (1998) Association of road-traffic accidents with benzodiazepine use. *Lancet.* **352**: 1331–1336.
23 Leveille SG *et al.* (1994) Psychoactive medications and injurious motor vehicle collisions involving older drivers. *Epidemiology.* **5**: 591–598.
24 Ray WA *et al.* (1992) Psychoactive drugs and the risk of injurious motor vehicle crashes in elderly drivers. *American Journal of Epidemiology.* **136**: 873–883.
25 Ramaekers JG (2003) Antidepressants and driver impairment: empirical evidence from a standard on-the-road test. *Journal of Clinical Psychiatry.* **64**: 20–29.
26 Dassanayake T *et al.* (2011) Effects of benzodiazepines, antidepressants and opioids on driving: a systematic review and meta-analysis of epidemiological and experimental evidence. *Drug Safety.* **34**: 125–156.
27 Hemmelgarn B *et al.* (1997) Benzodiazepine use and the risk of motor vehicle crash in the elderly. *Journal of the American Medical Association.* **278**: 27–31.
28 Ramaekers JG *et al.* (2004) Dose related risk of motor vehicle crashes after cannabis use. *Drug Alcohol Dependence.* **73**: 109–119.
29 UK Department for Transport (2000) Cannabis and driving: a review of the literature and commentary (No.12). Available from: http://www.dft.gov.uk/pgr/roadsafety/research/rsrr/theme3/cannabisanddrivingareviewoft4764
30 Twycross RG (1997) *Oral Morphine in Advanced Cancer* (3e). Beaconsfield Publishers, Beaconsfield.
31 Orriols L *et al.* (2009) The impact of medicinal drugs on traffic safety: a systematic review of epidemiological studies. *Pharmacoepidemiol Drug Safety.* **18**: 647–658.
32 Rapoport MJ and Banina MC (2007) Impact of psychotropic medications on simulated driving: a critical review. *CNS Drugs.* **21**: 503–519.
33 Kurzthaler I *et al.* (2005) The effect of nabilone on neuropsychological functions related to driving ability: an extended case series. *Human Psychopharmacology.* **20**: 291–293.

20: CONTINUOUS SUBCUTANEOUS INFUSIONS

CSCI in clinical practice

Continuous subcutaneous infusion (CSCI) is used extensively in palliative care in the UK, particularly in patients for whom swallowing medication has become increasingly difficult or impossible.[1,2] For most drugs, this route of administration is off-label (see p.xxiii).[3]

Ambulatory battery-powered infusion devices are commonly used to administer the CSCI.[2] These devices are also used to administer medication by spinal infusion (see p.681).

CSCI is as effective as continuous IV infusion (CIVI),[4] and at least as good as intermittent bolus injections.[5] In settings where it is difficult to be certain that intermittent regular injections will be administered on time, CSCI is likely to provide better round-the-clock comfort (Box 20.A).

Box 20.A Advantages and disadvantages of CSCI

Advantages

Saving of nursing time.
Round-the-clock comfort because plasma drug concentrations are maintained without peaks and troughs.
Less need for repeated injections.
Generally needs to be loaded once daily or less, depending on sterility guidelines.
Control of multiple symptoms with a combination of drugs.
Independence and mobility maintained because the device is lightweight and can be worn in a holster under or over clothes.
Patient preference.

Disadvantages

Initial cost of infusion devices.
Training of staff, together with need to maintain competency.
Lack of flexibility if more than one drug is being administered.
Lack of reliable compatibility data for some mixtures.
Possible inflammation and pain at the infusion site.
Although uncommon, problems with the infusion device can lead to break-through (episodic) pain (or other symptom) if the problem cannot be resolved quickly.

Indications for CSCI

CSCI should not just be thought of as the last resort but as a useful alternative route of administration in certain circumstances.[6] CSCI is *not* 'Step 4' on the analgesic ladder, but merely an alternative route of administration. Indications for using CSCI include:

- persistent nausea and vomiting
- dysphagia
- intestinal obstruction
- coma
- poor absorption of oral drugs (rare)
- patient preference.

Before setting up a CSCI, it is important to explain to the patient and family:

- the reason(s) for using this route
- how the infusion device works
- the advantages and possible disadvantages of CSCI (see Box 20.A).

Although often administered by CSCI, several drugs with a long duration of action, e.g. **dexamethasone**, **levomepromazine** can be given equally well as a bolus SC or IV injection once daily or b.d. (Table 20.1)[1] However, it should be noted that for **promethazine** and **phenobarbital** (see p.272), bolus SC injections should *not* be used because of the risk of severe irritation and tissue necrosis; IM and IV administration is possible as long as SPC guidance, e.g. regarding dilution, is followed.

Table 20.1 Drugs which can be given once daily or b.d. instead of by CSCI

Drug	*Plasma halflife (h)*	*Duration of action (h)*
Clonazepam[a]	20–60	≤12–24
Dexamethasone	3–4.5	36–54
Furosemide	0.5–2	6–8
Granisetron	10–11	≤24
Haloperidol	13–35	≤24
Levomepromazine[b]	15–30	≤24
Methadone[b]	8–75	≤12
Promethazine[c]	12	≥12

a. for SC/IV bolus doses, dilute each 1mg/mL amp with 1mL WFI
b. relatively irritant SC
c. severely irritant SC; give only by deep IM or IV injection.

Drug doses

If symptoms are controlled, start the CSCI 1–2h before the effect of the medication is due to wear off. If symptoms are uncontrolled, set up the CSCI immediately with stat doses of the same drugs.

Drugs are generally *more* bio-available by injection than PO. This means that the dose of a drug given by CSCI will be *less* than the dose previously given PO, generally between 1/3 and 2/3 of the PO dose. The bio-availability data given at the end of the pharmacology section in the individual drug monographs serve as a guide to the appropriate reduction. For example, the dose of a drug with oral bio-availability of 75% should be reduced by a quarter when given SC and, if 50% bio-available, the dose should be halved when given SC, and so on. The SC and IV routes are generally considered equipotent, and the respective doses are thus the same.[4,7]

Rescue medication

Appropriate doses of p.r.n. medication should always be prescribed. These are given via a separate small SC needle/cannula (and the latter flushed with compatible diluent, see p.667). To avoid potential issues with incompatibility and delaying the CSCI, do not give p.r.n. medication via a side-arm or port of a CSCI cannula or extension set.

TD patches

As a general rule, TD **buprenorphine** or **fentanyl** patches should be continued when the need for supplemental opioid via CSCI is short-term, e.g. in the last days of life (see Quick Practice

Guides, p.388 and p.398). It is simpler to supplement the patch with a CSCI of **morphine** or other opioid than to convert completely to a single alternative opioid.

Diluent

If a drug is licensed for CSCI use, the SPC will indicate the diluent to be used. This is unlikely to be the case for drugs *not* licensed for CSCI use. In any case, such information is of limited help when mixing drugs. Nonetheless, generally either WFI or 0.9% saline can be used. They both have advantages and disadvantages (Table 20.2).

In the UK, WFI is widely used as the first-line diluent because there is less chance of incompatibility with **cyclizine *lactate*** (see p.233) or higher concentrations of **haloperidol** (approaching 2mg/mL) or **diamorphine *hydrochloride*** (>40mg/mL), particularly when mixing drugs. There is also a wealth of supporting compatibility data and clinical experience for WFI (see Appendix 3, p.773).

However, in countries where **cyclizine *lactate*** is not available or not used, 0.9% saline is probably equally satisfactory. Indeed, for **granisetron**, **hydromorphone ketamine**, **ketorolac**, **octreotide** and **ondansetron**, there are more compatibility data for combinations diluted in 0.9% saline.

Some centres in the USA use 5% glucose in water as the standard diluent. However, this is acidic and unsuitable for very alkaline drugs, e.g. **dexamethasone**, **furosemide**, **ketorolac** and **phenobarbital**.

To avoid confusion, consistency of practice within individual units is important.[8] *PCF recommends that generally WFI is used as the standard diluent of choice*. However, 0.9% saline should be considered if there is a potential or actual problem with inflammatory reactions at the skin injection site (see p.671).

Table 20.2 Comparison of diluents

Advantages	*Disadvantages*
0.9% saline[9]	
Isotonic Less infusion site pain and skin reaction	*Incompatible* with some drugs, e.g. cyclizine; haloperidol at high concentrations approaching 2mg/mL; diamorphine >40mg/mL Generally less compatibility data available for commonly used drugs
WFI	
Less chance of incompatibility Generally more compatibility data available for commonly used drugs	Large volumes are hypotonic, which may cause infusion site pain and skin reaction (but generally not a problem in practice because infusion rates are so slow).

Volume

Factors influencing the volume of the CSCI include the infusion device being used, the total volume of the drugs, the maximum rate of delivery, the intended infusion time and local guidelines. Greater dilution reduces:
- the risk of incompatibility
- the impact of priming an extension set (less drug in the 'dead space')
- injection site skin reactions from the drug.

One approach, applicable to McKinley T34 syringe pumps, is to dilute the contents to a standard volume, e.g.:
- for total drug volumes <10mL, dilute to 15mL in a 20mL luerlock syringe
- for total drug volumes >10mL dilute to 20mL in a 30mL luerlock syringe.

Additional dilution may be necessary when mixing drugs where compatibility depends on the final drug concentrations, e.g. **cyclizine**, **dexamethasone**, **haloperidol**, **ketorolac** (see p.669, and footnotes of Charts A3.1–A3.7, p.776–789).

The total volume of drugs required may exceed the maximum volume/24h that an infusion device can deliver (e.g. about 34mL in a 50mL syringe for McKinley T34 syringe pump or 18mL in a 30mL syringe for Graseby syringe drivers). This is most likely with combinations which include higher doses of **metoclopramide**, **midazolam**, or **morphine**. This problem can generally be circumvented by:

- prescribing drugs for a shorter infusion time, e.g. 12h
- switching from **morphine** to **diamorphine** or **hydromorphone**
- using a different infusion device.[10]

When a cartridge/cassette/bag infusion system is used, a larger final volume is possible. Even so, some centres standardize to 50mL volume with a maximum rate of 2mL/h.

Drug stability and sterility

In the UK, CSCI syringes are generally timed to empty over 24h. The main reasons for this are:

- extrapolation of sterility guidelines for CIVI
- constraints of older syringe drivers
- stability data available
- standardization of practice (for safety reasons).

Generally, 24h is satisfactory in terms of both stability and sterility.[11,12] However, various factors can affect stability (Box 20.B) and potentially could lead to instances of incompatibility or poor symptom control. Thus, regular checks of the CSCI together with the patient's condition should be undertaken (see p.672).

For certain infusion devices, e.g. CADD pumps, elastomeric devices, stability and compatibility data may exist for a longer duration of infusion, e.g. 48–72h. Generally, these solutions are made up in aseptically controlled environments, e.g. pharmacy aseptic units to ensure sterility.

Box 20.B Factors which may affect drug stability and compatibility[13–15]

Drug concentration
Brand/formulation/strength[a] of the drug, e.g. differing or incompatible excipients
Concentration of drug(s)
Diluent
Duration of infusion
Temperature, ambient or local, e.g. infusion device worn under or over clothes
Exposure to light
Order of mixing, e.g. dexamethasone added first or last
Delivery system material[b,c]

a. compatibility data for oxycodone and cyclizine differs between the oxycodone 50mg/mL and 10mg/mL formulations (see p.790)[16]
b. some drugs adsorb onto the material of the container, e.g. up to 50% of a dose of clonazepam onto PVC tubing (see p.145)[17]
c. cloudiness can be caused by chemicals in the material of the syringe or tubing leaching into the solution.

Mixing drugs

The combination of two or more licensed drugs results in a new unlicensed product being formed. Doctors and other independent prescribers (nurse, pharmacist) can mix, and direct others to mix, drugs for administration to a particular patient. Supplementary prescribers can mix and direct others to mix when part of a Clinical Management Plan.[18] Also see p.xxiv.

Additional guidance on mixing drugs is available from the MHRA and the National Prescribing Centre.[18,19]

In the UK, it is common practice to administer 2–3 different drugs in the same infusion device.[1,2,20] Some centres mix four drugs. This is generally because of a decision to add **dexamethasone** or an antisecretory drug, e.g. **hyoscine *butylbromide***, **hyoscine *hydrobromide*** or **glycopyrronium**.

Drug compatibility

When mixing drugs it is essential to consider drug compatibility (Box 20.C).

Box 20.C Drug compatibility data

Physical compatibility

If mixing two or more drugs does not result in a physical change, e.g. discolouration, clouding or crystallization, they are said to be physically compatible.

Observational data

Data from many palliative care services about the visual appearance of various drug mixtures over the infusion period (generally 24h) have been collated for use in Appendix 3. However, observational data are subjective and imprecise; generally, only major incompatibilities can be identified in this way.

Laboratory data

These are generally derived from microscopic examination of a drug mixture under polarized light at specified concentrations and several time points when kept under controlled conditions. Although more robust, these are not definitive; a solution may remain physically clear even when there is chemical incompatibility.[21]

Chemical compatibility

If mixing two or more drugs does not result in a chemical change leading to loss or degradation of one or more of the drugs, the mixture is said to be chemically compatible. Chemical compatibility data are generally obtained by analyzing the drug mixture by high-performance liquid chromatography (HPLC) at specified concentrations and several time points when kept under controlled conditions.

Occasionally, a drug combination has been shown to be chemically compatible but physically incompatible. Thus, both physical and chemical compatibility should be checked.

Information on CSCI compatibility can be obtained from several sources:

- *for WFI:* charts A3.1–A.3.7 (see Appendix 3, p.773) summarize the compatibility data for the more commonly used 2- and 3-drug combinations. They have been compiled from clinical observations in palliative care services in the UK, New Zealand and Australia, and from published compatibility data
- *for 0.9% saline:* charts summarizing 2- and 3-drug combinations are available on www.palliativedrugs.com
- *Syringe Driver Survey Database* (SDSD) on www.palliativedrugs.com. This is a continually updated resource and contains observational compatibility data on mixing combinations of up to 4 drugs. For this to be of maximum benefit, health professionals are urged to donate information about both *successful* and *unsuccessful* combinations for which there are no previously published data. There is a particular need for information about **alfentanil** and **hydromorphone**.
- *The Syringe Driver: Continuous Subcutaneous Infusions in Palliative Care*[20]
- www.pallcare.info
- *Handbook on Injectable Drugs.*[13]

Many factors affect drug stability and compatibility (Box 20.B). Drug combinations may be compatible only at certain concentrations. Thus the *concentration* of each drug in the solution (the dose of each drug divided by the total final volume) should be compared with compatibility data, *not* the dose. The diluent used and the time period for which the infusion ran should also be checked because different diluents and longer infusion periods may also cause compatibility problems.

Other factors, which may not be specified in the compatibility data, may also affect drug stability and compatibility (Box 20.B), and these may explain conflicting anecdotal and published reports, e.g. **oxycodone** compatibility with **cyclizine** is different for **oxycodone** 50mg/mL and 10mg/mL. This may be due to different ratios of excipients in each formulation.[16] Health professionals should be aware that using a different strength and/or brand of any drug may affect compatibility.

If there is doubt about the relevance of the compatibility data to the situation in which a given drug combination is to be used, advice should be obtained from a clinical pharmacist.

When there is a lack of robust compatibility data for the prescribed drugs, the following general principles should be noted:

- generally, drugs with a similar pH are more likely to be compatible than those with widely differing ones (Table 20.3)
- most drugs are acidic in solution, however, **dexamethasone, diclofenac, furosemide**, **ketorolac** and **phenobarbital** are alkaline in solution and often cause compatibility problems (Table 20.3); **diclofenac**, **furosemide** and **phenobarbital** should not be mixed with other drugs
- the risk of precipitation with **dexamethasone** is reduced if it is added last to an already dilute drug mixture. On the other hand, as already noted, **dexamethasone** has a long duration of action. Thus, except when it is being given to reduce the risk of skin reactions (see p.671), there is no real need to give it by CSCI (Table 20.1)
- checks in use should be undertaken more regularly (see p.672) monitoring both the infusion and expected clinical outcome. Where incompatibilities are found e.g. crystal formation, details should be submitted to the SDSD, to help build a database of evidence for drug combinations.

Table 20.3 Approximate pH values of parenteral drugs[13]

Drug[a]	*pH*	*Drug*[a]	*pH*
Alfentanil	4–6	Hyoscine *hydrobromide*	5–7
Clonazepam	3.6	Ketamine	3.5–5.5
Clonidine	4–4.5	Ketorolac	6.9–7.9
Cyclizine lactate	3.3–3.7	Levomepromazine	4.5
Dexamethasone *sodium phosphate*	7–10.5	Lidocaine	5–7
Diamorphine[b]		Methadone	3–6.5
Diclofenac	7.8–9	Metoclopramide	4.5–6.5
Furosemide	8–9.3	Midazolam	3
Glycopyrronium	2–3	Morphine *sulphate*	2.5–6.5
Granisetron	4.7–7.3	Octreotide	3.9–4.5
Haloperidol	3–3.8	Ondansetron	3.3–4
Hydromorphone	4–5.5	Oxycodone	4.5–5.5
Hyoscine *butylbromide*	3.7–5.5	Phenobarbital	9.2–10.2

a. pH values may vary between each strength and different brands

b. powder for reconstitution; most stable when reconstituted so that the pH is 3.8–4.5.

Siting the CSCI

- avoid areas listed in Box 20.D
- choose a preferred site, commonly; anterior chest wall, anterolateral aspects of upper arms, sometimes; anterior abdominal wall, anterior surface of the thighs
- insert an 18-gauge butterfly needle at an angle of 30–45° into SC tissue
- alternatively, use a plastic cannula (always use in patients with a known metal allergy)
- where possible use fine bore tubing with a small priming volume (preferably less than 0.3mL)
- secure the tubing with a transparent semipermeable adhesive dressing (e.g. Tegaderm®), with a loop to reduce the likelihood of needle displacement.

Box 20.D Skin areas to avoid when siting a CSCI

Oedematous areas	Bony prominences
Skin folds	Near a joint
Breast	Anterior chest wall in cachectic patients
Broken, inflamed or infected skin	Upper arm in bedbound patients who need turning
Recently irradiated skin sites	Scarring
Cutaneous tumour sites	

Infusion site problems

Infusion site problems may be due to various causes (Box 20.E).[20,22,23]

Box 20.E Causes of infusion site problems

Irritant drugs
Tonicity of the solution
pH of the solution
Incompatible drug/diluent mixture
Glass particles from ampoules
Infection
Sterile abscess
Allergy to nickel needle
Infrequent resiting
Anatomical site

With non-irritant drugs an infusion site may be satisfactory for ≥1 week (and occasionally 2–3 weeks).[24] Site reactions can be reduced by:[23]

- use of a less irritant drug, e.g. **haloperidol** instead of **prochlorperazine** (Box 20.F)
- considering the use of 0.9% saline as a diluent, when compatibility data exists (see p.667)
- diluting the solution as much as practical, this may include changing the syringe q12h instead of q24h to permit further dilution
- using a plastic cannula instead of a butterfly needle[25,26] (always use in patients with a known metal allergy)
- changing the site prophylactically every 2–3 days
- applying **hydrocortisone** 1% cream to the skin around the needle entry site, and covering it with an occlusive dressing
- adding **dexamethasone** 1mg to the solution if compatibility data permits.[24]

Although the routine addition of **dexamethasone** has been recommended on the grounds that it extends the life of an infusion site by about 50%, the fact that some sites have lasted 2–3 weeks without **dexamethasone** suggests that routine use cannot be recommended.[24]

Box 20.F Drugs which are irritant SC

Strongly irritant, do *not* give by CSCI
Chlorpromazine
Diazepam
Prochlorperazine (sometimes given by SC bolus)

Relatively irritant by CSCI, precautions may be necessary[a]
Diclofenac
Ketamine
Ketorolac
Levomepromazine
Methadone
Octreotide[b]
Ondansetron
Phenobarbital[c]
Promethazine[c]

a. see text and respective monographs
b. painful if given as SC bolus; this is reduced if warmed to body temperature before injection
c. strongly irritant with risk of tissue necrosis if given by SC bolus injection

Converting from CSCI to PO

Some patients are able to revert from CSCI to PO medication, e.g. those being treated for nausea and vomiting. When this seems possible, convert the drugs sequentially rather than all at once. For example, convert the anti-emetic medication first and, if the nausea and vomiting do not recur, change the other medication 1–2 days later.

Remember: just as drug doses were reduced when starting CSCI, doses will generally need to be increased when reverting to PO. This is particularly the case with strong opioid analgesics, e.g. **morphine** 15mg/24h CSCI will need to be increased to **morphine** 30mg/24h PO (see p.666).

The CSCI is generally discontinued when the first dose of the PO medication is administered. It is important at this time to review p.r.n. medication, and to adjust it appropriately.

Ambulatory infusion devices

For CSCI in the UK, syringe drivers are the most commonly used devices. The use of cartridges/cassettes prepared by a pharmacist adds significantly to the cost.

Until recently in the UK, the Graseby MS16A and MS26 syringe drivers were widely used.[27] However, occasional serious errors occurred because of confusion over the different ways of calculating the rate of drug delivery and insufficient safety features. Consequently, NPSA issued an alert recommending that all ambulatory infusion devices should have the following safety features:

- rate setting in *millilitres* (mL) per hour
- a mechanism to stop the infusion if the syringe is not properly and securely fitted
- an alarm which activates if the syringe is removed before the infusion is stopped
- lock-box cover and/or lock-out controlled by password
- provision of internal log memory to record all infusion device events.[28]

As a result, Graseby syringe drivers are being phased out of use. Many centres have already switched to the McKinley T34 syringe driver, which complies with the required safety features.[29,30]

Setting up the infusion device

Full instructions can be found in the manufacturer's instruction manuals. For Quick Practice Guides on setting up the McKinley T34 and the Graseby MS16A and MS26A drivers, see p.673 and p.676 respectively.

Checks in use

Specific record charts should be used for checking a CSCI; examples are available in the Document Library on www.palliativedrugs.com. Checks should be documented within 1h of setting up the CSCI, and then q4h:

- is the device still working?
- is the correct rate still infusing?
- amount of time and/or solution left, and whether the infusion is running to time (based on the preceding 4h)
- appearance of the solution in the tubing and syringe/cartridge/bag
- condition of the skin site
- battery status.

Do not remove the syringe/cartridge/bag from the infusion device to perform these checks. If checking indicates a problem, action should be taken and then documented, e.g. if the infusion needs to be resited (and hence reprimed), the time, the new site and the new infusion volume/syringe length should be recorded. Other comments might include details of incompatibility and mention of any mishaps, e.g. the delivery device found disconnected.

Quick Practice Guide: Setting up a McKinley T34 syringe pump for CSCI

For full instructions, see the manufacturer's operation manual.

PCF recommends 'Lock on' mode for general use; this automatically provides an infusion duration of 24h.

PCF does *not* recommend the use of the automatic purge. Although designed to reduce the slack in the pump mechanism and achieve the correct flow rate more quickly (about 20min vs. 2h), it is more complex to set up and the clinical relevance of the time difference is unknown. Further, patients should have access to p.r.n. medication for the relief of any symptoms.

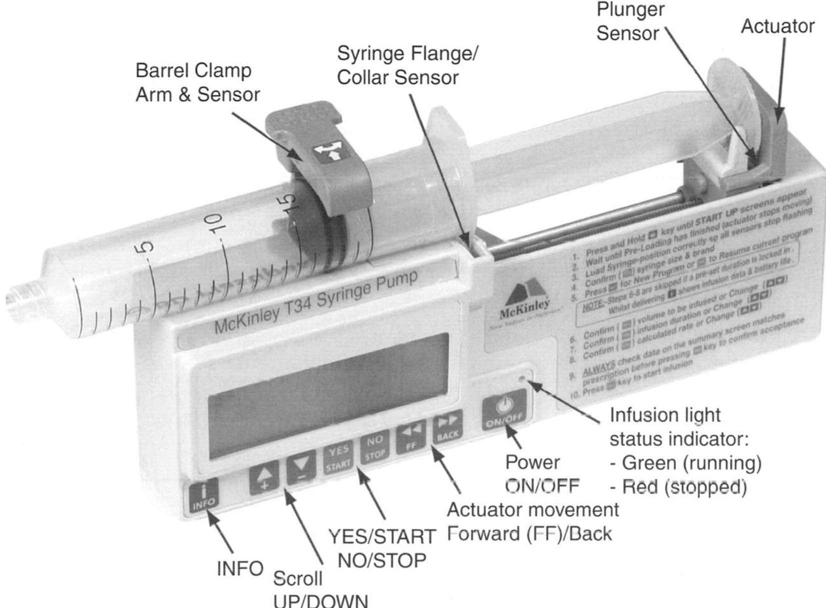

Figure The McKinley T34 syringe pump.

Additional equipment

- battery, PP3: 9V Alkaline/Lithium + spare battery (each lasts about 3–4 days)
- 20mL or 30mL luerlock syringe
- 100cm McKinley SC extension set with integrated anti-free flow and anti-siphon valve (0.3mL priming volume)
- lock-box and key.

1 A CSCI may take 4–6h to provide effective symptom control. SC bolus doses of the appropriate rescue medication should be available to relieve any symptoms.

2 Fill a luerlock syringe with the drugs and dilute the contents to a standard volume, e.g. 15mL in a 20mL syringe with WFI, or when the volume of the undiluted drugs is >10mL, to 20mL in a 30mL syringe. A larger final volume may also be required to ensure compatibility. For maximum fill volumes, see table below.

continued

Syringe size	*Maximum fill volume*
20mL syringe	17mL
30mL syringe	22mL
50mL syringe[a]	34mL

a. the lock-box will not accommodate a 50mL syringe; however, the pump itself is still locked and thus can be used.

Note: dexamethasone should be the last drug added to an already dilute combination of drugs in order to reduce the risk of incompatibility.

3 The syringe should be made up immediately before use, using strict aseptic technique. Ensure adequate mixing has occurred; the solution should be clear and free from crystals or precipitate.

4 Label the syringe, taking care not to completely obscure the solution. The label should be flat and unfolded to avoid obstructing the pump mechanism.

5 Attach the syringe to a McKinley extension set and prime manually (this uses about 0.3mL) and note the remaining volume.

6 Insert the battery into the syringe driver.

7 Ensure the barrel clamp is down and the syringe is *not* connected.

8 Press and hold the **black** ON/OFF key until START UP screens appear.

9 Wait until pre-loading has finished (actuator stops moving).

10 Check the battery capacity by pressing the **blue** INFO key (use +/− keys to scroll to the battery status option) and the **green** YES key to view battery status.

At least 40% battery capacity is required for 24 hours. Change the battery if necessary, e.g. for community use. Switch off by holding down the **black** ON/OFF key until the screen goes blank, discard the battery, insert a new one and repeat steps 7–10.

11 The actuator will move automatically to the size of the last syringe used. If a different size syringe is required, use the FF/BACK keys to move the actuator to the correct position for syringe loading. Once the actuator has stopped moving, lift and rotate the barrel clamp arm, load the syringe (ensuring the plunger and syringe barrel are in the correct slots) and rotate and replace the barrel arm clamp.

12 The display screen will show if any of the 3 positioning points are not aligned correctly. If this is the case, remove the syringe and repeat step 11.

13 Ensure the pump has detected the correct syringe type and size, press the **green** YES key to confirm or use +/− keys to scroll and select the correct option.

14 A new programme *must* be set for each new syringe. If the pump gives the option of resuming a previous programme, it has been set up incorrectly. Do *not* take this option (press **red** NO key). Turn off the pump, remove the syringe and start again.

15 Check the correct infusion volume (as documented after priming) and duration (24 hours) is shown on the display. The rate is automatically calculated, but it is good practice to double check this by dividing the volume by the time. Press the **green** YES key if settings are correct.

16 Insert the cannula subcutaneously in the patient in a suitable position; secure and attach the syringe and extension set to the cannula.

17 Press the **green** YES key to start the infusion.

The screen will continually show the time remaining for the infusion, the rate (mL/h) and the syringe selected.

continued

18 Lock the keypad by pressing and holding the **blue** INFO key until the display shows Keypad LOCK ON.

19 Secure the pump in the lockbox provided. This can not accommodate a 50mL syringe, but the pump itself can still be locked.

20 Protect the syringe from excessive sunlight and heat, e.g. electric blankets.

21 Regular checks on the progress, the visual appearance of the infusion and administration site should be performed and documented during the infusion. Do not remove the syringe from the pump to perform these checks. If checking indicates a problem, action should be taken and then documented. An infusion progress summary can be obtained whilst infusing by pressing the **blue** INFO key.

22 If there is a problem, an alert (short audible alarm and a screen message, infusion continues) or an alarm (continuous alarm, infusion stops and a red light appears above the **black** ON/OFF key) will activate. Refer to the trouble-shooting guide and manufacturer's operation manual for implications and actions.

23 Do not add drugs to a syringe or extension set once the infusion has been commenced. Additional bolus drugs needed should be administered by a separate cannula.

Temporarily stopping and disconnecting the infusion

The infusion may sometimes need to be temporarily stopped (e.g. to change the battery) or disconnected (e.g. when the patient bathes/showers):
- unlock the keypad by pressing and holding the **blue** INFO key until the display shows LOCK OFF
- press the **red** STOP key to stop the infusion
- press and hold the **black** ON/OFF key to switch the pump off; leave the syringe attached to the pump
- *when temporarily disconnecting the infusion*: disconnect the extension set at the cannula end; cap off both the extension set and the cannula
- store syringe and extension set safely; lock in a CD cupboard if it contains a CD.

After interruption:
- reconnect the extension set to the cannula
- turn on the pump by pressing and holding the **black** ON/OFF key
- confirm the syringe size and brand
- press the **green** YES key to resume the infusion
- check and confirm the volume, duration and rate
- press the **green** YES key to start the infusion.

24 When the infusion is completed an alarm will sound and the infusion will stop. Unlock the keypad by pressing and holding the **blue** INFO key until the display shows keypad LOCK OFF. Press the **red** STOP key. Press and hold the **black** ON/OFF key to switch the pump off.

25 *If the next prescription is to be repeated exactly*, the same extension set may be re-used as per local policy. Follow the guidance from step 1; at step 5 priming is not needed, remove the completed syringe from the pump, but leave it connected to the patient; at step 16, remove the old syringe from the extension set and reconnect the extension set to the new syringe; complete the remaining steps in the set up as before.

26 *If the next prescription is different (or changed mid-infusion)*, stop the infusion as in step 24, disconnect the extension set from the patient *before* removing the syringe from the pump. Set up the next prescription from step 1 of the guidelines, using a new syringe and new extension set.

Quick Practice Guide: Setting up a Graseby MS16A or MS26 syringe driver for CSCI

For full instructions, see the manufacturer's operation manual.

PCF does *not* recommend Graseby MS16A and MS26 syringe drivers because they do not have all of the safety features recommended by the UK NPSA.
PCF does *not* recommend the use of the MS26 boost facility because
- a single boost does not deliver an effective analgesic dose
- there is no lock-out period
- when multiple drugs are being infused, boosting is non-specific
- the infusion will run out before the scheduled changeover time.

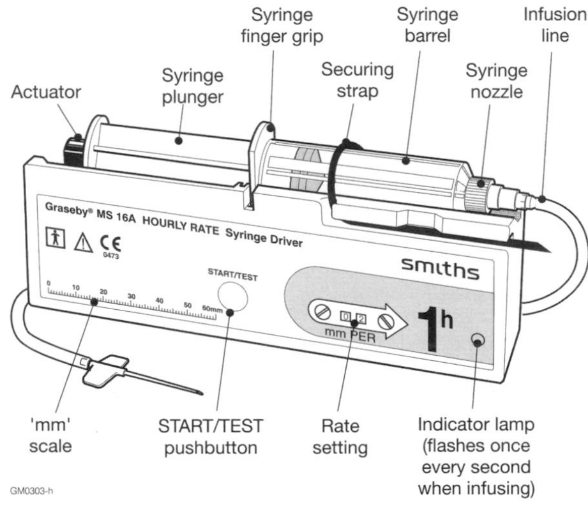

Figure The Graseby MS16A *hourly* rate syringe driver.

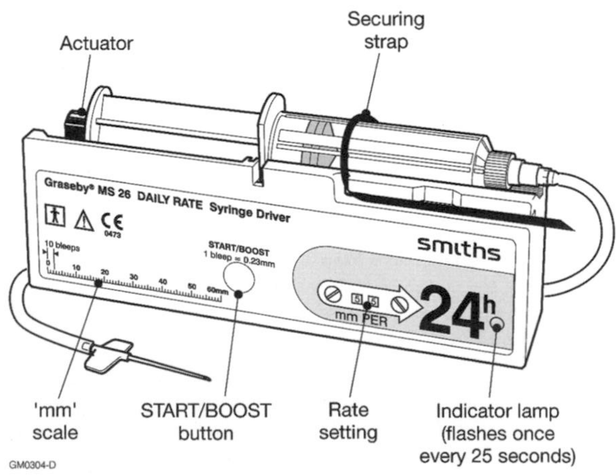

Figure The Graseby MS26 *daily* rate syringe driver.

Additional equipment

- battery: 9V Alkaline + spare battery
- 20mL luerlock syringe
- SC extension set with integrated anti-free flow and anti-siphon valve
- lock-box.

1 A CSCI may take 4–6h to provide effective symptom relief. SC bolus doses of the appropriate rescue medication should be available to relieve any symptoms.

2 Insert the battery and perform initial safety checks to ensure the correct syringe driver has been selected and is working correctly. Remove the battery until ready to commence the infusion.

3 Fill a luerlock syringe with the drugs and dilute the contents to the required volume using the millimetre length scale on the driver or ruler for reference. The MS16A and MS26 can deliver a maximum length of 60mm. However, many palliative care services standardize the length used at 48mm.

The rate of delivery is based upon *a length of fluid in millimetres per unit time*; this allows any brand of syringe to be used. The rate is calculated differently between the MS16A (an *hourly* rate driver, i.e. delivers in **millimetres per hour**) and the MS26 (a *daily* rate driver, i.e. delivers in **millimetres per 24h**). Great care must be taken to ensure the rate of delivery is calculated accurately.

Note: dexamethasone should be the last drug added to an already dilute combination of drugs in order to reduce the risk of incompatibility.

4 The syringe should be made up immediately before use, using strict aseptic technique. Ensure adequate mixing has occurred; the solution should be clear and free from crystals or precipitate.

5 Label the syringe, taking care not to completely obscure the solution. The label should be flat and unfolded to avoid obstructing the mechanism.

6 Calculate the delivery rate (see Box) and have it independently verified. Set the rate by adjusting the screws on the front of the driver using the tool provided. If using a standard delivery length of 48mm:

Graseby **MS16A** *hourly* rate driver delivers in **millimetres per hour**.
Set at **02** to run at 2mm/h over **24** hours.
Set at **04** to run at 4mm/h over **12** hours.

Graseby **MS26** *daily* rate driver delivers in **millimetres per 24 hours**.
Set at **48** to run at 2mm/h over **24** hours.
Set at **96** to run at 4mm/h over **12** hours.

7 Connect the syringe to the extension set and manually prime. Priming uses about 0.5mL and the contents of the delivery device will thus be delivered in less than the planned time, generally 24h. Re-measure and document this new length but do not adjust the set rate. Subsequent infusions which do not involve priming will last a full 24h.

8 Fit the flange of the syringe into the slot on the syringe driver and slide the end plate up to the plunger. Secure the syringe with the rubber strap.

9 Connect the syringe, primed extension set and butterfly cannula.

Box Setting the rate of a Graseby syringe driver

MS16A hourly rate driver

$$\text{Rate} = \frac{\text{measured 'length of volume' in mm}}{\text{delivery time in hours}}$$

e.g. $\frac{48\text{mm}}{24\text{h}}$ = 2mm/h (48mm is about 8mL in a 10mL BD plastikpak syringe)

MS26 daily rate driver

$$\text{Rate} = \frac{\text{measured 'length of volume' in mm}}{\text{delivery time in days}}$$

e.g. $\frac{48\text{mm}}{1\text{ day}}$ = 48mm/day

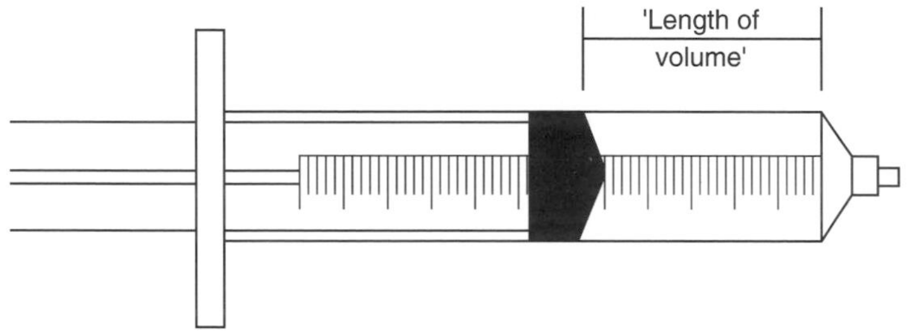

10 Re-insert the battery and an audible alarm sounds. Press and release start button to silence the alarm and to activate the driver. The syringe driver also makes this noise when:
- the syringe is empty
- the extension set is blocked
- the start/test button is held for 5sec (MS16A)
- the start/boost button is held for 10sec (MS26).

11 The light on the driver should start flashing (every second for MS16A, every 25sec for MS26). If it does not flash, consult manufacturer's guidelines regarding battery replacement.

12 The clear plastic cover or lock-box should be carefully placed over the syringe driver. Ensure it is placed the correct way round to prevent accidental pressing of the start/boost button.

13 Protect the syringe from excessive sunlight and heat, e.g. electric blankets.

14 Regular checks on the progress, the visual appearance of the infusion and administration site should be performed and documented during the infusion. Do not remove the syringe from the driver to perform these checks. If checking indicates a problem, action should be taken and then documented.

15 Do not add drugs to a syringe or extension set or increase the rate once the infusion has commenced. Additional bolus drugs needed should be administered by a separate cannula.

16 If the drug prescription is changed, discard the syringe in place and make up a new syringe. Use a new extension set and consider giving stat doses of appropriate medication if an immediate effect is needed by a separate cannula.

17 To stop a syringe driver, remove the battery. Always disconnect the extension set from the patient before removing the syringe from the driver.

1 Wilcock A *et al.* (2006) Drugs given by a syringe driver: a prospective multicentre survey of palliative care services in the UK. *Palliative Medicine*. **20**: 661–664.
2 O'Doherty CA *et al.* (2001) Drugs and syringe drivers: a survey of adult specialist palliative care practice in the United Kingdom and Eire. *Palliative Medicine*. **15**: 149–154.
3 Fonzo-Christe C *et al.* (2005) Subcutaneous administration of drugs in the elderly: survey of practice and systematic literature review. *Palliative Medicine*. **19**: 208–219.
4 Nelson KA *et al.* (1997) A prospective within-patient crossover study of continuous intravenous and subcutaneous morphine for chronic cancer pain. *Journal of Pain and Symptom Management*. **13**: 262–267.
5 Watanabe S *et al.* (2008) A randomized double-blind crossover comparison of continuous and intermittent subcutaneous administration of opioid for cancer pain. *Journal of Palliative Medicine*. **11**: 570–574.
6 Anderson SL and Shreve ST (2004) Continuous subcutaneous infusion of opiates at end-of-life. *Annals of Pharmacotherapy*. **38**: 1015–1023.
7 Moulin D *et al.* (1991) Comparisons of continuous subcutaneous and intravenous hydromorphone infusion for management of cancer pain. *Lancet*. **337**: 465–468.
8 Flowers C and McLeod F (2005) Diluent choice for subcutaneous infusion: a survey of the literature and Australian practice. *International Journal of Palliative Nursing*. **11**: 54–60.
9 Schneider J *et al.* (1997) A study of the osmolality and pH of subcutaneous drug infusion solutions. *Australian Journal of Hospital Pharmacy*. **27**: 29–31.
10 Fudin J *et al.* (2000) Use of continuous ambulatory infusions of concentrated subcutaneous (s.q.) hydromorphone versus intravenous (i.v.) morphine: cost implications for palliative care. *American Journal of Hospice and Palliative Care*. **17**: 347–353.
11 BNF (2011) Prescribing in palliative care and Appendix 6: Intravenous additives. In: *British National Formulary* (No. 61). British Medical Association and Royal Pharmaceutical society of Great Britain, London. Available from: www.bnf.org.
12 NPSA (National Patient Safety Agency) (2007) Patient safety alert 20: Promoting safer use of injectable medicines. Available from: www.npsa.nhs.uk/nrls/alerts-and-directives/alerts/injectable-medicines/
13 Trissel LA (2010) *Handbook on Injectable Drugs* (16e). American Society of Health System Pharmacists, Maryland, USA.
14 Kohut J, 3rd *et al.* (1996) Don't ignore details of drug-compatibility reports. *American Journal of Health System Pharmacy*. **53**: 2339.
15 Vermeire A and Remon JP (1999) Stability and compatibility of morphine. *International Journal of Pharmaceutics*. **187**: 17–51.
16 Napp (2010) *Personal communication*.
17 Schneider JJ *et al.* (2006) Effect of tubing on loss of clonazepam administered by continuous subcutaneous infusion. *Journal of Pain and Symptom Management*. **31**: 563–567.
18 Department of Health (2010) Mixing of medicines prior to administration in clinical practice: medical and non-medical prescribing. HMSO, London. Available from: www.dh.gov.uk/prod_consum_dh/groups/dh_digitalassets/@dh/@en/@ps/documents/digitalasset/dh_116360.pdf
19 National Prescribing Centre (2010) Mixing of medicines prior to administration in clinical practice – responding to legislative changes. Liverpool. Available from: www.npc.nhs.uk/improving_safety/mixing_meds/resources/mixing_of_medicines.pdf
20 Dickman A *et al.* (2005) *The Syringe Driver: Continuous Subcutaneous Infusions in Palliative Care* (2e). Oxford University Press, Oxford.
21 Good PD *et al.* (2004) The compatibility and stability of midazolam and dexamethasone in infusion solutions. *Journal of Pain and Symptom Management*. **27**: 471–475.
22 Oliver D (1991) The tonicity of solutions used in continuous subcutaneous infusions. The cause of skin reactions? *Hospital Pharmacy Practice*. **Sept**: 158–164.
23 Graham F (2006) Syringe drivers and subcutaneous sites: a review. *European Journal of Palliative Care*. **13**: 138–141.
24 Reymond L *et al.* (2003) The effect of dexamethasone on the longevity of syringe driver subcutaneous sites in palliative care patients. *Medical Journal of Australia*. **178**: 486–489.
25 Dawkins L *et al.* (2000) A randomized trial of winged Vialon cannulae and metal butterfly needles. *International Journal of Palliative Nursing*. **6**: 110–116.
26 Ross JR *et al.* (2002) A prospective, within-patient comparison between metal butterfly needles and Teflon cannulae in subcutaneous infusion of drugs to terminally ill hospice patients. *Palliative Medicine*. **16**: 13–16.
27 Palliativedrugs.com (2006) Syringe Driver Survey Results. In: *June/July 2006 newsletter*. Palliativedrugs.com Ltd. Available from: www.palliativedrugs.com
28 NPSA (National Patient Safety Agency) (2010) Safer ambulatory syringe drivers. In: Rapid Reponse Report RRR019. Available from: www.npsa.uk
29 Palliativedrugs.com (2011) Which syringe driver do you use? Available from: www.palliativedrugs.com
30 Freemantle A *et al.* (2011) Safer ambulatory syringe drivers: experiences of one acute hospital trust. *International Journal of Palliative Nursing*. **17**: 86–91.

21: SPINAL ANALGESIA

Indications

Spinal analgesia is commonly used for obstetric or peri-operative pain relief. In the case of cancer patients receiving specialist palliative care, about 2–4% proceed to spinal analgesia because of unsatisfactory pain relief with more standard systemic analgesia.[1–7] However, it is anecdotally reported that a progressive increase in the use of **ketamine** (see p.593) in palliative care has been associated with a decrease in the use of spinal analgesia.

Typical indications for spinal analgesia include:

- systemic opioid intolerance (i.e. an unacceptable balance between efficacy and toxicity)
- refractory neuropathic pain (e.g. visceral neuropathic pain, lumbosacral plexopathy)
- pathological fracture in a patient close to death.

Spinal analgesia is effective in ⩾50% of patients.[3,8–13] Good communication between palliative, pain and primary care teams is essential.

Contra-indications: Uncorrected coagulopathy, systemic or local infection, raised intracranial pressure.

Circumstances in which extra caution should be used include:

- spinal deformity
- incipient spinal cord compression
- myelosuppressive chemotherapy.

Route, placement and delivery device considerations

Analgesics are delivered to the intrathecal (IT) or epidural (ED) space via an indwelling catheter placed by an anaesthetist. Commonly, the tube is tunnelled subcutaneously to emerge at a distant site, e.g. the supraclavicular fossa or flank, on the basis that this will reduce the risk of displacement and infection. This can be done using local anaesthesia ± sedation, but general anaesthesia is more comfortable for the patient.[7] However, simple placement without tunnelling (and without general anaesthesia) appears to be equally satisfactory.[14]

The preferred route and delivery device are influenced by local custom and the likely duration of use (Table 21.1). Although ED catheters are sometimes left in place for several months,[15] IT is the preferred route for long-term spinal analgesia expected to be necessary for more than a few weeks.[3] Devices vary in relation to fixed vs. variable delivery rates, patient-controlled boluses, and cost.

Drugs delivered to the ED space diffuse through the meninges to reach the spinal cord and adjacent nerve roots. The level of the spinal cord at which the catheter is sited influences the area over which maximal analgesia is obtained. Migration or misplacement of ED catheters into the IT space (a rare event) will deliver an excessive dose resulting in significant toxicity, and may cause death secondary to respiratory arrest, unless recognized and treated urgently.

The IT route delivers drugs directly to the cerebrospinal fluid (CSF). Compared with the ED route, lower doses are required, thereby permitting the use of smaller devices and/or reducing the frequency of refilling (see below).[15] IT administration generally provides better pain relief than the ED route.[3,16,18,19] The area of analgesia is less dependent on the site of the catheter because drugs in the CSF automatically diffuse rostrally.

Table 21.1 Suggested route and delivery device

Likely duration of use	*Route and device*	*Comments*
≤3 weeks	External ED device (re-usable)	Fewer initial complications than IT (8% vs. 25%); less headache from CSF leakage[16]
3 weeks–3 months	External IT device (re-usable)	Fewer later complications than ED (5% vs. 55%); less catheter occlusion or migration[16]
≥ 3 months	Implantable IT device	More expensive initially, lower running costs; more cost-effective long-term[17]

Although the same delivery devices can theoretically be used for SC, IV and spinal infusion, for maximum safety it is best to use a device specifically designed for spinal delivery.[4] Distinct pumps and connectors will reduce the potential for confusion in a patient receiving concurrent spinal and SC/IV infusions.[3,20] However, such recommendations must be weighed against the considerable advantage of staff using a delivery device with which they are familiar from frequent SC/IV use.

Clinical services caring for patients receiving spinal analgesia require clear procedures to be in place to minimize risk at all stages of treatment. An added problem is maintaining staff competence where such approaches are required infrequently: clear clinical guidelines and 'refresher' training can be helpful.

Bolus vs. continuous infusion

Some centres give an initial bolus dose at the time of catheter placement before starting the infusion. This may lead to a transitory period of anaesthesia which the patient may find unpleasant. Others just insert the catheter and start the continuous infusion. There is no evidence to suggest any major benefit from an initial bolus dose.[21]

Choice of drugs

Diamorphine/morphine, **bupivacaine** and **clonidine** are the most commonly used (see below). In cancer pain, particularly neuropathic pain, opioids are generally combined from the outset with **bupivacaine** (or alternative local anaesthetic), and **clonidine** added subsequently if necessary. However, some units use **clonidine** from the outset.[22,23]

Health professionals should familiarize themselves with the guidance and supporting material relating to the legal implication of mixing medicines before administration[24,25] together with any local policy and practice.

Opioids

In the UK, **morphine** and **diamorphine** are widely used; the latter because of its solubility and lack of preservatives.[3,4,22,26–28] Because of concerns about precipitation with **diamorphine**, it has been recommended that **morphine** should always be used in Medtronic SynchroMed® pumps.[4] However, there has been no formal comment about the simpler implanted Isomed pump or the Codman Archimedes®. **Hydromorphone** is an alternative where **morphine** is poorly tolerated.[3–5,29,30]

Spinally administered opioids act locally and/or in the brain stem. The latter occurs through CSF diffusion and/or systemic redistribution. The advantages of spinal administration are greatest with hydrophilic opioids, e.g. **diamorphine**, **morphine** and **hydromorphone**. These are relatively slowly redistributed, i.e. will remain within the CSF for longer. However, respiratory depression secondary to rostral spread within the CSF can be a late onset feature.

In contrast, the fentanils are highly lipid-soluble, and are rapidly redistributed systemically. Thus, spinal administration has fewer advantages over systemic use.[31] However, the lower risk of catheter tip granuloma may benefit some patients (see p.689).

There is considerable uncertainty about dose equivalents between routes.[3,21,32] Although there is a wide variation in response[33] the conversion factors for **diamorphine** and **morphine** in Table 21.2 will generally provide a safe initial spinal dose. In the example in Table 21.2, the appropriate p.r.n. dose of SC **morphine** will be (as usual) 1/10–1/6 of the SC equivalent of the IT dose, i.e. 30–50mg SC.[3,21,30]

Table 21.2 Suggested starting doses for spinal diamorphine and morphine

Total 24h SC opioid	*Total 24h ED opioid dose*	*Total 24h IT opioid dose*
Diamorphine x mg	x divided by 10	x divided by 100
Morphine y mg	y divided by 10	y divided by 100
Example:		
morphine 300mg	morphine 30mg	morphine 3mg

For patients who have not been on an established systemic opioid regimen, recommendations for an appropriate starting IT dose are shown in (Table 21.3).

Table 21.3 Suggested IT total daily drug doses (when not converting from an established systemic opioid regimen)

Drug	*Starting doses*	*Typical range of final doses*
Diamorphine	1–2mg	1–30mg
Morphine	1–2mg	1–30mg
Bupivacaine	5–12mg	5–30mg
Clonidine	5–15microgram	15–30microgram

Maximum opioid concentrations and daily doses have been proposed to minimize the risk of catheter tip granuloma formation (Table 21.4). These are less applicable if short-term use is anticipated, although granulomas have been reported after just 27 days.[34]

Table 21.4 Recommended maximum long-term IT drug concentrations and doses

Drug	*Maximum concentration (mg/mL)*	*Maximum daily dose (mg)*
Morphine	20	15
Hydromorphone	10	4
Bupivacaine	40	30
Clonidine	2	1

Local anaesthetic

Bupivacaine is the most widely used local anaesthetic for spinal analgesia.[3–5,30] It has inherent bactericidal properties which theoretically reduces the probability of infection.[30] Undesirable effects include dose-dependent motor and sensory impairment, affecting 4–13% and ≤7% of patients respectively, generally at doses >15mg/day.[3,4,8–10,12]

Alternatives include **levobupivacaine** and **ropivacaine**. Both have similar efficacy and general tolerability to **bupivacaine**, and are less cardiotoxic.[35–38] On the other hand, they are not bactericidal; although, in practice, this appears not to result in more infections.

α-Adrenergic receptor agonist

Clonidine 15–30microgram/24h (IT) or 150–300microgram/24h (ED) is generally given with an opioid and a local anaesthetic. Benefit is seen particularly in neuropathic pain. Undesirable effects include dose-dependent hypotension and bradycardia (see p.67).[3,4,30] Abrupt cessation (e.g. because of pump failure) may cause severe rebound hypertension. Administer oral **clonidine** while seeking specialist advice.[5]

Other drugs
Baclofen is used for pain related to spasticity. An overdose can cause rostral progression of hypotonia, respiratory depression, coma and occasionally seizures.[39] Symptoms of underdosing are generally limited to a return of the patient's baseline spasticiy and rigidity. However, a life-threatening withdrawal syndrome can occur if IT **baclofen** is abruptly discontinued (Box 21.A).

Box 21.A IT baclofen withdrawal syndrome[39,40]

Cause
Sudden cessation of IT baclofen (e.g. delivery device failure; also see p.563).
Reported with a wide range of doses (50–1,500microgram/24h).

Clinical features
Symptoms evolve over 1–3 days:
- prodromal pruritus or paraesthesia; ± priapism
- seizures (early and/or late onset)
- tachycardia, hypotension or labile blood pressure
- fever (→ hyperthermia)
- dysphoria and malaise → decreased level of consciousness
- spasticity and rigidity greater than patient's baseline
- rhabdomyolysis → hepatic and renal failure, DIC
- coma (→ death).

Management
Restart the IT baclofen infusion as soon as possible.
Cardiopulmonary support as indicated.
High-dose baclofen PO or by enteral feeding tube (up to 120mg/24h).
If necessary, give a benzodiazepine by CSCI/CIVI (e.g. midazolam) titrated to achieve muscle relaxation, normothermia, stabilization of blood pressure and cessation of seizures.[a]

a. dantrolene is reported to improve spasticity but not other symptoms. Its use in this setting has been superseded by the benzodiazepines.

The use of spinal **ketamine** is associated with histological changes of uncertain significance within the cord.[5,41–44]

The spinal use of various other drugs is described or under investigation, including **adenosine**, **gabapentin**, **midazolam**, **ketorolac**, **ziconotide** and **octreotide**.[5,45]

Drug compatibility
Unlike acute pain, with chronic intractable pain, single drug spinal analgesia is often inadequate. Combinations of **morphine** or **diamorphine** with **bupivacaine** ± **clonidine** are widely used, particularly with external devices.[8–10,18] Long-term compatibility data for drug combinations in both external devices (at room temperature) and implanted pump reservoirs (at body temperature) are limited.[4] Several factors can affect drug stability and compatibility (see Box 20.B, p.668). It is important to ascertain if the compatibility data are relevant to the situation of intended use, and confirm what is the appropriate diluent, i.e. discuss with a pharmacist.

When mixing drugs for long periods it is important to consider the type of material the delivery device is made of because this can affect drug stability, e.g. **diamorphine** should not be used in SynchroMed® pumps because of reports of precipitation.

Compatibility data at room temperature
There are compatibility data on the following combinations at room temperature:
- **diamorphine** with **bupivacaine** 4 weeks[46]
- **morphine sulphate** with **bupivacaine** or **clonidine** 2 months[47,48]
- **morphine sulphate** with **ropivacaine** 1 month[37]
- **hydromorphone** with **bupivacaine** 3 days[49]
- **fentanyl** with **ropivacaine**[37]

- **sufentanil** with **ropivacaine**[37]
- **clonidine** with **bupivacaine** 2 weeks[50]
- **clonidine** with **ropivacaine** 1 month.[37]

Compatibility data at body temperature

There are compatibility data on the following combinations at body temperature:

- **morphine sulphate** with **clonidine** ± **bupivacaine** ≤3 months in a SynchroMed® pump[51,52]
- **hydromorphone** 4 months in a SynchroMed® pump[53]
- **clonidine** with **hydromorphone** 1.5 months (only stability of **clonidine** evaluated).[54]

Ideally, delivery devices with mixtures to be administered over >24h should be prepared in a sterile environment, e.g. a licensed pharmacy unit, and not on the ward/by the bedside. Drugs should be preservative-free.[4]

Undesirable effects and complications of spinal analgesia

MRI can cause some types of implantable pumps to malfunction, e.g. Medtronic SynchroMed®. This is related to the magnetic field strength of the scanner. Acccording to Medtronic Technical Services department, no problems have been seen with Isomed® implanted pumps subjected to MR field strengths of up to 1.5 tesla.

Although the Medtronic SynchroMed® implantable pump may stop during an MRI scan, it generally restarts spontaneously afterwards. However, delays in restarting or alterations in pump programming have occurred. The MHRA has issued guidelines for dealing with this, and advises that when consultation with staff responsible for managing the pump has not been possible:

- an alternative imaging technique should be considered *or*
- the patient should be observed closely until it has been confirmed that the pump has restarted.[55,56]

Generally, undesirable effects and complications relate to:[57]

- the drug(s) (Table 21.5)
- medical complications, e.g. bleeding, infection (Table 21.6)
- the delivery system (Table 21.6).

All health professionals caring for patients with spinal analgesia should at least be aware of the most serious undesirable effects and complications, and their management (Box 21.B). Respiratory failure can result from central depression of respiratory drive (opioids) or impaired motor output to the respiratory muscles at the spinal level (**bupivacaine**). Rate of onset varies: systemic redistribution of the spinally administered opioid causes respiratory depression within minutes or hours, whereas diffusion through the CSF causes a delayed onset, occurring after 6–48h. Both **bupivacaine** and **clonidine** cause hypotension, the latter also causing bradycardia.

The transient undesirable effects seen when commencing systemic opioids are also seen with spinal opioids (Box 21.C).[30,57] Clinical areas should have access to resuscitation equipment including IV fluids, **naloxone** and **ephedrine**. Before insertion of a spinal catheter, baseline blood tests will help to evaluate fitness and exclude, for example, a coagulopathy. A neurological and cardiopulmonary examination provides an essential baseline for future reference if a problem arises.

Suspected infection

Catheter-related infections can occur, often with coagulase + or −*Staphylococci*.

Exit site infection: transparent dressings allow the early identification of exit site erythema. Systemic and topical antibacterials should be started promptly; this reduces the incidence of deeper infection/meningitis.[3] However, prophylactic antibacterials should not be routinely used.

ED abscesses: present with fever, escalating pain (this is invariable; either the original pain and/or back pain at the ED site), and new neurological impairment (80%).[12] Evaluation includes blood cultures, aspiration of fluid from the spinal catheter for microscopy and culture, neurological examination, identification of other potential sources of fever and MRI (see warning about MRI above). Seek early advice from a microbiologist and spinal or neurosurgeon. The risk increases with time. Distant non-healing wounds may be a risk factor.[7]

Meningitis: presents with fever and/or meningeal irritation (neck stiffness, stretch signs). Evaluation includes blood and line microscopy and cultures, white cell count, neurological examination, and identification of other potential sources of fever. Consider also MRI, particularly if

Table 21.5 Drug-related undesirable effects

Drug	*Undesirable effect*	*Frequency (%)*	*Comment*
Early onset and/or after titration			
Withdrawal of systemic opioids	Diarrhoea and intestinal colic		Partly avoidable if laxatives stopped and then re-titrated after change to spinal route
Opioids	Nausea and vomiting	33%[3,12,58,59]	
Opioids	Pruritus	15%	*Rare* except in opioid-naïve patients[13,58,59]
Bupivacaine	Motor or sensory disturbance; dose-dependent	4–13%	Persistent motor impairment, overall frequency in palliative care series[3,9,12]
Opioids, bupivacaine	Urinary retention	8–43%[3,8,59]	
Opioids, bupivacaine	Respiratory depression	0.1–2%[3,60]	
Bupivacaine, clonidine	Cardiovascular compromise	5–20%	Symptomatic hypotension; clonidine also causes bradycardia[3]
Late onset (also see p.345)			
Opioids[a]	Catheter tip granulomas	0.1%[34]	MRI screening revealed granulomas in 3% of patients with long-term IT infusions; of these, >80% were asymptomatic (also see p.689);[61] more common with ED infusions
Opioids	Decreased libido, ± disturbed menstruation	70–95%[62]	Endocrine effect seen with IT opioids if given >1 year but may occur sooner. In patients with a long prognosis, measure testosterone and LH at baseline and annually in men, and estradiol, progesterone, LH and FSH in women[4]
Opioids	Hypocorticalism or growth hormone deficiency	15%[62]	
Opioids	Oedema	6–18%[4,11,63]	
Opioids	Immuno-modulation	Frequency uncertain[64]	Significance uncertain. May be more pronounced with systemic opioids

a. less commonly described with non-opioids.

Table 21.6 Non-drug complications of spinal analgesia

Undesirable effect	*Frequency (%)*	*Comment*
Traumatic catheter placement		
CSF leakage headache	25% of IT[19]	Less common in recent palliative series (0–7%), perhaps because of concurrent systemic analgesia[3,65] or more modern spinal needles[66]
ED haematoma	Rare	
Neurological tissue damage	≤0.004%[67,68]	
Infection		
Exit site infection	≤6%	In palliative care patients cared for at home or in palliative care units[3,9,65,69]
ED abscess	≤8%[3,7,12,69]	
Meningitis	≤3% [3,7,9,12]	
Delivery system		
Device-related complications	8–27%	E.g. catheter-related (fracture, kinking, displacement or withdrawal); pump failure (battery failure, mechanical failure, programming or refilling error). Rates, and propensity to human error, vary between pumps[3,57,58,63,70]

Box 21.B Emergency management of life-threatening complications

Stop spinal infusion.
Administer oxygen
Obtain IV access.
If patient arrests, follow local resuscitation procedures.

Respiratory depression (sedation often precedes bradypnoea)
Sit the patient up.
If respiratory rate ≤8 breaths/min, the patient is barely rousable, and/or cyanosed, administer 20microgram boluses of naloxone every 2min until respiratory status is satisfactory (see p.435).
Further boluses may be necessary because naloxone is shorter acting than morphine and other spinal opioids.

Hypotension[a] (systolic <80mmHg)
Lay patient flat (not head down).
Check heart rate: if <40 beats/min, treat bradycardia (below) *or*
If no evidence of fluid overload, give an IV fluid challenge, e.g. 500mL of a colloidal plasma expander over 30min.
Examine for alternative causes such as bleeding.
If no response to fluids, give ephedrine 6mg IV.

Bradycardia[a]
ECG monitoring, if available.
Administer atropine (0.6mg boluses IV, up to total 3mg).
If atropine ineffective, give ephedrine 6mg IV.

a. cardiovascular disturbance also occurs with IT baclofen withdrawal syndrome (see Box 21.A).

Box 21.C Management of undesirable effects of spinal analgesia

Opioid discontinuation (diarrhoea, colic, sweating, restlessness)
Spinal delivery results in a massive reduction in the patient's total opioid dose. Laxatives should be stopped and retitrated. If peripheral withdrawal symptoms occur, the pre-spinal opioid should be given p.r.n. in a dose approximately 25% of the former pain-related p.r.n. dose.

Opioid-induced pruritus
In palliative care, patients receiving spinal analgesia are generally *not* opioid-naïve (thus reducing the probability of pruritus) and most receive bupivacaine concurrently (this tends to restrict pruritus to the face).[71,72] If there is persistent pruritus, switching to an alternative opioid may help.[26]

In *opioid-naïve* patients receiving spinal morphine, e.g. for caesarian section, up to 80% develop pruritus. The following are effective:
- $5HT_3$ receptor antagonist, e.g. ondansetron 4mg IV, can be used prophylactically
- diphenhydramine 25mg IV (not UK), is as effective as ondansetron.[73,74]

Nonetheless, for both of the above, about 1/3 of patients either do not respond, or pruritus recurs after 1–12h. For these patients ultra-low dose naloxone has been used:[74]
- titrate to effect using repeat bolus doses of 40microgram IV
- if pruritus recurs, give 1microgram/kg/h by IVI (rarely necessary).

However, use of opioid antagonists (naloxone, naltrexone) risks reversing analgesia.[72,75–77]

Urinary retention
Drug-related urinary retention may be transient; removal of urinary catheter after 3–4 days is successful in 3/4 of patients.[8] If persistent, may be because of the underlying disease.

new neurological impairment is present (see warning about MRI above). Spinal catheters need not be automatically removed and allow a means of obtaining CSF for culture.[3] Mild meningeal irritation can be a normal phenomenon post-procedure, and patients can be safely observed while awaiting CSF cultures if they are systemically well and the above reveal no evidence of infection.[78] A prolonged operation time when placing the catheter is a risk factor for serious catheter-related infection.[79]

New neurological impairment
It can be difficult to distinguish between new neurological signs and symptoms caused by complications of spinal analgesia and those caused by disease progresssion (Box 21.D). Estimates of complication rates vary greatly, and often predominantly relate to peri-operative/obstetric spinal anaesthesia.[80] Disease-related neurological impairment is common: spinal cord compression occurs in ≤6% of patients receiving spinal analgesia.[3] ED metastases are present in ≤70% of patients with refractory cancer pain. They are associated with motor impairment, and higher **morphine** and **bupivacaine** dose requirements (although not higher pain scores). Those with spinal canal stenosis (58%) also have higher IT insertion complication rates.[81]

Catheter tip granulomas may present as catheter occlusion (manifesting as renewed and increasing pain) or local mass effects (spinal cord or cauda equina compression with associated pain). Generally occur 3 months–years after starting a spinal infusion; with the risk increasing with time.[61] Pain typically precedes neurological impairment, which develops gradually over days–weeks.[83]

Granulomas are more common with ED infusions than IT ones, and occur particularly with **morphine** or **hydromorphone** at higher concentrations.[5] The risk with **fentanyl** is probably lower. A granuloma caused by IT **baclofen** has been reported.[34] Granulomas often resolve spontaneously within a few months of discontinuing an infusion.

In the absence of neurological impairment, options include catheter tip relocation, opioid dose reduction and/or switching to **fentanyl** (but see p.682) or a non-opioid. Surgical excision may be necessary if symptoms persist or there is neurological impairment.[34]

Box 21.D Differential diagnosis of new neurological impairment in patients receiving spinal analgesia

Neurological damage caused by insertion of the catheter.
Bupivacaine-induced; dose-dependent, generally seen only when IT doses exceed 15mg/day,[4] but unmasking of incipient spinal cord compression can occur with lower doses.[4,82]
Disease progression, e.g. cauda equina or spinal cord compression.
Catheter complication, e.g. ED abscess or haematoma, catheter tip granuloma.

Evaluation

Neurological examination: to confirm the location of the problem: is it related to the catheter or could it be a separate second phenomenon?

Time of onset (after starting infusion):

- immediate: spinal medication, 'unmasking' of subclinical impairment, or neurological damage at insertion
- after days–weeks or longer: ED abscess, haematoma, or disease progression
- after several months–years: catheter tip granuloma.

Investigation: MRI = optimum (but see warning on p.685)

Exacerbation of pain

Increased pain may reflect:

- worsening of the original pain
- development of a new pain because of:
  - ▹ disease progression or co-morbidity
  - ▹ spinal catheter-related abscess, haematoma or granuloma
- reduced effect of the spinal infusion (delivery device malfunction).

Evaluation may reveal evidence of progression or new sites of disease, neurological impairment associated with spinal catheter-related mass, or infection. If external, the delivery system can be examined for disconnection, rate of delivery and contents.

A sudden increase in pain (e.g. as a result of catheter dislodgement) should be initially treated with p.r.n. opioid medication PO/SC while the cause is investigated. Alternatively, give **ketamine** 10–25mg PO/SC p.r.n. (see p.593), particularly if the pain is opioid poorly-responsive.

If the spinal infusion includes **baclofen**, and sudden failure of drug delivery is suspected, be alert to the presence of a severe life-threatening withdrawal syndrome (see Box 21.A). The sudden cessation of **clonidine** can cause severe rebound hypertension. Treat with oral **clonidine** while seeking specialist advice.[5]

Delivery device malfunction may involve:

- an empty syringe (problem with last refill, altered delivery rate or calendar error about next refill date)
- a problem with the pump itself (battery failure, mechanical failure)
- a problem with the catheter (kinking, fracture, displacement, occlusion).

Plain radiographs may show a kinked, dislodged or disconnected catheter. Catheter position and patency can be confirmed by injection of a radiological contrast agent *after first aspirating the catheter dead-space to avoid delivery of the dead-space contents as a bolus*. The contrast agent must be appropriate for CSF use: *IT delivery of inappropriate radiological contrast agents can cause arachnoiditis and death.*

Checks in use

It is recommended for spinal infusions that specific charts are used to monitor the delivery device, the infusion contents and patient's condition, comparable with those widely used for checking CSCI (see p.672). The use of a spinal chart should be cross-referenced on the patient's main prescription chart, and should list the drugs being infused.

1 Zech D *et al.* (1995) Validation of World Health Organization guidelines for cancer pain relief: a 10-year prospective study. *Pain*. **63**: 65–76.
2 Hanks G *et al.* (2001) Morphine and alternative opioids in cancer pain: the EAPC recommendations. *British Journal of Cancer*. **84**: 587–593.
3 Baker L *et al.* (2004) Evolving spinal analgesia practice in palliative care. *Palliative Medicine*. **18**: 507–515.
4 British Pain Society (2007) Intrathecal drug delivery for the management of pain and spasticity in adults; recommendations for best clinical practice. The British Pain Society. Available from: www.britishpainsociety.org
5 Deer T *et al.* (2007) Polyanalgesic consensus conference 2007: Recommendations for the management of pain by intrathecal (intraspinal) drug delivery; report of an interdisciplinary expert panel. *Neuromodulation*. **10**: 300–328.
6 Tei Y *et al.* (2008) Treatment efficacy of neural blockade in specialized palliative care services in Japan: a multicenter audit survey. *Journal of Pain and Symptom Management*. **36**: 461–467.
7 Burton AW *et al.* (2004) Epidural and intrathecal analgesia is effective in treating refractory cancer pain. *Pain Medicine*. **5**: 239–247.
8 Sjoberg M *et al.* (1991) Long-term intrathecal morphine and bupivacaine in 'refractory' cancer pain. Results from the first series of 52 patients. *Acta Anaesthesiologica Scandinavica*. **35**: 30–43.
9 Mercadante S (1994) Intrathecal morphine and bupivacaine in advanced cancer pain patients implanted at home. *Journal of Pain and Symptom Management*. **9**: 201–207.
10 Sjoberg M *et al.* (1994) Long term intrathecal morphine and bupivacaine in patients with refractory cancer pain. Results from a morphine:bupivacaine dose regimen of 0.5:4.75 mg/ml. *Anesthesiology*. **80**: 284–297.
11 Hassenbusch S *et al.* (1995) Long-term intraspinal infusions of opioids in the treatment of neuropathic pain. *Journal of Pain and Symptom Management*. **10**: 527–543.
12 Smitt PS *et al.* (1998) Outcome and complications of epidural analgesia in patients with chronic cancer pain. *Cancer*. **83**: 2015–2022.
13 Smith TJ *et al.* (2002) Randomized clinical trial of an implantable drug delivery system compared with comprehensive medical management for refractory cancer pain: impact on pain, drug-related toxicity, and survival. *Journal of Clinical Oncology*. **20**: 4040–4049.
14 Linklater GT and Macaulay L (2005) Epidural analgesia in advanced cancer patients. *Anesthesia and Analgesia*. **100**: 600; author reply 600–601.
15 Chambers WA (2008) Nerve blocks in palliative care. *British Journal of Anaesthesia*. **101**: 95–100.
16 Crul BJP and Delhaas EM (1991) Technical complications during long term subarachnoid or epidural administration of morphine in terminally ill cancer patients: A review of 140 cases. *Regional Anesthesia*. **16**: 209–213.
17 Hassenbusch SJ *et al.* (1997) Clinical realities and economic considerations: economics of intrathecal therapy. *Journal of Pain and Symptom Management*. **14**: S36–48.
18 Nitescu P *et al.* (1990) Epidural versus intrathecal morphine-bupivacaine: assessment of consecutive treatments in advanced cancer pain. *Journal of Pain and Symptom Management*. **5**: 18–26.
19 Dahm P *et al.* (1998) Efficacy and technical complications of long-term continuous intraspinal infusions of opioid and/or bupivacaine in refractory nonmalignant pain: a comparison between the epidural and the intrathecal approach with externalized or implanted catheters and infusion pumps. *Clinical Journal of Pain*. **14**: 4–16.
20 NPSA (National Patient Safety Agency) (2011) Safer spinal (intrathecal), epidural and regional devices. In: Patient Safety Alert Update PSA001. Available from: www.npsa.uk
21 Mercadante S (1999) Problems of long-term spinal opioid treatment in advanced cancer patients. *Pain*. **79**: 1–13.
22 Lee MA *et al.* (2001) A simple method of using epidural analgesia in palliative medicine. *Palliative Medicine*. **15**: 347–348.
23 Exner HJ *et al.* (2003) Epidural analgesia at end of life: facing empirical contraindications. *Anesthesia and Analgesia*. **97**: 1740–1742.
24 Department of Health (2010) Mixing of medicines prior to administration in clinical practice: medical and non-medical prescribing. HMSO, London. Available from: www.dh.gov.uk/prod_consum_dh/groups/dh_digitalassets/@dh/@en/@ps/documents/digitalasset/dh_116360.pdf
25 National Prescribing Centre (2010) Mixing of medicines prior to administration in clinical practice — responding to legislative changes. Liverpool. Available from: www.npc.nhs.uk/improving_safety/mixing_meds/resources/mixing_of_medicines.pdf
26 Hassenbusch SJ *et al.* (2004) Polyanalgesic Consensus Conference 2003: an update on the management of pain by intraspinal drug delivery — report of an expert panel. *Journal of Pain and Symptom Management*. **27**: 540–563.
27 Chrubasik J *et al.* (1993) The ideal epidural opioid–fact or fantasy? *European Journal of Anaesthesiology*. **10**: 79–100.
28 Stein C (ed) (1999) *Opioids in pain control. Basic and clinical aspects*. Cambridge University Press, Cambridge.
29 Dougherty PM and Staats PS (1999) Intrathecal drug therapy for chronic pain: from basic science to clinical practice. *Anesthesiology*. **91**: 1891–1918.
30 Bennett G *et al.* (2000) Evidence-based review of the literature on intrathecal delivery of pain medication. *Journal of Pain and Symptom Management*. **20**: S12–36.
31 Bernards CM (2002) Understanding the physiology and pharmacology of epidural and intrathecal opioids. *Best Practice and Research Clinical Anaesthesiology*. **16**: 489–505.
32 Sylvester R *et al.* (2004) The conversion challenge: from intrathecal to oral morphine. *American Journal of Hospice and Palliative Medicine*. **21 (2)**: 143–147.
33 Kedlaya D *et al.* (2002) Epidural and intrathecal analgesia for cancer pain. *Best Practice and Research Clinical Anaesthesiology*. **16**: 651–665.
34 Deer T *et al.* (2008) Management of intrathecal catheter-tip inflammatory masses: an updated 2007 consensus statement from an expert panel. *Neuromodulation*. **11**: 77–91.
35 Svedberg K *et al.* (2002) Compatibility of ropivacaine with morphine, sufentanil, fentanyl, or clonidine. *Journal of Clinical Pharmacy and Therapeutics*. **27**: 39–45.
36 Dahm P *et al.* (2000) Comparison of 0.5% intrathecal bupivacaine with 0.5% intrathecal ropivacaine in the treatment of refractory cancer and noncancer pain conditions: results from a prospective, crossover, double-blind, randomized study. *Regional Anesthesia and Pain Medicine*. **25**: 480–487.
37 Simpson D *et al.* (2005) Ropivacaine: a review of its use in regional anaesthesia and acute pain management. *Drugs*. **65**: 2675–2717.
38 Foster RH and Markham A (2000) Levobupivacaine: a review of its pharmacology and use as a local anaesthetic. *Drugs*. **59**: 551–579.

39 Coffey RJ *et al.* (2002) Abrupt withdrawal from intrathecal baclofen: recognition and management of a potentially life-threatening syndrome. *Archives of Physical Medicine and Rehabilitation.* **83**: 735–741.

40 Mohammed I and Hussain A (2004) Intrathecal baclofen withdrawal syndrome- a life-threatening complication of baclofen pump: a case report. *BMC Clinical Pharmacology.* **4**: 6.

41 Karpinski N *et al.* (1997) Subpial vacuolar myelopathy after intrathecal ketamine: report of a case. *Pain.* **73**: 103–105.

42 Benrath J *et al.* (2005) Long-term intrathecal S(+)-ketamine in a patient with cancer-related neuropathic pain. *British Journal of Anaesthesia.* **95**: 247–249.

43 Vranken JH *et al.* (2005) Neuropathological findings after continuous intrathecal administration of S(+)-ketamine for the management of neuropathic cancer pain. *Pain.* **117**: 231–235.

44 Vranken JH *et al.* (2006) Severe toxic damage to the rabbit spinal cord after intrathecal administration of preservative-free S(+)-ketamine. *Anesthesiology.* **105**: 813–818.

45 Deer T *et al.* (2008) Future directions for intrathecal pain management: a review and update from the interdisciplinary polyanalgesic consensus conference 2007. *Neuromodulation.* **11**: 92–97.

46 Mehta A and Kay E (1996) Admixtures' storage is extended. *Pharmacy in Practice.* **6**: 113–118.

47 Xu Quanyun A *et al.* (2002) Physical and chemical stability of low and high concentrations of morphine sulfate with clonidine hydrochloride packaged in plastic syringes. In: *International Journal of Pharmaceutical Compounding.* Available from: www.ijpc.com/editorial/SearchByIssue.cfm?PID = 100

48 Trissel Lawrence A *et al.* (2002) Physical and chemical stability of low and high concentrations of morphine sulfate with bupivacaine hydrochloride packaged in plastic syringes. In: *International Journal of Pharmaceutical Compounding.* Available from: www.ijpc.com/editorial/SearchByIssue.cfm?PID = 100

49 Christen C *et al.* (1996) Stability of bupivacaine hydrochloride and hydromorphone hydrochloride during simulated epidural coadministration. *American Journal of Health System Pharmacy.* **53**: 170–173.

50 Trissel LA (2010) *Handbook on Injectable Drugs* (16e). American Society of Health System Pharmacists, Maryland, USA.

51 Hildebrand KR *et al.* (2003) Stability and Compatibility of Morphine-Clonidine Admixtures in an Implantable Infusion System. *Journal of Pain and Symptom Management.* **25**: 464–471.

52 Classen AM *et al.* (2004) Stability of admixture containing morphine sulfate, bupivacaine hydrochloride, and clonidine hydrochloride in an implantable infusion system. *Journal of Pain and Symptom Management.* **28**: 603–611.

53 Hildebrand KR *et al.* (2001) Stability and Compatibility of Hydromorphone Hydrochloride in an Implantable Infusion System. *Journal of Pain and Symptom Management.* **22**: 1042–1047.

54 Rudich Z *et al.* (2004) Stability of clonidine in clonidine-hydromorphone mixture from implanted intrathecal infusion pumps in chronic pain patients. *Journal of Pain and Symptom Management.* **28**: 599–602.

55 MHRA (2008) Medical device alert MDA/2008/087: Implantable drug pumps manufactured by Medtronic — Synchro EL models 8626 and 8627 and SynchroMed II model 8637. Available from: www.mhra.gov.uk/home/idcplg?IdcService = GET_FILE&dDocName = CON033659&RevisionSelectionMethod = LatestReleased

56 MHRA (2009) Effects of MRI on implantable drug pumps. In: *Drug Safety Update.* Available from: www.mhra.gov.uk/home/idcplg?IdcService = GET_FILE&dDocName = CON041213&RevisionSelectionMethod = LatestReleased

57 Naumann C (1999) Drug adverse events and system complications of intrathecal opioid delivery for pain: origins, detection, manifestations and management. *Neuromodulation.* **2**: 92–107.

58 Paice JA *et al.* (1996) Intraspinal morphine for chronic pain: a retrospective, multicenter study. *Journal of Pain and Symptom Management.* **11**: 71–80.

59 Winkelmuller W *et al.* (1999) Intrathecal opioid therapy for pain: Efficacy and outcomes. *Neuromodulation.* **2**: 67–76.

60 Rawal N *et al.* (1987) Present state of extradural and intrathecal opioid analgesia in Sweden. A nationwide follow-up survey. *British Journal of Anaesthesia.* **59**: 791–799.

61 Deer TR (2004) A prospective analysis of intrathecal granulomas in chronic pain patients: a review of the literature and report of a surveillance study. *Pain Physician.* **7**: 225–228.

62 Abs R *et al.* (2000) Endocrine consequences of long-term intrathecal administration of opioids. *Journal of Clinical Endocrinology and Metabolism.* **85**: 2215–2222.

63 Winkelmuller M and Winkelmuller W (1996) Long-term effects of continuous intrathecal opioid treatment in chronic pain of nonmalignant etiology. *Journal of Neurosurgery.* **85**: 458–467.

64 Budd K and Shipton E (2004) Acute pain and the immune system and opioimmunosuppression. *Acute Pain.* **6**: 123–135.

65 Mercadante S *et al.* (2007) Intrathecal treatment in cancer patients unresponsive to multiple trials of systemic opioids. *Clinical Journal of Pain.* **23**: 793–798.

66 Moen V *et al.* (2004) Severe neurological complications after central neuraxial blockades in Sweden 1990–1999. *Anesthesiology.* **101**: 950–959.

67 Aromaa U *et al.* (1997) Severe complications associated with epidural and spinal anaesthesias in Finland 1987–1993. A study based on patient insurance claims. *Acta Anaesthesiologica Scandinavica.* **41**: 445–452.

68 Cook TM *et al.* (2009) Major complications of central neuraxial block: report on the Third National Audit Project of the Royal College of Anaesthetists. *British Journal of Anaesthesia.* **102**: 179–190.

69 Holmfred A *et al.* (2006) Intrathecal catheters with subcutaneous port systems in patients with severe cancer-related pain managed out of hospital: the risk of infection. *Journal of Pain and Symptom Management.* **31**: 568–572.

70 Nitescu P *et al.* (1995) Complications of intrathecal opioids and bupivacaine in the treatment of 'refractory' cancer pain. *Clinical Journal of Pain.* **11**: 45–62.

71 Asokumar B *et al.* (1998) Intrathecal bupivacaine reduces pruritus and prolongs duration of fentanyl analgesia during labor: a prospective, randomized, controlled trial. *Anaesthesia and Analgesia.* **87**: 1309–1315.

72 Reich A and Szepietowski JC (2010) Opioid-induced pruritus: an update. *Clinical Experimental Dermatology.* **35**: 2–6.

73 Bonnet MP *et al.* (2008) Effect of prophylactic 5-HT3 receptor antagonists on pruritus induced by neuraxial opioids: a quantitative systematic review. *British Journal of Anaesthesia.* **101**: 311–319.

74 Siddik-Sayyid SM *et al.* (2010) Ondansetron is as effective as diphenhydramine for treatment of morphine-induced pruritus after cesarean delivery. *Acta Anaesthesiologica Scandinavica.* **54**: 764–769.

75 Korbon G *et al.* (1985) Intramuscular naloxone reverses the side effects of epidural morphine while preserving analgesia. *Regional Anaesthesia.* **10**: 16–20.

76 Kjellberg F and Tramer M (2001) Pharmacological control of opioid-induced pruritus: a quantitative systematic review of randomized trials. *European Journal of Anaesthesiology.* **18**: 346–357.

77 Lockington PF and Fa'aea P (2007) Subcutaneous naloxone for the prevention of intrathecal morphine induced pruritus in elective Caesarean delivery. *Anaesthesia.* **62**: 672–676.

78 Paice JA *et al.* (1997) Clinical realities and economic considerations: efficacy of intrathecal pain therapy. *Journal of Pain and Symptom Management.* **14 (suppl)**: S14–26.
79 Byers K *et al.* (1995) Infections complicating tunneled intraspinal catheter systems used to treat chronic pain. *Clinical Infectious Diseases.* **21**: 403–408.
80 Bromage PR (1997) Neurological complications of subarachnoid and epidural anesthesia. *Acta Anaesthesiologica Scandinavica.* **41**: 439–444.
81 Appelgren L *et al.* (1997) Spinal epidural metastasis: implications for spinal analgesia to treat 'refractory' cancer pain. *Journal of Pain and Symptom Management.* **13**: 25–42.
82 van Dongen RTM *et al.* (1997) Neurological impairment during long-term intrathecal infusion of bupivacaine in cancer patients: a sign of spinal cord compression. *Pain.* **69**: 205–209.
83 Miele VJ *et al.* (2006) A review of intrathecal morphine therapy related granulomas. *European Journal of Pain.* **10**: 251–261.

22: DRUG ADMINISTRATION TO PATIENTS WITH SWALLOWING DIFFICULTIES OR ENTERAL FEEDING TUBES

General principles

Simplifying drug therapy by reducing the number of medications and frequency of administration is particularly important for patients who are not able to swallow solids or for whom administering drugs by an enteral feeding tube (EFT) is being considered.

Modifying a product in a way not specified in the manufacturer's SPC renders its use off-label, e.g. emptying out the contents of a capsule. Thus, if available, appropriate alternative formulations of those drugs still considered necessary should be used, e.g. a soluble tablet or an oral liquid instead of a solid tablet (or an alternative licensed drug).

Administering drugs by EFT is generally off-label, and consideration should also be given to using an alternative licensed route, e.g. PR, SC, IV.[1,2] However, administration by EFT may be preferable from a practical or personal point of view.

Drug therapy, the formulations used, and swallowing ability should be kept under review, particularly before inpatient discharge. Training and detailed written instructions regarding the supply, preparation and administration of each drug should be given to the patient and/or carer and primary care team.[3]

Guidance on minimizing wrong route errors when giving drugs by PO or other enteral route has been published by the UK National Patient Safety Agency (NPSA).[4] Only enteral syringes should be used to draw up and administer oral liquids. Many local guidelines stipulate once only use. NPSA has also produced guidance on testing the position of nasogastric tubes.[5]

The administration of drugs by EFT is considered a level 3 skill for care workers in care homes. Staff must be adequately trained.[6] General guidance for the administration of drugs by EFT is given in the Quick Practice Guide (see p.700).

Choosing a suitable formulation

When planning to change to an alternative formulation or administer a drug by EFT, guidance should be obtained from a pharmacist. For those with impaired swallowing a Speech and Language Therapist (SALT) should also be consulted in order to understand the degree of swallowing impairment and perform a risk assessment.[7] Taking into account the balance of risks and uncertainties for drug administration to these patients, the choice of formulation in descending order of preference generally comprises:

- soluble tablet or commercial oral liquid
- effervescent tablet or dispersed tablet (licensed or off-label)
- oral liquid prepared by local pharmacy or special order
- dispersed capsule contents or crushed tablet
- injection (given PO or by EFT).

However, there are considerations and disadvantages for each of these options which can vary according to the drug prescribed, the patient's clinical need and the practical situation. These issues are summarized in Table 22.1. Thus, every drug needs to be assessed individually to determine which would be the most appropriate formulation, i.e. do not simply convert all solid dose medication to oral liquids. Table 22.2, p.701 contains a list of the formulations available for palliative care drugs with licensed and off-label alternatives for patients with swallowing difficulties and EFT.

Table 22.1 Summary of the issues to consider when choosing a suitable formulation

Formulation	*Considerations / Disadvantages*
Soluble tablet	Availability Sodium content, often high Cost
Commercial oral liquid	Excipients causing undesirable effects Bio-availability and dosing frequency Viscosity and particle size Volume and palatability Cost
Effervescent tablet or dispersed tablet (licensed or off-label)	Sodium content, often high Particle size Practicality Cost of licensed formulations
Locally prepared or special order oral liquid	As for commercial oral liquid *plus*: shelf-life/expiry storage conditions continuity of supply reduced quality assurance variable formulations between special order manufacturers higher cost than commercial oral liquid
Dispersed capsule contents (licensed or off-label) or crushed tablet	Occupational exposure Particle size Practicality Risk of using an inappropriate formulation, e.g. m/r and causing destruction of m/r mechanism, more rapid absorption, and danger to patient
Injection given PO or by EFT	Osmolality/hypertonicity/unsuitable pH Excipients unsuitable for PO administration Risk of wrong route error Continuity of supply in the community Cost

Option 1: Licensed soluble tablet or commercial oral liquid

If available, soluble tablets are generally the preferred option. Soluble tablets dissolve *completely* when placed in 10mL water to give a solution of the drug in contrast to effervescent, dispersible or orodispersible tablets which disperse in water or in the mouth to give particles (see option 2 below).

Liquid formulations are not always suitable as direct substitutes for solid dosage forms for several reasons:

- *excipients causing undesirable effects:* many oral liquid formulations contain excipients which in large volumes can cause osmotic diarrhoea, particularly with jejunal administration, e.g. sorbitol ≥15g/24h. The normal osmolality of GI secretions is 100–400mosm/kg, but many liquid formulations are > 1,000mosm/kg.[8,9] Reduce osmolality by diluting with as much water as is practical. Some liquid formulations contain alcohol, e.g. Oramorph®, **loperamide, phenobarbital, ranitidine**

- *altered bio-availability and/or dosing frequency:* an oral liquid formulation may have a different bio-availability from the corresponding solid formulation, e.g. **citalopram**, **phenytoin**, **sodium fusidate**, necessitating a different dose. When converting from a m/r formulation to a normal-release oral liquid, the dose and/or frequency may need to be changed
- *viscosity and particle size of suspensions:* patients may be unable to swallow a highly viscous formulation or particulate suspension. EFT easily blocked by a highly viscous formulation, e.g. **amoxicillin-clavulanate**, mineral oil, syrups or by particles from a suspension, e.g. **ciprofloxacin**, **clarithromycin**. Viscosity may be reduced by diluting with 30–50mL water if practical[9]
- *large volumes:* from high doses or multiple drugs may be impractical, unpalatable and costly.

Option 2: Effervescent tablet or dispersed tablet (licensed or off-label)

Do not administer a formulation by EFT if it has not dispersed into non-visible particles or which has an oily residue. Sediment and oily films increase the risk of blocking the tube (Box 22.A).[9,10]

Effervescent tablets and licensed dispersible tablets disintegrate in water to particle/granule form. Depending on the degree of dispersion, this may not be suitable for patients unable to swallow biphasic preparations, i.e. solids and liquids together, and the particles may be too large for administration by fine-bore EFT.

Many standard tablets disperse sufficiently or dissolve when mixed with 10mL water even if not marketed as dispersible/soluble. Although off-label, this is often the most practical option for both patients with swallowing difficulties and those with EFT (Box 22.A). Fractional dosing from effervescent or dispersed tablets is not recommended due to inaccuracy.

Orodispersible tablets are designed to disperse on the tongue and are generally swallowed with the saliva without water. Some orodispersible formulations may be more suitable than others for patients with swallowing difficulties and may depend on the extent of dysphagia. The formulations, dose equivalences and administration of orodispersible tablets vary depending on the drug concerned. Individual product details should be consulted before using by EFT.

Buccal, sublingual and most oromucosal formulations are designed to be absorbed by the oral mucosa and not the GI tract, thus bypassing first-pass hepatic metabolism. These may be suitable alternatives for patients with swallowing difficulties but are unsuitable for EFT administration. Check if the formulation is intended for buccal or enteral administration to prevent wrong route errors.

Option 3: Locally prepared or special order oral liquid

An oral liquid formulation prepared locally or by special order (see Appendix 1, p.769) may be an alternative if a licensed product is not available or not suitable.[11] The same issues as for licensed oral liquids need to be considered (see Table 22.1). However, it may be possible for an experienced pharmacist to alter a formulation with careful consideration for quality, storage and shelf-life and thus make it more suitable.[11] Continuity of supply after a patient has returned home, short shelf-life, storage conditions (e.g. refrigeration), differences in formulation between manufacturers and higher cost often make this option impractical.

Option 4: Dispersed capsule contents or crushed tablet

Opening capsules in order to disperse the contents is generally off-label and risks topical and inhaled exposure of the contents to the health professional. It is not recommended for certain drugs, e.g. antibiotics, cytotoxics, prostaglandin analogues or hormone antagonists. There are also risks to the patient if unsuitable formulations are used, e.g. m/r formulations may be harmful if accidentally chewed or crushed, or if the contents are irritant, e.g. **demeclocycline**.

A few capsules contain liquid contents, e.g. **nifedipine**. Because of the small volume of the contents (which varies between brands), it is not recommended that these are used as a source of a drug for swallowing difficulties or EFT administration.

It is sometimes feasible to add the contents of some capsules to water for administration by EFT, or to soft food, fruit juice or other liquids to aid those with swallowing difficulties. The manufacturer's SPC should be consulted to ensure that this will not cause problems with absorption or cause undesirable effects. Small quantities of soft food or liquids, e.g. a tablespoon (15mL), should be used to ensure that the entire dose is administered.

Crushing tablet/capsule contents to facilitate dispersion is *not* generally necessary as many tablets and capsule contents will disperse sufficiently in water without crushing (see option 2). Crushing can be dangerous for certain formulations (Box 22.B) and care must be taken to ensure that this is safe for both the patient and health professionals. It should be considered a last resort and avoided unless specifically recommended by a pharmacist.[1]

Box 22.A Guidelines for preparation of dispersed formulations[1,3]

Information about the preparation of each medication should be documented on the prescription and in the patient's notes.

Prepare (and administer) each drug separately.

Place the tablet(s) or capsule contents into the barrel of a 50mL enteral syringe;
use a large container/drug pot for effervescent formulations.

Only if specifically recommended by a pharmacist, use a mortar and pestle or tablet crusher to crush tablet(s) or capsule contents (see text).

Add 10mL of tap water (50mL for effervescent formulations), allow to disperse, then mix well:
- *use sterile water for jejunal tubes or immunocompromised patients*
- if using a drug pot or other container, once dispersed, draw up the contents using a 50mL enteral syringe.

Ensure the drug is sufficiently dispersed into non-visible particles without residue, then administer by the EFT (see Quick Practice Guide, p.700).

If using a drug pot or other container, rinse with water, draw up with the same enteral syringe and administer the rinsings through the tube.

To ensure the patient receives the whole dose, use the same enteral syringe to draw up and administer the flush (see Quick Practice Guide, p.700).

Thoroughly clean any drug pots/containers/tablet crushers with hot soapy water according to local policy to avoid cross-contamination.

Do not:
- use hot water for drug dispersion as this may alter bio-availability
- leave dispersed medicines lying around unlabelled
- use plastic containers to crush tablets as the drug may adhere to the container.

Box 22.B Formulations which must not be crushed

Do not crush

M/r formulations (including m/r capsule contents) because this will destroy the m/r mechanism and result in dangerous dose peaks and troughs.[9,10,12–14]

E/c (gastro-resistant) formulations (including e/c capsule contents) because this will destroy the e/c properties of the formulation, may alter bio-availability, and may block the tube.[9,10,13,14]

Cytotoxics, prostaglandin analogues, hormone antagonists or antibiotics because there are risks to the staff through inhalation and/or topical absorption.[9,10,14]

Buccal or sublingual formulations because their bio-availability may be dramatically reduced if absorbed by the GI tract.[9,10,14]

Option 5: Injection (given PO or by EFT)

Formulations for injection are often unsuitable for enteral administration. This may be for one or more of several reasons:

- high osmolality or hypertonicity; the high solute concentration can cause osmotic diarrhoea
- unsuitable pH of the formulation or acidic conditions of the stomach chemically degrading the drug, e.g. **omeprazole**
- formulation with a different salt of unknown bio-availability
- an additive which is irritant to the GI tract, e.g. polysorbate 80 (Tween® 80) in **amiodarone**.[1,15]
- risk of IV administration by mistake[4]
- cost.

Generally, all injections suitable for enteral administration should be diluted before administration, e.g. with 30–50mL water by EFT. Bio-availability between the solid dose form and the injection solution may be different and alter clinical response, e.g. more rapid absorption and higher peak levels may occur.

Specific considerations for EFT

Testing of tube position

Correct tube placement should be confirmed following insertion. For NG tubes, test aspirate with CE marked pH paper.[5] A break in feeding of 1h is required before testing. Radiographic confirmation in accordance with specific NPSA guidance is necessary only when there is doubt.

Correct tube position should be confirmed before each feed, before each drug administration and at least once daily. However, for patients on continuous feeding, multiple drug administration times, or on acid-suppressing drugs (e.g. antacids, H_2 antagonists and PPIs) this is impractical. Providing initial tube placement has been correctly confirmed and there is no reason to suspect displacement, tube position should be confirmed by observation of the external tube length and positioning in accordance with NPSA guidelines.[5] Likewise for NJ tubes.

Site of drug delivery

The position of the tube may alter bio-availability, e.g. with jejunal tubes, absorption may be unpredictable because of the effects of pH or because the tube may extend beyond the main site of absorption of the drug, e.g. **cephalexin**, **ketoconazole**, **metronidazole benzoate**.[1,8] Care should also be taken with drugs that have a narrow therapeutic range, e.g. **digoxin**, **warfarin**, **phenytoin** and other anti-epileptics.[8] Drugs which undergo extensive first-pass hepatic metabolism may have greater systemic effects because of increased absorption from direct delivery to the jejunum, e.g. opioids, TCAs.[2] Undesirable effects may also be increased because of rapid delivery into the jejunum. The acid barrier of the stomach is bypassed with jejunal tubes, some centres use aseptic technique to reduce the risk of infective diarrhoea.

Function of the tube

Drugs should not be administered if the tube is on free drainage or suction.[9]

Number of lumens

Ensure the correct lumen is used with multilumen tubes; some tubes have one lumen terminating in the stomach and another in the jejunum. *Do not use an aspiration gastric decompression port for drug administration.*

Lumen size

The outer diameter of an EFT is measured by the French gauge (1 French unit = 0.33mm).[2] However, the internal diameter of equivalent French gauge tubes varies between manufacturers. The tube material also affects the internal lumen size, e.g. silicone and latex tubes have thicker walls and therefore narrower internal lumens. Narrow lumen, e.g. 5–12 French, or long tubes, e.g. NJ, are more likely to block, particularly with thick oral syrups and suspensions with large particles. Wide bore tubes require larger flush volumes.

Flushing the tube

This is essential to minimize drug interactions with the feeds. Water is the standard flush; use sterile water for jejunal tubes or immunocompromised patients because the acid barrier in the stomach is bypassed.[1] Tubes should be flushed before, in between drugs, and after drug administration ideally with 30mL water.[1,16] Use a 50mL enteral syringe to reduce the risk of tube rupture which can be caused by smaller syringes. Flush slowly with a push-pause technique to prevent leaving a coating of feed on the internal tube surface. Record the total flush and drug volume administered.

Feeding regimen

With continuous feeding and multiple drug administration periods, it may be necessary to adjust the feeding rate to compensate for the breaks in feed administration. If possible, the drug schedule should be rationalized, aiming for once daily drug administration to allow time for adequate nutrition.[2]

Bulk-forming laxatives

Do not administer by EFT because they may block the tube; use an enteral feed with a high-fibre content instead.[9]

Drug interactions and complications with EFT

Drugs can interact with food in many ways.[17,18] Enteral feeds can cause different problems associated with bio-availability, physical compatibility, and chemical interactions. Because they are in liquid form, the content, consistency and pH is very different to normal diet and variable between brands.

Drugs should *never* be added to enteral feeds because this increases the risk of incompatibility, microbial contamination, tube blockage, and underdosing or overdosing if the feed rate is altered.[19] However, complications can still arise from:

- *binding of drugs to the internal surface of the tube reducing absorption*, e.g. **carbamazepine**,[20] **clonazepam**, **diazepam**, **phenytoin**; minimize by diluting with 30–50mL water and flushing as per Quick Practice Guide (see p.700)
- *physical interaction with the feed causing coagulation*, particularly if the drug formulation is acidic, i.e. pH < 4.[9] This applies to many syrups,[2] and risks tube blockage and reduced drug absorption. Abdominal distension caused by excessive gas production from effervescence has been reported when sodium bicarbonate solutions, used to deliver PPI formulations, have come into contact with the feed[21]
- *chemical interaction between the drug and feed causing a non-absorbable drug-feed complex*, e.g. bezoar (insoluble concretion) formation with **sucralfate**, in the tube or in the stomach.[22,23] Do not prescribe **sucralfate** by EFT
- *chemical interaction between the drug and the feed resulting in reduced drug available for absorption*, e.g. **carbamazepine**, **ciprofloxacin**, **digoxin**, **penicillins**, **phenytoin**, **theophylline**, **warfarin**.[24] A feed break of at least 1h before and after each drug is recommended to minimize the risk of reduced absorption
- *indirect drug or nutrient interactions*, e.g. the **vitamin K** content of a feed affecting the action of **warfarin**[17]
- *the effects of malnutrition on drug pharmacokinetics*.

Usual considerations for physical and chemical drug-drug interactions must also be taken into consideration, particularly if rationalizing drug administration to once or twice a day.

Flushing the tube effectively, diluting potentially problematic formulations, inserting a feed break as outlined in the Quick Practice Guide (see p.700) and choosing an appropriate formulation will reduce the risk of dangerous interactions. Clinically, the most important interactions are those drugs with a narrow therapeutic range, e.g. **digoxin**, **theophylline**, **warfarin**, **phenytoin** and other anti-epileptics; these may warrant monitoring plasma concentrations. Clinical response should also be monitored closely. Appropriate precautionary measures may need to be taken if the feed is discontinued, particularly if dose adjustments were made because of an interaction.

Administration of e/c (gastro-resistant) and m/r formulations by EFT

Generally, these products should *not* be administered by EFT because of the risk of blocking the tube. However, some capsules/granules/compressed tablets contain e/c or m/r granules for which specific procedures have been developed to allow administration of the coated granules by EFT, e.g. **esomeprazole** gastro-resistant tablets and gastro-resistant granules for oral suspension (Nexium®), **lansoprazole** orodispersible tablets (Zoton FasTab®), certain m/r **morphine** formulations (MST Continus® suspension and Zomorph® capsules) **omeprazole** capsules

(Losec®) and **theophylline** m/r capsules (Slo-Phyllin®). See the manufacturer's SPC and/or specialist information for details (Table 22.2).[1] In order to avoid dangerous dose peaks and troughs or tube blockage, it is essential that:

- the recommended procedure is strictly adhered to and is used only for that *specific* formulation and brand
- the correct tube size and type is used
- extreme care is taken to avoid crushing the coated granules, thereby destroying the coating
- clinical response is monitored closely.

Unblocking EFTs

Tube blockage may be caused by the feed, e.g. stagnant or contaminated feed, or by incorrect drug administration, e.g. particle blockage or interaction between the feed and drug. It can be minimized by effective flushing and choosing an appropriate formulation. It is more likely with narrow lumens; a 35% incidence of blockage in patients with 8 French tubes has been cited.[25] Many tubes can be unblocked using 15–30mL water in a 50mL syringe and a push-pull action, although this may take 20–30min. Excessive force must not be used to unblock a tube because of the danger of perforation. Care must be taken as unblocking a tube may result in bolus drug administration from residual drug in the tube.

Various other agents have anecdotally been used to unblock tubes, e.g. carbonated drinks or cranberry juice. However, these are acidic solutions and can make the situation worse by causing feed coagulation,[9] and are no longer recommended.[1] Pancreatic enzymes help only if the blockage is caused by the feed. Sodium bicarbonate needs to be added to activate the enzymes, which may not be practical. Re-insertion of guide-wires is not advisable unless under specialist supervision.[1]

For blockages which do not resolve with water, consult a specialist nutrition nurse if available.

Quick Practice Guide: Administration of drugs by enteral feeding tube

Before drug administration

1. The administration of drugs by an enteral feeding tube (EFT) is considered a level 3 skill for care workers in care homes. Staff must be adequately trained.
2. Drug charts should state the specific route of administration, e.g. nasogastric (NG), nasojejunal (NJ), and specify the lumen to be used to prevent wrong route errors.
3. Check that there is documented confirmation that the EFT was correctly positioned following insertion. For NG tubes, use CE marked pH paper intended for testing human gastric contents (safe range pH1–5.5 after a 1h break in feeding) or, when there is doubt, by approved radiographic confirmation in accordance with NPSA guidelines.
4. If practical, reconfirm correct NG tube position before each drug administration. For patients on continuous feeding, multiple drug administration times or on acid-suppressants (antacids, H_2 antagonists, PPIs), if correct tube placement confirmed initially and there is no reason to suspect displacement, confirm tube position by observation of the external tube length (in accordance with NPSA guidelines); likewise for NJ tubes.
5. The patient should be in a sitting position to prevent regurgitation and pulmonary aspiration.
6. To prevent accidental parenteral administration, use enteral syringes, i.e. syringes which cannot be connected to IV catheters, ports or other parenteral devices. A 50mL enteral syringe reduces the risk of rupture of the EFT.
7. All EFT lumens should be clearly labelled.

Do not use 3-way taps or syringe tip adaptors because these can inadvertently result in connection safeguards being bypassed.

Drug administration

Do not add drugs to enteral feeds because this increases the risk of incompatibility, microbial contamination, tube blockage, and underdosing or overdosing if the feed rate is altered.

8. Stop the feed and ensure any other ports are closed and airtight.
9. Flush the EFT using a **push-pause** action with 15–30mL of water (*use sterile water throughout if jejunal tube or immunocompromised patient*). This helps to clear the tube and prevent physical interactions with the feed which could result in coagulation and blockage of the tube.
10. Check if a specific time interval is needed before and after administration to achieve maximal absorption and/or reduce the risk of chemical interactions.
11. Administer the most suitable formulation of each drug separately (see Choosing a suitable formulation, p.693, Box 22.A and Table 22.2):
    - a 50mL enteral syringe reduces the risk of rupture of the EFT; a 2mL or smaller enteral syringe can be used for very small quantities to accurately measure the dose.
    - flush between each drug with 15–30mL of water
12. After drug administration, flush the EFT using a **push-pause** action with 15–30mL of water.
13. Resume feeding after any necessary feed break (see point 10).

After drug administration

14. Document the total volume of fluid given (including flushes) on a fluid balance chart.
15. Monitor the clinical response, particularly if:
    - changing from m/r to normal-release formulations
    - the drug has a narrow therapeutic range
    - the bio-availability of the drug differs between solid dose form and liquid.

Table 22.2 Information on alternative enteral formulations available for administering drugs to patients with swallowing dffilulties or by EFT[1,26–29]

Drug	*Soluble tablet or commercial oral liquid available*	*Tablet/capsule contents may disperse sufficiently for 8Fr NG tube*[a,b]	*Oral liquid can be prepared by local pharmacy or special order*	*Injection can be diluted and administered PO or by EFT*	*Comments*
Acetylcysteine	No			Yes	
Amiloride	Yes	Yes (APS)			Sugar- and sorbitol-free oral solution
Aminophylline[a]	No	No	Yes	Yes	Consider discontinuing therapy due to dosing complexities. Give aminophylline injection orally as a diluted oral solution,[1] take care converting from m/r to immediate-release or convert oral aminophylline total daily dose to oral *unlicensed* theophylline liquid (aminophylline 250mg PO = theophylline 200mg PO) and split into t.d.s regimen (see theophylline below). Monitor blood levels
Amiodarone	No	No	Yes[f]	No	A 25mg/5mL suspension[f] or 200mg/5mL suspension can be prepared.[29] Injection contains irritant Tween 80
Amitriptyline	Yes	No	Yes[c,e]		Sugar- and sorbitol-free oral solution
Amlodipine	No	Yes (Istin®, IVAX and Norton)	Yes[e,f]		A 1mg/mL suspension can be prepared (90 day shelf-life)[f] or with 1% methylcellulose in syrup (56 day shelf-life).[1] Disperse tablet for intrajejunal administration
Amoxicillin	Yes			Yes	Dilute oral suspensions with an equal volume of water to reduce viscosity for EFT use
Antacids	Yes				Not recommended by EFT as can coagulate with feed; not needed with jejunal tube
Ascorbic acid	No	Yes (effervescent)			Add effervescent tablets to 50mL water
Aspirin	No	Yes (dispersible)			Use commercially available dispersible tablet

continued

Table 22.2 Continued

Drug	*Soluble tablet or commercial oral liquid available*	*Tablet/capsule contents may disperse sufficiently for 8Fr NG tube*[a,b]	*Oral liquid can be prepared by local pharmacy or special order*	*Injection can be diluted and administered PO or by EFT*	*Comments*
Baclofen	Yes	Yes (APS, takes 2min, Lioresal® takes 5min)	Yes[d]		Commercial oral liquids are viscous and contain sorbitol (2.75g/5mL Lioresal®) dilute with an equal volume of water for EFT use. Dispersing tablets is preferable particularly for intrajejunal administration
Bethanechol	No		Yes		A 5mg/mL suspension with cherry syrup can be prepared (60 day shelf-life)[1]
Calcium & vitamin D	No	Yes (effervescent)			Use effervescent granules or effervescent tablet and add to 50mL water. The solution can crystallize and calcium can bind to phosphate in enteral feed. Flush EFT well to avoid
Carbamazepine[a]	Yes				Commercial oral liquid contains sorbitol (1.25g/5mL Tegretol®). Dilute with an equal volume of water to reduce adherence to EFT. Monitor for increased undesirable effects particularly with intrajejunal administration
Carbocisteine	Yes				
Cefalexin	Yes				Dilute oral suspensions with equal volume of water to reduce viscosity for EFT use. Avoid opening capsules/crushing tablets due to risk of cephalosporin sensitization
Cefradine	Yes				Avoid opening capsules/crushing tablets due to risk of cephalosporin sensitization
Celecoxib	No	Yes			

continued

Table 22.2 Continued

Drug	*Soluble tablet or commercial oral liquid available*	*Tablet/capsule contents may disperse sufficiently for 8Fr NG tube*[a,b]	*Oral liquid can be prepared by local pharmacy or special order*	*Injection can be diluted and administered PO or by EFT*	*Comments*
Chlorphenamine	Yes				Dilute oral liquid with an equal volume of water for EFT use. Flush EFT well to prevent coagulation with feed.
Chlorpromazine	Yes	No	Yes[d]		Some oral liquids contain sorbitol. Handle with care to avoid contact sensitization; do not crush tablets
Cimetidine	Yes	Yes (effervescent)		Yes (Tagamet®)	Some oral liquids contain sorbitol (Dyspamet® 2.8g/5mL, Tagamet® negligible). Use effervescent tablet added to 30mL water, or diluted injection for intrajejunal administration. Tagamet® and Dyspamet® disperse but no information on suitability for EFT
Cinnarizine	No	Yes (Norton, takes 5min)			
Ciprofloxacin	Yes	Yes (Ranbaxy, Generics)	Yes[c]		Commercial oral suspension not recommended for EFT because too viscous and granular. Disperse tablet with 30–50mL sterile water *not tap water* (to avoid ion chelation). Stop feed for 1h before and 1–2h after dose. Do not administer with iron or zinc
Citalopram	Yes	Yes (Generics, takes 5min)			10mg of tablet equivalent to 8mg of oral liquid
Clarithromycin[a]	Yes			No	Dilute commercial oral liquid with an equal volume of water for EFT. Do not use EFT less than 9Fr gauge
Clindamycin	No	Yes (capsules)	Yes[e]		Avoid inhalation of the capsule contents

continued

Table 22.2 Continued

Drug	*Soluble tablet or commercial oral liquid available*	*Tablet/capsule contents may disperse sufficiently for 8Fr NG tube*[a,b]	*Oral liquid can be prepared by local pharmacy or special order*	*Injection can be diluted and administered PO or by EFT*	*Comments*
Clomipramine[a]	No	Yes (APS)			
Clonazepam	No	Yes (Rivotril® takes 5min)	Yes[d,e,f]	Yes	Unlicensed commercial oral liquid has 6 month shelf-life. 200microgram/5mL (3 month shelf-life)[l] and 500microgram/5mL formulations can be prepared.[f,29] Dilute all formulations with 30–50mL water to reduce risk of binding to the tube. Disperse tablets for intrajejunal administration. Injection contains alcohol and other excipients
Clonidine	No	Yes (100microgram Catapres®)	Yes[d]	Yes (Catapres®)	100microgram/mL formulation with simple syrup can be prepared (1 month shelf-life)[l]
Co-amoxiclav	Yes	No			Commercial oral liquid not recommended for EFT because too viscous
Co-codamol	No	Yes (efferevescent/ dispersible)			Add effervescent/dispersible tablet to 50mL water
Co-codaprin	No	Yes (dispersible)			Add dispersible tablet to 50mL water
Co-danthramer	Yes				Dilute commercial oral liquid 25mg/200mg in 5mL with an equal volume of water for EFT use
Co-danthrusate	Yes				No information on suitability via EFT
Codeine phosphate	Yes		Yes[d]		Dilute commercial oral liquid with an equal volume of water to reduce viscosity for EFT use. Tablets disperse but no information on suitability by EFT

continued

Table 22.2 Continued

Drug	*Soluble tablet or commercial oral liquid available*	*Tablet/capsule contents may disperse sufficiently for 8Fr NG tube*[a,b]	*Oral liquid can be prepared by local pharmacy or special order*	*Injection can be diluted and administered PO or by EFT*	*Comments*
Co-phenotrope	No	Yes (Lomotil® takes 5min)			
Co-trimoxazole	Yes				Commercial oral liquid (Septrin®) contains sorbitol and needs diluting 3 times to reduce viscosity for EFT use
Cyclizine	No	Yes (Valoid® takes 5min)	Yes[c]	Yes	
Cyproterone	No		Yes[d]		Tablets disperse but no information on suitability by EFT
Dantrolene	No		Yes[d]	No	Injection formulation may hydrolyse in the stomach. Capsule contents disperse but no information on suitability by EFT
Demeclocycline	No	No			Capsule contents are irritant and only sparingly soluble. Absorption is reduced by calcium
Desmopressin	No	Yes (Desmotabs, DDAVP® takes 5min)			DDAVP Melt® for SL use only, not for EFT administration
Dexamethasone	Yes	Yes (Organon)	Yes[d]	Yes	Commercial oral liquid contains sorbitol 500microgram/5mL
Diamorphine	No		Yes		
Diazepam	Yes	Yes (APS)	Yes[d,e]	Yes	Dilute commercial oral liquid with an equal volume of water to reduce viscosity and risk of binding to the EFT. Disperse tablets for intrajejunal administration. Anecdotal evidence of using injection enterally; drug loss may occur due to binding to tube

continued

Table 22.2 Continued

Drug	*Soluble tablet or commercial oral liquid available*	*Tablet/capsule contents may disperse sufficiently for 8Fr NG tube*[a,b]	*Oral liquid can be prepared by local pharmacy or special order*	*Injection can be diluted and administered PO or by EFT*	*Comments*
Diclofenac[a]	No	Yes (dispersible)	Yes[e]		Use commercially available dispersible tablet for EFT. Alternative unlicensed 10mg dispersible tablets or 50mg/5mL oral liquid (1 year shelf-life) available
Dicycloverine	Yes				Dilute oral liquid with an equal volume of water for EFT use
Digoxin	Yes				In theory 50microgram Lanoxin® oral liquid = 62.5microgram tablet, however in practice unlikely to be clinically important, monitor plasma concentrations if changing formulation or using a high-fibre feed. Commercial oral liquid may cause diarrhoea. Lanoxin® tablets disperse but no information on suitability by EFT
Dihydrocodeine[a]	Yes				Dilute oral liquid with an equal volume of water for EFT use
Docusate sodium	Yes				Dilute oral liquid with an equal volume of water for EFT use
Domperidone	Yes	Yes (Co-Pharma, CP)	Yes[d]		Dilute oral liquid with an equal volume of water for EFT use. Contains sorbitol 2.3g/5mL. Consider dispersing tablets for intrajejunal administration
Doxepin	No	Yes (Sinepin®)			
Doxycycline	No	Yes (dispersible)			Use dispersible tablets, do not open capsules as contents are irritant
Erythromycin[a]	Yes	No			Dilute oral liquid with an equal volume of water for EFT use, some brands contain sorbitol. Tablets and capsule contents are e/c therefore not suitable for EFT
Esomeprazole	No	Yes (Nexium®)			Nexium® is licensed for administration via a gastric tube. The tablet contains a compressed core of e/c microgranules which can be dispersed and flushed via an 8Fr gauge NG tube. Do not crush. Strictly follow the procedure in the SPC to prevent tube blockage

continued

Table 22.2 Continued

Drug	*Soluble tablet or commercial oral liquid available*	*Tablet/capsule contents may disperse sufficiently for 8Fr NG tube*[a,b]	*Oral liquid can be prepared by local pharmacy or special order*	*Injection can be diluted and administered PO or by EFT*	*Comments*
Etamsylate	No		Yes[d]		
Ferrous sulphate	No	No		No	Convert to an alternative iron salt oral liquid preparation. Ferrous sulphate 200mg = 3.3mL Niferex® *or* 7mL Fersamal® / Galfer® *or* 12mL Sytron® (contains sorbitol 2g/5mL) *or* 13mL Plesmet®; dilute with an equal volume of water for EFT use
Flecainide	No	Yes (Generics)	Yes[c,e]	Yes	Use de-ionized/sterile water, *not tap water*. Note crushed tablets have a local anaesthetic effect. *Do not* dilute the injection or mix with alkaline solutions, e.g. chlorides, phosphates, sulphates
Flucloxacillin	Yes	No		Yes (Berk, CP)	Dilute commercial oral liquid with an equal volume of water for EFT use. Stop feed for 1h before and after dose. Avoid opening capsules due to risk of sensitization
Fluconazole	Yes	Yes (50mg capsule)	Yes[d]	No	Do not use the 150mg capsule contents
Fludrocortisone	No	Yes (Florinef®)			
Fluoxetine	Yes				Capsule contents can be dispersed but no information on suitability via EFT
Furosemide	Yes		Yes[d]		Commercial oral liquid is alkaline and may coagulate with other acidic preparations. Flush EFT well to avoid. Lasix® tablets disperse but no information on suitability via EFT
Gabapentin	No	Yes (Neurontin®)			
Glibenclamide	No	Yes (APS)	Yes[d]		Daonil® tablets disperse but no information on suitability via EFT

continued

Table 22.2 Continued

Drug	*Soluble tablet or commercial oral liquid available*	*Tablet/capsule contents may disperse sufficiently for 8Fr NG tube*[a,b]	*Oral liquid can be prepared by local pharmacy or special order*	*Injection can be diluted and administered PO or by EFT*	*Comments*
Gliclazide[a]	No	Yes (Alpharma, CP, Generics) takes 5min	Yes[d]		When administering dispersed tablets by EFT, there may be residue left in the syringe, which is unlikely to be active drug due to high solubility. Flush EFT well to avoid blockage
Glycopyrronium	No	Yes[e]	Yes[e]	Yes	Tablets disperse coarsely and may leave sediment. A 1mg/mL and 1mg/5mL unlicensed formulation are available. A 1mg/10mL solution can be made from glycopyrronium powder (see p.11). Cost of bulk powder may be prohibitive
Granisetron	No	Yes (Kytril®) takes 5min	Yes[f]	Yes	250microgram/5mL suspension can be prepared[f,29]
Haloperidol	Yes				Dilute oral liquid with an equal volume of water. Serenace® tablets disperse but no information on suitability by EFT
Hydrocortisone	No	Yes (MSD)		Yes (Efcortesol®)	Injection contains significant amounts of phosphate
Hydromorphone[a]	No				Do not administer contents of m/r capsules by EFT due to high risk of blockage
Hyoscine *butylbromide*	No	No		Yes	Injection may be stored for 24h in a refrigerator once opened
Hyoscine *hydrobromide*	No			Yes	
Ibuprofen[a]	Yes	No			Commercial oral liquid contains sorbitol 500microgram/5mL, dilute with an equal volume of water (more for intrajejunal administration) to reduce viscosity for EFT use

continued

Table 22.2 Continued

Drug	*Soluble tablet or commercial oral liquid available*	*Tablet/capsule contents may disperse sufficiently for 8Fr NG tube*[a,b]	*Oral liquid can be prepared by local pharmacy or special order*	*Injection can be diluted and administered PO or by EFT*	*Comments*
Imipramine	No		Yes[c]		Tofranil® disperse but particles may be too large for EFT use
Ispaghula husk					Do not administer due to high risk of blockage, consider using a high-fibre feed
Itraconazole	Yes				Stop the feed for 2h before and after dose. Commercial oral liquid contains sorbitol and is acidic. Flush EFT well to avoid coagulation. Absorption via jejunum may be reduced
Ketamine	No		Yes	Yes	A 50mg/5mL oral solution using the injection formulation can be prepared by pharmacy, 7 day shelf-life (see p.593)
Ketoconazole	No	Yes (Nizoral®)	Yes[f]		Stop feed for 0.5h before and 2h after dose. Jejunal administration not recommended; low pH needed for absorption. A 100mg/5mL suspension can be prepared[f,29]
Ketorolac	No	Yes (Toradol®) takes 5min			
Lactulose	Yes				Dilute commercial oral liquid with 2–3 times volume of water
Lamotrigine	No	Yes	Yes[d,f]		Use commercially available dispersible tablet. A 5mg/5mL suspension can be prepared[f,29]
Lansoprazole	No	Yes	Yes		Add commercially available orodispersible tablet (FasTab®) to 10mL of water and administer by EFT using a push-pull technique to keep the granules suspended. *Do not crush.* For tubes smaller than 8Fr, open capsules and mix e/c granules with 10mL of 8.4% sodium bicarbonate, (14 day shelf-life in a refrigerator if locally prepared by pharmacy)[l]

continued

Table 22.2 Continued

Drug	*Soluble tablet or commercial oral liquid available*	*Tablet/capsule contents may disperse sufficiently for 8Fr NG tube*[a,b]	*Oral liquid can be prepared by local pharmacy or special order*	*Injection can be diluted and administered PO or by EFT*	*Comments*
Levomepromazine	No	Yes (Nozinan®)	Yes[d]	Yes	Tablet dispersion is coarse and may block tubes smaller than 8Fr
Lofepramine	Yes				Dilute oral liquid with an equal volume of water for EFT use; contains sorbitol 1.4g/5mL
Loperamide	Yes				Oral solution contains alcohol
Loratadine	Yes				Dilute oral liquid with an equal volume of water for jejunal administration to reduce osmolarity
Lorazepam	No	No	Yes[d]		Tablets do not disperse easily. Tablets (Genus brand) and injection can be used sublingually
Macrogols	Yes				May not be suitable for EFT use due to the large volume required to dissolve the powder
Magnesium glycerophosphate	No		Yes[e]		Unlicensed oral liquid 1mmol/mL available. Various unlicensed tablets available, some will disperse but no information on suitability by EFT
Mebeverine[a]	Yes				135mg tablet = 15mL oral liquid 50mg/5mL. Most effective when given 20min before food
Medroxy-progesterone acetate	No	Yes (Provera® 5mg, 100mg) takes 5min	Yes[d]		Farlutal® 500mg tablets disperse but no information on suitability by EFT
Megestrol acetate	No	Yes (Megace®) takes 5min	Yes[d,e]		
Menadiol sodium phosphate	No		Yes[d]		Tablets disperse but no information on suitability by EFT

continued

Table 22.2 Continued

Drug	*Soluble tablet or commercial oral liquid available*	*Tablet/capsule contents may disperse sufficiently for 8Fr NG tube*[a,b]	*Oral liquid can be prepared by local pharmacy or special order*	*Injection can be diluted and administered PO or by EFT*	*Comments*
Metformin[a]	Yes	Yes (Glucophage® sachets)	Yes[d]		Sachets disperse fully in 20mL of water for EFT, (manufacturer recommends 150mL for PO use)
Methadone	Yes				No information on suitability via EFT
Methyl-prednisolone	No	Yes (Medrone®)			
Metoclopramide[a]	Yes			Yes	Dilute oral liquid with an equal volume of water for intrajejunal administration to reduce osmolarity, some liquids may contain sorbitol. Maxolon® tablets disperse but no information on suitability by EFT
Metronidazole	Yes	No	Yes		Dilute commercial oral liquid with an equal volume of water for NG use and stop feed for 1h before the dose to allow gastric pH to recover to metabolize the benzoate salt. The benzoate salt is metabolized in the stomach, therefore *not* suitable for jejunal use. A 50mg/mL suspension with cherry syrup can be prepared (60 day shelf-life);[1] it does not require a break in feeding and is more suitable for intrajejunal administration
Midazolam	No			Yes	Solution for *buccal* use available from specials manufacturers. Injection can be used via PO, buccal, intranasal and PR routes[30]
Mirtazapine	Yes	No			Commercial orodispersible tablets (Zispin SolTab®) not recommended for EFT use because too granular; use commercial oral liquid
Misoprostol	No	No			

continued

Table 22.2 Continued

Drug	*Soluble tablet or commercial oral liquid available*	*Tablet/capsule contents may disperse sufficiently for 8Fr NG tube*[a,b]	*Oral liquid can be prepared by local pharmacy or special order*	*Injection can be diluted and administered PO or by EFT*	*Comments*
Moclobemide	No	Yes (APS) takes 5 min			
Morphine[a]	Yes				Commerical oral liquid can be used; 10mg/5mL contains alcohol. Dilute with an equal volume of water, or use unit dose vials for intrajejunal administration to reduce osmolarity. The m/r granules in Zomorph® capsules are licensed for gastric administration via a 16Fr tube (internal diameter 2.5mm) with an open distal end or lateral pores (see SPC). Certain tubes have been found to cause problems.[g] The m/r granules should be mixed (*do not crush*) with 30mL water. Take great care to ensure that all the m/r granules are administered and are not crushed with the syringe plunger. Add extra water if necessary. There is some anecdotal data on using 8Fr tubes.[1] The m/r granules in MST Continus® suspension sachets have been administered as above in tubes with 8Fr gauge or minimum internal diameter 1.05mm. The m/r granules in Morcap SR® capsules have been administered as above via 16Fr gastric tubes.[26] The granules will block tubes 12Fr gauge or smaller. The m/r granules in MXL® capsules are *not* suitable for EFT administration[28]
Nabilone	No				The capsule contents disperse but no information on suitability by EFT
Nabumetone	Yes	No			Commercial oral liquid contains sorbitol 1.25mg/5mL
Naproxen[a]	No				Naprosyn® and Synflex® disperse but no information on suitability by EFT

continued

Table 22.2 Continued

Drug	*Soluble tablet or commercial oral liquid available*	*Tablet/capsule contents may disperse sufficiently for 8Fr NG tube*[a,b]	*Oral liquid can be prepared by local pharmacy or special order*	*Injection can be diluted and administered PO or by EFT*	*Comments*
Nefopam	No	Yes (Acupan®) takes 3–4min			High risk of sediment when dispersing tablets, may not be suitable for EFT
Nifedipine[a]	No		Yes[f]		Consider an alternative product e.g. amlodipine. Drawing up contents of liquid capsules *not* recommended, volumes vary between manufacturers, liquid is light sensitive, and risk of profound hypotension, particularly if converting from m/r preparation. A 20mg/5mL suspension can be prepared using capsule contents[f,29]
Nitrazepam	Yes		Yes[e]		Dilute commercial oral liquid to reduce osmolality for intrajejunal use
Nitrofurantoin[a]	Yes	Yes (Alpharma, APS) takes 5min	Yes[d]		Dilute commercial oral liquid with an equal volume of water for EFT use
Olanzapine	No	Yes (Zyprexa Velotab®)			
Omeprazole	No	Yes (Alpharma or Dexcel tablets)	Yes	Yes	A 2mg/mL formulation with 20mg capsule contents and 10mL 8.4% sodium bicarbonate can be prepared by pharmacy (45 day shelf-life in a refrigerator).[l] Commercially available orodispersible tablet (Losec MUPS®) can be added to 25mL of water and administered by EFT using a push-pull technique to keep the granules suspended. *Do not crush*. Suitable for 8Fr gauge. Commercially available *tablets* (Alpharma, Dexcel) disperse in 5min, larger doses may be required in gastric administration as this method destroys the e/c coating. Contact Astra Zeneca for details of use of injection or infusion via EFT

continued

Table 22.2 Continued

Drug	*Soluble tablet or commercial oral liquid available*	*Tablet/capsule contents may disperse sufficiently for 8Fr NG tube*[a,b]	*Oral liquid can be prepared by local pharmacy or special order*	*Injection can be diluted and administered PO or by EFT*	*Comments*
Ondansetron	Yes			Yes	Commercial oral liquid contains sorbitol 3g/5mL. Zofran® tablets disperse but no information on suitability by EFT or of the commercially available orodispersible tablet (Zofran Melt®). The injection is acidic, flush well to avoid coagulation with feed
Orphenadrine	Yes		Yes[c]		Commercial oral liquids contain sorbitol, 0.45g/5mL (Rosemont) and 1.75g/5ml (Biorphen®). Disipal® tablets disperse but no information on suitability by EFT
Oxybutynin[a]	Yes	Yes (Tillomed) takes 5min	Yes[d,e]		Commercial oral liquid contains sorbitol 1.3g/5mL. Ditropan® may disperse but no information on suitability by EFT. Cystrin® may leave sediment and be unsuitable for EFT use. Transdermal patch available
Oxycodone[a]	Yes				Significant anecdotal reports of use of liquid preparation by EFT
Paracetamol	Yes	Yes (dispersible/ effervescent)			Add commercially available dispersible tablet to 50mL of water; consider sodium content
Paroxetine	Yes				Dilute oral liquid with an equal volume of water for EFT use, contains sorbitol
Phenobarbital	Yes		Yes[d,e,f]		Commercially available elixir contains alcohol 38%. An unlicensed alcohol-free preparation can be obtained. Tablets may disperse but no information on suitability by EFT. A Phenobarbital 50mg/5mL suspension can be prepared[f,29] Dilute oral liquids with an equal volume of water for intrajejunal administration to reduce osmolarity
Phenoxymethyl-penicillin	Yes				Stop feed for 2h before and 1h after dose

continued

Table 22.2 Continued

Drug	*Soluble tablet or commercial oral liquid available*	*Tablet/capsule contents may disperse sufficiently for 8Fr NG tube*[a,b]	*Oral liquid can be prepared by local pharmacy or special order*	*Injection can be diluted and administered PO or by EFT*	*Comments*
Phenytoin	Yes	Yes (Epanutin® capsules) takes 5min	Yes[e]		Stop feed for 2h before and after dose and flush tube with 50mL water to minimize interaction with feed. Convert to once daily dose. Phenytoin *base* 30mg/5mL oral suspension (Epanutin®); 90mg (15mL) = 100mg phenytoin *sodium* tablet/capsule, shake liquid well, then dilute dose with 30–50mL water, administer and flush. An unlicensed concentrated oral liquid 90mg/5mL is available. Epanutin® capsule contents will disperse after 5min. Monitor plasma levels and adhere to a consistent protocol. Jejunal absorption is poor
Phytomenadione	No			Yes (Konakion MM®)	The injection is incompatible with certain types of siliconized syringes. Braun syringes are known to be compatible
Piroxicam	No				Add commercially available dispersible tablet (Feldene Melt®) to 50mL water, no information on suitability by EFT
Pilocarpine	No		Yes		
Potassium supplements[a]	Yes	Yes (effervescent)			Flush EFT well to prevent physical interaction with feed. Add effervescent tablets to 50mL water. Commercial oral liquid contains sorbitol 2g/5mL and may cause diarrhoea, dilute with 50–100mL water, not recommended for intrajejunal administration
Prednisolone[a]	Yes	No	Yes[d]		
Pregabalin	No	Yes (Lyrica® capsules)			

continued

Table 22.2 Continued

Drug	*Soluble tablet or commercial oral liquid available*	*Tablet/capsule contents may disperse sufficiently for 8Fr NG tube*[a,b]	*Oral liquid can be prepared by local pharmacy or special order*	*Injection can be diluted and administered PO or by EFT*	*Comments*
Prochlorperazine	Yes	Yes (APS, Meridian)			Dilute commercial oral liquid with an equal volume of water for EFT use. Use effervescent granules or disperse tablets for intrajejunal administration. Stemetil® tablets disperse but no information on use by EFT
Promethazine	Yes	Yes (Phenergan®) takes 5min			Dilute commercial oral liquid with an equal volume of water for EFT use
Propantheline	No		Yes[e]		
Ranitidine	Yes	Yes (effervescent)	Yes[d]	Yes	Add effervescent tablets to 30mL water, consider sodium content. Commercial oral liquid contains alcohol 8% and sorbitol
Rifampicin	Yes		Yes[f]		Stop feed for 2h before and 30min after dose. Dilute commercial oral liquid with equal volume of water. Do not open capsules; risk of contact sensitization. A 125mg/5mL suspension can be prepared (7 day shelf-life)[f,29]
Risperidone	Yes	Yes (Risperdal®) takes 5min			No information on suitability of orodispersible tablets (Quicklet®) via EFT
Senna	Yes		Yes[d]		Granules not suitable for administration by EFT
Sertraline	No	Yes (Lustral®) takes 5min	Yes[e]		Coarse tablet dispersion may block tube, consider alternative drug. Note crushed tablets have a local anaesthetic effect
Sodium clodronate	No	Yes (Bonefos®)			Stop feed for 1h before and after dose. Both capsule contents and tablets disperse in water
Sodium fusidate	Yes				Sodium fusidate tablets 500mg = 750mg oral suspension. Commercial oral liquid contains sorbitol

continued

Table 22.2 Continued

Drug	*Soluble tablet or commercial oral liquid available*	*Tablet/capsule contents may disperse sufficiently for 8Fr NG tube*[a,b]	*Oral liquid can be prepared by local pharmacy or special order*	*Injection can be diluted and administered PO or by EFT*	*Comments*
Sodium valproate[a]	Yes	Yes (Epilim® Crushable) takes 5min		No	Dilute commerical oral liquid with an equal volume of water for EFT use. Some formulations contain sorbitol. Consider dispersing crushable tablets for intrajejunal administration or dilute oral liquid 3–4 times
Spironolactone	No	Yes (Most generics, Aldactone®) takes 5min	Yes[d,e,f]		Dilute commercial oral liquid with an equal volume of water for EFT use. Disperse tablet for intrajejunal administration. A 125mg/5mL suspension can be prepared.[c] Other suspension formulae are also available[29]
Sucralfate	Yes				Do not use sucralfate via EFT. Commercial oral liquid *not* recommended due to high viscosity, bezoar formation and binding with feed; likely to block tube. Need to stop feed for 1h before and after dose; impractical for q4h schedule
Temazepam	Yes				Commercial oral liquid contains sorbitol
Tetracycline	No		Yes[f]		A 125mg/5mL suspension can be prepared (7day shelf-life)[f,29]
Theophylline[a]	No		Yes[e]		Convert total daily dose of m/r preparations to oral *unlicensed* liquid and split into t.d.s. regimen. Stop feed for 1h before and 1h after dose. Dilute oral liquid with an equal volume of water. Monitor plasma levels closely. The m/r granules of Slo-phyllin® capsules can be administered via EFT, although may block smaller tubes. Take care not to crush. There is some information on giving aminophylline injection orally[l]
Tolbutamide	No	No	Yes[d]		

continued

Table 22.2 Continued

Drug	*Soluble tablet or commercial oral liquid available*	*Tablet/capsule contents may disperse sufficiently for 8Fr NG tube*[a,b]	*Oral liquid can be prepared by local pharmacy or special order*	*Injection can be diluted and administered PO or by EFT*	*Comments*
Topiramate	No	Yes (Topamax® tablets) takes 5min			Do not use Topamax® Sprinkle capsules by EFT as the beads stick to the tube causing blockage
Tramadol[a]	No	Yes (Ranbaxy capsules, Zydol® soluble, Zamadol Melt®)	Yes[f]		Use commercially available dispersible tablets. Zydol® capsule contents may disperse but no information on suitability by EFT. A 25mg/5mL suspension can be prepared[f,29]
Tranexamic acid	No	Yes (Cyklokapron®, Manx)	Yes[d]	Yes	
Trimethoprim	Yes		Yes[d]		Administer the dose during a break in feeding if practical. Dilute commercial oral liquid with an equal volume of water for EFT use, some formulations contain sorbitol
Vancomycin	No	No		Yes	Use reconstituted injection orally (24h shelf-life time in fridge for enteral use). Vancocin® is licensed for NG tube use
Venlafaxine[a]	No	Yes (Efexor®) takes 5 min			
Warfarin	Yes	Yes	Yes[d]		Stop feed for 1h before and 1–2h after dose. INR may be affected by the varying content of vitamin K in feeds
Zinc	No	Yes (effervescent)			Add effervescent tablet to 10mL water. Jejunal administration may reduce bioavailability

a. do not use m/r or e/c preparations unless specifically indicated. Take care if converting from m/r to normal-release preparations because dose, frequency and clinical effect may be different
b. use the brand or manufacturer specified; different brands may not disperse equivalently
c. a simple suspension using Diluent C suspending agent can be prepared by some local pharmacies with a 7 day shelf-life
d. a simple suspension using Keltrol (Diluent A) suspending agent can be prepared by some local pharmacies with a 7 day shelf-life
e. unlicensed product, available from 'specials' manufacturers or imported (see Obtaining unlicensed products, p.769)
f. a simple suspension using 1:1 mixture of Ora-Plus and Ora-Sweet as a vehicle can be prepared by some local pharmacies, 28 day shelf-life unless otherwise stated[29]
g. tubes which should *not* be used for administration of Zomorph® capsules include; Mallinkrodt enral 205-09-1, Bioser 1147221, Vygon 39110 and Vygon 2395.09. Tubes known to be successful in administering Zomorph® capsules include Pharma Plast LEVIN CH/FG 18, Vygon 391.16, Ventrol 15016IT 85753, Ventrol 82316 16A, Bioser 1147239 and Sherwood 90L100A.

1 White R and Bradnam V (2010) *Handbook of Drug Administration via Enteral Feeding Tubes* (2e). Pharmaceutical Press, London.
2 Williams NT (2008) Medication administration through enteral feeding tubes. *American Journal of Health-System Pharmacy.* **65**: 2347–2357.
3 BAPEN (British Association of Parenteral and Enteral Nutrition) (2004) Administering drugs via enteral feeding tubes. A practical guide. BAPEN. Available from: www.bapen.org.uk/res_drugs.html
4 NPSA (National Patient Safety Agency) (2007) Promoting safter measurement and administration of liquid medicines via oral and other enteral routes. In: *Patient safety alert 19.* Available from: www.npsa.nhs.uk/public/alerts
5 NPSA (National Patient Safety Agency) (2011) Reducing the harm caused by misplaced nasogastric feeding tubes in adults and infants. In: Patient safety alert 002 and supporting information. Available from: www.npsa.nhs.uk
6 UKMI (2009) Therapeutic options for patients unable to take solid oral dosage forms. 294.1. In: *Drugs Q&As*. Available from: www.nelm.nhs.uk
7 Jackson LD *et al.* (2008) Safe medication swallowing in dysphagia: a collaborative improvement project. *Healthcare Quarterly.* **11**: 110–116.
8 Adams D (1994) Administration of drugs through a jejunostomy tube. *British Journal of Intensive Care.* **4**: 10–17.
9 Thomson F *et al.* (2000) Enteral and parenteral nutrition. *Hospital Pharmacist.* **7**: 155–164.
10 Gilbar P (1999) A guide to drug administration in palliative care (review). *Journal of Pain and Symptom Management.* **17**: 197–207.
11 Royal Pharmaceutical Society of Great Britain (2010) Good Practice Guidance on the procurement and supply of pharmaceutical specials. Available from: www.rpharms.com
12 Schier JG *et al.* (2003) Fatality from administration of labetalol and crushed extended-release nifedipine. *Annals of Pharmacotherapy.* **37**: 1420–1423.
13 Cornish P (2005) "Avoid the crush": hazards of medication administration in patients with dysphagia or a feeding tube. *Canadian Medical Association Journal.* **172**: 871–872.
14 Wright DN *et al.* (2006) Consensus guideline on the medication management of adults with swallowing difficulties. *Guidelines London Connect Medical.*
15 Sanofi Aventis (2008) *Medical information. Data on file.*
16 Phillips NM and Nay R (2008) A systematic review of nursing administration of medication via enteral tubes in adults. *Journal of Clinical Nursing.* **17**: 2257–2265.
17 Baxter K (2011) Stockley's Drug Interactions (online edition). Pharmaceutical Press, London. Available from: www.medicinescomplete.com
18 Schmidt LE and Dalhoff K (2002) Food-drug interactions. *Drugs.* **62**. 1481–1502.
19 Engle KK and Hannawa TE (1999) Techniques for administering oral medications to critical care patients receiving continuous enteral nutrition. *American Journal of Health System Pharmacy.* **56**: 1441–1444.
20 Clark-Schmidt AL *et al.* (1990) Loss of carbamazepine suspension through nasogastric feeding tubes. *American Journal of Hospital Pharmacy.* **47**: 2034–2037.
21 Freeman KL and Trezevant MS (2009) Interaction between liquid protein solution and omeprazole suspension. *American Journal of Health System Pharmacy.* **66**: 1901–1902.
22 Garcia-Luna PP *et al.* (1997) Esophageal obstruction by solidification of the enteral feed: a complication to be prevented. *Intensive Care Medicine.* **23**: 790–792.
23 Chugai Pharma UK (2010) Summary of product characteristics for Antepsin suspension. Available from: www.medicines.org.uk accessed 15/11/2010
24 Wohlt PD *et al.* (2009) Recommendations for the use of medications with continuous enteral nutrition. *American Journal of Health System Pharmacy.* **66**: 1458–1467.
25 Marcuard SP and Stegall KS (1990) Unclogging feeding tubes with pancreatic enzyme. *Journal of Parenteral Enteral Nutrition.* **14**: 198–200.
26 Jones R *et al.* (1996) 'Kapanol' capsules:pellet formulation provides alternative methods of administration of sustained-release morphine sulphate. *Clinical drug investigations.* **12**: 88–93.
27 Nottingham City Hospital NHS Trust Pharmacy (1998) Administering drugs to patients by artifical enteral methods. Data on file.
28 Palliativedrugs.com (2003) July Newsletter. Available from: www.palliativedrugs.com
29 Smyth J (2010) *The NEWT guidelines for administration of medication to patients with enteral feeding tubes or swallowing difficulties* (2e). Pharmacy Department, North East Wales NHS Trust.
30 BNF for Children (2010–2011). Available from: www.bnfc.org

23: NEBULIZED DRUGS

Nebulizers are used in asthma and COPD for both acute exacerbations and long-term prophylaxis (see Bronchodilators, p.97).[1–3] Other uses include the pulmonary delivery of antimicrobial drugs for cystic fibrosis, bronchiectasis and AIDS-related pneumonia. Nebulizers are also used in palliative care (see below). The aim is to deliver a therapeutic dose of a drug as an aerosol in particles small enough to be inspired within 5–10min. A nebulizer is preferable to a hand-held metered dose inhaler (MDI) when:

- a large drug dose is needed
- co-ordinated breathing is difficult
- MDIs + a spacer are ineffective
- a drug is unavailable in an inhaler.

By improving drug delivery, a nebulizer can result in better symptom relief.[4] However, nebulizers are noisy, more expensive and less convenient than an MDI; they are also ineffective in patients with shallow breathing, and if unable to sit semi-upright or more. The higher doses administered also increase the risk of undesirable effects and use should be carefully monitored to ensure ongoing efficacy and tolerability. Commonly used nebulizers are:

Jet: the aerosol is generated by a flow of gas from, for example, an electrical compressor or an oxygen cylinder. At least 50% of the aerosol produced at the recommended driving gas flow should be particles small enough to inhale.

Ultrasonic: the aerosol is generated by ultrasonic vibrations of a piezo-electric crystal.

Aerosol output (the mass of particles in aerosol form produced/min) is not necessarily the same as drug output (the mass of drug produced/min as an aerosol). Ideally, the drug output should be known for each drug given. Various factors affect the drug output and deposition:

- gas flow rate (generally air at 6–8L/min but oxygen if treating acute asthma)
- chamber design
- volume (commonly 2–2.5mL, up to 4mL)
- residual volume (commonly 0.5mL)
- physical properties of the drug in solution
- breathing pattern of the patient.

The choice of nebulizer can be crucial, particularly when trying to produce an aerosol small enough to deliver a drug to the alveoli. Services which provide nebulizers will generally offer information, education and support for patients (Box 23.A). Information should include:

- a description of the equipment and its use
- drugs used, doses and frequencies
- equipment maintenance/cleaning
- action to take if treatment becomes less effective
- action to take and emergency telephone number to use if equipment breaks down.

Patients should be instructed to take steady normal breaths (interspersed with occasional deep ones) and nebulization time should be less than 10min or 'to dryness'. Because there is always a residual volume, 'dryness' should be taken as 1min after spluttering starts. In general, whereas a mask can be used for bronchodilators, a mouthpiece should be used for other drugs to limit environmental contamination and/or contact with the patient's eyes. However, a mask may be preferable in patients who are acutely ill, fatigued or very young, regardless of the nature of the drug.

Nebulizers in palliative care

A number of drugs have been given by nebulizer to ease cough and breathlessness in advanced cancer (Table 23.1 and Table 23.2). However, apart from the use of bronchodilators for reversible airflow obstruction, it should be noted that there is often little evidence to support such use.

Box 23.A Advice about using a nebulizer at home

To help your breathing, your doctor has prescribed a drug to be used with a nebulizer. The nebulizer converts the drug into a fine mist which you inhale.

The apparatus

Your nebulizer system consists of the following parts:

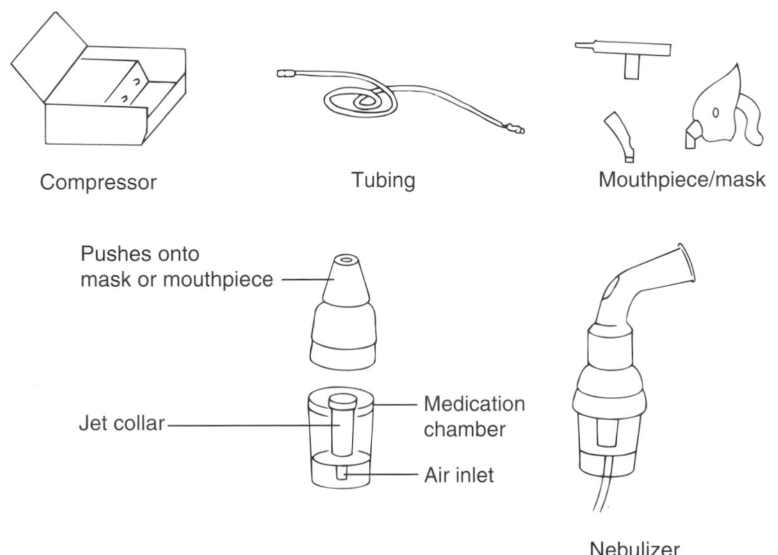

The compressor is the portable pump which pumps air along the tubing into the nebulizer. The nebulizer is a small chamber for the liquid medicine, through which air is blown to make a mist.

The nebulizer has a screw-on top onto which the mask or mouthpiece is attached.

How to use your nebulizer

Place the medication in the nebulizer, replace the screw-on top and turn the compressor on. Inhale by mouthpiece or mask while breathing at a normal rate. Stop 1 minute after the nebulizer contents start spluttering or after a maximum of 10 minutes.

General advice

If you have a cough, the nebulizer may help you to expectorate, so have some tissues nearby. You may wish to use the nebulizer before attempting an activity which makes you feel out of breath.

If the effects of the nebulizer wear off or you have any questions or concerns about it, please speak to your doctor or nurse.

Cleaning

Wash the mouthpiece/mask and nebulizer in warm water and detergent, then rinse and dry well. Ideally this should be done after every use, but *once a day as a minimum*. Attach the tube and run the nebulizer empty for a few moments after cleaning it to make sure the equipment is dry. Once a week, unplug and wipe the compressor and tubing with a damp cloth.

Table 23.1 Nebulized drugs and cancer-related cough or breathlessness[2,13]

Class of drug	*Indications*	*Scientific evidence*	*Comments*
0.9% saline	Loosening of tenacious secretions	None	Probably underused in this setting; may also help breathlessness
Mucolytic agents e.g. hypertonic saline, acetylcysteine	To thin viscous sputum	Conflicting evidence	May result in copious liquid sputum which the patient may still not be able to cough up
Corticosteroids e.g. budesonide	Stridor, lymphangitis, radiation pneumonitis, cough after the insertion of a stent	None	Very limited clinical experience only; may not be more beneficial than use of inhaler or oral routes
Local anaesthetics e.g. lidocaine, bupivacaine	Cough, particularly if caused by lymphangitis carcinomatosa	Conflicting evidence for both breathlessness[14,15] and cough[16]	Risk of bronchospasm; reduces gag reflex[5,6]
Opioids e.g. morphine, fentanyl	Breathlessness associated with diffuse lung disease	Despite supportive anecdotal evidence,[17] a systematic review indicates no advantage compared with 0.9% saline[18]	Not recommended; risk of bronchospasm
Bronchodilators e.g. salbutamol	Treatment of severe reversible airway obstruction	Extrapolated from patients with asthma and COPD	Try MDI + spacer first.[19,20] Use nebulizers only if trial of therapy shows real benefit
Furosemide	Breathlessness	Despite anecdotal reports of benefit (see Furosemide, p.55), an RCT was not supportive of its use[21]	Not recommended

Table 23.2 Recommended uses of nebulized drugs in palliative care

Indication	*Drug*	*Initial regimen*	*Dose titration*	*Comments*
Tenacious secretions	Saline 0.9%	5mL q6h	Up to q2h	
Reversible airway obstruction	Salbutamol	2.5mg q6h–q4h	Up to 5mg q4h	Risk of sensitivity to cardiac stimulant effects
Cough	*†Lidocaine 2%	5mL p.r.n.	Up to q6h	Risk of bronchospasm; fast for 1h after nebulization
	*†Bupivacaine 0.25%	5mL p.r.n.	Up to q8h	

Thus, some drugs are not recommended by *PCF* for routine use; the remainder should be considered only when other avenues have failed, and reviewed after 2 days to check effectiveness (Table 23.1 and Table 23.2).

When using **lidocaine** or **bupivacaine** for a dry cough (not recommended for breathlessness), in patients with asthma, pretreat with **salbutamol** because of the risk of initial bronchospasm.[5,6] After treatment with a local anaesthetic, patients should be advised not to eat or drink for 1h because the reduced gag/cough reflex increases the risk of aspiration (also see Antitussives, p.128).

Because of lack of data, e.g. physio-chemical compatibility, and aerodynamic properties, manufacturers generally do not recommend mixing nebulizer solutions; thus most mixtures are off-label. However: [7–12]

- some ready-mixed combinations are commercially available, e.g. **salbutamol** + **ipratropium bromide** (generic and Combivent®)
- there are limited data indicating that 2-drug mixtures comprising one drug from any two of the classes below will be physically and chemically compatible (for all strengths):
  - ▷ *β_2-adrenergic receptor agonists (β_2 agonists)*, **salbutamol** (Ventolin® nebules) or **terbutaline** (Bricanyl®)
  - ▷ *antimuscarinic*, **ipratropium bromide** (Atrovent®)
  - ▷ *corticosteroids*, **budesonide** (Pulmicort®) or **fluticasone** (Flixotide®)
- solutions should be mixed immediately before use, using aseptic technique; if colour changes or cloudiness/precipitation occur, the mixture should be discarded
- if dilution is necessary, sterile 0.9% saline is generally best.

There is no information on 3-drug mixtures, and these cannot be recommended.

1 The Nebulizer Project Group of the British Thoracic Society Standards of Care Committee (1997) Current best practice for nebuliser treatment. *Thorax.* **52 (suppl 2)**: s1–3.

2 European Respiratory Society (2001) Guidelines on the use of nebulizers. *European Respiratory Journal.* **18**: 228–242.

3 NICE (2010) Chronic obstructive pulmonary disease: management of chronic obstructive pulmonary disease in adults in primary and secondary care. London: National Clinical Guideline Centre. Available from: http://guidance.nice.org.uk/CG101/Guidance

4 Tashkin DP *et al.* (2007) Comparing COPD treatment: nebulizer, metered dose inhaler, and concomitant therapy. *American Journal of Medicine.* **120**: 435–441.

5 McAlpine L and Thomson N (1989) Lidocaine-induced bronchoconstriction in asthmatic patients. Relation to histamine airway responsiveness and effect of preservative. *Chest.* **96**: 1012–1015.

6 Groeben H *et al.* (2000) Combined lidocaine and salbutamol inhalation for airway anesthesia markedly protects against reflex bronchoconstriction. *Chest.* **118**: 509–515.

7 Woodland G (2009) Which commonly used nebuliser solutions are compatible? Medicines Q&As 100.4. Welsh Medicines Information Centre and UK Medicines Information. Available from: www.nelm.nhs.uk/en/NeLM-Area/Evidence/Medicines-Q–A/Which-nebuliser-solutions-are-compatible/

8 Roberts G and Rossi S (1993) Compatibility of nebuliser solutions. *Australian Journal of Hospital Pharmacy.* **23**: 35–37.

9 McKenzie JE and Cruz-Rivera M (2004) Compatibility of budesonide inhalation suspension with four nebulizing solutions. *Annals of Pharmacotherapy.* **38**: 967–972.

10 Burchett DK *et al.* (2010) Mixing and compatibility guide for commonly used aerosolized medications. *American Journal of Health System Pharmacy.* **67**: 227–230.

11 Joseph JC (1997) Compatibility of nebulizer solution admixtures. *Annals of Pharmacotherapy.* **31**: 487–489.

12 Harriman A-M *et al.* (1996) Can we mix nebuliser solutions? Stability of drug admixtures in solutions for nebulisation. *Pharmacy in Practice*. **Oct**: 347–348.
13 Ahmedzai S and Davis C (1997) Nebulised drugs in palliative care. *Thorax*. **52 (suppl 2)**: s75-s77.
14 Winning A *et al.* (1988) Ventilation and breathlessness on maximal exercise in patients with interstitial lung disease after local anaesthetic aerosol inhalation. *Clinical Science*. **74**: 275–281.
15 Wilcock A *et al.* (1994) Safety and efficacy of nebulized lignocaine in patients with cancer and breathlessness. *Palliative Medicine*. **8**: 35–38.
16 Gaze M *et al.* (1997) Pain relief and quality of life following radiotherapy for bone metastases: a randomised trial of two fractionation schedules. *Radiotherapy and Oncology*. **45**: 109–116.
17 Young IH *et al.* (1989) Effect of low dose nebulized morphine on exercise endurance in patients with chronic lung disease. *Thorax*. **44**: 387–390.
18 Jennings A *et al.* (2002) A systematic review of the use of opioids in the management of dyspnoea. *Thorax*. **57**: 939–944.
19 Congleton J and Muers MF (1995) The incidence of airflow obstruction in bronchial carcinoma, its relation to breathlessness, and response to bronchodilator therapy. *Respiratory Medicine*. **89**: 291–296.
20 Colacone A *et al.* (1993) A comparison of albuterol administered by metered dose inhaler (and holding chamber) or wet nebulizer in acute asthma. *Chest*. **104**: 835–841.
21 Wilcock A *et al.* (2008) Randomised, placebo-controlled trial of nebulised furosemide for breathlessness in patients with cancer. *Thorax*. **63**: 872–875.

24: PROLONGATION OF THE QT INTERVAL IN PALLIATIVE CARE

The QT interval has attained greater clinical significance since it became apparent that various factors which prolong the QT interval, particularly drugs, predispose to a potentially fatal ventricular arrhythmia, *torsade de pointes.*

An accurate diagnosis of *torsade de pointes* is important because its management differs from other forms of ventricular tachycardia. Indeed, conventional drug treatments for ventricular tachycardia can exacerbate the underlying electrochemical derangement and perpetuate *torsade de pointes.*

Palliative care clinicians caring for patients with cardiac disease, or using **methadone**, need to be particularly aware of this phenomenon.

The QT interval lies on the electrocardiograph (ECG) between the beginning of the QRS complex (which marks the start of ventricular depolarization) and the end of the T wave (which marks the end of ventricular repolarization) (Figure 24.1).

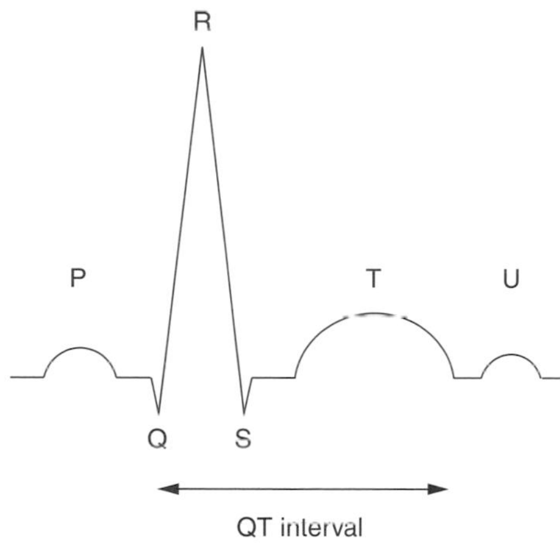

Figure 24.1 The QT interval.

The QT interval tends to be longer with slower heart rates. For comparative purposes, it is important to adjust ('correct') the observed QT interval to take account of this. The corrected value is designated QTc. Some ECG machines automatically calculate QTc, and this is a useful guide. However, automatic calculations can be inaccurate, particularly in the presence of atrial fibrillation, frequent ventricular ectopics, or a noisy trace. Thus, manual calculation of QTc is more accurate (Box 24.A).[1] There are several ways of doing this, and local practice varies.[1,2]

Box 24.A Measuring the QT interval and calculating QTc[1]

ECG

A 12-lead ECG at 25mm/sec at 10mm/mV amplitude is generally adequate.

Measure the QT interval together with the preceding RR interval in 3–5 heart beats from leads II and V5/V6.

Calculate the mean QT and RR interval from these 3–5 measurements.

Calculate QTc using one of the following formulas:

- Bazett's (exponential square root):

$$QTc = \frac{QT\,(sec)}{\sqrt{RR}\,(sec)}$$

- Fridericia's (exponential cube root):

$$QTc = \frac{QT\,(sec)}{\sqrt[3]{RR}\,(sec)}$$

Although Bazett's formula is the most widely used, Fridericia's may be more accurate at the extremes of heart rate.

Interpretation

QTc (msec)	*Male*	*Female*
Normal	<430	<450
Borderline	430–450	450–470
Abnormal	>450	>470

Note: These limits are to a certain extent arbitrary, and given a lack of international consensus, they vary between sources.

Obtain advice

Obtain cardiology advice if:

- the end of the T wave is difficult to determine, e.g. because of a U wave
- there is bundle branch block
- there is atrial fibrillation.

A prolonged QT interval is a pro-arrhythmic state associated with an increased risk of ventricular arrhythmia, particularly *torsade de pointes* (Figure 24.2); this is a form of polymorphic ventricular tachycardia of varying polarity which appears to wind around the baseline and hence its name. Short runs may cause palpitation, longer ones syncope (generally without warning) or seizure-like activity; it can settle spontaneously within seconds or degenerate into fatal ventricular fibrillation.[3]

Additional premonitory ECG signs of *torsade de pointes* include TU wave distortion (more exaggerated in a beat after a pause), T-wave alternans (marked alternate variation in size), new ventricular ectopics or couplets, and nonsustained polymorphic ventricular tachycardia initiated in the beat after a pause.[4]

Treatment includes cardioversion when haemodynamically compromised and **magnesium sulphate** IV (2g bolus followed by an infusion of 2–4mg/min).[3] The risk of *torsade de pointes* grows as the QT interval increases, particularly >500msec. A drug which leads to an increase in QTc interval of 20–60msec should also raise concern and, if by >60msec, serious concern about the risk of arrhythmia.[5]

Drugs prolong the QT interval mainly through potassium-channel blockade (particularly I_{Kr} 'rapid' subtype) by interfering with potassium currents in (enhanced) and out (reduced) of the cardiac myocytes, modifying their repolarization and prolonging the duration of the action potential.[6] The resulting dispersion of intramural repolarization may promote triggered activity and re-entry, the electrophysiological substrate for *torsade de pointes*. Several drugs have been

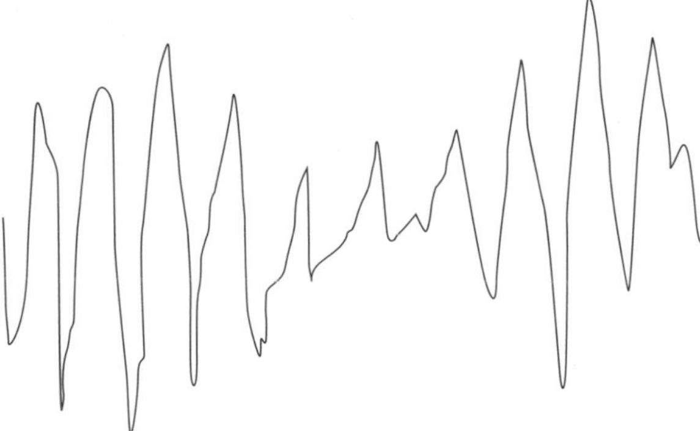

Figure 24.2 *Torsade de pointes*. Twisting complexes of ventricular tachycardia.

definitely linked with *torsade de pointes* (Box 24.B). Concerns about safety have resulted in certain drugs being withdrawn from the UK market, e.g. **astemizole**, **cisapride**, **terfenadine**, **thioridazine**.

The incidence of *torsade de pointes* is greatest with cardiac anti-arrhythmics, particularly those with class III activity. For some drugs, the risk is present only with:[7,8]

- high doses
- IV administration
- a pharmacokinetic drug interaction, e.g. **ketoconazole** inhibits CYP3A4 and thereby impairs the metabolism of **methadone** (see Cytochrome P450, p.735)
- impaired metabolism:
  - ▷ congenital, e.g. CYP2D6 poor metabolizers may be exposed to dangerously high plasma concentrations of risk-related drugs which are substrates for CYP2D6, even with normal doses
  - ▷ acquired, e.g. hepatic or renal impairment.

Thus, the degree of prolongation of the QT interval is not only dose-related. The risk of drug-induced *torsade de pointes* is increased by the concurrent use of two or more drugs which prolong the QT interval, and is more likely to occur in the presence of other risk factors (Box 24.C).[8] Some patients have a subclinical congenital long QT syndrome unmasked by a QT-prolonging drug.[3]

Box 24.B Drugs available in the UK associated with a prolonged QT interval and *torsade de pointes*[a]

Anti-arrhythmic drugs
Amiodarone
Disopyramide
Sotalol

Antimicrobial drugs
Macrolides
e.g. clarithromycin, erythromycin
Pentamidine

Antimalarial drugs
Chloroquine

Psychotropic drugs
Chlorpromazine
Droperidol
Haloperidol
Pimozide

Miscellaneous
Arsenic trioxide
Domperidone
Methadone
Saquinavir
Toremifene

a. see www.azcert.org for a longer list of drugs to be avoided by patients with congenital long QT syndrome. The website also includes other drugs which have been suspected of causing *torsade de pointes* but for which the evidence is inconclusive.

Box 24.C Main additional risk factors in drug-induced *torsade de pointes*

Female gender
Congenital long QT syndrome
Baseline prolonged QT interval
Electrolyte imbalance:
- hypokalaemia
- hypomagnesaemia

Cardiac disease, e.g.:
- bradycardia <50 beats/min
- left ventricular hypertrophy
- heart failure
- recent conversion from atrial fibrillation
- ventricular arrhythmia

An additional contributory factor may be central sleep apnoea, which is associated with bradycardia and QT prolongation, and is reported to occur in 30% of patients on **methadone** maintenance.[9]

Implications for practice

General recommendations to guide practice are given in Box 24.D.[2]

Box 24.D A clinical approach to drug-induced QT prolongation

When using drugs known to prolong the QT interval, a prescriber needs to:
- understand the pharmacology of the drug, in particular factors which may lead to accumulation, e.g. drug–drug interaction, impaired elimination
- whenever possible, avoid the concurrent use of more than one drug which prolongs the QT interval
- use the lowest effective dose of the QT-prolonging drug
- evaluate and balance the potential benefit against the potential risk, taking into account the specific circumstances of the patient and the presence of other risk factors (see Box 24.C), e.g.:
  - ▹ in patients with a known (pre-existing) prolonged QT interval, avoid the use of all QT-prolonging drugs except under specialist guidance (see Box 24.B)
  - ▹ in patients with cardiac disease, drugs which prolong the QT interval should generally be avoided unless no suitable alternative exists
  - ▹ in patients with cardiac disease, if a cardiac anti-arrhythmic known to prolong the QT interval is prescribed, consider undertaking an ECG before and after starting the drug, and regular monitoring of plasma potassium and magnesium concentrations to ensure these remain well within their normal ranges
  - ▹ in patients without cardiac disease but with other risk factors, consider similar monitoring to above when using a QT-prolonging drug
  - ▹ for advice about patients at the end of life and also methadone, see text
- explain to the patient (and family) the risk involved and the reasons for using the drug in question, to allow an informed decision to be made
- report instances of drug-related QT prolongation to the MHRA through the yellow card scheme at www.mhra.gov.uk/index.htm
- consider *torsade de pointes* as a possible cause of palpitations, syncope or seizure-like activity.

Palliative care patients in general may be at higher risk of a prolonged QT interval given the high prevalence of multiple drug use and metabolic disturbance. Polypharmacy is the norm in palliative care,[10] and using more than one drug concurrently increases the risk of drug interactions.[11–13] However, of 300 patients referred to a specialist palliative care unit who were not imminently dying, although 48 (16%) had a prolonged QT interval, only 2 (0.7%) had a severely prolonged uncorrected QT interval of >500msec (Figure 24.3).[5,14] Both patients had ischaemic heart disease and, if being considered for a QT-prolonging drug such as **methadone**, would have been

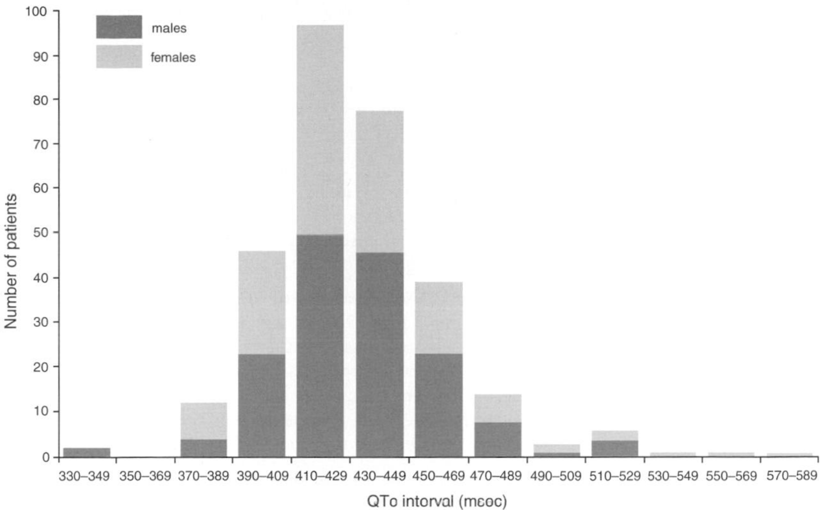

Figure 24.3 Distribution of the QT interval in 300 palliative care patients.[14]

identified by following the guidance to undertake an ECG in patients with one or more risk factors.

Nonetheless, a commonsense approach should prevail and the benefit of certain drugs used in the last days of life, e.g. **haloperidol**, is likely to far outweigh any risk, and an ECG is not required.[15]

Methadone

There have been longstanding concerns relating to the occurrence of serious adverse events with **methadone**, including deaths, from apparent unintentional overdose, particularly in the first 2 weeks of administration. As the use of **methadone** has increased, for both **methadone** maintenance and chronic pain, so has the number of deaths, disproportionately more than with other opioids, resulting in the US FDA issuing an alert to health professionals in 2006.[9] A major factor is considered to be a lack of knowledge among clinicians about the need to carefully monitor the use of **methadone**, particularly during the first 2–4 weeks (see **methadone**, p.416). Although many of these deaths are likely to be a result of respiratory depression, *torsade de pointes* may be a contributing factor (Box 24.E).

Guidelines to minimize the risk of cardiac toxicity with **methadone** are based largely on expert opinion, and recommendations vary.[15] Although some suggest routine ECG screening, this is debatable. However, most advise an ECG in the presence of other risk factors for QT interval prolongation.[15] For example, since 2006, the SPC for **methadone** has recommended that it is used with caution in patients with any of the following risk factors for QT prolongation:

- a history of cardiac conduction abnormalities
- advanced heart disease or ischemic heart disease
- liver disease
- a family history of sudden death
- electrolyte abnormalities
- concurrent treatment with drugs which:
  - ▷ may cause electrolyte abnormalities
  - ▷ have a potential to prolong QT
  - ▷ inhibit CYP3A4 (see p.735).

ECG monitoring is recommended in such patients before starting **methadone** and when the dose is stabilized. ECG monitoring is also recommended in patients without recognized risk

Box 24.E Methadone, prolonged QT and *torsade de pointes*

The association between methadone and prolonged QT was first reported in 1973.[16] The link with *torsade de pointes* was made in 2002 when it was described in 17 patients receiving a median dose of methadone of 330mg/day PO; all had QT >500msec and most had other risk factors.[17]

Subsequently, methadone has been found to block ion channels associated with QT prolongation, and to increase the QT interval and the risk of *torsade de pointes* generally in a dose-dependent manner. However, QTc >500msec and *torsade de pointes* have been reported with daily doses as low as 30–40mg PO.[18]

A review of 59 reports (five fatal) to the FDA confirmed that *torsade de pointes* is generally seen with higher daily doses (median 345mg, range 29–1,680mg). However, *torsade de pointes* was a confirmed cause of death in only one case, and for most reports other risk factors were present, e.g. multiple QT-prolonging drugs, drug interaction, hypokalaemia, hypomagnesaemia, or heart disease.[19] The frequent co-existence of other risk factors makes it difficult to quantify the risk from methadone alone and may explain the inconsistent dose-relationship seen between methadone and QT prolongation.

Although slight prolongation of the QT interval by methadone appears to be common, the clinical significance of this is unclear. A marked increase in QTc to >500msec is seen in a small proportion of patients given methadone (generally about 2%, but 16% in one report).[18,20] The incidence of *torsade de pointes* and of *fatal torsade de pointes* is hard to quantify, but both are likely to be rare, e.g.:

- of the 400 adverse drug events for methadone reported to the MHRA between 1964 and 2009, 13 (3 fatal) were classified as cardiac; these included only one report each of *torsade de pointes* or ventricular fibrillation, both non-fatal; the deaths occurred after cardiopulmonary arrest or an unspecified fatal arrhythmia[21]
- the maximum mortality attributable to prolonged QT has been estimated to be 0.06 per 100 patient-years, based on the examination of deaths of patients receiving methadone maintenance therapy in Norway.[22]

IV methadone has been considered high-risk. In cancer patients receiving median IV doses of 430mg/day (range 2.4mg–2.4g):[23]

- two patients with prolonged QT died suddenly (although a definite link with *torsade de pointes* was not proven)
- QTc >500msec occurred in a patient receiving as little as 10mg/day.

However, the formulation of methadone contained the QT-prolonging preservative chlorbutanol; this works synergistically with methadone to prolong the QT interval.
Note: None of the methadone injections marketed in the UK contain chlorbutanol.

factors for QT prolongation, before dose titration above 100mg/day PO and 1 week after such up-titration (an arbitrary dose, based on expert opinion). Monitoring of serum electrolytes, e.g. potassium, magnesium, is generally recommended in patients taking diuretics or at risk of hypokalaemia, e.g. because of vomiting or diarrhoea.

Other guidelines also suggest an ECG if other risk factors develop during treatment and highlight the importance of educating patients taking **methadone** to avoid where possible the use of other drugs which can prolong QT or inhibit **methadone** metabolism, and to urgently report cardiac symptoms, e.g. palpitation, dizziness, fainting spells, seizures.[24]

Specific guidance from a palliative care perspective is limited. In the USA, an expert group has developed a guideline for the use of *parenteral* **methadone** for chronic pain and in the palliative/hospice setting. Partly because of the increased risk presented by the preservative **chlorbutanol** (Box 24.E), an ECG is recommended:

- before starting IV therapy and after 1 and 4 days of treatment
- when the dose is significantly increased
- if an additional risk factor for QT prolongation develops.[25]

Monitoring serum electrolytes in high risk patients and discussing the potential risks of prolonged QT and *torsade de pointes* with the patient and carers are also recommended. However, consideration of burden vs. benefit is paramount and, in those with life-limiting illness, the potential benefit of controlling otherwise refractory pain may far outweigh the risks, even when monitoring for arrhythmia is impractical.[25] A commonsense approach should prevail: ECG monitoring is generally irrelevant in the last days of life.[15]

On the other hand, for a patient with a reasonable prognosis, it may be appropriate to identify any risk factors for QT prolongation and consider ECG monitoring as recommended in the SPC. Nonetheless, research is required to establish the magnitude of the risk of *torsade de pointes* with **methadone** and the overall value of adopting such an approach in the palliative care setting.

If the baseline QT is prolonged, an alternative opioid should be considered. Further, if the QT interval increases to >500msec while on **methadone**, generally it should be discontinued and an alternative used. However, there has been a report of the successful use of parenteral **methadone** for analgesia in a patient with a prolonged QT interval.[26] Implantable cardioverter-defibrillators have also been used in addicts with *torsade de pointes* who needed to remain on **methadone**.[27]

Generally, **methadone** is available only as a racemic mixture. (*S*)-**methadone** is a more potent blocker of the potassium channels in the cardiac myocytes than (*R*)-**methadone**. CYP2B6 also displays stereoselectivity for the metabolism of (*S*)-**methadone**, and initial findings suggest that CYP2B6 poor metabolizers (found in about 6% of Caucasians and African-Americans) have higher levels of (*S*)-**methadone** and may thus be at greater risk of prolonged QTc.[28] The use of (*R*)-**methadone** may thus be safer in this respect but, at present, it is available only in Germany.[29]

1 Goldenberg I *et al.* (2006) QT interval: how to measure it and what is 'normal'. *Journal of Cardiovascular Electrophysiology.* **17**: 333–336.
2 Al-Khatib SM *et al.* (2003) What clinicians should know about the QT interval. *Journal of the American Medical Association.* **289**: 2120–2127.
3 Gupta A *et al.* (2007) Current concepts in the mechanisms and management of drug-induced QT prolongation and torsade de pointes. *American Heart Journal.* **153**: 891–899.
4 Drew BJ *et al.* (2010) Prevention of torsade de pointes in hospital settings: a scientific statement from the American Heart Association and the American College of Cardiology Foundation. *Circulation.* **121**: 1047–1060.
5 Committee for Proprietary Medicinal Products (1996) Points to consider: the assessment of the potential for QT interval prolongation by non-cardiovascular medicinal products. *European Agency for the Evaluation of Medicinal Products (EMEA).* **CPMP/986/96**.
6 Haverkamp W *et al.* (2000) The potential for QT prolongation and proarrhythmia by non-antiarrhythmic drugs: clinical and regulatory implications. Report on a policy conference of the European Society of Cardiology. *European Heart Journal.* **21**: 1216–1231.
7 Idle JR (2000) The heart of psychotropic drug therapy. *Lancet.* **355**: 1824–1825.
8 Zipes DP *et al.* (2006) ACC/AHA/ESC 2006 guidelines for management of patients with ventricular arrhythmias and the prevention of sudden cardiac death: a report of the American College of Cardiology/American Heart Association Task Force and the European Society of Cardiology Committee for Practice Guidelines (Writing Committee to Develop guidelines for management of patients with ventricular arrhythmias and the prevention of sudden cardiac death) developed in collaboration with the European Heart Rhythm Association and the Heart Rhythm Society. *Europace.* **8**: 746–837.
9 Andrews CM *et al.* (2009) Methadone-induced mortality in the treatment of chronic pain: role of QT prolongation. *Cardiology Journal.* **16**: 210–217.
10 Twycross RG *et al.* (1994) Monitoring drug use in palliative care. *Palliative Medicine.* **8**: 137–143.
11 Bernard SA and Bruera E (2000) Drug interactions in palliative care. *Journal of Clinical Oncology.* **18**: 1780–1799.
12 Davies SJ *et al.* (2004) Potential for drug interactions involving cytochromes P450 2D6 and 3A4 on general adult psychiatric and functional elderly psychiatric wards. *British Journal of Clinical Pharmacology.* **57**: 464–472.
13 Wilcock A *et al.* (2005) Potential for drug interactions involving cytochrome P450 in patients attending palliative day care centres: a multicentre audit. *British Journal of Clinical Pharmacology.* **60**: 326–329.
14 Walker G *et al.* (2003) Prolongation of the QT interval in palliative care patients. *Journal of Pain and Symptom Management.* **26**: 855–859.
15 Wilcock A and Beattie JM (2009) Prolonged QT interval and methadone: implications for palliative care. *Current Opinion in Supportive and Palliative Care.* **3**: 252–257.
16 Stimmel B *et al.* (1973) Electrocardiographic changes in heroin, methadone and multiple drug abuse: a postulated mechanism of sudden death in narcotic addicts. *Proceedings of the National Conference on Methadone Treatment.* **1**: 706–710.
17 Krantz MJ *et al.* (2002) Torsade de pointes associated with very-high-dose methadone. *Annals of internal medicine.* **137**: 501–504.
18 Stringer J *et al.* (2009) Methadone-associated QT interval prolongation and torsades de pointes. *American Journal of Health System Pharmacy.* **66**: 825–833.
19 Pearson EC and Woosley RL (2005) QT prolongation and torsades de pointes among methadone users: reports to the FDA spontaneous reporting system. *Pharmacoepidemiology Drug Safety.* **14**: 747–753.
20 Reddy S *et al.* (2010) The effect of oral methadone on the QTc interval in advanced cancer patients: a prospective pilot study. *Journal of Palliative Medicine.* **13**: 33–38.
21 MHRA (2009) Personal communication.

22 Anchersen K *et al.* (2009) Prevalence and clinical relevance of corrected QT interval prolongation during methadone and buprenorphine treatment: a mortality assessment study. *Addiction.* **104**: 993–999.
23 Kornick CA *et al.* (2003) QTc interval prolongation associated with intravenous methadone. *Pain.* **105**: 499–506.
24 Office of Alcoholism and Substance Abuse Services (2009 March) Medical advisory panel position on QTc interval screening in methadone treatment. Available from: http://www.oasas.state.ny.us/Admed/cme/QTCinterval.cfm
25 Shaiova L *et al.* (2008) Consensus guideline on parenteral methadone use in pain and palliative care. *Palliative and Supportive Care.* **6**: 165–176.
26 Sekine R *et al.* (2007) The successful use of parenteral methadone in a patient with a prolonged QTc interval. *Journal of Pain and Symptom Management.* **34**: 566–569.
27 Patel AM *et al.* (2008) Role of implantable cardioverter-defibrillators in patients with methadone-induced long QT syndrome. *American Journal of Cardiology.* **101**: 209–211.
28 Eap CB *et al.* (2007) Stereoselective block of hERG channel by (S)-methadone and QT interval prolongation in CYP2B6 slow metabolizers. *Clinical Pharmacology and Therapeutics.* **81**: 719–728.
29 Gaertner J *et al.* (2008) Methadone: a closer look at the controversy. *Journal of Pain and Symptom Management.* **36**: e4–7.

25: CYTOCHROME P450

Cytochrome P450 is a super-family of enzymic proteins with a major responsibility for the oxidative metabolism of many drugs and other hydrophobic endogenous and exogenous chemicals. It is estimated that up to 60% of all currently used drugs are metabolized to some extent by cytochrome P450, which may lead to inactivation of the pharmacological response or the production of a pharmacologically or toxicologically active metabolite. Given this extensive involvement in the metabolic elimination of drugs and because of genetic variation or interaction with other drugs/chemicals, it is not surprising that variation in activity of the cytochrome P450 system can have a major impact on drug action. This is most likely to occur if an individual P450 enzyme is the sole or predominant determinant of the elimination of a drug from the body.

Cytochrome P450 enzymes exist in virtually all tissues, but their highest concentration is in the liver. In humans, 18 families (>40% identical amino acid sequence) with 44 active subfamilies (>55% identical amino acid sequence) have been identified. Cytochrome P450 enzymes have been assigned the root symbol CYP, followed by:

- a number designating the enzyme family
- a capital letter designating the subfamily
- a number designating the individual enzyme.

In genetic studies, the individual enzyme number is followed by an asterisk with a further number and letter to designate specific variants with normal, increased or decreased activity. For example, CYP2D6*1A has normal activity, whereas CYP2D6*10B contains minor mutations associated with reduced enzyme activity.[1,2]

The mammalian P450 families can be divided into two major classes, comprising those involved in the synthesis and degradation of endogenous substances, e.g. fatty acids, eicosanoids, steroids and bile acids (CYP4 to CYP51), and those which primarily metabolize foreign substances (xenobiotics), e.g. drugs and toxins (CYP1 to CYP3; Table 25.1).[3] The vast majority of hepatic P450-mediated reactions are mediated by CYP1A2, CYP2B6, CYP2C8/9, CYP2C19, CYP2D6, CYP2E1, and CYP3A4/5, each of which has a broad but overlapping substrate specificity (see Table 25.2 for a selected list). Together, these CYPs account for 70% of the total P450 content of the liver. CYP3A4/5 is also present in the wall of the GI tract, where it can affect the bio-availability of substrate drugs and pro-drugs through first-pass metabolism.[1] Drugs responsible for interactions act either as *inhibitors* or *inducers*.

Table 25.1 Routes of elimination for the 200 most commonly prescribed drugs in the USA[4]

Route	*Proportion of drugs eliminated (%)*
CYP3A4/5	27
Renal	25
CYP2C8/9	16
CYP2D6	10
CYP2C19	7
CYP1A2	6
Other CYP	4
Unknown	5

Inhibition

Inhibition of drug biotransformation begins within a few hours of the administration of the inhibitor drug, leading to an increase in the plasma substrate drug concentration, drug response and toxicity, *except pro-drugs which will have a corresponding reduced effect* (see below). The

Table 25.2 Selected list of CYP substrates, inhibitors and inducers

Enzyme	*Substrates*	*Inhibitors*	*Inducers*
CYP1A2	Amitriptyline Caffeine Clomipramine Clozapine Ethinyloestradiol Imipramine Olanzapine Paracetamol Propranolol Theophylline Tizanidine Trimipramine	Cimetidine Ciprofloxacin[a] Diltiazem Erythromycin (weak) Fluoxetine (weak)[b] Fluvoxamine[b] Mexiletine Norfloxacin (weak)[a] Paroxetine (weak)[b] Sertraline (weak)[b] Verapamil	Brassicas Charbroiled beef Smoking Omeprazole Phenobarbital Phenytoin
CYP2B6	Bupropion Ketamine Methadone Propofol		Phenobarbital Rifampicin
CYP2C8/9	Amitriptyline Diclofenac Fluvastatin Glipizide Ibuprofen Imipramine Losartan Naproxen Phenytoin Piroxicam Tolbutamide Torsemide Warfarin Zafirlukast	Amiodarone Cimetidine Cranberry juice (may significantly inhibit CYP2C9 at >600mL/24h; see text) Fluconazole[c] Fluvastatin (possibly) Metronidazole Miconazole Ritonavir Sulfamethoxazole Trimethoprim Zafirlukast	Barbiturates Carbamazepine Rifampicin St John's wort
CYP2C19[d]	Amitriptyline Citalopram Clomipramine Clopidogrel Diazepam Fluoxetine Imipramine Lansoprazole Moclobemide Nelfinavir Omeprazole Pantoprazole Pentamidine Phenytoin Proguanil Propranolol Sertraline	Cimetidine Esomeprazole Fluoxetine[b] Fluvoxamine[b] Ketoconazole[c] Lansoprazole Moclobemide Omeprazole Rabeprazole	Carbamazepine Phenytoin Rifampicin (possibly)

continued

Table 25.2 Continued

Enzyme	*Substrates*	*Inhibitors*	*Inducers*
CYP2D6[e]	Amitriptyline Carvedilol Clomipramine Clozapine Codeine Desipramine Dextromethorphan Dextropropoxyphene Flecainide Fluoxetine Haloperidol Hydrocodone Imipramine Metoprolol Mexiletine Nortriptyline Ondansetron Oxycodone Paroxetine Perphenazine Propafenone Propranolol Quinidine Risperidone Ritonavir Sertraline Timolol Tramadol Venlafaxine	Amiodarone Cimetidine Clomipramine Flecainide Fluoxetine[b] Fluvoxamine (weak)[b] Haloperidol Levomepromazine Paroxetine[b] Perphenazine Propafenone Quinidine[f] Sertraline (weak)[b] Tramadol[g]	
CYP2E1	Alcohol Caffeine Isoniazid Paracetamol Theophylline	Disulfiram Isoniazid	Alcohol Isoniazid
CYP3A4/5[h]	Alfentanil Alprazolam Amiodarone Amitriptyline Atorvastatin Bromocriptine Carbamazepine Cisapride Clarithromycin Clomipramine Clopidogrel Clozapine Codeine Corticosteroids Ciclosporin Diazepam Diltiazem	Bromocriptine Cimetidine Clarithromycin Ciclosporin Danazol Delavirdine Dextropropoxyphene Diltiazem Ergotamine Erythromycin Ethinylestradiol Fluconazole[c] Fluoxetine[b] Fluvoxamine[b] Grapefruit juice Indinavir Itraconazole[c]	Carbamazepine Dexamethasone Efavirenz Nevirapine Phenobarbital Phenytoin Rifabutin Rifampicin St John's wort

continued

Table 25.2 Continued

Enzyme	*Substrates*	*Inhibitors*	*Inducers*
	Erythromycin	Ketoconazole[c]	
	Ethinyloestradiol	Miconazole	
	Felodipine	Midazolam	
	Imipramine	Nicardipine	
	Indinavir	Nifedipine	
	Lidocaine	Omeprazole	
	Losartan	Paroxetine (weak)[b]	
	Lovastatin	Progesterone	
	Methadone	Quinidine	
	Midazolam	Ritonavir	
	Nelfinavir	Saquinavir	
	Nifedipine	Sertraline (weak)[b]	
	Omeprazole	Testosterone	
	Paracetamol	Verapamil	
	Phenytoin	Zafirlukast	
	Pimozide		
	Propafenone		
	Quinidine		
	Ritonavir		
	Saquinavir		
	Sertraline		
	Sildenafil		
	Simvastatin		
	Tamoxifen		
	Theophylline		
	Triazolam		
	Venlafaxine		
	Verapamil		
	Warfarin		

a. relative inhibitory potency of fluoroquinolones: ciprofloxacin > norfloxacin > ofloxacin (almost none)
b. *in vitro* data suggest only moderate inhibition of SSRIs. CYP1A2 inhibition: fluvoxamine > all other SSRIs; CYP2D6 inhibition: paroxetine and fluoxetine > sertraline > fluvoxamine (almost none); CYP3A4 inhibition: fluvoxamine > fluoxetine > paroxetine and sertraline (almost none)
c. relative inhibitory potency of imidazoles: ketoconazole ≈ itraconazole > fluconazole (and possibly clotrimazole)
d. genetic polymorphism. Autosomal recessive inheritance: 2% of white Caucasians and 20% of orientals do not express this enzyme and are 'slow metabolizers'
e. genetic polymorphism. Autosomal recessive inheritance: 5–10% of white Caucasians and 1–2% of blacks and orientals do not express this enzyme and are 'slow metabolizers'
f. most potent CYP2D6 inhibitor
g. significant competitive inhibition of quinidine and propafenone metabolism has been documented with tramadol administration
h. expressed in GI mucosa resulting in substantial first-pass metabolism during absorption of some drugs.

mechanism of enzymatic inhibition is either reversible or irreversible. In reversible inhibition, the inhibitor drug (e.g. **cimetidine**, **ketoconazole**, macrolide antibacterials) binds to the P450 enzyme and prevents the metabolism of the substrate drug. The extent of inhibition of one drug by another depends on their relative affinities for the P450 enzyme, and the relative doses. In irreversible inhibition, the enzyme is destroyed or inactivated by the inhibitor drug or its metabolites (e.g. **chloramphenicol**, **spironolactone**).

The occurrence of serious cardiac arrhythmias when **ketoconazole** (an inhibitor) and **terfenadine** are given concurrently is an example of a non-competitive inhibitory drug interaction involving CYP3A4/5 (Box 25.A).[5,6] Because of similar interactions, **terfenadine** and **astemizole** have been withdrawn in various parts of the world (see Prolongation of the QT interval in palliative care, p.727).

Box 25.A Ketoconazole-induced terfenadine cardiotoxicity[5]

A 39-year-old woman began a course of terfenadine and, 1 week later, ketoconazole. After a further two days she experienced several episodes of light-headedness and syncope. ECG showed prolongation of the QT interval and *torsade de pointes*. High concentrations of terfenadine and reduced concentrations of its main metabolite were found, suggesting inhibition of metabolism. It was concluded that ketoconazole-induced inhibition of terfenadine metabolism was responsible for the cardiotoxicity

Clopidogrel is a pro-drug activated by CYP2C19. PPIs can reduce the level of the active metabolite through inhibition of this enzyme, and thus reduce its antithrombotic effect. Individual PPIs vary in the extent to which they inhibit CYP2C19 but the general advice is to avoid concurrent use.[7–10]

Box 25.B gives examples of enhanced drug effects resulting from enzyme inhibition, and Table 25.2 gives numerous examples of cytochrome P450 enzyme inhibitors which may increase the plasma concentrations of various substrate drugs.[1,11,12]

Box 25.B Examples of drug interactions based on enzyme inhibition

Cimetidine reduces diazepam clearance → increased effect.[13]
Ciprofloxacin reduces theophylline clearance by 18–113% → increased effect.[14]
Diltiazem prolongs the halflife of propranolol and metoprolol → increased effect.[15]
Fluvoxamine increases warfarin concentration by 65% → increased effect.[16]
Quinidine inhibits biotransformation of codeine to morphine → *decreased* analgesic effect.[17]
SSRIs reduce clearance of TCAs → increased plasma concentrations by 50–350% → increased effect.[18–20]

Food–drug interactions

A particular form of drug interaction centred around inhibition of cytochrome P450 enzymes is a food–drug interaction involving grapefruit juice and substrates of CYP3A enzymes, including some benzodiazepines (**diazepam**, **midazolam**, **triazolam**), some statins (**atorvastatin**, **lovastatin**, **simvastatin**), **buspirone**, **ciclosporin**, **felodipine**, **nifedipine**, **saquinavir** and **terfenadine**.[1,21–24] Grapefruit juice contains several bioflavonoids (naringenin, naringin, kaempferol and quercetin) and furanocoumarins (bergamottin) which non-competitively inhibit oxidation reactions mediated by CYP3A enzymes in the wall of the GI tract.[23,25,26] The effect is variable because the quantity of these components in grapefruit products varies considerably.[27,28]

The effect is maximal when grapefruit juice is ingested 30–60min before the drug. A single 250mL glass of grapefruit juice can inhibit CYP3A for 24–48h and regular intake continually suppresses GI CYP3A.[1,23] Thus, patients taking many drugs metabolized by CYP3A are warned to avoid grapefruit juice, particularly if the drug has a narrow therapeutic index, e.g. **ciclosporin**. Pomelo, Seville orange and lime juices may also inhibit CYP3A, although confirmation is required.[29,30] Apple juice has not been implicated.

Besides inhibiting CYP3A, naringin (and thus grapefruit juice) inhibits organic anion-transporting polypeptide 1A2 (OATP1A2), a carrier protein in the wall of the GI tract which is responsible for the uptake of several drugs. Orange juice (through its major flavonoid, hesperidin) has a similar effect.[31] Preliminary research suggests that apple juice also inhibits OATP1A2.[32] Drugs which may have their absorption reduced by this inhibition include some β-blockers (**atenolol**, **celiprolol**, **talinolol**), **ciclosporin**, **etoposide**, **fexofenadine**, **itraconazole**, and quinolone antibacterials (**ciprofloxacin**, **levofloxacin**).[31,32]

There is also some concern that ingestion of cranberry juice may also modify drug action, mediated through flavonoids which specifically inhibit CYP2C9. **Warfarin** is an example of a drug which might be affected by this interaction and, indeed, early reports linked cranberry juice with adverse events associated with **warfarin**.[33–36] However, recent reports suggest that this interaction is unlikely to occur with the amounts of cranberry juice recommended for prophylaxis against UTIs (see Cranberry juice, p.531).[37–40]

Nonetheless, an interaction with **warfarin** cannot be ruled out, particularly when large volumes of cranberry juice are drunk regularly, or when cranberry products other than juice are taken.[37,38,41] Thus, the INR should be monitored more closely in patients on **warfarin** if they consume large amounts of cranberry juice or take other cranberry supplements for prophylaxis against UTIs.[37]

Induction

Induction of the rate of drug biotransformation results in a decrease in the parent drug plasma concentrations and *decreased effect*, but *increased toxicity* if active metabolites are formed or if the administered drug is an inactive pro-drug. The onset and offset of enzyme induction is gradual, e.g. 2–3 weeks, because:

- onset depends on drug-induced synthesis of new enzyme
- offset depends on elimination of the enzyme-inducing drug and the decay of the increased enzyme stores.

Sequential dose adjustments, either up or down, may be necessary to maintain the desired clinical effect of the affected drug during a progressive change in CYP activity.[1]

Several molecular mechanisms for enzyme induction have been characterized, including increased DNA transcription (the most common), increased RNA processing and mRNA stabilization.

Some anti-epileptics (including **carbamazepine**, **phenobarbital**, **phenytoin**), and other drugs such as **dexamethasone**, **griseofulvin**, **rifampicin** induce members of the CYP3A subfamily. **Rifampicin** is the most potent clinically used inducer of cytochrome CYP3A. Some oestrogens are metabolized by CYP3A4/5, and induction by **rifampicin** (or another enzyme inducer) can cause oral contraceptive failure. Failure of protease inhibitor treatment for HIV infection has also occurred when **St John's wort** was taken concurrently.[42–44] Box 25.C gives examples of decreased drug effects as a result of enzyme induction, and Table 25.2 gives numerous examples of cytochrome P450 enzyme inducers which may decrease the plasma concentrations of various substrate drugs.

Box 25.C Examples of drug interactions based on enzyme induction

Carbamazepine and phenytoin increase midazolam metabolism → decreased effect.[45]
Phenytoin increases carbamazepine metabolism → possible therapeutic failure.
Rifampicin increases phenytoin clearance (halflife halved) → decreased effect.[46]

Carbamazepine can potentially decrease the effect of many other drugs by decreasing their plasma concentrations (or can expedite the biotransformation of a drug to an active metabolite). For example, **carbamazepine** increases **diazepam** metabolism but, in this case, there may be no detectable clinical effect because of active metabolites.

Genetic polymorphism

Genetic differences in the amount of drug metabolized by an enzymatic pathway has resulted in the classification of individuals into slow (poor) metabolizers and rapid (extensive) metabolizers.[47] More recently, intermediate and ultra-rapid metabolizers have been identified for some pathways.[1] Inevitably, even within the general population of rapid metabolizers, there is a normal distribution of enzyme activity ranging from well below-average to well above-average. However, the slow metabolizers (and ultra-rapid ones) form a discontinuous genetically distinct group; they are *not* just one end of a spectrum. Slow metabolizer status is generally linked to only one enzyme in any one individual, and is inherited as an autosomal recessive trait (Table 25.3). The inherited allele may encode an inactivated enzyme or one with reduced activity. Ultra-rapid metabolism may result from inheriting a more active form of the enzyme or multiple copies of an allele encoding an enzyme with normal activity.[1]

Table 25.3 Genetic polymorphism and slow (poor) metabolizer status[1,48,49]

Pathway	*A selection of drugs affected*	*Population affected*
CYP2D6 (debrisoquine hydroxylase)	β-Blockers Codeine Debrisoquine Flecainide Oxycodone Phenothiazines SSRIs (some) TCAs (some) Tramadol	Whites 5–10% Asians 1–2%
CYP2C9	Glipizide Phenytoin Tolbutamide Warfarin	Europeans <1%
CYP2C19	Diazepam PPIs S-mephenytoin	Whites 2–5% Blacks 4% Asians 10–25%

Other modifiers of cytochrome P450 activity

Non-genetic circumstances in which drug metabolism may become relatively slower include liver damage (with an associated decrease in cytochrome P450 enzyme activity) and old age. In general, age-related decreases in liver mass, liver enzyme activity and hepatic blood flow result in a decrease in the overall metabolic capacity of the liver in the elderly. This is of particular importance in relation to drugs which have a high 'hepatic extraction ratio', e.g. **amitriptyline**, **lidocaine**, **propranolol**, **verapamil**. The risk of toxicity from these drugs will be significantly higher in patients with liver damage and in the elderly.

Drug–drug interactions involving CYP enzymes in palliative care

Many patients receiving palliative care are elderly and take multiple drugs, often for several chronic conditions. This increases the likelihood of drug interactions involving CYP enzymes.

An audit of 160 patients attending palliative care day centres in the UK found that patients were taking a median of 7 drugs (range 1–17). About 20% were receiving a combination likely to produce a definite or potential clinically important CYP-mediated interaction (Table 25.4). Approximately 50% of these interactions involved corticosteroids, and 25% analgesics. The two definite clinically important interactions were between **omeprazole** and **diazepam** (which could result in drowsiness from increased **diazepam** concentrations) and between **phenytoin** and **dexamethasone** (which could result in a reduced **dexamethasone** effect).[50] Thus, it is important to consider the possibility of interactions when adding drugs to a patient's existing medication.

Table 25.4 Drug combinations likely to produce definitely or potentially clinically important CYP-mediated interactions in 160 patients attending palliative care day centres in the UK[50]

Category	*Drug combination*	*Number of times prescribed*	*Likely outcome of the interaction*[a]
Definitely important	Omeprazole + diazepam	3	Diazepam ↑
	Phenytoin + dexamethasone	2	Dexamethasone ↓
Potentially important	Dexamethasone + temazepam	5	Temazepam ↓
	Haloperidol + oxycodone	4	Oxycodone ↓
	Levomepromazine + oxycodone	3	Oxycodone ↓
	Prednisolone + diazepam	3	Diazepam ↓
	Dextropropoxyphene + tramadol	2	Tramadol ↑
	Carbamazepine + zopiclone	1	Zopiclone ↓
	Co-proxamol + codeine	1	Codeine ↓
	Dexamethasone + amitriptyline	1	Amitriptyline ↓
	Dexamethasone + fentanyl	1	Fentanyl ↓
	Dexamethasone + quinine	1	Quinine ↓
	Dexamethasone + simvastatin	1	Simvastatin ↓
	Dexamethasone + tacrolimus	1	Tacrolimus ↓
	Dexamethasone + zopiclone	1	Zopiclone ↓
	Fluoxetine + codeine	1	Codeine ↓
	Haloperidol + codeine	1	Codeine ↓
	Levomepromazine + haloperidol	1	Levomepromazine ↑ Haloperidol ↑
	Levomepromazine + tamoxifen	1	Tamoxifen ↓
	Prednisolone + amlodipine	1	Amlodipine ↓
	Prednisolone + fentanyl	1	Fentanyl ↓
	Prednisolone + trazodone	1	Trazodone ↓
	Prednisolone + zopiclone	1	Zopiclone ↓
	Verapamil + zopiclone	1	Zopiclone ↑
	Total	39	
	Number of patients prescribed ≥1 combination likely to produce a definitely or potentially clinically important interaction	34 (21%)	

a. ↑ = drug effect increased; ↓ = effect decreased.

1 Wilkinson GR (2005) Drug metabolism and variability among patients in drug response. *New England Journal of Medicine*. **352**: 2211–2221.

2 Sim SC (2005) Human Cytochrome P450 (CYP). Allele Nomenclature Committee. Available from: www.imm.ki.se/CYPalleles

3 Nebert DW and Russell DW (2002) Clinical importance of the cytochromes P450. *Lancet*. **360**: 1155–1162.

4 Zanger UM *et al.* (2008) Functional pharmacogenetics/genomics of human cytochromes P450 involved in drug biotransformation. *Analytical and Bioanalytical Chemistry*. **392**: 1093–1108.

5 Monaham B (1990) Torsades de Pointes occurring in association with terfenadine. *Journal of the American Medical Association*. **264**: 2788–2790.

6 Honig P *et al.* (1993) Terfenadine-ketoconazole interaction. Pharmacokinetic and electrocardiographic consequences. *Journal of the American Medical Association*. **269**: 1513–1518.

7 MHRA (2009) Interactions between the use clopidogrel and proton pump inhibitors. Available from: http://www.mhra.gov.uk/home/idcplg?IdcService=SS_GET_PAGE&ssDocName=CON051743

8 Society for Cardiovascular Angiography and Interventions (2009) A national study of the effect of individual proton pump inhibitors on cardiovascular outcomes in patients treated with clopidogrel following coronary stenting: The Clopidrogrel Medco Outcomes Study. Available from: http://www.scai.org/drlt1.aspx?PAGE_ID=5870

9 Juurlink DN *et al.* (2009) A population-based study of the drug interaction between proton pump inhibitors and clopidogrel. *Canadian Medical Association Journal*. **180**: 713–718.

10 Ho M *et al.* (2009) Risk of adverse outcomes associated with concomitant use of clopidogrel and proton pump inhibitors following acute coronary syndrome. *Journal of the American Medical Association*. **301**: 937–944.

11 Aeschlimann J and Tyler L (1996) Drug interactions associated with cytochrome P-450 enzymes. *Journal of Pharmaceutical Care in Pain and Symptom Control*. **4**: 35–54.

12 Johnson MD *et al.* (1999) Clinically significant drug interactions. *Postgrad Med*. **105**: 193–222.

13 Klotz U and Reimann I (1980) Delayed clearance of diazepam due to cimetidine. *New England Journal of Medicine*. **302**: 1012–1014.

14 Nix D *et al.* (1987) Effect of multiple dose oral ciprofloxacin on the pharmacokinetics of theophylline and indocyanine green. *Journal of Antimicrobial Chemotherapy*. **19**: 263–269.

15 Tateishi T *et al.* (1989) Effect of diltiazem on the pharmacokinetics of propranolol, metoprolol and atenolol. *European Journal of Clinical Pharmacology*. **36**: 67–70.

16 Tatro D (1995) Fluvoxamine drug interactions. *Drug Newsletter*. **14**: 20ff.

17 Sindrup S *et al.* (1992) The effect of quinidine on the analgesic effect of codeine. *European Journal of Clinical Pharmacology*. **42**: 587–591.

18 Vandel S *et al.* (1992) Tricyclic antidepressant plasma levels after fluoxetine addition. *Neuropsychobiology*. **25**: 202–207.

19 Finley P (1994) Selective serotonin reuptake inhibitors: pharmacologic profiles and potential therapeutic distinctions. *Annals of Pharmacotherapy*. **28**: 1359–1369.

20 Pollock B (1994) Recent developments in drug metabolism of relevance to psychiatrists. *Harvard Reviews of Psychiatry*. **2**: 204–213.

21 Benton R *et al.* (1996) Grapefruit juice alters terfenadine pharmacokinetics, resulting in prolongation of repolarization on the electrocardiogram. *Clinical Pharmacology and Therapeutics*. **59**: 383–388.

22 Maskalyk J (2002) Grapefruit juice: potential drug interactions. *Canadian Medical Association Journal*. **167**: 279–280.

23 Dahan A and Altman H (2004) Food-drug interaction: grapefruit juice augments drug bioavailability-mechanism, extent and relevance. *European Journal of Clinical Nutrition*. **58**: 1–9.

24 MHRA (2004) Statins and cytochrome P450 interactions. *Current Problems in Pharmacovigilance*. **30 (Oct)**: 1–2.

25 Rouseff RL (1988) Liquid chromatographic determination of naringin and neohesperidin as a detector of grapefruit juice in orange juice. *Journal – Association of Official Analytical Chemists*. **71**: 798–802.

26 Gibaldi M (1992) Drug interactions. Part II. *Annals of Pharmacotherapy*. **26**: 829–834.

27 Tailor S *et al.* (1996) Peripheral edema due to nifedipine itraconazole interaction: a case report. *Archives of Dermatology*. **132**: 350–352.

28 Fukuda K *et al.* (2000) Amounts and variation in grapefruit juice of the main components causing grapefruit-drug interaction. *Journal of Chromatography B, Biomedical Sciences and Applications*. **741**: 195–203.

29 Savage I (2008) Forbidden fruit: interactions between medicines, foods and herbal products. *Pharmaceutical Journal* **281**: f17.

30 Baxter K (2008) Drug interactions and fruit juices. *Pharmaceutical Journal*. **281**: 333.

31 Bailey DG *et al.* (2007) Naringin is a major and selective clinical inhibitor of organic anion-transporting polypeptide 1A2 (OATP1A2) in grapefruit juice. *Clinical Pharmacology and Therapeutics*. **81**: 495–502.

32 Sampson M (2008) New reasons to avoid grapefruit and other juices when taking certain drugs. Report from the 236th National Meeting of the American Chemical Society. Philadelphia, August 19th 2008. Available from: www.eurekalert.org/pub_releases/2008-08/acs-nrt072308.php

33 Grant P (2004) Warfarin and cranberry juice: an interaction? *Journal of Heart Valve Disease*. **13**: 25–26.

34 CSM (Committee on Safety of Medicines) (2004) Interaction between warfarin and cranberry juice: new advice. *Current Problems in Pharmacovigilance*. **30 (October)**: 10.

35 MHRA (2003) Possible interaction between warfarin and cranberry juice. *Current Problems in Pharmacovigilance*. **29 (Sept)**: 8.

36 Suvarna R *et al.* (2003) Possible interaction between warfarin and cranberry juice. *British Medical Journal*. **327**: 1454.

37 O'Mara N (2007) Does a cranberry juice-warfarin interaction really exist? Detail document. *Pharmacist's Letter/Prescriber's Letter*. **23**: 1–3.

38 Aston JL *et al.* (2006) Interaction between warfarin and cranberry juice. *Pharmacotherapy*. **26**: 1314–1319.

39 Lilja JJ *et al.* (2007) Effects of daily ingestion of cranberry juice on the pharmacokinetics of warfarin, tizanidine, and midazolam–probes of CYP2C9, CYP1A2, and CYP3A4. *Clinical Pharmacology and Therapeutics*. **81**: 833–839.

40 Li Z *et al.* (2006) Cranberry does not affect prothrombin time in male subjects on warfarin. *Journal of the American Dietetic Society*. **106**: 2057–2061.

41 Welch J and Forster K (2007) Probable elevation in international normalized ratio from cranberry juice. *Journal of Pharmacy Technology*. **23**: 104–107.

42 Piscitelli SC *et al.* (2000) Indinavir concentrations and St John's wort. *Lancet*. **355**: 547–548.

43 Henderson L *et al.* (2002) St John's wort (Hypericum perforatum): drug interactions and clinical outcomes. *British Journal of Clinical Pharmacology*. **54**: 349–356.

44 Flexner C (2000) Dual protease inhibitor therapy in HIV-infected patients: pharmacologic rationale and clinical benefits. *Annual Review of Pharmacology and Toxicology*. **40**: 649–674.

45 Backman J *et al.* (1996) Concentrations and effects of oral midazolam are greatly reduced in patients treated with carbamazepine or phenytoin. *Epilepsia*. **37**: 253–257.

46 Kay L *et al.* (1985) Influence of rifampicin and isoniazid on the kinetics of phenytoin. *British Journal of Clinical Pharmacology*. **20**: 323–326.

47 Meyer U (1991) Genotype or phenotype: the definition of a pharmacogenetic polymorphism. *Pharmacogenetics*. **1**: 66–67.

48 Riddick D (1997) Drug biotransformation. In: H Kalant and W Roschlau (eds) *Principles of Medical Pharmacology* (6e). Oxford University Press, New York.

49 Poulsen L *et al.* (1996) The hypoalgesic effect of tramadol in relation to CYP2D6. *Clinical Pharmacology and Therapeutics*. **60**: 636–644.

50 Wilcock A *et al.* (2005) Potential for drug interactions involving cytochrome P450 in patients attending palliative day care centres: a multicentre audit. *British Journal of Clinical Pharmacology*. **60**: 326–329.

26: DRUG-INDUCED MOVEMENT DISORDERS

Drug-induced movement disorders (extrapyramidal reactions) encompass:

- parkinsonism
- acute dystonia
- acute akathisia
- tardive dyskinesia.

The features of the various syndromes are listed in Box 26.A.[1] Most extrapyramidal reactions are caused by drugs which block dopamine receptors in the CNS; these include all antipsychotics and **metoclopramide**.[2,3] The risk is associated with dose, pre-existing extrapyramidal signs, dementia and a genetic predisposition.[4,5] To minimize the risk, always use the lowest effective dose for the shortest duration possible.

Box 26.A Movement disorders associated with dopamine-receptor antagonists[1]

Parkinsonism
Coarse resting tremor of limbs, head, mouth and/or tongue
Muscular rigidity (cogwheel or lead pipe)
Bradykinesia, notably of face
Sialorrhoea (drooling)
Shuffling gait

Acute dystonias
one or more of
Abnormal positioning of head and neck (retrocollis, torticollis)
Spasms of jaw muscles (trismus, gaping, grimacing)
Tongue dysfunction (dysarthria, protrusion)
Dysphagia
Laryngopharyngeal spasm
Dysphonia
Eyes deviated up, down or sideways (oculogyric crisis)
Abnormal positioning of limbs or trunk

Acute akathisia
one or more of
Fidgety movements or swinging of legs
Rocking from foot to foot when standing
Pacing to relieve restlessness
Inability to sit or stand still for several minutes

Tardive dyskinesia
Exposure to antipsychotic medication for >3 months (>1 month if >60 years of age)
Involuntary movement of tongue, jaw, trunk or limbs:

- choreiform (rapid, jerky, non-repetitive)
- athetoid (slow, sinuous, continual)
- rhythmic (stereotypic)

Antipsychotic drugs differ in their propensity for causing extrapyramidal reactions (see p.150). A lower risk is associated with lower affinity for the D_2-receptor, D_2 partial agonism and/or $5HT_{2A}/5HT_{2C}$ antagonism.[6–8] Thus the risk is a spectrum (in descending order):

- **haloperidol** (the highest risk)
- phenothiazines (e.g. **levomepromazine**)
- **risperidone**
- **olanzapine**
- **quetiapine**, **clozapine** (the lowest risk).

However, their overall tolerability is comparable because lower rates of extrapyramidal reactions are offset by increased rates of sedation and/or undesirable metabolic effects (see p.150).[9]

Numerous other drugs have been implicated,[10–12] including most classes of antidepressants, **carbamazepine**, **diltiazem**, **5-hydroxytryptophan**, **levodopa**, **lithium**, **methyldopa**, **ondansetron** and **valproate**.[13–15]

The link between extrapyramidal reactions and the serotoninergic system is partly caused by $5HT_{2A}$- and $5HT_{2C}$-receptors inhibiting dopaminergic neurones.[6] Thus, increased inhibition is seen in the propensity of SSRIs to induce such disorders, including akathisia,[16] whereas $5HT_{2A}$- and $5HT_{2C}$ antagonism reduces this propensity among some antipsychotics (see above).

Parkinsonism

Parkinsonism develops in 30–60% of patients treated long-term with antipsychotics.[4] It is most common in those over 60 years of age. It can develop at any stage but, except in patients with dementia, generally not before the second week.[4] There may be asymmetry in the early stages. The tremor of drug-induced parkinsonism typically:

- has a frequency of <8 cycles per second
- is worse at rest
- is suppressed during voluntary movements
- is associated with rigidity and bradykinesia (Box 26.A).

This is different from drug-induced tremors of the hands, head, mouth or tongue which have a frequency of 8–12 cycles per second, and are best observed with hands held outstretched or mouth held open (Box 26.B).

Treatment

- if possible, reduce or stop causal drug
- if caused by:
  - **metoclopramide**, substitute **domperidone**
  - an antipsychotic, switch to an alternative with a lower rate of extrapyramidal reactions (e.g. **quetiapine**)

Box 26.B Drug-induced (non-parkinsonian) tremor[17]

Anti-epileptics
- valproate

Antidepressants
- SSRIs
- TCAs

Antipsychotics
- butyrophenones
- phenothiazines

β_2 Agonists
- salbutamol
- salmeterol

Lithium

Methylxanthines
- caffeine
- aminophylline
- theophylline

Psychostimulants
- dexamfetamine
- methylphenidate

- prescribe an antimuscarinic antiparkinsonian drug, e.g.:
  - ▹ **orphenadrine** SR 100mg once daily *or*
  - ▹ **procyclidine** 2.5–5mg t.d.s. *or*
  - ▹ **trihexyphenidyl** 2–5 mg once daily–t.d.s.

Acute dystonia

Acute dystonias occur in up to 10% of patients treated with antipsychotics.[4,18] They are most common in young adults. They develop abruptly within days of starting treatment, and are accompanied by anxiety (Box 26.A).

Treatment

- if possible, discontinue or reduce the dose of the causal drug
- if caused by **metoclopramide**, substitute **domperidone**
- if caused by an antipsychotic, switch to an alternative with a lower rate of extrapyramidal reactions (e.g. **quetiapine**).

For immediate relief, give an injection of:

- **diazepam** 5mg IV[19] *or*
- an antimuscarinic, e.g. **procyclidine** 5–10mg IV/IM *or*
- an antihistaminic antimuscarinic drug, e.g. **dimenhydrinate** or **diphenhydramine** 25–50mg IV/IM (both not UK).

With antimuscarinic drugs, benefit is typically seen in 10–20min. If necessary, repeat the injection after 30min. Continue treatment PO for 1 week with:

- SR **orphenadrine** 100mg once daily *or*
- **dimenhydrinate** or **diphenhydramine** 25–50mg b.d.–q.d.s. (both not UK).

Acute akathisia

Akathisia is a form of motor restlessness in which the subject is compelled to pace up and down or to change the body position frequently (Box 26.A).[20] It occurs in 20% or more of patients receiving typical antipsychotics.[4] The prevalence is no longer considered to be age-related, but younger patients may respond better to treatment than elderly ones.[4]

Akathisia can develop within days of starting treatment, and generally resolves within a week of stopping the causal drug. If the drug is continued, it may progress to parkinsonism. **Haloperidol** and **prochlorperazine** carry the highest risk.[21,22] It is uncommon for **metoclopramide** to cause akathisia.

Treatment

- if possible, discontinue or reduce the dose of the causal drug
- switch to an alternative antipsychotic with a lower rate of extrapyramidal reactions (e.g. **quetiapine**)
- if necessary, add **propranolol** 10mg t.d.s., increasing if necessary every few days to a maximum daily dose of 120mg (further benefit above this level is unlikely)[23]
- if the patient is very distressed, a benzodiazepine can be prescribed in addition for a few days, e.g. **diazepam** 5–10mg/24h,[19] **clonazepam** 0.5–1mg/24h, **lorazepam** 1–3mg/24h.

Although **propranolol**, a highly lipophilic non-selective β-adrenergic receptor antagonist (β-blocker), has a proven anti-akathisia effect, selective β_1-adrenergic receptor antagonists such as **atenolol** and **metoprolol** are either less or not effective.[23] This suggests that the effect is a central one, and/or that both β_1- and β_2-receptor antagonism is necessary to reduce akathisia.

Antimuscarinic antiparkinsonian drugs are sometimes helpful.[23] However, response in **haloperidol**-induced akathisia is less likely.[24] It has been suggested that benefit from antimuscarinic antiparkinsonian drugs occurs only if akathisia is associated with drug-induced parkinsonism.[25]

Diphenhydramine (not UK) may also be of benefit.[19] Other possible treatments include **amantidine**, **buspirone** and **clonidine**.[23,26]

Tardive dyskinesia

Tardive (late) dyskinesia is caused by the long-term administration of drugs that block dopamine receptors, particularly D_2-receptors.[27] It occurs in 20% of patients receiving a typical antipsychotic for >3 months, particularly in the elderly and in those on high doses, e.g. **chlorpromazine** 300mg/24h or more.[4,28] It is less common in patients receiving atypical antipsychotics (see p.150).[28] Tardive dyskinesia is also associated with the long-term use of **metoclopramide**.[29]

Tardive dyskinesia typically manifests as involuntary stereotyped chewing movements of the tongue and orofacial muscles (Box 26.A). The involuntary movements are made worse by anxiety and reduced by drowsiness and during sleep.

Tardive dyskinesia is associated with akathisia in 25% of cases. In younger patients, tardive dyskinesia may present as abnormal positioning of the limbs and tonic contractions of the neck and trunk muscles causing torticollis, lordosis or scoliosis. In younger patients, tardive dyskinesia may occur if antipsychotic treatment is stopped abruptly.

Early diagnosis

'Open your mouth and stick out your tongue.'

The following indicate a developing tardive dyskinesia:
- worm-like movements of the tongue
- inability to protrude tongue for more than a few seconds.

Treatment

- if possible, discontinue or reduce the dose of the causal drug
- if caused by **metoclopramide**, substitute **domperidone**
- if caused by a typical antipsychotic, switch to an atypical antipsychotic
- withdraw antimuscarinics (it is exacerated by antimuscarinic antiparkinsonian drugs).[30]

Withdrawal of the causal drug leads to resolution in 30% in 3 months and a further 40% in 5 years. However, it is sometimes irreversible, particularly in the elderly. Seek specialist advice before initiating other drug treatments:
- **tetrabenazine**, depletes presynaptic dopamine stores and blocks post-synaptic dopamine receptors; best not used in depressed patients; start with 12.5mg b.d., increasing the dose slowly to 25mg t.d.s. to avoid troublesome hypotension
- **levodopa**, may produce long-term benefit after causing initial deterioration
- **clonidine** 50–200microgram/24h
- **baclofen**, **clonazepam**, **diazepam** and **valproate**, all act by potentiating GABA inhibition, but all give inconsistent results
- **pyridoxine** up to 400 mg/24h
- **branched-chain amino acids** (Tarvil®) 222mg/kg t.d.s.

Paradoxically, increasing the dose of the causal drug may help temporarily, but should be considered only in desperation because it could subsequently exacerbate the dyskinesia.[30]

1 APA (American Psychiatric Association) (1994) Neuroleptic-induced movement disorders. In: *Diagnostic and Statistical Manual of Mental Disorders* (4e). American Psychiatric Association, New York, pp. 736–751.

2 Tonda M and Guthrie S (1994) Treatment of acute neuroleptic-induced movement disorders. *Pharmacotherapy*. **14**: 543–560.

3 Jackson N *et al.* (2008) Neuropsychiatric complications of commonly used palliative care drugs. *Postgraduate Medical Journal*. **84**: 121–126.

4 Caligiuri MR *et al.* (2000) Antipsychotic-Induced movement disorders in the elderly: epidemiology and treatment recommendations. *Drugs Aging*. **17**: 363–384.

5 Tang S *et al.* (2009) MDPD: an integrated genetic information resource for Parkinson's disease. In: *Nucleic Acids Research*. Available from: http://nar.oxfordjournals.org/cgi/content/full/37/suppl_1/D858

6 Stahl SM (2008) Psychosis and schizophrenia. In: *Essential Psychopharmacology: Neuroscientific Basis and Practical Applications* (3e). Cambridge University Press, USA, pp. 247–325.

7 Lieberman JA (2004) Dopamine partial agonists: a new class of antipsychotic. *CNS Drugs*. **18**: 251–267.

8 Kapur S and Mamo D (2003) Half a century of antipsychotics and still a central role for dopamine D2 receptors. *Progress in Neuro-psychopharmacology and Biology Psychiatry*. **27**: 1081–1090.

9 Lieberman JA *et al.* (2005) Effectiveness of antipsychotic drugs in patients with chronic schizophrenia. *New England Journal of Medicine*. **353**: 1209–1223.

10 Tarsy D and Simon DK (2006) Dystonia. *New England Journal of Medicine*. **355**: 818–829.

11 Anonymous (1994) Drug-induced extrapyramidal reactions. *Current Problems in Pharmacovigilance*. **20**: 15–16.

12 Zubenko G *et al.* (1987) Antidepressant-related akathisia. *Journal of Clinical Psychopharmacology*. **7**: 254–257.

13 Anonymous (2009) Neuroleptic-induced extrapyramidal reactions. In: *Drugdex®Consults* Micromedex, Thompson Healthcare. Available from: http://www.micromedex.com/products/drugdex/

14 Matthews H and Tancil C (1996) Extrapyramidal reaction caused by ondansetron. *The Annals of Pharmacotherapy*. **30**: 196.

15 Arya D (1994) Extrapyramidal symptoms with selective serotonin reuptake inhibitors. *British Journal of Psychiatry*. **165**: 728–733.

16 Lane R (1998) SSRI-induced extrapyramidal side-effects and akathisia: implications for treatment. *Journal of Psychopharmacology*. **12**: 192–214.

17 APA (American Psychiatric Association) (1994) Medication-induced postural tremor. In: *Diagnostic and Statistical Manual of Mental Disorders* (4e). American Psychiatric Association, New York, pp. 749–751.
18 Launer M (1996) Selected side-effects: 17. Dopamine-receptor antagonists and movement disorders. *Prescribers' Journal.* **36**: 37–41.
19 Gagrat D *et al.* (1978) Intravenous diazepam in the treatment of neuroleptic-induced acute dystonia and akathisia. *American Journal of Psychiatry.* **135**: 1232–1233.
20 White C and Jackson N (2005) Acute akathisia in palliative care. *European Journal of Palliative Care.* **12 (1)**: 5–7.
21 Kawanishi C *et al.* (2007) Unexpectedly high prevalence of akathisia in cancer patients. *Palliative and Supportive Care.* **5**: 351–354.
22 Gattera J *et al.* (1994) A retrospective study of risk factors of akathisia in terminally ill patients. *Journal of Pain and Symptom Management.* **9**: 454–461.
23 Miller CH and Fleischhacker WW (2000) Managing antipsychotic-induced acute and chronic akathisia. *Drug Safety.* **22**: 73–81.
24 Van Putten T *et al.* (1984) Akathisia with haloperidol and thiothixene. *Archives of General Psychiatry.* **41**: 1036–1039.
25 Braude W *et al.* (1993) Clinical characteristics of akathisia: a systematic investigation of acute psychiatric in-patient admission. *British Journal of Psychiatry.* **143**: 139–150.
26 Poyurovsky M and Weizman A (1997) Serotonergic agents in the treatment of acute neuroleptic-induced akathisia: open-label study of buspirone and mianserin. *International Clinical Psychopharmacology.* **12**: 263–268.
27 APA (American Psychiatric Association) (1992) *Tardive dyskinesia: a task force report of the American Psychiatric Association.* American Psychiatric Association, Washington, DC.
28 Jeste D (2000) Tardive dyskinesia in older patients. *Journal of Clinical Psychiatry.* **61 (suppl 4)**: 27–32.
29 Sewell DD and Jeste DV (1992) Metoclopramide-associated tardive dyskinesia: An analysis of 67 cases. *Archives of Family Medicine.* **1**: 171–278.
30 Margolese HC *et al.* (2005) Tardive dyskinesia in the era of typical and atypical antipsychotics. Part 2: Incidence and management strategies in patients with schizophrenia. *Canadian Journal of Psychiatry.* **50**: 703–714.

27: ANAPHYLAXIS

Anaphylaxis is a life-threatening systemic allergic reaction. It manifests as a constellation of features but there is disagreement about which are essential. The confusion arises partly because systemic allergic reactions can be mild, moderate or severe. In practice, the term 'anaphylaxis' is best reserved for cases where there is:

- respiratory difficulty (related to laryngeal oedema or bronchoconstriction) *or*
- hypotension (presenting as fainting, collapse or loss of consciousness) *or*
- both.[1]

Urticaria, angioedema or rhinitis alone are best not described as anaphylaxis because neither respiratory difficulty nor hypotension is present.[1]

Causes

In anaphylaxis, an allergic reaction results from the interaction of an allergen with specific IgE antibodies bound to mast cells and basophils. This leads to activation of the mast cell with release of chemical mediators (including bradykinins, histamine, leukotrienes, prostaglandins) stored in granules as well as rapidly synthesized additional mediators. A rapid major systemic release of these mediators causes capillary leakage, vasodilation, mucosal oedema and bronchoconstriction, resulting in shock and respiratory difficulty.[1]

In contrast, anaphylactoid reactions are caused by activation of mast cells and release of the same mediators, but without the involvement of IgE antibodies. For example, certain drugs act directly on mast cells. In terms of management, it is not necessary to distinguish anaphylaxis from an anaphylactoid reaction. This difference is relevant only when investigations are being considered.

Anaphylaxis is rare in palliative care and is generally associated with antibacterials, **aspirin** or another NSAID. A possible case has been recorded in a woman with known peanut allergy who received an **arachis** (peanut) **oil** enema.[7] Anaphylaxis is:

- specific to a given drug or chemically-related class of drugs
- more likely after parenteral drug administration
- more frequent in patients taking β-adrenergic receptor blocking drugs (β-blockers, see p.753), or who have **aspirin**-induced asthma or systemic lupus erythematosus.

Clinical features

No single set of criteria will identify all anaphylactic reactions, but anaphylaxis is likely when all three of the following criteria are met:

- sudden onset and rapid progression of symptoms
- life-threatening respiratory or circulatory problems
- skin and/or mucosal changes.

Anaphylaxis causes a range of signs and symptoms (Box 27.A).[3] Bronchospasm occurs in only 10% of patients. Skin and mucosal changes occur in 80% of patients, but may be subtle. Angioedema may develop anywhere in the body but often involves the lips, eyes, hands or feet. Oedema of the larynx may lead to stridor and acute airway obstruction.[4]

Management

National guidelines vary slightly; the advice included here is based primarily on guidance published by the UK Resuscitation Council.[3,5] Anaphylaxis requires urgent treatment with **adrenaline** (epinephrine) followed by an antihistamine and **hydrocortisone** (Box 27.B). However, corticosteroids are only of secondary value because their impact is not immediate.

Adrenaline (epinephrine) is a direct-acting sympathomimetic. Through its α_1-receptor agonist effects, it causes vasoconstriction, increases peripheral vascular resistance and reduces mucosal

Box 27.A Clinical features of anaphylaxis

Essential
Sudden onset of life-threatening circulatory and/or respiratory problems, e.g.

Circulatory problems
Tachycardia
Hypotension
Shock
Decreased consciousness
Cardiac arrest

Respiratory problems
Airway
- pharyngeal/laryngeal oedema
- hoarse voice
- stridor

Breathing
- breathlessness
- wheeze/bronchospasm
- cyanosis
- respiratory arrest

Probable
Skin/mucosal changes:
- flushing or pallor
- erythema of skin
- urticaria
- angioedema[a]

Possible
Agitation
Confusion
Abdominal pain
Vomiting
Diarrhoea
Incontinence
Tingling of the extremities
Rhinitis
Conjunctivitis

a. angioedema is swelling in the dermis, subcutaneous and submucosal tissues.

Box 27.B Management of anaphylaxis in adults

1 Discontinue administration of any causal agent, e.g. IVI of antibacterial or blood product.

2 Oxygen (>10L/min) is of primary importance.

3 Adrenaline (epinephrine) every 5min until blood pressure, pulse and breathing are satisfactory:
- 1:1,000 (1mg/1mL), 500microgram (0.5mL) IM *or*
- 300microgram (0.3mL) if an adrenaline (epinephrine) auto-injector is used.

4 Chlorphenamine to counter histamine-induced vasodilation and bronchoconstriction:
- 10mg IM or IV over 1min
- if necessary, repeat up to a maximum of 40mg/24h
- 4–8mg PO q6h for 1–3 days to prevent relapse.[6]

5 Hydrocortisone sodium succinate 200mg IM or slowly IV for patients with bronchospasm, and for all severe or recurrent reactions to prevent further deterioration. Note: may take up to 6h to act.

6 If still shocked, give 1–2L of IV fluid; a crystalloid, e.g. 0.9% saline, may be safer than a colloid.[7]

7 If bronchospasm has not responded to the above, give a nebulized β_2 agonist, e.g. salbutamol 5mg.

8 Also prescribe prednisolone 40–50mg once daily for 3–4 days to prevent relapse.[8]

oedema. As a β_1 agonist, it increases the rate and force of myocardial contraction. As a β_2 agonist, it dilates bronchial airways, increases glycogenolysis and suppresses activity of mast cells, reducing histamine and leukotriene release. Thus, **adrenaline** (epinephrine) is effective in attenuating anaphylaxis if given early and in sufficient dose.[3]

The best site for IM injections is the anterolateral aspect of the middle third of the thigh.[3] If there is doubt about the adequacy of the circulation, **adrenaline** (epinephrine) can be given as a dilute IV solution, i.e. 1 in 10,000 (1mg/10mL), *using 50microgram (0.5mL) boluses, titrated to response*. However, because injecting **adrenaline** (epinephrine) IV too rapidly can cause ventricular arrhythmias, IV administration is discouraged unless given by a specialist, and intensive care facilities are available.[3,9]

If bronchospasm does not respond to nebulized **salbutamol**, consider IV **salbutamol** 250microgram, or a nebulized antimuscarinic bronchodilator, e.g. **ipratropium bromide** 250–500mg q.d.s–q4h.[3,9] Occasionally, emergency tracheotomy and assisted respiration are necessary.

Some centres also give an H_2-receptor antagonist, e.g. ranitidine 50mg IV stat or 150mg PO stat.[6,10] However, H_2-receptors are involved only to a limited extent in anaphylaxis, and the use of an H_2-receptor antagonist in this situation is not essential.[3,11]

β-Adrenergic receptor blocking drugs (β-blockers) and anaphylaxis

Patients taking β-blockers, particularly non-cardioselective ones, are at increased risk of severe anaphylaxis because the β-receptor-mediated effects of **adrenaline** (epinephrine) are blunted. Further, unopposed stimulation of α-receptors, with reflex vagotonic effects, may lead to bradycardia, coronary artery constriction, *hypertension* and intracerebral haemorrhage. TCAs and MAOIs potentiate **adrenaline** (epinephrine) and increase the risk of cardiac arrhythmias.

Previous UK anaphylaxis guidelines recommended halving the dose of **adrenaline** (epinephrine) given to patients on β-blockers, TCAs and MAOIs.[12] However, current guidelines note the large inter-individual variation in response to **adrenaline** (epinephrine), and this recommendation has been withdrawn. Patients on these drugs should be given a full initial dose of **adrenaline** (epinephrine), and further doses titrated according to the initial response.[3]

For patients taking β-blockers and unresponsive to **adrenaline** (epinephrine), give **glucagon** 1–2mg IM or IV every 5min, or as an IV infusion. **Glucagon** has β-receptor independent inotropic, chronotropic and vaso-active effects.[3,5,13] These patients in particular may not respond to nebulized **salbutamol** and may require IV **salbutamol** or nebulized **ipratropium bromide** (see above).[3,9]

1 Ewan P (1998) ABC of allergies: anaphylaxis. *British Medical Journal*. **316**: 1442–1445.
2 Pharmax (1998) *Data on file*.
3 Resuscitation Council (UK) (2008) Emergency treatment of anaphylactic reactions: Guidelines for healthcare providers. Available from: www.resus.org.uk/pages/reaction.pdf
4 CKS (2007) Angio-oedema and Anaphylaxis (Topic Review). In: *Clinical Knowledge Summary Service*. Available from: www.cks.library.nhs.uk/angio_oedema_and_anaphylaxis
5 Soar J (2009) Emergency treatment of anaphylaxis in adults: concise guidance. *Clinical Medicine*. **9**: 181–185.
6 Ellis AK and Day JH (2003) Diagnosis and management of anaphylaxis. *Canadian Medical Association Journal*. **169**: 307–311.
7 Schierhout G and Roberts I (1998) Fluid resuscitation with colloid or crystalloid solutions in critically ill patients: a systematic review of randomised trials. *British Medical Journal*. **316**: 961–964.
8 Poon M and Reid C (2004) Best evidence topic reports. Oral corticosteroids in acute urticaria. *Emergency Medical Journal*. **21**: 76–77.
9 BNF (2010) Section 3.4.3 Anaphylaxis. In: *British National Formulary* (No. 60). British Medical Association and the Royal Pharmaceutical Society of Great Britain, London. Current BNF available from www.bnf.org.
10 Mayumi *et al*. (1987) Intravenous cimetidine as an effective treatment for systemic anaphylaxis and acute allergic skin reaction. *Annals of Allergy*. **58**: 447–450.
11 Ellis AK and Day JH (2003) Anaphylaxis Treatment: The details. *Canadian Medical Association Journal* **169**: 1148–1149.
12 McLean-Tooke AP *et al*. (2003) Adrenaline in the treatment of anaphylaxis: what is the evidence? *British Medical Journal*. **327**: 1332–1335.
13 Thomas M and Crawford I (2005) Best evidence topic report. Glucagon infusion in refractory anaphylactic shock in patients on beta-blockers. *Emergency Medical Journal*. **22**: 272–273.

28: ORAL NUTRITIONAL SUPPLEMENTS

This section provides an overview of cachexia and the use of oral nutritional supplements in adults with cancer. It does not address nutritional supplements in children, patients with renal or hepatic failure, tube feeding or parenteral nutrition.

Introduction

Weight loss is a common adverse feature of cancer, associated with increased morbidity, poorer treatment tolerability and outcomes, and reduced survival. It generally occurs in the context of cancer cachexia, a multifactorial syndrome characterized by an ongoing loss of *skeletal muscle* mass (± fat), leading to progressive functional impairment.[1] There is negative protein and energy balance driven by a variable combination of reduced food intake and abnormal metabolism, with no standard treatment available for the latter. Nutritional support alone can prevent or slow the rate of weight loss in patients with an inadequate intake, but this appears to be via an effect on fat rather than skeletal muscle mass.[2]

Screening

Whatever the cause of malnutrition, early detection and intervention is preferable and requires a multiprofessional pro-active approach. NICE guidance suggests that all patients should be screened for malnutrition when:

- admitted to hospital, and weekly thereafter
- admitted to care homes, and repeated if there is clinical concern
- first seen in outpatients, and repeated if there is clinical concern
- registering with a general practice.

As a minimum, screening should evaluate:

- the body mass index (BMI):

$$\text{BMI} = \frac{\text{weight(kg)}}{\text{height}^2\text{(m)}}$$

- percentage unintentional weight loss
- time over which nutrient intake has been unintentionally reduced and/or the likelihood of future impaired intake.[3]

Screening tools include the Malnutrition Universal Screening Tool (MUST) and the Nutritional Risk Screening Tool 2002.[4,5] Although not validated specifically for use in patients with cancer, they are easy to complete.[5,6] The Patient Generated Subjective Global Assessment is a specific tool for patients with cancer but requires more training and takes longer to complete.[7,8]

NICE guidance suggests nutritional support should be considered for patients with:

- BMI $<18.5\text{kg/m}^2$
- unintentional weight loss of $>10\%$ in the last 3–6 months
- BMI $<20\text{kg/m}^2$ and unintentional weight loss of $>5\%$
- inadequate oral intake for >5 days
- malabsorption, increased nutrient losses, increased catabolism.[3]

Using these criteria, 30% and 60% of patients with thoracic or upper GI cancers respectively are malnourished even at the time of diagnosis.[9,10] Further, it could be argued that the remainder are at risk of malnutrition because of increased catabolism.

Recent cancer-specific recommendations have suggested lower thresholds for the diagnosis of cachexia, i.e. *any* of the following:

- weight loss $>5\%$ over past 6 months

- BMI $<20kg/m^2$ and weight loss $>2\%$
- sarcopenia and weight loss $>2\%$.[1]

Ideally, patients identified by the screening process should then have their nutritional status assessed by an appropriately trained health professional (typically a dietitian) in order to produce an individualized nutrition care plan, which includes monitoring.[6,11] The assessment would take into account the patient's physical condition and prognosis, state of hydration, dietary intake, estimation of nutritional requirements, identification of underlying symptoms contributing to malnutrition (e.g. poor oral health or dentition, nausea, early satiety), and other psychosocial and dietary considerations.

Assessment and management

Guidelines on assessment and use of enteral nutrition in (Box 28.A) are based on The European Society for Clinical Nutrition and Metabolism (ESPEN) guidelines on enteral nutrition (non-surgical oncology).[2]

Box 28.A Guidelines on enteral nutrition by mouth or by tube

Nutritional assessment should be performed and nutritional support started when:
- malnutrition exists
- a patient is losing weight due to insufficient nutritional intake
- it is anticipated that the patient will be unable to eat for >7 days
- it is anticipated that food intake will be inadequate for >10 days
  - $<60\%$ of estimated energy requirements *or*
  - estimated as $<50\%$ of usual pre-illness intake (based on 24h recall of intake).

Daily energy requirements
When resting energy expenditure cannot be measured, daily total energy expenditure (TEE) can be estimated:
- ambulant patient: 30–35kcal/kg/day
- bedbound patient: 20–25kcal/kg/day.

These estimates are less accurate in patients who are severely underweight (underestimates TEE) or obese (overestimates TEE).

Daily protein
Generally 1–2g/kg/day.

Daily fluid requirement
Generally 30–40mL/kg/day, but consider losses caused by pyrexia, malabsorption, fistulas, high output stomas.

Goals of therapy
- prevent and treat malnutrition
- enhance effectiveness and reduce undesirable effects of anticancer treatment
- improve quality of life.

Route
The enteral route (PO or tube feeding when PO not feasible) is preferred to the parenteral route.[12]

Tube feeding can be delivered via transnasal or percutaneous (e.g. gastrostomy, jejunostomy) routes.

Tube feeding is preferable in patients with head and neck or oesophageal cancers causing dysphagia, or when severe radiotherapy-induced oral or oesophageal mucositis is anticipated (when the percutaneous route may need to be used).

The parenteral route is preferred when there is an increased risk of bleeding or infections from tube placement, e.g. in neutropenic or thrombocytopenic patients, or when the GI tract is not functioning.

continued

Box 28.A Continued

Formula
Standard nutrient composition formulas (1–1.5kcal/mL) should generally be used.
For patients with early satiety or increased nutritional requirements, high-energy high-protein formulas may be preferable.

Peri-operatively, ESPEN recommend formulas that provide immune-modulating substrates, e.g. arginine, ω-3 fatty acids, nucleotides. However, the evidence is contradictory.[13,14]

Drug treatment
In the presence of chronic systemic inflammation (evidenced by a raised CRP), drug treatments are recommended in addition to nutritional support. The anti-inflammatory effects of corticosteroids and progestogens can enhance appetite, improve metabolic derangements and quality of life.[15] They should be used for short periods only, weighing their benefits against their undesirable effects, particularly the risk of thrombosis with progestogens (see p.513).

There are contradictory findings with the ω-3 fatty acid, eicosapentanoic acid (EPA), but benefit appears most likely when given in sufficient quantities (1.5–2g EPA/day) in combination with a high-protein and high-energy nutritional supplement.[16–19]

Peri-operative
All patients undergoing major abdominal surgery benefit from 5–7 days of nutritional support containing immune-modulating substrates, independent of their nutritional status.

Patients at severe nutritional risk benefit from 1–2 weeks of nutritional support before major surgery.

Radiotherapy, chemotherapy, or stem cell transplant
Enteral nutrition support should be prescribed when general indications are met (see above). Patients undergoing head and neck or GI radiation should receive nutritional support to increase dietary intake and prevent therapy-associated weight loss.

End of life
Generally, hunger and the urge to eat are much diminished or absent in the last weeks/days of life.[20,21] Because cachexia is considered 'refractory' in patients with a limited prognosis, i.e. <3 months, the focus of care is on providing symptom relief, addressing patient and family eating-related distress, and the use of appetite stimulants when appropriate.[1] Small amounts of food can be offered as desired by the patient to alleviate hunger, and for pleasure and social purposes.[22]

Provision of oral nutrition support

Correct the correctable

If oral intake is to be improved, attention must be paid to:

- the ability to obtain and prepare food
- oral problems, e.g. xerostomia, mucositis, oral candidosis
- uncontrolled nausea and vomiting
- dysphagia.

Particularly in relation to neurogenic dysphagia, simple measures such as adding thickeners to liquids and to semi-solid foods may be enough. Generally, patients with swallowing difficulties which put them at risk of aspiration should be assessed by a speech and language therapist (SALT).

General advice

This includes:

- meal patterns, e.g. eat small amounts frequently
- substitute water-based drinks, e.g. tea, coffee with milk-based drinks, e.g. hot chocolate, malted drinks, milky coffee
- dietary fortification, e.g. use full-fat milk and cream, extra butter, margarine, oil and sugar (fats are the most concentrated source of energy)
- consider relaxing pre-imposed dietary restrictions, e.g. diabetic diet
- making use of microwave meals and convenience foods; quick and easy to prepare, often small portions, high in fat and salt. The latter may help patients with a reduced sense of taste.

Generally, weight gain is more likely with dietary advice and nutritional supplements than with dietary advice alone in patients with illness-related malnutrition.[23]

Appetite stimulants

See Progestogens (p.513) and Systemic corticosteroids (p.483).

Oral nutritional supplements

Oral nutritional supplements should be considered when a patient is unable to improve their nutritional intake by diet alone. Generally, they should supplement existing intake rather than replace it, e.g. 1–2 cartons/day of a 1.5kcal/mL milk-based nutritional supplement. However, some products are nutritionally complete and, if ingested in sufficient quantities, can be used as a sole source of nutrition (e.g. see Table 28.2, p.760).

Oral nutritional supplements are available in liquid, semi-solid or powder formulations. General prescribing guidelines are contained in Box 28.B and product details in Table 28.1–Table 28.13, including thickeners and thickened drinks for use in patients with dysphagia.

Box 28.B Guidelines for prescribing oral nutritional supplements

1 Ensure correctable underlying problems are addressed and general nutritional advice has been given.

2 Guided by the patient's preferences, provide a variety of formulations and flavours either separately or in commercially available starter packs, e.g.:
- Fortisip® Range (Nutricia) contains Fortisip®, Fortijuce® and Fortisip Yoghurt Style® in various flavours
- Ensure Plus Commence® (Abbott) contains Ensure Plus® in various flavours.

3 Provide information on how to use the supplements together with any special instructions, e.g.:
- keep supplements chilled to improve palatability
- use the straw provided with supplement to minimize unpleasant odour
- use supplement as a between-meal snack, not as a meal replacement
- maintenance of good oral hygiene
- once opened, supplements can be stored in a refrigerator for up to 24h.

4 Review patient after one week:
- prescribe the required number of cartons/units per day of the formulation and flavour(s) which are acceptable to the patient
- if none are acceptable, try an alternative, e.g. juice-based or milkshake powder.

continued

Box 28.B Continued

5 Review patient after 4 weeks of supplement use. If weight loss continues, seek advice from a dietitian. Monitoring should continue on a monthly basis until supplements are no longer required.

6 Patients with renal or hepatic failure, malabsorption, dysphagia, or at risk of refeeding syndrome should be referred to a dietitian.

Energy content is given per unit and per mL and the protein content per unit. For other supplements, the nutritional content is given per 100mL or 100g as appropriate. Flavours frequently alter; check availability with the manufacturer. Unless otherwise stated, all products listed are Advisory Committee on Borderline Substances (ACBS) approved for patients with disease related malnutrition.

The oral nutritional supplements listed are gluten-free and most are suitable for vegetarians. Those containing fish oils (EPA) and micronutrients or colourings derived from animal sources may not be acceptable to strict vegetarians. If uncertain with patients who have specific dietary restrictions, consult a dietitian or the manufacturers for advice.

Ingesting sufficient quantities orally may be difficult for patients with anorexia or taste changes and various strategies, including recipes suggested by the manufacturers, can be tried to aid compliance (Box 28.C).

Box 28.C Aiding compliance with milk- and juice-based supplements

Milk-based
Serve chilled ± ice
Add extra full-fat milk
Make a smoothie by adding fresh fruit and ice cream
Make into a jelly
Use instead of milk on cereals and in puddings (unflavoured)
Use to make custard/rice pudding (vanilla flavour)
Further recipes are available from:
www.abbottnutritionuk.com
www.fresenius-kabi.co.uk
www.nestlenutrition.co.uk
www.nutricia.co.uk

Juice-based
Serve chilled ± ice
Add extra fruit juice
Make a spritzer by adding soda water/lemonade/carbonated water
Make into a jelly
Pour over fresh or tinned fruit
Freeze to make an ice lolly or ice cubes

Table 28.1 Milkshake-style nutritional supplements (suitable as a sole source of nutrition)[a,b]
Included for completeness: generally supplements with higher energy and protein content should be used.

Product	*Unit size*	*Energy content*	*Protein content*	*Flavours/comments*
Ensure® (Abbott)	250mL Can	250kcal (1.0kcal/mL)	10g	Chocolate, coffee, vanilla
Fresubin Original® (Fresenius)	200mL Bottle	200kcal (1.0kcal/mL)	8g	Blackcurrant, chocolate, mocha, nut, peach, vanilla

a. avoid acidic citrus/tangy flavours in patients with a sore mouth
b. best served chilled.

Table 28.2 High-energy milkshake-style nutritional supplements (suitable as a sole source of nutrition)[a,b]

Product	*Unit size*	*Energy content*	*Protein content*	*Flavours/comments*
Fortisip Compact® (Nutricia)	125mL Bottle	300kcal (2.4kcal/mL)	12g	Banana, mocha, strawberry, vanilla
Ensure Plus Milkshake Style® (Abbott)	220mL Bottle	330kcal (1.5kcal/mL)	14g	Banana, blackcurrant, caramel, chocolate, coffee, fruits of the forest, orange, peach, raspberry, strawberry, vanilla, unflavoured
Fortisip Bottle® (Nutricia)	200mL Bottle	300kcal (1.5kcal/mL)	12g	Banana, chocolate, orange, strawberry, toffee, tropical, vanilla, unflavoured
Fresubin Energy® (Fresenius)	200mL Bottle	300 kcal (1.5kcal/mL)	11g	Banana, blackcurrant, cappuccino, chocolate, lemon, strawberry, tropical fruit, vanilla, unflavoured
Resource Energy® (Nestle)	200mL Bottle	300kcal (1.5kcal/mL)	11g	Apricot, banana, chocolate, coffee, strawberry-raspberry, vanilla

a. avoid acidic citrus/tangy flavours in patients with a sore mouth
b. best served chilled.

Table 28.3 Savoury nutritional supplements[a]

Product	*Unit size*	*Energy content*	*Protein content*	*Flavours/comments*
Ensure Plus Savoury® (Abbott)	250mL Can	375kcal (1.5kcal/mL)	16g	Suitable as a sole source of nutrition; chicken, mushroom
Fortisip Savoury Multifibre® (Nutricia)	200mL Cup	300kcal (1.5kcal/mL)	15g	Contains 5g (60:40 soluble:insoluble) fibre. Suitable as a sole source of nutrition; chicken, tomato
Provide Extra ® (Fresenius)	200mL Bottle	300kcal (1.5kcal/mL)	8g	Tomato

a. best served warmed, do not boil.

Table 28.4 Milkshake-style nutritional supplements with fibre (suitable as a sole source of nutrition)[a,b]

Product	*Unit size*	*Energy content*	*Protein content*	*Flavours/comments*
Resource 2.0 Fibre® (Nestle)	200mL Bottle	400kcal (2.0kcal/mL)	18g	Contains 5g soluble fibre (50:50 FOS:GOS); apricot, coffee, strawberry, summer fruit, vanilla, unflavoured
Ensure Plus Fibre® (Abbott)	200mL Bottle	305kcal (1.5kcal/mL)	13g	Contains 5g fibre and fructo-oligosaccharides; banana, chocolate, fruits of the forest, raspberry, strawberry, vanilla
Fortisip Multifibre® (Nutricia)	200mL Bottle	300kcal (1.5kcal/mL)	12g	Contains 4.6g (60:40 soluble:insoluble) fibre; banana, chocolate, orange, strawberry, vanilla
Fresubin Energy Fibre® (Fresenius)	200mL Bottle	300kcal (1.5kcal/mL)	11g	Contains 4g mixed fibre blend; banana, caramel, cherry, chocolate, strawberry, vanilla

a. useful for patients with constipation
b. shake well before use.

Table 28.5 Yoghurt-style nutritional supplements (suitable as a sole source of nutrition)[a,b]

Product	*Unit size*	*Energy content*	*Protein content*	*Flavours/comments*
Ensure Plus Yoghurt Style® (Abbott)	220mL Bottle	330kcal (1.5kcal/mL)	14g	Orange, peach, pineapple, strawberry
Fortisip Yoghurt Style® (Nutricia)	200mL Bottle	300kcal (1.5kcal/mL)	12g	Peach-orange, raspberry, vanilla-lemon

a. can be more palatable in patients with taste change (citrus/tangy flavours vs. sweet)
b. avoid acidic citrus/tangy flavours in patients with a sore mouth.

Table 28.6 Fruit juice-style nutritional supplements (not suitable as a sole source of nutrition)[a,b]

Product	*Unit size*	*Energy content*	*Protein content*	*Flavours/comments*
Fortijuce® (Nutricia)	200mL Bottle	300kcal (1.5kcal/mL)	8g	Apple, blackcurrant, forest fruit, lemon, orange, strawberry, tropical
Ensure Plus Juce® (Abbott)	220mL Bottle	330kcal (1.5kcal/mL)	11g	Apple, fruit punch, lemon and lime, orange, peach, strawberry
Provide Extra® (Fresenius)	200mL Bottle	300kcal (1.5kcal/mL)	8g	Apple, blackcurrant, cherry, citrus-cola, lemon and lime, melon, orange and pineapple
Resource Fruit® (Nestle)	200mL Bottle	250kcal (1.3kcal/mL)	8g	Apple, orange, pear-cherry, raspberry-blackcurrant

a. may be preferable for patients with a dry mouth
b. avoid acidic citrus/tangy flavours in patients with a sore mouth.

Table 28.7 High protein milkshake-style nutritional supplements[a,b]

Product	*Unit size*	*Energy content*	*Protein content*	*Flavours/comments*
Fresubin 2kcal® (Fresenius)	200mL Bottle	400kcal (2kcal/mL)	20g	Not suitable as a sole source of nutrition; apricot-peach, cappuccino, fruits of the forest, toffee, vanilla
Fresubin 2kcal Fibre® (Fresenius)	200mL Bottle	400kcal (2kcal/mL)	20g	Not suitable as a sole source of nutrition. Contains 3g fibre; cappuccino, chocolate, lemon, vanilla
Fortisip Extra® (Nutricia)	200mL Bottle	320kcal (1.6kcal/mL)	20g	Not suitable as a sole source of nutrition; chocolate, forest fruit, mocha, strawberry, vanilla, unflavoured
Fresubin Protein Energy Drink® (Fresenius)	200mL Bottle	300kcal (1.5kcal/mL)	20g	Not suitable as a sole source of nutrition; cappuccino, chocolate, strawberry, tropical fruits, vanilla
Fortimel Regular ® (Nutricia)	200mL Bottle	200kcal (1kcal/mL)	20g	Not suitable as a sole source of nutrition; chocolate, forest fruits, strawberry, vanilla
Resource Protein® (Nestle)	200mL Bottle	250kcal (1.25kcal/mL)	19g	Suitable as a sole source of nutrition. apricot, chocolate, forest fruits, strawberry, vanilla
Ensure Twocal® (Abbott)	200mL Bottle	400kcal (2kcal/mL)	17g	Suitable as a sole source of nutrition. Contains 2g FOS; banana, strawberry, vanilla, unflavoured

a. consider in patients with high protein loss or wounds when overall energy intake is adequate
b. caution required when renal function impaired (seek advice).

Table 28.8 Semi-solid nutritional supplements (suitable as a sole source of nutrition)[a]

Product	*Unit size*	*Energy content*	*Protein content*	*Flavours/comments*
Fresubin Creme® (Fresenius)	125g Pot	225kcal (1.8kcal/g)	13g	Cappuccino, chocolate, praline, strawberry, vanilla
Forticreme Complete® (Nutricia)	125g Pot	200kcal (1.6kcal/g)	12g	Banana, chocolate, forest fruit, vanilla
Resource Dessert Energy® (Nestle)	125g Pot	200kcal (1.6kcal/g)	6g	Caramel, chocolate, vanilla
Resource Dessert Fruit® (Nestle)	125g Pot	200kcal (1.6kcal/g)	6g	Apple, apple-peach, apple-strawberry
Ensure Plus Creme® (Abbott)	125g Pot	171kcal (1.4kcal/g)	7g	Banana, chocolate, vanilla, unflavoured
Fortisip Fruit Dessert® (Nutricia)	150g Pot	200kcal (1.3kcal/g)	11g	Apple, strawberry

a. useful for patients with dysphagia.

Table 28.9 Powdered milkshake- and soup-style nutritional supplements (not suitable as a sole source of nutrition)[a,b,c]

Product	*Unit size*	*Energy content*	*Protein content*	*Flavours/comments*
Enshake® (Abbott)	96.5g Sachet	434kcal (4.5kcal/g)	8g	600kcal and 16g protein when reconstituted with full-fat milk (240mL); banana, chocolate, strawberry, vanilla, in boxes of 6
Calshake® (Fresenius)	87g Sachet	431kcal (5kcal/g)	4g	588kcal and 12g protein when reconstituted with full-fat milk (240mL); banana, chocolate, strawberry, unflavoured, vanilla, in boxes of 7
Scandishake Mix® (Nutricia)	85g Sachet	431kcal (5kcal/g)	4g	600kcal and 12g protein when reconstituted with full-fat milk (240mL); banana, caramel, chocolate, strawberry, vanilla, unflavoured, in boxes of 6
Foodlink Complete (Foodlink)	450g Box	270kcal (4kcal/g)	12g	1 serving = 3 to 4 heaped dessert spoons. Reconstitute with full-fat milk or water (250mL); banana, chocolate, strawberry, vanilla with fibre, unflavoured
Complan Shake® (Complan Foods Ltd.)	57g Sachet	250kcal (4kcal/g)	9g	385kcal and 16g protein when reconstituted with full-fat milk (200mL); With added vitamins and minerals; banana, chocolate, strawberry, vanilla, unflavoured
Vitasavoury® (Vitaflo)	33g Cup 50g Sachet	200kcal (6kcal/g) 300kcal (6kcal/g)	4g 6g	Reconstitute with hot water; chicken, golden vegetable, leek and potato, mushroom

a. high palatability
b. lower in some vitamins and minerals compared with other supplements
c. milkshake style should be reconstituted using full-fat milk to optimize energy content.

Table 28.10 OTC nutritional supplements (not suitable as a sole source of nutrition)

Product	*Unit size*	*Energy content*	*Protein content*	*Comments*
BuildUp Nutrition Shake® (Nestle)	38g Sachet	127kcal	8g	Reconstitute with 200mL full-fat milk; contains 3g soluble fibre; banana, chocolate, strawberry, vanilla, in boxes of 4
BuildUp Nutrition Soup® (Nestle)	49g Sachet	200kcal	8g	Reconstitute with 200mL hot water/full-fat milk; chicken, potato and leek, tomato, vegetable
BuildUp Original® (Nestle)	400g Tub	360kcal/ 100g	24g/ 100g	Use to fortify foods or as a drink; unflavoured
Complan® (Complan Foods Ltd)	57g Sachet	250kcal (4 kcal/g)	9g	Reconstitute with 200mL hot or cold water/ full-fat milk; banana, chocolate, strawberry, vanilla, unflavoured, in boxes of 4
Complan Savoury® (Complan Foods Ltd)	57g Sachet	250kcal (4 kcal/g)	9g	Reconstitute with 200mL hot water/full-fat milk; chicken, vegetable, in boxes of 4

Table 28.11 Special application nutritional products[a]

Product	*Unit size*	*Energy content*	*Protein content*	*Flavours/comments*
Supportan® (Fresenius)	200mL Bottle	300kcal	20g	For use in patients with cachexia (pancreatic cancer and lung cancer undergoing chemotherapy). Contains eicosapentanoic acid (EPA) and docosahexanoic acid (DHA), anti-oxidants and fibre. Recommended dose 3 bottles/day (providing 2.85g EPA and DHA); cappuccino, tropical fruits
Prosure® (Abbott)	240mL Tetrapak	295kcal	16g	For use in patients with cachexia (pancreatic cancer and lung cancer undergoing chemotherapy). Contains eicosapentanoic acid (EPA) and anti-oxidants. An intake of 1.5–2 cartons/day is required for benefit; not nutritionally complete at this dose; vanilla
Forticare® (Nutricia)	125mL Carton	200kcal	11g	For use in patients with cachexia (pancreatic cancer and lung cancer undergoing chemotherapy). Contains EPA, fibre and anti-oxidants. Recommended dose 3 cartons/day (providing 2.2g EPA); not nutritionally complete at this dose; cappuccino, orange-lemon, peach-ginger
Oral Impact® (Nestle)	74g Sachet	303kcal	17g	Contains immune-modulating substrates and soluble fibre (e.g. ω-3 fatty acids, arginine, nucleotides). Pre-operatively, 2–4 sachets a day recommended for 5–7 days; not nutritionally complete at this dose; citrus, coffee, tropical

continued

Table 28.11 Continued

Product	*Unit size*	*Energy content*	*Protein content*	*Flavours/comments*
Respifor® (Nutricia)	125mL Bottle	188kcal	9g	For early intervention use in patients with COPD. Recommended dose 125mL t.d.s in combination with activity plan for 3 months; chocolate, strawberry, vanilla
Elemental E028 Extra Liquid® (SHS)	250mL Tetrapak	215kcal	6g	A liquid elemental feed for patients with intractable malabsorption or radiation enteritis. Protein source is a mixture of essential and non-essential amino acids. Nutritionally complete; grapefruit, orange and pineapple, summer fruits
Elemental E028 Extra® (SHS)	100g Sachet	427kcal/ 100g	13g/100g	An elemental feed for patients with intractable malabsorption or radiation enteritis. Protein source is a mixture of essential and non-essential amino acids. Nutritionally complete. Reconstitute with 100g powder in 500mL water; banana, citrus, orange, unflavoured
Peptamen® (Nestle)	200mL Cup vanilla	200kcal	8g	For patients with impaired GI function. Contains protein source as peptides and fat is 70% medium-chain triglycerides to improve digestion and absorption. Nutritionally complete. Can be flavoured with 2 scoops of Nestle Nutrition Flavour Mix/100mL to improve palatability; banana, chocolate, coffee, lemon and lime, strawberry
Resource OptiFibre® (Nestle)	250g Tub (5g per scoop) 10g Sachet	–	–	For use with patients who have constipation. Each scoop contains 4g and each sachet 6g of soluble fibre (partially hydrolyzed guar gum) which is mixed into hot or cold liquids and foods. Introduce gradually; begin with 1 scoop or 1/2 sachet and increase by 1 scoop or 1/2 sachet every 3 days. Recommended dose is 2 sachets/3 scoops/day, maximum 32g/day
Forceval® (Alliance)	15, 30, 45 and 90 Cap pack	–	–	Multivitamin and mineral supplement given as 1 capsule daily. Capsule can be opened and contents mixed, for example, with a teaspoon of jam

a. use with dietetic supervision.

Table 28.12 Modular carbohydrate, protein and fat supplements (not suitable as a sole source of nutrition)[a]

Product	*Unit size*	*Energy Source*	*Energy content*	*Comments*
Caloreen® (Nestle)	500g Tub	Carbohydrate	385kcal/100g	Glucose polymer powder to add to food and drinks; unflavoured
Polycal Powder® (Nutricia)	400g Tub	Carbohydrate	384kcal/100g	Glucose polymer powder to add to food and drinks; unflavoured
Maxijul Super Soluble Powder® (SHS)	132g Sachet, 200g, 2.5kg, 25kg Tub	Carbohydrate	380kcal/100g	Glucose polymer powder to add to food and drinks; unflavoured
Vitajoule® (Vitaflo)	500g, 2.5kg, 25kg Tub	Carbohydrate	380kcal/100g	Glucose syrup powder to add to food and drinks; unflavoured
Polycal Liquid® (Nutricia)	200mL Tetrpak	Carbohydrate	247kcal/100mL	Glucose polymer solution; can be used in drinks diluted; orange, unflavoured
Protifar® (Nutricia)	225g Tub	Protein	380kcal/100g 89g protein/100g	High-protein powder supplement to add to food and drinks; unflavoured
Vitapro® (Vitaflo)	250g, 2kg Tub	Protein	360kcal/100g 75g protein /100g	High-biological value powdered protein supplement to add to food and drinks; unflavoured
Fresubin 5kcal Shot® (Fresenius)	120mL Bottle	Fat	500kcal/100mL	Medium-chain triglyceride fat emulsion. Recommended dose 30mL t.d.s–q.d.s; lemon, unflavoured
Liquigen® (SHS)	250mL, Bottle	Fat	450kcal/100mL	Medium-chain triglyceride fat emulsion; unflavoured
Calogen® (Nutricia)	250mL, 500mL Bottle	Fat	450kcal/100mL	Long-chain triglyceride fat emulsion. Recommended dose 30mL t.d.s; banana, strawberry; unflavoured
Calogen Extra® (Nutricia)	200mL Bottle	Fat, carbohydrate	400kcal/100mL 5g protein/100mL	High energy fat emulsion with protein, carbohydrate, vitamins and minerals. Recommended dose 30mL q.c.s; strawberry, unflavoured
Super Soluble Duocal® (SHS)	400g Tub	Fat, carbohydrate	492kcal/100g	Fat and glucose polymer powder to add to food and drinks; unflavoured
Duocal Liquid® (SHS)	250mL	Fat, carbohydrate	166kcal/100mL	Fat and carbohydrate emulsion; unflavoured
ProSource Liquid® (Nutrinovo)	100 × 30mL Sachet	Protein and carbohydrate	333kcal/100mL 33g protein/100mL	Protein and energy liquid supplement to add to food and drinks or take as a shot
Pro-Cal® (Vitaflo)	25 × 15g Sachet 510g, 1.5kg, 12.5kg, 25kg Tub	Protein, fat, carbohydrate	667kcal/100g 14g protein /100g	Energy and protein powder to add to food and drinks; unflavoured
Pro-Cal Shot® (Vitaflo)	250mL Bottle	Protein, fat, carbohydrate	334/100mL 7g protein/100mL	Fat, protein and carbohydrate emulsion; unflavoured
Quickcal® (Vitaflo)	25x13g Sachet	Protein, fat, carbohydrate	780kcal/100g 5g protein /100g	High-energy powder to add to food and drinks; unflavoured

a. use with dietetic supervision.

Table 28.13 Thickeners and thickened drinks[a]

Product	*Unit size*	*Energy content*	*Comments*
Fresubin Thickened® (Fresenius)	200mL Bottle	150kcal/100mL 20g protein/100mL	Texture modified supplement drink in stage 1 and stage 2 consistency; strawberry, vanilla
Resource Thickened Drinks® (Nestle)	114mL Cup	89kcal/100mL	Ready to use, available in syrup and custard consistency; apple, orange
Thick and Easy Thickened Juices® (Fresenius)	118mL Pot 1420mL Bottle	58–73kcal/100mL	Ready to use, available in honey consistency; apple, apple and orange (Pot only), blackcurrant, cranberry, kiwi-strawberry, orange
Nutilis® (Nutricia)	225g Can	333kcal/100g	Modified maize starch. Can be used to thicken fluids and food
Resource Thicken Up (Nestle)	4.5g Sachet 227g Can	368kcal/100g	Modified maize starch. Can be used to thicken fluids and food
Resource Thicken Up Clear® (Nestle)	1.2g Sachet 125g Can	310kcal/100g	Maltdextrin, xanthangum and potassium chloride. Can be used to thicken fluids and food. Fluids remain clear
Thick and Easy Instant Food Thickener® (Fresenius)	9g Sachet 225g, 4.5kg Tub	373kcal/100g	Modified maize starch. Can be used to thicken fluids and food
Vitaquick® (Vitaflo)	300g, 2.5kg, 6kg Tub	380kcal/100g	Pre-gelatinized modified starch. Can be used to thicken fluids and food

a. for patients with dysphagia.

Cautions

The high sugar content and acidity of some nutritional supplement drinks can encourage dental caries and patients should be advised on good oral hygiene, e.g. ingest the supplement relatively quickly and then clean teeth. However, sipping the supplement over a prolonged period may be unavoidable in patients with early satiety.

Generally, patients with diabetes can use nutritional supplements without problem. However, monitoring of blood sugars may be required when using supplements with a high carbohydrate content, e.g. carbohydrate modular supplements. Rarely, and generally in patients already taking large doses of additional vitamins, nutritional supplements have contributed to ingestion of harmful amounts of vitamins, e.g. vitamin B6 leading to sensory neuropathy. Drug-nutrient interactions may occur with:

- vitamin K, present in significant quantities in the nutritional supplement drinks, and **warfarin** → reduced anticoagulation
- eicosapentanoic acid, in Forticare®, Oral Impac®, Prosure®, and Supportan®, and **warfarin** → enhanced anticoagulation.[24,25]

Refeeding syndrome

Refeeding syndrome is a potentially fatal condition caused by major shifts in fluids and electrolytes in malnourished patients who are started too rapidly on enteral or parenteral nutritional supplements.[26,27] Biochemically, refeeding syndrome is characterized primarily by hypophosphataemia.

During a period of starvation, the body adapts in various ways to cope with the lack of readily available carbohydrate, and switches to using fat and protein as the main source of energy. If malnutrition is prolonged, there are further hormonal and metabolic changes aimed at preventing protein and muscle breakdown. Several intracellular minerals become severely depleted (although plasma concentrations may remain normal).

During refeeding, glycaemia leads to increased insulin secretion and a series of sequential effects, including decreases in the plasma concentrations of phosphate, potassium, magnesium, and thiamine. If unrecognized and untreated, refeeding syndrome can result in life-threatening complications, including cardiac arrhythmia and multi-organ failure.[27] It is thus important that high risk patients should be managed by appropriately trained health professionals.

Although a regimen of rapid refeeding is unlikely in patients with advanced cancer and chronic oligophagia and/or cachexia, palliative care clinicians should be aware of the syndrome, and have a basic understanding of its management (Box 28.D).

Box 28.D Risk factors for and management of refeeding syndrome[28]

Refeeding syndrome is associated with high morbidity and mortality. Its management requires appropriately trained health professionals.

High risk patients

Those with one or more of the following:
- BMI $<16\text{kg/m}^2$
- unintentional weight loss of $>15\%$ in the last 3–6 months
- little or no nutritional intake for >10 days
- low plasma concentrations of PO_4^-, K^+, Mg^{2+} before restarting feeding.

Or two or more of the following:
- BMI $<18.5\text{kg/m}^2$
- unintentional weight loss $>10\%$ within the last 3–6 months
- little or no nutritional intake for >5 days
- a history of alcohol abuse or drugs, including insulin, chemotherapy, antacids and diuretics.

Management

For the first 2 days, patients who have had little or nothing to eat for ≥ 5 days should only be offered/given nutritional support estimated to meet $\leq 50\%$ of their ideal requirements. After this, if biochemical parameters are satisfactory, it is safe to provide full nutrition.

If high risk:
- ensure adequate hydration
- before feeding, and for the next 10 days, administer:
  - ▹ thiamine 200–300mg once daily
  - ▹ strong compound vitamin B 1–2 tablets t.d.s. (or IV vitamin B once daily)
  - ▹ multivitamin and mineral supplement once daily
- start nutritional support at ≤ 10kcal/kg/day (5kcal/kg/day in extreme cases)
- increase intake progressively to achieve full nutritional requirements after 4–7 days
- if pre-feeding plasma concentrations are low, prescribe biochemical supplements:
  - ▹ magnesium (e.g. 0.2mmol/kg/day IV, 0.4mmol/kg/day PO)
  - ▹ phosphate (e.g. 0.3–0.6mmol/kg/day)
  - ▹ potassium (e.g. 2–4mmol/kg/day).

Monitoring

Daily until stable, and then 2–3 times weekly: fluid balance, nutritional intake, biochemical parameters, and general physical and psychological condition.

1 Fearon K *et al.* (2011) Definition and classification of cancer cachexia: an international consensus. *Lancet Oncology.*
2 Arends J *et al.* (2006) ESPEN Guidelines on Enteral Nutrition: Non-surgical oncology. *Clinical Nutrition.* **25**: 245–259.
3 National Collaborating Centre for Acute Care (2006) *Nutrition Support in Adults: Oral nutrition support, enteral tube feeding and parenteral nutrition* (No. 32). National Institute for Clinical Excellence, London.
4 Malnutrition Advisory Group (2003) The Malnutrition Universal Screening Tool. BAPEN, UK. Available from: www.bapen.org.uk/must_tool.html
5 Kyle UG *et al.* (2006) Comparison of tools for nutritional assessment and screening at hospital admission: a population study. *Clinical Nutrition.* **25**: 409–417.
6 Davies M (2005) Nutritional screening and assessment in cancer-associated malnutrition. *European Journal of Oncology Nursing.* **9 (suppl 2)**: S64–73.
7 Ottery FD (1996) Definition of standardized nutritional assessment and interventional pathways in oncology. *Nutrition.* **12**: S15–19.
8 Bauer J *et al.* (2002) Use of the scored Patient-Generated Subjective Global Assessment (PG-SGA) as a nutrition assessment tool in patients with cancer. *European Journal of Clinical Nutrition.* **56**: 779–785.
9 Chauhan A *et al.* (2007) NICE guidance for screening for malnutrition: implications for lung cancer services. *Thorax.* **62**: 835.
10 Halliday V *et al.* (2010) Screening for malnutrition: implications for upper gastrointestinal cancer services. *Journal of Surgical Oncology.* **102**: 543–544.
11 Thoresen L and de Soysa AK (2006) The nutritional aspects of palliative care. *European Journal of Palliative Care.* **13**: 194–197.
12 Bozzetti F *et al.* (2009) ESPEN Guidelines on Parenteral Nutrition: non-surgical oncology. *Clinical Nutrition.* **28**: 445–454.
13 Lobo DN *et al.* (2006) Early postoperative jejunostomy feeding with an immune modulating diet in patients undergoing resectional surgery for upper gastrointestinal cancer: a prospective, randomized, controlled, double-blind study. *Clinical Nutrition.* **25**: 716–726.
14 Heyland DK *et al.* (2001) Should immunonutrition become routine in critically ill patients? A systematic review of the evidence. *Journal of the American Medical Association.* **286**: 944–953.
15 Yavuzsen T *et al.* (2005) Systematic review of the treatment of cancer-associated anorexia and weight loss. *Journal of Clinical Oncology.* **23**: 8500–8511.
16 Fearon KC *et al.* (2003) Effect of a protein and energy dense N-3 fatty acid enriched oral supplement on loss of weight and lean tissue in cancer cachexia: a randomised double blind trial. *Gut.* **52**: 1479–1486.
17 Wilcock A (2005) Cachexia and omega-3 polyunsaturated fatty acids: the beginning of the end or the end of the beginning? *Palliative Medicine.* **19**: 500–502.
18 Mazzotta P and Jeney CM (2009) Anorexia-cachexia syndrome: a systematic review of the role of dietary polyunsaturated Fatty acids in the management of symptoms, survival, and quality of life. *Journal of Pain and Symptom Management.* **37**: 1069–1077.
19 van der Meij BS *et al.* (2010) Oral nutritional supplements containing (n-3) polyunsaturated fatty acids affect the nutritional status of patients with stage III non-small cell lung cancer during multimodality treatment. *Journal of Nutritrion.* **140**: 1774–1780.
20 McCann RM *et al.* (1994) A comfort care for terminally ill patients: the appropriate use of nutrition and hydration. *Journal of the American Medical Association.* **272**: 179–181.
21 Sarhill N *et al.* (2003) Evaluation of nutritional status in advanced metastatic cancer. *Supportive Care in Cancer.* **11**: 652–659.
22 Antoun S *et al.* (2006) Artificial nutrition at the end of life: is it justified? *European Journal of Palliative Care.* **13**: 194–197.
23 Baldwin C and Weekes C (2008) Dietary advice for illness-related malnutrition in adults. *Cochrane Database of Systematic Reviews.* **1**: CD002008.
24 Baxter K (2011) Stockley's Drug Interactions (online edition). Pharmaceutical Press, London. Available from: www.medicinescomplete.com
25 Holbrook AM *et al.* (2005) Systematic overview of warfarin and its drug and food interactions. *Archives of Internal Medicine.* **165**: 1095–1106.
26 Mehanna HM *et al.* (2008) Refeeding syndrome: what it is, and how to prevent and treat it. *British Medical Journal.* **336**: 1495–1498.
27 Boateng AA *et al.* (2010) Refeeding syndrome: treatment considerations based on collective analysis of literature case reports. *Nutrition.* **26**: 156–167.
28 NICE (2006) Nutrition support in adults. Clinical guidelines CG32. Available from: **http://guidance.nice.org.uk/CG32**

Appendix 1: Obtaining Unlicensed Products

The Department of Health recommends that licensed products should be used whenever possible. The MHRA is responsible for ensuring that medicines and medical devices are effective, safe and of appropriate quality. Generally, medicinal products must have a marketing authorisation (MA), previously known as a product licence, before they can be marketed. However, in the UK there is an exemption to the regulations, whereby an unlicensed medicine can be prescribed if there is a clear, clinical need which cannot be satisfied by an existing licensed product.[1] (This is not the same as off-label use, in which a licensed medicine is used outside the clinical indications of its MA; see p.xxiii.) These unlicensed products are generally termed 'specials' or 'named patient supplies'.

Specials

The term 'special' is generally used to include the following:

- a medicine manufactured by a specials manufacturer holding a manufacturer's specials licence (MS), produced in multiple quantities with end product analytical testing, e.g. some prefilled opioid syringes
- a bespoke medicine produced by a specials manufacturer holding an MS, without end product analytical testing, e.g. some TPN and chemotherapy
- a locally prepared (extemporaneous) unlicensed medicine made in a pharmacy under a pharmacist's direct supervision, e.g. dilution of creams or ointments.

Named patient supplies

The term 'named patient supplies' generally includes the following:

- a medicine licensed in another country but not in the UK and which is imported into the UK by a specialist importing company
- a medicine which may be available from a UK manufacturer before an MA has been issued, e.g. if a patient wishes to continue an investigational medicine after a clinical trial
- a medicine which has had its MA withdrawn but special provision has been made by the MHRA for a continued supply, where the clinical need of the patient cannot be satisfied by any other licensed product, e.g. co-proxamol.

Prescribers should be aware or made aware of the unlicensed nature of any 'special' or 'named patient' medicine prescribed. With the exception of locally prepared (extemporaneous) supplies, pharmacists must keep records of the source, quantity obtained and supplied, batch numbers of the medicines, prescriber and patient details. They must also record and report any adverse reactions associated with their use.[1,2]

Suppliers

The MHRA maintains a register of specials manufacturers and specialist importing companies (http://tinyurl.com/cdslke). Licensed NHS hospital manufacturing units may also manufacture specials as unlicensed medicines. A list of these units is included in the BNF. A database (*Pro-File*; www.pro-file.nhs.uk) provides information on medicines manufactured in the NHS but access is restricted to NHS pharmacy staff. The Association of Commercial Specials Manufacturers may also be able to provide information about commercial companies (www.acsm.uk.com).

1 MHRA (2008) The supply of unlicensed relevant medicinal products for individual patients. In: *MHRA Medicines and Healthcare Regulatory Authority Guidance Note 14*. Available from: www.mhra.gov.uk (accessed 24 Feb 2011)

2 Anonymous (2010) Good practice guidance on the procurement and supply of pharmaceutical specials. *Pharmacy Professional*. **June**: 27–32.

Appendix 2: Taking controlled and prescription drugs to other countries

For patients living in the UK, because the regulations may change, it is advisable to check for the latest Home Office guidance by contacting them directly or visiting their website:

The Home Office
Drugs Licensing and Compliance
4th Floor, Fry Building
2 Marsham Street
London SW1P 4DF
Tel: 020 7035 0484
Fax: 020 7035 6161
e-mail: licensing_enquiry.aadu@homeoffice.gsi.gov.uk
www.homeoffice.gov.uk/drugs/licensing/personal/

Some patients receiving palliative care travel to other countries and need to take medication with them. Two sets of laws need to be considered, those of the UK and those of the country or countries to which they are travelling. Detailed advice can be obtained from the regulatory authorities, embassies or consulates in the relevant countries. A list of embassy contact details is available from the Home Office drugs website.

The UK customs regulations were simplified in 2008. For UK residents, the main limitation is likely to be the legislation of the countries to which they are travelling, e.g. some countries do not allow the importation of **codeine**, **dihydrocodeine** or **diamorphine**.

Away for <3 months

A letter from the prescribing doctor is sufficient, even for **CD**. A list of drug classes and schedules is included in the BNF (www.bnf.org.uk/bnf/). The letter should state:

- the patient's name, address and date of birth
- the destination(s) and dates of outward and return travel
- the names, forms, strengths, doses and total amounts of the drugs being carried.

Away for ≥3 months or carrying more than three months supply

If a patient is planning to stay away for 3 months or longer, they should be advised to make contact with a doctor in the country in which they will be staying, and to obtain prescriptions for further supplies from that doctor. Otherwise they will need a personal import or export licence and a letter from their UK prescribing doctor. The licence application form can be downloaded from the Home Office website. They must apply for this at least 10 working days before the intended travel date, providing the same information as outlined above.

CD should be kept in their original packaging and carried in the patient's hand luggage (together with the covering letter or licence) in case Customs want to examine them. Air passengers are generally allowed to carry up to 100mL of liquid in their hand luggage. To carry more than 100mL may require prior approval from the airline and the departure airport; the medication should be presented at security for x-ray inspection and possible verification.

Travelling to or through other countries

It is important to fulfil the **CD** requirements for all the countries which the patient will visit, otherwise entry may be refused. The International Narcotics Control Board has produced a list of suggested maximum quantities for personal import/export of internationally controlled substances (Table A2.1), and a model import/export certificate (Box A2.A). It is also advisable to carry a duplicate copy of the prescription, preferably stamped by the pharmacy from which the drugs were obtained. *However, patients should check the exact legal details and the quantities they are allowed to import with the relevant embassies or consulates before travelling.*

Table A2.1 Suggested maximum quantities of controlled substances for international travellers[a,b]

Drug	*Quantity*
Buprenorphine	300mg
Codeine	12g
Diazepam	300mg
Dihydrocodeine	12g
Fentanyl transdermal patches[b]	100mg
Fentanyl (other formulations)	20mg
Hydromorphone	300mg
Lorazepam	75mg
Methadone	2g
Morphine	3g
Oxycodone	1g

a. this is not a complete list; see referenced source for more details
b. approximately, this adds up to 6 fentanyl 100microgram/h patches, and 8, 12, 24, 48 of the 75, 50, 25, 12microgram/h patches, respectively.

Box A2.A Model certificate for personal import/export of internationally controlled substances[1]

Country and place of issue
Country of issue
Place of issue
Date of issue
Period of validity[a]

Prescribing physician
Last name, first name
Address
Telephone (including country code)
Professional licence number

Patient
Last name, first name
Sex
Place of birth
Date of birth
Home address
Passport or identity card number
Intended country of destination

Prescribed medical preparation
Trade name of drug (or composition)
Formulation (ampoules, tablets, etc.)
Number of tablets, etc.
rINN of the active substance
Concentration of the active substance
Total quantity of the active substance
Instructions for use
Duration of prescription in days
Remarks

Issuing authority
Official name of the authority
Address
Telephone (country code, local code, number)
Official seal of the authority
Signature of the responsible officer

a. the recommended duration is 3 months.

1 International Narcotics Control Board (2004) Guidelines for travellers. Available from: www.incb.org/incb/guidelines_travellers.html

Appendix 3: Compatibility charts

PCF recommends that generally water for injection (WFI) is used as the standard diluent of choice because there is less likelihood of incompatibility. However, 0.9% saline should be considered when there is actual or potential for inflammation at the injection site (see p.667).

Charts A3.1–A3.7 and Table A3.1 summarize the compatibility data available for the more commonly used 2-drug and 3-drug combinations given by CSCI in WFI. Charts summarizing the compatibility data available for the more commonly used 2-drug and 3-drug combinations given by CSCI in 0.9% saline can be found on www.palliativedrugs.com.

The charts have been compiled from clinical observations in palliative care services submitted to the www.palliativedrugs.com Syringe Driver Survey Database (SDSD) from the UK, New Zealand and Australia, and from published compatibility data (see reference list). The SDSD is a continually updated resource and contains more detailed observational compatibility data on mixing up to four drugs in either WFI or 0.9% saline.

A traffic light system has been devised for use in the clinical setting as a practical summary of the data available:

- *red* = do not use (available information indicates a compatibility problem)
- *amber* = proceed with caution (possible compatibility problem, depending on the order of mixing or drug concentrations)
- *green* = reported compatible (data may be observational, physical or chemical, i.e. may be practice- or evidence-based).

Multiple factors affect drug stability and compatibility, including drug concentration, brand/formulation of the drug (e.g. compatibility for oxycodone 10mg/mL and 50mg/mL formulations differ), diluent, infusion time, exposure to light, ambient temperature, order of mixing and delivery system material (see p.668). These factors probably explain why conflicting reports occur. *Regular monitoring of all CSCI drug combinations is essential*, even for those coded green. If there is doubt about the relevance of the compatibility data in any particular situation, e.g. at the extremes of dose and concentration, advice should be obtained from a clinical pharmacist.

Dexamethasone often causes compatibility problems. It should always be the last drug to be added to an already dilute combination of drugs, thus reducing the risk of precipitation. However, because **dexamethasone** has a long duration of action, it can generally be given as a bolus SC injection once daily.

Health professionals are urged to contact hq@palliativedrugs.com if their experience indicates that the code for a combination should be changed. Submissions to the SDSD of details of successful combinations for which there are no published data are also welcome.

Most of the information in these charts relates to the use of drugs outside the scope of their Marketing Authorization and health professionals using this information must satisfy themselves as to its appropriateness in any given clinical situation (also see p.xxii). Further, health professionals should familiarize themselves with the guidance and supporting material relating to the legal implications of mixing medicines before administration (Department of Health, 2010 and National Prescribing Centre, 2010) together with any local policy and practice (also see p.xxiv).

Allwood M (1984) Diamorphine mixed with antiemetic drugs in plastic syringes. *British Journal of Pharmaceutical Practice*. **6**: 88–90.
Allwood M (1991) The stability of diamorphine alone and in combination with anti-emetics in plastic syringes. *Palliative Medicine*. **5**: 330–333.
Allwood M *et al.* (1994) Stability of injections containing diamorphine and midazolam in plastic syringes. *International Journal of Pharmacy Practice*. **3**: 57–59.
Back I (2006) *Syringe driver database*. Available from: www.pallcare.info
Department of Health (2010) Mixing of medicines prior to administration in clinical practice: medical and non-medical prescribing. Department of Health Gateway reference14330. Available from www.dh.gov.uk.
Dickman A *et al.* (2005) *The Syringe Driver: Continuous Subcutaneous Infusions in Palliative Care* (2e). Oxford University Press, Oxford.
Fawcett J *et al.* (1994) Compatibility of cyclizine lactate and haloperidol lactate. *American Journal of Hospital Pharmacy*. **51**: 2292–2294.
Fielding H *et al.* (2000) The compatibility and stability of octreotide acetate in the presence of diamorphine hydrochloride in polypropylene syringes. *Palliative Medicine*. **14**: 205–207.
Frimley Park Hospital NHS Trust (1998) *Personal communication*.
Gardiner P (2003) Compatibility of an injectable oxycodone formulation with typical diluents, syringes, tubings, infusion bags and drugs for potential co-administration. *Hospital Pharmacist*. **10**: 354–361.
Good PD *et al.* (2004) The compatibility and stability of midazolam and dexamethasone in infusion solutions. *Journal of Pain and Symptom Management*. **27**: 471–475.
Grassby P and Hutchings L (1997) Drug combinations in syringe drivers: the compatibility and stability of diamorphine with cyclizine and haloperidol. *Palliative Medicine*. **11**: 217–224.
Grassby PF (1995) *UK stability database (Apr 1995 and Jul 1997)*. Welsh Pharmaceutical Services, St. Mary's Pharmaceutical Unit, Corbett Road, Penarth, South Glamorgan.
Hines S and Pleasance S (2009) Compatibility of an injectable high strength oxycodone formulation with typical diluents, syringes, tubings, infusion bags and drugs for potential co-administration. *European Journal of Hospital Pharmacy Practice* **15**: 32–38.
Huang E and Anderson RP (1994) Compatibility of hydromorphone hydrochloride with haloperidol lactate and ketorolac tromethamine. *American Journal of Hospital Pharmacy*. **51**: 2963.
Hughes A *et al.* (1997) Ketorolac: continuous subcutaneous infusion for cancer pain. *Journal of Pain and Symptom Management*. **13**: 315–317.
Ingallinera TS *et al.* (1979) Compatibility of glycopyrrolate injection with commonly used infusion solutions and additives. *American Journal of Hospital Pharmacy*. **36**: 508–510.
Lau M-H *et al.* (1998) Compatibility of ketamine and morphine injections. *Pain*. **75**: 389–390.
Lawson WA *et al.* (1991) Stability of hyoscine in mixtures with morphine for continuous subcutaneous administration. *Australian Journal of Hospital Pharmacy*. **21**: 395–396.
LeBelle MJ *et al.* (1995) Compatibility of morphine and midazolam or haloperidol in parenteral admixtures. *Canadian Journal of Hospital Pharmacy*. **48**: 155–160.
Mendenhall A and Hoyt DB (1994) Incompatibility of ketorolac tromethamine with haloperidol lactate and thiethylperazine maleate. *American Journal of Hospital Pharmacy*. **51**: 2964.
Napp (2010) *Personal communication*.
National Prescribing Centre (2010) Mixing of medicines prior to administration in clinical practice – responding to legislative changes. Available from www.npc.co.uk/policy/resources/mixing_of_medicines.pdf.
NHS Argyll and Clyde (2005) *Syringe driver guidelines for Graseby MS26 (mm/24h)* Available from: www.palliativedrugs.com
NUH (Nottingham University Hospitals) NHS Trust (2002) *Data on file*. Hayward House, Nottingham.
Palliativedrugs.com (2006) *Syringe Driver Survey Results*. In: June/July 2006 newsletter. Palliativedrugs.com Ltd. Available from: www.palliativedrugs.com
Pesko LJ *et al.* (1988) Physical compatibility and stability of metoclopramide injection. *Parenterals*. **5**: 1–3, 6–8.
Pinguet F *et al.* (1995) Compatibility and stability of granisetron, dexamethasone, and methylprednisolone in injectable solutions. *Journal of Pharmaceutical Sciences*. **84**: 267–268.
Regnard C *et al.* (1986) Antiemetics/diamorphine mixture compatibility in infusion pumps. *British Journal of Pharmaceutical Practice*. **8**: 218–220.
Schneider JJ (2001) *Personal communication*.
SIGN (2000) *Control of pain in patients with cancer*. Scottish Intercollegiate Guidelines Network. Guideline 44. Available from: www.sign.ac.uk/guidelines/fulltext/44/index.htmlSign
Smith JC *et al.* (2000) The stability of diamorphine and glycopyrrolate in PCA syringes. *Pharmaceutical Journal*. **265(suppl)**: R69.
Storey P *et al.* (1990) Subcutaneous infusions for control of cancer symptoms. *Journal of Pain and Symptom Management*. **5**: 33–41.
Trissel LA (2010) *Handbook on Injectable Drugs* (16e). American Society of Health System Pharmacists, Maryland, USA.
Walker SE *et al.* (1991) Compatibility of dexamethasone sodium phosphate with hydromorphone hydrochloride or diphenhydramine hydrochloride. *American Journal of Hospital Pharmacy*. **48**: 2161–2166.

General key for charts

	Do *not* use, *incompatible* at usual concentrations
	Use with caution, compatibility may depend on order of mixing or drug concentrations
a,b,c, etc.	Some reports of *incompatibility*, but may be compatible at other concentrations (see footnotes)
	Reported compatible (data may be observational, physical or chemical, i.e. practice- or evidence-based)
?	No data. Please provide information on this combination to the Syringe Driver Survey Database (SDSD), www.palliativedrugs.com
	Not applicable or not generally recommended, e.g. seek specialist advice when combining multiple anti-emetics
#	Use non-PVC tubing; up to 50% of a dose of clonazepam is adsorbed by PVC tubing
##	Dexamethasone sodium phosphate can generally be given once daily by SC bolus injection. If given by CSCI, to minimize the risk of incompatibility, always add it last to a maximally diluted syringe
###	Compatibility data for oxycodone 10mg/mL formulation only; for 50mg/mL formulation, see Table A3.1

Alf	Alfentanil
Clzm	Clonazepam
Cyc	Cyclizine
Dex/Dexamethasone	Dexamethasone sodium phosphate
Dia	Diamorphine
Gly	Glycopyrronium
Gra	Granisetron
Hal	Haloperidol
HBBr	Hyoscine butylbromide
HHBr	Hyoscine hydrobromide
Hyd	Hydromorphone
Keta	Ketamine
Ketor	Ketorolac
Levo	Levomepromazine
Meto	Metoclopramide
Mid	Midazolam
MS	Morphine sulphate
MT	Morphine tartrate
Oct	Octreotide
Ond	Ondansetron
Oxy	Oxycodone 10mg/mL

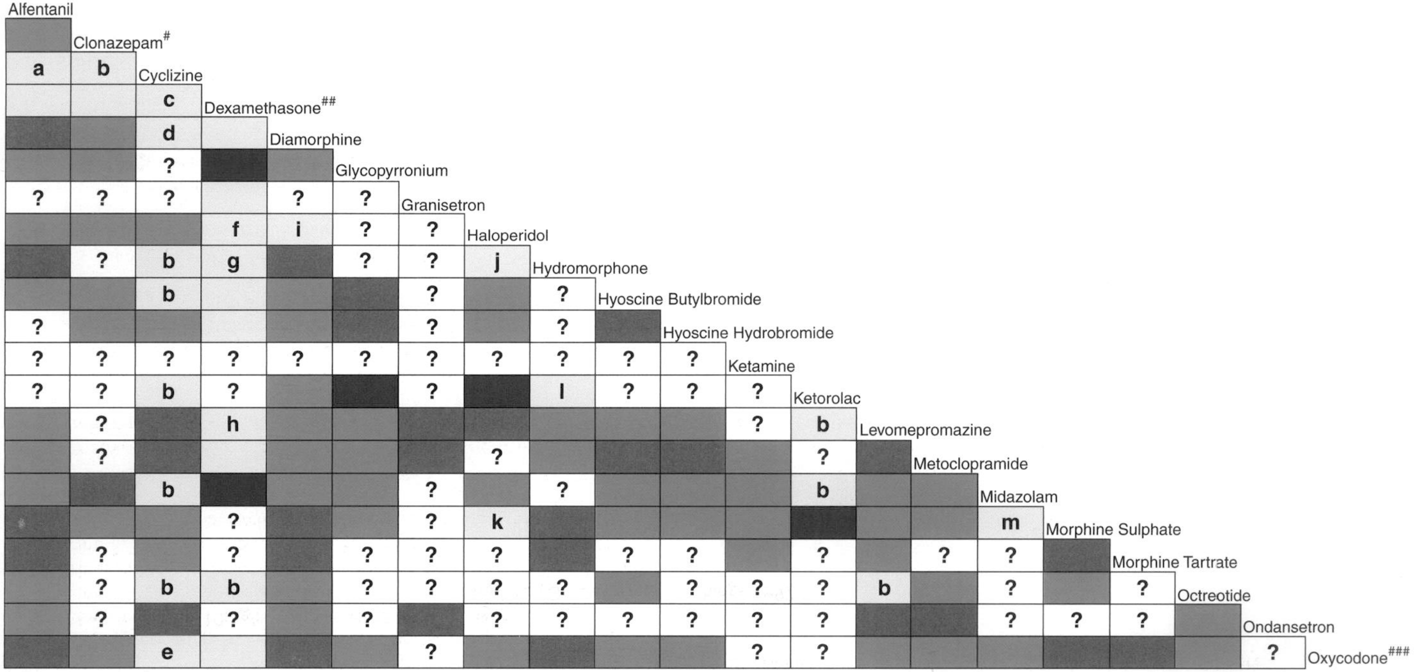

	Alfentanil	Clonazepam#	Cyclizine	Dexamethasone##	Diamorphine	Glycopyrronium	Granisetron	Haloperidol	Hydromorphone	Hyoscine Butylbromide	Hyoscine Hydrobromide	Ketamine	Ketorolac	Levomepromazine	Metoclopramide	Midazolam	Morphine Sulphate	Morphine Tartrate	Octreotide	Ondansetron
Clonazepam#	a																			
Cyclizine		b																		
Dexamethasone##			c																	
Diamorphine			d																	
Glycopyrronium			?																	
Granisetron	?	?	?		?	?														
Haloperidol				f	i	?	?													
Hydromorphone		?	b	g		?	?	j												
Hyoscine Butylbromide			b				?		?											
Hyoscine Hydrobromide	?						?		?											
Ketamine	?	?	?	?	?	?	?	?	?	?	?									
Ketorolac	?	?	b	?			?		l	?	?	?								
Levomepromazine		?		h								?	b							
Metoclopramide		?						?					?							
Midazolam			b				?		?				b							
Morphine Sulphate				?			?	k								m				
Morphine Tartrate		?		?		?	?	?		?	?		?		?	?				
Octreotide		?	b	b		?	?	?	?		?	?	?	b		?		?		
Ondansetron		?		?		?		?	?	?	?	?	?			?	?	?		
Oxycodone###			e				?					?	?							?

Note: This chart summarizes the compatibility information available for drug combinations in **WFI** used for CSCI over 24h in palliative care units and in the literature (see p.774). It includes compatibility data for oxycodone 10mg/mL formulation only; for 50mg/mL, see p.790. It should be used in conjunction with the key and footnotes. Further information about each combination may be found at www.palliativedrugs.com on the Syringe Driver Survey Database (SDSD). Charts with drug combinations diluted in 0.9% saline can also be found on the SDSD.

Chart A3.1 Compatibility chart for *two* drugs in ***WFI***.

Chart A3.1 footnotes

All drug concentration values (mg/mL) specified below are the *final* concentrations of each drug in the syringe after mixing and dilution. For full references, see p.774.

a. alfentanil 0.24mg/mL + cyclizine 8.8mg/mL reported compatible (Dickman *et al.* 2005)
   alfentanil 4.25mg/mL + cyclizine 7.5mg/mL reported *incompatible* (Dickman *et al.* 2005)

b. observational reports of *incompatibility* from miscellaneous sources

c. cyclizine 8.33mg/mL + dexamethasone sodium phosphate 0.33mg/mL reported compatible; *incompatibility* may occur at higher concentrations (Dickman *et al.* 2005)

d. cyclizine + diamorphine *incompatible* at higher concentrations, the maximum final concentrations that have been found to be compatible are:
   cyclizine up to 20mg/mL + diamorphine up to 20mg/mL
   cyclizine maximum 10mg/mL + diamorphine >20mg/mL
   cyclizine >20mg/mL + diamorphine maximum 15mg/mL (Grassby and Hutchings 1997)

e. cyclizine 3mg/mL + oxycodone 9mg/mL reported compatible (SFC)
   cyclizine 6.25mg/mL + oxycodone 8.75mg/mL reported *incompatible*
   for practical purposes, cyclizine concentrations between 3mg/mL and 8mg/mL may be used as long as the oxycodone concentration is reduced to below 3mg/mL by diluting with WFI (Napp 2010)

f. dexamethasone sodium phosphate 0.15mg/mL + haloperidol 0.38mg/mL reported compatible (Dickman *et al.* 2005)
   dexamethasone sodium phosphate 0.6mg/mL + haloperidol 0.25mg/mL reported *incompatible* (Dickman *et al.* 2005)

g. dexamethasone sodium phosphate + hydromorphone *incompatible* at higher concentrations, the maximum final concentrations that have been found to be compatible are:
   dexamethasone sodium phosphate 2mg/mL + hydromorphone 20mg/mL
   dexamethasone sodium phosphate >2mg/mL + hydromorphone 10mg/mL (Walker *et al.* 1991)

h. dexamethasone sodium phosphate 0.11mg/mL + levomepromazine 2.78mg/mL reported compatible
   dexamethasone sodium phosphate 0.14mg/mL + levomepromazine 1.79mg/mL reported *incompatible* (Dickman *et al.* 2005, palliativedrugs.com 2006)

i. diamorphine + haloperidol *incompatible* at very high concentrations, the maximum final concentrations that have been found to be compatible are:
   diamorphine up to 50mg/mL + haloperidol 4mg/mL max
   diamorphine 50–100mg/mL + haloperidol 3mg/mL max (Grassby 1995)

j. haloperidol 2.5mg/mL + hydromorphone 5mg/mL reported compatible (Huang and Anderson 1994)
   haloperidol 2mg/mL + hydromorphone 10mg/mL reported *incompatible* (Storey et *al.* 1990)

k. haloperidol 2mg/mL + morphine sulphate 20mg/mL reported *incompatible* (Storey *et al.* 1990, Trissel 2006, LeBelle *et al.* 1995); observational reports of compatibility at lower usual concentrations (palliativedrugs.com 2006)

l. hydromorphone 0.5mg/mL + ketorolac 15mg/mL reported compatible (Huang and Anderson 1994)
   hydromorphone 5mg/mL + ketorolac 15mg/mL reported *incompatible* (Huang and Anderson 1994)

m. midazolam + morphine sulphate subvisual microprecipitation may occur (LeBelle *et al.* 1995); observational reports suggest may be compatible at some concentrations (palliativedrugs.com 2006).

	Alf + Clzm[#]	Alf + Cyc	Alf + Dex[##]	Alf + Gly	Alf + Gra	Alf + Hal	Alf + HBBr	Alf + HHBr	Alf + Keta	Alf + Ketor	Alf + Levo	Alf + Meto	Alf + Mid	Alf + Oct
Cyclizine	a													
Dexamethasone[##]	?	?												
Glycopyrronium		?	?											
Granisetron	?	?	?	?										
Haloperidol			?		?									
Hyoscine Butylbromide	?	?	?		?	?								
Hyoscine Hydrobromide		?	?		?	?								
Ketamine	?	?	?	?	?	?	?	?						
Ketorolac	?	?	?	?	?	?	?	?	?					
Levomepromazine	?		?					?	?	?				
Metoclopramide	?		?			?			?	?				
Midazolam		b	?	?	?		?	?	?	?				
Octreotide	?	?	?	?	?	?	?	?	?	?			?	
Ondansetron	?	?	?	?		?	?	?	?	?			?	?

Note: This chart summarizes the compatibility information available for drug combinations in **WFI** used for CSCI over 24h in palliative care units and in the literature (see p.774). It should be used in conjunction with the key and footnotes. Further information about each combination may be found at www.palliativedrugs.com on the Syringe Driver Survey Database (SDSD). Charts with drug combinations diluted in 0.9% saline can also be found on the SDSD.

Chart A3.2 Compatibility chart for alfentanil: *three* drugs in ***WFI***.

Chart A3.2 footnotes

All drug concentration values (mg/mL) specified below are the *final* concentrations of each drug in the syringe after mixing and dilution. For full references, see p.774.

a. alfentanil 0.53mg/mL + clonazepam 0.24mg/mL + cyclizine 8.82mg/mL reported compatible; *incompatibility* may occur at higher concentrations (Dickman *et al.* 2005)

b. alfentanil 3mg/mL + cyclizine 6mg/mL + midazolam 1.2mg/mL reported compatible; *incompatibility* may occur at higher concentrations (Dickman *et* al. 2005).

	Dia + Clzm[#]	Dia + Cyc	Dia + Dex[##]	Dia + Gly	Dia + Gra	Dia + Hal	Dia + HBBr	Dia + HHBr	Dia + Keta	Dia + Ketor	Dia + Levo	Dia + Meto	Dia + Mid	Dia + Oct
Cyclizine														
Dexamethasone[##]		a												
Glycopyrronium		?												
Granisetron	?	?	?	?										
Haloperidol		b	d											
Hyoscine Butylbromide			?		?	h								
Hyoscine Hydrobromide	?				?									
Ketamine		?	?	?	?	?	?	?						
Ketorolac	?	?	?		?	?	?	?	?					
Levomepromazine									?	?				
Metoclopramide	?		e						?	?				
Midazolam		c	f		?					i				
Octreotide	?		?	?	?			?	?	?				
Ondansetron	?	?	g	?		?	?	?	?	?			?	?

Note: This chart summarizes the compatibility information available for drug combinations in **WFI** used for CSCI over 24h in palliative care units and in the literature (see p.774). It should be used in conjuction with the key and footnotes. Further information about each combination may be found at www.palliativedrugs.com on the Syringe Driver Survey Database (SDSD). Charts with drug combinations diluted in 0.9% saline can also be found on the SDSD.

Chart A3.3 Compatibility chart for diamorphine: *three* drugs in ***WFI***.

Chart A3.3 footnotes

All drug concentration values (mg/mL) specified below are the *final* concentrations of each drug in the syringe after mixing and dilution. For full references, see p.774.

a. diamorphine 5.88mg/mL + cyclizine 8.82mg/mL + dexamethasone sodium phosphate 0.71mg/mL reported compatible; *incompatibility* may occur at higher concentrations (Dickman *et al.* 2005)

b. diamorphine 56mg/mL + cyclizine 13mg/mL + haloperidol 2.1mg/mL reported compatible (Grassby 1995); *incompatibility* may occur at higher concentrations (Dickman *et al.* 2005)

c. diamorphine 37mg/mL + cyclizine 8.82mg/mL + midazolam 2.35mg/mL reported compatible; *incompatibility* may occur at higher concentrations (Dickman *et al.* 2005)

d. diamorphine 25mg/mL + dexamethasone sodium phosphate 0.35mg/mL + haloperidol 0.59mg/mL reported compatible; *incompatibility* may occur at higher concentrations (Dickman *et al.* 2005)

e. diamorphine 3.53mg/mL + dexamethasone sodium phosphate 0.59mg/mL + metoclopramide 2.35mg/mL reported compatible; *incompatibility* may occur at higher concentrations (Dickman *et al.* 2005)

f. diamorphine 2.94mg/mL + dexamethasone sodium phosphate 0.24mg/mL + midazolam 1.18mg/mL reported compatible (Dickman *et al.* 2005)
diamorphine 1mg/mL + dexamethasone sodium phosphate 0.53mg/mL + midazolam 0.67mg/mL reported *incompatible* (palliativedrugs.com 2006, SIGN 2000)

g. diamorphine 35mg/mL + dexamethasone sodium phosphate 0.06mg/mL + ondansetron 1.41mg/mL reported compatible; *incompatibility* may occur at higher concentrations (Dickman *et al.* 2005)

h. diamorphine 10.7mg/mL + haloperidol 0.33mg/mL + hyoscine butylbromide 6.67mg/mL reported compatible (palliativedrugs.com 2006); *incompatibility* may occur at higher concentrations (NUH 2002)

i. diamorphine + ketorolac + midazolam generally regarded as *incompatible* (Hughes *et al.* 1997); may be compatible at very low concentrations (Back 2006).

	Hyd + Clzm[#]	Hyd + Cyc	Hyd + Dex[##]	Hyd + Gly	Hyd + Gra	Hyd + Hal	Hyd + HBBr	Hyd + HHBr	Hyd + Keta	Hyd + Ketor	Hyd + Levo	Hyd + Meto	Hyd + Mid	Hyd + Oct
Cyclizine	?													
Dexamethasone[##]	?	?												
Glycopyrronium	?	?	?											
Granisetron	?	?	?	?										
Haloperidol	?	?	?	?	?									
Hyoscine Butylbromide	?	?	?		?	?								
Hyoscine Hydrobromide	?	?	?		?	?								
Ketamine	?	?	?	?	?	?	?	?						
Ketorolac	?	?	?	?	?		?	?	?					
Levomepromazine	?		?	?			?	?	?	?				
Metoclopramide	?		?			?			?	?				
Midazolam		?	a	?	?	a	?	?	?	?				
Octreotide	?	a	?	?	?	?	?	?	?	?	?		?	
Ondansetron	?	?	?	?		?	?	?	?	?			?	?

Note: This chart summarizes the compatibility information available for drug combinations in **WFI** used for CSCI over 24h in palliative care units and in the literature (see p.774). It should be used in conjunction with the key and footnotes. Further information about each combination may be found at www.palliativedrugs.com on the Syringe Driver Survey Database (SDSD). Charts with drug combinations diluted in 0.9% saline can also be found on the SDSD.

Chart A3.4 Compatibility chart for hydromorphone: *three* drugs in ***WFI***.

Chart A3.4 footnote

All drug concentration values (mg/mL) specified below are the *final* concentrations of each drug in the syringe after mixing and dilution. For full references, see p.774.

a. incompatibility has been reported with 2 of the drugs in this combination, see 2-drug charts for further details and use with caution.

	MS + Clzm#	MS + Cyc	MS + Dex##	MS + Gly	MS + Gra	MS + Hal	MS + HBBr	MS + HHBr	MS + Keta	MS + Ketor	MS + Levo	MS + Meto	MS + Mid	MS + Oct
Cyclizine														
Dexamethasone##	?													
Glycopyrronium	?	?	?											
Granisetron	?	?	?	?										
Haloperidol	?		?	?	?									
Hyoscine Butylbromide	?	a	?		?									
Hyoscine Hydrobromide	?	?	?		?	?								
Ketamine	?	?	?	?	?	?	?	?						
Ketorolac	?	?	?	?	?	?	?	?	?					
Levomepromazine	?		?	?				?	?	?				
Metoclopramide	?		?						?	?				
Midazolam			?		?				?	?				
Octreotide	?	?	?	?	?		?	?	?	?	?		?	
Ondansetron	?	?	?	?		?	?	?	?	?			?	?

Note: This chart summarizes the compatibility information available for drug combinations in **WFI** used for CSCI over 24h in palliative care units and in the literature (see p.774). It should be used in conjunction with the key and footnotes. Further information about each combination may be found at www.palliativedrugs.com on the Syringe Driver Survey Database (SDSD). Charts with drug combinations diluted in 0.9% saline can also be found on the SDSD.

Chart A3.5 Compatibility chart for morphine sulphate: *three* drugs in ***WFI***.

Chart A3.5 footnote

All drug concentration values (mg/mL) specified below are the *final* concentrations of each drug in the syringe after mixing and dilution. For full references, see p.774.

a. morphine sulphate 4.44mg/mL + cyclizine 8.33mg/mL + hyoscine butylbromide 3.33mg/mL reported *incompatible* (palliativedrugs.com 2006); observational reports of *incompatibility* with 2-drug combinations of cyclizine and hyoscine butylbromide.

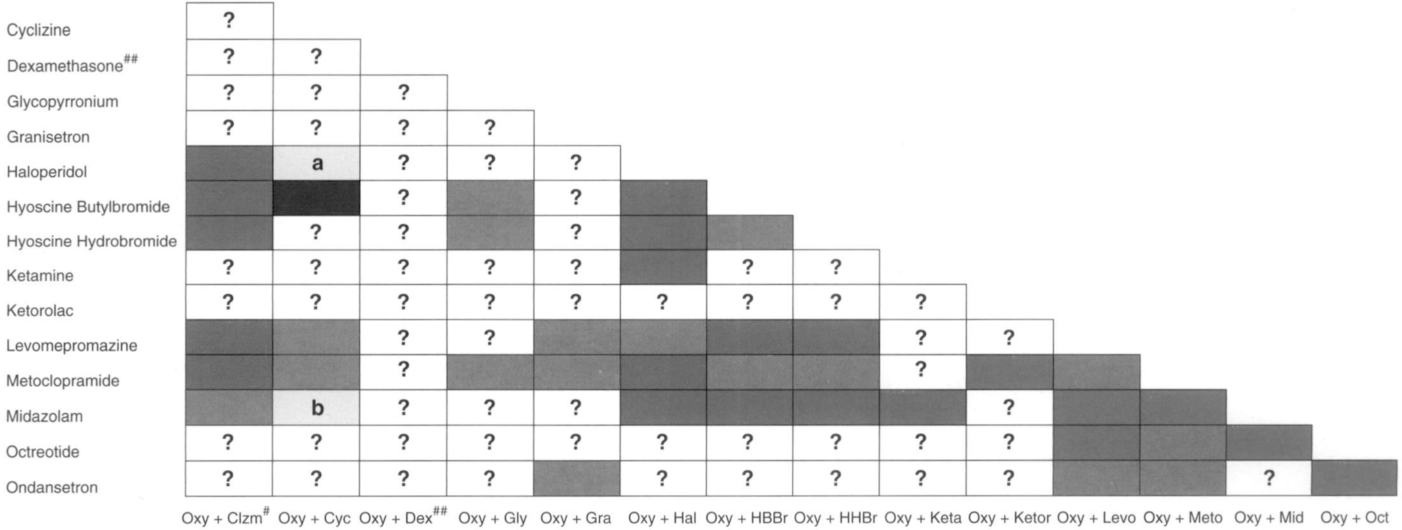

	Oxy + Clzm#	Oxy + Cyc	Oxy + Dex##	Oxy + Gly	Oxy + Gra	Oxy + Hal	Oxy + HBBr	Oxy + HHBr	Oxy + Keta	Oxy + Ketor	Oxy + Levo	Oxy + Meto	Oxy + Mid	Oxy + Oct
Cyclizine	?													
Dexamethasone##	?	?												
Glycopyrronium	?	?	?											
Granisetron	?	?	?	?										
Haloperidol		a	?	?	?									
Hyoscine Butylbromide			?		?									
Hyoscine Hydrobromide		?	?		?									
Ketamine	?	?	?	?	?		?	?						
Ketorolac	?	?	?	?	?	?	?	?	?					
Levomepromazine			?	?					?	?				
Metoclopramide			?						?					
Midazolam		b	?	?	?					?				
Octreotide	?	?	?	?	?	?	?	?	?	?				
Ondansetron	?	?	?	?		?	?	?	?	?			?	

Note: Compatibility data for oxycodone 10mg/mL formulation only; for 50mg/mL formulation, see p.790. This chart summarizes the compatibility information available for drug combinations in **WFI** used for CSCI over 24h in palliative care units and in the literature (see p.774). It should be used in conjunction with the key and footnotes. Further information about each combination may be found at www.palliativedrugs.com on the Syringe Driver Survey Database (SDSD). Charts with drug combinations diluted in 0.9% saline can also be found on the SDSD.

Chart A3.6 Compatibility chart for oxycodone 10mg/mL formulation: *three* drugs in ***WFI***.

Chart A3.6 footnotes

All drug concentration values (mg/mL) specified below are the *final* concentrations of each drug in the syringe after mixing and dilution. For full references, see p.774.

a. oxycodone 1.9mg/mL + cyclizine 7.14mg/mL + haloperidol 0.95mg/mL reported compatible (palliativedrugs.com 2006); *incompatibility* may occur at higher concentrations (Dickman *et al.* 2005); concentration dependent *incompatibility* with 2-drug combination of oxycodone + cyclizine (Napp 2010)

b. oxycodone 2.22mg/mL + cyclizine 8.33mg/mL + midazolam 0.28mg/mL reported compatible (palliativedrugs.com 2006); *incompatibility* may occur at higher concentrations; concentration dependent *incompatibility* with 2-drug combinations of oxycodone + cyclizine (Napp 2010) and *incompatibility* with cyclizine + midazolam reported (Back 2006).

	Clzm[#] + Meto	Cyc + Dex[##]	Cyc + Hal	Cyc + HBBr	Dex[##] + Mid	Gly + Keta	Gly + Levo	Hal + Mid	HBBr + Ketor	Levo + Mid
Haloperidol		?		b	d	?				
Hyoscine Butylbromide		a	b							
Hyoscine Hydrobromide		?	?		?					
Ketamine	?	?	?	?	?		?		?	?
Ketorolac	?	?	?	?	?	?	?			?
Metoclopramide					?	?			?	
Midazolam		?		c			?			
Octreotide	?	?	?	?	?	?		?	?	?

Note: This chart summarizes the compatibility information available for drug combinations in **WFI** used for CSCI over 24h in palliative care units and in the literature (see p.774). It should be used in conjuction with the key and footnotes. Further information about each combination may be found at www.palliativedrugs.com on the Syringe Driver Survey Database (SDSD). Charts with drug combinations diluted in 0.9% saline can also be found on the SDSD.

Chart A3.7 Compatibility chart for non-opioids: *three* drugs in ***WFI***.

Chart A3.7 footnotes

All drug concentration values (mg/mL) specified below are the *final* concentrations of each drug in the syringe after mixing and dilution. For full references, see p.774.

a. cyclizine 8.82mg/mL + dexamethasone sodium phosphate 0.71mg/mL + hyoscine butylbromide 2.35mg/mL reported compatible; *incompatibility* may occur at higher concentrations (Dickman *et al.* 2005)

b. cyclizine + haloperidol + hyoscine butylbromide generally regarded as *incompatible* (NUH 2002); one observational report of compatibility (Back 2006)

c. cyclizine + hyoscine butylbromide + midazolam observational reports of *incompatibility* (NUH 2002)

d. dexamethasone sodium phosphate 0.44mg/mL + haloperidol 0.14mg/mL + midazolam 0.14mg/mL reported compatible (Dickman *et al.* 2005); observational reports of *incompatibility* (NUH 2002); *incompatibility* with 2-drug combinations of dexamethasone sodium phosphate and midazolam (Good *et al.* 2004).

Compatibility information for oxycodone 50mg/mL formulation

When mixed with other drugs some differences in compatibility have been demonstrated for the 10mg/mL and 50mg/mL formulations of oxycodone solution for injection, e.g. with cyclizine (Gardiner 2003, Hines and Pleasance 2009). This may be due to the different ratios of excipients in each formulation. The manufacturer recommends that the compatibility information for each formulation is considered separately and not extrapolated from one formulation to another.

Chemical compatibility data between oxycodone 50mg/mL solution for injection and other drugs over 24h at room temperature are summarized inTable A3.1. Full details are available on the SDSD on www.palliativedrugs.com. Please submit details to the SDSD of successful combinations containing oxycodone 50mg/mL and, more important, details of combinations which were incompatible.

Table A3.1 Oxycodone 50mg/mL formulation compatibility with other drugs (Hines and Pleasance 2009)

	Oxycodone 250mg diluted[a]		*Oxycodone 500mg undiluted*	
	Dose (mg)	*Concentration (mg/mL)*	*Dose (mg)*	*Concentration (mg/mL)*
Cyclizine[b,c,d]	150	8.8	50	4.5
Dexamethasone sodium phosphate	20	1.2	40	2
Glycopyrronium	1.2	0.07	2.4	0.1
Haloperidol	7.5	0.4	15	1.2
Hyoscine butylbromide	30	1.8	60	4.6
Hyoscine hydrobromide	1.2	0.07	2.4	0.15
Ketamine	400	23.5	800	44.4
Levomepromazine	100	5.9	200	11.1
Metoclopramide	50	2.9	100	3.3
Midazolam	50	2.9	100	3.3

a. oxycodone 50mg/mL formulation, 5mL (250mg) mixed with the drug and diluted to 17mL with WFI or 0.9% saline; oxycodone final concentration 14mg/mL

b. use WFI only, *incompatible* with 0.9% saline

c. maximum concentrations found compatible for cyclizine and oxycodone 50mg/mL formulation; concentration dependent *incompatibility* found above this

d. for practical purposes, a cyclizine concentration of >4mg/mL to a maximum of 8mg/mL may be used if the oxycodone concentration is kept <14mg/mL by diluting with WFI (Napp, 2010).

Drug Index

Note: Main references are in **bold**.

Supplementary Topic Index

A textbook on pain and symptom management should be consulted for a full discussion of these topics.

Note: **words** in **bold type** indicate a chapter or an appendix.
Bold numbers indicate the more important references.